Principles of Sports Medicine
& Exercise Science

Principles of Sports Medicine & Exercise Science

Editor
Michael A. Buratovich, PhD

SALEM PRESS
A Division of EBSCO Information Services, Inc.
Ipswich, Massachusetts

GREY HOUSE PUBLISHING

Cover photo: AJ_Watt/iStock.

Copyright © 2022, by Salem Press, A Division of EBSCO Information Services, Inc., and Grey House Publishing, Inc.

Principles of Sports Medicine & Exercise Science, published by Grey House Publishing, Inc., Amenia, NY, under exclusive license from EBSCO Information Services, Inc.

All rights reserved. No part of this work may be used or reproduced in any manner whatsoever or transmitted in any form or by any means, electronic or mechanical, including photocopy, recording, or any information storage and retrieval system, without written permission from the copyright owner. For information, contact Grey House Publishing/Salem Press, 4919 Route 22, PO Box 56, Amenia, NY 12501.

∞ The paper used in these volumes conforms to the American National Standard for Permanence of Paper for Printed Library Materials, Z39.48 1992 (R2009).

Publisher's Cataloging-In-Publication Data
(Prepared by Parlew Associates, LLC)

Names: Buratovich, Michael A., editor.
Title: Principles of sports medicine & exercise science / editor, Michael A. Buratovich, PhD.
Description: Ipswich, MA : Salem Press, a division of EBSCO Information Services, Inc. ; Amenia, NY : Grey House Publishing, 2022. | Series: [Principles of science]. | Includes bibliographic references and index. | Includes b&w photos and illustrations.
Identifiers: ISBN 9781637003794 (hardback)
Subjects: LCSH: Sports medicine. | Kinesiology. | Sports injuries. | Movement — physiology. | Exercise — Physiological aspects. | BISAC: MEDICAL / Sports Medicine. | HEALTH & FITNESS / General. | SPORTS & RECREATION / Health & Safety.
Classification: LCC RC1210 B87 2022 | DDC 613.7—dc23

FIRST PRINTING
PRINTED IN THE UNITED STATES OF AMERICA

Contents

Publisher's Note ix
Introduction xi
Contributors xiii

Anatomy 1
Anatomy 3
Bones and the Skeleton 8
Brain Structure 15
Cartilage 23
Circulation 26
Connective Tissue 30
Fascia 33
Heart 36
Hippocampus 42
Human Respiratory System 45
Knee 50
Ligaments 52
Lower Extremities 55
Muscles 62
Prefrontal Cortex (PFC) 68
Upper Extremities 71

Physiology/Pathophysiology 79
Bone Disorders 81
Brain 86
Exercise Physiology 92
Glycolysis 98
Haller Establishes Physiology as a Science 105
Hypertrophy 108
Inflammation 113
Iron-Deficiency Anemia 116
Lactate Threshold 121
Metabolism 124
Motor Control 135
Motor Skill Development 139
Neuroplasticity 144
Osmosis 147
Osteoarthritis 150
Pain 152
Steroids 157

Exercise Training 167
Aerobics 169
Autogenic Training 171
Blood Flow Restriction (BFR) Training 174
Cross-training 175
Endurance Training 177
Ergogenic Aids 181
High-Intensity Interval Training (HIIT) 184
Progressive Muscle Relaxation 186
Static Stretching 189
Stretching 191
Stress Reduction 194
Weight Training 196

Nutrition and Supplements 199
Amino Acids 201
Anti-Inflammatory Diet 205
Biotin 207
Branched-Chain Amino Acids 209
Carbohydrates 211
Cetylated Fatty Acids 213
Creatine 214
Essential Nutrients 219
Fatty Acid 222
Glucosamine 225
Iron 228
Lecithin 233
Nicotinamide Adenine Dinucleotide (NAD) . . . 234
Nutrition 235
Protein 241
Sports and Energy Drinks 242
Sports and Fitness Performance 245
Supplements 255
Vitamins and Minerals 257

Injuries 265
Back Pain 267
Bruises 269
Chronic Traumatic Encephalopathy (CTE) 270
Common Shoulder Injuries 273
Concussion 276

Fracture and Dislocation 279
Injuries, Minor 285
Muscle Sprains, Spasms, and Disorders 287
Post-Concussion Syndrome 292
Repetitive Strain Injury (RSI) 294
Soft Tissue Pain 297
Sports-Related Wrist and Hand Injuries 298
Strength Training 301
Tendinitis 304
Tendon Disorders 307
Tennis Elbow (Lateral Epicondylitis) 309
Traumatic Brain Injury 312
Wounds 321

Diagnostic Techniques 325
Genetic Testing 327
Genomics 331
Magnetic Resonance Imaging (MRI) 336
Single-Photon Emission Computed
    Tomography (SPECT) 338
Ultrasonography 341

Injury Treatments—Standard 347
Advances in Spinal Cord Injury Research 349
Arthroplasty 351
Astym® Therapy 354
Braces, Orthopedic 356
Casts and Splints 359
Constraint-Induced Movement
    Therapy (CIMT) 361
Exercise-Based Therapies 364
Hyaluronic Acid Injections 367
Kneecap Removal 369
Physical Rehabilitation 371
Rotator Cuff Surgery 376
Tendon Repair 380
Tommy John Surgery 382

Injury Treatments—Alternative/Experimental . . 385
Acupressure 387
Acupuncture 390
Applied Kinesiology 395
Cupping 397
Diet-Based Therapies 399

Homeopathic Remedies for Sports-Related
    Injuries 402
Magnet Therapy 403
Prolotherapy 414
Sports and Fitness Recovery 416
Sports Injuries and Homeopathy 418
Tissue Engineering 420

Medications 425
Anti-Inflammatory Drugs 427
Baclofen 430
Carisoprodol 431
Codeine 432
Fentanyl 434
Ketamine 436
Morphine 438
Nonsteroidal Anti-inflammatory Drugs
    (NSAIDs) 439
Oxycodone 445
Pain Management 447
Prescription NSAIDs 449
Tramadol 451
Valium (diazepam) 452

Drug Doping 455
Athlete Drug Testing 457
Blood Doping 458
Lance Armstrong Stripped of Tour de
    France Titles 461
Erythropoietin 463
Mark McGwire Evades Congressional
    Questions on Steroid Use 466
Genetic Engineering 468
Gymnast Andreea Raducan Loses Her
    Olympic Gold Medal 475
Olympic Athlete Marion Jones Admits
    Steroid Use 478
Olympic Champion Lasse Virén Is Accused
    of Blood Doping 481
Performance-Enhancing Drugs 483
Russian Sports Doping Scandal 486
Soccer Star Diego Maradona Is Expelled
    from World Cup 489
Steroid Abuse 492

Steroids: HGH and PEDS................ 494
Steroids in Baseball..................... 496
Track-and-Field Champion Heike
    Dreschler Doping Scandal 500

Sports in General 503
Benefits of Playing Sports................ 505
Exercise Addiction 508
Exercise and Mental Health 510
Health Risks to Student Athletes 512
Intramural Sports 516
Overtraining Syndrome 521
Sociology of Sport....................... 523
Sports Engineering...................... 528
Sports Psychology 533
Transgender Athletes: Overview........... 539
Transgender College Athletes 542

Careers 549
Athletic Training........................ 551
Cardiology 557
Exercise Science 564
Kinesiology............................ 570
Neuroscience........................... 575
Occupational Therapist 578
Orthopedics 582
Personal Trainer 588
Physical Medicine and Rehabilitation (PM&R) .. 592
Physical Therapist...................... 595
Podiatry............................... 600
Sports Medicine 604

Bibliography........................... 613
Glossary............................... 651
Organizations 677
Subject Index 679

Publisher's Note

Sports Medicine & Exercise Science is the next volume in *Salem's Principles of Science* series, which includes *Microbiology, Energy, Marine Science, Geology, Information Technology,* and *Mathematics*.

This new resource explores the world of sports fitness, injury, and rehabilitation, introducing readers to important topics in easy-to-understand language. Achieving optimum fitness levels, whether for the professional athlete or for the amateur enthusiast, requires knowledge of human anatomy and a basic understanding of the effects of exercise, injury, and nutrition on the body. Treatments, diagnostic tools, sports-related careers, and athlete doping scandals round out the discussion of this perennially popular topic. This volume offers amateur athletes and students who want to learn about the complexities of sports medicine and exercise science a solid and accessible introduction.

This work begins with a comprehensive Editor's Introduction to the topic written by Michael A. Buratovich.

Following the Introduction, *Principles Sports Medicine & Exercise Science* includes 163 entries organized into 12 convenient sections.

The Anatomy section discusses the complex organization of the human body, while Physiology topics delve into how the body works and what happens when things go wrong. The Exercise and Nutrition and Supplements segments discuss the importance of balance to training for optimal fitness levels and to rehabilitating injuries. Sports- and exercise-related damage to the human body is covered in detail in the Injuries, Diagnostic Techniques, Injury Treatments (both Standard and Alternative/Experimental), and Medications sections. Unfair and illegal competitive advantage is discussed in the Drug Doping section, while sports psychology and sociology topics take the lead in Sports in General. The final section discusses possible careers in sports medicine as well as necessary study topics for these fields.

Entries begin by specifying Specialties and Related Fields, followed by a brief description and then a list of Key Terms summarizing important points; all entries end with a helpful Further Reading section. Numerous photographs and illustrations throughout enhance the categories.

This work also includes helpful appendices, including:
- Bibliography;
- Glossary;
- Organizations;
- Subject Index

Salem Press extends appreciation to all involved in the development and production of this work. Names and affiliations of contributors to this work follow the Editor's Introduction.

Principles of Sports Medicine & Exercise Science, as well as all Salem Press reference books, is available in print and as an e-book. Please visit www.salempress.com for more information.

Introduction

Americans love sports. They spend inordinate amounts of time watching it and patronizing the organizations that sponsor professional sports teams. According to The Motley Fool website, the sports channel ESPN made the Disney corporation $24.6 billion in 2021. The National Football League made $1.8 billion that same year. The National Basketball Association made $8.3 billion during the 2019-2020 season. Major League Baseball made almost ten million dollars in 2021. European love of football (soccer in American parlance) is even more passionate. European football clubs netted $33 billion during the 2018-2019 season.

Behind the athletes who wow us on the field is a veritable army of coaches, athletic trainers, personal trainers, strength and conditioning specialists, physical therapists, orthopedists, sports doctors, nutritionists, masseuses, and other experts. Sports medicine and exercise science are integral components of the colossal sports machine.

In addition to our infatuation with professional sports, Americans spend $155 per month on health and fitness. Amateur athletes play hours of soccer, softball, and football, or spend time running, biking, swimming, boating, or hiking. We also shell out over $30 billion for dietary supplements each year. Websites and YouTube videos advertise quick fixes for everything from sore knees to constipation. Amateur athletes do not have a pool of experts to help them make informed decisions about their diet, exercise, and training regimens. Where can they go for reliable information?

Salem Press's *Principles of Science* series offers readers reliable starting points to learn more about complex subjects, and we are pleased to offer *Principles of Sports Medicine & Exercise Science* to help amateur athletes and students who want to learn about the complexities of sports medicine and exercise science.

Before learning about how the human body works, students must learn how it is constructed. This volume begins with a summary of human anatomy. Articles in this section provide a foundational understanding of the structure of the human body. The second section examines human physiology or function and pathophysiology, or what happens when function goes awry. Readers will discover that the structure and function of the human body are intimately interrelated. Since steroids represent a drug class at the center of drug doping, one article lays out the normal physiological role of steroid hormones in our bodies. This entry sets up later discussions on drug doping.

The third section introduces the principles of exercise training strategies. While elite athletes may push the boundaries of their performance to gain a competitive edge, most amateurs want to keep fit or just have fun. Fortunately, scientific studies of exercise provide deep insight into the benefits and pitfalls of certain workout programs. These entries give trustworthy information about what works for whom and what does not. This section provides guidance for everyone.

The fourth section dives into the prickly subject of diet, nutrition, and dietary supplements. Many outlandish claims for dietary supplements far outstrip the evidence for those claims. These articles take a careful look at several popular supplements and their caveats. Others provide a foundational understanding of what a healthy diet looks like for all athletes, professional and elite.

The fifth section examines what happens when athletes are injured. These articles examine the nature of injuries and how they are diagnosed, addressed, and rehabilitated. The goal is to understand how structural damage causes abnormal function and how restoring human structure brings human function into normal homeostatic ranges. A natural extension of this section is the following one; the sixth section explains those diagnostic technologies that accurately identify the site, nature, and severity of various injuries.

The seventh and eighth sections identify strategies for treating sports injuries. The seventh section examines standard surgical and rehabilitation procedures to heal athletic injuries (e.g., casts and splints, knee and hip replacement, rotator cuff surgery, and others). The eighth section illustrates some alternative (e.g., acupuncture, acupressure, magnet therapy, and others) and experimental (e.g., tissue engineering, prolotherapy) procedures for addressing athletic injuries. Some standard injury treatments are technically complicated, but these entries provide excellent introductions. The eighth section takes a critical look at the evidence base for alternative healing techniques and, in many cases, finds them wanting.

The ninth section illustrates those medications that treat athletic injuries. Muscle relaxants, pain relievers, and anti-inflammatory medicines aid in rehabilitation and mitigate pain. Unfortunately, some of these medicines are abused by athletes, and these articles stress the adverse effects and potential for abuse of each medicine.

The tenth section summarizes the tragedy of doping. Athletes use various drugs to enhance their performance, including anabolic steroids, stimulants, and human growth hormone. This section examines each drug class used for doping and presents vignettes of athletes caught doping and stripped of their awards.

The penultimate section examines sports participation in general. This section examines the benefits and risks of sports participation. Topics include sports psychology, sociology, the participation of transgender athletes in sports, and sports engineering.

The final, twelfth, section covers careers in sports medicine and kinesiology, such as sports medicine, orthopedics, podiatry, physical therapy, occupational therapy, and others. Anyone interested in sports can find advice for pursuing such a career in sports medicine and exercise training.

Sports—whether professional or amateur—is an important part of many people's lives. *Principles of Sports Medicine & Exercise Science* provides a wealth of current information on how the human body functions, what can go wrong while participating in sports and exercise, and how injuries and conditions are treated, as well as highlighting the many careers that are related to this fascinating field. This volume contains relevant content for readers of every profession, level, and interest.

—*Michael A. Buratovich, PhD*

Contributors

Richard Adler, PhD
University of Michigan-Dearborn

Michael Aeurbach, MA
Marblehead, Massachusetts

Oluwatoyin O. Akinwunmi, PhD
Muskingum College

Adriel Barrios-Anderson
Brown University

Samar Aslam, MD
South Nassau Communities Hospital

Mihaela Avramut, MD, PhD
Verlan Medical Communications, American Medical Writers Association

Barbara C. Beattie
Sarasota, Florida

Paul F. Bell, PhD
Heritage Valley Health System

Allison C. Bennett, PharmD
Duke University

Alvin K. Benson, PhD
Utah Valley State College

Matthew Berria, PhD
Weber State University

Zuzana Bic, MD, DPH
University of California, Irvine

Nyla R. Branscombe
University of Kansas

Howard Bromberg, JD
University of Michigan Law School

Amy Webb Bull, DSN, APN
Tennessee State University School of Nursing

Michael A. Buratovich, PhD
Spring Arbor University

Rosslynn S. Byous, DPA, PA-C
University of Southern California, Keck School of Medicine

Jeffrey R. Bytomski, DO
Duke University Medical Center

Cait Caffrey
Independent Scholar

Josephine Campbell
Independent Scholar

Richard P. Capriccioso, MD
University of Phoenix

Christine M. Carroll, RN, BSN, MBA
American Medical Writers Association

Donatella M. Casirola, PhD
University of Medicine and Dentistry, New Jersey Medical School

Karen Chapman-Novakofski, RD, LDN, PhD
University of Illinois

Paul J. Chara Jr., PhD
Northwestern College

Rose Ciulla-Bohling, PhD
Independent Scholar

Julien M. Cobert
Duke University

Tisha Davidson, AM
Fremont, California

LeAnna DeAngelo, PhD
Arizona State University

Tracey M. DiLascio-Martinuk, JD
Framingham, Massachusetts

Lillian Dominguez
Brown University

Mark Dziak
Northeast Editing, Inc.

Patricia Stanfill Edens, PhD, RN, FACHE
The Oncology Group, LLC

Jack Ewing
Independent Scholar

Elisabeth Faase, MD
Athens Regional Medical Center

C. Richard Falcon
Roberts and Raymond Associates, Philadelphia

L. Fleming Fallon Jr., MD, PhD, MPH
Bowling Green State University

Nick Feo
South Nassau Communities Hospital

Fernando J. Ferrer, PhD
Carlsbad, California

K. Thomas Finley, PhD
State University of New York, Brockport

Simone Isadora Flynn, PhD
Yale University

Anthony J. Fonseca
Nicholls State University

M. A. Foote, PhD
M. A. Foote Associates

Joanne R. Gambosi, BSN, MA
Gold Canyon, Arizona

Justin D. García
Indiana University, Bloomington

Jason Georges
Glendale, California

Soraya Ghayourmanesh, PhD
City University of New York

Jennifer L. Gibson, PharmD
Marietta, Georgia

Lenela Glass-Goodwin, MWS
Texas A&M University

James S. Godde, PhD
Monmouth College

Joy Goldsmith, PhD
University of Memphis

Daniel G. Graetzer, PhD
University of Montana

Jodi L. Guy, BSN, RN, CMSRN
Spring Arbor University

Gina Hagler
Rare Math

Angela Harmon
Independent Scholar

Liam Hooper
Independent Scholar

Daniel Horowitz
Independent Scholar

Ryan C. Horst
Eastern Mennonite University

Mary Hurd
East Tennessee State University

Misa Hyakutake, MD
New York, NY

Micah L. Issitt
St. Louis, MO

Bruce E. Johansen
University of Nebraska at Omaha

Walter Klyce
Brown University

Jeffrey A. Knight, PhD
Mount Holyoke College

Ernest Kohlmetz, MA
Independent Scholar

Bill Kte'pi
Independent Scholar

Jeanne L. Kuhler, MS, PhD
Auburn University, Montgomery

Jeffrey P. Larson, PT, ATC
Northern Medical Informatics

Jack Lasky
Independent Scholar

Jacob F. Lee
Filson Historical Society

Leon Lewis
Appalachian State University

Martha Oehmke Loustaunau, PhD
New Mexico State University

Eric V.D. Luft, PhD, MLS
SUNY, Upstate Medical University

L. L. Lundin, MA
Independent Scholar

Bonita L. Marks, PhD
University of North Carolina, Chapel Hill

Geraldine Marrocco, EdD, APRN, CNS, ANP-BC
Yale University School of Nursing

Trudy Mercadal, PhD
Florida Atlantic University

Michael R. Meyers
Pfeiffer University

Roman J. Miller, PhD
Eastern Mennonite College

Shari Parsons Miller, MA
Accenture

Eli C. Minkoff, PhD
Bates College

Elizabeth Mohn
Northeast Editing, Inc.

Tinker D. Murray
Southwest Texas State University

Bryan Ness, PhD
Pacific Union College

Caryn E. Neumann, PhD
Miami University of Ohio

Marsha M. Neumyer
Pennsylvania State University College of Medicine

Derek T. Nhan
University of Colorado, Denver

Jane C. Norman, PhD, RN, CNE
Tennessee State University

Kelly Owen, Esq.
Independent Scholar

Mario Pacheco, PhD
Buffalo State College

Ellen E. Anderson Penno, BS, MS, MD, FRCSC
Western Laser Eye Associates

Elizabeth Peterson
Independent Scholar

Nancy Piotrowski, PhD
University of California, Berkeley

Marichelle Pita
NYITCOM

Victoria Price, PhD
Lamar University

Jason Pyon
Independent Scholar

Jerome L. Rekart, PhD
Rivier University

Richard M. Renneboog, MSc
Independent Scholar

Lauren Ruvo
Harvard University Graduate School of Education

David K. Saunders, PhD
Emporia State University

Elizabeth D. Schafer, DO
South Nassau Communities Hospital

Jason J. Schwartz, PhD, JD
Los Angeles, California

Thomas L. Sevier, MD, FACSM, FACP
Performance Dynamics, Inc., Astym Program

Richard Sheposh
Penn State University

R. Baird Shuman, PhD
University of Illinois, Urbana-Champaign

Sanford S. Singer, PhD
University of Dayton

Genevieve Slomski, PhD
New Britain, Connecticut

Shelby L. Hinkle Smith
University of Vermont

Lisa Levin Sobczak, RNC
Santa Barbara, California

Sharon W. Stark, RN, APRN, DNSc
Monmouth University

Susan E. Thomas, MLS
Indiana University South Bend

Marcella Bush Trevino
Florida SouthWestern State College

Janine Ungvarsky
Independent Scholar

John V. Urbas, PhD
Kennesaw State College

Mikhail Varshavski, OMS-IV
New York Institute of Technology

Charles Vigue, PhD
University of New Haven

James Waddell, PhD
University of Minnesota

Edith K. Wallace, PhD
Heartland Community College

C. J. Walsh, PhD
Mote Marine Laboratory

Daniel L. Wann
Murray State University

Bradley R. A. Wilson, PhD
University of Cincinnati

Bonnie Wolff
Pacific Coast Cardiac and Vascular Surgeons

George D. Zgourides, MD, PsyD
John Peter Smith Hospital

Scott Zimmer, MLS, MS, JD
Alliant International University

Rebecca Zukauskas
Northeast Editing, Inc.

ANATOMY

"Think little of thy flesh: blood, bones, and a skin; a pretty piece of knit and twisted work, consisting of nerves, veins and arteries; think no more of it, than so."

—Marcus Aurelius, *Meditations*

Since the time of this great Roman emperor/philosopher, we have learned much more about the human body. It is more than "a pretty piece of knit and twisted work." Instead, the human body is a highly organized, complicated organism that works as a functional unit. Understanding the structure of human anatomy is key to training for optimal fitness levels and to rehabilitating injuries. Topics discussed in this section include: bones and the skeleton, brain structure, the heart, the respiratory system, and muscles.

Anatomy

Specialties and related fields: All
Definition: the structure of the human body—its parts, systems, and organs

KEY TERMS

abdomen: the rib-free part of the trunk, below the diaphragm
head: the part of the body containing the major sense organs (such as the eyes and ears) and the brain
lower extremities: the thigh, lower leg, and foot
thorax: the part of the trunk above the diaphragm, containing the ribs; the chest
trunk: the central part of the body to which the extremities are attached
upper extremities: the arm, forearm, and hand

STRUCTURE AND FUNCTIONS

The body's parts can be categorized either regionally or functionally. Regionally, the body consists of a trunk attached to two upper extremities, two lower extremities, and a head attached through a neck. Functionally, the body consists of a digestive system, a circulatory system, an excretory system, a respiratory system, a reproductive system, a nervous system, an endocrine system, an integument (skin), a skeleton, and a series of muscles.

The trunk can be divided into an upper portion called the "chest" (or thorax), containing ribs, and a lower, rib-free portion called the "abdomen." Internally, the thorax and abdomen are separated by a muscular sheet called the "diaphragm." The upper extremities of the trunk include the arms, forearms, and hands; the lower extremities include the thighs, lower legs, and feet. The head includes the brain and the major sense organs such as the eyes and ears; the neck is the narrower, flexible part that connects the head to the trunk. The abdomen's ventral (front) surface is often divided around the umbilicus into upper-left, upper-right, lower-left, and lower-right quadrants.

Functionally, the body consists of several organ systems. The digestive system breaks down foods into simpler substances and absorbs them. The circulatory system transports oxygen and other materials around the body. The excretory system rids the body of many waste products. In contrast, the respiratory system rids the body of carbon dioxide and adds oxygen to the blood. The reproductive system produces sex cells and, in females, provides an environment for the development of an embryo. The nervous system sends signals in the form of nerve

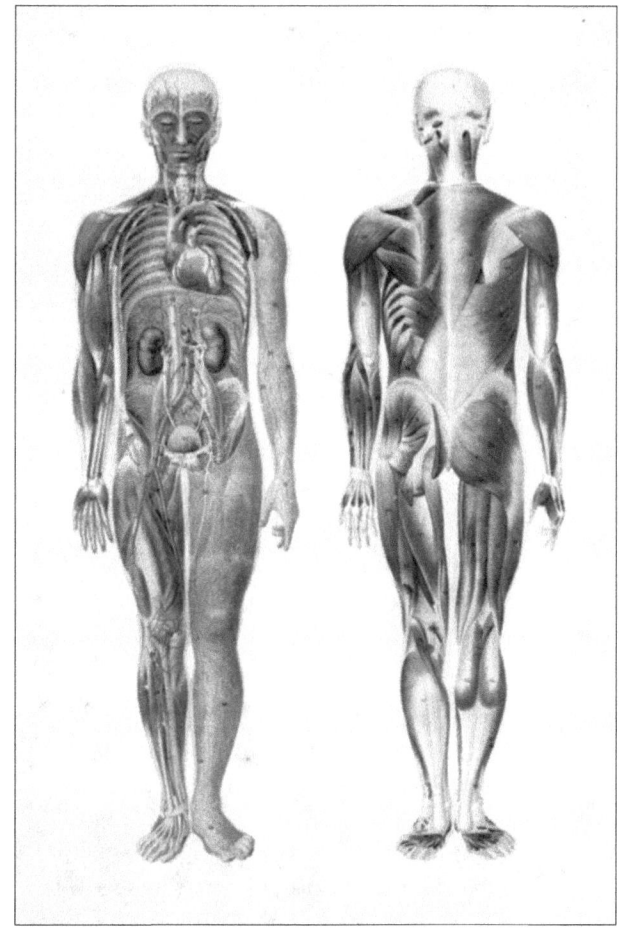

Image via iStock/Grafissimo. [Used under license.]

impulses from one part of the body to another. The endocrine organs send chemical messengers (hormones) through the bloodstream. The integument, or skin, protects the outer surface of the body from infection, injury, and drying out (desiccation); it also maintains the body's internal temperature by providing insulation and preventing the body from overheating during exercise through sweating. The skeleton serves as the body's framework and consists of 206 separate bones; these bones support the body's other organs and protect the heart, the lungs, and especially the central nervous system (including the brain and the spinal cord). The muscles contract and produce movements.

DIRECTIONAL TERMS FOR THE BODY
superior: upward; toward the top of the head
inferior: downward; toward the ground or the feet
cranial: toward the head; the same as superior in humans
caudal: toward the tail
dorsal: toward the back
ventral: toward the belly surface
medial: toward the midline
lateral: away from the midline
radial: on the medial side (or thumb side) of the arm, forearm, and hand
ulnar: on the lateral side (or little finger side) of the arm, forearm, and hand; the same side that contains the ulna
anterior: forward, in the customary direction of motion; equivalent to ventral in humans, but the same as cranial in other animals
posterior: toward the rear, opposite to the customary direction of motion; equivalent to dorsal in humans, but the same as caudal in other animals

Each major organ system is constructed of several major organs. The major organs contained within the thorax, for example, are the heart, lungs, and thymus body. The major organs contained within the abdomen include the stomach, spleen, liver, pancreas, small intestine (consisting of the duodenum, ileum, and jejunum), large intestine (consisting of the cecum, colon, and rectum, with the colon further divided into an ascending colon, transverse colon, descending colon, and sigmoid colon), and bladder. The kidneys and urinary ducts lie along the dorsal body wall of the abdomen. Also contained within the lower abdomen are the uterus, ovaries, and Fallopian tubes in the female and the vas deferens and prostate gland in the male. In males, two downward extensions of the abdominal cavity form the scrotal sacs surrounding the testes.

The thoracic and abdominal cavities (and the scrotal cavities in males) are considered part of the general body cavity or coelom. Each part of the coelom is lined on all sides with a thin, single layer of flat (squamous) cells known as the "peritoneum." The peritoneum forming the outer wall of these cavities is called the "parietal peritoneum"; the peritoneum on the outer surface of the internal organs, or viscera, is called the "visceral peritoneum.

Each type of organ is made of several different tissues. The four major types of tissues are epithelial tissues, connective tissue, muscle tissue, and nervous tissue. Epithelial tissues (or epithelium) include those tissues that originate in broad, flat surfaces; their functions include protection, absorption, and secretion. Epithelia can be one-layered (simple) or many-layered (stratified). Their cells can be flat (squamous), tall and skinny (columnar), or equal in height and width (cuboidal). Some simple epithelia have nuclei at two different levels, giving the false appearance of different layers; these tissues are called "pseudostratified." Some simple squamous epithelia have special names: The inner lining of most blood vessels is called the "endothelium." In contrast, the lining of the body cavities (including all parts of the coelom) is called the "mesothelium." Kidney tubules and most small ducts are also lined with simple squamous epithelia. The pigmented layer of the eye's retina and the front surface of the lens are examples of simple cuboidal epithelia. Simple columnar epithelia form the inner lining of most digestive organs and the small bronchi and gallbladder linings. The epithelia lining the Fallopian tubes, nasal cavities, and bronchi are ciliated, meaning that the cells have small, hairlike extensions called "cilia."

The outer layer of skin is a stratified squamous epithelium. Stratified squamous epithelia also line the inside of the mouth, esophagus, and vagina. Sweat glands and other glands in the skin are lined with stratified cuboidal epithelia. Most of the urinary tract is lined with a special kind of stratified cuboidal epithelium, known as "transitional epithelium," that allows a large amount of stretching. Parts of the pharynx, the larynx, the urethra, and the ducts of the mammary glands are lined with stratified columnar epithelium.

Glands are composed of epithelial tissues that are highly modified for secretion. They may be either exocrine glands (in which the secretions exit by ducts to targets nearby) or endocrine glands (in which the secretions are carried by the bloodstream to targets some distance away). The salivary glands in the mouth, the glandular lining of the stomach, and the sebaceous glands of the skin are examples of exocrine glands. The thyroid gland, adrenal gland, and pituitary gland are examples of endocrine glands. The pancreas has both exocrine and endocrine portions: The exocrine parts secrete digestive enzymes, while the endocrine parts, referred to as the islets of Langerhans, secrete the hormones insulin and glucagon.

Connective tissues contain large amounts of material called the "extracellular matrix" located outside the cells. The matrix may be a liquid (such as blood plasma), a solid interlaced with collagen fibers and related proteins, or an inorganic solid containing calcium salt (as in bone). Blood and lymph are connective tissues with a liquid matrix (plasma) that can solidify when the blood clots. In addition to plasma, blood contains red cells (erythrocytes), white cells (leukocytes), and tiny platelets that help form clots. The many kinds of leukocytes include granular types (basophils, neutrophils, and eosinophils, all named according to the staining properties of their granules), the monocytes, and the several types of lymphocytes. Lymph contains lymphocytes and plasma only.

Most connective tissues have a solid matrix, which includes fibrous proteins such as collagen and elastic fibers in some cases. Suppose all the fibers are arranged in the same direction, as in ligaments and tendons. In that case, the tissue is called "regular connective tissue." The dermis of the skin is an example of an irregular connective tissue in which the fibers are arranged in all directions. Loose connective tissue and adipose (fat) tissue have very few fibers. The simplest type of loose connective tissue with the fewest fibers is sometimes called "areolar connective tissue." Adipose tissue is a connective tissue in which the cells are filled with fat deposits.

Hematopoietic (blood-forming) tissue occurs in the bone marrow and the thymus. It contains the immature cell types that develop into most connective tissue cells, including blood cells. Cartilage tissue matrix contains a shock-resistant complex of protein and sugar-like (polysaccharide) molecules. Cartilage cells usually become trapped in this matrix and eventually die, except for those closest to the surface. Bone tissue gains its supporting ability and strength from a calcium salts matrix. Its typical cells, called "osteocytes," contain many long strands. These cells exchange nutrients and waste products with other osteocytes and, ultimately, the bloodstream. Bone also contains osteoclasts, large cells responsible for bone resorption and calcium release into the bloodstream.

Mesenchyme is an embryonic connective tissue made of wandering, amoeba-like cells. During embryological development, the mesenchyme cells develop into many different cell types, including hemocytoblasts, which give rise to most blood cells, and fibroblasts, which secrete protein fibers and then usually differentiate into other cell types.

Muscle tissues are specially modified for contraction. When a nerve impulse is received, overlapping fibers of the proteins actin and myosin slide against one another to produce the contraction. The three types of muscle tissue are smooth muscle, cardiac muscle, and skeletal muscle. The term "striated muscle" is sometimes used to refer to cardiac and skeletal muscle, both of which have cylindrical fibers marked by cross-bands, also called "cross-striations." The striations are caused by the parallel arrangement of the contractile proteins actin and myosin. Smooth muscle contains cells with tapering ends and centrally located nuclei. Muscular contractions are smooth, rhythmic, and involuntary, usually not subject to fatigue. The cells are not cross-banded.

Smooth muscle occurs in many digestive organs, reproductive organs, skin, and many other organs. Cardiac muscle occurs only in the heart. Its cross-striated fibers branch and come together repeatedly. Contractions of these fibers are involuntary, rhythmic, and without fatigue. Nuclei are near the center of each cell; cell boundaries are marked by dark-staining structures called "intercalated disks." Skeletal muscle occurs in the voluntary muscles of the body. Their cylindrical, cross-striated fibers contain many nuclei but no internal cell boundaries; a multinucleated fiber of this type is called a "syncytium." Skeletal muscle is capable of rapid, forceful contractions, but it fatigues easily. Skeletal muscle tissue always attaches to connective tissue structures.

Nervous tissues contain specialized nerve cells (neurons) that respond rapidly to stimulation by conducting nerve impulses. All neurons contain ribonucleic acid (RNA)-rich granules, also referred to as "Nissl granules," in the cytoplasm. Neurons with a single long extension of the cell body are called unipolar. Those with two long extensions are called "bipolar," and neurons with more than two long extensions are called "multipolar." There are two extensions: Dendrites conduct impulses toward the cell body. In contrast, axons generally conduct impulses away from the cell body. Many axons are surrounded by a multilayered fatty substance called the "myelin sheath," composed of many layers of cell membrane wrapped around the axon.

Nervous tissues also contain several types of neuroglia, cells that hold nervous tissue together. Many neuroglia cells have projections that wrap around the neurons and help nourish them. The many types of neuroglia include the tiny microglia and the larger protoplasmic astrocytes, fibrous astrocytes, and oligodendroglia.

Two major tissue types make up most of the brain and spinal cord, or central nervous system. The first type, gray matter, contains the cell bodies of many neurons, along with smaller amounts of axons, dendrites, and neuroglia cells. The second type, white matter, contains mostly the axons (and sometimes also the dendrites) of neurons whose cell bodies lie elsewhere along with the myelin sheaths surrounding many axons. Clusters of cell bodies found within the brain are called "nuclei" and "ganglia" when they occur elsewhere. Bundles of axons are known as "tracts" within the central nervous system and nerves when they appear peripherally.

Anatomists describe the body using directional terms, defined relatively according to the location of a given body part or segment. Some important directional terms are superior, inferior, cranial, caudal, dorsal, ventral, medial, lateral, radial, ulnar, anterior, and posterior.

DISORDERS AND DISEASES

Diseases or disorders that affect the entire body are systemic or multisystem. For example, fevers or febrile diseases raise the body's temperature. Many fevers are caused by infectious diseases such as influenza (a series of different viral infections). Influenzas cause fever, sore throat, muscle aches, coughs, headache, fatigue, and a general feeling of malaise.

Edema, or tissue swelling, is marked by an increase in extracellular fluid in several parts of the body at once. In the case of pulmonary edema, the fluid stains pink and fills the usually empty lung spaces (alveoli).

Most cancers are recognized by abnormalities of the cells in which they occur. Large tumors mark the most dangerous cancers with ill-defined, irregular margins. If the cancer tumor is well-defined, small, and has a smooth, circular margin, it is much less of a threat. Cancers are especially dangerous when they undergo metastasis, a process by which they produce wandering cells that spread throughout the body.

Juvenile diabetes mellitus (also referred to as diabetes mellitus, type 1, and insulin-dependent diabetes mellitus, or IDDM), like most endocrine disorders, has systemic consequences throughout the body, including damage to nearly all the blood vessels. The primary defect in this disorder is a lack of insulin, which impairs the body's ability to use glucose. Another endocrine disorder with systemic consequences is Addison's disease, which is caused by a deficiency of the hormone adrenocorticotropic hormone (ACTH) that normally stimulates the cortex of the adrenal gland. Symptoms include weakness, loss of appetite, fatigue, weight loss, and reduced tolerance to cold. These symptoms result from imbalances in glucose and mineral salts throughout the body.

Systemic lupus erythematosus, a connective tissue disease, often produces red skin lesions marked by degeneration and flattening of the lower layers of the epidermis, drying and flaking of the outermost layer, dilation of the blood vessels under the skin, and the leakage of red blood cells out of these vessels, adding to the red color. (The word *erythematosus* means "red.")

Muscular dystrophy has several forms; the most common is marked in its advanced stages by enlarged muscles in which a fatty substance replaces the muscle tissue. Another muscular disease, myasthenia gravis, is often marked by overall enlargement of the thymus and an increase in the number of thymus cells. Myocardial infarction, a form of heart disease marked by damage to the heart muscle, is noticed in histological sections by dead, fibrous scar tissue replacing the muscle tissue in the heart wall. In patients with arteriosclerosis, the usually elastic walls of the arteries become thicker and more fibrous and rigid; many of the same patients also have atherosclerosis, a buildup of deposits on the inside of the blood vessel, partially or completely blocking blood flow.

In nervous tissue, damage to peripheral nerves often results in a process referred to as chromatolysis in the cell bodies of the neurons from which these axons arise. The nuclei of these cells enlarge and become displaced to one side while the Nissl granules disperse, and the cell body swells. Increased deposits of fibrous tissue characterize multiple sclerosis and certain other disorders of the nervous system. Some of these diseases are also marked by a degeneration of the myelin sheath around nerve fibers. In the case of a cerebrovascular stroke, impaired blood supply to the brain causes degeneration of the neuroglia. It is followed by general tissue death and the replacement of the neuroglia by fibrous tissue. Cranial hematoma (abnormal bleeding) results in blood clots (complete with blood cells and connective tissue fibers) in abnormal locations. Granules of a protein-like substance mark Alzheimer's disease called "amyloid," sometimes containing aluminum, surrounded by additional concentric layers of similar composition.

PERSPECTIVE AND PROSPECTS

The Latin names used today for most body parts are derived in large measure from the writings of Galen, or Claudius Galenus, the physician to the Roman army in the second century. The study of anatomy was furthered in the Renaissance by artists such as Leonardo da Vinci (1452-1519) and Michelangelo (1475-1564). They dissected human corpses illegally to gain further knowledge of the anatomical structures visible on the body's surface. Such studies were followed by the well-illustrated anatomical texts of Andreas Vesalius (1514-64). He corrected many of Galen's errors regarding the structure of the human body.

A medical understanding of the circulatory system began with the studies of the Renaissance physician William Harvey (1578-1657). He examined the veins in the arms of many patients. Harvey first described the presence of valves in the veins and proved that the blood circulates outward from the heart, throughout the body, and then back again to the heart.

Microscopes were first developed around 1700 by Antoni van Leeuwenhoek (1632-1723) and others. Electron microscopes first became commercially available in the 1950s. Microscopy using instruments of these two types was widely used for distinguishing between healthy and diseased tissue taken either from bodies at autopsy or from biopsies of living patients. Modern diagnostic radiology began with the discovery of X-rays by Wilhelm Conrad Röntgen (1845-1923). Computed tomography (CT) scanning, developed in the 1960s and 1970s, creates a three-dimensional X-ray picture.

—*Eli C. Minkoff*

Further Reading

Abrahams, Peter H., Johannes M. Boon, and Jonathan D. Spratt. *McMinn's Color Atlas of Human Anatomy*. 6th ed., Mosby/Elsevier, 2008.

Agur, Anne M. R., and Arthur F. Dalley. *Grant's Atlas of Anatomy*. 13th ed., Wolters Kluwer Health/Lippincott Williams & Wilkins, 2013.

Crouch, James E. *Functional Human Anatomy*. 4th ed., Lea & Febiger, 1985.

Marieb, Elaine N. *Essentials of Human Anatomy and Physiology*. 10th ed., Pearson Education, 2012.

Moore, Keith L., and Anne M. R. Agur. *Essential Clinical Anatomy*. 4th ed., Lippincott Williams & Wilkins, 2011.

Netter, Frank H. *The CIBA Collection of Medical Illustrations*. CIBA Pharmaceutical, 1995.

Poewe, Werner, and Joseph Jankovic, editors. *Movement Disorders in Neurologic and Systemic Disease*. Oxford UP, 2014.

Preston, David C., and Barbara Ellen Shapiro. *Electromyography and Neuromuscular Disorders: Clinical-electrophysiologic Correlations*. 3rd ed., Elsevier/Saunders, 2013.

Rohen, Johannes W., Chihiro Yokochi, and Elke Lütjen-Drecoll. *Color Atlas of Anatomy: A Photographic Study of the Human Body*. 7th ed., Lippincott Williams & Wilkins, 2006.

Rosse, Cornelius, and Penelope Gaddum-Rosse. *Hollinshead's Textbook of Anatomy*. 5th ed., Lippincott-Raven, 1997.

Standring, Susan, et al., editors. *Gray's Anatomy*. 40th ed., Churchill Livingstone/Elsevier, 2008.

Wright, Thomas. *William Harvey: A Life in Circulation*. Oxford UP, 2013.

BONES AND THE SKELETON

Category: Anatomy

Specialties and related fields: Exercise physiology, orthodontics, orthopedics, osteopathic medicine, podiatry, sports medicine

Definition: bones are hard tissues that form the skeleton, the structure underlying the softer tissues of the body; they provide support while allowing flexibility

KEY TERMS

calcitonin: a hormone made and released by the thyroid gland that lowers the level of calcium in the blood by stimulating the formation of bone

collagen: a protein found in bone and other connective tissues; collagen fibers are well suited for support and protection because they are sturdy, flexible, and resist stretch

hormones: molecules made in the body and released into the blood that act as chemical messengers for the regulation of specific body functions

matrix: in bone, the matrix is a solid nonliving material that is a composite of protein fibers and mineral crystals

osteoblast: a bone cell that can produce and form bone matrix; osteoblasts are responsible for new bone formation

osteoclast: a large bone cell that can destroy bone matrix by dissolving the mineral crystals

osteocyte: the primary living cell of mature bone tissue

tissue: a collection of similar cells that perform a specific function

STRUCTURE AND FUNCTIONS

Bones are active throughout life: the 206 bones of the skeleton establish the size and proportions of the body and interact with all other organ systems. Disorders of the skeleton can have profound effects on the other organ systems and serious health consequences for the organism.

Bone, or osseous tissue, contains specialized cells and a solid, stony matrix. The living cells found in bone account for less than 2 percent of the total bone mass. The unique hardened quality of the matrix results from layers of calcium salt crystals such as calcium phosphate, which is responsible for about two-thirds of a bone's weight, and calcium carbonate.

Despite the great strength of the calcium salts, their inflexible nature means that they can fracture when exposed to sufficiently great bending or twisting forces or sharp impacts. Because the calcium crystals exist as minute plates positioned on a framework of collagen protein fibers, the resulting composite structure does lend a certain degree of flexibility to the bone matrix.

Based on the internal organization of its matrix, bone is classified as either compact (dense) bone or cancellous (spongy) bone. Compact bone is internally more solid, while cancellous bone is made from bony filaments (trabeculae) whose branching interconnections form a three-dimensional network. The bone marrow usually fills the cavities of the cancellous bone network, the primary location for blood cell formation in adults.

Both types of bone contain bone cells (osteocytes) living in small chambers called "lacunae," found periodically between the matrix plates. Osteocytes provide the collagen fibers and the conditions for proper maintenance of the mineral crystals of the matrix. Microscopic channels (canaliculi) connect neighboring lacunae and permit the exchange of nutrients and wastes between osteocytes and accessible blood vessels.

Atypical skeletal bone has a central marrow cavity bordered by cancellous bone. The bone is enclosed by compact bone, and the outer surface is covered by periosteum. Periosteum consists of a fibrous outer layer and a cellular inner layer. The periosteum plays an important part in the growth and repair of bone, and it is the attachment site for muscles. Collagen protein fibers from the periosteum interconnect with the collagen fibers of the bone.

The marrow cavity inside the bone is lined by endosteum. Endosteum is an incomplete layer covering the trabeculae of cancellous bone and contains various types of cells. The endosteum also plays important roles during bone growth and repair.

The bone matrix is not an unchanging, permanent structure. The bone matrix is constantly dissolved during a person's life while the new matrix is synthesized and deposited. Approximately 18 percent of bone protein and mineral constituents are replaced each year. Such bone remodeling can result in altered bone shape or internal rearrangement of the trabeculae. It may also result in a change in the total amount of minerals stored in the skeleton. These processes of bone demineralization (osteolysis) and new bone production (osteogenesis) are precisely regulated in the healthy individual.

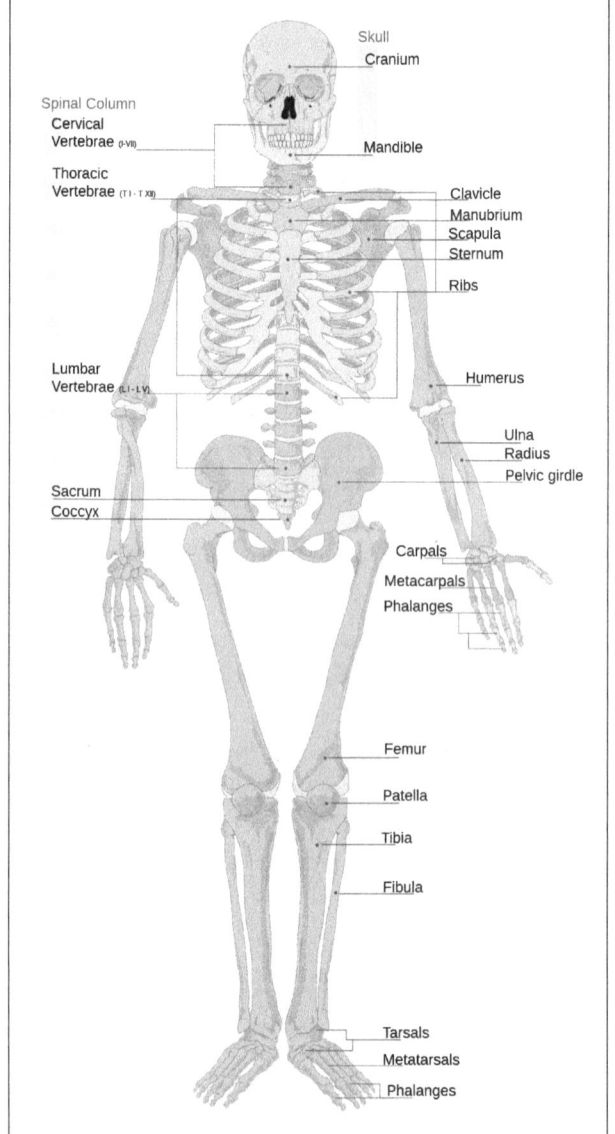

Image via Wikimedia Commons. [Public domain.]

An osteoclast is the type of bone cell responsible for dissolving the mineralized matrix. The osteoblasts are the cells that produce the materials that later become the bony matrix. The activities of these cells are influenced by several hormones and the physical stress forces to which a bone may be exposed, such as when a particular muscle becomes stronger as the result of weight training and pulls more strongly on the bones to which it is attached. Increased stress forces on a bone result in that bone becoming thicker and stronger, thereby allowing the bone to withstand the stresses better and reducing the risks of bone fracture. When bones are not subjected to ordinary stresses, such as in persons confined to bed or in astronauts living in microgravity conditions during space flight, there is a corresponding loss of bone mass, with the unstressed bones becoming thinner and more brittle. After several weeks in an unstressed state, a bone can lose nearly a third of its mass. Following the resumption of normal loading stresses, the bone can regain its mass just as quickly.

The skeleton has five major functions: support for the body; protection of the soft tissues and organs; leverage to change the direction and size of the muscular forces; blood cell production, which occurs within the red marrow residing in the marrow cavities of many bones; and storage of both minerals (to maintain the body's important reserves of calcium and phosphate) and fats (in yellow marrow to serve as an important energy reserve for the body).

The human skeleton contains 206 bones. These are distributed between two subdivisions of the skeleton: the axial skeleton and the appendicular skeleton. The axial skeleton contains eighty bones distributed among the skull (twenty-nine bones), the chest (twenty-five bones), and the spinal (vertebral) column (twenty-six bones). The remaining 126 bones are found in the appendicular skeleton's components: four bones in the shoulder (pectoral) girdles, sixty bones in the arms (including the fifty-four bones located in both of the hands and wrists), two bones in the hip (pelvic) girdle, and sixty bones in the legs (including the fifty-two bones found in the ankles and feet).

Skeletal bones are classified according to their shape. Short bones are cuboid in shape and are found in the wrist and the ankle. Long bones occur in the upper arm, the forearm, the thigh, the lower leg, the palm, the fingers, the sole of the foot, and the toes. Flat bones form the top of the skull, the shoulder blade, the breastbone, and the ribs. Sesamoid bones are typically small, round, and flat. They are found near some joints, such as the kneecap on the front of the knee joint. Irregular bones have shapes that are difficult to describe because of their complexity. Examples of irregular bones are found in the spinal column and the skull.

Learning to name the bones solely by their appearance is made somewhat easier because each one has a definitive form and distinctive surface features. Where blood vessels and nerves enter a bone or lie along its surface are commonly discernible as indentations, grooves, or holes. The locations where muscles are connected to bones by tendons or where a bone is tethered to another bone by ligaments are often visible as elevations, projections, or ridges of the bony matrix or as roughened areas on the surface of the bone. Finally, the areas of the bone that are involved in forming joints (articulations) with other bones have characteristic shapes that impart specific properties to the joint. Various specialized terms are used to name these features.

The joint's anatomy determines its functional capability, and the parts of the bones that form the joint have distinctive structural features. Articulations are found wherever one bone meets another. The amount of motion permitted between the bones forms an articulation range from none (for example, between the skull bones) to considerable (as at the shoulder joint).

DISORDERS AND DISEASES

Among the skeleton disorders, several of them occur during the growth and development of the bones. The problems usually result in abnormal (most often decreased) stature or abnormal shape of the bones. The aberrations may alter the entire skeleton or be restricted to a portion of it. The basis of the pathology is to be found in a disruption of the normal, orderly sequence of events that take place during the growth and remodeling of the bones.

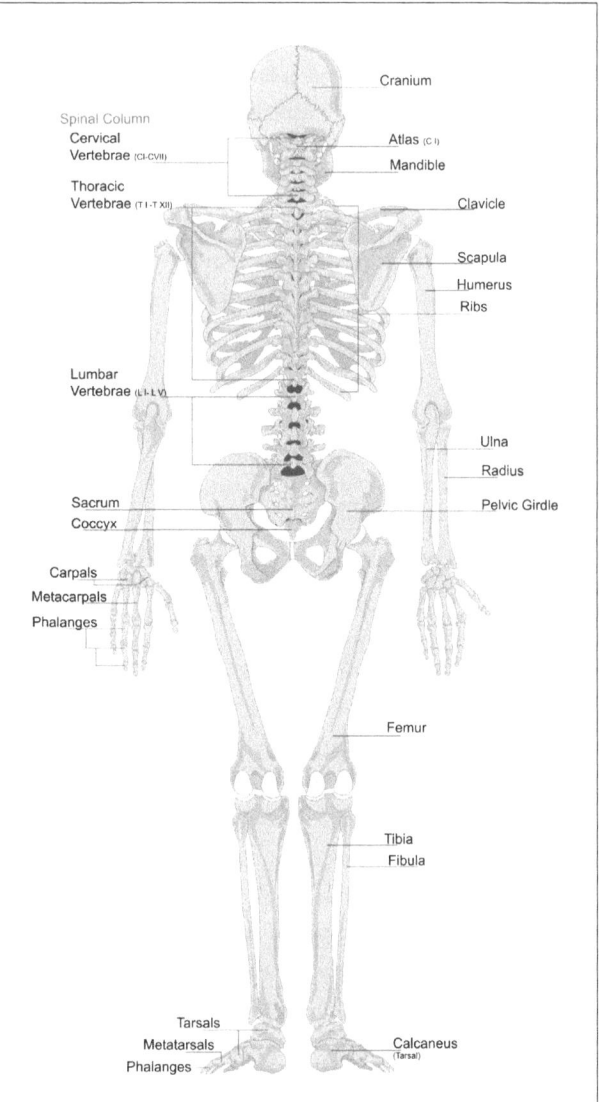

Image via Wikimedia Commons. [Public domain.]

Osteopetrosis belongs to this class of disturbance. It is an inherited condition in which abnormal remodeling increases bone density. Osteopetrosis seems to result from a reduced activity level by the cells responsible for dissolving the bone matrix—the osteoclasts. There is a precisely regulated relationship between osteoclast and osteoblast activity in healthy, normal individuals. Depending on the body's current needs, or merely those of a single bone, the rate of bone matrix formation by osteoblasts may be greater than, equal to, or less than the rate of bone resorption by osteoclasts.

Osteoclasts are derived from cells that are made in the bone marrow. For this reason, bone marrow transplantation has been tried as a treatment for osteopetrosis; however, this approach is risky and not always successful. There has also been improvement in the condition of some osteopetrosis patients following treatment with a hormone related to vitamin D. This particular hormone can increase bone resorption and thereby may prevent the increase in bone density that characterizes this condition.

Another member of this category of disturbance is congenital hypothyroidism. This condition can be caused by an insufficient supply of the element iodine in the pregnant mother, or it may result from inherited errors in producing the thyroid hormones. The basic problem in this condition is underactivity of the thyroid gland during the development of the fetus, resulting in a decrease in the production of thyroid hormones in the fetus.

Among the organ systems seriously affected by this condition is the skeleton. The bones do not develop correctly; consequently, the bones are shorter and thicker than normal, with corresponding changes in the child's appearance. Early diagnosis of the condition and timely treatment with drug forms of thyroid hormones can halt the disease. Otherwise, the adult skeleton has stubby arms and legs, a somewhat flattened face, and a disproportionately large chest and head.

A pituitary gland disorder can result in skeletal development abnormalities that are opposite to those observed in congenital hypothyroidism: namely, excessive growth in the length of bones. This condition is called "giantism" (or gigantism). It results from the overproduction of growth hormone by the pituitary gland before normal adult stature has been achieved. Cases are known of people attaining heights of more than eight feet tall. Unfortunately, because of complications involving other organ systems due to the excessive production of growth hormone, the persons suffering from this disorder usually die before the age of thirty. The most common cause of this situation is a tumor in the pituitary gland.

Surgical removal of the pituitary tumor is often attempted. Successful tumor removal stops growth hormone overproduction. In other cases, radiation treatments are used to destroy the tumor. It is also possible to combine both treatment techniques. Drug therapy is also possible. Because of the high doses necessary and the accompanying side effects of high drug dosages, however, the reduction of growth hormone levels through drug treatment is usually applied only in conjunction with one or both other therapies.

Some disorders afflict adult bone. Most of the remodeling disorders involve a loss of bone mass. The group of disorders known as "osteoporosis" (porous bone) is a rather common example; according to the International Osteoporosis Foundation, by 2013, osteoporosis affected more than 200 million people worldwide. The reduction in bone mass is sufficient to result in increased fragility and ease of breakage. There is also slower healing of bone fractures. In advanced cases, bones have been known to break when the person sneezes or rolls over in bed.

Loss of bone mass is a normal feature of aging, becoming quite marked after seventy-five, particularly in the hip and leg bones. Because of the normal decrease in bone mass with aging, there is no clear distinction between normal, age-related skeletal changes and the clinical condition of osteoporosis. The occurrence of excessive fragility at a relatively early age is an indication that osteoporosis is developing. Normally, between the ages of thirty and forty, the activity of the osteoblast cells (those that form the bone matrix) begins to decrease. In contrast, the osteoclast cells (those that dissolve the matrix) maintain their previous activity level. This imbalance between osteoclast and osteoblast activities results in the loss of about 8 percent of the total bone mass each decade for women and about 3 percent for men. Because of unequal loss in the different skeletal regions, the outcome is gradual height reduction, teeth loss, and fragile limb development.

Osteoporotic bones are indistinguishable from normal bones concerning their bone composition. The problem is too little of the strength-imparting matrix, with both compact and spongy bone being affected.

There are multiple causes of osteoporosis. Some cases have no known cause (idiopathic osteoporosis), some are inherited, and others are brought about because of hormonal (endocrine) disorders, vitamin or mineral deficiency, or effects of the long-term use of certain drugs.

The fact that women are more often affected than men and that the process is most conspicuous in women beyond menopause has implicated the female sex hormones (and, specifically, their decreased production) in the initiation of the osteoporotic process. One form of therapy is the administration of certain female sex hormones (specifically estrogens) to postmenopausal women (who have decreased production of estrogens). This treatment slows their loss of bone mass. While hormone therapy has been the mainstay of osteoporosis treatment for many years, controversy regarding the risks of hormone therapy has caused many women to stop using this treatment altogether. In 2002, two major studies found that the risks associated with hormone therapy outweigh the benefits. Following these studies, doctors began to look closer at the roles that high-impact exercise and the use of calcium and vitamin D play in decreasing bone density loss.

Other osteoporosis treatments include specific medications, such as bisphosphonates, recombinant parathyroid hormones, and monoclonal antibodies that influence bone deposition and resorption. The five main bisphosphonates are alendronate, ibandronate, pamidronate, risedronate, and zoledronate. These drugs bind to the hydroxyapatite matrix in the bone. When osteoclasts degrade bone, they also take in the bisphosphonates, which poison the osteoclast's metabolism. Bisphosphonates, therefore, diminish bone resorption. Daily subcutaneous injections of parathyroid hormone mimics stimulate bone formation. These drugs include Teriparatide (Forteo and others) and abaloparatide (Tymlos). Both medications are Food and Drug Administration (FDA)-approved to treat osteoporosis for up to two years in postmenopausal women at high risk for fracture. Denosumab is a human monoclonal antibody that binds the RANKL protein, preventing RANKL from binding to RANK receptors on the surface of osteoclasts precursors. RANKL inhibition prevents the activation and maturation of osteoclasts, which limits bone breakdown. Denosumab (Prolia, Xgeva) is injected subcutaneously every six months to treat postmenopausal osteoporosis. This drug also treats cancers that metastasize to bone, but it is administered once a month in such cases. The newest osteoporosis medicine is romosozumab (Evenity). This monoclonal antibody binds to and inhibits a bone-specific signaling protein called "sclerostin." Sclerostin inhibition increases bone formation and decreases bone resorption. The FDA approved romosozumab for the once-monthly subcutaneous treatment of osteoporosis. The newness of this drug caused the FDA to only approve its use for up to one year in osteoporotic women who did not respond to or could not tolerate other drugs.

Women at risk for osteoporosis and breast cancer have other options for their treatment. Raloxifene (Evista and generics) is a selective estrogen receptor modulator (SERM). This drug has estrogen-like effects on bones but antiestrogen effects on the uterus and breast. Raloxifene reduces the risk of invasive breast cancer and increases bone density. It provides a good treatment option for women with osteoporosis who have a high risk for invasive breast cancer.

Regular exercise is a means both of preventing the onset of osteoporosis and slowing its progression. Because muscular activity is critical for maintaining bone mass, extended periods of inactivity or immobilization can induce osteoporosis. For women, it is known that the amount and regularity of their exercise during their teenage years is strongly associated with their chances of developing osteoporosis thirty and more years later. The exercise need only be of moderate intensity to significantly decrease the risk of developing osteoporosis. Indeed, exercise at a level of intensity so high that it interferes with the normal female menstrual cycle (stopping the occurrence of menstruation completely or causing irregular cycle lengths) can increase the risk of developing osteoporosis later in life.

PERSPECTIVE AND PROSPECTS

One of the bone's primary functions is the protection of softer, more vulnerable tissues and organs. The physical properties of bone—it is as strong as cast iron but only weighs as much as an equally large piece of pinewood—make it ideal for this job. This combination of strength and lightness derives from the bony matrix of mineral crystals and the architecture of the bone, which unites compact and spongy bone.

The physical and chemical properties of the mineral crystals also result in the permanency of bone following death. Often the only trace of a dead body is the skeleton. Because of the resistance of bone to the processes of decomposition that befall the other tissues of the body following death, investigators are often able to determine the sex of the person whose skeleton has been found, even though all other tissues have long since disappeared. This identification is possible because of the characteristic differences between male and female adult skeletons. Racial differences in the detailed structure of the skull and pelvis, age-related changes in the skeleton, signs of healed bone fractures, and the prominence of ridges where muscles attach (giving clues about the degree of muscular development) are also valuable sources of information when attempting to identify skeletal remains.

The sexual differences in the human skeleton are most obvious in the adult pelvis. These are genetically determined differences that are structural adaptations for childbearing. For example, the pelvis is smoother and wider in females than in males. Other differences include a lighter and smoother female skull, a more sloping male forehead, a larger and heavier male jawbone, and generally heavier male bones that typically possess more prominent markings.

Among the common age-related changes found in skeletons are a general reduction in the mineral content and less prominent bone markings, which become more obvious after about age fifty. Various bones in the skull fuse together at characteristic ages ranging from one to thirty years of age. Examination of other bones throughout the body can also provide more accurate estimates of the age of a skeleton at the time of death.

Another consequence of the permanent nature of bone is that it provides a record of the changes in the skeletal anatomy of humans that have occurred during the hundreds of thousands of years of human evolution. Expert examination of skeletal remains can reveal an amazing wealth of information concerning the health and even the deceased's lifestyle.

—*John V. Urbas, Michael A. Buratovich*

Further Reading

Ballard, Carol. *Bones*. Heinemann Library, 2002.

"Bone Health for Life: Health Information Basics for You and Your Family." *NIH Osteoporosis and Related Bone Diseases National Resource Center*, Apr. 2018, www.bones.nih.gov/health-info/bone/bone-health/bone-health-life-health-information-basics-you-and-your-family. Accessed 29 May 2022.

"Bones, Muscles, and Joints." *KidsHealth*, Jan. 2019, kidshealth.org/en/parents/bones-muscles-joints.html. Accessed 29 May 2022.

Campbell, Barbara, J., and Stuart J. Fischer. "Bone Health Basics." *OrthoInfo*, May 2020, orthoinfo.aaos.org/en/staying-healthy/bone-health-basics/. Accessed 29 May 2022.

Currey, John D. *Bones: Structures and Mechanics*. Princeton UP, 2002.

"Drugs for Postmenopausal Osteoporosis." *Medical Letter on Drugs and Therapeutics*, vol. 62, no. 1602, 2020, pp. 105-12.

"Epidemiology of Osteoporosis and Fragility Fractures." *International Osteoporosis Foundation*, 2022, www.osteoporosis.foundation/facts-statistics/epidemiology-of-osteoporosis-and-fragility-fractures. Accessed 29 May 2022.

Fox, Stuart, and Krista Rompolski. *Human Physiology*. 16th ed., McGraw-Hill, 2021

Joyce, Christopher, and Eric Stover. *Witnesses from the Grave: The Stories Bones Tell*. Little Brown & Co., 1991.

Marieb, Elaine N., and Suzanne Keller. *Essentials of Human Anatomy and Physiology*. 13th ed., Pearson, 2021.

VanPutte, Cinnamon, Jennifer Regan, and Andrew Russo. *Seeley's Anatomy and Physiology*. 13th ed., McGraw-Hill, 2022.

BRAIN STRUCTURE

Category: Anatomy

Specialties and related fields: Emergency medicine, medical imaging, neurology, neurosurgery, occupational therapy, physical therapy, psychiatry, psychology, radiology

Definition: different brain areas have specialized functions that control activities ranging from basic biological processes to complex psychological operations; understanding the distinctive features of different neurological areas provides insight into why people and other animals act, feel, and think as they do

KEY TERMS

brain lobes: structural divisions of the cerebrum into four divisions or lobes—the frontal, parietal, temporal, and occipital lobes—each with distinct functions; the frontal lobe houses cognitive functions and control of voluntary movement or activity; the parietal lobe processes temperature, taste, touch, and movement information; the occipital lobe is primarily responsible for vision; and the temporal lobe processes memories, integrating them with taste, sound, sight, and touch sensations

cerebral cortex: the outer layer of the cerebrum. composed of folded gray matter and plays an important role in consciousness

cerebral hemispheres: either of the rounded halves of the cerebrum of the brain, divided laterally by a deep fissure and connected at the bottom by the corpus callosum

forebrain: the anterior of the three primary divisions of the brain in the embryo of a vertebrate, or the part of the adult brain derived from this tissue, including the diencephalon and telencephalon; the prosencephalon

hindbrain: the most posterior of the three primary divisions of the brain in the embryo of a vertebrate or the part of the adult brain derived from this tissue, including the cerebellum, pons, and medulla oblongata; rhombencephalon

midbrain: the middle of the three primary divisions of the brain in the embryo of a vertebrate or the part of the adult brain derived from this tissue; mesencephalon

neural tube: a tube formed by the closure of ectodermal tissue in the early vertebrate embryo that later develops into the brain, spinal cord, nerves, and ganglia

neurons: nerve cells that produce, carry, and transmit neural impulses throughout the nervous system

INTRODUCTION

About two weeks after conception, a fluid-filled cavity called the "neural tube" begins to form on the back of the human embryo. This neural tube will sink under the embryo's surface, and the two major structures of the central nervous system (CNS) will begin to differentiate. The top part of the tube will enlarge and become the brain; the bottom part will become the spinal cord. The cavity will persist through development and become the fluid-filled central canal of the spinal cord and the brain's four ventricles. The ventricles and the central canal contain cerebrospinal fluid. This clear plasma-like fluid supports and cushions the brain and provides nutritional and eliminative functions for the CNS. At birth, the average human brain weighs approximately twelve ounces (350 grams), a quarter of the size of the average adult brain, which is about three pounds (1,200 to 1,400 grams). Development of the brain in the first year is rapid, with the brain doubling in weight in the first six months.

The development of different brain areas depends on intrinsic and extrinsic factors. Internally, chemicals called "neurotrophins" promote the survival of neurons, the basic cells of the nervous system that are specialized to communicate electrochemically with one another and help determine

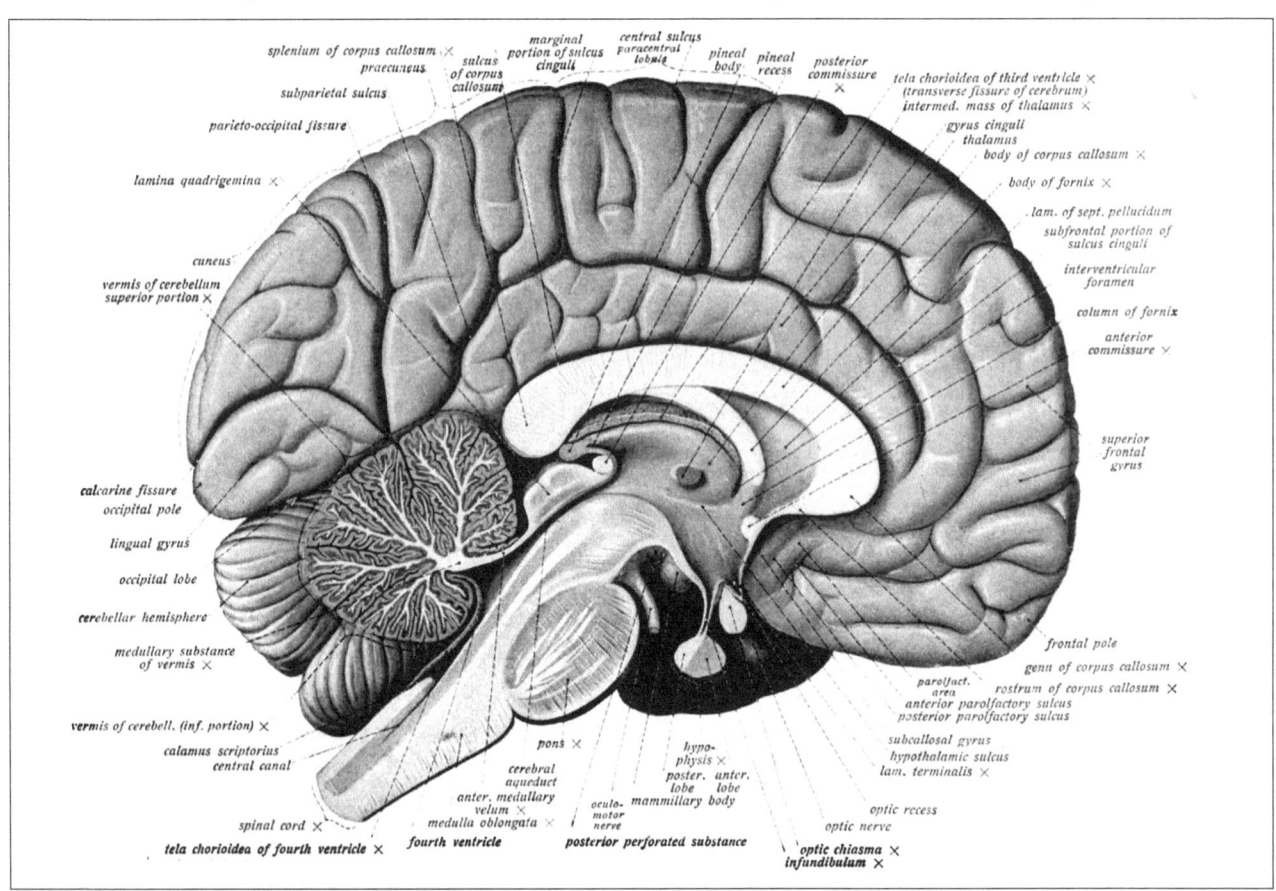

Brain structure. Image via Wikimedia Commons. [Public domain.]

where and when those neurons will form connections and become diverse neurological structures. Externally, diverse experiences enhance the survival of neurons and play a major role in the degree of development of different neurological areas. Research has demonstrated that the greater the exposure a child receives to a particular experience, the greater the development of the neurological area involved in processing that type of stimulation. Although this phenomenon occurs throughout the life span, the greatest impact of environmental stimulation in restructuring and reorganizing the brain occurs in the earliest years of life.

Experience can alter the shape of the brain, but its basic architecture is determined before birth. The brain consists of three major subdivisions: the hindbrain (rhombencephalon, or "parallelogram-brain"), the midbrain (mesencephalon, or "midbrain"), and the forebrain (prosencephalon, or "forward brain"). The hindbrain is further subdivided into the myelencephalon ("marrow-brain") and the metencephalon ("after-brain"). At the same time, the forebrain is divided into the diencephalon ("between-brain") and the telencephalon ("end-brain"). To visualize these brain areas' locations in a person, one can hold an arm out, bend the elbow ninety degrees, and make a fist. If the forearm is the spinal cord, where the wrist enlarges into the base of the hand corresponds to the hindbrain, with the metencephalon farther up than the myelencephalon. The palm, enclosed by the fingers, would be the midbrain. The fingers would be analogous to the forebrain, with the topmost surface parts of the fingers being the telencephalon.

One can take the analogy a step further. If a fist is made with the fingers of the other hand and placed next to the fist previously made, each fist would represent the two cerebral hemispheres of the forebrain, with the skin of the fingers representing the forebrain's cerebral cortex, the six layers of cells that cover the two hemispheres. Finally, the meninges cover the cortex like close-fitting gloves. The three layers of the meninges play a protective and nutritive role for the brain.

The more advanced the species, the greater the development of the forebrain, particularly the cortex. The emphasis here is placed on a neuroanatomical examination of the human brain, beginning with a look at the hindbrain and progressing to an investigation of the cerebral cortex. The terms "anterior" (toward the front) and "posterior" (toward the back) will be used frequently in describing the location of different brain structures. Additionally, the words "superior" (above) and "inferior" (below) will be used to describe vertical locations.

THE HINDBRAIN

As the spinal cord enters the skull, it enlarges into the bottommost structure of the brain, the medulla oblongata, often called the "medulla." The medulla controls many of the most basic physiological functions necessary for survival, particularly breathing and the beating of the heart and reflexes such as vomiting, coughing, sneezing, and salivating. It is sensitive to opiate and amphetamine drugs, and overdoses of these drugs can impair its normal functioning. Severe impairment can lead to a fatal shutdown of the respiratory and cardiovascular systems.

Above the medulla lie the pons, parts of the reticular formation, the raphe system, and the locus coeruleus. All these structures play a role in arousal and sleep. The pons plays a major role in initiating rapid eye movement (REM) sleep. Rapid eye movement sleep is characterized by repeated horizontal eye movements, increased brain activity, and frequent dreaming. The reticular system, sometimes called the reticular activating system (RAS), stretches from the pons through the midbrain to projections into the cerebral cortex. There must be activation from the reticular formation for the brain to pay attention to something. Activation of the reticular system by sensory stimulation or thinking increases arousal and alertness in diverse brain areas. Like the reticular system, the raphe system can increase the brain's readiness to respond to stimuli. However, unlike the reticular formation, the raphe system can decrease alertness to stimulation, decrease sensitivity to pain, and initiate sleep. Raphe system activity is modulated by an adjacent structure called the "locus coeruleus." The abnormal functioning of this structure has been linked with depression and anxiety.

The largest structure in the metencephalon is the cerebellum, which branches off from the base of the brain and occupies a considerable space in the back of the head. The cerebellum's primary function is to learn and control coordinated perceptual-motor activities. Learning to walk, run, jump, throw a ball, ride a bike, or perform any other complex motor activity causes chemical changes in the cerebellum that construct a program for controlling the muscles involved in the particular motor skills. Activation of specific programs enables the performance of particular motor activities. The cerebellum is also involved in other types of learning and performance. Learning language, reading, shifting attention from auditory to visual stimuli, and timing, such as in music or finger tapping, are just a few tasks for which normal cerebellar functioning is essential. Children diagnosed with learning disabilities often are found to have abnormalities in the cerebellum.

THE MIDBRAIN

The superior and posterior part of the midbrain is called the "tectum." There are two enlargements on both sides of the tectum known as the "colliculi." The superior colliculus controls visual reflexes, such as tracking a ball's flight. In contrast, the inferior colliculus controls auditory reflexes such as turning toward the sound of a buzzing insect. Above and between the colliculi lies the pineal gland, which contains melatonin. This hormone greatly influences the sleep-wake cycle. Melatonin levels are high when it is dark and low when light. High levels of melatonin induce sleepiness, which is why people sleep better when it is darker. Another structure near the colliculi is the ventricular system's periaqueductal gray (PAG) area. Stimulation of the PAG helps to block the sensation of pain.

Beneath the tectum is the tegmentum, which includes some structures involved in movement. Red nucleus activity is high during twisting movements, especially of the hands and fingers. The substantia nigra smooths out movements and is influential in maintaining good posture. The characteristic limb trembling and posture difficulties of Parkinson's disease are attributable to neuronal damage in the substantia nigra.

THE FOREBRAIN

In the center of the brain, right above the midbrain, lies the thalamus, the center of sensory processing. All incoming sensory information except for the sense of smell goes to the thalamus first before it is sent to the cerebral cortex and other brain areas. Anterior to and slightly below the thalamus is the hypothalamus.

Hypothalamic activity is involved in numerous motivated behaviors such as eating, drinking, sexual activity, temperature regulation, and aggression, largely through its regulation of the pituitary gland, which is attached beneath the hypothalamus. The pituitary gland controls the release of hormones that circulate in the endocrine system.

Subcortical structures. Numerous paired structures lie beneath the cerebral cortex, one in each hemisphere. Many of these structures are highly interconnected and are therefore seen as part of a system. Furthermore, most subcortical structures can be categorized as belonging to one of two major systems. Surrounding the thalamus is one system called the "basal ganglia," which is most prominently involved in movements and muscle tone. The basal ganglia deteriorate in Parkinson's and Huntington's diseases, both disorders of motor activity. The three major structures of the basal ganglia are the caudate nucleus and putamen, which form the striatum, and the globus pallidus. The activities of the basal ganglia extend beyond motor control. The striatum, for instance, plays a significant role in the learning of habits as well as in obsessive-compulsive disorder, a disorder of excessive habits. In addition, disorders of memory, attention, and emotional expression (especially depression) frequently involve abnormal functioning of the basal ganglia.

While not considered part of the basal ganglia, the nucleus basalis is nevertheless highly interconnected with those structures (and the hypothalamus) and receives direct input from them. Nucleus basalis activity is essential for attention and arousal.

The other major subcortical system is the limbic system, which was originally thought to be involved in motivated or emotional behaviors and little else. Later research, however, demonstrated that many of these structures are crucial for memory formation. The fact that people have heightened recall for emotionally significant events is likely a consequence of the limbic system's strong involvement in memory and motivation or emotion.

Two limbic structures are essential for memory formation. The hippocampus plays a key role in making personal events and facts into long-term memories. For a person to remember information of this nature for more than thirty minutes, the hippocampus must be active. In people with Alzheimer's disease, deterioration of the hippocampus is accompanied by memory loss. Amnesias, indecisiveness, and confusion result from brain damage involving the hippocampus. The hippocampus takes several years to develop fully. The gradual development of the hippocampus might explain why adults remember very little from their first five years of life; a phenomenon called "infantile amnesia."

The second limbic structure essential for learning and memory is the amygdala, which provides the hippocampus with information about the emotional context of events. It is also crucial for emotional perception, particularly determining how threatening events are. When a person feels threatened, their amygdala will become very active. Early experiences in life can fine-tune how sensitive a person's amygdala will be to potentially threatening events. A child raised in an abusive environment will likely develop an oversensitive amygdala, predisposing that person to interpret too many circumstances as threatening. Two additional limbic structures work with the amygdala to interpret threatening events, the septal nuclei and the cingulate gyrus. High activity in the former structure inclines one to interpret events as nonthreatening. In contrast, activity in the latter structure is linked to positive or negative emotional expressions such as worried, happy, or angry looks.

Other major structures of the limbic system include the olfactory bulbs and nuclei, the nucleus accumbens, and the mammillary bodies. The olfactory bulbs and nuclei are the primary structures for smell perception. Experiencing pleasure involves the nucleus accumbens, which is also often stimulated by anything that can become addictive. The mammillary bodies are involved in learning and memory.

Cortical Lobes. The most complex thinking abilities are primarily attributable to the thin layers covering the two cerebral hemispheres, known as the "cortex." This covering of the brain makes for the greatest differences between the intellectual capabilities of humans and those of other animals. Both hemispheres are divided into four main lobes, the distinct cortical areas of specialized functioning. There are, however, many differences between people, not only in the relative size of different lobes but also in how much cerebral cortex is not directly attributable to any of the four lobes.

The occipital lobe is located at the back of the cerebral cortex. The most posterior tissue of this lobe is called the striate cortex due to its distinctive striped appearance. The striate cortex is also called the "primary visual cortex" because it is where most visual information is eventually processed. Each of the layers of this cortical area is specialized to analyze different features of visual input. The synthesis of visual information and the interpretation of that result involves other brain lobes. The occipital lobe also plays a primary role in various aspects of spatial reasoning. Activities such as spatial orientation, map reading, or knowing what an object will look like if rotated to a certain degree depend on this lobe.

A deep groove called the "central sulcus" can be seen roughly in the middle of the brain if the brain is viewed from above. Between the central sulcus and the occipital lobe is the parietal lobe. The parietal lobe's principal function is processing bodily sensations: taste, touch, temperature, pain, and kinesthesia (feedback from muscles and joints). A parietal band of tissue called the "postcentral gyrus" adjacent to the central sulcus (posterior and runs parallel to it) contains the somatosensory cortex. In the somatosensory cortex, the body's surface is represented upside down in a maplike fashion. Each location along this cortical area corresponds to sensations from a different body part. Furthermore, the left side of the body is represented on the right hemisphere and vice versa. Damage to the right parietal cortex usually leads to sensory neglect of the left side of the body—the person ignores sensory input from that side. However, damage to the left parietal cortex causes no or little sensory neglect of the right side of the body.

The parietal lobe is involved with some aspects of distance sensation. The posterior parietal lobe plays a role in the visual location of objects and the bringing together different types of sensory information, such as coordinating sight and sound when a person looks at someone who just called their name. Some aspects of learning languages also engage the operation of the parietal cortex.

On the sides of each hemisphere, next to the temples of the head, reside the temporal lobes. The lobes closest to the ears are the primary sites of the interpretation of sounds. This task is accomplished in the primary auditory cortex, tucked into a groove in each temporal lobe called the "lateral sulcus." Low-frequency sounds are analyzed on the outer part of this sulcus; higher-pitched sounds are represented deeper inside this groove. Closely linked with auditory perception are two other major functions of the temporal lobe: language and music comprehension. Posterior areas, particularly Wernicke's area, play key roles in word understanding and retrieval. More medial areas are involved in different aspects of music perception, especially the planum temporale. The planum temporale is just lateral and behind the auditory cortex (a region known as "Heschl's gyrus") within the Sylvian fissure. It is a triangle-shaped region that forms the heart of Wernicke's area. With Broca's area (posterior part of the inferior frontal gyrus), Wernicke's area is among the most important functional brain areas for language.

The temporal cortex is the primary site of two important visual functions. Recognition of visual objects is dependent on inferior temporal areas. These areas of the brain are very active during visual hallucinations. One area in this location, the fusiform gyrus, is very active in perceiving faces and complex visual stimuli. A superior temporal area near the conjunction of the parietal and occipital lobes is essential for reading and writing.

The temporal lobe is near and shares strong connections with the limbic system. Thus, it is not surprising that the temporal lobe plays a significant role in memory and emotions. Damage to the temporal cortex leads to major deficits in the ability to learn and in maintaining a normal emotional balance.

The largest cerebral lobe, comprising one-third of the cerebral cortex, is the frontal lobe. It is involved in the greatest variety of neurological functions. The frontal lobe consists of several anatomically distinct and functionally distinguishable areas that can be grouped into three main regions. Starting at the central sulcus, which divides the parietal and frontal lobes, and moving toward the anterior limits of the brain, one finds, in order, the precentral cortex, the premotor cortex, and the prefrontal cortex. Each of these areas is responsible for different types of activities.

In 1870, German physicians Gustav Fritsch and Eduard Hitzig were the first to stimulate the brain electrically. They found that stimulating different regions of the precentral cortex resulted in different parts of the body moving. Subsequent research identified a "motor map" that represents the body in a fashion similar to the adjacent and posteriorly located somatosensory map of the parietal lobe. Therefore, the precentral cortex can be considered the primary area for the execution of movements.

The premotor cortex is more responsible for planning the operations of the precentral cortex. In other words, the premotor cortex generates the plan to pick up a pencil. In contrast, the precentral cortex directs the arm to do so. Thinking about picking up the pencil but not doing so involves more activity in the premotor cortex than in the precentral cortex. An inferior premotor area essential for speaking was discovered in 1861 by Paul Broca and has since been named for him. Broca's area, usually found only in the left hemisphere, is responsible for coordinating the various operations necessary for speech production.

The prefrontal cortex is the part of the brain most responsible for various complex thinking activities, foremost among them being decision making and abstract reasoning. Damage to the prefrontal cortex often leads to an impaired ability to make decisions, rendering the person lethargic and greatly lacking in spontaneous behavior. Numerous aspects of abstract reasoning, such as planning, organizing, keeping time, and thinking hypothetically, are also greatly disturbed by injuries to the prefrontal cortex.

Research with patients with prefrontal disturbances has demonstrated the important role of this neurological area in personality and social behavior. Patients with posterior prefrontal damage exhibit many symptoms of depression, such as apathy, restlessness, irritability, lack of drive, and lack of ambition. Anterior abnormalities, particularly in an inferior prefrontal region called the "orbitofrontal area," result in numerous symptoms of psychopathy, including lack of restraint, impulsiveness, egocentricity, lack of responsibility for one's actions, and indifference to others' opinions and rights.

The prefrontal cortex also contributes to the emotional value of decisions, smell perception, working memory (the current ability to use memory), and the capacity to concentrate or shift attention. Children correctly diagnosed with attention-deficit hyperactivity disorder (ADHD) often have prefrontal abnormalities.

Hemispheric differences. A large band of fibers connects the two cerebral hemispheres called the "corpus callosum" and several small connections called "commissures." In the early 1940s, American surgeon William van Wagenen, to stop epileptic seizures from crossing from one hemisphere to the other, performed the first procedure of cutting the 200 million fibers of the corpus callosum. However, the results were mixed, and it was not until the 1960s that two other American surgeons, Joe Bogen and Philip Vogel, decided to try the operation again, this time also including some cutting of commissure fibers. The results reduced or stopped the seizures in most patients. However, extensive testing by American psychobiologist Roger Sperry and his colleagues demonstrated notable behavioral changes in the patients, called the "split-brain syndrome." Research on split-brain syndrome and less invasive brain imaging techniques, such as computed tomography (CT) and positron emission tomography (PET) scans, has demonstrated many anatomical and functional differences between the left and right hemispheres.

The degree of differences between the two cerebral hemispheres varies greatly depending on several factors. Men develop greater lateralization—larger differences between the hemispheres—and develop the differences sooner. Those with a dominant right hand have greater lateralization than left- or mixed-handers. Therefore, when there is talk of "left brain" versus "right brain," it is important to remember that a greater degree of difference exists in right-handed men. A minority of people, usually left-handers, show little difference between the left and right hemispheres.

The right hemisphere tends to be larger and heavier than the left hemisphere, with the greatest difference in the frontal lobe. Conversely, several other neurological areas are larger in the left hemisphere, including the occipital lobe, the planum temporale, Wernicke's area, and the Sylvian fissure. One gender difference in hemispheric operation is that the left-hemisphere amygdala is more active in women, and the right-hemisphere amygdala is more active in men.

The left-brain/right-brain functional dichotomy has been the subject of much popular literature. Although there are many differences in operation between the two hemispheres, it is important to realize that many of the differences are subtle. In many regards, both hemispheres are involved in a given psychological function, only to different degrees. The most striking difference between the two hemispheres is that the right hemisphere is responsible for sensory and motor functions of the left side of the body. The left hemisphere controls those same functions for the body's right side. This contralateral control is found to a lesser degree for hearing and, due to the optic chiasm, not at all for vision.

Categorical decisions, understanding metaphors, and the symbolic aspects of language involve both hemispheres. In sound and communication, the left hemisphere plays a greater role in speech production, language comprehension, phonetic and semantic analysis, visual word recognition, grammar, verbal learning, lyric recitation, musical performance, and rhythm keeping. A greater right-hemisphere contribution is found in interpreting nonlanguage sounds, reading Braille, using emotional tone in language, understanding humor and sarcasm, expressing and interpreting nonverbal communication (facial and bodily expressions), and perceiving music.

The right hemisphere plays a greater role in mathematical operations. Still, the left hemisphere is essential for remembering numerical facts and reading and writing numbers. Visually, the right hemisphere contributes more to mental rotation, facial perception, figure-ground distinctions, map reading, and pattern perception. Detail perception draws more on left-hemisphere resources. The right hemisphere is linked more with negative emotions, such as fear, anger, pain, and sadness. At the same time, positive affect is associated more with the left hemisphere. There are exceptions to this; however, schizophrenia, anxiety, and panic attacks are related more to increased left-hemisphere activity.

SUMMARY

It has been estimated that the adult human brain contains 100 billion neurons forming more than 13 trillion connections with one another. These connections are constantly changing, depending on the brain's health and how much learning is taking place. In this dynamic system of different neurological areas concerned with diverse functions, the question arises of how a sense of wholeness and stability emerges. In other words, where is the "me" in the mind? While some areas of the brain, such as the frontal lobe, appear more closely linked with such intimate aspects of identity as planning and making choices, no single structure or particular function can likely be equated with the self. It may take the activity of the whole brain to give a sense of wholeness to life. Moreover, the self is not found in any single brain structure. Instead, what the whole brain does—its activity patterns—defines the self.

—Paul J. Chara Jr.

Further Reading

Evans, Amanda, and Patricia Coccoma. *Trauma-Informed Care: How Neuroscience Influences Practice*. Routledge, 2014.

Gazzaniga, Michael S. *The Consciousness Instinct: Unraveling the Mystery of How the Brain Makes the Mind*. Farrar, Straus and Giroux, 2018.

Getz, Glen E. *Applied Biological Psychology*. Springer, 2014.

Goldberg, Stephen. *Clinical Neuroanatomy Made Ridiculously Simple*. 4th ed., MedMaster, 2010.

Hendleman, Walter J. *Atlas of Functional Neuroanatomy*. 2nd ed., CRC, 2006.

Kalat, James W. *Biological Psychology*. 11th ed., Wadsworth, 2013.

Ornstein, Robert. *The Right Mind: Making Sense of the Hemispheres*. Harcourt, 1997.

Ornstein, Robert, and Richard F. Thompson. *The Amazing Brain*. Houghton, 1984.

Swaab, D. F. *We Are Our Brains: A Neurobiography of the Brain, from the Womb to Alzheimer's*. Translated by Jane Hedley-Prôle. Random, 2014.

Thaler, Alison I., and Malcolm S. Thaler. *The Only Neurology Book You'll Ever Need*. Lippincott Williams & Wilkins, 2022.

CARTILAGE

Category: Biology
Specialties and related fields: Geriatrics, orthopedics, otolaryngology, radiology, rheumatology
Definition: versatile connective tissue with several functions, most prominently strength and flexibility, found in many structures throughout the body

KEY TERMS

chondrocyte: the cell type responsible for secreting the collagen and elastin components of the cartilage matrix

proteoglycan: a compound found in connective tissue, and other places in the body, composed of a protein to which chains of sugar-based groups are attached

STRUCTURE AND FUNCTION

Cartilage represents a vital tissue component of the human body. It is responsible for numerous functions ranging from structural support to shock absorption. It is a subtype of the broader category of connective tissues. It thus embodies many of the features of this class. Like other connective tissues, cartilage does not receive any innervation from neurons or nerve cells, nor does it receive a blood supply like muscle or epithelial tissue. In addition, connective tissue is composed of an extracellular matrix—a conglomeration of fibers that provides the structural backbone and ground substance, which helps the tissue retain water. In the case of cartilage, these components are collagen fibers, a triple helix of protein fibrils that helps provide strength against resistance and various types of proteoglycans.

Chondrocytes are the cells primarily responsible for the production of the cartilage matrix. They are diverse in their function of maintaining the flexible yet resilient nature of cartilage. During development, chondrocytes develop from the line of embryonic stem cells, specifically the subsequent mesenchymal cells that hold the ability to become fibroblasts or precursors to bone. Chondrocytes secrete two primary elements of cartilage: collagen, which is a protein building block that provides strength, and elastin, which allows for flexibility. Unlike other similar tissues made of an extracellular matrix, cartilaginous cells themselves make up only about 10 percent of the overall structure of cartilage, a much lower percentage than other connective tissues. One hypothesis for the low cellular population is that cartilage relies heavily on diffusion for its nutrition. It does not have a blood or immunologic supply.

Three types of cartilage exist: hyaline, elastic, and fibrous. Each one has its histologic structure and unique function. Hyaline cartilage is the most abundant type and includes articular cartilage, which is the cartilage found on joint surfaces. Its major role is to help reduce friction and maintain the composition of joints since these surfaces are under constant motion throughout the day. Hyaline cartilage is located in the throat, larynx, nose, and costal carti-

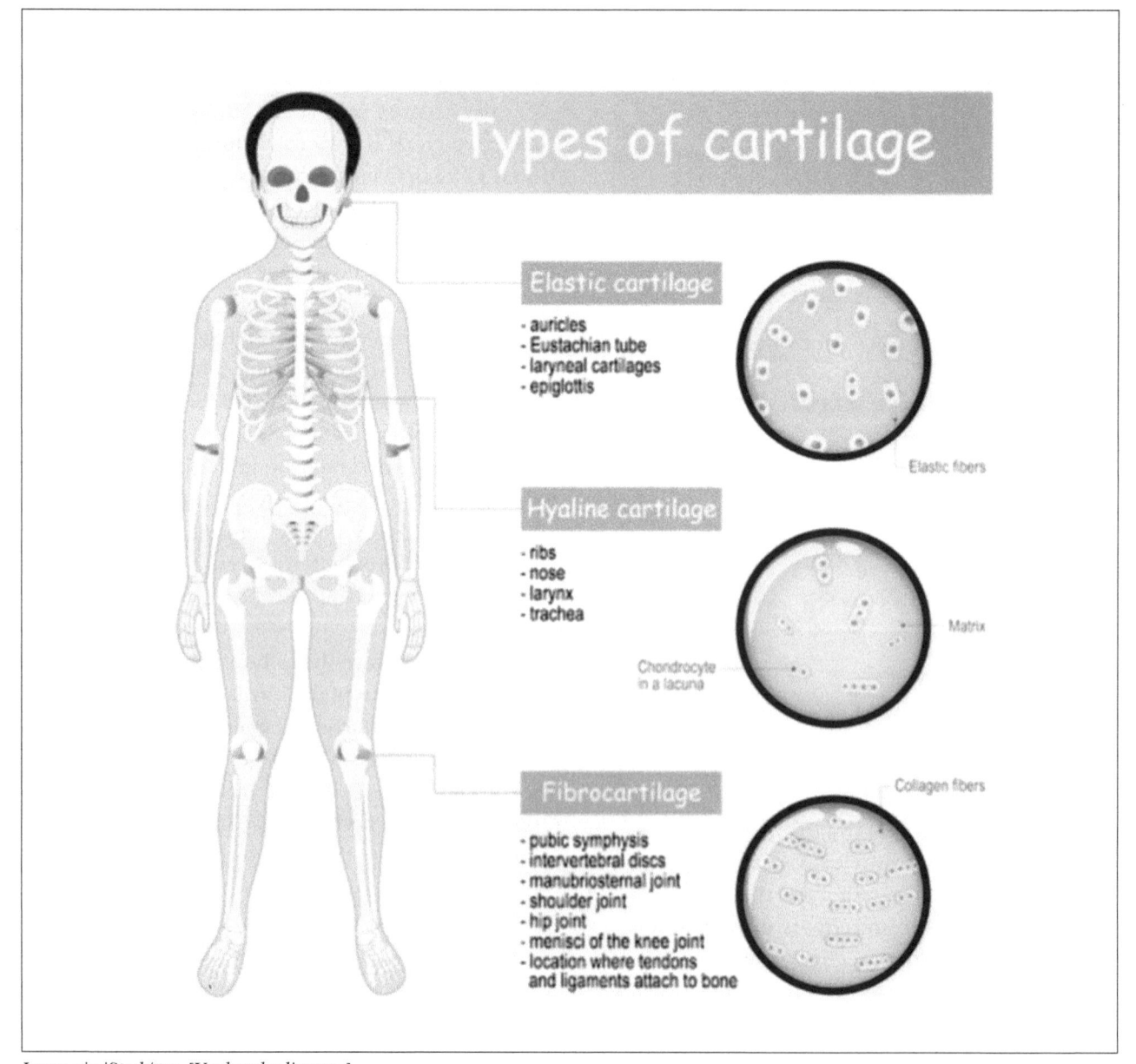

Image via iStock/ttsz. [Used under liscense.]

lages that attach the ribs to the sternum. Hyaline cartilage allows ribs to bounce back to their original position with respiration. Structurally, hyaline cartilage is about 5 to 10 percent chondrocytes. Approximately 70 percent of the remaining mass of cartilage is made up of water. The remaining 20 to 25 percent of cartilage is comprised of various proteins and extracellular components, such as type 2 collagen and proteoglycans.

The remaining 90 to 95 percent is composed of various proteins such as type 2 collagen and proteoglycans, that is, proteins with sugar groups, which help to retain the approximately 70 percent water component.

The pubic symphysis, which fuses the pubic bones, maintains structure against the turning forces from the two halves of the pelvis that articulates with the legs. On the other hand, fibrous cartilage, located in the disks that sit between vertebrae and in the structure that fuses the two pubic bones, functions primarily to provide rigidity and resist compressive forces. The fibrous cartilage helps resist and cushion the continuous downward compressive forces from walking and gravity in the spine. The structure of fibrous cartilage is distinct from hyaline in that the chondrocytes, while similar in quantity, secrete much thicker collagen fibers, thus resisting compression.

Elastic cartilage, the third type, is even more distinct from hyaline cartilage. It is located in the ears and epiglottis. It helps to spring the tongue back into its resting position with each swallow. This type of cartilage contains a much larger cell population than either hyaline or fibrous cartilage. The chondrocytes here produce many more elastic fibers, providing the necessary flexibility.

DISORDERS AND DISEASES

Diseases associated with cartilage can arise in several forms, including degeneration, congenital problems, and inflammatory conditions. While the list can be extensive, the most common disorders affecting cartilage include osteoarthritis (OA), costochondritis, spinal disc herniation, and disc degeneration. In general, these diseases result from disruptions in cartilage production and maintenance. Because of the vast number of structures in the body reliant on cartilage, these effects can potentially be devastating.

Osteoarthritis is a widespread disease affecting as many as 3 million people worldwide. Osteoarthritis has been linked to local inflammatory changes that can occur with increases in body fat and the metabolic changes of aging. Such changes alter the fine balance between the cartilage-producing chondrocytes and various catabolic or destructive elements, such as oxygen atoms with unpaired electrons. Because articular cartilage in weight-bearing joints, such as the knees and hips, is particularly affected in OA, individuals with this condition report joint discomfort worse at the end of the day. Radiologic findings include narrowing the joint space from loss of the cartilage, sclerosis or stiffening of the joint capsule, and bony cyst formation. Treatment involves a combination of medications targeted to reduce this inflammation, including nonsteroidal anti-inflammatory drugs (NSAIDs), like naproxen or ibuprofen, and steroid injections directly into the joint space. Rheumatoid arthritis, a close cousin of OA, likewise involves degradation of the cartilage's extracellular matrix but is associated with an autoimmune phenomenon. The body develops a reaction to its cartilage, leading to cellular destruction.

Costochondritis is a contributing cause of extracardiac chest pain. It is due primarily to inflammation of the hyaline cartilage at the costochondral junctions. Like OA, costochondritis is primarily controlled by NSAIDs and possible steroid injections.

Spinal disc herniation occurs when the nucleus pulposus, or the central component of a vertebral disc, begins to herniate or leak into the surrounding annulus fibrosus and cause swelling that irritates nearby nerves. On a similar note, disc degeneration involves weakening both layers, starting from the hyaline-type pulposus, and extending to the fibrous annulus. Studies have shown early loss of the proteoglycan component within both layers as a contributing factor.

PERSPECTIVE AND PROSPECTS

Cartilage damaged by degenerative, inflammatory, and traumatic etiologies has shown a limited ability to regenerate, thus afflicting millions of people. The future of managing such conditions will rely on restorative and regenerative technologies to restore or reduce the damage to the cartilage. Current research has ranged from implementing template-like devices to laying a foundation for various proteins. Some research has also considered carbohydrate polymer gels that mimic the extracellular matrix. Other tools include the injection of growth factors to stimulate the proliferation of chondrocytes and even the injection of mesenchymal stem cells to increase the chondrocyte population.

Of these research techniques, the field of cartilage tissue engineering has advanced significantly over the last five to ten years. Despite the proliferation of technologies, significant challenges persist, as none of these methods have been proven to replicate the structure and function of original cartilage fully. In addition, various obstacles exist, including regulatory concerns and ethical liabilities associated with embryonic stem cell-based products.

—*Derek T. Nhan, Walter Klyce*

Further Reading

Firestein, Gary S., et al., editors. *Kelley's Textbook of Rheumatology.* 8th ed., Elsevier, 2008.

Grassel, Susanne, and Attila Aszodi, editors. *Cartilage: Pathophysiology.* Springer, 2017.

Pham, Phuc Van, editor. *Bone and Cartilage Regeneration.* Springer, 2016.

CIRCULATION

Specialties and related fields: Cardiology; hematology; vascular medicine

Definition: the continuous movement of blood throughout the body by an organ system called the "circulatory system" that consists of the heart, lungs, arteries, and veins

KEY TERMS

aneurysm: a localized enlargement of a vessel, usually an artery

atherosclerosis: accumulation of plaque within the arteries

calcification: the deposit of lime salts in organic tissue, leading to calcium in the arterial wall

capillaries: hairlike vessels that connect the ends of the smallest arteries to the beginnings of the smallest veins

claudication: muscle cramps that occur when arterial blood flow does not meet the muscles' demand for oxygen

diastole: the period of relaxation in the cardiac cycle

hypertension: a blood pressure higher than what is normal

lumen: the space within an artery, vein, or other tubes

stenosis: the constriction or narrowing of a passage

systole: the period of contraction in the cardiac cycle

thrombus: a blood clot that commonly obstructs a vein but may also occur in an artery or the heart

vasoconstriction: a decrease in the diameter of a blood vessel

vasodilation: an increase in the diameter of a blood vessel

STRUCTURE AND FUNCTIONS

The cardiovascular system comprises the heart, arteries, veins, capillaries, and lungs. The heart serves as a pump to deliver blood to the arteries for distribution throughout the body. The veins bring the blood back to the heart, and the lungs oxygenate the blood before returning it to the arterial system.

Contraction of the heart muscle forces blood out of the heart. This period of contraction is known as "systole." The heart muscle relaxes after each contraction, allowing blood to flow into the heart. This period of relaxation is known as "diastole." A typical blood pressure taken at the upper arm provides a pressure reading during two phases of the cardiac cycle. The first number is known as the "systolic pressure" and represents the pressure of the heart during peak contraction. The second number is the diastolic pressure and represents the pressure while the heart is at rest. A typical pressure reading for a young adult would be 120/80. When blood pressure is abnormally elevated, it is commonly referred to as high blood pressure or hypertension.

The heart is separated into two halves by a muscle wall known as the "septum." The two halves are known as the "left and right heart." The left side of the heart is responsible for high-pressure arterial distribution. It is larger and stronger than the right side. The right side of the heart is responsible for accepting the low-pressure venous return and redirecting it to the lungs.

Strong construction of the arterial wall allows tolerance of significant pressure elevations from the left heart. Because of these pressure differences from one side of the heart to the other, the arteries and veins' vessel wall constructions differ. As with the artery, the vein's wall is made up of three distinct tissue layers. The arterial wall comprises three major tissue layers, known as "tunics." Secondary layers of tissue that provide strength and elasticity to the artery are known as "elastic and connective tissues." Compared to an artery, the wall of a vein is thinner and less elastic, which allows the wall to be easily compressed by surrounding muscle during contraction.

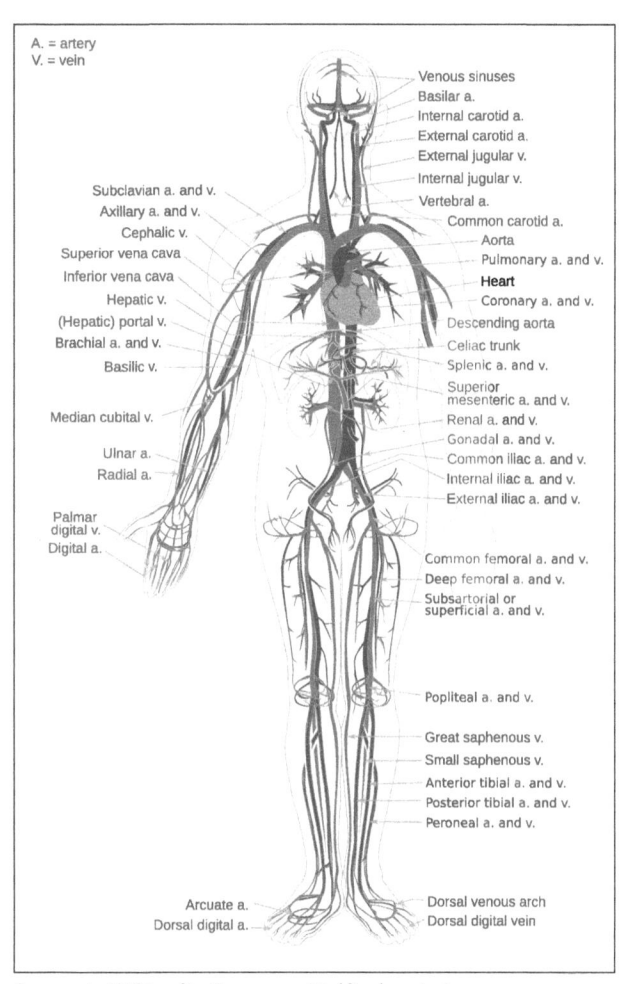

Image via Wikimedia Commons. [Public domain.]

While the heart is at rest, newly oxygenated arterial blood passes from the lungs between contractions and enters the left heart. Each time the heart contracts, blood is forced from the left heart into a major artery known as the "aorta." From the aorta, blood is distributed throughout the body. Once depleted of nutrients and oxygen, arterial blood passes through an extensive array of minute vessels known as "capillaries." A significant pressure drop occurs as blood is dispersed throughout the immense network of capillaries. The capillaries empty into the venous system, which carries the blood back to the heart.

The primary responsibility of the venous system is to return deoxygenated blood to the lungs and heart. Much more energy is required from the body to move venous flow than arterial flow. Unlike the artery, the vein does not depend on the heart of gravity for energy to move blood. The venous system has a unique means of blood transportation known as the "venous pump," which moves blood toward the heart.

The components making up the venous pump include muscle contraction against the venous wall, intra-abdominal pressure changes, and one-way venous valves. Compression against the walls of a vein induces the movement of blood. Muscle contraction against a vein wall occurs throughout the body during periods of activity. Activity includes every movement, from breathing to running. Variations in respiration cause fluctuations in the pressure within the abdomen, which produces a siphon-like effect on the veins, pulling venous blood upward. Valves are located within the veins of the extremities and pelvis. A venous valve has two leaflets, which protrude inward from opposite sides of the vein wall and meet in the center. Valves are necessary to prevent blood from flowing backward, away from the heart.

The venous system is divided into two groups known as the "deep and superficial veins." The deep veins are located parallel to the arteries. In contrast, the superficial veins are located just beneath the skin surface and are often visible through the skin.

DISORDERS AND DISEASES

Numerous variables may affect the flow of blood. The autonomic nervous system is connected to muscle within the artery's wall by way of neurological pathways known as "sympathetic branches." Various drugs or conditions can trigger responses in the sympathetic branches and constrict the smooth muscle in the arterial wall (vasoconstriction) or relaxation of the arterial wall (vasodilation). Alcohol consumption and a hot bath are examples of conditions that produce vasodilation. Exposure to cold and cigarette smoking are examples of conditions that produce vasoconstriction. Various drugs used in the medical environment are capable of producing similar effects. The diameter of the lumen of an artery influences the pressure and the flow of blood through it.

Another condition that alters the arterial diameter is atherosclerosis, a disease primarily of the large arteries, which allows the formation of fat (lipid) deposits to build on the inner layer of the artery. Lipid deposits are more commonly known as "atherosclerotic plaque." Plaque is similar to rust accumulation within a pipe that restricts water flow. Plaque accumulation reduces the arterial lumen diameter, causing various degrees of flow restriction. A restriction of flow is referred to as stenosis. The majority of stenotic lesions occur where arteries divide into branches, also known as "bifurcations." In the advanced stages of plaque development, plaque may become calcified. Calcified plaque is hard and may become irregular, ulcerate, or hemorrhage, providing an environment for new clot formation and release of small pieces of plaque debris downstream. When pieces of plaque break off, they may move downstream into smaller blood vessels, causing a blockage and restricting the flow of oxygenated blood; this can cause tissue death, stroke, and heart attack.

An arterial wall may become very hard and rigid, commonly known as the "hardening of the arteries." Hardened arteries may eventually become twisted, kinked, or dilated due to the hardening process of the arterial wall. A hardened artery, which has become dilated, is known as an "aneurysm."

Normal arterial flow is undisturbed. When blood cells travel freely, they move together at a similar speed with very little variance (laminar flow). Nonlaminar (turbulent) flow is seen when irregular plaque or kinks in the arterial wall disrupt the smooth flow of cells. Plaque with an irregular surface may produce mild turbulence. In contrast, narrow stenosis produces significant turbulence immediately downstream from the stenosis.

Many moderate or severe stenoses can be heard using a standard stethoscope over the vessel of interest. The physician can hear a high-pitched sound consequent of the increased velocity of the blood cells moving through a narrow space. (A similar effect is produced when a standard garden hose is kinked to create a spray and a hissing sound is heard.) Medically, this sound is often referred to as a bruit. Bruit (pronounced "broo-ee") is a French word meaning noise.

Patients with significant lower extremity arterial disease will consistently experience calf pain and occasionally experience thigh discomfort with exercise. The discomfort is relieved when the patient stands still for a few moments. This condition, vascular claudication, results from a pressure drop due to a severely stenotic (reduced in diameter by greater than 75 percent) or occluded artery. If the muscle cannot get enough oxygen due to reduced blood flow, it will cramp, forcing the patient to stop and rest until blood supply has caught up to muscle demand. Alternate pathways around an obstruction prevent pain at rest when muscle demand is low. Alternate pathways are also referred to as collateral pathways. Small, otherwise insignificant branches from the main artery become important vessels when the body uses them as collateral pathways around an obstruction. Time and exercise help to collateralize arterial branches into larger, more prominent arterial pathways. Suppose collateral pathways do not provide enough flow to prevent the patient from experiencing painful muscle cramps while performing daily exercise routines. It may be necessary to perform either a surgical bypass around the obstruction or another interventional procedure such as angioplasty, atherectomy, or laser surgery.

Claudication may also occur in the heart. The main coronary arteries lie on the surface of the heart and distribute blood to the heart muscle. Patients who have coronary artery disease (CAD) may experience tightness, heaviness, or pain in the chest after flow restriction to the heart muscle due to atherosclerotic plaque within the coronary arteries. These symptoms are known as "angina pectoris," or simply "angina," usually occurring with exercise and relieved by rest. The intensity of the symptoms is relative to the extent of the disease. A myocardial infarction (heart attack) results from a coronary artery occlusion.

Unlike the arteries, the venous system is not affected by atherosclerosis. The primary diseases of the veins include blood clot formation and varicose veins. A varicose vein is an enlarged and meandering vein with poorly functioning valves. Varicosity typically involves the veins near the skin surface, the superficial veins. It is often visualized as an irregular or raised segment through the skin surface. Varicosities are most common in the lower legs.

Valve leaflets are common sites for the development of a thrombus. Thrombosis is the formation of a clot within a vein, which occurs when blood flow is delayed or obstructed for many hours. Several conditions that may induce venous clotting include prolonged bed rest (postoperative patients), prolonged sitting (long airplane or automobile rides), and the use of oral contraceptives. Cancer patients are at high risk of clot formation secondary to a metabolic disorder that affects the natural blood-thinning process.

Because numerous tributaries are connected to the superficial system, it is easy for the body to compensate for a clot in this system by rerouting blood through other branches. However, the deep venous system has fewer branches, which promotes the progression of a thrombus toward the heart. A thrombus in the deep venous system is more serious because the risk of pulmonary emboli, commonly known as "blood clots" in the lungs, is much higher than superficial vein thrombosis. The further a thrombus propagates, the higher the risk to the patient.

Lower extremity venous return must take an alternate route via the superficial venous system when a thrombus obstructs the deep system. These alternative circulatory routes are known as "compensatory flow" around an obstruction.

PERSPECTIVE AND PROSPECTS
Historically, physicians evaluated the vasculature of the human body by placing one's fingers on the skin, palpating for the presence or absence of a pulse, and making notes of the patient's symptoms. Before the 1960s, treatment of the circulatory system was very limited or nonexistent, resulting in a high death rate and large numbers of amputations, strokes, and heart attacks. The development of arteriography (the angiogram) revealed more about the vasculature and the nature of the diseases involved. In conjunction with arteriography came corrective bypass surgery.

Vast improvements followed this development period in diagnostics, treatment, and preventive maintenance knowledge. Today, synthetic bypass grafts are commonplace and are used to reroute flow around an obstruction. In many cases, procedures such as atherectomy and angioplasty are often performed as outpatient procedures in which plaque or a thrombus is removed through a catheter inserted into the vessel. In cases where an artery has been seriously narrowed or weakened, a stent, a small mesh tube, may be inserted into the blood vessel to keep it open and unobstructed following the angioplasty procedure.

Diagnostic imaging of the cardiovascular system and the study of hemodynamics using ultrasound have been useful for patient screening, the monitoring of disease progression, and the postoperative evaluation of surgical/interventional procedures. Ultrasound is a particularly valuable diagnostic tool because, compared to X-rays or arteriography, it is less expensive; it is also quick, painless, and noninvasive (no radiation, needle, or dye is required).

Much new information has been made available to improve the general public's knowledge regarding diet, exercise, and the avoidance of unhealthy habits such as cigarette smoking as the way to create and maintain a healthier cardiovascular system. In addition to technological advances, new medications have been made available to reduce the risk of graft rejection, hypertension, and clotting and lower blood cholesterol. However, preventive measures such as a healthy diet, weight maintenance, and regular exercise constitute the most effective approach to good cardiovascular health.

—*Bonnie L. Wolff*

Further Reading
Ford, Earl S. "Combined Television Viewing and Computer Use and Mortality from All-Causes and Diseases of the Circulatory System among Adults in the United States." *BMC Public Health*, vol. 12, no. 1, 2012, pp. 70-79.
Guyton, Arthur C., and John E. Hall. *Human Physiology and Mechanisms of Disease*. 6th ed., B. Saunders, 1997.
Marder, Victor J., et al., editors. *Disorders of Thrombosis and Hemostasis: Basic Principles and Clinical Practice*. 6th ed., Lippincott Williams & Wilkins, 2012.
Marieb, Elaine N., and Katja Hoehn. *Human Anatomy and Physiology*. 9th ed., Pearson/Benjamin Cummings, 2012.
Saltin, Bengt, et al., editors. *Exercise and Circulation in Health and Disease*. Human Kinetics, 2000.
Strandness, D. Eugene, Jr. *Duplex Scanning in Vascular Disorders*. 4th ed., Lippincott Williams & Wilkins, 2009.

CONNECTIVE TISSUE

Category: Anatomy
Specialties and related fields: Biochemistry, hematology, orthopedics, rheumatology
Definition: a tissue category composed of adipose (fat), blood, bone, cartilage, ligaments, and tendons; the function of connective tissue is to connect, support, bind, protect, and store materials

KEY TERMS

adipocyte: a cell whose specific function is to store fats and associated nutrients, hormones, etc.

fascia: a thin layer of connective tissue that surrounds each structural component of a body like a protective coating

intracellular: refers to the space between cells in a tissue structure

sclera: the white part of the eyeball that is visible when the eyelids are withdrawn

STRUCTURE AND FUNCTION

Cells, the structural and functional units of life, are organized into tissues, a group of different types of cells and their nonliving intracellular matrix, or glue, that performs a specialized function. The four groups of tissues are: epithelial (covering and lining tissue; also glands); connective (adipose, blood, bone, cartilage, ligament, and tendon); muscle (skeletal, cardiac, and smooth); and nervous (brain and spinal cord).

Connective tissue typically has cells widely scattered throughout a large amount of intracellular matrix (that is, a substance in which the cells are embedded), unlike epithelial tissue, which typically has cells arranged in an orderly manner and has a limited amount of intracellular matrix.

Connective tissues are categorized as loose (areolar), dense, and specialized. Some connective tissues are difficult to classify, with the distinction between "loose" and "dense" not clearly defined. Dense connective tissue may also be called "fibrous connective tissue" because of the large quantity of collagen or elastin fibers.

Because tissues are defined as a collection of different cells, several types of cells may be found in various types of connective tissue: fibroblasts, which secrete collagen and other elements of the extracellular matrix, thereby creating and maintaining the matrix; adipocytes, which store excess caloric energy in the form of fat; and mast cells, macrophages, leukocytes, and plasma cells, which have immune functions and, therefore, an active role in inflammation. The matrix components are different in the various types of connective tissue. They may include fibers, amorphous ground substances (glycoproteins, proteins, and proteoglycans), and tissue fluid. Each type of connective tissue has a characteristic pattern of cells and a specific amount and type of matrix. For example, a bone matrix includes minerals, while blood has plasma for a matrix.

Loose connective tissue is the most common type of connective tissue; it holds organs in place and attaches epithelial tissue to underlying tissues. Loose connective tissue can be further categorized based on the type of fibers and how the fibers are arranged: collagenous fibers, which are composed of collagen and are arranged as coils; elastic fibers, which are composed of elastin and can stretch; and reticular fibers, which join connective tissue to other tissues. Loose connective tissue has a relatively large number of cells, matrix, or both, and a relatively small amount of fibers. Loose connective tissue is found in the hypodermis and fascia (the connective tissue that loosely binds structures to one another).

Dense connective tissue is identified by the high density of fibers in the tissue and a low density of cells and matrix. The type of fiber that predominates determines the type of dense connective tissue. Dense collagenous connective tissue, for example, contains an abundance of collagen fibers and is found in structures where tensile strength is needed, such as the sclera (white) of the eye, tendons, and ligaments. Dense elastic connective tissue contains an abundance of elastin fibers in structures where elasticity is needed (for example, the aorta).

Specialized connective tissues include adipose tissue, cartilage, bone, and blood. Adipose tissue is a form of loose connective tissue that stores fat. It is found in the fatty layer around the abdomen, in bone marrow, and surrounding the kidneys. Carti-

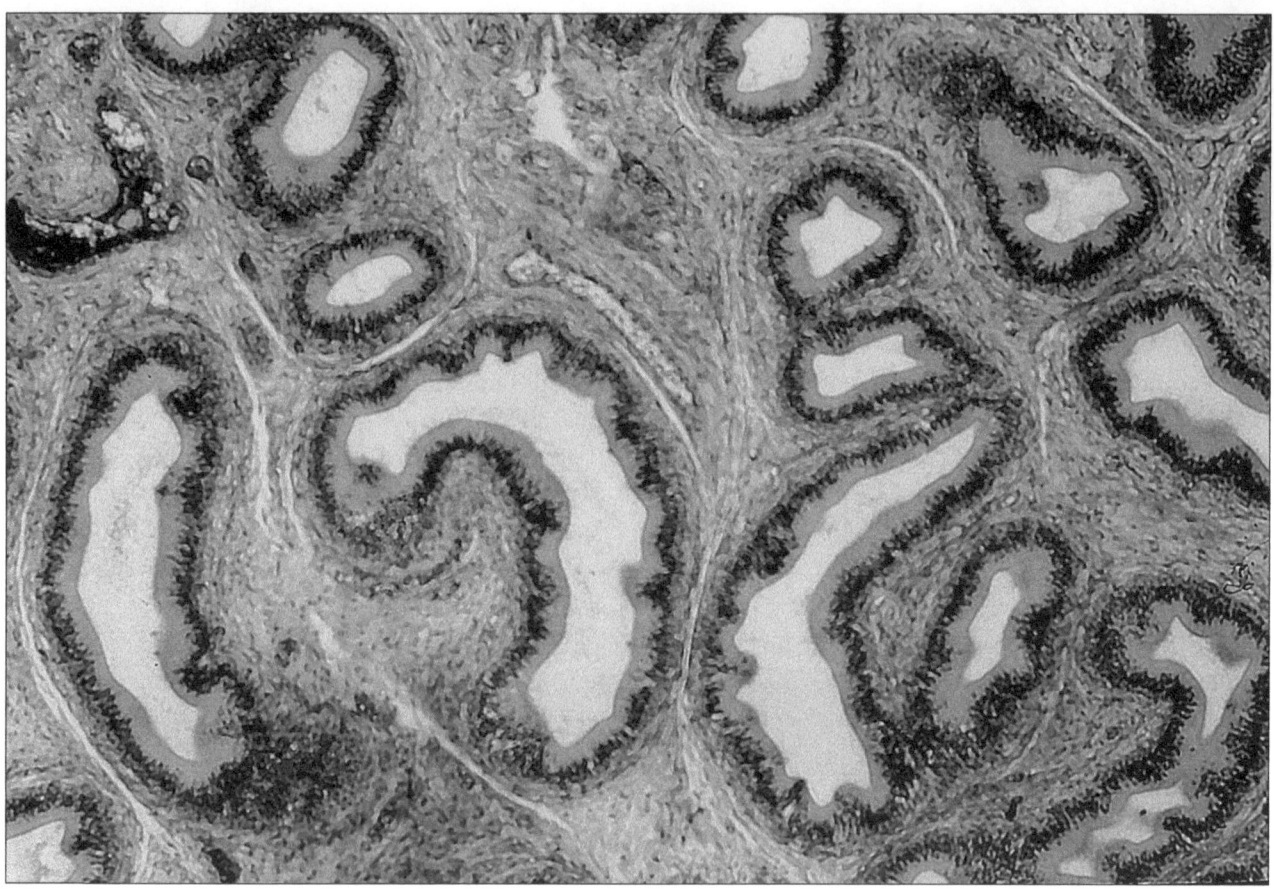

Collagenous connective tissue. Photo by Rollroboter, via Wikimedia Commons.

lage is a form of fibrous connective tissue. It comprises closely packed collagenous fibers embedded in a gelatinous intracellular matrix called "chondrin." While the skeleton of human embryos is composed of cartilage, cartilage does not become bone but rather is replaced by bone. The replacement is not universal; cartilage provides flexible support for the ears (external pinnae), nose, and trachea. Bone is a type of mineralized connective tissue containing collagen and calcium phosphate. Cells found in bone include osteoblasts, which form new bone for growth, repair, or remodeling, and osteoclasts, which break down the bone for growth and remodeling. The living cells are found in spaces in the calcified matrix. These spaces are lacunae interconnected by small channels called "canaliculi" that eventually join up with blood vessels in the bone organ. Thus, living cells can obtain nutrients and expel wastes even in a solidified matrix.

Blood, too, is a type of specialized connective tissue. Blood may seem to be an unlikely connective tissue. Still, it fits the definition: different cells widely dispersed in an intracellular matrix, working together to perform a specific function. Unlike other connective tissues, blood has no fibers. Blood does have several types of cells: red blood cells or erythrocytes, white blood cells or leukocytes (with subdivisions of monocytes, macrophages, eosinophils, lymphocytes, neutrophils, and basophils), and platelets or thrombocytes. The matrix is liquid and contains enzymes, hormones, proteins, carbohydrates, and fats.

DISORDERS AND DISEASES

Like any other tissue, connective tissue is subject to disorders and diseases. Some disorders are inherited (passed from one generation to the next through deoxyribonucleic acid (DNA) in chromosomes). In contrast, other disorders are related to environmental factors (such as deficiencies of specific nutrients).

Some inherited connective tissue disorders are Marfan syndrome and osteogenesis imperfecta. In Marfan syndrome, connective tissue grows outside the cell, having harmful effects on the lungs, heart valves, aorta, eyes, central nervous system, and skeletal system. People with Marfan syndrome are often unusually tall with long, slender arms, legs, and fingers. In osteogenesis imperfecta or brittle bone disease, the quantity and quality of collagen are insufficient to produce healthy bones. People with this disorder have multiple spontaneous bone breaks. Other connective tissue diseases are environmental, such as scurvy, caused by a lack of vitamin C required for the production and maintenance of collagen. Without sufficient vitamin C in the diet and subsequent lack of collagen, the patient will develop spots on the skin, particularly the legs and thighs, will be tired and depressed, and may lose teeth. Osteoporosis has many factors, but a lack of vitamin D and calcium in the diet will lead to thinning the bone, subjecting the patient to fractures, primarily of the hip, spine, and wrist.

Connective tissue diseases may also be classified as systemic autoimmune diseases and may have genetic and environmental causes. Examples of systemic autoimmune diseases include systemic lupus erythematosus and rheumatoid arthritis. Systemic lupus erythematosus can damage the heart, joints, skin, lungs, blood vessels, liver, kidneys, and nervous system. The immune system is spontaneously overactivated in these situations and produces autoantibodies that attack the body's cells. More women than men are diagnosed with lupus and more black women than other groups. Rheumatoid arthritis is caused when immune cells attack the membrane around joints and destroy the joint's cartilage; it can also affect the heart and lungs and interfere with vision.

—*M. A. Foote*

Further Reading

Gordon, Caroline, and Wolfgang Gross. *Connective Tissue Diseases: An Atlas of Investigation and Management.* Clinical Publishing, 2011.

"Hereditary Connective Tissue Disorders." *University of Miami Health System*, 2022, umiamihealth.org/en/treatments-and-services/genetics/hereditary-connective-tissue-disorders.

Lundon, Katie. *Orthopedic Rehabilitation Science: Principles for Clinical Management of Nonmineralized Connective Tissue.* Butterworth-Heinemann, 2003.

"Mixed Connective Tissue Disease." *Mayo Clinic*, 25 May 2022, www.mayoclinic.org/diseases-conditions/mixed-connective-tissue-disease/symptoms-causes/syc-20375147.

Price, Sylvia Anderson, and Lorraine McCarty Wilson, editors. *Pathophysiology: Clinical Concepts of Disease Processes.* Mosby, 2003.

Royce, Peter M., and Beat Steinmann, editors. *Connective Tissue and Its Heritable Disorders: Molecular, Genetic, and Medical Aspects.* Wiley-Liss, 2002.

"What Are Heritable Connective Tissue Disorders?" *The ILC Foundation*, 2022, www.theilcfoundation.org/what-are-heritable-connective-tissue-disorders/.

FASCIA

Category: Anatomy

Specialties and related fields: Exercise physiology, neurology, orthopedics, osteopathic medicine, physical therapy

Definition: a network of connective tissue that extends throughout the body; it functions as a shock absorber, a structural component of the body, and a medium that permits intracellular communication

KEY TERMS

connective tissue: the tissue in the body that binds and supports body parts

parasympathetic nervous system: part of the autonomic nervous system that restores and conserves the body's resources

synovial: related to or producing a fluid that fills a saclike structure surrounding a joint and provides lubrication

STRUCTURE AND FUNCTIONS

There are three layers of fascia: the superficial fascia, the deep fascia, and the visceral fascia. The superficial fascia, also known as the "subcutaneous tissue," is a layer of adipose or fatty tissue under the skin. The deep fascia is a layer of dense, fibrous tissue under the superficial fascia, surrounding and penetrating the muscles, bones, nerves, body organs, and blood vessels. The deep fascia has extensions that stretch from the tendons that attach muscles to bone and lie in broad, flat sheets, called "aponeurosis." The deep fascia is so strong that it is rarely damaged, even in traumatic injuries. The visceral fascia surrounds the body organs, suspends them, and wraps them in a protective layer of connective tissue.

The superficial fascia can stretch to accommodate pregnancy and weight gain. Usually, it slowly reverts to its normal tension level after pregnancy or weight loss. The visceral fascia lacks the elastic properties of the superficial fascia since its role is to protect the body organs. It provides for limited movement of the organs within their cavities while not constricting the organs. The deep fascia contains many sensory receptors that can report pain and changes in body movement, pressure, and vibration within the body, in the chemicals produced by the body, and in body temperature.

The deep fascia contracts when the body responds to a threat, which is part of the "fight-or-flight" reflex. This increased tension increases its strength.

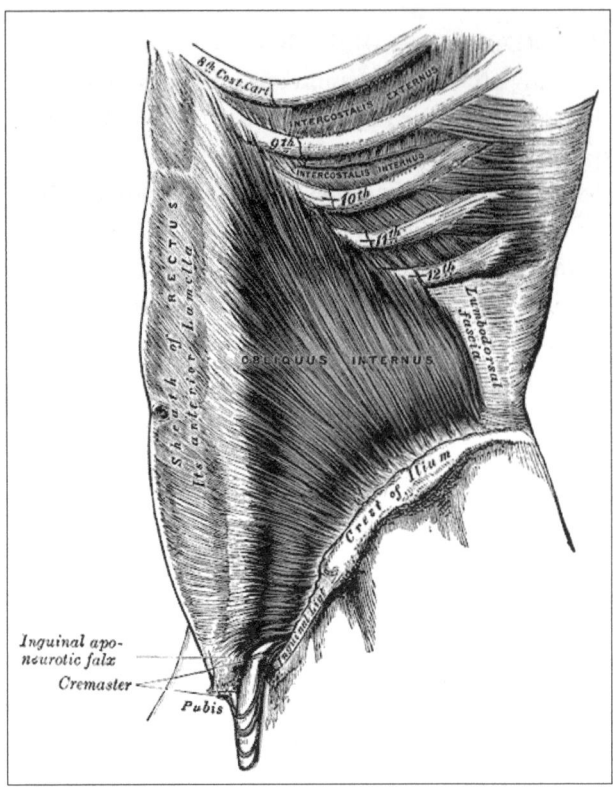

The rectus sheath (extensive vertical darker gray at left), an example of a fascia. Image via Wikimedia Commons. [Public domain.]

The deep fascia relaxes at times when the body is stressed beyond what it can tolerate and when the body is put in a relaxing position. Suppose the tension on the deep fascia persists. In that case, it responds by adding collagen and other proteins, which bind to the existing proteins. While this increases the strength of the body, it can restrict the structures that it is supposed to protect. Hormones produced by the body can relax the deep fascia. For example, parasympathetic nervous system hormones can trigger its relaxation.

DISORDERS AND DISEASES

Due to the presence of fascia throughout the body, many conditions can be caused by its disorders. Some examples are adhesions, carpal tunnel syndrome, compartment syndrome, fibromyalgia, hernia, Marfan syndrome, meningitis, mixed connective tissue disease, myofascial pain syndrome, necrotizing fasciitis, pericardial effusion, plantar fasciitis, pleural effusion, polyarteritis nodosa, rheumatoid arthritis, scleroderma, and tendinitis.

Common conditions affecting fascia are carpal tunnel syndrome, inguinal hernia, plantar fasciitis (heel spur), rheumatoid arthritis, and tendonitis. Carpal tunnel syndrome affects a small opening through the wrist into the hand. The median nerve and the carpal ligament pass through this opening. Narrowing the opening pinches these structures and causes pain and numbness in the hand. The treatment includes physical therapy, wrist splints, and possibly surgery. An inguinal hernia is the protrusion of part of the bowel through an opening in the fascia. It protrudes through the openings in the abdominal aponeurosis for the two saphenous veins. Inguinal hernias are treated by surgery to support the aponeurosis in these openings. Plantar fasciitis is caused by chronic inflammation of the fascia that supports the arch of the foot, leading to calcification on the bottom of the heel. This condition is treated with orthotics or surgery. Rheumatoid arthritis is an autoimmune condition that affects symmetric joints in the body and causes chronic inflammation of the synovial membranes in the joints, leading to joint damage. Many medications are available to treat rheumatoid arthritis. Still, they suppress the body's immune response and so have risks. Tendinitis is inflammation of a tendon, often due to injury or repetitive use, such as "tennis elbow." This condition is treated with corticosteroid injections into the joint, the application of ice or heat, and rest.

PERSPECTIVE AND PROSPECTS

The importance of the fascia has been embraced by practitioners other than doctors of traditional medicine. The fascia forms the basis for therapies such as Rolfing, massage, chiropractic, physical therapy, osteopathy, yoga, and Tai Chi Chuan. In the late 1800s, Sweden's Pehr Henrik Ling, with his associates, wrote of the relationship between mind and body. His therapy aimed to improve the mental status of a person by improving their ability to move their body. In 1984, Raymond Nimmo wrote of the importance of treating the fascia and trigger points in the body.

Ida P. Rolf (1896-1979) was a notable pioneer in understanding the importance of the body fascia. Rolf felt that the medical community had largely ignored the fascia and developed a technique centered on structural integrity and the importance of gravity. Structural integrity deals with the property of the fascia that causes it to adapt to changes in the body, even when the change puts the body off balance, out of alignment, or causes pain. Rolf devoted much of her life to treating those disabled who had not responded to medical treatment. Her therapy is called "Rolfing."

Medical doctors specializing in exercise physiology, neurology, and orthopedics are becoming more aware of the role of the fascia in the body. However, chiropractors continue to hold the primary role in dealing with fascia problems that do not respond to medical treatment. In 2007, the first International Fascia Research Congress was held in Boston, Massachusetts.

—*Christine M. Carroll*

Further Reading

"Bones, Joints, and Muscles." *Healthdirect*, Sept. 2021, www.healthdirect.gov.au/bones-muscles-and-joints

"Carpal Tunnel Syndrome." *Mayo Clinic*, 25 Feb. 2022, www.mayoclinic.org/diseases-conditions/carpal-tunnel-syndrome/symptoms-causes/syc-20355603. Accessed 8 June 2022.

Hecht, Marjorie. "Understanding Tendinopathy." *Healthline*, 8 Nov. 2018, www.healthline.com/health/tendinopathy. Accessed 8 Jun. 2022.

"Inguinal Hernia," *Johns Hopkins Medicine*, n.d., www.hopkinsmedicine.org/health/conditions-and-diseases/hernias/inguinal-hernia.

Leach, Robert E., and Teresa Briedwell. "Tendinopathy." *Health Library*, 18 Mar. 2013.

Lesondak, David. *Fascia: What it is and Why it Matters*. Handspring Pub. Ltd., 2017.
Lindsay, Mark. *Fascia: Clinical Applications for Health and Human Performance*. Delmar Cengage Learning, 2008.
Paoletti, Serge. *The Fasciae: Anatomy, Dysfunction, and Treatment*. Eastland Press, 2006.
"Plantar Fasciitis." *MedlinePlus*, 20 Jan. 2022, www.mayoclinic.org/diseases-conditions/plantar-fasciitis/symptoms-causes/syc-20354846. Accessed 8 Jun. 2022.
"Rheumatoid Arthritis." Cleveland Clinic, 18 Feb. 2022, my.clevelandclinic.org/health/diseases/4924-rheumatoid-arthritis. Accessed 8 June 2022.
Schleip, Robert. *Fascia in Sport and Movement*. 2nd ed., Handspring Publishing, 2021.

HEART

Category: Anatomy
Specialties and related fields: Cardiology, emergency medicine, exercise physiology, family medicine, hematology, rheumatology, vascular medicine
Definition: the muscular pump that moves blood through the body through rhythmic contractions

KEY TERMS

arteries: vessels that take blood away from the heart and toward the tissues

atria: the upper receiving chambers of the heart that lie above the ventricles

atrioventricular (A-V) node: a small region of specialized heart muscle cells that receives the electrical impulse from the atria and begins its transmission to the ventricles

coronary arteries: the arteries that supply blood to the heart muscle

diastole: the period of relaxation of the heart between beats

sinoatrial (S-A) node: a small region of specialized heart muscle cells that spontaneously generates and sends an electrical signal that gives the heart an automatic rhythm for contraction

systole: the period of contraction of the heart when blood moves out of the heart chambers and into the arteries

veins: vessels that take blood to the heart and from the tissues

ventricles: the lower pumping chambers of the heart located below the atria; they force blood into the arteries

STRUCTURE AND FUNCTIONS

All the cells in the human body depend on the blood in the cardiovascular system (the heart and blood vessels) to transport gases, nutrients, hormones, and other factors. Likewise, the tissues must have a way to dispose of waste products, so they do not build to harmful levels. All these substances are dissolved in the blood, but something must provide the force to transport the blood to all body parts at all times—the heart. This organ must beat continuously from early in development until death. It beats without conscious control and can vary how quickly it moves blood throughout the body depending on the needs and activities of the tissues.

In humans, an individual's heart is about the size of a fist and is enclosed in the center of the chest cavity between the lungs. The heart contains specialized muscle cells known as "cardiac muscle." These cardiac cells make up most of the thickness of the heart's walls; they are responsible for moving blood out of the heart and are also involved in maintaining the rhythm of the heartbeat. This heavily muscled layer is referred to as the myocardium. The heart's inner lining is called the "endocardium"; it is continuous with the lining of all the blood vessels in the body. The outermost layer of the heart is the epicardium, which covers the myocardium. The heart moves as it beats and is contained within a fluid-filled bag called the "pericardial sac." The rhythmically beating heart has the potential to rub against adjacent structures (such as the lungs), harming itself and those structures. Therefore, the heart must be encased in the pericardial sac with its lubricating fluid.

The human heart has four separate chambers. These internal cavities can be identified by their location and function. The upper pair of smaller chambers are "atria," and the lower larger chambers are called "ventricles." Because the atria and ventricles have a muscular wall that separates them into right and left halves, one can refer to the individual chambers as the right atrium and left atrium, and the right ventricle and left ventricle. The wall that separates the right and left halves of the heart is called the "septum." The septum prevents any mixing of blood from the right and left sides of the heart. However, the atria and ventricles on the same side must allow blood to pass through them in a single direction. This action is accomplished by one-way valves between the atria and ventricles. The valve that allows blood to pass from the right atrium to the right ventricle is called the "tricuspid valve" because it is made of three flaps. On the left side of the heart is the "bicuspid valve" (with two flaps), also known as the "mitral valve." The bicuspid valve allows blood from the left atrium to flow only into the left ventricle. This rather complex anatomy is necessary because the heart must pump blood in one direction and into two separate systems.

The heart's anatomy often makes more sense if one understands its function or physiology. For example, one may consider an active cell in the body, perhaps a muscle cell that moves the foot. This cell utilizes oxygen to help metabolize food for energy. Carbon dioxide is produced as a waste product during this process, and high carbon dioxide levels can harm cells. Therefore, one of the jobs of the cardiovascular system is to deliver oxygen and take away carbon dioxide. Once the blood picks up the carbon dioxide, it travels back to the heart via veins and enters the right atrium. The blood passes through the tricuspid valve and enters the right ventricle. The right ventricle sends the blood past a one-way

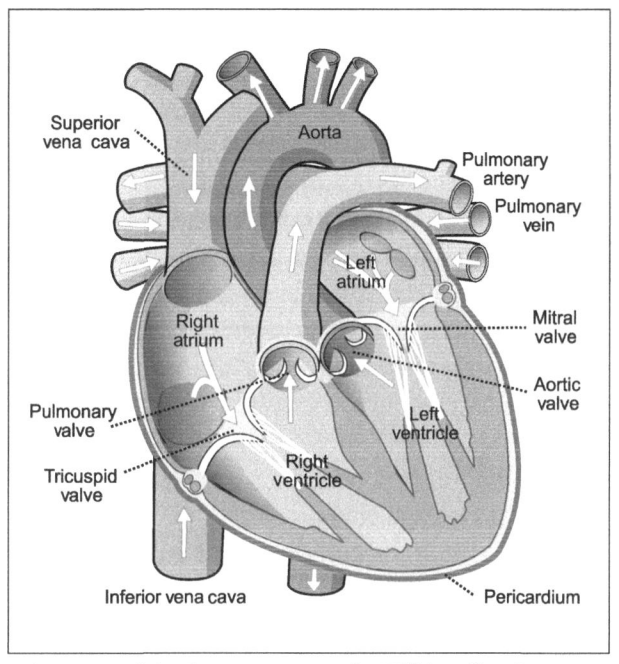

Diagram of the heart. Image via Wikimedia Commons. [Public domain.]

semilunar valve called the "pulmonic valve" into blood vessels that transport it to the lungs. In the lungs, the blood loses carbon dioxide and picks up oxygen. The oxygenated blood returns to the heart through pulmonary veins that empty into the left atrium. The heart pushes the from the left atrium, past the bicuspid mitral valve, into the left ventricle. The blood is pumped from the powerful left ventricle through another semilunar valve (the aortic) into the blood vessels that will carry the blood to all the body's tissues, including the heart itself. The blood vessels that feed the heart directly are known as "coronary vessels."

The orderly pattern by which blood flows through the heart, lungs, and body requires the heart's chambers to work in a coordinated fashion. The atria contract together to help send blood into the ventricles. The ventricles then contract together so that blood flows through the lungs from the right ventricle and through the tissues of the body from the left ventricle. The tricuspid and bicuspid valves prevent a backflow of blood into the atria when the ventricles contract. The semilunar valves prevent blood from returning to the ventricles after they have contracted.

Something must coordinate the heart's contraction so that the atria contract together before the ventricles do so. Highly specialized myocardium cells can rapidly conduct electrical impulses and discharge spontaneously at a certain rate. These properties allow the heart to be stimulated synchronously and generate its rate and rhythm. One region of the right atrium is known as the sinoatrial (S-A) node; it functions as the heart's pacemaker. The S-A node can spontaneously generate an electrical signal with a relatively rapid rhythm. Therefore, it "paces" the heart rate—the atria contract when the S-A node sends its electrical impulse throughout the atria. There is a slight delay before the impulse reaches the ventricles, which allows the atria to contract fully before the ventricles. The atrioventricular (A-V) node will pick up the electrical signal and send it through both ventricles via specialized conductive heart muscle fibers known as "Purkinje's fibers."

Purkinje's fibers transmit the electrical signal, ensuring that all the ventricular muscle cells contract nearly simultaneously. The ventricles contract so that the bottom tip of the heart (apex) contracts slightly before the region of the ventricles next to the atria (base). Additionally, the ventricles contract in a somewhat twisting motion that causes the heart to "wring out" the blood.

This rather complex system allows the heart to contract at its rate and highly synchronously. Nevertheless, one's heart rate varies depending on one's physical activity or emotional state. For example, during exercise or when an individual is under stress, the heart rate goes up. When one is relaxed, the heart does not beat as rapidly. Therefore, the body must have a way to regulate the rate at which the S-A node signals the heart to contract.

The autonomic nervous system, which functions without one's conscious control, regulates the heart rate. It is divided into two systems: parasympathetic and sympathetic. The parasympathetic nervous system is active during rest periods and can slow the heart. During periods of physical or emotional stress, the sympathetic nervous system stimulates the heart to contract more forcefully and rapidly. The parasympathetic and sympathetic systems communicate with the heart via chemical messengers known as "neurotransmitters." The parasympathetic nervous system uses the neurotransmitter acetylcholine to slow the heart. At the same time, norepinephrine and epinephrine are the neurotransmitters used by the sympathetic nervous system to increase the heart rate and the force of heart contractions.

DISORDERS AND DISEASES

Even though the heart seems adaptable to various situations throughout one's life, it can malfunction. Heart and blood vessel diseases are the number-one killer in the United States. One common disease that affects the heart directly is coronary artery disease, which can lead to life-threatening heart attacks. Although medical researchers are still investigating the causes of coronary artery disease, most evidence points to hypertension (high blood pressure) and atherosclerosis (a buildup of fatty plaque in the walls of arteries).

Hypertension is usually defined as a blood pressure greater than 140/90 millimeters of mercury (mmHg) at rest. Typical blood pressure for a young, healthy adult is 120/80 mmHg. The top number measures the force of blood against an artery wall during the heart's contraction, referred to as systolic pressure. The bottom number, the diastolic pressure, is a measured force when the heart is relaxed. The patient is considered hypertensive if either systolic or diastolic pressure exceeds 130/90 mmHg. The cause of hypertension has not been determined. Still, it is known that with hypertension, the heart must work harder to push the blood through the arteries, including the coronary arteries. Physicians treat hypertension by prescribing drugs that block the effect of the sympathetic nervous system on the heart, such as metoprolol (Lopressor). They may also prescribe drugs such as hydralazine or hydralazine/isosorbide dinitrate (BiDil) that dilate arteries and prevent them from becoming too narrow.

Hypertension is also seen in patients who have atherosclerosis. This buildup of fatty materials such as cholesterol under the lining of the artery causes the plaque to protrude, narrowing the diameter of the vessel. Atherosclerosis can lead to blood clot formation on artery walls that are irregular. This clot, also known as a "thrombus," may dislodge and travel in the bloodstream. Eventually, it may block a small artery, thereby preventing blood flow to the tissue. If this happens in a coronary artery, a myocardial infarction (heart attack) will result.

A heart attack occurs when a portion of the heart dies because of a lack of oxygen or a buildup of waste products. Heart muscle cannot repair itself, and the resulting damage is permanent. Suppose the patient is transported to the hospital immediately. In that case, the emergency room physician may give drugs to prevent further blood clot formation (aspirin and heparin) and help dissolve the clot (tissue plasminogen activator or TPA derivatives such as alteplase, reteplase, or tenecteplase). Suppose the coronary artery is only partially blocked. In that case, the patient may suffer from angina pectoris, a chest pain that radiates down the left arm. These patients usually take drugs such as nitroglycerin, which help dilate (widen) blood vessels, reestablishing adequate flow to the heart.

Another devastating disease of the heart is congestive heart failure, a condition in which the heart fails to pump enough blood to meet the demands of the body's tissues. The heart becomes enlarged because of the resulting excessive increase in blood volume. There are several causes of heart failure, most of which stem from the fact that the heart loses its ability to pump efficiently. For example, a patient who has had a heart attack may have lost significant function because of heart damage. Even without a heart attack, some individuals may have malfunctioning heart valves or other problems that cause an inefficient ejection of blood and thus heart failure.

The cardiovascular system attempts to compensate for heart failure in several ways. The sympathetic nervous system increases the heart rate, and the kidneys retain more fluid to increase blood volume. These compensatory mechanisms help to reestablish adequate blood flow for a while. Because of the increase in blood volume, however, more blood enters the chambers of the heart and causes them to stretch. At some point, the ventricles can no longer force out the increased amount of blood entering them, and they enlarge. This increase in the size of the heart chamber further enlarges the heart and strains the heart muscle. The heart will continue to weaken, unable to keep up with the body's demands. Compensatory mechanisms attempt to meet the body's need for continuous blood flow but further overload the heart. This vicious cycle may lead to complete heart failure and death.

Congestive heart failure may involve only one side of the heart, perhaps because of a heart attack that affected that side. If heart failure occurs on the left side, the right ventricle pumps blood to the lungs efficiently. Still, the left ventricle cannot pump all the blood returning from the lungs. Therefore, blood backs up and pools in the lung tissues. Similarly, if the right ventricle begins to fail and the left ventricle is normal, blood begins to pool throughout the body since the right side of the heart cannot keep up with its pumping.

Physicians can slow the progression of congestive heart failure by prescribing drugs according to how they classify their patient's heart failure. The New York Heart Association (NYHA) Heart Failure classification scheme is the most widely used classification schema for heart failure. This scheme is so popular that the European Society of Cardiology adopted it. The NYHA classification has four classes. Class I patients experience symptoms like shortness of breath only after extreme exertion. Class II patients experience symptoms with moderate exertion. Class III patients become short of breath during mild exertion. Class IV patients suffer heart failure symptoms at rest.

Cardiologists treat heart failure according to the New York Heart Association classification. Regardless of their NYHA class, all people with heart failure must reduce daily sodium intake to less than 2 grams. They must also decrease their daily fluid intake to less than 2 liters. Sodium and fluid restriction reduce blood volume and pressure, reducing heart strain. All heart failure patients have prescribed a beta-blocker and an angiotensin-converting enzyme (ACE) inhibitor or an angiotensin II receptor blocker (ARB). Alternatively, heart failure patients may receive a combination medication, Entresto, containing sacubitril, and the ARB, valsartan. Entresto has proven remarkably effective for some heart failure patients. As the patient's heart failure worsens, more medicines are prescribed. Patients with class II NYHA heart failure are additionally prescribed a loop diuretic, like furosemide, bumetanide, torsemide, or ethacrynic acid, or a thiazide diuretic like hydrochlorothiazide, chlorthalidone, indapamide, or metolazone. Diuretics increase water elimination by the kidneys, reduce fluid overload and relieve symptoms. Those with class III heart failure receive a prescription for aldosterone antagonists like spironolactone or eplerenone and BiDil to maintain healthy potassium levels and further reduce blood pressure. People with class IV heart failure are given digoxin to increase the strength of heart muscle contractions to reduce symptoms. If possible, those with type IV heart failure are also candidates for a heart transplant.

In the heart, specialized heart muscle cells that provide the heart's rhythm and conduct the electrical signals necessary for a coordinated heartbeat may be affected by the disease. The heart normally beats about seventy to eighty times per minute in the resting adult. Several conditions exist whereby the heart loses control of its normal rate and rhythm, a serious condition.

For example, suppose the heart begins to beat too rapidly. In that case, the ventricles do not have enough time to fill, and blood movement to the heart muscle and the rest of the body is impaired. The atria or ventricles may contract at a high rate and lose their coordinated contraction sequence; this is referred to as atrial or ventricular fibrillation. Atrial fibrillation may be tolerated under some circumstances; ventricular fibrillation is a medical emergency. The patient will die if immediate action is not taken to reestablish the normal rate and conduction sequence. Emergency measures such as electrical defibrillation may shock the heart into reestablishing its normal rhythm and conduction pathways. It is easy to understand how these abnormal patterns of heart activity occur if one imagines more than one pacemaker attempting to control heart function. The cause of these and other, less severe heart rhythms may be heart damage affecting the conductive pathway, drugs, or even psychological distress.

Heart disease is a major cause of death, but most experts agree that many heart problems are preventable. High blood pressure and high blood levels of fat and cholesterol are associated with an increased incidence of coronary artery disease. Cigarette smoking and excessive weight are also correlated with heart disease. Additionally, exercise seems critical in maintaining a healthy heart, as sedentary individuals have a twofold increase in their risk of heart disease compared to active people.

Individuals at risk can likely lessen the probability of having heart problems by adopting a more healthful lifestyle, including stopping smoking, reducing excessive weight and mental stress, and engaging in enjoyable physical activities (with their physician's permission).

PERSPECTIVE AND PROSPECTS

The ancient Egyptians questioned the role of the heart in the functioning of the human body and attributed breathing to the heart. The Chinese first documented that the heart is responsible for the pulse and movement of blood. They also believed that the heart was the seat of happiness. The ancient Greeks had a different idea about the heart's function, believing that it was the region where thinking originated.

When William Harvey (1578-1657), an English physiologist, published his experiments on the heart and circulation, scientists believed blood was pumped continuously by the heart. He observed that both the heart's ventricles contracted and expanded simultaneously. Harvey also noted that when he removed the heart from an animal, it continued to contract and relax; that is, it had an automatic rhythm.

Over one hundred years after Harvey published his work, Stephen Hales made the first blood pressure measurements. He did so by inserting a tube into the neck artery of a horse and watching the blood rise 9 feet (3 meters) above the animal. Then early in the twentieth century, Willem Einthoven invented an instrument to measure electrical currents. Thomas Lewis used this instrument to measure the electrical activity in the heart, the first electrocardiograph (ECG).

By the mid-twentieth century, heart surgeries were being performed to correct heart defects. These early surgeries had to be done with the heart still beating. In 1953, Dr. John Gibbon used the heart-lung machine to take over the heart's pumping function during surgery so that the surgeon could stop the heart. In 1967, Christiaan Barnard performed the first heart transplantation on a human. Heart transplants were performed during the next ten years with no long-term survivors, usually because of tissue rejection. In 1982, a completely artificial heart was implanted into a patient. This patient died in the spring of 1983.

Scientists are making comparable strides in finding ways to prevent heart disease by treating already existing conditions. Heart transplants have become much more successful, however, mainly because of the use of immunosuppressive drugs that help prevent rejection of the transplanted heart. In January 2012, the US National Heart, Lung, and Blood Institute reported that heart transplant patients had a one-year survival rate of 88 percent, a five-year survival rate of 75 percent, and a ten-year survival rate of 56 percent. Newer drugs and procedures such as coronary bypass surgery, angioplasty, and atherectomy are more effective in treating heart disease. Likewise, breathtaking advances in imaging the heart while it pumps have revolutionized heart disease diagnosis. Nevertheless, perhaps the best approach to maintaining a healthy heart is to practice preventive medicine.

—*Matthew Berria, Michael A. Buratovich*

Further Reading

"About Heart Valves." *American Heart Association*, 7 May 2020, www.heart.org/en/health-topics/heart-valve-problems-and-disease/about-heart-valves. Accessed 8 June 2022.

Gersh, Bernard J. *The Mayo Clinic Heart Book: The Ultimate Guide to Heart Health.* 2nd ed., William Morrow, 2000.

Hales, Dianne. *An Invitation to Health Brief.* Updated ed., Wadsworth/Cengage Learning, 2010.

"Heart Diseases." *MedlinePlus*, 31 Dec. 2020, medlineplus.gov/heartdiseases.html. Accessed 8 July 2022.

"Heart Treatments." *NIH National Heart, Lung, and Blood Institute*, 24 Mar. 2022, www.nhlbi.nih.gov/health/heart-treatments-procedures. Accessed 8 June 2022.

"Heart Valves and Circulation." *American Heart Association*, 7 May 2020, www.heart.org/en/health-topics/heart-

valve-problems-and-disease/about-heart-valves/heart-valves-and-circulation. Accessed 8 June 2022.
Mackenna, B. R., and R. Callander. *Illustrated Physiology*. 6th ed., Churchill Livingstone, 1997.
Marieb, Elaine N., and Katja Hoehn. *Human Anatomy and Physiology*. 9th ed., Pearson, 2022.
Park, Myung K., and Mehrdad Salamat. *Park's the Pediatric Cardiology Handbook*. 6th ed., Mosby/Elsevier, 2021.
Tortora, Gerard J., and Bryan Derrickson. *Principles of Anatomy and Physiology*. 16th ed., John Wiley & Sons, 2020.
"What Is a Total Artificial Heart?" *NIH National Heart, Lung, and Blood Institute*, 24 Mar. 2022, www.nhlbi.nih.gov/health/total-artificial-heart. Accessed 8 June 2022.

HIPPOCAMPUS

Category: Anatomy
Specialties and related fields: Neurology, psychology
Definition: a bilateral structure in the cerebral hemispheres that plays a central role in learning and memory

KEY TERMS

episodic memory(relational): memory of events, the associated temporal and spatial relationships, and the context in which an event occurs

grid cells: specialized cells found in the entorhinal cortex that encode a specific region in space and are involved in allowing for spatiotemporal navigation

neurodegeneration: the death and destruction of neurons and neuronal fibers that often occurs as a direct result of many diseases that target the nervous system

neurogenesis: the development or growth of new neuronal cells

place cells: specialized cells found in the hippocampus that encode a specific point in space and seem to encode an animal's position or perceived position in a given setting

synaptic plasticity: the cellular process in the nervous system where connections between neurons, known as "synapses," strengthen or weaken in an activity-dependent manner; this process is believed to underlie learning in the brain

telencephalon: an early embryological structure in the developing nervous system that ultimately develops into the cortex, basal ganglia, and hippocampus, among other mature brain regions

STRUCTURE AND FUNCTIONS

The hippocampus is a neural structure that plays a critical role in key brain functions, including learning and memory, synaptic plasticity, and spatial navigation. There are two bilateral hippocampi, one in each hemisphere, that are mirror images of one another and are located deep in the brain's medial temporal lobe. The hippocampus is named after the Greek word for "seahorse" due to its gross anatomical appearance. It has been an area of active neuroscience research for the past several decades.

The hippocampus is found in the brains of all mammals, and its general connectivity and functional anatomy are well-conserved across different species. The hippocampus is formed around midgestation in humans from the early cerebral structure known as the "telencephalon." The fully developed hippocampus or hippocampal formation consists of the dentate gyrus, the cornu ammonis (CA) regions, and the subiculum. The predominant neuronal cell types in the hippocampus include pyramidal cells, which populate the CA regions, and granule cells found in the dentate gyrus. The neurons in these regions form pathways that lead from the hippocampus, beginning at the dentate, and exiting through the subiculum, to a host of other brain regions, including the cingulate cortex, amygdala, and prefrontal cortices. The hippocampus also receives input signals from various brain regions, including sensory association areas, the olfactory bulb, and feedback from the prefrontal cortex, making hippocampal activity an integral component of many complex brain processes.

No behavior is more readily attributable to proper brain function than learning and forming memories. Extensive behavioral neuroscience research in animals and humans has illustrated the hippocampus's critical role in forming and consolidating memories. For instance, in 1997, Fried and others showed that hippocampal neurons in humans exhibited increased responses when individuals were shown a familiar stimulus instead of an unfamiliar one. These findings were notable because they indicated that some neurons were actually "remembering" whether or not they had encountered a stimulus before. Some of the most convincing studies have been lesion studies in which the hippocampi of animals were selectively destroyed. In studies where rats must learn to navigate a maze to reach a food reward, those animals with hippocampal lesions are not able to learn to navigate the maze. Whereas healthy rats learn to navigate the maze after successive trials, those rats that lacked hippocampi had to go through a process of trial and error even after repeated exposure to the same maze. The rats with hippocampal lesions behaved as if it was the first time navigating the maze each time.

Since these preliminary studies, it has been well established that subsets of neurons in the hippocampus are responsible for encoding and retrieving specific memories. Contemporary research that lends the most credibility to this hypothesis includes studies using optogenetics. Using optogenetics, neuroscientists can selectively stimulate specific populations of neurons by shining a light on them. In 2013, Ramirez and colleagues used optogenetic stimulation of hippocampal CA1 neurons to "create a false memory" in mice. By timed stimulation of hippocampal neurons that as-

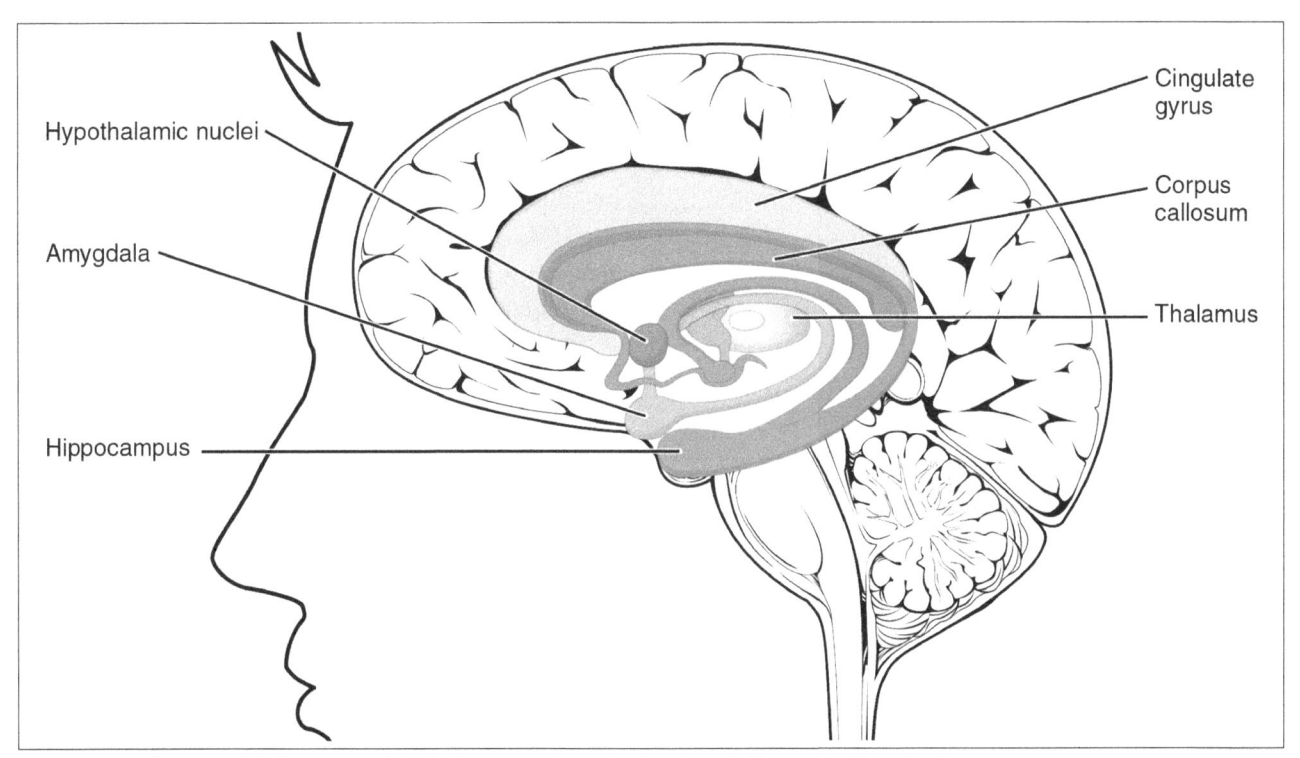

Hippocampus (lowest pink bulb) as part of the limbic system. Image by OpenStax College, via Wikimedia Commons.

sociated a specific context with a fear response, researchers made mice behave as if they were afraid in a context that had previously elicited no fear response. This research has helped convince neuroscientists that hippocampal neurons may encode a memory of place, time, and general context, known as "relational or episodic memory." Precisely how hippocampal neurons encode memory or information about context is an active area of research. The predominant hypothesis is that mechanisms of synaptic plasticity in the hippocampus underlie memory formation.

Neurons in the hippocampus also play a critical role in spatial navigation. In 1971, O'Keefe discovered the existence of place cells in the hippocampus. Place cells are unique neurons in the hippocampus that encode the location of a given animal in space. O'Keefe and his colleagues found that certain neurons in the hippocampi of rats fired in conjunction with a rat's particular perceived location in its environment.

Further research by May-Britt Moser and Edvard Moser in 2005 led to the discovery of "grid cells" in the entorhinal cortex. This adjacent brain region sends input to the hippocampus. Grid cells are neurons that are responsive within a regular, repeated grid-like pattern and function like a neural GPS aiding spatial navigation. O'Keefe, May-Britt Moser, and Edvard Moser shared the Nobel Prize in 2014 for their combined work uncovering the hippocampus' role in spatial navigation. While place and grid cells are not known to exist in the human brain, human brain imaging studies have shown significant hippocampal involvement when individuals are asked to complete tasks involving navigation. One brain imaging study found that London taxi drivers had greater hippocampal volume than non-taxi drivers and that those taxi drivers with more experience had larger hippocampal volumes than those with less, further supporting the hippocampal role in spatial navigation.

More recent research has also uncovered that the hippocampus is one of the few brain regions that continue to exhibit neurogenesis, the production of new brain cells, throughout adulthood. Studies have shown that the hippocampus can be stimulated to produce new neurons by various animal activities and interventions, including exercise, learning, environmental enrichment, and treatment with certain psychopharmaceuticals. The function and molecular mechanisms of hippocampal neurogenesis remain unclear.

DISORDERS AND DISEASES

Severe damage or lesions to the hippocampus have been associated with amnesia or memory loss. One well-known case was that of patient HM, who underwent a bilateral temporal lobectomy in the 1950s to treat seizures and, in the process, had nearly all of his hippocampal tissue removed. While HM's personality, neurophysiological functioning, and intelligence were virtually unchanged due to the procedure, he suffered from severe memory deficits. HM experienced retrograde amnesia, or severe memory loss in the years preceding his surgery. He also notably exhibited anterograde amnesia, marked by an inability to form and consolidate new memories. It was HMs case that led researchers to suspect the involvement of the hippocampus in making and consolidating memories.

While surgical lesions or removal of the hippocampus no longer takes place, pathologically induced hippocampal damage is a common feature of many neurological diseases. The hippocampus is particularly vulnerable to damage caused by neuroinflammation and neurodegeneration in stroke and Alzheimer's Disease (AD). Neurons in the CA1 and CA3 of the hippocampus undergo programmed cell death (apoptosis) in response to inflammatory and cytotoxic factors released during stroke, AD, and other neuropathologies. Memory loss and difficulty forming new short and long-term memories are commonplace symptoms in many neurological diseases, partly because of pathologically induced hippocampal damage.

The hippocampus has also been implicated in pathological neural circuitry associated with psychiatric pathologies, including schizophrenia, affective disorders, and anxiety disorders.

PERSPECTIVE AND PROSPECTS
The hippocampus is a deceptively small brain structure with an incredibly big role in brain processes that remains to be fully understood. Research efforts aim to understand further the hippocampus' precise roles and mechanisms in learning, memory, and navigation processes. The hippocampus is a common locus of injury in neuropathology, so research to explore treatments to preserve and protect this critical brain region is of the utmost importance.

—*Adriel Barrios-Anderson*

Further Reading
Berkowitz, Aaron. *Lange Clinical Neurology and Neuroanatomy: A Localization-Based Approach.* McGraw Hill / Medical, 2016.
Bear, M. F., et al. *Neuroscience: Exploring the Brain.* Lippincott Williams & Wilkins, 2007.
Felten, D. L., et al. *Netter's Atlas of Neuroscience.* Elsevier Health Sciences, 2015.
Groh, J. M. *Making Space: How the Brain Knows Where Things Are.* Harvard UP, 2014.
Kandel, E. R., et al. *Principles of Neural Science.* McGraw Hill, 2012.
Morris, R. G. M., and Richard G. M. *Elements of a Neurobiological Theory of the Hippocampus: The Role of Activity-Dependent Synaptic Plasticity in Memory.* Amsterdam UP, 2005.
Moser, E. I., et al. "Place Cells, Grid Cells, and the Brain's Spatial Representation System." *Annual Review of Neuroscience*, vol. 31, 2008, pp. 69-89.
O'Keefe, J., and L. Nadel. *The Hippocampus as a Cognitive Map.* Clarendon Press, 1978.
Ramirez, S., et al. "Creating a False Memory in the Hippocampus." *Science*, vol. 341, 2013, pp. 387-91.
Ropper, Allan H., et al. *Adams and Victor's Principles of Neurology.* 11th ed., McGraw Hill / Medical, 2019.
Rosenberg, Roger N., and Juan Pascual, editors. *Rosenberg's Molecular and Genetic Basis of Neurological and Psychiatric Disease.* 6th ed., Academic Press, 2020.
Sahay, A. et al. "Increasing Adult Hippocampal Neurogenesis Is Sufficient to Improve Pattern Separation." *Nature*, vol. 472, 2011, pp. 466-70.
Scoville, W. B., and Milner, B. "Loss of Recent Memory After Bilateral Hippocampal Lesions." *Journal of Neurology, Neurosurgery, and Psychiatry*, vol. 20, no. 1, Feb. 1957, pp. 11-21.

HUMAN RESPIRATORY SYSTEM

Category: Anatomy
Specialties and related fields: Emergency medicine, critical care, pulmonology, respiratory therapy
Definition: an organ system that consists of the set of tissues and organs responsible for exchanging oxygen from the surrounding environment with carbon dioxide produced in the body

KEY TERMS
alveoli: the tiny, clustered, air-filled sacs in the lungs where the exchange of oxygen and carbon dioxide takes place
bronchioles: branches of the primary bronchus
pleura: a pair of moist and slippery membranes that surround the lungs; the outer, or parietal, pleura lines the inside of the rib cage and the diaphragm, and the inner, or visceral, pleura covers the lungs; the space between the two pleura is the intrapleural space that contains fluid secreted by the pleura
surfactant: compounds that reduce the surface tension of fluid into which they are dissolved
thoracic cavity: the space within the body between the diaphragm and the neck; it contains the lungs and heart and is enclosed by the ribs

Human Respiratory System

Principles of Sports Medicine & Exercise Science

STRUCTURE AND FUNCTIONS

Since gas exchange occurs inside the body, air from the atmosphere must be carried from the surrounding space and into the body. Air flows into the lungs through conducting passages that connect different parts of the respiratory system and allow the air to flow in and out. These passages are called "airways" and are usually divided into upper and lower airways; the division between the two systems is designated as the point where the esophagus and the tra-

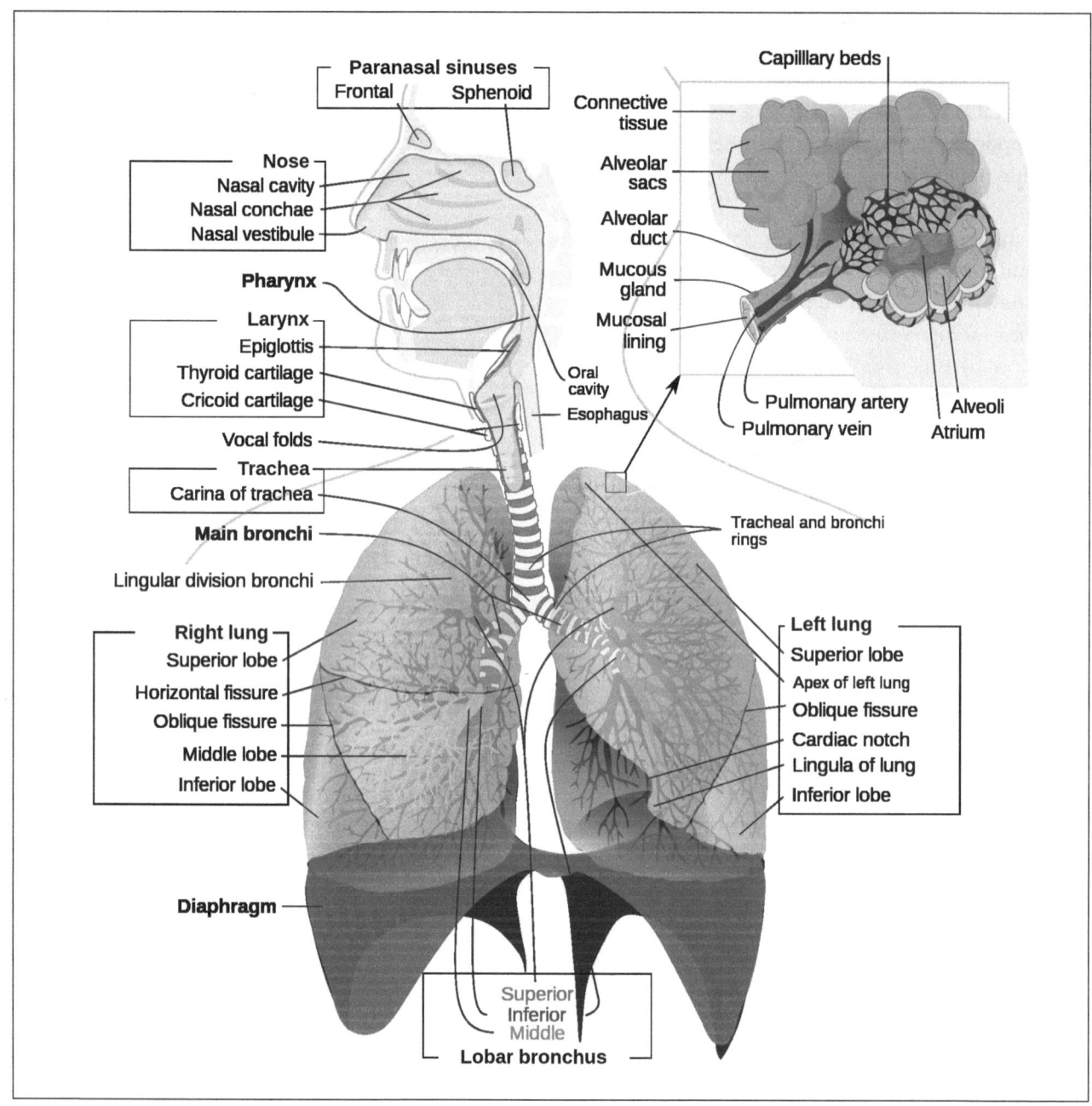

Image via Wikimedia Commons. [Public domain.]

chea branch off from one another at the top of a person's throat. The upper airways are the parts above this point and include the nose, the mouth, the sinuses, the pharynx, or the upper part of the throat. The lower airways include the larynx (also called the "voice box"), the trachea, and the bronchi, which connect the trachea to the lungs.

The inner functions of the lungs are the central feature of the process of respiration. Air breathed in travels into the body through the nose or mouth, flows down the trachea, and enters the bronchi. There are two bronchi, one leading from the trachea to each lung. After leaving the bronchi, the air flows into the lungs, reaching smaller, narrower passages known as "bronchioles." Small, clustered air sacs called "alveoli" are at the end of the bronchioles. The alveoli are exquisitely thin, delicate sacs made of a set of cells called "type 1 alveolar cells" that provide the interface between the many capillaries that line the wall of the gases in the alveoli. Molecular oxygen (O_2) diffuses across these type 1 alveolar cells and into the surrounding capillaries. Once the oxygen enters the capillaries, it is carried by hemoglobin in the red blood cells throughout the body by the network of blood vessels.

Pressure changes within the lungs move air into the lungs (inspiration) or drive air from the lungs (expiration). These pressure changes result from changes in lung volume. Gas molecules exert pressure on their containers by colliding with the sides of the container. The smaller the volume of the gas, the more frequently the gas molecules strike the sides of the container, which results in greater pressure. Therefore, as the volume of a gas decreases, the pressure of that gas increases. To change the volume of the lungs, a large, parachute-shaped muscle underneath the lungs, called the "diaphragm," moves down as it contracts and rises as it relaxes. During inspiration, the diaphragm lowers as it contracts, increasing the lung volume and decreasing pressure within the lungs. When the pressure in the lungs decreases below atmospheric pressure, air from the atmosphere flows into the lungs in response to this pressure disparity. During expiration, the diaphragm rises as it relaxes, which decreases the volume of the lungs and increases the pressure within the lungs. When the pressure within the lungs exceeds atmospheric pressure, the gases within the lungs move into the atmosphere in response to these pressure differences.

The lungs must expand and contract as air is inhaled and then exhaled. Hence, they require an enclosure that allows them to maintain their position in the body while still being able to increase and decrease in volume. The lungs are also quite delicate structures, so they need protection from outside forces that might be directed against the body. The design of the thoracic cavity in which the lungs are situated accommodates these competing needs for strength and flexibility. The ribs that make up the ribcage encase the lungs in a lattice of sturdy bone to protect them from injury. However, to keep this structure from being too rigid and potentially even damaging the lungs it is supposed to protect, the ribs are attached to the thoracic vertebrae in the spinal column by articulated facets and to the sternum by cartilage. Cartilage is firm tissue that is more flexible than bone yet stronger than the softer tissue of which organs are composed. This means that the ribs encircling the lungs can move slightly to allow the lungs to function while keeping them safe. The lungs expand and contract within the thoracic cavity, protected by two membranes called "pleurae." One pleura, called the "visceral pleura," encases the lung itself; the other, the parietal pleura, coats the inside of the thoracic cavity. A small amount of fluid flows between the two pleurae to prevent the lungs from rubbing against the inside of the thoracic cavity.

The expansion and contraction of the lungs are aided by the presence of large amounts of a protein called "elastin," which acts like a molecular rubber band that can stretch and snaps back repeatedly. This ability of the lungs to stretch and distend is called "lung compliance." However, the inner side of the alveoli is quite wet, and the cohesive properties of water would cause the contracting alveoli to collapse during expiration and not reinflate upon inspiration. To prevent their collapse during expiration, the walls of the alveoli contain a second cell type called "type 2 alveolar cells" that secrete a detergent-like concoction called "surfactant." Surfactant decreases water's cohesive properties and reduces the alveoli's surface tension. Consequently, the lungs require less energy to expand, and surfactant discourages alveolar collapse during expiration.

A good way of seeing the human respiratory system in action is to follow how the body responds to strenuous exercise while the activity occurs. During exercise, the body's need for energy increases because it moves more quickly and forcefully than it normally would. This means there is a greater need for oxygen to enter the bloodstream and for carbon dioxide to be removed from the blood. To provide additional oxygen, the rate of breathing increases so that more breaths are taken per minute, and each breath is deeper than it would be if the person were at rest. This increases the amount of oxygen entering the body. However, this extra oxygen still needs to reach all the body's different parts. To help accomplish this, the heart rate increases along with the increase in the rate of breathing. As the heart beats faster and stronger, it pushes the oxygenated blood out to the body's extremities much more quickly, ensuring they receive the oxygen-rich blood they need to sustain the exercise.

Measuring the increase in breathing rate is quite straightforward. One only needs to count the number of breaths in a specific time frame during exercise and compare it with the number counted without exercise. Measuring how deep a breath is can be a more complicated undertaking because it requires using a special apparatus called a "spirometer." To use a spirometer, the person being evaluated must place their lips around a straw-like device and inhale through it. The spirometer measures the volume of air being removed from it and drawn into the lungs. These devices are used not only to monitor and measure respiration but also as a type of respiratory therapy for patients who have had surgery or are recovering from some trauma affecting their respiration. A frequent consequence of these experiences is that the lungs become partially deflated and must be conditioned to return to their full capacity. This can be challenging, especially with children, because breathing is often painful during recovery. For this reason, doctors will often use breathing devices to encourage patients to inhale as much as possible to expand their lungs. Most devices have a straw one must breathe through, and a ball that rises along an enclosed tube as air is pulled out of its chamber. Patients are told to use this device several times per hour and to use their breath to pull hard enough to raise the ball to a designated level.

One of the major vulnerabilities of the human respiratory system is the possibility of contaminants entering the body in the same way that air does. This could be very dangerous because small particles of matter carried by air could damage the delicate structures inside the lungs, cause an infection, or both. The body has several systems in place to help prevent these harms from occurring. Very small hairs grow inside the nose to filter out larger particles such as dust and pollen. Particles that are too small to be captured this way may become stuck in the layer of mucus that lines the nasal passages and other airflow conduits. There is also an organ at the back of the throat called the "epiglottis," which ensures that food and liquids go down the esophagus to the stomach rather than traveling down the trachea and potentially into the lungs. Upon swallowing, the epiglottis reflexively folds over the trachea to close it off. After the solid or liquid has been swallowed, the epiglottis pulls back from covering the trachea.

DISORDERS AND DISEASES

Several diseases and disorders can afflict the human respiratory system. One of the most common is pneumonia, an infection of the alveoli caused by bacteria. The infection causes fluid to build up in the alveoli, which interferes with the ability of oxygen to pass through the walls of the alveoli and enter the bloodstream. If this process continues long enough, the person may suffer from oxygen deprivation and require supplemental oxygen from an oxygen tank, delivered through a face mask. While not generally fatal, pneumonia can cause death in patients who are very old, very young, or immunocompromised in some fashion.

One of the symptoms exhibited by a person suffering from pneumonia is coughing, which is one of the primary ways the human respiratory system has to clear up materials or conditions that are interfering with regular breathing. Coughing occurs when a person inhales a volume of air, closes the glottis (the opening between the vocal folds in the larynx, not to be confused with the epiglottis), forces the inhaled air against the closed glottis under pressure, and then opens the glottis to allow the inhaled air to blast outward. Coughing is used to expel foreign matter that has entered the respiratory system, such as when a person takes a sip of a beverage, and the liquid goes down the trachea instead of the esophagus. Coughing can be initiated voluntarily or as a reflex. Voluntary coughing may occur when people wish to clear out obstructing matter from their airways—involuntary coughing results from situations that cause the body to expel matter in the airway to prevent choking. An example of involuntary coughing occurs when a person ingests water while drowning.

Some illnesses can cause the pleurae to become inflamed, which can make it extremely painful to breathe. The lungs are so delicate that they can collapse in much the same way a balloon collapses when punctured. This can happen when air or fluid enters the thoracic cavity due to an injury known as "pneumothorax"; the air or fluid presses on the lung and prevents it from fully inflating.

Fetal lungs do not make surfactant until the last two months of fetal life. Premature babies born before their lungs make sufficient quantities of surfactant cannot keep their alveoli inflated between breaths and suffer from infant respiratory distress syndrome (IRDS, also called "hyaline membrane disease"). A lack of sufficient airway causes the lungs to completely or partially collapse, a condition called "atelectasis." Atelectasis triggers inflammation and swelling of the lung tissue (pulmonary edema). Blood that passes through capillaries in the atelectatic portions of the lung does not receive adequate oxygen, and the infant suffers from oxygen-deficient (hypoxemia). Infant respiratory distress syndrome is treated by aerosolizing synthetic surfactant into the respiratory passages of the baby. In severe cases, mechanical respiration may be needed.

PERSPECTIVE AND PROSPECTS

Many people are unaware of the role played by the human respiratory system in the everyday activity of speech. Human beings communicate in many ways, but speech is the most common, barring conditions that prevent a person from speaking. Speech is the act of creating sounds to signify specific concepts. The respiratory system is critical to producing vocalized speech because to produce intelligible sounds; one vibrates the vocal cords in the larynx while exhaling to cause air to pass over them. By varying the type of vibration, people can change the tone and volume of their speech, producing anything from a whisper to a shout. If the vocal cords become damaged or paralyzed, or if a person has trouble breathing, speech can be problematic or even impossible. Some injuries and illnesses can cause the muscles that control the vibration of the vocal cords to become paralyzed, such as throat cancer, vocal-cord infections, or accidents affecting the neck and throat.

—Scott Zimmer

Further Reading

Green, Robert J. *Green's Respiratory Therapy: A Practical and Essential Tutorial on the Core Concepts of Respiratory Care.* Aventine Press, 2017.

Hickin, Sarah, et al. *Respiratory System.* 4th ed., Mosby, 2015.

Kaminsky, David. *The Netter Collection of Medical Illustrations: Respiratory System.* 2nd ed., Saunders, 2011.

Knapp, Rose. *Respiratory Care Made Incredibly Easy.* 2nd ed., Lippincott Williams & Wilkins, 2018.

Martini, Frederic H., et al. *Fundamentals of Anatomy & Physiology.* 11th ed., Pearson, 2017.

Maury, Bertrand. *The Respiratory System in Equations.* Springer, 2013.

McKinley, Michael P., et al. *Human Anatomy.* 4th ed., McGraw, 2015.

VanPutte, Cinnamon L., Jennifer Regan, and Andrew Russo. *Seeley's Essentials of Anatomy & Physiology.* 11th ed., McGraw-Hill Education, 2021.

Ward, Jeremy P. T., Jane Ward, and Richard M. Leach. *The Respiratory System at a Glance.* 4th ed., Wiley, 2015.

Welsh, Charles, and Cynthia Prentice-Craver. *Hole's Human Anatomy & Physiology.* 16th ed., McGraw-Hill Education, 2021.

KNEE

Category: Anatomy
Specialties and related fields: Orthopedics, orthopedic surgery, physical therapy, sports medicine
Definition: a large and complex joint that connects the lower leg with the upper leg, or thigh, by several tendons that bind the joint together

KEY TERMS

condyle: a rounded protuberance at the end of a bone that is part of an articulated joint

eminence: a projection or prominence in the shape of a bone

fibrocartilage: a type of cartilage in which the matrix contains thick bundles of collagen fibers, making it appear white

hyaline cartilage: a type of cartilage that is smooth and glassy in appearance

meniscus: a crescent- or lens-shaped structure composed of fibrocartilage found especially in the knee joint

tuberosity: an elevated round process in the shape of a bone

STRUCTURE AND FUNCTION

The knee is a synovial joint that allows for flexion, extension, and rotation of the lower leg. The femur, tibia, and patella are the three bones involved in the structure of this joint. The knee has three separate points of contact: the medial condyle of the femur will interact with the medial plateau of the tibia. The lateral condyle of the femur will interact with the lateral tibial plateau, and the patella will glide over the femur in the femoral trochlear groove.

Since the knee is a synovial joint, a capsule encases the femorotibial articulations and the patella to contain fluid. Hyaline cartilage covers the surfaces of the distal femur, proximal tibia, and posterior patella, protecting these articulating surfaces. In addition to the hyaline cartilage, the knee also has wedge-shaped medial and lateral menisci that are made up of fibrocartilage, protecting the articular cartilage of the knee and providing extra support. Two main sets of ligaments connect the femur to the tibia. The collateral ligaments are on the lateral edges of the knee joint. The medial collateral ligament (MCL) attaches at the medial condyle of the femur and the tibia. This ligament resists lateral forces on the knee. The lateral collateral ligament (LCL) connects from the lateral condyle of the femur to the tibia. This ligament resists medial forces on the knee. The cruciate ligaments are located within the joint capsule but are considered extra synovial structures. The anterior cruciate ligament

(ACL) attaches the posterior medial femoral condyle to the anterior tibial eminence.

The ACL prevents anterior movement of the tibia. The posterior cruciate ligament (PCL) joins the lateral aspect of the medial femoral condyle to the posterior proximal tibia. The PCL prevents posterior displacement of the tibia. The posterior of the knee joint is supported primarily by the capsule fibers. However, the oblique popliteal ligament (OPL) and arcuate ligament provide secondary support. The OPL inserts on the semimembranosus tendon and attaches to the posterior capsule. The arcuate ligament also attaches to the posterior capsule but inserts onto the fibular head instead. The patellar ligament is the only ligament supporting the pallatofemoral joint. This ligament connects the tibial tuberosity to the inferior pole of the patella.

Bursae are synovial fluid-filled structures located superficial to the ligaments of the knee. The role of bursae is to decrease the friction between the tendons and the muscles of the knee when they cross over bony protuberances during motion. There are four bursae in the anterior knee: suprapatellar, subcutaneous prepatellar, subcutaneous infrapatellar, and deep infrapatellar. These four bursae help the patella move across the patellofemoral joint during leg flexion and extension. Two bursae are located between the MCL tendons that aid in leg flexion. The first bursa is between the MCL and the pes anserine tendon, and the second is between the semimembranosus tendon and the MCL. Two lateral bursae are located between the LCL and the biceps femoris tendon, the LCL, and the popliteus muscle. These structures also help with leg flexion. Lastly, the posterior bursae are located under the gastrocnemius muscle. Two bursae are under the medial head of the gastrocnemius, and the other two are under the lateral head. These bursae may communicate with the synovial capsule in some patients and help with deep knee flexion. Two primary muscle groups extend and flex the lower leg through the knee. The chief extensor of the lower leg is the quadriceps muscle group (rectus femoris, vastus medialis, vastus lateralis, and vastus intermedius.) The rectus femoris will become the quadriceps tendon as it approaches the patella. This tendon inserts onto the superior pole of the patella. It will work with the patellar ligament to extend the lower leg.

The hamstring muscles are the primary muscle group involved in leg flexion. The biceps femoris inserts on the head of the fibula and the lateral condyle of the tibia. The other primary flexor of the leg is the semimembranous muscle, which inserts on the medial condyle of the tibia. There are also secondary movers of the lower leg. The pes anserinus is the union of semitendinosus, gracilis, and sartorius tendons that insert onto the tibia's medial tuberosity. These muscles stabilize the knee and are weak flexors of the leg. The iliotibial band attaches to the lateral aspect of the leg and inserts onto the lateral tibia and the patella. This muscle and fascia stabilize the lateral knee and is a secondary flexor of the lower leg.

INJURIES

Several injuries can affect the integrity of the knee joint. Any form of trauma can alter the bony structure of the knee. High-speed trauma can dislocate the tibia from the femur. Patients with this injury

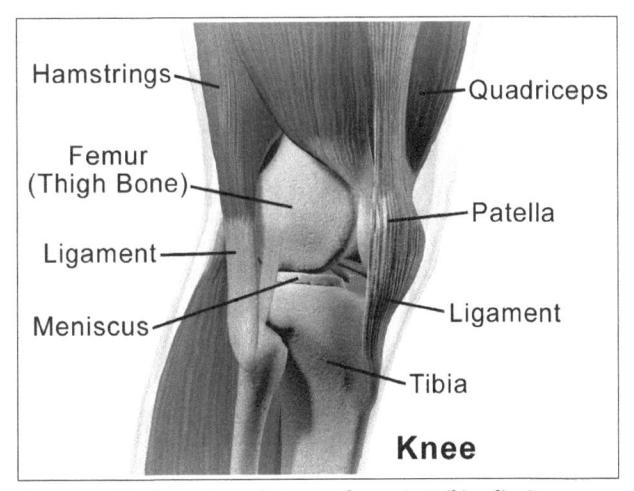

Anatomy of the knee. Image by BruceBlaus, via Wikimedia Commons.

will need immediate orthopedic evaluation to realign the knee. Another consequence of high-speed impact is the possibility of fractures. The femur, patella, and tibia can fracture secondary to high-impact trauma. Depending on the extent of the injury and the amount of displacement of the bones, immediate surgical intervention might be needed. Injuries at lower velocities have the potential for ligament and meniscal damage.

Forceful impacts on a planted foot can lead to sprains or tears of either the medial or lateral collateral ligaments. The cruciate ligaments can be injured as well. Twisting on a hyperextended knee can tear the ACL, or a direct blow to a flexed knee can rupture the PCL. Depending on the severity of the sprain, the patient might need surgery to repair the ligament. A twisting motion of a planted foot can create a shearing force that would shear a meniscus. A partially detached meniscus would need to have a surgical correction. A surgeon decides if the tear needs to be removed or is large enough to reattach to the rest of the meniscus.

Aside from meniscectomy, osteoarthritis can occur from chronic knee wear and tear, resulting in degenerative changes to the meniscus or cartilage. These changes will lead to direct contact between the femur and the tibia, causing pain. The final type of injury to the knee can result from inflammation. Since the knee is a synovial joint, bacteria or other pathogens can enter the joint and cause an infection. Patients will present with a red, painful, and swollen joint. The infected fluid can be aspirated and analyzed; the patient will be started on antibiotics or another treatment. The bursae that help the knee articulate can also become inflamed and cause pain with associated motion. Treatment can involve rest and ice in mild cases. However, in more refractory cases, steroids can be used to thwart any inflammation.

—*Nick Feo*

Further Reading

"Meniscus Tears." *OrthoInfo*, Mar. 2021, orthoinfo.aaos.org/topic.cfm?topic=A00358.

Morton, David, et al. *The Big Picture: Gross Anatomy*. 2nd ed., McGraw Hill/Medical, 2018.

Murphy, Andrew. "Knee Bursae." *Radiopaedia*, 9 Nov. 2021, radiopaedia.org/articles/knee-bursae.

Thompson, Jon C. *Netter's Concise Orthopaedic Anatomy*. 2nd ed., Saunders Elsevier, 2015.

LIGAMENTS

Category: Anatomy

Specialties and related fields: Orthopedics, physical therapy, physical medicine and rehabilitation

Definition: type of connective tissue that connects a bone to one or more other bones to provide stability around a joint

KEY TERMS

connective tissue: tissue throughout the body that develops from mesoderm, the middle embryological layer, and serves various functions in stability and anatomic structure

fascia: type of connective tissue that either connects one group of muscles to another or encircles an organ, separating parts of the body into different compartments

sprain: injury to a ligament, typically from overstretching it along its length that may cause pain, swelling, and instability

strain: injury to a muscle tendon, either from overstretching it along its length or forcefully contracting it, that may cause bruising, pain, swelling, and weakness

tendon: type of connective tissue that connects a muscle or muscle group to one or more bones, providing an anchor for the muscle fibers to pull against

Ligaments

STRUCTURE AND FUNCTIONS

In a healthy human body, the normal function of joints requires a balance between flexibility and structural strength: the joint must be pliable enough to glide easily through the planes in which it functions but rigid enough to stabilize nearby structures and not translate or veer into undesired angles or translations. Whereas muscles are the structures that pull joints back and forth in their plane of motion, just as the quadriceps and hamstring flex and extend the knee, ligaments are the structures that provide stability around this joint, such as the anterior cruciate ligament (ACL) and posterior cruciate ligament (PCL), which prevent the tibia from dislocating forward or backward with motion about the knee. Like muscles, bones, and fascia, ligaments are connective tissue. They are thus derived from the middle layer of the embryo known as the "mesoderm."

The role of skeletal muscles around a joint is fairly straightforward. By either contracting or relaxing, they shorten or lengthen longitudinally and force the joint to move in one direction. Tendons are the thin part of the muscle that connect the body of the muscle, the portion which actively contracts, to the bone. Ligaments, in contrast, have a fixed length and cannot actively contract. Instead, they provide passive resistance against extraneous motion around the joint and prevent it from moving into an unintended configuration. Ligaments have diverse shapes and sizes, ranging from thin and ropelike, as in the ACL, or flat and sheetlike, as in the longitudinal ligaments that vertically line the spinal canal, to fan-shaped, as in the talofibular ligaments in the ankle.

Like most connective tissue, ligaments are composed primarily of collagen—in this case, type 1 collagen, which makes up 70 percent of most liga-

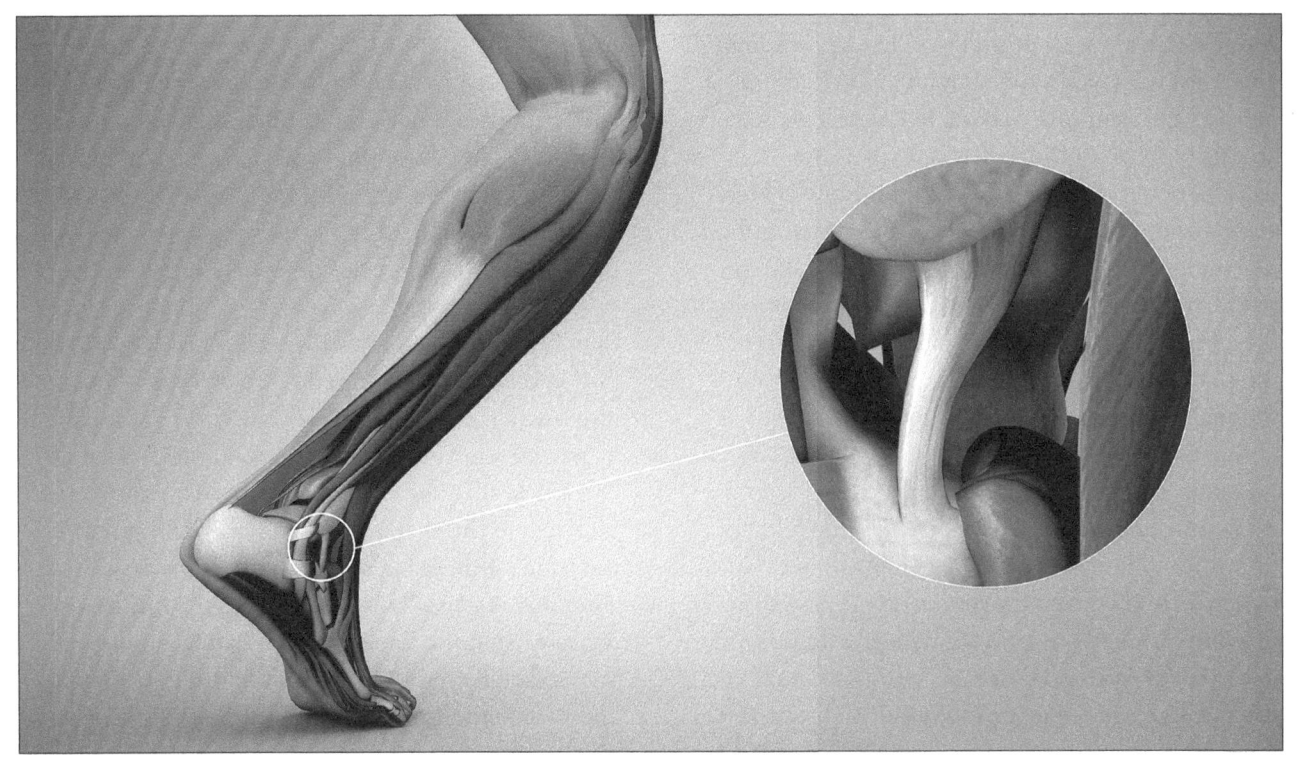

Articular ligament. Image by www.scientificanimations.com, via Wikimedia Commons.

ments. Since ligaments must provide a flexible resistance to motion rather than rigid stability, they also contain a higher amount of elastin than tendons, allowing them to stretch slightly to compensate for lengthwise force. The remainder of a ligament is composed of a small amount of fat cells and proteoglycans or proteins whose surfaces are covered with bound sugars. Variations in ligament thickness, length, and composition partly explain why some individuals have more natural flexibility, or "ligamentous laxity," than others. Although ligaments are not as metabolically active as muscles or bones, they contain some important sensory structures. In particular, they have nerve endings called Pacinian corpuscles—"little bodies of Pacini"—that detect vibration and pressure, allowing the body to sense the position and tension of ligaments and help protect them from injury.

Outside the context of joints, ligaments also play an important role in stabilizing organs and their surrounding structures within the pelvic, abdominal, and chest cavities. In the abdomen, for example, numerous ligaments are needed to create a normal anatomic position of the gut tube, such as the hepatoduodenal ligament, which houses the blood vessels and ducts that run between the liver and upper small intestine, and the gastrocolic ligament, which anchors the transverse colon to the bottom of the stomach. A similar array of ligaments is found in the pelvis, such as the many ligaments that hold a woman's ovaries and uterus in place.

In a few cases, ligaments also refer to the vestigial remnants of fetal structures that previously served other functions in the neonate or unborn child but transformed into fibrous, collagenous connective tissue once they were no longer needed. These structures are primarily seen in the digestive and circulatory systems since these are two systems that differ most between the fetus and the adult. The urachus, for example, is a duct that connects the fetal bladder to the maternal placenta to help excrete nitrogenous waste. In children, the duct seals off and regresses into a fibrous structure called the "median umbilical ligament." Similarly, the fetal cardiac system has additional blood vessels, called the "ductus venosus" and "ductus arteriosus," to help it to bypass the liver and lungs, respectively. This is useful because those structures do not perform their functions in the fetus. After birth, the ductus venosus seals up to become the ligamentum venosum, and the ductus arteriosus seals up to become the ligamentum arteriosum.

DISEASES AND DISORDERS

Ligaments are distributed throughout the human body, and thus any one of them presents a potential area for injury. The most classic ligamentous injuries occur at joints, typically due to excessive, inappropriately directed force or motion, such as hyperflexion, hyperextension, or twisting around a joint. Whereas strain is the term used to refer to a hyperextension muscle injury, such as a strained hamstring, a sprain is a hyperextension ligament injury, such as a sprained ankle or sprained knee. These injuries usually cause immediate pain, typically followed by swelling, reduced range of motion, and potential bruising. Although the body can often repair ligamentous sprains, these injuries can sometimes take even longer to heal than a fracture, in part since these regions are less metabolically active than bone and have a smaller blood supply.

If enough force is placed on them, ligaments can also break partly along their transverse plane, called a "partial tear," or completely dissociate, called a "complete tear" or "rupture." The ACLs and PCLs intersect in the shape of a cross or crux, representing some of the most serious injuries for an athlete. The ACL is typically injured through a rapid twisting inward of the knee and can lead to significant knee instability in the forward direction. If injured badly enough, it may require complete surgical replacement, which can take up to a year to return to full function. While this is the most important example of ligamentous injury, ligaments may potentially tear and require surgery anywhere in the body, including the hips, ankles, feet, shoulders, elbows, hands, and spine.

While some degree of joint laxity is necessary for normal function, a pathological amount of laxity may also be seen in people with certain genetic conditions. People with Down syndrome, for example, have been found to have more flexible joints, presumably because one of the genes for collagen is found on chromosome 21 a. Similarly, people with inherited connective tissue diseases such as Marfan syndrome, Ehlers-Danlos syndrome, and Loeys-Dietz syndrome are all known to have increased ligamentous laxity because of the altered composition of their ligaments.

The internal ligaments of the chest, abdomen, and pelvis are less likely to be injured during normal human activity. However, they still represent potential areas for injury. Those ligaments containing blood vessels, such as the stomach, ovaries, and uterus, must be carefully protected during nearby surgeries, as they can result in dangerous bleeding. Meanwhile, those vestigial ligaments that connect to blood vessels can be devastating when injured. In particular, the ligamentum arteriosum can tear a hole in the aorta during rapid deceleration, such as a car crash, and may lead to life-threatening bleeding and rapid loss of life.

PERSPECTIVE AND PROSPECTS
The realm of orthopedics makes frequent advances in treating injury to joint ligaments. As such, it represents a field of medicine that is rapidly changing. For many years, the standard of care for complete ACL tear was reconstructing the ligament with a surgical graft using the person's hamstring or patellar tendon. However, advances in molecular biology have pointed toward potential evolutions in this field. Using stem cells reduces the recovery time for athletes hoping to return rapidly to function. If current scientists can induce the ACL to recover entirely using nonoperative, biochemical therapies, surgery for complete ACL reconstruction may soon become obsolete.

While the internal ligaments of the abdomen and pelvis are less frequent targets for surgery, they can lead to nonnegligible complications when damaged incidentally. As laparoscopic surgery has risen in popularity over the past few decades, the precision possible in abdominal and pelvic surgeons has increased, leading to less blood loss intraoperatively. Robotic surgeries using technologies such as the Da Vinci Surgical System have increased precision and reduced the complication rate of abdominal and pelvic surgery. They likely represent the next stage in the standard of care for these operations.

—*Walter Klyce, Derek T. Nhan*

Further Reading
Mulcahey, Mary K. "Sprains, Strains and Other Soft-Tissue Injuries." *OrthoInfo*, June 2020, orthoinfo.aaos.org/en/diseases—conditions/sprains-strains-and-other-soft-tissue-injuries/.
Norkin C. C. *Joint Structure and Function*. 4th ed., F. A. Davis, 2005.
Scuderi, Giles R. *Sports Medicine: A Comprehensive Approach*. 2nd ed., Mosby/Elsevier, 2005.
Vorvick, Linda J. "Tendon vs. Ligament." *MedlinePlus*, 13 Aug. 2020, medlineplus.gov/ency/imagepages/19089.htm.

Lower Extremities

Category: Anatomy
Specialties and related fields: Neurology, occupational therapy, orthopedics, physical therapy, podiatry
Definition: the lower extremities of the human body comprise the thighs, lower legs, and feet; they are attached to the pelvis at the hip joint and consist of muscles, bones, blood vessels, lymph vessels, nerves, skin, and toenails

KEY TERMS

distal: farther away from the base or attached end

femur: the long bone extending from the hip joint to the knee

fibula: the smaller of the two bones in the lower leg, on the lateral side

knee: the complex articulated joint between the thigh and the lower leg

lateral: on the outer side; toward the little toe when in reference to the leg

leg: the lower extremity, excluding the foot; the lower leg runs from the knee to the ankle

medial: on the side toward the midline of the body; toward the big toe when in reference to the leg

proximal: closer to the base or attached end

tarsus: the ankle

thigh: the upper segment of the leg, from the hip joint to the knee

tibia: the larger of the two bones in the lower leg, on the medial side

STRUCTURE AND FUNCTIONS

The lower extremities consist of the thighs, lower legs, and feet. Each extremity attaches to the pelvis (innominate bone) at the hip joint. The lower extremity is made mostly of bones and muscles. Still, it also contains blood vessels, lymphatics, nerves, skin, toenails, and other structures. Important directional terms for the lower extremity include proximal (closer to the base or attached end), distal (further from the base or attached end), medial (on the same side as the tibia and big toe), and lateral (on the same side as the fibula and little toe). Along the foot, the lower surface is called "plantar"; the upper surface is called "dorsal." The lower extremity is clothed in the skin (or integument). The sole or plantar surface of the foot is unusual, along with the palm, in being completely hairless; it also contains the thickest outer skin layer (the stratum corneum) of any part of the body. Each toe has a hardened toenail on its dorsal surface.

The pelvic girdle that supports the lower extremity develops as three separate bones: the ilium, ischium, and pubis. All three help form the acetabulum, a socket into which the femur fits. Below the acetabulum, the ischium and pubis surround a large opening called the "obturator foramen." The right and left pubis meet to form a pubic symphysis. The lower extremity bones include the femur, tibia, fibula, tarsals, metatarsals, and phalanges. The femur (thigh bone) is the largest bone in the body. Its rounded upper end, or head, fits into the acetabulum and is attached by a short neck. A rough-surfaced greater trochanter lies just beyond this neck and serves for the attachment of many muscles. The lesser trochanter, also for muscle attachments, lies below the neck. The knee joint is covered and protected by the kneecap, or patella, the largest of the sesamoid bones formed within tendons at stress points. The lower leg, from the knee to the ankle, contains two bones: the tibia on the medial side and the slenderer fibula on the lateral side. The tarsus, or ankle, includes the talus, calcaneus, and five smaller bones. The talus (or astragalus) has a pulley-like facet for the tibia and other curved surfaces for articulation with the calcaneus and navicular. The calcaneus, or heel bone, is vertically enlarged in humans; the Achilles tendon attaches to its roughened lower tuberosity. Smaller tarsal bones include the navicular, the medial (or inner) cuneiform, the intermediate cuneiform, the lateral (or outer) cuneiform, and the cuboid. Beyond the tarsal bones, the foot is supported by five metatarsal bones. The big toe, or hallux, contains two phalanges; each of the remaining toes contains three phalanges.

The lower extremity muscles include extensors, which straighten joints, and flexors, which bend joints. Abductor muscles move the limbs sideways, away from the midline, while adductors pull the limbs back toward the midline. The muscles of the iliac region attach the lower extremity to the body.

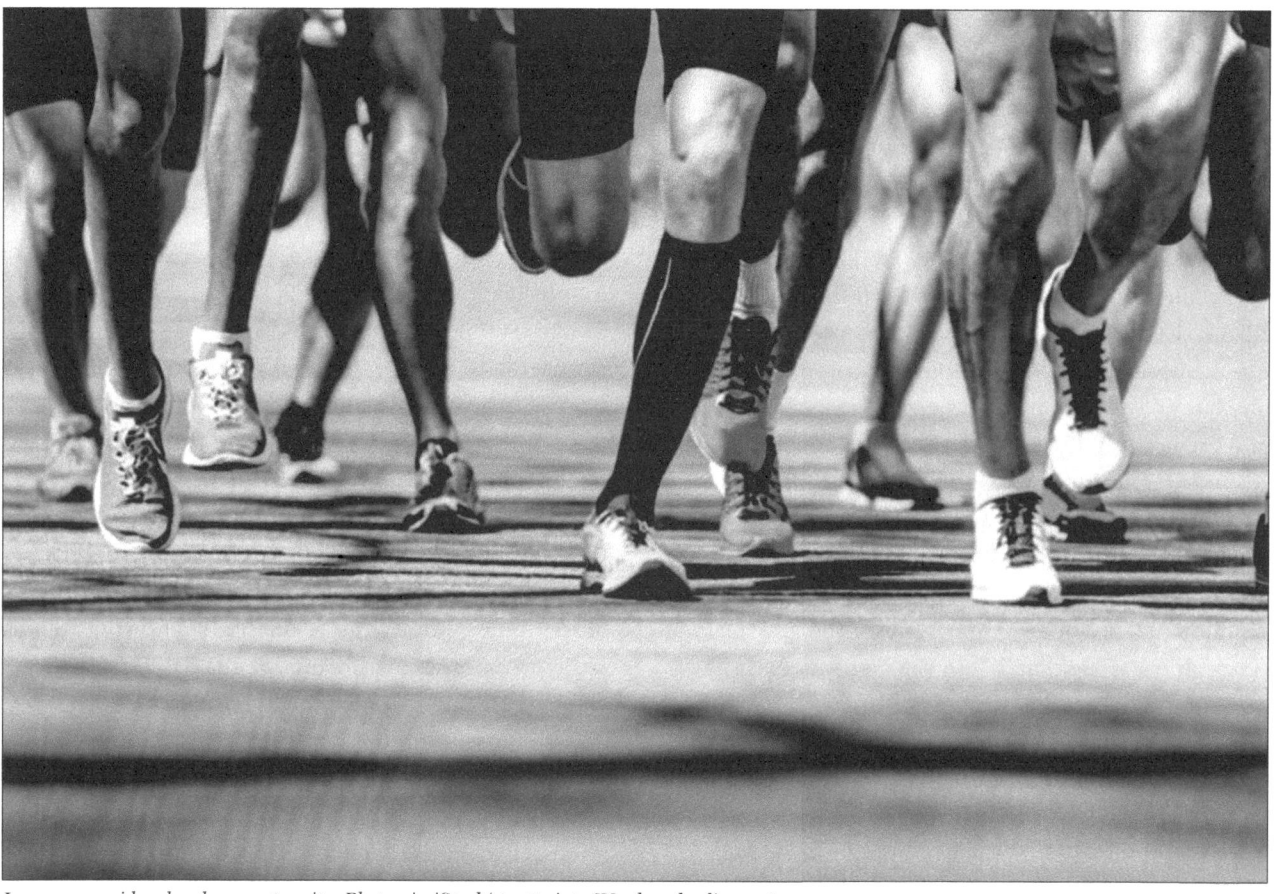

Legs are considered a lower extremity. Photo via iStock/sportpoint. [Used under license.]

The psoas major runs from the lumbar vertebrae to the lesser trochanter of the femur. The iliacus runs from the ilium and part of the sacrum to the femur, including the lesser trochanter. The anterior muscles of the thigh include the sartorius, the quadriceps femoris, and the articularis genus. The sartorius, the longest muscle in the body, flexes both hip and knee joints. It runs obliquely from the anterior border of the ilium across the front of the thigh to insert onto the medial side of the knee at the upper end of the tibia. The quadriceps femoris consists of the rectus femoris and the three vastus muscles; all four are strong knee extensors. The rectus femoris originates from the region surrounding the acetabulum. The vastus lateralis, vastus medialis, and vastus intermedius muscles all originate along the shaft of the femur. All four quadriceps muscles insert onto a common tendon that runs over the knee and inserts onto the top of the tibia. The patella is a sesamoid bone enclosed within this tendon, where it runs over the front of the knee. The smaller articularis genus muscle originates on the anterior side of the shaft of the femur; it inserts onto the kneecap.

The hip and thigh extensor muscles help maintain an upright posture. The gluteus maximus, the largest of these muscles, originates from the posterior portion of the ilium and inserts high on the femur, especially onto the greater trochanter. The gluteus medius and gluteus minimis originate from the ilium's outer surface and insert onto the greater trochanter. The tensor fasciae latae originates along the iliac crest; it inserts onto a broad, sheet-like tendon (the fascia lata) covering much of the thigh's lateral surface. The piriformis runs from the sacrum to the greater trochanter of the femur. The obturator internus runs from the inner surface of the pelvis through the obturator foramen to the greater trochanter of the femur. The gemellus superior and the gemellus inferior originate from the rear margin of the ischium; they both insert onto the greater trochanter. The quadratus femoris originates from the lateral surface of the ischium; it inserts between the greater and lesser trochanters of the femur. The obturator externus originates along the outer surface of the pelvis below the obturator foramen and inserts near the greater trochanter.

The muscles on the medial (or inner) side of the thigh are all abductors of the thigh. The gracilis is a long, thin muscle that originates from the pubis, runs along the medial side of the thigh, and inserts high on the tibia. The pectineus originates anteriorly on the pubis and inserts onto the shaft of the femur below the lesser trochanter. The adductor longus originates from the pubis and inserts onto the posterior edge of the femur. The adductor brevis originates from the pubis and inserts onto the posterior edge of the femur. The adductor magnus is a large, triangular muscle that originates from the lower portion of the ischium and pubis; it expands to a long, thin insertion along the posterior edge of the femur.

The hamstring muscles run along the posterior side of the femur; they flex the knee and extend the hip joint. The biceps femoris originates from the posterior portion (the tuberosity) of the ischium and separately from the posterior edge of the femur. Both portions converge onto a common tendon that inserts primarily onto the top of the fibula. The semitendinosus originates from the posterior end of the ischium; it inserts by a long tendon onto the medial side of the tibia. The semimembranosus runs from the ischium to the posterior surface of the tibia.

The muscles on the lower leg's front (anterior) side raise the foot by flexing it dorsally. At the ankle, their tendons are held in place by two transverse bands, the extensor retinacula. The tibialis anterior originates along the anterior edge of the tibia; it inserts by a tendon onto the medial cuneiform and the base of the first metatarsal. The extensor hallucis longus originates from the anterior surface of the fibula; its tendon passes beneath the extensor retinacula to insert onto the distal phalanx of the big toe. The extensor digitorum longus originates near the top of the tibia and along the anterior side of the fibula. Its tendon passes beneath the extensor retinacula and splits into four tendons, inserted onto the second and third phalanges of the second through fifth digits. The peroneus tertius originates along the anterior edge of the fibula and runs alongside the extensor digitorum longus. It inserts onto the base of the fifth metatarsal bone.

The muscles on the lower leg's posterior surface are mostly foot extensors; some also flex the knee. The gastrocnemius originates in two heads from opposite sides of the femur. It inserts onto the Achilles tendon, which attaches to the calcaneus. The soleus originates from the posterior surface of the fibula; it inserts onto the Achilles tendon. The plantaris originates from the posterior surface of the femur and inserts onto the posterior portion of the calcaneus. The popliteus runs from the lateral side of the femur across the back of the knee to insert onto the tibia. The flexor hallucis longus originates along the posterior surface of the fibula; its tendon runs around to the medial side of the ankle and inserts onto the base of the big toe. The flexor digitorum longus originates from the posterior surface of the tibia; its tendon crosses the sole obliquely and divides into four tendons that insert onto the distal phalanges of the second through fifth toes. The tibialis posterior originates from the posterior surfaces of the tibia, the fibula, and the interosseous membrane that joins them; its tendon passes around to insert onto the navicular bone. The peroneus longus originates along the lateral surface of the fibula; its tendon runs along a groove on the bottom of the cuboid to insert obliquely onto the base of the first metatarsal. The peroneus brevis originates along the lateral margin of the fibula; its tendon inserts onto the fifth metatarsal. The extensor digitorum brevis originates from the calcaneus and runs obliquely across the dorsal side of the foot, dividing into four tendons. One tendon inserts onto the base of the big toe; the remaining tendons insert onto the tendons of the extensor digitorum longus.

Several flexor muscles of the foot are attached to the plantar aponeurosis. This flat ligament runs from the calcaneus along the sole of the foot to the bases of the toes and several flexor tendons. The abductor hallucis originates from the calcaneus and the plantar aponeurosis; it inserts onto the base of the big toe. The flexor digitorum brevis originates from the plantar aponeurosis and the calcaneus; it divides into four portions, each giving rise to a tendon. These tendons run into the second through fifth toes, each splitting in half to insert onto opposite sides of the second phalanx, separated by the tendons of the flexor digitorum longus, which emerge between them. The abductor digiti quinti originates from the calcaneus and the plantar aponeurosis; it inserts onto the base of the fifth toe. The quadratus plantae originates from the calcaneus and inserts onto the tendons of the flexor digitorum longus. The four small lumbricals run from the tendons of the flexor digitorum longus to the corresponding tendons of the extensor digitorum longus. The flexor hallucis brevis originates from the cuboid and lateral cuneiform bones; its two portions insert onto the big toe from opposite sides. The adductor hallucis originates from the second through fourth metatarsals and the bases of the third through fifth toes. Its tendon inserts onto the base of the big toe. The flexor digiti quinti originates from the fifth metatarsal base and inserts onto the base of the fifth toe. The four dorsal interossei originate from the bases of the metatarsal bones; they insert onto the bases of the second through fourth toes. The three plantar interossei originate from the third through fifth metatarsals and run beneath these bones to insert onto the bases of the corresponding toes.

Blood vessels of the lower extremity include both arteries and veins. The common iliac arteries arise from the dorsal aorta; each divides into an internal and an external iliac. The internal iliac artery supplies many muscles of the thigh region and pelvis. The external iliac artery branches into an inferior epigastric artery and a deep iliac circumflex artery; it then continues along the femur as the femoral artery. The femoral artery gives rise to a deep femoral artery running to the medial and posterior regions of the thigh; the base of this artery also gives rise to two circumflex arteries that send branches upward into many thigh muscles. Near the knee, the femoral artery branches into a descending geniculate artery to the knee, then continues as the popliteal artery, forming several branches to the thigh muscles and other small branches to the knee before splitting into anterior and posterior tibial arteries.

The anterior tibial artery descends along the front of the tibia, forming several small branches. It then continues into the foot as the dorsalis pedis artery, giving rise to a lateral tarsal artery and an arcuate artery, both of which form arches by joining with branches of the peroneal artery. The deep plantar artery and hallucis dorsalis artery also branch from the dorsalis pedis artery. In contrast, individual arteries to the second through fourth metatarsals arise from the arcuate artery. Arterial branches to all the toes arise from the individual metatarsal arteries, including the hallucis dorsalis, forming a system of collateral circulation in which multiple alternate routes permit blood flow even if one of the routes is temporarily blocked.

The posterior tibial artery gives rise to a peroneal artery; the two arteries then run down the posterior side of the lower leg, forming small branches to the muscles of the lower leg and nutrient arteries to the tibia and fibula. The posterior tibial artery branches to the calcaneus before it splits into a medial plantar artery that runs along the medial margin of the foot into the big toe and a much larger lateral plantar artery. The lateral plantar artery runs across the foot obliquely to the lateral side, then turns and runs obliquely in the other direction to the base of the big toe, where it runs into the deep plantar artery to form a loop. From this loop arise a series of plantar metatarsal arteries to all five toes. Blood can reach each toe from either side. The arch that supplies this blood can receive its blood either through the posterior tibial and lateral plantar arteries or through the anterior tibial and deep plantar arteries, providing another example of collateral circulation.

There are several important veins draining the lower extremity. The deep veins originate from a series of plantar digital veins draining the individual toes into a deep plantar venous arch. This arch is drained in either direction by a lateral plantar vein and a medial plantar vein, which later unite to form a posterior tibial vein; this vein and the peroneal vein run parallel to the corresponding arteries along the posterior side of the lower leg. An anterior tibial vein drains the lower leg's anterior side and the foot's dorsal side. Near the knee, the peroneal vein and the anterior and posterior tibial veins unite to form the popliteal vein, which continues into the thigh as the femoral vein. The femoral vein receives the deep femoral vein as a tributary, then the saphenous vein. The femoral vein then continues as the external iliac vein.

The lower extremity is also covered with a network of superficial veins that lie beneath the skin. The vessels of this network are drained along the medial side of the lower leg and thigh by the great saphenous vein, which runs into the femoral vein just below the groin. The lateral side of the foot and the posterior surface of the lower leg are drained by the small saphenous vein, which drains into the popliteal vein.

The nerves to the lower extremity arise from two series of complex branchings, the lumbar plexus, and sacral plexus. The largest nerve formed from the lumbar plexus is the femoral nerve, supplying muscles on the anterior side of the thigh and part of the lower leg. Other branches to the muscles include the obturator nerve to the adductor muscles and separate muscular branches to the psoas and iliacus muscles. Cutaneous sensory nerves to the skin include the lateral femoral cutaneous nerve to the lateral side of the thigh, the anterior cutaneous branches of the femoral nerve to the medial side of the thigh, and the saphenous nerve, a branch of the femoral nerve to the medial side of the lower leg.

The sacral plexus gives rise to the very large sciatic nerve and several smaller nerves, including the superior gluteal and inferior gluteal nerves to the gluteal muscles and separate muscular branches to the piriformis, quadratus femoris, obturator internus, and gemelli. Cutaneous branches such as the posterior femoral cutaneous nerve supply sensory fibers to the skin on the posterior surface of the thigh. The sciatic nerve, the largest nerve in the body, branches off to the hamstring muscles before splitting into the tibial and peroneal nerves. The tibial nerve supplies the muscles on the posterior side of the lower leg. It then runs onto the sole, splitting into the medial and lateral plantar nerves, which supply cutaneous sensation and muscular innervation to the sole. The peroneal nerve divides into deep and superficial portions. The deep peroneal nerve supplies the muscles on the anterior side of the lower leg and the dorsal surface of the foot. The superficial peroneal nerve supplies cutaneous sensation to the lateral surface of the lower leg and the dorsal surface of the foot.

DISORDERS AND DISEASES

Many medical conditions and disorders affect the lower extremity; these include animal bites (including snakebites), injuries, fungus infections such as athlete's foot, contact dermatitis (including poison ivy), and an assortment of neuromuscular disorders, including nerve paralyses, muscular atrophies, and muscular dystrophies. Nerve paralyses of the lower extremities usually arise from traumatic injury. Muscular atrophies are diseases in which muscle tissues become progressively weaker and smaller, usually beginning after the age of forty. Spastic movements sometimes occur. The small muscles of the hands and feet are usually affected sooner and more severely compared to the larger muscles of the legs and thighs. Amyotrophic lateral sclerosis (ALS), commonly known as "Lou Gehrig's disease," is one such disease that usually begins with weakness and deterioration of the distal muscles. The disease affects the rest of the extremities, then other parts of the body; it is usually fatal within three to five years after onset. A rarer type of atrophy, myelopathic muscular atrophy (or Aran-Duchenne atrophy), affects both upper and lower extremities and eventually spreads to the trunk. A degenerative gray matter lesion in the spinal cord's cervical region is usually responsible.

Muscular dystrophy is a series of inherited diseases that begin in early childhood, affecting males more often than females. The most common type, Duchenne muscular dystrophy, is caused by a sex-linked recessive trait that impairs the body's ability to synthesize a large protein called "dystrophin." Muscular dystrophy primarily affects the large muscles of the thigh and lower leg, impairing the ability to stand unassisted or walk. The affected muscles become very weak but remain approximately normal in size and may even increase as muscle tissue is replaced by fatty and fibrous tissue. Progressive weakening makes walking and similar motor functions impossible, but patients can live for decades with proper care.

Sports injuries often occur in the lower extremities and are generally treated by orthopedic specialists. Fractured bones are generally set in casts and kept immobile until they heal. Injured or ruptured ligaments often require surgical treatment. Snakebites and other animal bites occur more often to the lower extremities than to other parts of the body. The bites of poisonous snakes must be treated quickly before the venom reaches the heart. The patient must be kept calm and quiet, and experienced medical attention should be sought as soon as possible.

PERSPECTIVE AND PROSPECTS

The major muscles and bones of the lower extremities were studied in ancient societies by such individuals as Galen (or Caius Galenus), the physician to the Roman army in the second century. The science of anatomy took many great strides because of artists who studied the human body to create realistic sculptures and paintings. During the Renaissance, Leonardo da Vinci (1452-1519) and Michelangelo (1475-1564) dissected human corpses illegally in their quest for this knowledge. Andreas Vesalius (1514-64) produced the first well-illustrated anatomical texts containing information that corrected many of the errors made by Galen.

Injuries to the leg are generally treated surgically. Whenever possible, broken bones are set in place, immobilized in a cast, and then allowed to heal. Muscles (or their tendons) must be sewn together. Nerve endings must be matched with their former locations to grow back correctly. Gangrene, or tissue death from lack of circulation, occurs more often in the lower extremities than in the upper extremities. Amputation is often performed when the lower extremity is gangrenous or is injured beyond repair. Artificial legs or partial legs are sometimes attached to the lower extremity.

—*Eli C. Minkoff*

Further Reading

Agur, Anne M. R., and Arthur F. Dalley. *Grant's Atlas of Anatomy*. 15th ed., Lippincott Williams & Wilkins, 2020.

Brummett, Chad M., and Steven P. Cohen. *Managing Pain: Essentials of Diagnosis and Treatment*. Oxford UP, 2013.

Carr, Kevin, and Mary Kate Feit. *Functional Training Anatomy*. Human Kinetics, 2021.

Currey, John D. *Bones: Structures and Mechanics*. 2nd ed., Princeton UP, 2006.

Iyer, K. Mohan. *Orthopedics of the Upper and Lower Limb*. 2nd ed., Springer, 2020.

Kim, Daniel H., et al. *Atlas of Peripheral Nerve Surgery*. Elsevier/Saunders, 2013.

Marieb, Elaine N. *Essentials of Human Anatomy and Physiology*. 13th ed., Pearson, 2021.

Rosse, Cornelius, and Penelope Gaddum-Rosse. *Hollinshead's Textbook of Anatomy*. 5th ed., Lippincott-Raven, 1997.

Standring, Susan, et al., editors. *Gray's Anatomy*. 40th ed., Churchill Livingstone/Elsevier, 2008.

Van De Graaff, Kent M. *Human Anatomy*. 6th ed., McGraw-Hill, 2002.

MUSCLES

Category: Anatomy

Specialties and related fields: Cardiology, exercise physiology, orthopedics, osteopathic medicine, physical therapy, sports medicine

Definition: specialized tissues composed of tissues that can contract, making possible body movement, peristalsis (the movement of food through the gastrointestinal system), and blood circulation throughout the body

KEY TERMS

cardiac muscle: a type of muscle found only in the heart that makes up the major portion of the heart; involved in the movement of blood through the body

muscle contraction: the shortening of a muscle, which may result in the movement of a particular body part

muscle fibers: elongated muscle cells that make up skeletal, cardiac, and smooth muscles

musculature: the arrangement of skeletal muscles in the body

skeletal muscle: a type of muscle that attaches to bone and causes movement of body parts; the only type that is under conscious, voluntary control

smooth muscle: a type of muscle found in the walls of internal organs such as the stomach, intestines, and urinary bladder; involved in the movement of food through the digestive tract

STRUCTURE AND FUNCTIONS

More than half of the body weight of humans is made up of muscle. Three types of muscles are found in the body: skeletal muscle, cardiac muscle, and smooth muscle. These muscles are composed of different types of muscle cells and perform different functions within the body. The characteristics and functions of these three muscle types will be discussed separately, starting with skeletal muscle.

Skeletal muscles attach to and cover bones. This type of muscle is often referred to as voluntary muscle because it is the only muscle type that can be controlled or made to move by consciously thinking about it. Skeletal muscles perform four important functions: bringing about body movement, helping to maintain posture, helping to stabilize joints such as the knee, and generating body heat.

Nearly all body movement is dependent upon skeletal muscle. Skeletal muscle is needed not only to run and jump but also to speak, write, and move and blink the eyes. These movements are brought about by the contraction or shortening of skeletal muscles. These muscles are attached to two bones or other structures by tough, thin strips or cords of tissue known as "tendons." When a muscle contracts or shortens, it pulls the tendons, which then pull on the bones or other structures to which they are connected. In this way, the desired movement is brought about.

Skeletal muscles also aid in the maintenance of posture. Posture is defined as the ability to maintain a position of the body or body parts: for example, the ability to stand or sit erect. The body must overcome the constant force of gravity to maintain a standing or seated posture. Small adjustments to the force of gravity are constantly being made through slight contractions of skeletal muscle.

Skeletal muscles—or, more appropriately, their tendons—help to maintain joint stability. Many of the tendons that connect muscles to bones cross movable joints such as the knee and the shoulder. These tendons are kept taut by the constant contraction of the muscles to which they are attached. As a result, they act as walls to prevent the joints from dislocating or shifting out of their normal positions.

More than 40 percent of the human body is composed of skeletal muscle. Skeletal muscles generate heat as they contract. As a result, skeletal muscles are extremely important in maintaining normal body temperature. When the body is exposed to cold temperatures, it begins to shiver. This shivering results from muscle contractions, which generate body heat and maintain the body's normal temperature.

Skeletal muscles are made up of skeletal muscle cells. These cells are long and tube-shaped and therefore are referred to as skeletal muscle fibers. In some instances, these muscle fibers may be a foot long. When individual skeletal muscle fibers are viewed under a microscope, they display bands referred to as striations. For this reason, skeletal muscle is often called "striated muscle."

Each skeletal muscle, depending upon its size, is made up of hundreds or thousands of skeletal muscle fibers. These muscle fibers are surrounded by a tough connective tissue that holds the muscle fibers together. These muscle fibers and their surrounding connective tissue form a skeletal muscle. In the human body, there are more than 600 skeletal muscles.

The arrangement of these muscles in the body is referred to as the musculature, or muscle system.

Smooth muscles are often referred to as involuntary muscles because they cannot be made to contract by conscious effort. Smooth muscles are typically found in the walls of internal organs such as the esophagus, stomach, intestines, and urinary bladder. The primary function of smooth muscles in these organs is to enable the passage of material through a tube or tract. For example, the contraction of smooth muscles in the intestines helps move digested materials through the digestive system.

Smooth muscle is composed of smooth muscle cells. These cells differ from skeletal muscle fibers in that they are short and spindle-shaped. They also differ from skeletal muscle cells in that they are not striated. Furthermore, smooth muscle cells usually are not surrounded by a tough connective tissue to form a muscle; instead, they are arranged in layers.

Cardiac muscle is found only in the heart. Like smooth muscle, cardiac muscle cannot contract through conscious effort. Like skeletal muscle, however, cardiac muscle is striated. Cardiac muscle contraction causes the heart to beat. Each heartbeat results from cardiac muscle contraction, which pumps blood throughout the body.

Although many differences exist among skeletal, smooth, and cardiac muscles, all have one thing in common—their ability to contract. However, the methods by which this contraction is brought about in skeletal muscle differ from those used by smooth muscle and cardiac muscle.

For skeletal muscles to contract, they must first be electrically stimulated. This electrical stimulation is brought about by nerves closely associated with the muscle fibers. Each muscle fiber has a branch of a nerve, an axon terminal, that lies very close to it. This axon terminal does not touch the muscle fiber but is separated from it by a tiny space known as the "synaptic cleft" (or gap). An electrical impulse from the nerve causes the release of a chemical called a "neurotransmitter" into the synaptic cleft. The specific type of neurotransmitter for skeletal muscle is known as acetylcholine. Acetylcholine passes through the synaptic cleft to the muscle fiber membrane, where it will bind to a particular site on a membrane protein known as a "nicotinic receptor." When the neurotransmitter binds to the receptor, it causes an electrical impulse, or depolarization, to travel down the muscle fiber. Depolarization brings calcium into the muscle cell, which induces muscle

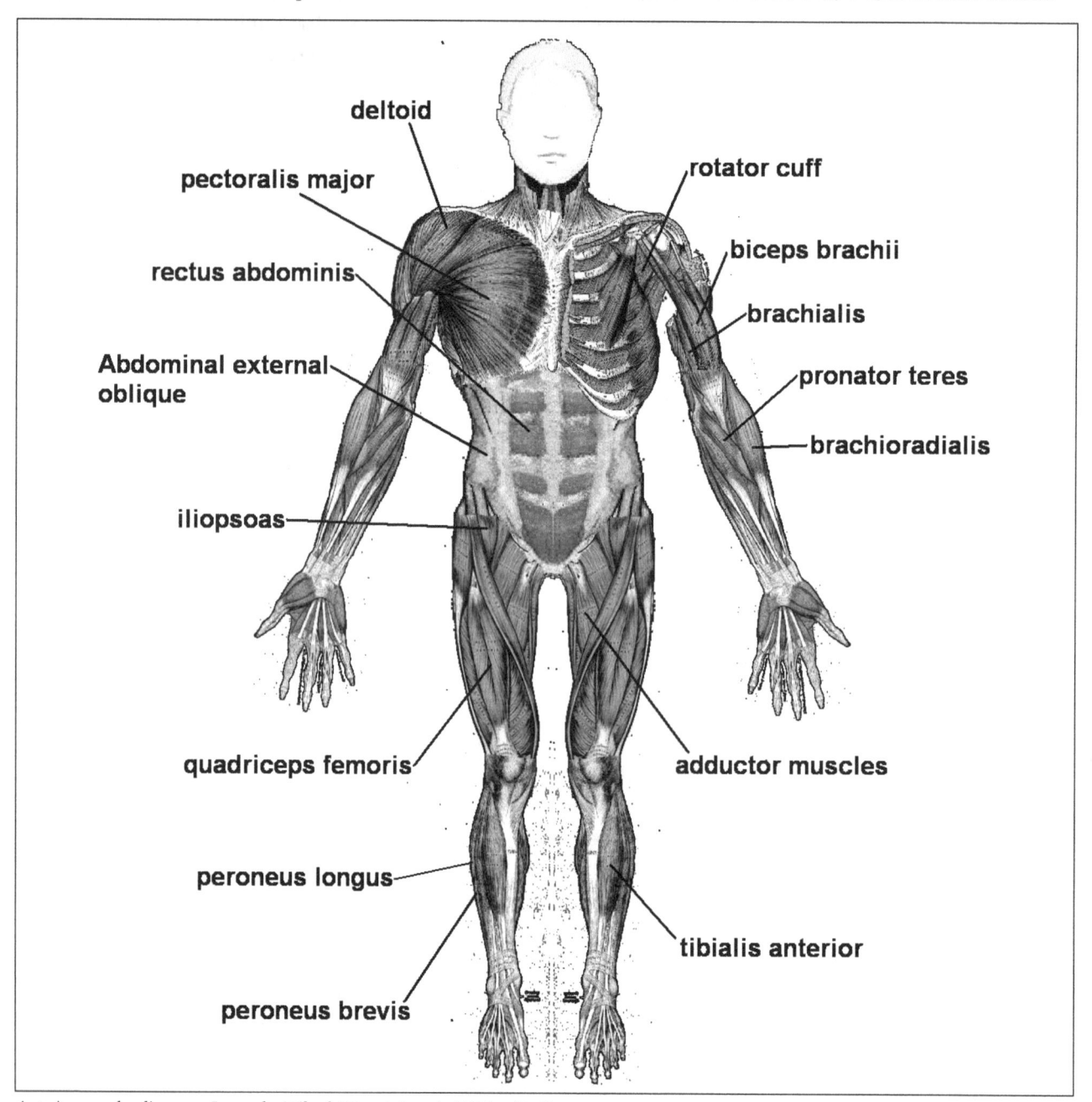

Anterior muscles diagram. Image by Mikael Häggström, via Wikimedia Commons.

fiber contraction. When most or all of the muscle fibers contract, the result is the contraction of the entire muscle.

The muscle fibers and muscle will remain contracted as long as the neurotransmitter is bound to the receptor on the muscle fiber membrane. The nicotinic receptor must release its bound acetylcholine for the muscle fiber to relax. The enzyme cholinesterase destroys unbound acetylcholine. This enzyme is called "acetylcholinesterase" in skeletal

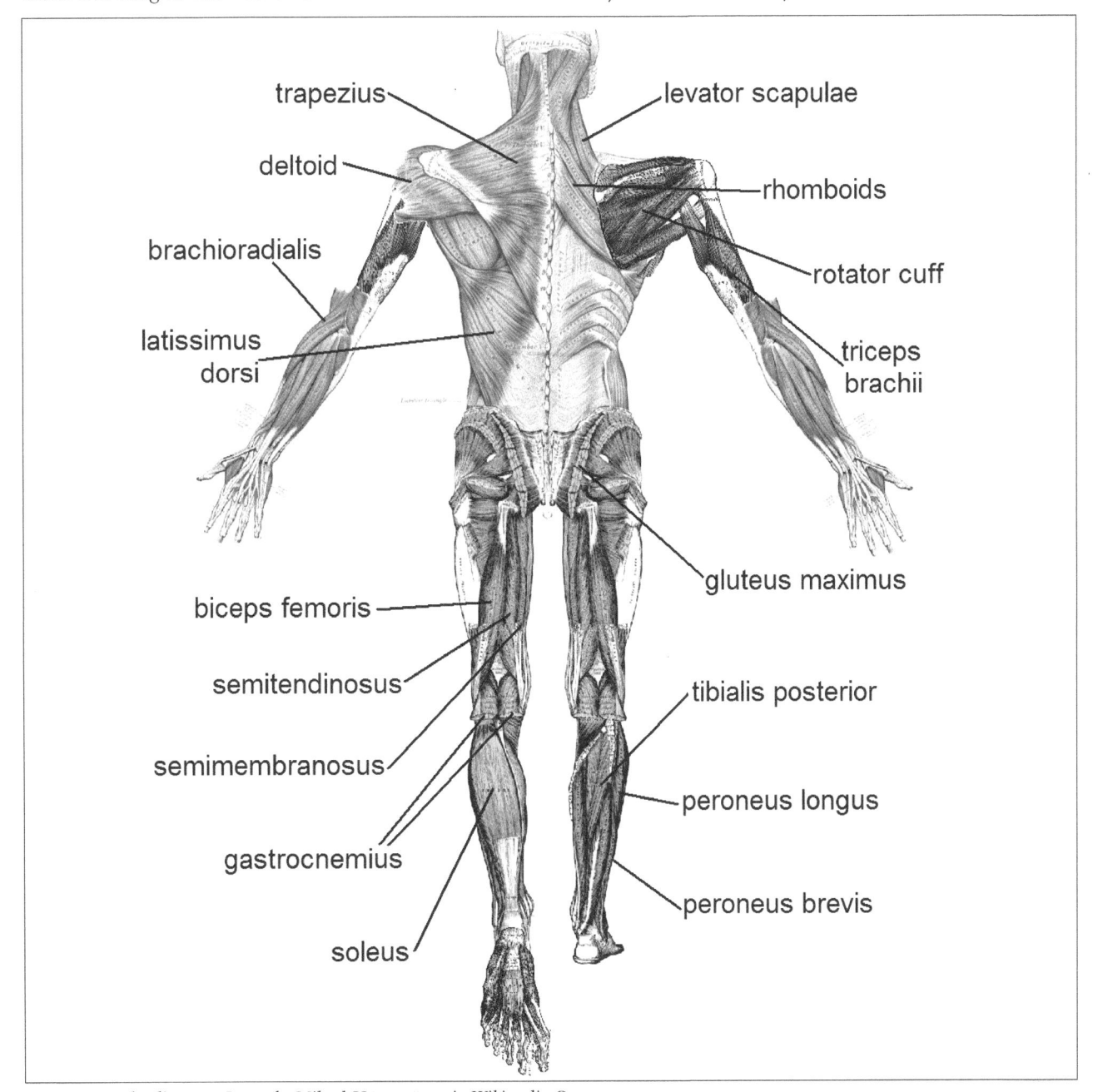

Posterior muscles diagram. Image by Mikael Häggström, via Wikimedia Commons.

muscle because it destroys the neurotransmitter acetylcholine.

The contraction of cardiac muscle differs from skeletal muscle in that motor neuron axons do not innervate each cardiac muscle fiber. Cardiac muscles can make their own electrical impulse; nerves do not need to initiate the electrical impulse for every cardiac muscle fiber. An impulse is started in a particular place in the heart, called the atrioventricular (A-V) node. This impulse spreads from muscle fiber to muscle fiber. Thus, each cardiac muscle fiber stimulates those fibers next to it. The electrical impulse spreads so fast that nearly all the cardiac muscle fibers contract at the same time. As a result, the single impulse that begins in the A-V node causes the entire heart to contract.

DISORDERS AND DISEASES

Any muscle disorder can disrupt the normal functions performed by muscles. Skeletal muscle disorders can disrupt body movement and the ability to maintain posture. If these disorders affect the diaphragm, the principal breathing muscle, they can also be fatal.

Perhaps the most common and least detrimental muscle disorder is disuse atrophy. When muscles are not used, the muscle fibers will become smaller, a process called "atrophy." As a result of the decrease in the diameter of the muscle fibers, the entire muscle also becomes smaller and, therefore, weaker.

Disuse atrophy occurs in such circumstances as when an individual is sick or injured and must remain in bed for prolonged periods. As a result, the muscles are not used and begin to atrophy. Disuse atrophy is also fairly common in astronauts because of the lack of gravity against which the muscles must work. If a muscle does not work against a load or force, such as gravity, it will tend to decrease in size.

In general, disuse muscle atrophy is easily treated. The primary treatment is to exercise the unused muscle. Physical activity, particularly in which the muscle must work to lift or pull a weight, will increase the diameter of the skeletal muscle fibers and thus of the entire muscle. The increase in the muscle fibers and muscle diameter is referred to as hypertrophy.

Another common muscle disorder is a muscle cramp. A muscle cramp is a spasm in which the muscle undergoes strong involuntary contractions. These involuntary contractions, which may last as short as a few seconds or as long as a few hours, are extremely painful. Muscle cramps appear to occur more frequently at night or after exercise. Treatment for cramps involves rubbing and massaging the affected muscle.

Muscles are often overused or overstretched. When this is the case, the muscle fibers can tear. When the muscle fibers are torn, the result is a muscle strain, more often called a "pulled muscle." Although pulled muscles may be painful, they are usually not serious. Treatment for pulled muscles most often involves the resting of the affected muscle. If the muscle fibers are torn completely apart, surgery may be required to reattach the muscle fibers.

Among the more serious skeletal muscle disorders is muscular dystrophy. The term "muscular dystrophy" is used to define those muscle disorders that are genetic or inherited. These diseases often begin in childhood, but a few cases have been reported to begin during adulthood—muscular dystrophy results in progressive muscle weakness and muscle atrophy. The most common form of muscular dystrophy is known as "Duchenne muscular dystrophy." This form of muscular dystrophy primarily affects males. In those affected with Duchenne muscular dystrophy, muscular weakness and atrophy appear at three to five years of age. There is a progressive loss of muscle strength and muscle mass such that, by the age of twelve, those afflicted with the disorder use a wheelchair. Usually, between the ages of fourteen and eighteen, the patients develop serious and sometimes fatal respiratory diseases due to the impairment of the diaphragm, the primary breathing muscle. The progressive deterioration of the muscles cannot be stopped. Still, it may be slowed by exercising the affected muscles.

Myasthenia gravis is also a severe muscle disorder. This disease results in excessive weakness of skeletal muscles, a condition known as "muscle fatigue." Those with myasthenia gravis complain of fatigue even after performing everyday body movements. Although severe, myasthenia gravis is usually not fatal unless the diaphragm is affected.

Myasthenia gravis results from a decrease in the availability of nicotinic receptors for acetylcholine. If fewer acetylcholine receptors are available on the muscle fibers, less acetylcholine binds to the muscle fiber receptors; this binding is needed for contraction. As a result, fewer muscle fibers within the muscle contract. The fewer muscle fibers within the entire muscle that contract, the weaker the muscle.

Myasthenia gravis affects about one in every ten thousand individuals. Unlike Duchenne muscular dystrophy, myasthenia gravis may affect any group, and, overall, women are affected more frequently than men. Myasthenia gravis is usually first detected in the facial muscles, particularly those of the eyes and eyelids. Those afflicted have droopy eyelids and experience difficulty in keeping their eyes open. Other symptoms are weakness in those muscles involved in chewing and difficulty swallowing because of weakening of the tongue muscles. In most patients, there is also some weakening of the legs and arms muscles.

The prognosis for the treatment of myasthenia gravis is very good. The most important treatment for the disorder is the use of anticholinesterase drugs. These drugs inhibit the breakdown of acetylcholine. As a result, there is a large amount of acetylcholine in the neuromuscular junction to bind with the limited number of acetylcholine receptors. This, in turn, increases the ability and number of the muscle fibers that can contract, increasing muscle strength and the ability to use the muscles without fatigue.

Also of interest is the effect of pesticides and how they affect muscle function. Some pesticides are classified as organic pesticides that inhibit the enzyme acetylcholinesterase. If acetylcholinesterase is inhibited, it will no longer break down the acetylcholine bound to the receptor on the skeletal muscle membrane. Suppose the acetylcholine is not removed from the receptor. In that case, the muscle cannot relax and is in a constant state of contraction. As a result, the respiratory muscles cannot contract and relax, a process required for breathing. Thus, organic pesticides function to prevent the respiratory muscles from working, and an affected animal will die as a result of not being able to breathe.

Muscle fibers also require a blood supply to keep them alive. If the blood supply to the muscle fibers is inhibited, death of the muscle fibers can result. If enough muscle fibers are affected, death of the muscle can result. Cardiac must is particularly sensitive to oxygen deprivation. Suppose the blood supply to the cardiac muscle making up the heart is reduced or cut off. In that case, the result is decreased cardiac muscle's ability to contract, leading to heart failure.

PERSPECTIVE AND PROSPECTS
The study of muscles and musculature is as old as the study of anatomy itself. Galen of Pergamum did the first well-documented study of muscles in the first century. Galen made drawings of muscles and described their functions. Galen described more than 300 muscles in the human body, almost half of all the muscles now known.

In the late fifteenth century, anatomists made some of the first refined drawings and descriptions of the body's skeletal muscles. Among those who stood out as muscle anatomists during this period was Leonardo da Vinci, whose drawings of the skeletal muscles of the body were magnificent. His chief interest in the body's muscles, like Galen's, was their function. He accurately described, among many other muscles, the muscles involved in the movement of the lips and cheeks.

A major step to understanding muscle physiology did not occur until the late eighteenth century. In 1791, Luigi Galvani discovered the relationship between muscle contraction and electricity when he found that an electrical current could cause the contraction of a frog leg. The use of electrical stimulation to study muscle contraction and function was fully utilized in the mid-nineteenth century by Duchenne de Boulogne. The actual measurement of the electrical activity in a muscle came about in 1929 with the invention by Edgar Douglas Adrian and Detlev Wulf Bronk of the needle electrode, which could be placed into the muscle to record the muscle's electrical activity. This recording of the electrical activity of the muscle is known as an "electromyogram," or EMG. Electromyograms are important in evaluating the electrical activity of resting and contracting muscles. Since the discovery of EMGs, they have been used by anatomists, muscle physiologists, exercise physiologists, and orthopedic surgeons to study and diagnose muscle diseases. Furthermore, the knowledge gained from EMGs has led to the making of artificial limbs that can be controlled by the electrical impulses of the existing muscles.

Knowledge of muscle names, muscle anatomy, and movement, as well as muscle physiology, is needed in many medical fields. These fields include kinesiology, the study of movement; physical and occupational therapy; the treatment and rehabilitation of those who are disabled by injury; exercise physiology and sports medicine, in which the effects of exercise on muscles and the damage of muscle as a result of sports injuries are studied; and, finally, orthopedic surgery, which is the surgical repair of damaged bones, joints, and muscles.

—*David K. Saunders*

Further Reading

Blakey, Paul. *The Muscle Book*. Himalayan Institute, 2000.
Burke, Edmund. *Optimal Muscle Performance and Recovery*. Rev. ed., Putnam, 2003.
Cash, Mel. *Pocket Atlas of the Moving Body*. Crown, 2000.
Clarkson, Hazel M. *Musculoskeletal Assessment: Joint Motion and Muscle Testing*. Wolters Kluwer Health/Lippincott Williams & Wilkins, 2013.
Fox, Stuart, and Krista Rompolski. *Human Physiology*. 16th ed., McGraw Hill, 2021.
Hall, John E., and Michael E. Hall. *Guyton and Hall Textbook of Medical Physiology*. 14th ed., Elsevier, 2020.
Marieb, Elaine N., and Suzanne Keller. *Essentials of Human Anatomy and Physiology*. 13th ed., Pearson, 2021.
Tortora, Gerard J., and Bryan Derrickson. *Principles of Anatomy and Physiology*. 16th ed., John Wiley & Sons, 2020.
Welsh, Charles. *Hole's Essentials of Human Anatomy and Physiology*. 14th ed., McGraw-Hill, 2020.
Willems, Mark. *Skeletal Muscle: Physiology, Classification, and Disease*. Nova Biomedical, 2013.

PREFRONTAL CORTEX (PFC)

Category: Anatomy
Specialties and related fields: Anatomy, neuroanatomy, neuroanatomy, psychiatry, psychology
Definition: the gray matter of the anterior part of the frontal lobe that is highly developed in humans and plays a role in the regulation of complex cognitive, emotional, and behavioral functioning

KEY TERMS

brain: an organ of soft nervous tissue contained in the skull of vertebrates, functioning as the coordinating center of sensation and intellectual and nervous activity

cerebral hemispheres: either of the rounded halves of the brain's cerebrum, divided laterally by a deep fissure and connected at the bottom by the corpus callosum

cerebral lobes: cerebral cortex is divided lengthways into two cerebral hemispheres connected by the corpus callosum; each hemisphere is divided into four lobes: frontal, parietal, temporal, and occipital

cerebrum: the largest part of the brain, divided into two hemispheres, or halves, called the "cerebral hemispheres"

INTRODUCTION

The prefrontal cortex (PFC) is part of the brain that helps regulate decision-making, planning, and speaking. The PFC is part of the frontal lobe—one of the last parts of the brain to develop in humans. The PFC helps regulate emotion and executive function, including complicated mental processes such as planning and decision-making. Scientists have been able to study the PFC through imaging and observations of people who have illnesses or injuries that affect that section of the brain. Scientists believe that the PFC is an important factor in several mental illnesses and disorders, such as depression, bipolar disorder, and Alzheimer's disease.

BACKGROUND

The prefrontal cortex is part of the cerebrum, the largest part of the human brain. The brain acts as the body's control center, directing the operations of the organs and processes necessary for the body to function. The cerebrum controls functions such as sight, hearing, speech, and moto control. The cerebrum is split into left and right hemispheres, further broken down into four lobes—the frontal lobe, the parietal lobe, the occipital lobe, and the temporal lobe. Cracks, wrinkles, or fissures separate the lobes. Although they are separate, different parts of the brain work together to perform tasks. Even areas of the brain that are suited to one task generally work with other parts to complete other tasks. Different brain parts can also "learn" to perform different functions if parts of the brain are damaged by injury or illness.

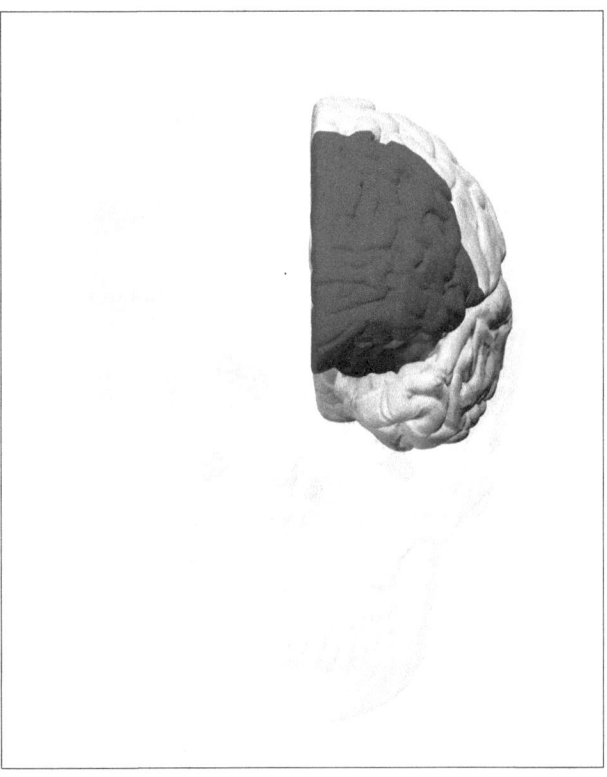

Anterior view of the left cerebral hemisphere. Image by DataBase Center for Life Science, via Wikimedia Commons.

OVERVIEW

The prefrontal cortex (PFC) is part of the brain of mammals. The PFC is located directly behind the skull at the front of the forehead. The frontal lobe, of which the PFC is a part, extends front the front of the skull to about the middle of the brain; the PFC is the largest section of the frontal lobe. It is itself broken down into different parts, though the exact parts and names are debated among scientists. The PFC is well-developed in humans, but it is very small in animals such as rats, making some brain studies challenging in rodents and other animals.

The PFC is vital to daily life because of its role in cognitive function. The PFC is responsible for executive function, high-order thinking that includes decision-making and planning for the future. This part of the brain helps humans develop and produce speech and also helps in abstract reasoning. People use the PFC to understand others' emotions and thoughts, making it important for feelings of empathy. It can also give people insight into themselves, their thoughts, and their judgments. Because the PFC regulates so many cognitive functions, an injury or illness that affects that section of the brain can greatly influence vital day-to-day actions.

Scientists have developed a basic understanding of how the PFC works. However, they still do not understand the majority of how the brain functions. They do know the PFC collects information from other parts of the brain. This information can include visual or auditory information. The PFC uses this input and then sends commands back to other brain parts based on the input. For example, the PFC can send signals to control motor function or focus the attention of the senses.

The PFC develops over the early course of a human lifetime and is the last part of the brain to develop fully. This development continues into a person's twenties. Scientists theorize that this results in young adults and teenagers not always making the best possible decisions or planning for the future. However, adults with a fully developed prefrontal cortex can also face problems if their PFC does not always function at the most efficient level.

Brain arousal also affects the performance of the PFC. For example, a person could experience weak PFC function if they are tired or only partially awake. A person can also be affected by too much brain arousal, such as experiencing a great amount of stress or trauma. Scientists believe this may explain why people sometimes make poor decisions when tired or overly stressed. Scientists believe brains that maintain healthy arousal levels can create strong neural pathways from the PFC to other parts of the brain. Increased cerebral connectivity allows the PFC to regulate thoughts, actions, and emotions better. When a person experiences stress, the PFC's function weakens, and other brain parts are activated. Scientists believe a weakened PFC could activate the brain's more primitive parts, such as the amygdala. When a person uses these less-developed sections, it can lead to overreactions instead of thoughtful action. Furthermore, if these more primitive parts are overused, the brain will begin to rely on them more often.

Scientists have also found a link between the PFC and common mental illnesses and disorders. For example, depression is a mental illness that can cause sadness, loss of interest, and hopelessness. Imaging studies have shown decreased activity in parts of the PFC in people suffering from depression. Bipolar disorder is a condition that can cause manic and depressive episodes. During manic episodes, people become less inhibited, more active, and more distractible. Imaging studies have shown that the part of the PFC that helps regulate inhibitions has decreased activity during manic episodes. Scientists still do not fully understand the connections between the PFC and mental illness. Still, they hope that by studying the PFC, they can someday help people with these disorders.

—Elizabeth Mohn

Further Reading
Antonio H. Lara, and Jonathan D. Wallis. "The Role of Prefrontal Cortex in Working Memory: A Mini Review." *Frontiers in Systems Neuroscience*, 18 Dec. 2015, www.frontiersin.org/articles/10.3389/fnsys.2015.00173/full. Accessed 4 May 2020.
Arnsten, Amy F. T. "Stress Signaling Pathways that Impair Prefrontal Cortex Structure and Function." *Nature Reviews Neuroscience*, vol. 10, no. 6, 2009, pp. 410-22.
"Brain Map Frontal Lobes." *Queensland Government*, 18 Apr. 2017, www.health.qld.gov.au/abios/asp/bfrontal. Accessed 4 May 2020.
Clark, Luke, and D. Phil. "Cognitive Neuroscience and Brain Imaging in Bipolar Disorder." *Dialogues in Clinical Neuroscience*, vol. 10, no. 2, 2008, pp. 153-65.
Dolan, Eric W. "In Depressed People, the Medial Prefrontal Cortex Exerts More Control over Other Parts of the Brain." *PsyPost*, 19 June 2017, www.psypost.org/2017/06/depressed-people-medial-prefrontal-cortex-exerts-control-parts-brain-49168. Accessed 4 May 2020.

Fetterman, Anne, Joseph Campellone, and Raymond Kent Turley. "Understanding the Teen Brain." *University of Rochester Medical Center Rochester*, 2020, www.urmc.rochester.edu/encyclopedia/content.aspx?ContentTypeID=1&ContentID=3051. Accessed 4 May 2020.

"Get To Know Your Brain Series—The Frontal Lobe." *UPMC HealthBeat*, 1 Dec. 2014, share.upmc.com/2014/12/ get-know-brain-series-frontal-lobe/. Accessed 4 May 2020.

Leibenluft, Ellen. "Neuropathology of Bipolar Disorder." *Cold Spring Harbor Laboratory*, www.cshl.edu/dnalcmedia/neuropathology-of-bipolar-disorder/. Accessed 4 May 2020.

"Parts of the Brain That Slow Down or Speed up in Depression." *McGill University*, thebrain.mcgill.ca/flash/i/i_08/i_08_cr/i_08_cr_dep/i_08_cr_dep.html. Accessed 4 May 2020.

UPPER EXTREMITIES

Category: Anatomy

Specialties and related fields: Neurology, occupational therapy, orthopedics, physical medicine and rehabilitation, physical therapy, sports medicine

Definition: the upper extremities include the arms (upper arms, forearms, and hands), which are attached to the shoulder blade at the shoulder joint and which consist of muscles, bones, blood vessels, lymph vessels, nerves, skin, and fingernails

KEY TERMS

carpus: the wrist

distal: farther away from the base or attached end

elbow: the joint between the upper arm and the forearm

forearm: the region from the elbow joint to the wrist; also called the "antebrachium"

humerus: the bone that forms the structural beam of the upper arm

proximal: closer to the base or attached end

radial: toward the edge of the forearm and hand containing the radius and thumb

radius: the shorter of the two forearm bones on the thumb side

ulna: the larger of the two forearm bones, forming the principal part of the elbow joint with the humerus

ulnar: toward the edge of the forearm and hand containing the ulna and little finger

upper arm: the region from the shoulder joint to the elbow joint; also called the "brachium"

STRUCTURE AND FUNCTIONS

The upper extremities consist of the upper arms, forearms, and hands. Each extremity is attached to the shoulder blade (or scapula) at the shoulder joint. The upper extremity is made mostly of bones and muscles but also contains blood vessels, lymphatics, nerves, skin, fingernails, and other associated structures. Important directional terms associated with the upper extremity include proximal (closer to the base or attached end), distal (farther from the base or attached end), radial (on the same side as the radius and the thumb), and ulnar (on the same side as the ulna and the little finger). Along the forearm and hand, the palm's surface is called "palmar"; the opposite surface is called "dorsal."

The bones and muscles of the shoulder provide support structures for the upper extremity. Beyond the shoulder, the major parts of the upper extremity include the upper arm (or brachium), from the shoulder joint to the elbow; the forearm, from the elbow to the wrist; the carpus, or wrist; and the manus, or hand. The hand's five fingers are numbered one through five, beginning with the thumb. Digit two is also called the "index finger," digit three the middle finger, digit four the ring finger, and digit five the little finger.

Like other body parts, the upper extremity is clothed in skin or integument. The skin covering the armpit (or axilla) has more hair and glands (especially the apocrine sweat glands) than most other body parts. The palm of the hand is unusual, along with the sole of the foot, in being completely hairless and having a very thick outermost layer called the "stratum corneum." Each finger has on its dorsal surface a fingernail; the thin crescent of semitransparent skin covering the base of the fingernail is called the "eponychium." The ridges on the palm and fingers form individually characteristic patterns called "dermatoglyphics," both fingerprints and palm prints.

The upper extremity bones include the scapula, clavicle, humerus, radius, ulna, carpals, metacarpals, and phalanges. The scapula, or shoulder blade, develops as part of the skeleton of the upper extremity and remains more strongly attached to the upper arm than to the body's trunk. The outer (superficial) surface of the scapula is marked by a ridge called the "spine," perpendicular to the scapular blade; the outer tip of this blade is called the "acromion." The sculpted area above the spine is called the "supraspinous fossa"; the larger sculpted area below the spine is called the "infraspinous fossa." The flat undersurface of the scapula is the subscapular fossa. The hook-like coracoid process marks the superior border of the scapula. At the shoulder joint, the scapula has a nearly spherical glenoid cavity into which the head of the humerus fits. The clavicle, or collarbone, runs from the upper end of the sternum (the manubrium) to the edge of the glenoid cavity of the scapula. It strengthens the shoulder region and provides additional support to the upper extremity.

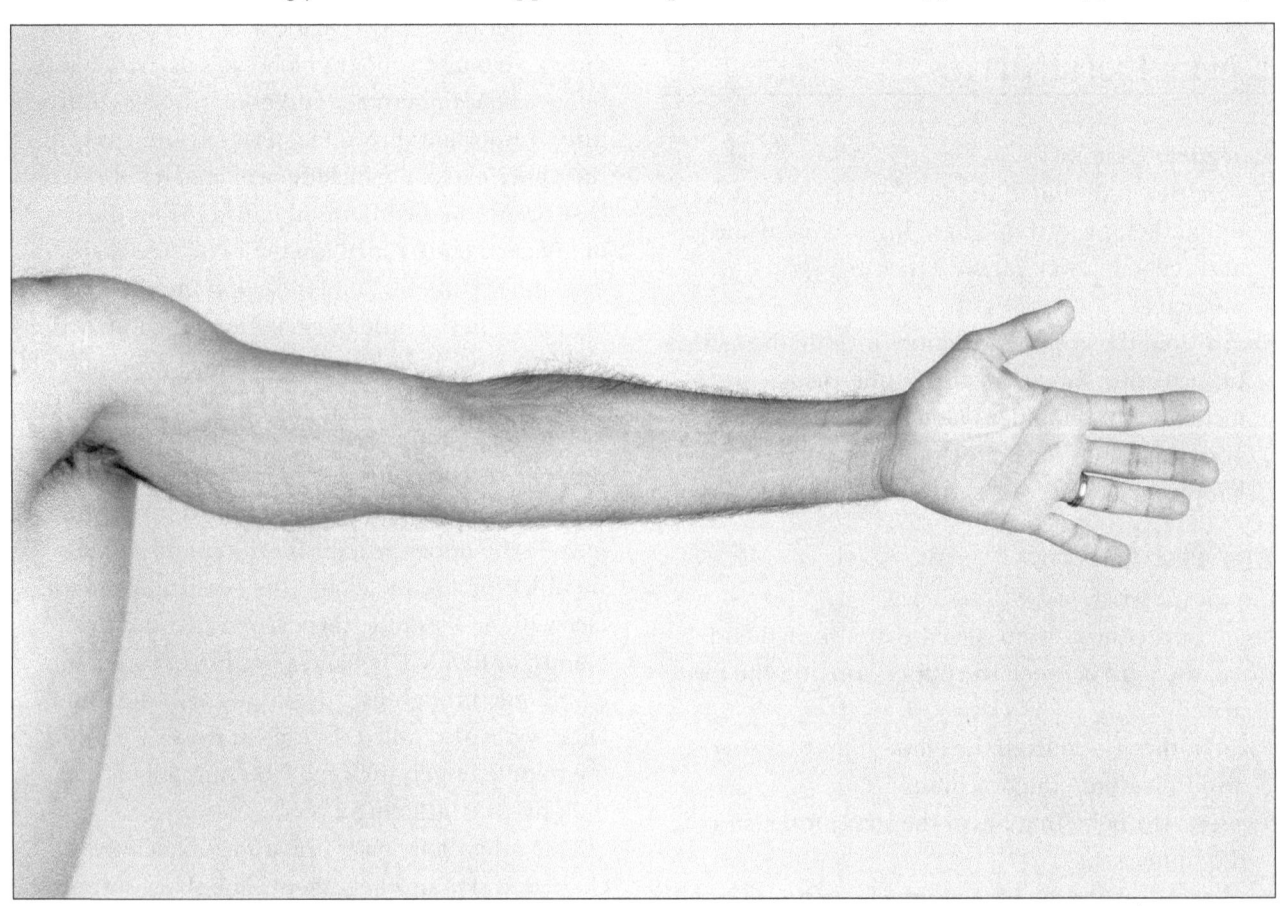

Arms are considered an upper extremity. Photo by Genusfotografen & Wikimedia Sverige, via Wikimedia Commons.

The humerus runs from the shoulder joint to the elbow. At the shoulder joint, it attaches to the scapula through a rounded head that fits into the glenoid cavity of the scapula. The head is flanked by two protruding structures, the greater and lesser tuberosities, to which various muscles attach. The humerus attaches to the ulna at the elbow joint through a pulley-like structure called the "trochlea." The humerus also attaches to the radius by a smaller, rounded structure called the "capitulum." Areas for muscle attachment on the lower end of the humerus include the lateral epicondyle (on the outer side) and the medial epicondyle (on the inner side).

The forearm contains two bones, the radius, and ulna. The smaller of the two forearm bones is the radius, which articulates loosely with the humerus and more strongly with the wrist and hand. The ulna is the larger of the two. It forms the principal attachment with the humerus through a semilunar notch. Part of the ulna extends proximally beyond this semilunar notch to form a projection known as the olecranon process (the hard structure on which one rests the elbows).

The carpus, or wrist, includes two rows of small bones. The proximal row includes (in order from the radial side to the ulnar) the scaphoid, lunate, cuneiform (triquetrum), and pisiform bones. The distal row includes the trapezium, trapezoid, capitate, and hamate bones, also in order from radial to ulnar. The trapezium supports the thumb, the trapezoid supports the index finger, the capitate supports the middle finger, and the hamate supports the two remaining digits. An important ligament called the "transverse carpal ligament" (or flexor retinaculum) runs across the palmar side of the wrist, forming a tunnel through which the tendons of the flexor muscles run. A similar ligament, the dorsal carpal ligament (or dorsal retinaculum), crosses the back of the wrist, forming a similar tunnel through which the tendons of the extensor muscles run. Beyond the wrist, the palm is supported by five bones called "metacarpals," numbered one through five. The thumb contains two finger bones or phalanges; each of the remaining fingers contains three phalanges.

The upper extremity muscles are divided into extensors (which straighten joints) and flexors (which bend joints). The shoulder muscles attaching the upper extremity to the body's trunk include the trapezius, pectoralis major, pectoralis minor, deltoideus, coracobrachialis, subscapularis, supraspinatus, infraspinatus, teres major, teres minor, and latissimus dorsi. The trapezius, deltoideus, and supraspinatus are extensors; the coracobrachialis, latissimus dorsi, and the two pectoralis muscles are flexors; and the remaining muscles are primarily responsible for rotational movements. The trapezius originates from the cervical and thoracic vertebrae, including the adjoining ligaments and the adjacent part of the skull; its fibers converge mostly onto the spine and acromion of the scapula, but some also insert onto the clavicle. The pectoralis major is triangular; it originates from the sternum, costal cartilages, and a portion of the clavicle, from which its fibers converge toward an insertion on the greater tuberosity of the humerus. The pectoralis minor originates from the third through fifth ribs and inserts onto the coracoid process of the scapula. The deltoideus is a triangular muscle that originates from the clavicle and the spine and acromion of the scapula; its fibers converge to insert through a strong tendon onto the shaft of the humerus. The coracobrachialis runs from the coracoid process to an insertion along the shaft of the humerus. The subscapularis originates from the subscapular fossa and inserts onto the lesser tuberosity of the humerus. The supraspinatus originates along the supraspinous fossa and inserts onto the greater tuberosity of the humerus. The infraspinatus originates from the infraspinous fossa and inserts onto the greater tuberosity of the humerus. The teres major and teres minor originate from the scapula's lower (inferior) border; the teres major inserts onto the lesser tubercle of the humerus, and the teres minor inserts onto the greater tubercle. The latissimus dorsi is a broad, flat muscle that originates from the lower half of the vertebral column (and part of the ilium) by a tough tendinous sheet (the lumbar aponeurosis); it inserts high on the humerus.

The major flexors of the upper arm include the biceps brachii and the brachialis. The biceps brachii originates in two heads, one from the coracoid process of the scapula and one from the shoulder joint capsule. Both heads insert through a strong tendon onto a raised tuberosity of the radius. The brachialis originates from the shaft of the humerus and inserts high on the ulna.

The major extensor of the upper arm is the three-part triceps brachii. The long head of the triceps originates from the scapula just below the armpit; the other two heads originate along the shaft of the humerus. All three heads insert onto the olecranon process through a strong tendon. The anconeus (or subanconeus) is not always present; its fibers run directly from the shaft of the humerus to that of the ulna. Still, a smaller anconeus and an epitrochlearis are sometimes present as well. The epitrochlearis (or dorsoepitrochlearis), also variably present, may be viewed as a connecting band of muscle tissue from the latissimus dorsi onto the triceps brachii.

Flexors of the forearm include the flexor carpi radialis, palmaris longus, flexor carpi ulnaris, pronator teres, flexor digitorum superficialis, flexor digitorum profundus, flexor pollicis longus, and pronator quadratus. Many of these muscles have long, thin tendons that run in the tunnel formed beneath the transverse carpal ligament. The first five of these muscles originate from the medial epicondyle of the humerus. The pronator teres runs at an angle and inserts onto the shaft of the radius. The flexor carpi radialis inserts by a long, thin tendon onto the base of the second metacarpal. The palmaris longus ends in a broad tendon that spreads over the palm to form the palmar aponeurosis, a sheet that sends tendinous branches into the fingers. The flexor carpi ulnaris inserts by a tendon onto the pisiform bone; the tendon then continues onto the hamate bone. The flexor digitorum superficialis originates from parts of the radius and ulna as well as the humerus; its strong tendon passes beneath the transverse carpal ligament, then divides into four branches to each of digits two through five. Each of these branches splits and then reunites to allow a tendon of the flexor digitorum to penetrate. The flexor digitorum profundus originates mostly from the shaft of the ulna. It gives rise to four strong tendons that run beneath the transverse carpal ligament, separates from one another over the palm, runs into the second through fifth fingers, penetrates through the openings in the tendons of the flexor digitorum superficialis, and inserts onto the base of the terminal phalanx of each finger except the thumb. The flexor pollicis longus arises from the radius alongside the previous muscle; its tendon runs beneath the transverse carpal ligament and inserts onto the base of the distal phalanx of the thumb. The pronator quadratus consists of a muscular sheet running between the distal portions of the radius and ulna.

The forearm's more superficial (shallower) extensors include the brachioradialis, extensor carpi radialis longus, extensor carpi radialis brevis, extensor carpi ulnaris, extensor digitorum communis, and extensor digiti minimi. The brachioradialis originates from a ridge on the shaft of the humerus and inserts onto the radius at its distal end. The extensor carpi radialis longus originates from the shaft of the humerus; its tendon passes beneath the dorsal carpal ligament to insert near the base of the second metacarpal. The next four muscles originate together from the lateral epicondyle of the humerus. The extensor carpi radialis brevis gives rise to a tendon that passes beneath the dorsal carpal ligament to insert onto the base of the third metacarpal. The extensor carpi ulnaris gives rise to a tendon that passes beneath the dorsal carpal ligament and inserts onto the base of the fifth metacarpal. The extensor digitorum communis gives rise to four tendons that pass beneath the dorsal carpal ligament, then diverge to run into each finger except the thumb, where they each insert onto the base of the second phalanx, the base of the terminal phalanx, and a tendinous sheath covering the first phalanx. The extensor digiti minimi gives rise to a tendon that runs beneath the dorsal carpal ligament and unites over the first phalanx of the fifth finger with the tendon to that digit of the extensor digitorum communis.

The deeper extensors of the forearm include the supinator, abductor pollicis longus, extensor pollicis brevis, extensor pollicis longus, and extensor indicis. The supinator originates mostly from the proximal end of the ulnar shaft. Still, some of this muscle originates from the elbow joint capsule and the humerus's lateral epicondyle. Its fibers spiral toward the body's midline and insert onto the shaft of the radius. The abductor pollicis longus originates beneath the supinator from the shaft of the radius; it inserts through a tendon onto the base of the first metacarpal. The extensor pollicis brevis originates from the shaft of the radius and inserts through a tendon onto the base of the first phalanx of the thumb. The extensor pollicis longus originates from the middle portion of the shaft of the ulna; it gives rise to a tendon that runs beneath the dorsal carpal ligament to insert onto the base of the distal phalanx of the thumb. The extensor indicis arises beside the preceding muscle from the shaft of the ulna; its tendon passes beneath the dorsal carpal ligament and eventually attaches to the tendon going to the index finger from the extensor digitorum communis.

The flexor muscles that are "intrinsic" to the hand—that is, those confined to the hand—include the flexor pollicis brevis, abductor pollicis brevis, adductor pollicis, opponens pollicis, palmaris brevis, flexor digiti minimi, abductor digiti minimi, opponens digiti minimi, the lumbricales, and the interossei. There are no intrinsic extensor muscles in the hand.

The upper extremity can move in various ways. At the shoulder joint, possible movements include extension (or protraction) of the shoulder, which raises the arms; flexion (or retraction) of the shoulder, which lowers the arms; adduction of the arms, bringing them closer together; and abduction of the arms, pulling them farther apart. The two movements possible at the elbow joint are extension (straightening) and flexion (bending). Two special movements are possible within the forearm: Pronation is an inward rotation of the radius upon the ulna in such a way that the palms face downward; supination is an outward rotation of the radius upon the ulna in such a way that the palms face upward. Various movements are possible at the wrist, including flexion (bending), extension (straightening), hyperextension (bending the hand upward), radial abduction (twisting the hand toward the thumb side), and ulnar abduction (twisting the hand toward the little finger side). Movements of the phalanges include flexion (bending), extension (straightening), abduction (spreading the fingers), and adduction (bringing the fingers back together).

Blood vessels of the upper extremity include both arteries and veins. The brachial artery is the major continuation of the subclavian and axillary arteries into the upper arm; as it approaches the elbow, it divides into the radial and ulnar arteries, which supply most of the forearm. Near the wrist, each of these last two arteries divides into a branch that runs closer to the palm and another that runs closer to the back of the hand. The two palmar branches then connect to form a loop called the "palmar digital arch"; the other two branches also connect, forming a loop called the "dorsal digital arch." From these two digital arches arises a secondary digital arch running into each finger, connecting to the palmar arch at one end and the dorsal arch at the other. This type of arrangement, called "collateral circulation," uses multiple alternate routes to permit blood flow even if one of the routes is temporarily blocked.

There are several important veins draining the upper extremity. Several of these veins run just beneath the skin: the cephalic vein, running along the radial margin of the forearm and upper arm; the median antebrachial vein, draining the palmar surface of the hand and forearm; and the basilic vein, continuing the median antebrachial vein along the inner side of the upper arm. The deep veins of the arm all drain into the brachial vein. As it flows into the shoulder, the brachial vein joins with the basilic vein to form the axillary vein, which then becomes the subclavian vein when it reaches the rib cage.

The major nerves to the upper extremity arise from a series of complex branchings, known as the brachial plexus, originating mostly from the fifth through eighth cervical nerves and the first thoracic nerve. The major nerves of the brachial plexus are a lateral cord (formed from branches of the fifth, sixth, and seventh cervical nerves), a medial cord (formed from branches of the last cervical and first thoracic nerves), and a posterior cord (formed from branches of the sixth, seventh, and eighth cervical nerves). The major nerves of the arm include a musculocutaneous nerve arising from the lateral cord, an axillary nerve and a radial nerve arising from the posterior cord, an ulnar nerve and a medial antebrachial cutaneous nerve arising from the medial cord, and a median nerve arising from both the lateral and the medial cords. The musculocutaneous, ulnar, and median nerves constitute the main nerve supply to the arm and hand flexor muscles. In contrast, the axillary nerve supplies the deltoid muscle, and the radial nerve supplies the remaining extensor muscles. In addition, the radial nerve supplies sensory branches to the skin of the dorsal side of the forearm and hand (except for the fifth finger and part of the fourth). In contrast, the musculocutaneous and medial antebrachial cutaneous nerves supply sensory branches to the skin over the palmar or flexor side of the arm and forearm. The median nerve sends sensory branches to the skin over most of the hand's palmar surface from the thumb up to the middle of the fourth finger. In contrast, the ulnar nerve sends sensory branches to the skin on the palmar and dorsal sides of the fifth finger and the ulnar half of the fourth. At the elbow, the ulnar nerve passes around the olecranon process just under the skin, where it is easily subject to accidental pressure; the tingling that results from such pressure is the source of the term "funny bone."

DISORDERS AND DISEASES

Many types of medical conditions and disorders can affect the upper extremities. For example, many types of contact dermatitis, from poison ivy to "dishpan hands," are first noticed on the surface of the hands and forearms. Other medical problems of the upper extremity include animal bites, injuries, and an assortment of neuromuscular disorders.

Neuromuscular disorders involving the upper extremity include nerve paralyses, uncontrolled shaking (choreic) movements, muscular atrophies, and muscular dystrophies. Nerve paralyses may arise from traumatic injury, but cerebral palsy is the most common type of paralysis. Cerebral palsy is a group of paralytic disorders that begin at birth or during early childhood. The extent of the paralysis may vary, often involving large groups of muscles while sparing others. In addition to the lack of muscular control of the limbs, other symptoms may include spasms, athetoid (slow, rhythmic, and wormlike) movements, or muscular rigidity. Some types of cerebral palsy may result from injuries at birth or early infancy.

Uncontrolled, purposeless, and irregular shaking movements of the extremities are called "choreic movements." These disorders, which involve the upper extremities more often than the lower, include both Sydenham's chorea and Huntington's chorea. Sydenham's chorea (true chorea) typically begins in children and young adults, with maximum disability occurring two to three weeks after symptoms begin. Choreic symptoms typically diminish and disappear in a few months but may recur later. Drugs like deutetrabenazine (Austedo) or tetrabenazine (Xenazine) can control these uncontrollable movements. Huntington's chorea, also known as Huntington's disease, seldom begins before the age of forty. It typically begins with uncontrolled choreic movements of the hands. The disease progressively worsens and ultimately causes death about fifteen years after onset. A single dominant gene causes the disease.

Muscular atrophies are a variety of diseases in which muscle tissues become progressively weaker and smaller, usually beginning between forty and sixty years of age. Spastic movements may sometimes occur. The small muscles of the hands are usually affected sooner and more severely compared to the large muscles of the arms and shoulders. Amyotrophic lateral sclerosis (ALS), commonly known as Lou Gehrig's disease, is a progressive muscular atrophy that usually begins with weakness and deterioration of the hand muscles. The disease affects the rest of the extremities, then other parts of the body; it is usually fatal within three to five years after onset. A rarer type of atrophy, myelopathic muscular atrophy (or Aran-Duchenne atrophy), also begins in the small hand muscles and slowly spreads to the arms, shoulders, and trunk muscles, in that order. A degenerative gray matter lesion in the spinal cord's cervical region is usually responsible. Weakness and wasting of the muscles of the hands and forearms also characterize syringomyelia, a disorder of the glial cells in the cervical region of the spinal cord. Impairment of the cutaneous senses often occurs with this disease. It frequently results in burns and other injuries to the hand when the patient, unaware of a threat, fails to withdraw or take other countermeasures.

Muscular dystrophy is an inherited disease—actually several related diseases—that usually begins in early childhood and affects males more often than females. The most common type, Duchenne muscular dystrophy, is believed to be caused by a sex-linked recessive trait. Spastic movements do not occur, and the disease affects the large muscles of the shoulder, arm, and thigh more than the small muscles of the hand. The affected muscles become very weak but remain approximately normal in size or increase as fatty and fibrous tissue replaces muscle. Progressive weakening makes walking impossible, but patients can live for decades with proper care.

Repetitive motion injuries of the upper extremity may occur at the elbow joint (tennis elbow) or in the vicinity of the wrist. Some repetitive wrist movements can produce carpal tunnel syndrome, an injury of the tendons running through the tunnel beneath the transverse carpal ligament.

PERSPECTIVE AND PROSPECTS

The first well-illustrated anatomical texts were produced by Belgian physician Andreas Vesalius (1514-64); along with the rest of the human body, they showed the major muscles and bones of the upper extremities. An accurate medical understanding of the circulatory system began with the studies of the English physician William Harvey (1578-1657). He examined the veins in the arms of many patients. Harvey noticed the valves in the veins and proved that the blood circulates outward from the heart, throughout the body, and then back again to the heart.

Injuries to the arm are generally treated surgically. Whenever possible, broken bones are set in place, immobilized in a cast, and then allowed to heal. Torn muscles (or tendons) must be sewn together, and nerve endings must be placed in their former positions to grow back correctly. If the whole hand is severed at the wrist, many tendons and blood vessels must be reattached; such an operation is very difficult. When a portion of the upper extremity must be amputated, the stump is generally covered with a flap of skin. Sometimes an artificial hand is attached to the muscles that are still usable.

—*Eli C. Minkoff*

Further Reading

Agur, Anne M. R., and Arthur F. Dalley. *Grant's Atlas of Anatomy*. 15th ed., Lippincott Williams & Wilkins, 2020.

"Arm Injuries and Disorders." *MedlinePlus*, 3 Jan. 2017, medlineplus.gov/arminjuriesanddisorders.html.

"Hand Injuries and Disorders." *MedlinePlus*, 31 Aug. 2016, medlineplus.gov/handinjuriesanddisorders.html.

Marieb, Elaine N., and Suzanne M. Keller. *Essentials of Human Anatomy and Physiology*. 13th ed., Pearson, 2021.

Rosse, Cornelius, and Penelope Gaddum-Rosse. *Hollinshead's Textbook of Anatomy*. 5th ed., Lippincott-Raven, 1997.

Standring, Susan, et al., editors. *Gray's Anatomy*. 40th ed., Churchill Livingstone/Elsevier, 2008.

Physiology/Pathophysiology

This section is all about how the body works and what happens when things go wrong. It is incumbent on any student who wants to understand what causes an injury or disease to understand how the body works in the absence of these conditions. Research into exercise physiology provides information on the effects of exercise on the body's cells, systems, and tissues, in addition to the role of exercise in subcellular, molecular, and chemical processes. Among the subjects discussed in this section are: metabolism, motor control, pain, inflammation, and bone disorders.

Bone Disorders

Category: Disease/Disorder
Specialties and related fields: Geriatrics and gerontology, oncology, orthopedics, rheumatology
Definition: the various traumatic events or inherited conditions that can affect bones and the tissues surrounding them, such as fractures, dislocations, degenerative processes, infections, osteoporosis, and cancer

KEY TERMS

acute: referring to the sudden onset of a disease process
cartilage: connective tissue between bones that forms a pad or cushion to absorb weight and shock
chronic: referring to a lingering disease process
osteoblast: bone-forming cells that secrete the matrix that mineralizes into bone
osteoclast: large, multinucleated cells that resorb bone
pathogen: any disease-causing microorganism

CAUSES AND SYMPTOMS

Bones are usually studied together with their surrounding structures because many of the disorders to which bones are subjected also involve the muscular, connective, and cartilaginous tissues to which they are joined. Hence, a common term for this medical category is "musculoskeletal and connective tissue disorders."

Two hundred six bones in the human body serve three functions. Some form protective housing for body organs and structures; these include the skull, which encloses the brain, and the rib cage, which encloses the heart and lungs. Some support the body's posture and weight, including the spine and the bones of the hips and legs. The third function is motion: most of the bones in the body are involved in movement. These bones include those of the hands, wrists, arms, hips, legs, ankles, and feet.

> **INFORMATION ON BONE DISORDERS**
>
> **Causes**: Fractures, dislocations, degenerative processes, infections, cancer
>
> **Symptoms**: Varies widely; may include porous and brittle bones, impaired movement, pain, inflammation, numbness, and tingling
>
> **Duration**: Acute to chronic
>
> **Treatments**: Setting and immobilization of bones in cast or splint, surgery, medications (antirheumatic drugs, corticosteroids), supplements (vitamin D, calcium, hormone therapy), orthopedic support, lifestyle changes

Bone consists of three sections: an outer layer called the "periosteum"; the hard, bony tissue itself, composed of widely mineralized networks of collagen and other proteins that form rigid skeletal structures; and the interior, a spongy mass of cancellous (chambered) tissue, where blood marrow and some fat cells are stored. Bone is living tissue. It is a depository for calcium, phosphate, and other minerals vital to many body processes. Calcium and phosphate are constantly being deposited in and withdrawn from bone tissue to be used throughout the body.

Inherited bone disorders are collectively known as "skeletal dysplasias." These genetic diseases constitute a highly heterogeneous group of conditions. Skeletal dysplasias are estimated to occur in 15.7 per 100,000 births.

Achondroplasia is the most common skeletal dysplasia in humans and results from mutations in the *FGFR3* (fibroblast growth factor receptor 3) gene. Achondroplasia causes short stature (dwarfism) due to long bone shortening that affects the upper and lower extremities.

Dysostosis multiplex results from metabolic storage disorders. The body cannot degrade complex macromolecules like complex carbohydrates, glycoproteins, or glycolipids. The progressive accumulation of these waste products affects cartilage and bones, and the vertebrae flatten, and the ribs show "paddle rib deformities." The long bones are affected, as are the bones of the hands.

Disorders that cause low bone density include osteogenesis imperfecta and hypophosphatasia. Osteogenesis imperfecta results from mutations that cause abnormal deposition, formation, and secretion of bone-specific collagen (type I collagen) Because type I collagen is both a highly complex protein with three polypeptide chains wound about in a triple-helical structure that is cross-linked to form tight, strong cable-like structures, and the major organic component of bone, mutations in either the type I collagen structural genes (*COLA1* and *COLA2*), or genes that encode proteins necessary for processing, folding, synthesis, or secretion (*FKBL10*, *CRTAP*, *LEPRE1*, *PPIB*, *SERPINF1*, *SERPH1*, and *IFITM5*) of type I collagen result in various forms of osteogenesis imperfecta. Mutations in the tissue-nonspecific alkaline phosphatase gene (*TNSALP*) cause hypophosphatemia, which starves the forming bones for phosphate and inhibits bone mineralization.

Other skeletal dysplasias cause excessively high bone density. Bone equilibrium relies on bone deposition by osteoblasts and bone resorption by cells called "osteoclasts." Skeletal dysplasias that cause high bone densities, known as "osteopetroses," are caused by poor osteoclast activity. Pyknodysostosis is caused by mutations in the *CTSK* gene, which encodes the cathepsin K protein, an enzyme used by osteoclasts to degrade bone. This condition causes short stature, abnormal teeth, skull, face, and hand structure. Infantile malignant osteopetrosis is caused by mutations in the carbonic anhydrase type II (*CA2*) gene and is associated with early mortality. Autosomal dominant osteopetrosis type II (also known as "Albers-Schönberg disease") is caused by mutations in the *CLCN7* gene, which encodes a chloride channel, and results in deformities to the base of the skull, spine, and pelvis.

Finally, metaphyseal dysplasias cause disproportionately short statues with short limbs. These include cartilage-hair hypoplasia (caused by mutations in the *RMRP* gene), Schmid metaphyseal chondrodysplasia (caused by mutations in the *COL10A1* gene), Jansen type metaphyseal chondrodysplasia (caused by mutations in the *PTHR1* gene), and Schwachman-Diamond syndrome (caused by mutations in the *SBDS* gene).

Other maladies can also adversely affect bones. Bone can be broken or dislocated; the processes by which they form, grow, and maintain themselves can be compromised; pathogens can attack them; they can be subject to a series of degenerative diseases that impede function and even destroy bone tissue, and they can become cancerous.

Dislocations occur when the bones of a joint are forced out of alignment. They may occur in the elbows of young children whose arms are forcibly pulled. Fractures are more common. They arise from sports activities, accidents, falls, or hundreds of possible causes, including various diseases.

Bone infection is called "osteomyelitis"; it occurs most often in children. Infection can be introduced to the bone by fracture or other exposure or carried to the bone in the blood. The most prevalent long-term bone disorders are those in the general class of diseases called "arthritis." Osteoarthritis, a common form, is sometimes called "wear-and-tear arthritis" because it usually surfaces in older people after years of work have constantly challenged certain joints. It often occurs in contact sports such as football, where years of rough-and-tumble activity can accelerate its progression. Pads of cartilage cushion joints. Eventually, this cartilage can wear down and become rough. It cannot protect the bones of the joint, and little nodes form at the ends of the bones. Bones of the neck and back are often affected, as are the hips and knees.

Osteoarthritis is painful and debilitating, but it is rarely crippling. More painful and far more serious is rheumatoid arthritis, a progressive disease. It often starts with inflammation in the joints of the hands or feet. It is usually bilateral, for example affecting both hands, both feet, or both knees. While rheumatoid arthritis may start with relatively mild inflammation, it can progress to severe deformity and even destruction of the joint. Fingers and toes can become grossly twisted; the joint can become completely fused and immobile. There are other relatively common forms of arthritis. People with the skin condition psoriasis can develop psoriatic arthritis. Reiter's syndrome is a form of arthritis that can be transmitted through sexual contact. Ankylosing spondylitis is a form of arthritis that can affect any of the joints in the torso, such as the shoulders and hips. Still, it is most often found in the neck and spine. Patients with inflammatory bowel disease (IBD) may also develop concomitant arthritis in the joints of the hands or feet.

The bone condition called "gout" can affect many joints, but it often appears in the big toe. The body produces a substance called "uric acid." If for any reason, too much is produced, or if it is not properly eliminated, uric acid crystals can form around joints and trigger inflammation. Gout is extremely painful, and an attack may last for weeks.

The spine is subject to a wide range of disorders. One of the most common is the prolapsed (slipped) disk. The individual vertebrae of the spine are separated and cushioned by pads of cartilage called "discs." For various reasons, a disk can bulge out and impinge on the nerves of the spinal column. The result can be severe pain, numbness, and loss of movement. The spine fails to grow correctly in some individuals or becomes misaligned or curved. Lateral curvature of the spine causes scoliosis. The curvature of the spine can cause the ribs on one side of the body to separate as those on the other side are pushed together. Over time, this separation can cause severe heart and lung problems.

Many cases of joint pain are attributable to inflammation of the tissues surrounding the bony structures. An example is bursitis, in which the bursa, a saclike membrane enclosing many joints, becomes inflamed. Repetitive activities, such as throwing a baseball, hitting a tennis ball, or scrubbing the floor on one's knees, can irritate the membrane and cause inflammation.

Osteomalacia is a disorder of bone mineralization that occurs at newly formed bone sites. This disorder causes bone pain and tenderness, higher rates of fractures, difficulty walking and changes in gait, muscle weakness, spasms, cramps and numbness, and tingling. Poor bone mineralization results from inadequate calcium, phosphate, or alkaline phosphatase levels, severe vitamin D deficiencies, hyperthyroidism, and inherited kidney conditions that cause excessive phosphate loss (type 2 renal tubular acidosis).

Paget disease of bone occurs in about three percent of patients forty and up to nine percent of older patients. Paget disease is characterized by localized overgrowth of bone at various sites. Most of these overgrowths cause no symptoms (asymptomatic). Some boney overgrowths impinge on nearby organs and cause pain or compromise the function of compressed organs. Paget disease results from osteoclast malfunction.

Bone cancers or tumors can be benign or malignant. Cancer rarely begins in the bone; it usually spreads there from a tumorous site elsewhere in the body. Of the cancers that arise directly within bone tissue, the most common is multiple myeloma. Cancer originates in plasma (white) cells and affects the body's ability to produce proteins and fight infection, and osteosarcoma, in which the cancerous tumor originates within the bone.

TREATMENT AND THERAPY

In treating a fractured bone, the most important thing is to realign the segments and keep them immobile until they can fuse. The physician will often X-ray the fracture, set the bones correctly, and immobilize the limb in a cast. If injury to the spinal column is suspected, the physician may also order computed tomography (CT) scanning. Surgery is sometimes required to set the bones, and the surgeon may join the bone segments together with pins, plates, or screws. It is possible to cement bone fragments together with special glue in some cases. Casts and splints can easily immobilize broken arms, legs, fingers, and toes. In cases of accidents, falls, or other trauma, it is critical not to move the patient if there is any suspicion of injury to the spinal column. Movement can worsen the injury and even cause permanent paralysis.

Dislocations, like fractures, should be X-rayed. CT scanning may be required if the spinal column appears to be involved. The misaligned bones are put back in their proper positions, and the joint is immobilized, often with a splint. Osteoporosis requires both preventive and therapeutic care. Suppose the physician recognizes that an individual, usually a postmenopausal woman, is at high risk for osteoporosis. In that case, supplementary calcium will be prescribed and, in some patients, estrogen replacement therapy. When osteoporosis has begun, supplementary calcium, vitamin D, and hormone therapy may check the progress of the disease. Bisphosphonates, which inhibit osteoclast activity, stabilize bone density and reduce the risk of osteoporotic fractures of the spine, wrist, hip, humerus, and pelvis. Unfortunately, these drugs do not help increase bone density. To increase bone density, teriparatide (Forteo) or abaloparatide (Tymlos) shortened, recombinant forms of parathyroid hormone, an anti-RANK monoclonal antibody called denosumab (Prolia, Xgeva) or the antisclerostin monoclonal antibody romosozumab (Evenity) can increase bone density in patients with osteoporosis or decrease bone loss in patients with bone cancer. Teriparatide and abaloparatide tend to increase osteoblast activity. Denosumab inhibits the maturation of preosteoblasts into mature osteoblasts. Romosozumab increases bone formation and decreases bone resorption. A disadvantage of these drugs is that the patient loses bone density once they are discontinued. Finally, in women at high risk of invasive breast cancer, the selective estrogen receptor modulator, raloxifene (Evista and generics), can reduce the risk of osteoporotic fractures and invasive breast cancer. This drug has estrogen-like effects on bone and antiestrogen effects on the uterus and breast.

A patient may suffer from acute back pain because of crushed vertebrae in the spine. Patients with back pain may require pain relievers such as aspirin and orthopedic support. Gentle exercise is recommended to strengthen back muscles. In osteomalacia, vitamin D, phosphorus, and calcium supplements are the mainstays of therapy. In osteomyelitis, antibiotics will usually eradicate the infection, but surgery is required to remove infected tissue in some cases. In other cases, amputation is the only option. The first line of therapy for osteoarthritis and rheumatoid arthritis is the relief of pain and inflammation. The physician may recommend rest and immobilization of the joint; heating pads and hot baths may give some relief. Exercise can maintain motility in the joints and help the patient avoid stiffness. Most patients are given over-the-counter pain relievers such as aspirin, ibuprofen, or acetaminophen. In many patients, however, these drugs are either not adequate to manage the pain or, as in the case of aspirin, ibuprofen, and others (so-called nonsteroidal anti-inflammatory drugs or NSAIDs), may irritate the gastrointestinal tract. Gastrointestinal disturbances are also common with the drugs proscribed for arthritis. Gastric and duodenal ulcers are often reported and are sometimes so severe that the patient requires surgery. The outcome is fatal in a small but significant number of patients who develop such ulcers.

Because rheumatoid arthritis is a crippling disease that worsens over the years, the physician has an additional goal: to prevent the progress of the disease and avoid bone deterioration and degeneration. These patients may use a group of drugs called disease-modifying antirheumatic drugs (DMARDs) in conjunction with pain relievers. Conventional DMARDs include methotrexate, hydroxychloroquine, sulfasalazine, and leflunomide. Corticosteroids are also used to alleviate acute episodes of pain and inflammation. They can be very effective, but they cannot be used over the long term and may have severe side effects. Suppose conventional DMARDs fail to provide satisfactory treatment. The physician may prescribe biologic DMARDs like tumor necrosis factor inhibitors (adalimumab, infliximab, etanercept, golimumab, or certolizumab) or interleukin-6 inhibitors (tocilizumab or sarilumab). Biologic DMARDs are usually effective, but they have significant side effects.

Surgery is often required for arthritis patients. Synovectomy is a procedure in which part or all the synovial membrane surrounding the diseased joint is removed. It gives temporary relief to inflammation and may help preserve joint function. The physician may recommend joint replacement therapy (arthroplasty) when a joint has deteriorated severely. In this procedure, the degenerated bone and joint structures are surgically removed and replaced with an orthopedic device of metal or plastic. This procedure is most effective in hip replacement, although it is also used in the knee. Relief of pain is the main goal of therapy in other arthritic conditions such as psoriatic arthritis and Reiter's syndrome. In ankylosing spondylitis, exercise is also an important facet of treatment to help avoid stiffening of the spine. Gout tends to recur. Therefore, there are medications for acute episodes, such as pain relievers (NSAIDs, corticosteroids, and colchicine), to control uric acid levels (such as allopurinol) and prevent attacks. Benign bone tumors sometimes require surgery. Malignant tumors can be treated surgically and may also require radiation and chemotherapy.

PERSPECTIVE AND PROSPECTS

Osteoarthritis, rheumatoid arthritis, and other forms of arthritis continue to afflict vast populations worldwide. Radical new therapies for bone disorders are evolving, with exciting possibilities: bone regeneration, bone cement, and glues to knit fractures and replace bone destroyed by diseases. Current medical treatment is significantly flawed by the incidence of side effects, especially gastrointestinal effects, from the medications used. The search for safer medications is ongoing, as is the search for treatment modalities that halt the degenerative processes of rheumatoid arthritis.

Orthopedic implants are now quite successful in the hip, sometimes successful in the knee, but otherwise not universally useful in elbows, fingers, toes, and other joints that diseases can destroy. Orthopedic implant materials and surgical techniques remain an area of intense research. Operating techniques and instrumentation improve constantly. Many orthopedic surgeons use robotic techniques for hip arthroplasties. Many procedures are now done with the aid of arthroscopic instruments. Rather than an extensive incision to reveal the joint and surrounding tissues, the surgeon works through a tiny hole, through which they can inspect the inflamed joint and even perform minor surgery. Operations on prolapsed spinal disks once entailed long incisions and laborious, careful removal of disk tissue. Fusion of the involved vertebrae was often necessary, limiting spinal movement. Healing time could be extensive. Today, simpler, less painful procedures may be as successful and far less traumatic.

In one procedure, an enzyme is injected into the prolapsed disk, causing it to shrink, reducing pressure on nearby nerves. In another procedure, disk material is removed with a needle inserted through the skin into the disk. Overall, progress in the treatment of bone disorders has been significant: Many people who would have lived with deformities and disabilities are being helped with modern medical and surgical techniques, medications, and instrumentation.

—*C. Richard Falcon, Michael A. Buratovich*

Further Reading

Bilezikian, John P. *Primer on the Metabolic Bone Diseases and Disorders of Mineral Metabolism*. 9th ed., Wiley-Blackwell, 2018.

"Bone Diseases." *MedlinePlus*, 15 Mar. 2016, medlineplus.gov/bonediseases.html. Accessed 28 May 2022.

"Bone Infections." *MedlinePlus*, 21 Mar. 2016, medlineplus.gov/boneinfections.html. Accessed 28 May 2022.

Bunta, Andrew D., and Joseph M. Lane. "Bone Health Lifetime Challenges." *AAOS*, 1 June 2016, www.aaos.org/aaosnow/2016/jun/clinical/clinical07/. Accessed 28 May 2022.

Fox, Barry, and Nadine Taylor. *Arthritis for Dummies*. 3rd ed., For Dummies, 2022.

Lane, Nancy E., and Daniel J. *All About Osteoarthritis: The Definitive Resource for Arthritis Patients and Their Families*. Oxford UP, 2002.

Nelson, Miriam E., and Sarah Wernick. *Strong Women, Strong Bones: Everything You Need to Know to Prevent, Treat, and Beat Osteoporosis*. Rev. ed., Berkley Books, 2006.

Neuwirth, Michael, and Kevin Osborn. *The Scoliosis Sourcebook*. 2nd ed., McGraw-Hill, 2008.

Peterson, Lynne S. *Mayo Clinic Guide to Arthritis: Managing Joint Pain for an Active Life*. Mayo Clinic Press, 2020.

Porter, J. L., and M. Varacallo. "Osteoporosis." *StatPearls*, 12 Feb. 2022, www.ncbi.nlm.nih.gov/books/NBK441901/. Accessed 28 May 2022.

Shlotzhauer, Tammi L. *Living with Rheumatoid Arthritis*. 3rd ed., Johns Hopkins UP, 2014.

Brain

Category: Anatomy
Specialties and related fields: Neurology, psychiatry, psychology
Definition: the most complex organ in the body, which is used for thinking, learning, remembering, seeing, hearing, and many other conscious and subconscious functions

KEY TERMS

action potential: an electrochemical event that nerve cells use to send signals along their cellular extensions in the nervous system

axon: a nerve cell extension used to carry action potentials from one place to another in the nervous system

dendrite: a branching nerve cell extension that receives and processes the effects of action potentials from other nerve cells

dyskinesia: a neurologic disorder causing difficulty in the performance of voluntary movements

nucleus: a collection of nerve cell bodies in the brain, separable from other groups by their cellular form or by surrounding nerve cell extensions

soma: the body of a cell, where the cell's genetic material and other vital structures are located

synapse: an area of close contact between nerve cells that is the functional junction where one cell communicates with another

tract: a collection of nerve fibers (axons) in the brain or spinal cord that all have the same place of origin and the same place of termination

STRUCTURE AND FUNCTIONS

The human brain is a complex structure composed of two major classes of individual cells: nerve cells (or neurons) and neuroglial cells (or glial cells). It has been estimated that the adult human brain has around 100 billion neurons and an even larger number of glial cells. An average adult brain weighs about 1,400 grams and has a volume of 1,200 milliliters. These values vary directly with the person's body size; therefore, males have a typically 10 percent larger brain than females. However, there is no correlation between intelligence and brain size, as witnessed by brains as small as 750 milliliters or larger than 2,000 milliliters still show normal functioning.

Neurons process and transmit information. The usual structural features of a neuron include a cell body (or soma), anywhere from several to several hundred branching dendrites that are extensions from the soma, and a typically longer extension known as the "axon" with one or several synaptic terminals at its end.

The information processed and transmitted in the brain takes the form of very brief electrochemical events, with a typical duration of shorter than two milliseconds, called "action potentials" or "nerve impulses." These impulses most often originate near the point at which the axon and soma are joined and then travel at speeds of up to 130 meters per second along the axon to the synaptic terminals.

At the synaptic terminals, one neuron communicates its information to other neurons in the brain. These specialized structural points of neuron-to-neuron communication are called "synapses." Most synapses are found on the dendrites and soma of the neuron that is to receive the nerve signal. A neuron may have as many as fifty thousand synapses on its surface. However, the average seems to be

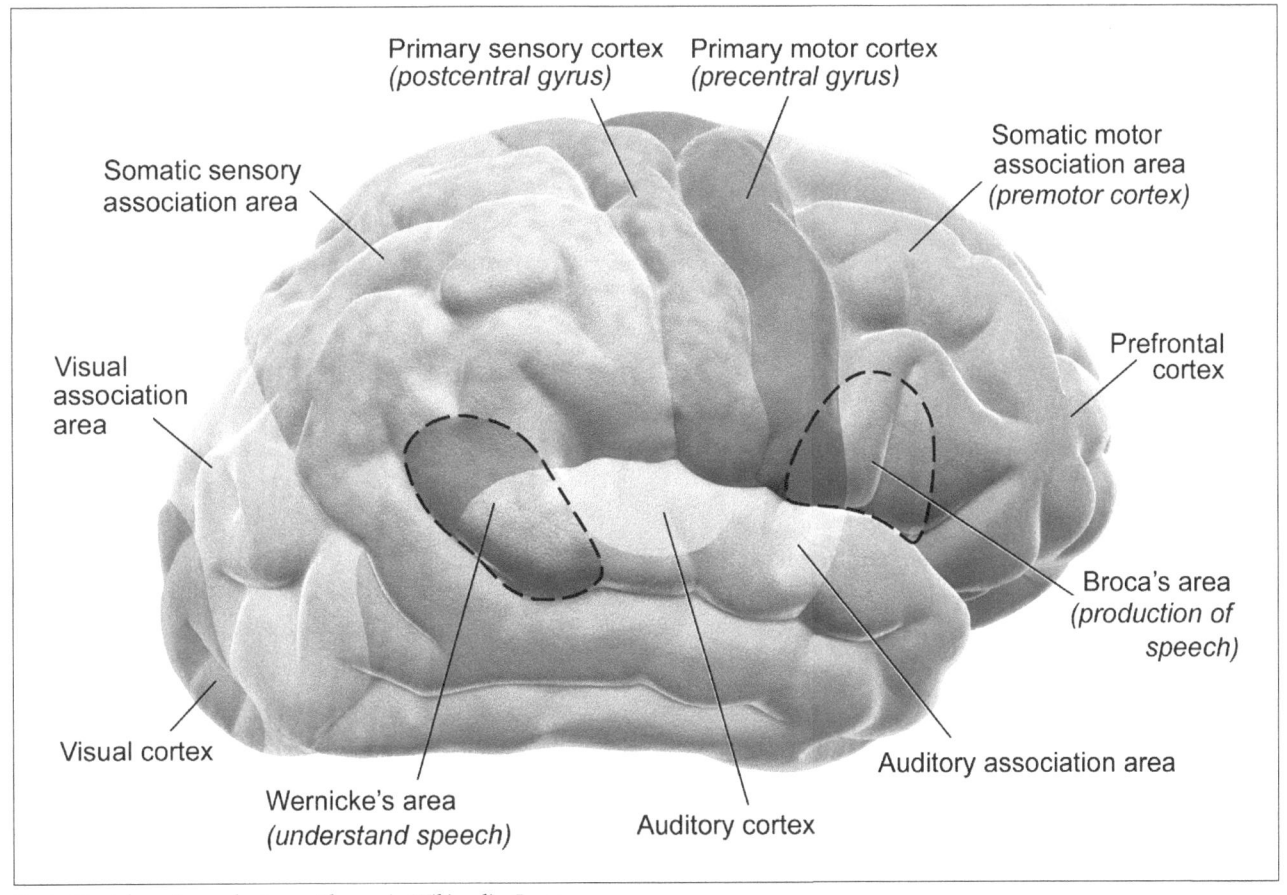

Brain physiology. Image by Bruce Blaus, via Wikimedia Commons.

around three thousand. It is thought that as many as 300 trillion synapses may exist in the adult brain.

Neuroglia function as supporting cells. They have a variety of important duties that include acting as a supporting framework for neurons, increasing the speed of impulse conduction along axons, acting as removers of waste or cellular debris, and regulating the composition of the fluid environment around the neurons to maintain optimal working conditions in the brain. Neuroglia make up about half of the brain's total volume.

The brain can be divided into two major components: gray matter and white matter, both named for their general appearance. The gray matter consists primarily of neural soma, dendrites, and axons that transmit information at relatively slow speeds. The white matter is made of collections of axons that have layers of specialized glial cells wrapped around them. This glial cell-synthesized insulation, called a "myelin sheath," enables much faster information transfer along these axons.

The brain has six major regions. Beginning from the top of the spinal cord and moving progressively upward, these regions are the medulla oblongata, the pons, the cerebellum, the mesencephalon (or midbrain), the diencephalon, and the cerebrum.

The initial lower portion of the medulla oblongata resembles the spinal cord. The medulla has a variety of functions besides the simple relaying of various categories of sensory information to higher brain centers. Several centers within the medulla are important for executing and regulating basic survival and maintenance duties. These duties are called "visceral functions" and include regulating the heart rate, breathing, digestive actions, and blood pressure.

The term *pons* comes from the Latin word meaning "bridge." The pons serves as a bridge from the medulla oblongata to the cerebellum, which is situated on the backside of the brain stem. The pons contains tracts and nuclei that permit communication between the cerebellum and other nervous system structures. Some pontine nuclei facilitate the control of such voluntary and involuntary muscle actions as chewing, breathing, and moving the eyes; other nuclei process information related to the sense of balance.

The cerebellum is itself a small brain. The two main functions of the cerebellum are to make fast and automatic adjustments to the muscles of the body that assist in maintaining balance and posture and in coordinating the activities of the skeletal muscles involved in movements or sequences of movements, thereby promoting smooth and precise actions. These functions are possible because of the sensory information input to the cerebellum from position sensors in the muscles and joints, from visual, touch, and balance organs; and even from the sense of hearing. There are also many communication channels to and from the cerebellum and other brain areas concerned with generating and controlling movements. While the cerebellum is not the origin of commands that initiate movements, it stores the memories of how to perform patterns of muscle contractions used to execute learned skills, such as serving a tennis ball.

The mesencephalon, or midbrain, is located just above the pons. The midbrain contains pathways carrying sensory information upward to higher-brain centers and transmitting motor signals from higher regions down to lower-brain and spinal cord areas involved in movements.

The nucleus known as the "substantia nigra" operates with nuclei in the cerebrum to generate the patterns and rhythms of activities like walking and running. Two important pairs of nuclei, the inferior and superior colliculi, are found on the backside of the mesencephalon. They coordinate visual and acoustic reflexes involving eye and head movements, such as eye focusing and orienting the head and body toward a sound source. Additional mesencephalic nuclei are important for the involuntary control of muscle tone, posture maintenance, and the control of eye movements.

The diencephalon, located above the midbrain, contains the two important brain structures known as the "thalamus" and "hypothalamus." The thalamus is the final relay for all sensory signals (except the sense of smell) before arriving at the cerebral cortex (the cerebrum's outer covering of gray matter). The hypothalamus is important for regulating drives and emotions. It serves as a master link between the nervous and endocrine systems.

The thalamus is a collection of different nuclei. Some cooperate with nuclei in the cerebrum to process memories and generate emotional states. Other nuclei have complex involvement in the interactions of the cerebellum, cerebral nuclei, and motor areas of the cerebral cortex.

The relatively small hypothalamus plays many crucial roles that help to maintain stability in the body's internal environment. It regulates food and liquid intake, blood pressure, heart rate, breathing, body temperature, and digestion. Other significant duties encompass the management of sexual activity, rage, fear, and pleasure.

The final major brain region is the cerebrum, the largest of the six regions and the seat of higher intellectual capabilities. Sensory information that reaches the cerebrum also enters into a person's conscious awareness. Voluntary actions originate in cerebral neural activities.

The cerebrum is divided into two cerebral hemispheres, each covered by the gray matter known as the "cerebral cortex." Below the cortex is the white matter, which consists of massive bundles of axons carrying signals between various cortical areas, down from the cortex to lower areas, and up into the cortex from lower areas. Embedded in the white matter are also several cerebral nuclei.

The cerebral cortex has the primary sensory areas for each of the senses and other areas whose major duties deal with the origin and planning of motor activities. The association areas of the cortex integrate and process sensory signals, often resulting in the initiation of appropriate motor responses. Cortical integrative centers receive information from different association areas. The integrative centers perform complex information analyses (such as predicting the consequences of various possible responses) and direct elaborate motor activities (such as writing).

The cerebral nuclei, also called the "basal nuclei" or "basal ganglia," form components of brain systems that have complex duties such as the regulation of emotions, the control of muscle tone, the coordination of learned patterns of movement, and the processing of memories.

The electrochemical signal that constitutes an action potential in a neuron sent along the neuron's axon to the synaptic contacts formed with other neurons in the brain is the basic unit of activity in neural tissue. Although the electrical voltage generated by a single action potential is very small and difficult to measure, the tremendous number of neurons active at any moment results in voltages large enough to be measured at the scalp with appropriate instruments called "electroencephalographs." The recorded signals are known as an electroencephalogram (EEG).

Although interpreting an EEG can be compared to standing outside a football stadium filled with screaming fans and trying to discern what is happening on the playing field by listening to the crowd noises, it still provides clinically useful information. It is used regularly in clinics around the world each day. The typical EEG signal appears as a series of wavy patterns whose size, length, shape, and location of best recording on the head provide valuable indications concerning the conditions of brain regions beneath the recording electrodes placed on the scalp.

DISORDERS AND DISEASES
One of the most useful applications of the EEG is in the diagnosis of epilepsy. Epilepsy is a group of dis-

orders originating in the brain. There are multiple possible causes. Epilepsy is characterized by malfunctions of the brain's motor, sensory, or even psychic operations, and there are often accompanying convulsive movements during the attack.

The most common type is idiopathic epilepsy, so-called because the cause of these attacks is unknown. The usual episode occurs suddenly as a large group of neurons begins to produce action potentials in a very synchronized fashion (called a "seizure"), which is not the typical mode of action in neural tissue. The seizure may be restricted to a localized area of brain tissue or may spread over the entire brain. When areas of the brain that generate or control movements become involved, the patient will exhibit varying degrees of involuntary muscle contractions or convulsions. There may be no impairment of consciousness or a complete loss of consciousness.

Some cases of epilepsy can be traced to definite causes such as brain tumors, brain injuries, drug abuse, adverse drug reactions, or infections that have entered the brain. Regardless of the cause, the diagnosis is often made by examining the EEG. A trained examiner can quickly identify the EEG abnormalities characteristic of epilepsy.

The usual treatment is directed toward preventing the synchronized bursts of neural activity. Administering anticonvulsive drugs such as phenobarbital or phenytoin usually achieves this result. These agents block the transmission of neural signals in the epileptic regions and thereby suppress the explosive episodes of synchronized neuronal discharges that induce the seizures. This approach successfully treats many people with epilepsy. They can lead normal, productive lives, free from uncontrollable seizures. Some patients can even discontinue their antiepileptic medications and, in some cases, never suffer another seizure.

Unfortunately, there are also cases where even the strongest medications do not prevent the seizures or only do so with debilitating side effects. In the most severe cases, the patients may have dozens of seizures each day, making any form of normal existence impossible. In addition, the large number of seizures eventually can lead to permanent brain damage. The most extreme form of treatment has been used for some of these patients: surgical removal of the brain tissue responsible for the seizures. This technique is accompanied by great risk because of the danger that removing a portion of brain tissue may leave the patient unable to speak or to speak intelligently, unable to understand spoken words, unable to interpret visual information, or suffering from any of a wide variety of behavioral disturbances, depending on the precise area of the brain that has been removed.

Although this approach is not appropriate in all cases, it has successfully treated many different cases. For these patients, success is usually defined as the possibility, following surgery, to control or prevent future seizures using anticonvulsive drugs and resume a normal life or a life that is much more normal than it was before surgery.

A varied group of disorders known as "dyskinesias" causes difficulty performing voluntary movements. The movements look like normal body movements or portions of normal movements. Dyskinesia often results from problems involving the basal nuclei. When the basal nuclei are affected, the dyskinesias usually do not occur during sleep. They are reduced during periods of emotional tranquility. However, anxiety, emotional tension, and stressful conditions cause dyskinesia to worsen. These observations can be explained by the fact that neural pathways are known to connect the brain centers involved with the generation of emotional states to the basal nuclei.

One example of dyskinesia affecting the basal nuclei is the inherited condition of Huntington's disease (or Huntington's chorea), for which no cure exists. Chorea is a dyskinesia in which the patient's movements are quick and irregular. Huntington's chorea first makes its appearance when the patient is in middle age. It results in the progressive degeneration of the basal nuclei, known as the "corpus striatum," in the cerebrum. Some common symptoms are involuntary facial grimacing, jaw and tongue movements, twisting and turning movements of the torso, and speaking difficulties. As the brain atrophy (degeneration) progresses, the patients become disabled. Death usually results in ten to fifteen years following the appearance of the first symptoms.

A category of generalized disturbances of higher-brain function is known as "dementia." Dementia is characterized by a generalized deficiency of intellectual performance, mental deterioration, memory impairment, and limited attention span. These are often accompanied by changes in personality, such as increased irritability and moodiness.

Various diseases can cause dementia. Alzheimer's disease is one of the most frequently observed dementias. It is a progressive condition that usually develops between forty and sixty. The disease is marked by the death of neurons in the cerebral cortex and the deep cerebral regions known as the "nucleus basalis" and the "hippocampus." The exact cause of neural death in Alzheimer's disease is unknown. While some cases are inherited, other instances appear without any family history of the disease. Death usually occurs within ten years after the appearance of the first symptoms, and no cure exists.

The areas of the brain showing neural degeneration also have abnormal collections of a specific type of protein. The appearance of this protein in the blood and the fluids surrounding the brain is a clinical sign of Alzheimer's disease. The areas of the brain that deteriorate during the progression of this disease illustrate the functional roles played by these regions. The hippocampus, in particular, is crucial for learning, the storage of long-term memories, the memory of recent events, and the sense of time. Therefore, hippocampal neuronal death helps explain the memory disturbances and related behavioral changes seen in Alzheimer's patients.

PERSPECTIVE AND PROSPECTS

Given the complexity of the human brain, understanding its structure and function is the ultimate challenge to medical science. Physicians and neuroscientists must understand how the brain functions to treat brain disorders. An appreciation of this can be gleaned by studying the history of some approaches used to treat brain disorders.

For example, in the Middle Ages, it was common to treat people with epilepsy by cutting open the patient's scalp and pouring salt into the wound (all of which was performed without anesthesia since anesthetics were not yet known). This treatment aimed to poison the spirits possessing the patient, forcing them to leave.

As modern science discovered the cellular basis of life, physicians gradually replaced such measures with treatments directed toward the biochemical imbalances, infections, or interruptions of blood flow that cause many brain disorders. The development of nonsurgical techniques permitting the visualization of the brain regions that are active or inactive during various tasks or illnesses greatly advanced the understanding of brain function and improved diagnosis, the planning of effective treatments, and the tracking of either the improvement or the deterioration of patients.

Late in the 1970s, the disease known as acquired immunodeficiency syndrome (AIDS) attracted the attention of the world's scientists. AIDS is caused by the human immunodeficiency virus (HIV). A significant portion of AIDS patients experience various neurological problems, including movement difficulties, memory loss, and cognitive disturbances. Although HIV cannot infect neurons or the neuroglia that make the myelin sheath (oligodendrocytes), these cells suffer extensive cell death. Half of the neurons may die in some cerebral cortical areas. Paradoxically, the two neuroglial that HIV can infect, microglia and astrocytes, produce HIV particles that move into the bloodstream but show little cell death. The HIV-infected astrocytes shed several HIV-specific proteins (e.g., Tat, Nef, and Rev). These viral proteins cause cell damage and promote inflammation, resulting in the death of nearby neurons and oligodendrocytes. HIV, therefore, transforms astrocytes, cells that normally support and protect neurons, into poisoning centers that damage nearby neurons and oligodendrocytes.

—*John V. Urbas*

Further Reading

Bear, Mark F., et al. *Neuroscience: Exploring the Brain*. 4th ed., Jones and Bartlett Learning, 2020.

Bloom, Floyd E., M. Flint Beal, and David J. Kupfer, editors. *The Dana Guide to Brain Health*. Dana Press, 2006.

"Brain Basics: Know Your Brain." *National Institute of Neurological Disorders and Stroke*, 2022, www.ninds.nih.gov/health-information/patient-caregiver-education/brain-basics-know-your-brain. Accessed 30 May 2022.

"Brain Diseases." *MedlinePlus*, 28 June 2018, medlineplus.gov/braindiseases.html. Accessed 30 May 2022.

"Brain Diseases from A-Z." *American Brain Foundation*, 2022, www.americanbrainfoundation.org/diseases/. Accessed 30 May 2022.

Davis, Joel. *Mapping the Mind: The Secrets of the Human Brain and How It Works*. Replica Books, 1999.

Fox, Stuart, and Krista Rompolski. *Human Physiology*. 16th ed., McGraw-Hill, 2021.

Horstman, Judith. *The Scientific American Day in the Life of Your Brain: A Twenty-four-Hour Journal of What's Happening in Your Brain*. Jossey-Bass, 2009.

Marieb, Elaine N., and Suzanne Keller. *Essentials of Human Anatomy and Physiology*. 13th ed., Pearson, 2021.

Vanderah, Todd, and Douglas Gould. *Nolte's The Human Brain: An Introduction to its Functional Anatomy*. 8th ed., Elsevier, 2020.

VanPutte, Cinnamon, et al. *Seeley's Anatomy and Physiology*. 13th ed., McGraw Hill, 2022.

Woolsey, Thomas A., et al. *Brain Atlas: A Visual Guide to the Human Central Nervous System*. 4th ed., Wiley, 2017.

Exercise Physiology

Category: Specialty

Specialties and related fields: Cardiology, family medicine, nutrition, physical therapy, preventive medicine, sports medicine

Definition: science that studies the effects on the body of various intensities and types of physical activity, including cellular metabolism, cardiovascular responses, respiratory responses, neural and hormonal adaptations, and muscular adaptations to exercise

KEY TERMS

adenosine triphosphate (ATP): a high-energy compound found in the cell that provides energy for all bodily functions

aerobic: metabolism involving the breakdown of energy substrates using oxygen

anaerobic: metabolism involving the breakdown of energy substrates without using oxygen

electrocardiogram (ECG): a graphic record of electrical currents of the heart

glycogen: the form that glucose takes when it is stored in the muscles and liver

heart rate: the number of times the heart contracts, or beats, per minute

maximal oxygen uptake: the maximum rate of oxygen consumption during exercise

metabolic equivalent (MET): a unit used to estimate the metabolic cost of physical activity; 1 MET is equal to 3.5 milliliters of oxygen consumed per kilogram of body weight per minute

SCIENCE AND PROFESSION

The primary aim of research in the field of exercise physiology is to gain a better understanding of the quantity and type of exercise needed for health maintenance and rehabilitation. A major goal of professionals in exercise physiology is to find ways to incorporate appropriate levels of physical activity into the lifestyles of all individuals.

Physiology is the science of the physical and chemical factors and processes involved in the function of living organisms. The study of exercise physiology examines these factors and processes as they relate to physical exertion. The physical responses that occur are specific to the intensity, duration, frequency, and type of exercise performed.

Exercise of low or moderate intensity relies on oxygen to release energy for work. This process is often referred to as aerobic exercise. In the muscles, carbohydrates and fats are broken down to produce adenosine triphosphate (ATP), the basic molecule used for energy. Aerobic exercise can be sustained for several minutes to several hours.

Higher-intensity exercise is predominantly fueled anaerobically (in the absence of oxygen) and can be sustained for up to two minutes only. Muscle glycogen is broken down without oxygen to produce ATP. Anaerobic metabolism is much less efficient at producing ATP than is aerobic metabolism.

During anaerobic metabolism, a byproduct called "lactic acid" begins to accumulate in the blood as

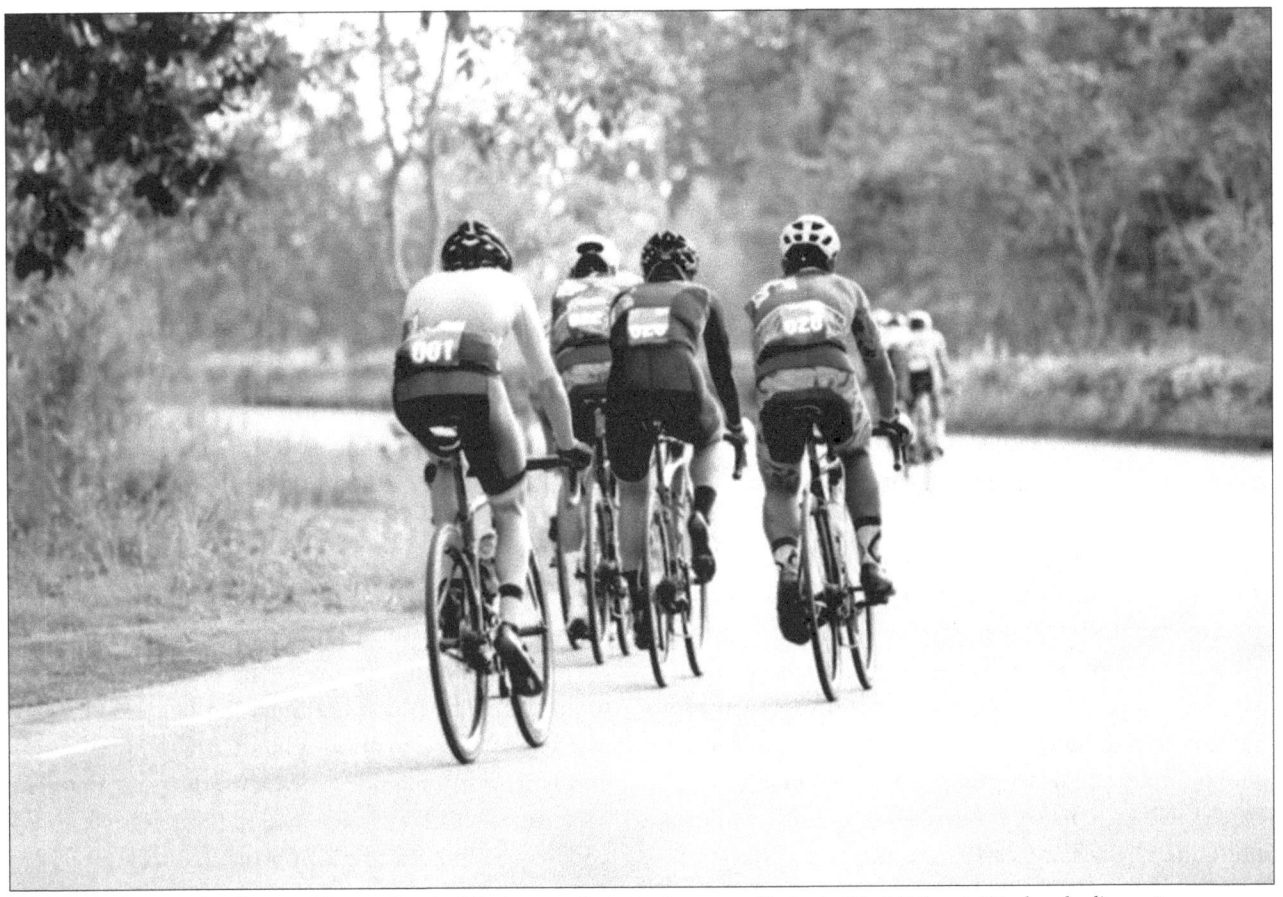

Cyclists may be trained and assessed by exercise physiologists to optimize performance. Photo via iStock/Adkasai. [Used under license.]

blood lactate. The point at which this accumulation begins is called the "anaerobic threshold" (AT), or the onset of blood lactate accumulation (OBLA). Blood lactate can cause muscle soreness and stiffness, but it also can be used as fuel during aerobic metabolism.

A third and less often used energy system is the creatine phosphate (ATP-CP) system. Using the very limited supply of ATP that is stored in the muscles, phosphate molecules are exchanged between ATP and CP to provide energy. This system provides only enough fuel for a few seconds of maximum effort.

The type of muscle fiber recruited to perform a specific type of exercise is also dependent on exercise intensity. Skeletal muscle is composed of "slow-twitch" and two types of "fast-twitch" muscle fibers. Slow-twitch fibers are more suited to using oxygen than are fast-twitch fibers, and they are recruited primarily for aerobic exercise. One type of fast-twitch fiber also functions during aerobic activity. The second type of fast-twitch fiber serves to facilitate anaerobic, or high-intensity, exercise.

Exercise mode is also a factor in people's physiological responses to exercise. Dynamic exercise (alternating muscular contraction and relaxation through a range of motion) using many large muscles requires more oxygen than does activity using smaller and fewer muscles. The greater the oxygen requirement of the physical activity, the greater the cardiorespiratory benefits.

Many bodily adaptations occur over a training period of six to eight weeks, and other benefits are gradually manifested over several months. The positive adaptations include reduced resting and working heart rates. As the heart becomes stronger, there is a subsequent increase in stroke volume (the volume of blood the heart pumps with each beat), which allows the heart to beat less frequently while maintaining the same cardiac output (the volume of the blood pumped from the heart each minute). Another beneficial adaptation is increased metabolic efficiency. This is partially facilitated by an increase in the number of mitochondria (the organelles responsible for ATP production) in the muscle cells.

One of the most recognized representations of aerobic fitness is the maximum volume of oxygen (VO_{2max}) an individual can use during exercise. VO_{2max} is improved through habitual, relatively high-intensity aerobic activity. After three to six months of regular training, levels of high-density lipoproteins (HDLs) in the blood increase. HDL molecules remove cholesterol (a fatty substance) from the tissues to aid in protecting the heart from atherosclerosis.

Various internal and external factors influence the metabolic processes that take place during and after exercise. Internally, nutrition, degree of hydration, body composition, flexibility, sex, and age are some of the variables that play a role in the physiological responses. Other internal variables include medical conditions such as heart disease, diabetes, and hypertension (high blood pressure). Externally, environmental conditions such as temperature, humidity, and altitude alter how the exercising body functions.

Various modes of exercise testing and data collection are used to study the physiological responses of the body to exercise. Treadmills and cycle ergometers (instruments that measure work and power output) are among the most common methods of evaluating maximum oxygen consumption. During these tests, special equipment and computers analyze expired air, heart rate is monitored with a heart rate monitor or an electrocardiograph (ECG), and blood pressure is taken using a sphygmomanometer. Blood and muscle-fiber samples can also be extracted to aid in identifying the fuel system and type of muscle fibers being used. Other data sometimes collected, such as skin temperature and body-core temperature, can provide pertinent information.

Metabolic equivalent units, or METs, are often used to translate a person's capability into workloads on various pieces of exercise equipment or into everyday tasks. For every 3.5 milliliters of oxygen consumed per kilogram of body weight per minute, the subject is said to be performing at a workload of one MET. One MET is approximately equivalent to 1.5 kilocalories per minute for each kilogram of body weight, or the amount of energy expended per kilogram of body weight in one minute when a person is at rest.

Another factor greatly affecting the physical response to exercise is body composition. The three major structural components of the body are muscle, bone, and fat. Body composition can be evaluated using a combination of anthropometric measurements. These measurements include body weight, standard height, measurements of circumferences at various locations using a tape measure, measurements of skeletal diameters using a sliding metric stick, and measurements of skinfold thicknesses using calipers.

Body fat can be estimated using several methods, the most accurate of which is based on a calculation of body density. This method, called "hydrostatic weighing," involves weighing the subject under water while taking into account the residual volume of air in the lungs. The principle underlying this measurement of body density is based on the fact that fat is less dense than water and thus will float, whereas bone and muscle, which are denser than water, will sink. One biochemical technique often used to determine levels of body fat is based on the relatively constant level of potassium-40 naturally existing in lean body mass. Another method uses ultrasound waves to measure the thickness of fat layers. X-rays and computed tomography (CT) scanning can be used to provide images from which fat and bone can be measured. Bioelectrical impedance analysis (BIA) is a method of estimating body composition based on the resistance imposed on a low-voltage electrical current sent through the body. The most widely used and easily assessable method, however, involves measurement of skinfolds at various sites on the body using calipers. In all cases, mathematical formulas have been devised to interpret the collected data and provide the best estimate of an individual's body composition.

Other tests have been developed to determine muscular strength, muscular endurance, and flexibility. Muscular strength is often measured by performance of one maximal effort produced by a selected muscle group. Muscular endurance of a muscle or muscle group is often demonstrated by the length of time or number of repetitions a particular submaximal workload or skill can be performed.

Two major types of flexibility have been identified. One type consists of the ability to move a muscle group or joint through its full range of motion at low speeds or hold a part of the body still at the extent of its range of motion. This is called "static flexibility," and it can be measured using a metric stick or a protractor-type instrument called a "goniometer." Dynamic flexibility, the other major identified type of flexibility, is the flexibility through the full range of motion of a muscle group or joint at normal or high speeds. Measuring dynamic flexibility is much more difficult.

Overlapping the science of exercise physiology are the studies of biomechanics or kinesiology (sciences dealing with human movement) and nutrition. Only through an understanding of efficient body mechanics and proper nutrition can the physiological responses of the body to exercise be identified correctly.

DIAGNOSTIC AND TREATMENT TECHNIQUES

Exercise prescription is the primary focus in the application of exercise physiology. General health maintenance, cardiac rehabilitation, and competitive athletics are three major areas of exercise prescription.

Before making recommendations for an exercise program, an exercise physiologist must evaluate the physical limitations of the exerciser. In a normal health-maintenance setting, often called a "wellness" program, a health-related questionnaire can reveal relevant information. Such a questionnaire should include questions about family medical history and the subject's history of heart trouble or chest pain, bone or joint problems, and high blood pressure. The presence of any of these problems suggests the need for a physician's consent prior to exercising. After the individual has been deemed eligible to participate, an assessment of the level of physical fitness should be performed. Determining or estimating VO_{2max}, muscular strength, muscular endurance, flexibility, and body composition is usually part of this assessment. It is then possible to design a program best suited to the needs of the individual.

For the healthy adult participant, the American College of Sports Medicine (ACSM), a widely recognized authoritative body on exercise prescription, recommends three to five sessions of aerobic exercise weekly. Each session should include a five- to ten-minute warm-up period, twenty to sixty minutes of aerobic exercise at a predetermined exercise intensity, and a five- to ten-minute cool-down period.

To recommend an appropriate aerobic exercise intensity, the exercise physiologist must determine an individual's maximum heart rate. The best way to obtain this maximum heart rate is to administer a maximal exercise test. Such a test can be supervised by an exercise physiologist or an exercise-test technician; it is advisable, especially for the older participant, that a cardiologist also be in attendance. An ECG is monitored for irregularities as the subject walks, runs, cycles, or performs some dynamic exercise to exhaustion or until the onset of irregular symptoms or discomfort.

Exercise prescription using heart rate as a measure can be achieved by various methods. A direct correlation exists between exercise intensity, in terms of oxygen consumption, and heart rate. From data collected during a maximal exercise test, a target heart-rate range of 40 to 89 percent of functional capacity can be calculated. Another method used to determine an appropriate heart-rate range is based on the difference between an individual's resting heart rate and maximum heart rate, called the "heart-rate reserve" (HRR). Values representing 40 percent and 89 percent of the HRR are calculated and added to the resting heart rate, yielding the individual's target heart-rate range. A third method involves calculating 70 percent and 85 percent of the maximum heart rate. Although this method is less accurate than the other two methods, it is the simplest way to estimate a target heart-rate range.

Intensity of exercise can also be prescribed using METs. This method relies on the predetermined metabolic equivalents required to perform activities at various intensities. Activity levels reflecting 40 to 85 percent of functional capacity can be calculated.

The rating of perceived exertion (RPE) is another method of prescribing exercise intensity. Verbal responses by the participant describing how an exercise feels at various intensities are assigned to a numerical scale, which is then correlated to heart rate. Through practice, the participant learns to associate heart rate with the RPE, reducing the necessity of frequent pulse monitoring in the healthy individual.

Adequate physical fitness can be defined as the ability to perform daily tasks with enough reserve for emergency situations. All aspects of health-related fitness direct attention toward this goal. Aerobic exercise often provides some conditioning for muscular endurance, but muscular strength and flexibility need to be addressed separately.

The ACSM recommends resistance training using the "overload principle," which involves placing habitual stress on a system, causing it to adapt and respond. For this training, it is suggested that eight to twelve repetitions of eight to ten strengthening exercises of the major muscle groups be performed a minimum of two days per week.

Flexibility of connective tissue and muscle tissue is essential to maximize physical performance and limit musculoskeletal injuries. At least one stretching exercise for each major muscle group should be executed three to four times per week while the muscles are warm. Four methods of stretching that have been designed to improve flexibility are ballistic stretching, dynamic stretching, static stretching, and proprioceptive neuromuscular facilitation (PNF). Ballistic stretching incorporates a bouncing motion and is generally prescribed only in sports that replicate this type of movement whereas dynamic stretching uses slow, controlled movements. During a static stretch, the muscles and connective tissue are actively or passively stretched to their maximum lengths and held for ten to thirty seconds. PNF involves a contract-relax sequence of the muscle.

In addition to exercise prescription for cardiorespiratory fitness, muscular fitness, and flexibility, it is appropriate for the exercise physiologist to make recommendations concerning body composition. Exercise is an effective tool in fat loss. Dietary caloric restriction without exercise results in a greater loss of muscle mass along with fat than if exercise is part of a weight loss program.

For persons with special health concerns, such as diabetes mellitus or high blood pressure, the exercise physiologist works with the participant's physician. The physician prescribes necessary medications and often decides which modes of exercise are contraindicated (i.e., should be avoided).

A second application, cardiac rehabilitation, takes exercise prescription a step further. Participation of a heart patient in cardiac rehabilitation is more individualized than in wellness programs. The conditions of the circulatory system, pulmonary system, and joints are only a few of the special concerns. Secondary conditions such as obesity, diabetes, and hypertension must also be considered. The responsibilities of exercise physiologists in cardiac rehabilitation include monitoring blood sugar in diabetic patients and blood pressure in all patients, especially those with hypertension. Many drugs affect heart rate or blood pressure, and most of these participants are taking more than one type of medication. Patients with heart damage caused by a heart attack may display atypical heart rhythms, which can be seen on an ECG monitor. Furthermore, the stage of recovery of the postsurgical patient is a major factor in recommending the type, frequency, intensity, and duration of exercise.

Patient education is also important. Lifestyle is usually the main factor in the development of heart disease. Cardiac patients often have never participated in a regular exercise program. They may smoke, be overweight, or have poor eating habits. Helping them to identify and correct destructive health-related behaviors is the focus of education for the heart patient.

A third application of the study of exercise physiology involves dealing with the competitive athlete sports medicine. In this case, findings from the most recent research are constantly applied to yield the best athletic performance possible. A delicate balance of aerobic training, anaerobic training, strength training, endurance training, and flexibility exercises are combined with the optimum percentage of body fat, proper nutrition, and adequate sleep. The program that is designed must enhance the athletic qualities that are most beneficial to the sport in which the athlete participates.

The competitive athlete usually pushes beyond the boundaries of general exercise prescription in terms of intensity, duration, and frequency of exercise performance. As a result, the athlete risks suffering more injuries than the individual who exercises for health benefits. If the athlete sustains an injury, the exercise physiologist may work in conjunction with an athletic trainer or sports medicine physician to return the athlete to competition as soon as possible.

PERSPECTIVE AND PROSPECTS

The modern study of exercise physiology developed out of an interest in physical fitness. In the United States, the concern for development and maintenance of physical fitness was well established by the end of the twentieth century. As early as 1819, Stanford and Harvard Universities offered professional physical-education programs. At least one textbook on the physiology of exercise was published by that time.

Much of the pioneering work in this field, however, was done in Europe. Nobel Prize-winning European research on muscular exercise, oxygen utilization as it relates to the upper limits of physical performance, and production of lactic acid during glucose metabolism dates back to the 1920s.

In the early 1950s, poor performance by children in the United States on a minimal muscular fitness test helped lead to the formation of what became known as the President's Council on Physical Fitness and Sport. Concurrently, a significant number of deaths of middle-aged American males were found to be caused by poor health habits associated with coronary artery disease. A need for more research in the areas of health and physical activity was recognized by the mid-1960s. The subsequent research was facilitated by the existence of fifty-eight exercise physiology research laboratories in colleges and universities throughout the country. Organizations such as the American Physiological Society (APS), the American Alliance of Health, Physical Education, Recreation and Dance (AAHPERD), and the American College of Sports Medicine (ACSM) were established by the mid-1950s. In an effort to ensure that well-trained professionals were involved in cardiac-rehabilitation programs, the ACSM developed a certification program in 1975. Certifications for fitness personnel were added later.

Increasingly sophisticated testing equipment should lead to a better understanding of fundamental physiological mechanisms, allowing practitioners to be more effective in measuring physical fitness and prescribing exercise programs. Health maintenance has become a priority as the number of adults over the age of fifty continues to increase. Advances in medical techniques also increase the survival rate of victims of heart attacks, creating a need for more cardiac-rehabilitation programs and practitioners. Health-care professionals and the general population need to be made more aware of the benefits of exercise for the maintenance of good health and the rehabilitation of individuals with medical problems.

—*Bradley R. A. Wilson*

Further Reading

American College of Sports Medicine. *ACSM's Guidelines for Exercise Testing and Prescription*. 11th ed., Wolters Kluwer, 2022.

———. *ACSM's Resources for the Exercise Physiologist*. 3rd ed., Wolters Kluwer, 2022.

McArdle, William, Frank I. Katch, and Victor L. Katch. *Exercise Physiology: Nutrition, Energy, and Human Performance*. 9th ed., Wolters Kluwer, 2022.

Powers, Scott K., and Edward T. Howley. *Exercise Physiology: Theory and Application to Fitness and Performance*. 11th ed., McGraw-Hill, 2021.

US Department of Health and Human Services. *Physical Activity Guidelines for Americans*. 2nd ed., US Department of Health and Human Services, 2018.

GLYCOLYSIS

Category: Biochemistry

Anatomy or system affected: Blood, cells, muscles, musculoskeletal system

Specialties and related fields: Biochemistry, cytology, exercise physiology, pharmacology, sports medicine

Definition: the chemical process of splitting a glucose molecule to obtain energy for other cellular processes; at times of intense activity, glycolysis produces most of the energy used by muscles

KEY TERMS

adenosine triphosphate (ATP): an important biological molecule that represents the energy currency of the cell; the energy in a special high-energy bond in ATP is used to drive almost all cellular processes that require energy

aerobic: occurring in the presence of oxygen

anaerobic: occurring in the absence of oxygen

cellular respiration: a complex series of chemical reactions by which chemical energy stored in the bonds of food molecules is released and used to form ATP

chemical energy: the energy locked up in the chemical bonds that hold the atoms of a molecule together; food molecules, such as glucose, contain much energy in their bonds

creatine phosphate: an energy-containing molecule present in significant quantities in muscle tissue; energy is stored in a high-energy bond like that of ATP

enzyme: a biological catalyst that speeds up a chemical reaction without itself being used up; enzymes are made of protein, and a single enzyme can usually only catalyze a single chemical reaction

nicotinamide adenine dinucleotide (NAD): a molecule used to hold pairs of electrons when they have been removed from a molecule by some biological process; the empty molecule is denoted by NAD+, while it is denoted as NADH when it is carrying electrons

STRUCTURE AND FUNCTIONS

Glycolysis is the first step in the process that cells use to extract energy from food molecules. Although energy can be extracted from most types of food molecules, glycolysis is usually considered to begin with glucose. The term "glycolysis" actually means the splitting (*lysis*) of glucose (*glyco*). Therefore, glycolysis is a good description of the process since the glucose molecule is split into two halves. The glucose molecule consists of a backbone of six carbon atoms attached, in various ways, to twelve hydrogen atoms and six oxygen atoms. The glucose molecule is inherently stable and unlikely to split spontaneously at any appreciable rate.

When the energy is extracted from a glucose molecule, it is stored, for the short term, in a much less stable molecule called "adenosine triphosphate" (ATP). The ATP molecule consists of a complex organic molecule (adenosine), to which are attached three simple phosphate groups.

Adenosine triphosphate consists of a five-carbon sugar called "ribose," linked to the nitrogenous base adenine and on the other side to a linear chain of phosphate groups. The molecule formed by the attachment of adenine to ribose is called "adenosine," and the linkage of three phosphates generates adenosine triphosphate. The first phosphate is attached to the ribose sugar through a chemical bond whose energy is no greater than those bonds found anywhere else in the molecule. While the first phosphate is attached by what one could call a "normal" chemical bond, the second and third phosphates are attached by high-energy bonds. These are chemical bonds that require a considerable amount of energy to create. Thus, ATP is an ideal energy storage molecule that provides readily available energy for the biosynthetic reactions of the cell and other energy-requiring processes.

When one of the high-energy bonds of ATP is broken, a large amount of energy is released. Usually, only the bond holding the last phosphate is broken, producing a molecule of adenosine diphosphate (ADP) and a free phosphate group. The phosphate group is only split from ATP at the precise moment when some other process in the cell requires energy. This breaking of ATP provides the energy to drive cellular processes. The processes include synthesizing molecules, the movement of molecules, and muscle contraction. The third phosphate can be reattached to ADP using the energy released from glycolysis or by other components of cellular

Glycolysis

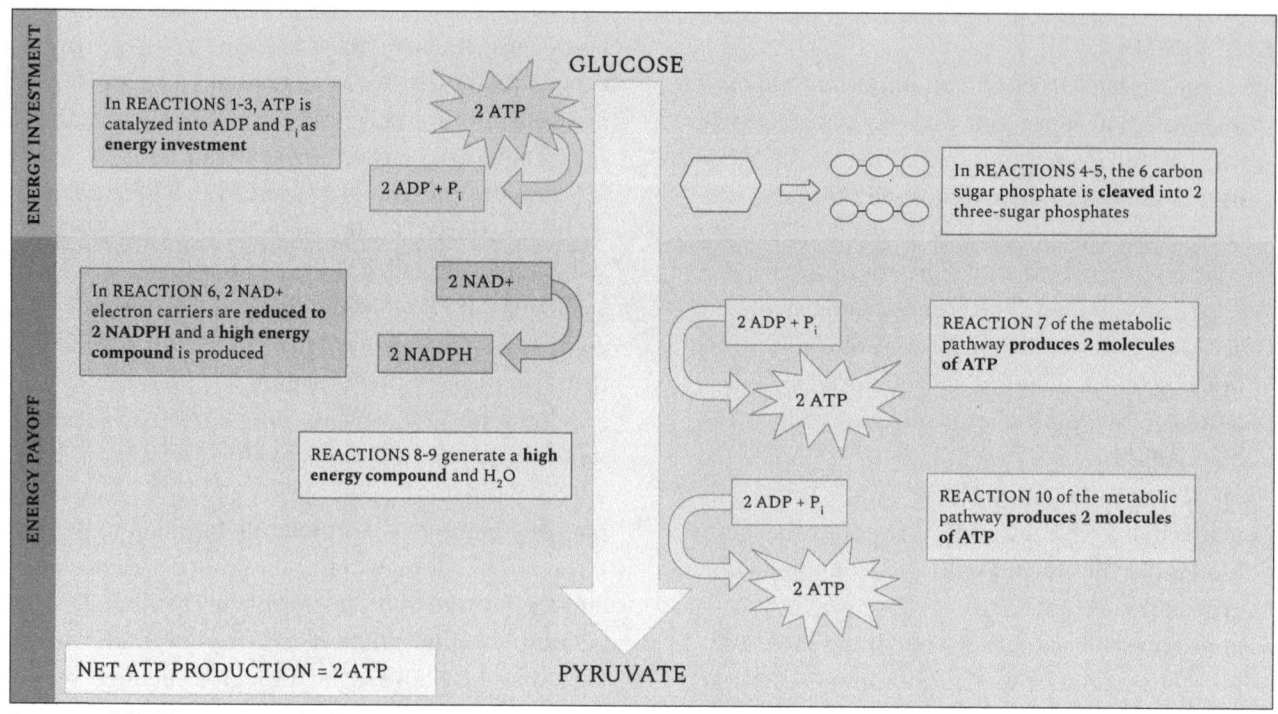

Principles of Sports Medicine & Exercise Science

ENERGY INVESTMENT

GLUCOSE

In REACTIONS 1-3, ATP is catalyzed into ADP and P$_i$ as **energy investment**

2 ATP → 2 ADP + P$_i$

In REACTIONS 4-5, the 6 carbon sugar phosphate is **cleaved** into 2 three-sugar phosphates

ENERGY PAYOFF

In REACTION 6, 2 NAD+ electron carriers are **reduced to 2 NADPH** and a **high energy compound** is produced

2 NAD+ → 2 NADPH

2 ADP + P$_i$ → 2 ATP

REACTION 7 of the metabolic pathway **produces 2 molecules of ATP**

REACTIONS 8-9 generate a **high energy compound** and H$_2$O

2 ADP + P$_i$ → 2 ATP

REACTION 10 of the metabolic pathway **produces 2 molecules of ATP**

NET ATP PRODUCTION = 2 ATP

PYRUVATE

Summary of the 10 reactions in glycolysis. Image by Sylvie Loh, via Wikimedia Commons.

respiration. The production of ATP can be diagrammed as follows: "energy from glycolysis + ADP + phosphate ATP. Similarly, the breakdown of ATP can be diagrammed as "ATP → ADP + phosphate + usable energy." With this understanding of how ATP works, one can look at how glycolysis generates it in the cell.

The first step in producing energy from sugar is an energy-consuming process. Since glucose is inherently a stable molecule, it must be activated before it will split. It is activated by attaching a phosphate group to each end of the six-carbon backbone. ATP supplies these phosphate groups. Therefore, glycolysis begins by using the energy from two ATP molecules. The atoms of the glucose molecule are also rearranged during the activation process so that it is changed into a very similar sugar, fructose. A fructose molecule with a phosphate group on either end is called "fructose 1,6-diphosphate." Thus, one can summarize the activation process as "glucose + 2 ATP → fructose 1,6-diphosphate + 2 ADP."

Fructose 1,6-diphosphate is a much more reactive molecule. It can be readily split by an enzyme called "aldolase" into two three-carbon compounds called "dihydroxyacetone phosphate" (DHAP) and "glyceraldehyde 3-phosphate" (G3P). DHAP is converted into G3P by an enzyme called "triose phosphate isomerase," making G3P the starting point for all the following steps of glycolysis. Each G3P undergoes several reactions, but only the more consequential reactions will be mentioned. Glyceraldehyde 3-phosphate undergoes an oxidation reaction catalyzed by an enzyme called "glyceraldehyde 3-phosphate dehydrogenase." Oxidation reactions involve the loss of high-energy electrons. Electrons are highly energetic and have a negative electrical charge. They are picked up and carried by molecules specially designed for this purpose.

These energy-carrying molecules are called "nicotinamide adenine dinucleotide" (NAD). Biologists have agreed on a conventional notation for this molecule to allow the reader to know whether the molecule is carrying electrons or is empty. Since the empty molecule has a net positive charge, it is denoted as NAD$^+$. When full, it holds a pair of electrons. One electron would neutralize the positive charge, while two result in a negative charge. The negative charge attracts one of the many hydrogen ions (H$^+$) in the cell. Thus, when carrying electrons, the molecule is denoted NADH. Glyceraldehyde 3-phosphate surrenders two high-energy electrons to NAD$^+$. The G3P molecule also picks up a free phosphate group at the end opposite, where one is already attached to form 1,3-bisphosphoglycerate. One can summarize the reaction as "2 Glyceraldehyde 3-phosphate + 2 NAD$^+$ + 2 inorganic phosphates → 2 1,3-bisphosphoglycerate + NADH + H$^+$." The following reactions merely transfer the energy in these chemical bonds to high-energy bonds by transferring these phosphate groups to ADP molecules to produce ATP. Since each G3P eventually produces two ATPs, and two G3Ps are produced from each original glucose molecule, glycolysis produces four ATP molecules. However, since two ATPs were used to activate the glucose, the cell has a net gain of two ATP molecules for each glucose molecule used.

The rearrangement of the atoms leaves them in a form called "pyruvate." Pyruvate still contains much energy locked up in its chemical bonds. In most of the body's cells, and most of the time, pyruvate will be further broken down and all of its energy released. This further breakdown of pyruvate requires oxygen and is beyond the scope of this topic. However, the complete breakdown of two pyruvate molecules can produce more than thirty additional ATP molecules. With the addition of oxygen, the end products are the simple molecules of carbon dioxide and water.

The oxidative pathways that completely break down pyruvate are limited by the lack of oxygen in very active muscles. The ability to deal with electrons from NADH is also drastically reduced. Glycolysis can continue even in the absence of oxygen, but the electrons produced by glycolysis must be dealt with.

There is a minimal amount of NAD$^+$ in each cell. Nicotinamide adenine dinucleotide + hydrogen is designed to hold electrons briefly while they are transferred to some other system. In the absence of oxygen, the electrons are transferred to pyruvate. Since pyruvate cannot be broken down without oxygen, there is an ample supply. Transferring electrons from NADH to pyruvate allows the empty NAD$^+$ to pick up more electrons produced by glycolysis. Therefore, glycolysis can continue producing two ATP molecules from each glucose molecule used. While two ATPs per glucose molecule is small compared to the more than thirty ATPs produced by oxidative metabolism, it is better than none.

The process of generating energy (ATPs) in the absence of oxygen is called "fermentation." Most people are familiar with the fermentation of grapes to produce wine. Yeast has the enzymes to transfer electrons from NADH to a pyruvate derivative and convert the resulting molecule into alcohol and carbon dioxide. No further energy is obtained from this process, and alcohol still contains much of the energy that was in glucose. Humans and other mammals have different enzymes than yeast cells. These enzymes transfer the electrons from NADH to pyruvate, producing lactate.

GLYCOLYSIS AND MUSCLE ACTIVITY

When yeast is fermented anaerobically (without oxygen), it will continue producing alcohol until it poisons itself. Most yeast cannot tolerate more than 12 percent alcohol, the concentration found in most wine. The lactate produced by fermentation in humans is also poisonous. People, however, do not respire completely anaerobically. The two ATPs produced per glucose molecule used are not enough to supply the energy needs of most human cells. Muscle cells have to be somewhat of an exception. One asks the muscle cells to use energy much faster than one can supply them with oxygen. One may consider a muscle working under various physical activity levels and examine its oxygen requirements and waste products.

At rest, a muscle requires very little ATP energy. Energy demands are minimal for an individual sitting on the couch watching television. The lungs inhale and exhale slowly and take in enough oxygen to keep their concentration in the blood high. A relatively slow heart rate can pump enough of this oxygen-rich blood to the muscles to supply their very minimal needs. However, as soon as one uses a muscle, its ATP consumption increases dramatically. Even if an individual walks as far as the refrigerator, large quantities of ATP are required to cause the leg muscles to contract. Muscle cells maintain a constant level of ATP so that, as soon as one asks a muscle to contract, it can do so. The broken-down ATP is almost instantly regenerated from an additional energy store peculiar to muscle cells. Creatine phosphate is a molecule similar to ATP in that it also has a high-energy phosphate bond. There is more creatine phosphate in muscle cells than ATP. As soon as ATP is broken down, phosphates, and their high-energy bonds, are transferred from creatine phosphate. Within the first few seconds of activity, the ATP concentration in a muscle cell remains almost constant. However, the creatine phosphate level begins to drop.

The aerobic (oxygen-requiring) respiratory processes speed up when the creatine phosphate concentration drops. These processes completely break down glucose to carbon dioxide and water and release plenty of ATP. This ATP can then be used for muscle contraction. If the muscle has now stopped contracting, the new ATP produced will be used to rebuild the store of creatine phosphate.

Within the first minute or so of muscle contraction, the use of oxygen can be pretty high. The circulatory system has not yet responded to this increased oxygen demand. Muscle tissue, however, has a reserve of oxygen. The red color of most mammalian muscles is attributable to myoglobin, which is similar to hemoglobin in that it has a strong affinity for oxygen. The myoglobin stores oxygen directly in the muscle so that the muscle can operate aerobically. At the same time, the circulatory and respiratory systems adjust to the increased oxygen demand.

At low or moderate muscle activity, the carbon dioxide produced by aerobic respiration in muscles will increase the activity of both the circulatory and the respiratory systems. An increased blood flow supplies the increased demand for oxygen by the muscles. Jogging around a track or participating in aerobic exercises would be considered low to moderate muscular activity. Respiration rate and pulse rate both increase with jogging. This increase in oxygen supply to the muscles provides all that they need. The level of creatine phosphate will be lower than that in resting muscles. However, it will soon be replenished when the activity is stopped. The muscle cells have a good supply of food molecules in the form of glycogen. Glycogen is simply a long string of glucose molecules connected for convenient storage. The glycogen supply can last for hours at a rate of activity such as that created by jogging. Even after it is used up, glycogen stored in the liver can be broken down to glucose and carried to the muscles by the blood. Individuals will probably want to stop jogging before their muscles want to quit.

High levels of muscular activity pose a different set of problems. After more than a minute of vigorous exercise, the muscles begin to use ATP faster than the bloodstream can supply oxygen to regenerate it. The additional ATP is supplied by lactic acid fermentation. Glucose is only broken down as far as pyruvate, then converted to lactate by adding electrons from NADH. Lactate begins to accumulate in the muscle tissue. Since the body is still using large amounts of ATP but not taking in enough oxygen, it is said to enter a state of oxygen debt.

When the muscular activity ends, the oxygen debt is repaid.

One can use an example of someone running to catch a bus, sprinting for fifty yards at full speed. That is not enough time for the circulation and lungs to respond to the increased demand for oxygen. The muscles have made up the difference between supply and demand with lactic acid fermentation. The individual now sits on the bus and pants to repay their oxygen debt.

Some of the oxygen will go to replenish the store in muscle myoglobin. Some will be used in oxidative metabolism in the muscle to replenish creatine phosphate reserves. The rest deals with the accumulated lactate. The lactate is not all dealt with in the muscle where it was produced. Being a small molecule, it quickly enters the bloodstream. In muscles throughout the body, it is converted back to pyruvate. Pyruvate can then re-enter the oxidative pathway and be used to generate ATP with the use of oxygen. The lactate, then, is being used as a food molecule to supply the needs of resting muscle. Much of the lactate is metabolized in the liver. Some of it will be metabolized with oxygen to produce the energy to convert the rest of it back to glucose. The glucose can then be circulated in the blood or stored as glycogen in the liver or muscles. A minimal amount of lactate is excreted in the urine or sweat.

If the subject of the preceding example missed the bus and ran to the office, lactate would build up in the muscles and the blood. If the office were far enough away, the subject would eventually reach the point of exhaustion and stop running. At that point, the level of lactate in the leg muscles would be high enough to inhibit the enzymes of glycolysis. Glycolysis would slow down so that lactate would not become any more concentrated. The muscles' supply of creatine phosphate would be almost exhausted. Still, the ATP supply would be slightly lower than in a resting muscle. The body is protected from damaging itself: Too much lactate would lower the pH to dangerous levels. The absolute lack of ATP causes muscles to lock, as in rigor mortis. The body's self-protection mechanisms force one to stop before either of these conditions exists. Once the subject stops running and pants long enough, they can continue. The additional oxygen taken in by increased respiration will have metabolized a sufficient amount of lactate to allow the muscles to start working again.

Muscles, which depend heavily on glycolysis when operating under conditions of oxygen debt, fail to perform well if any of the glycolytic enzymes are defective. In cases where an individual has an inherited deficiency of particular enzymes of glycolysis, the consequences for muscle tissue are rather dire. Symptoms include frequent muscle cramps, easy fatigability, and evidence of heavy muscle damage after strenuous exertion.

GLYCOLYSIS AND RED BLOOD CELL FUNCTION

Red blood cells are the oxygen-ferrying units of the bloodstream. They are filled with an iron-containing protein called "hemoglobin." Hemoglobin binds oxygen tightly when oxygen concentrations are high and releases oxygen when there are low oxygen concentrations. Red blood cells must maintain the health and functionality of their hemoglobin stores to perform their task successfully, and glycolysis helps them do that. Approximately 90 to 95 percent of the glucose that enters the cell is metabolized to lactate through glycolysis and lactate dehydrogenase in red blood cells. The ATP generated by glycolysis brings charged atoms into the cell, such as calcium, potassium, and others. The NADH generated by glycolysis is also used to maintain the iron found in hemoglobin in a state that allows it to bind oxygen. Glycolysis is also used to form the metabolite 2,3-DPG (2,3-Diphosphoglycerate). 2,3-DPG binds to hemoglobin and forces it to release oxygen more readily with low oxygen concentrations. Thus, 2,3-DPG aids hemoglobin delivery of oxygen to the tissues.

Abnormalities in the enzymes that catalyze the reactions of glycolysis are inherited. Individuals who inherit two copies of a gene that encodes a glycolytic enzyme's mutant form experience uncontrolled red blood cells' uncontrolled destruction (hemolysis). The red blood cell destruction that results from defects in glycolytic enzymes is chronic and not eased by drugs. An enlarged spleen is a typical symptom of glycolytic enzyme abnormalities. The spleen tends to fill with dying red blood cells. Removal of the spleen reduces red blood cell destruction. The red blood cell destruction can be so severe that blood transfusions might be necessary.

INSULIN, DIABETES, AND GLYCOLYSIS
The hormones insulin and glucagon heavily regulate glycolysis. Insulin, a hormone made and released by the beta cells of the pancreatic islets, stimulates the insertion of the GLUT4 glucose transporter into the membranes of cells. People with type 1 diabetes mellitus, who are incapable of making sufficient quantities of insulin, tend to have very high blood sugar readings. Without insulin, their cells do not receive the signal to insert GLUT4 into their membranes and remove glucose from the circulating blood. Consequently, in type 1 diabetics, the blood glucose level climbs to abnormally high levels. GLUT4 allows the uptake of glucose without the input of energy. Therefore, glycolysis occurs as fast as the cells can take up glucose.

Insulin also stimulates the synthesis of a metabolite called "fructose 2,6-bisphosphate." Fructose 2,6-bisphosphate is a potent activator of phospho-fructokinase, and activation of this enzyme ensures the activation of glycolysis. Insulin also activates the expression of genes that encode the protein involved in glycolysis. In liver cells, reduced glycolytic gene expression and attenuation of the levels of fructose 2,6-bisphosphate reduce glycolysis. During uncontrolled diabetes, reduced glucose transport in muscle diminishes muscle cell glycolysis. Decreased muscle glycolysis contributes to voluntary muscle weakness, liver dysfunction, and heart problems sometimes observed in diabetics.

GLYCOLYSIS AND CANCER
Glucose uptake and its degradation by glycolysis occur ten times faster in tumor cells than in nontumor cells. This phenomenon, called the "Warburg effect," seems to benefit tumor cells since they lack an extensive capillary network to feed them oxygen and rely on anaerobic glycolysis to generate ATP.

Oxygen-poor conditions also induce the synthesis of a protein called the "hypoxia-inducible factor" (HIF). Hypoxia-inducible factor is a transcription factor that helps turn on the expression of specific genes that help cells survive oxygen-poor conditions. HIF activates the synthesis of at least eight glycolytic enzymes. These fundamental observations of cancer cells have shown that glycolytic enzymes are excellent potential drug targets for anticancer agents.

PERSPECTIVE AND PROSPECTS
Cellular respiration is how organisms harvest usable energy in the form of ATP molecules from food molecules. Lactic acid fermentation is used by human muscles when oxygen is in a limited supply. Glycolysis is the energy-producing component of lactic acid fermentation, which is much less efficient than aerobic cellular respiration. Fermentation harvests only two molecules of ATP for every glucose molecule used. In comparison, aerobic respiration produces more than thirty molecules of ATP. The yield of two molecules of ATP for each glucose molecule used is not enough to sustain their high energy demand. Most life forms will resort to fermentation only when oxygen is absent or in short supply. While

multicellular organisms, such as humans, can obtain energy by fermentation for short periods, they incur an oxygen debt that the organism must eventually repay.

Nevertheless, lactic acid fermentation is an essential source of ATP for humans during strenuous physical exercise. Even though it is an inefficient use of glucose, it can provide enough ATP for a short burst of activity. After the activity is over, the lactate produced must be dealt with, which requires oxygen.

Most popular exercise programs focus on aerobic activity. Aerobic exercises do not stress muscles to the point where the blood cannot supply enough oxygen. These exercises are designed to improve the efficiency of the oxygen delivery system so that there is less need for anaerobic metabolism. Training programs attempt to tune the body to reduce the need for lactic acid fermentation. They concentrate on improving oxygen delivery to the muscles, storing oxygen in the muscles, or increasing muscular contraction efficiency.

Insulin signaling activates glycolysis, whereas another pancreatic peptide hormone, glucagon, inhibits glycolysis. People with diabetes can suffer from inadequate glycolytic activity in particular organs, resulting in organ dysfunction. The expression of mutant forms of various glycolytic enzymes or supporting enzymes in transgenic mice has elucidated the link between abnormalities in glycolysis and the pathology of diabetes mellitus.

In the 1920s, the German biochemist Otto Warburg demonstrated that cancer cells voraciously take up glucose and metabolize it to lactate. Glycolysis is very active in cancer cells and helps them flourish under low-oxygen conditions. The development of new glycolytic inhibitors may constitute a new class of anticancer drugs with wide-ranging therapeutic applications.

—*James Waddell, Michael A. Buratovich*

Further Reading

Da Poian, Andrea T., and Miguel A. R. B. Castanho. *Integrative Human Biochemistry: A Textbook for Medical Biochemistry*. 2nd ed., Springer, 2021.

Denniston, Katherine, et al. *General, Organic, and Biochemistry*. 10th ed., McGraw-Hill Education, 2019.

Fox, Stuart Ira, and Krista Rompolski. *Human Physiology*. 16th ed., McGraw-Hill, 2021.

Glycolysis. Physiopedia, n.d., www.physio-pedia.com/Glycolysis. Accessed 14 Apr. 2022.

"Glycolysis Pathway Made Simple!! Biochemistry Lecture on Glycolysis." *YouTube*, uploaded by MEDSimplified, 24 Nov. 2016, www.youtube.com/watch?v=8qij1m7XUhk.

Lodish, Harvey, et al. *Molecular Cell Biology*. 9th ed., W. H. Freeman, 2021.

Nelson, David L., and Michael A. Cox. *Lehninger Principles of Biochemistry*. 8th ed., New York: W. H. Freeman, 2021.

Reece, Jane B., et al. *Campbell Biology: Concepts & Connections*. 8th ed., Pearson, 2020.

HALLER ESTABLISHES PHYSIOLOGY AS A SCIENCE

Category: History of physiology

Specialties and related fields: History and philosophy of science, physiology

Definition: between 1757 and 1766, Haller published his textbook *Elementa physiologiae corporis humani*, a comprehensive work that established physiology as a science independent of anatomy; his discoveries that contractility is a quality inherent in muscles, while sensitivity and pain perception characterize nerve function, laid the foundation of modern neurology

KEY TERMS

contraction: the process in which a muscle becomes or is made shorter and tighter

physiology: a branch of biology that deals with the normal functions of living organisms and their parts

SUMMARY OF EVENT

The development of human physiology as a science required an accurate anatomical understanding of the human body. Scholars, physicians, and artists gained anatomical knowledge through the dissection of cadavers, a practice that began in Europe in the fourteenth century and gradually gained recognition in the fifteenth and especially the sixteenth century. Scientific developments of the seventeenth century led scientists to regard humans as machines, and this mechanical approach dominated research at that time. Albrecht von Haller, a former student of the Dutch mechanist Herman Boerhaave, coined the term *anatomia animata*, or living anatomy.

Boerhaave viewed the human being as a machine composed of hollow and solid elements. Influenced by the teachings of Boerhaave, Haller furthered physiologic understanding by carrying out numerous animal experiments. His areas of interest were multiple: He studied the development of chicken embryos and adopted the preformationist standpoint that the ovum contains a miniature being—a homunculus (little human)—that starts to grow once activated by semen. His work in the field of pulmonology demonstrated that lung expansion requires an airless pleural space. His research correctly ascribed digestive properties to saliva and pancreatic juices, and his understanding of the process of hearing approached that of modern science.

Haller designed hundreds of animal experiments to study muscle and nerve action. Denuded anatomical areas were exposed to thermal, chemical, or mechanical injury. The different reactions of the animal to the noxious stimuli allowed Haller to differentiate between "irritable" and "sensible" tissues. Muscles exhibited "irritability," a contraction of muscle fibers upon stimulation, whereas nerves displayed "sensibility" and were responsible for pain perception. The term "irritability" had been used a century earlier by British physician Francis Glisson,

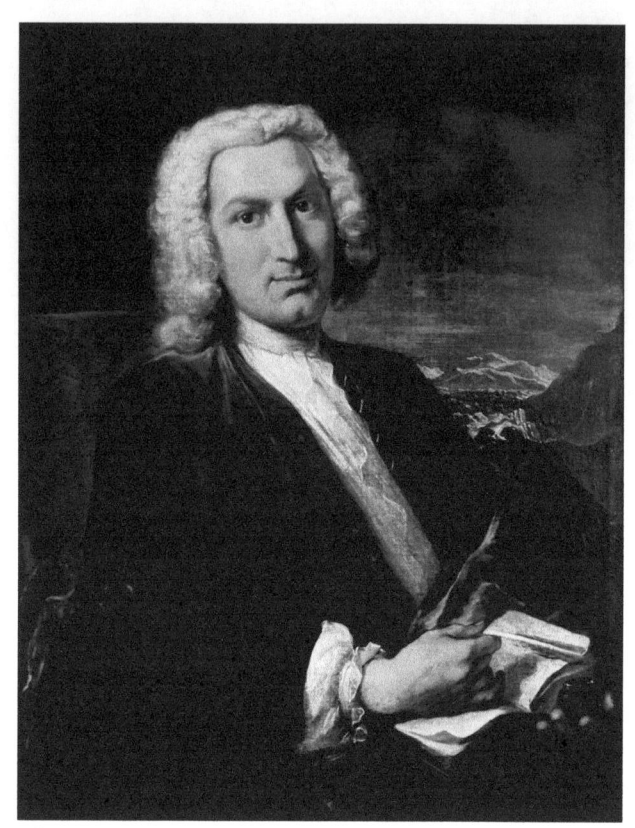

Albrecht von Haller. Portrait by Johann Rudolf Huber, 1736. Image via Wikimedia Commons. [Public domain.]

who presumed that all tissues could contract. Haller, however, showed through careful experimentation that irritability was restricted to muscle fibers.

Having observed that compression of the spinal cord and specific brain areas interfered with the transmission of nerve impulses, Haller could only speculate on the mode of communication between nerve and muscle. He discarded the possibilities of electrical conduction and vibration, hypothesizing that "juice" flowing from the central nervous system through the peripheral nerves led to muscle contraction. The concepts of irritability and sensibility, which Haller first announced in 1739, were discussed again in his monograph *De Partibus Corporis Humani Sensibilibus et Irritabilibus* (1753; *A Dissertation on the Sensible and Irritable Parts of Animals*, 1755). The full development of Haller's concept of nerve and muscle function was published in *Elementa Physiologiae Corporis Humani* (1757-66; *Elements of Human Physiology*).

During his lifetime, Haller published three textbooks of physiology, including a heavily annotated edition of professor Boerhaave's lectures, a text entitled *Primae lineae physiologiae* (1747; Dr. Albert Haller's Physiology, 1754), and the multivolume set *Elementa Physiologiae Corporis Humani*, in which he systematically presents the complete anatomic and physiologic knowledge of the human body. *Elementa Physiologiae Corporis Humani* not only contained macro- and microanatomical information on organ systems but also encompassed their physical and chemical properties. Haller discussed each organ structure and the experiments leading to understanding specific organ functions in minute detail. He provided references for the theories and experiments cited and credited scientists who had contributed to the data.

Haller critically analyzed the available information and avoided drawing unfounded conclusions. In addition to offering a critical analysis of the existing body of knowledge about human physiology, he discussed those contexts in which insufficient or inconclusive data were available to draw firm or meaningful conclusions. His text, therefore, stood as a complete, well-researched scientific work of experimental physiology, detailing the entire state of the field as it then existed and emphasizing what now is the golden rule of medical science: Knowledge and understanding of the human body must be based on valid, well-conceived experiments and reflect the efforts of each contributing researcher.

Haller, who had conducted most of his experimental work during the seventeen years he taught as a professor of anatomy, botany, and surgery at the University of Göttingen, began writing *Elementa Physiologiae Corporis Humani* upon his return to Switzerland in 1753. The first volume, *Fibra, Vasa, Circuitus Sanguinus* (*Fibers, Vessels, The Circulation of Blood*), was published in 1757. He completed the work in 1766, when the eighth volume, *Fetus hominisque vita* (*The Human Fetus and the Life of Man*), came out in print. Like the first volume, the second volume, *Sanguis, Ejus Motus, Humorum Separatio* (1760; *Blood, Its Motion, and the Separation of Fluids*), was dedicated to Frederick V of Denmark.

In the preface to volume 5, *Sensus Externi Interni* (1763; *External and Internal Senses*), Haller defended his theory of irritability and sensibility. The third volume (1761) treated respiratory function and voice, and volume 4, which appeared in 1762, discussed the brain, nerves, and muscles. Volume 6, *Deglutitio, Ventriculus, Omenta, Lien, Pancreas, Hepar* (*Swallowing, Stomach, Omenta, Spleen, Pancreas, Liver*), and volume 7, *Intestina, Chylus, Urina, Semen, Muliebra* (*Intestine, Juice, Urine, Seminal fluid, Female Organs*), were published in 1764 and 1765, respectively.

A complete German translation of Haller's monumental work appeared between 1759 and 1776. Portions of the work have also been translated into French and Dutch but very little into English. In 1774, the first eight pages of *Fibra, Vasa, Circuitus Sanguinus* were translated into English and published in *The Medical Magazine, Or, General Repository of Practical Physic and Surgery* under the title *Elements of Physiology*. Other translations were published in subsequent numbers.

Haller's support of preformationism may have delayed progress in understanding embryology. Still, his breakthrough work in neurology spurred scientists to explore how the transmission of nervous impulses occurred. Luigi Galvani and Alessandro Volta, drawing inspiration from Haller, later demonstrated that muscles would contract when electrically stimulated and paved the way for the development of electrophysiology.

SIGNIFICANCE

Albrecht von Haller's contributions to modern physiology facilitated the understanding of pathologic processes and ultimately led to progress in the treatment and prevention of disease. A mechanistic understanding of life evolved from the simplistic view of bodies as compositions of "beams and levers" and "pipes and vessels" to Haller's realization that living tissues are characterized by their specific functions: The intrinsic property of muscle is to contract, and that of nerves is to feel.

The discovery that the reaction to a stimulus depended on the tissue's organizational makeup—that is, the discovery that tissue was specialized or programmed to act a certain way—was entirely new. Haller's perception that tissues possess "vital properties" stimulated scientific thinking, leading to the concepts of an "internal milieu" and "body homeostasis." In the nineteenth century, it led to the further discovery that even nerves were specialized, as the same stimulus applied to different nerves could produce sight, smell, touch, taste, or sound.

It became increasingly apparent that the harmonious functioning of living organisms required an intricate messenger system: The role of the binding of hormones to their receptors in initiating the informational cascade between different organs has been elucidated, as well as the role of three-dimensional protein structures, play in cellular functioning.

—Elisabeth Faase

Further Reading

Hall, Thomas. *Ideas of Life and Matters*. Vol. 1. U of Chicago P, 1969.

Piccolino, Marco. "Biological Machines: From Mills to Molecules." *Nature Reviews: Molecular Cell Biology*, vol. 1, 2000, pp. 149-53.

Porter, Roy. *Blood and Guts: A Short History of Medicine*. W. W. Norton, 2002.

———. *The Greatest Benefit to Mankind*. W. W. Norton, 1998.

Roe, Shirley. *The Natural Philosophy of Albrecht von Haller*. Arno Press, 1981.

Rothschuh, Karl. *History of Physiology*. Robert E. Krieger, 1973.

Simmons, John. *The Scientific One Hundred: A Ranking of the Most Influential Scientists, Past and Present*. Carol, 1996.

Steinke, Hubert, and Claudia Profos. *Bibliographia Halleriana*. Schwabe Verlag, 2004.

Hypertrophy

Category: Biology
Specialties and related fields: Endocrinology, family medicine, internal medicine
Definition: the growth of a tissue or organ as the result of an increase in the size of the existing cells within that tissue or organ; this process is responsible for the growth of the body as well as for increases in organ size caused by increased workloads on particular organs

KEY TERMS

atrophy: the wasting of tissue, an organ, or an entire body as the result of a decrease in the size or number of the cells within that tissue, organ, or body

compensatory hypertrophy: an increase in the size of a tissue or an organ in response to an increased workload placed upon it

growth: the increase in the size of an organism or any of its parts during the developmental process; caused by increases in both cell numbers and cell size

hyperplasia: the increase in size or growth of a tissue or an organ as a result of an increase in cell numbers, with the size of the cells remaining constant

PROCESS AND EFFECTS

The growth and development of the human body and all its parts require an increase in the number of body cells as the body grows, a process known as "hyperplasia," but also an increase in the size of the existing cells, a process known as "hypertrophy." As humans grow, they increase the number of cells in their bodies, increasing the size of tissues, organs, systems, and the body. For some tissues, organs, and systems, however, the number of cells is genetically set; therefore, the number of cells will increase minimally, if at all, after birth. Thus, if growth occurs in those tissues, organs, and systems, it must occur through an increase in the size of the existing cells.

The hypertrophy process occurs in nearly all tissues in the body but is most common in those tissues where the number of cells is set at the time of birth. Among such tissues are adipose tissue, composed of fat cells and nervous tissue, found in the brain, the spinal cord, and skeletal muscle tissue. Other tissues, such as cardiac and smooth muscle tissue, also show the ability to undergo hypertrophy.

An increase in the amount of fat consumed in the diet increases the amount of fat placed inside a fat cell, increasing the fat cell's size. It is generally true that the number of fat cells within the human body is set at birth. Therefore, an increase in body fat is thought to result primarily from increased fat storage within the fat cells.

The number of nerve cells within the brain and spinal cord also is set at birth. The cerebellum of the human brain, however, increases in size about twentyfold from birth to adulthood. This increase is brought about by an increase in the size of the existing nerve cells, particularly by an increase in the number of extensions protruding from each nerve cell and the length to which the extensions grow. Furthermore, there is an increase in the number of components within the cell. Specifically, there is an increase in the number of mitochondria within the cell, which provide a usable form of energy so that the cell can grow.

The number of skeletal muscle cells is also, in general, preset at the time of birth. The skeletal muscle mass of the human body increases dramatically from birth to adulthood. This increase is accomplished primarily through individual skeletal muscle cell hypertrophy. This increase in the diameter of the individual muscle cells is brought about by increases in the amounts of the contractile proteins, myosin, and actin, as well as increases in the amount of glycogen and the number of mitochondria within individual cells. As each muscle cell increases in size, it causes an increase in the size of the entire muscle of which it is a part.

Each of the examples mentioned above occurs naturally as part of the growth process of the human body. Some tissues, however, are capable of increasing in size as the result of an increased load or demand being placed upon them. This increased load or demand is usually brought about by increased muscle use. This increase in the size of cells in response to increased demand or use is called "compensatory hypertrophy." The skeletal, cardiac, and smooth muscles are the most common tissues that show the phenomenon of compensatory hypertrophy.

Skeletal muscle is particularly responsive to being utilized. However, this response depends on how the skeletal muscle is used. It is well-known that such exercises as weight lifting can increase skeletal muscle size. Lifting heavy weights or objects requires strong contractions of the skeletal muscle doing the lifting. Suppose this lifting continues over a long period. In that case, it eventually increases the size of the existing muscle fibers, increasing the size of the exercised muscle. Since muscle strength depends on its size, increased muscle size causes increased muscle strength. The extent to which the muscle's size increases depends upon the amount of time spent lifting the objects and the weight of the objects. The size that a muscle can reach is, however, limited.

Unlike weight lifting, endurance types of exercise, such as walking, jogging, and aerobics, do not result in larger skeletal muscles. These types of exercise do not force the skeletal muscles to contract forcibly enough to produce muscle hypertrophy.

In the same way that an increased load or use will cause compensatory hypertrophy in skeletal muscle, a decreased use of skeletal muscle will shrink or waste away. This process is referred to as muscle atrophy. This type of atrophy commonly occurs when limbs are broken or injured and must be immobilized. After six weeks of limb immobilization, there is a marked decrease in muscle size. A similar type of atrophy occurs in the limb muscles of astronauts since there is no gravity present in space to provide resistance against which the muscles must work. If the muscles remain unused for more than a few months, there can be a loss of about one-half of the muscle mass of the unused muscle.

Cardiac muscle, like skeletal muscle, can also be caused to hypertrophy by increasing the resistance against which it works. Although endurance exercise does not cause hypertrophy in skeletal muscle, it does increase the heart's size because of the hypertrophy of the existing cardiac muscle cells in this organ. The heart mass of marathon runners enlarges by about 40 percent due to the increase in endurance training. This increase occurs because the heart must work harder to pump more blood to the rest of the body when the body is endurance exercising. Only endurance forms of exercise result in the hypertrophy of the cardiac muscle. Weight lifting, which causes skeletal muscle hypertrophy, does not affect the cardiac muscle.

Smooth muscle also is capable of compensatory hypertrophy. Increased pressure or loads on the smooth muscle within arteries can result in the hypertrophy of the muscle cells. This, in turn, causes a thickening of the arterial wall. Smooth muscle, unlike skeletal and cardiac muscle, is capable of hyperplasia and hypertrophy.

COMPLICATIONS AND DISORDERS

Hypertrophy also occurs as a result of some pathological and abnormal conditions. The most common pathological hypertrophy is an enlargement of the heart due to cardiovascular disease. Most cardiovascular diseases put an increased workload on the heart, making it work harder to pump the blood throughout the body. In response to the increased workload, the heart increases its size, a form of compensatory hypertrophy.

The left ventricle of the heart can hypertrophy to such an extent that its muscle mass may increase four- or fivefold. This increase results from improper functioning of the valves of the left heart. The valves of the heart work to prevent the backflow of blood from one chamber to another or from the arteries back to the heart. Suppose the valves in the left heart are not working properly. In that case, the left ventricle contracts, and blood that should leave the ventricle to go out to the body instead returns to the left ventricle. The enlargement of the left ventricle increases the force with which it can pump the blood out to the body, thus reducing the amount of blood that comes back to the left ventricle despite the damaged heart valves. However, there is a point at which the enlargement of the left ventricle can no longer help keep the needed amount of blood flowing through the body. At that point, the left ventricle finally tires out, and left heart failure occurs.

The same type of hypertrophy can and does occur in the right side of the heart. Again, this is the result of damaged valves that are supposed to prevent the backflow of blood into the heart. Should the valves of both sides of the heart be damaged, hypertrophy can occur on both sides of the heart.

High blood pressure, also known as "hypertension," may lead to hypertrophy of the heart's ventricles. With high blood pressure, the heart must work harder to deliver blood throughout the body because it must pump blood against increased pressure. The cardiac muscle hypertrophies to pump more blood because of the increased demand upon the heart.

The hypertrophy of the heart muscle is beneficial in pumping blood to the body in individuals with valvular disease and hypertension; however, extreme hypertrophy sometimes leads to heart failure. One of the reasons this may occur is the inability of the heart's blood supply to keep up with the growth of the cardiac muscle. As a result, the cardiac cells outgrow their blood supply, resulting in the loss of blood and thus a loss of oxygen and nutrients needed for the cardiac cells to survive.

Smooth muscle, like cardiac muscle, may also hypertrophy under the condition of high blood pressure. Smooth muscle makes up the bulk of many arteries and smaller arterioles in the body. The increased pressure on the arterial walls due to high blood pressure may cause the hypertrophy of the smooth muscles within the walls of the arteries and arterioles. This increases the thickness of the walls of the arteries and arterioles but also decreases the size of the hollow spaces within those vessels, known as the "lumina." In the kidneys, the narrowing of the lumina of the arterioles may result in a decreased blood supply to these organs. The reduced blood flow to the kidneys may eventually cause the kidneys to shut down, leading to renal failure.

Smooth muscle may also hypertrophy under some unique conditions. During pregnancy, the uterus will undergo dramatic hypertrophy. The uterus is a smooth muscle organ involved in housing and nurturing the developing fetus during pregnancy. Immediately before the birth of the fetus, there is marked hypertrophy of the smooth muscle within this organ. This increase in the size of the uterus is beneficial in providing the strong contractions of this organ that are needed for childbirth.

Skeletal muscle also may be caused to hypertrophy in some diseases in which there is an increase in the secretion of male sex hormones, particularly testosterone. Men's higher levels of testosterone, a potent stimulator of muscle growth, are responsible for the fact that males have a larger muscle mass than females. Furthermore, synthetic testosterone-like hormones have been used by some athletes to increase muscle size. These synthetic hormones are called "anabolic steroids." The use of these steroids does result in the hypertrophy of skeletal muscle. Still, anabolic steroids have been shown to have harmful side effects.

Obesity is another condition that results largely from the hypertrophy of existing fat cells. In adults, when weight is lost, it results from a decrease in the size of the existing fat cells; the number of fat cells remains constant. In children, however, obesity is thought to result not only from an increase in the size of fat cells but also from an increase in their number. Thus, it is important to prevent further weight increases in overweight children to prevent the creation of fat cells that will never be lost.

At the onset of diseases that result in muscle degeneration, such as muscular dystrophy, affected muscles undergo hypertrophy. This hypertrophy differs from other forms of muscle hypertrophy in that the muscle cells do not increase in size because of an increase in the contractile protein, mitochondria, or glycogen but because the muscle cells are being filled with fat. As a result of the contractile protein being replaced with fat, the affected muscles are no longer useful.

PERSPECTIVE AND PROSPECTS
The exact mechanisms that control the hypertrophy of cells and tissues are not well understood. During the growth and developmental periods, however, the hypertrophy of many tissues is thought to be under the control of blood-borne chemicals known as "hormones." Among these hormones is one that promotes growth and is thus called "growth hormone." Growth hormone brings about an increase in the number and size of cells. Growth hormone causes the hypertrophy of existing cells by increasing their protein-making capa-

bility. Thus, there is an increase in the number of organelles, such as mitochondria, within the cell, which leads to an increase in cell size.

Growth hormone also causes the release of chemicals known as "growth factors." There are several different growth factors, but one of particular importance is nerve growth factor. Nerve growth factor is involved with the increase in the number of cell processes of single nerve cells. Such chemicals have been shown to enhance the growth of damaged nerve cells in the brains of animals. As a result, nerve growth factor could be used in treating nerve damage in humans by causing the nerves to grow new cell processes and form new connections to replace those damaged. This may be of great importance for treating those suffering from brain or spinal cord damage.

Other hormones may have similar effects on tissues other than nervous tissue. For example, the hypertrophy of the smooth muscle in the uterus is thought to be hormonal. Immediately before birth, when uterine hypertrophy occurs, there is an increased amount of estrogen, the primary female hormone, in the blood. This increase in estrogen is thought to lead to the great enlargement of the uterus during this time. Other hormones have the effect of preventing or inhibiting the hypertrophy of body tissues. The enlargement of the uterus before birth is brought about not only by an increase in estrogen but also by a decrease in another hormone known as "progesterone." Progesterone levels are high in the blood throughout pregnancy. Immediately before birth, however, there is a dramatic decrease in the level of progesterone in the blood. The high level of progesterone prevents or inhibits the hypertrophy of the smooth muscle cells in the uterus since the hypertrophy of this organ will not occur until estrogen levels are high and progesterone levels are low.

It has been suggested that compensatory hypertrophy, such as that which occurs in skeletal, smooth, and cardiac muscle, occurs due to the stretching of the muscle. Some studies have shown that stretching skeletal, cardiac, and smooth muscle leads to hypertrophy. However, American astronauts and Russian cosmonauts showed a loss in muscle mass even though they exercised and stretched their muscles for as much as three hours per day, seven days per week. This suggests that mechanisms other than the stretching of muscles may be involved in compensatory muscle hypertrophy.

By understanding the mechanisms involved in muscle hypertrophy, it may one day be possible to prevent the atrophy that occurs during space flights, prolonged bed rest, and immobilization necessitated by the injury of limbs. Furthermore, understanding the mechanisms that control hypertrophy may help alleviate the effects of disabling diseases such as muscular dystrophy by reversing the effects of muscle atrophy.

—*David K. Saunders*

Further Reading

Barresi, Michael J. F., and Scott F. Gilbert. *Developmental Biology*. 12th ed., Sinauer Associates, 2022.

Hall, John E., and Michael E. Hall. *Guyton and Hall Textbook of Medical Physiology*. 14th ed., Elsevier, 2020.

Marieb, Elaine N., and Suzanne Keller. *Essentials of Human Anatomy and Physiology*. 13th ed., Pearson, 2021.

Melmed, Schlomo, et al. *Williams Textbook of Endocrinology*. 14th ed., Elsevier, 2019.

"Muscular Dystrophy." *Mayo Clinic*, 11 Feb. 2022, www.mayoclinic.org/diseases-conditions/muscular-dystrophy/symptoms-causes/syc-20375388. Accessed 8 June 2022.

Pietrangelo, Ann. "What Causes Muscle Wasting?" *Healthline*, 23 Aug. 2019, www.healthline.com/health/muscle-atrophy. Accessed 8 Jun. 2022.

Tortora, Gerard J., and Bryan Derrickson. *Principles of Anatomy and Physiology*. 16th ed., Wiley, 2020.

Welsh, Charles, and Cynthia Prentice-Craver. *Hole's Human Anatomy & Physiology*. 16th ed., McGraw-Hill Education, 2021.

INFLAMMATION

Category: Disease/Disorder
Specialties and related fields: Family medicine, internal medicine, pathology, rheumatology
Definition: the reaction of blood-filled living tissue to injury

KEY TERMS

chemotaxis: movement of white blood cells toward a gradient of increasing or decreasing concentration of a particular substance

histamine: a small molecule released by cells in response to injury and allergic and inflammatory reactions, causing contraction of smooth muscle and dilation of capillaries

interleukins: members of a class of glycoproteins produced by leukocytes that regulate immune responses

leukocytes: colorless, nucleated, amoeboid cells that circulate throughout the blood and body fluids and destroy or isolate foreign substances and infectious agents, including lymphocytes, granulocytes, monocytes, and macrophages

CAUSES AND SYMPTOMS

In inflammation, the following changes are seen locally: redness, swelling, heat, pain, and loss of function. These changes are chemically mediated. Inflammation may be caused by microbial infection; physical agents such as trauma, radiation, and burns; chemical toxins; caustic substances such as strong acids or bases; decomposing or necrotic tissue; and immune system reactions. Acute inflammation is of relatively short duration (from a few minutes to a day), while chronic inflammation lasts longer. The local changes associated with inflammation include the outflow of fluid into the spaces between cells and the inflow or migration of white blood cells (leukocytes) to the area of injury. Chronic inflammation is characterized by the presence of leukocytes and macrophages and the proliferation of new blood vessels and connective tissue.

Inflammation is a protective mechanism for the body. Inflammation produces heat through increased blood flow and heat-yielding chemical reactions in the local area. Redness is attributable to increased blood flow to the injured area. Swelling is caused by the flow of fluid into the spaces between cells. Swelling stretches the tissue producing pain, but the release of two main chemicals into the bloodstream, prostaglandins and bradykinin, augments pain sensation. Loss of function results from pain (the body limits movement to reduce discomfort) and swelling (interstitial fluid limits movement).

Acute inflammation. Many chemicals are involved in acute inflammation. Mediators of inflammation originate from blood plasma and both damaged and normal cells. Vasoactive amines are a class of chemicals that increase the permeability of blood vessels and cell walls. The most well-studied of these are histamine and serotonin. Histamine is stored in granules in mast cells found in both tissue and basophils, the latter being a type of cell found in the blood. Serotonin is found in mast cells and platelets, another type of cell found in the bloodstream. These substances cause vasodilation (expansion of the walls of blood vessels) and increased vascular permeability (leakage through the walls of small vessels, especially veins). Histamine and serotonin can be released by trauma or exposure to cold. Other chemicals that circulate in the blood can release histamine. Two are part of the complement system; another is called "interleukin-1." The effects of histamine diminish after approximately one hour.

INFORMATION ON INFLAMMATION

Plasma proteases comprise three interrelated systems that explain much about inflammation: the complement, kinin, and clotting systems. The complement system comprises twenty different proteins involved in reactions against microbial agents that invade the body. The various chemicals act in a cascade, like falling dominoes: Each sets off another in sequence. These chemical factors increase vascular permeability, promote chemotaxis (the attraction of living cells to specific chemicals), engulf invading microorganisms, and destroy pathogens through a process called "lysis."

The kinin system releases bradykinin, a chemical substance that causes contraction of smooth muscle tissue, dilation of blood vessels, and pain. The duration of action for bradykinin is brief because the enzyme kininase inactivates it. Bradykinin does not promote chemotaxis.

The clotting system is made up of a series of chemicals that form a solid mass. The most encountered example is the scab that forms at a cut in the skin. Like the complement system, the clotting system is a cascade of thirteen distinct proteins. In addition to producing a solid mass, the clotting system also increases vascular permeability and promotes chemotaxis for white blood cells.

Other substances are involved in acute inflammation. Among the most important of these is a class called "prostaglandins." Several different prostaglandin molecules have been isolated; they are derived from the membranes of most cells. Prostaglandins cause pain, vasodilation, and fever. Aspirin counteracts the effects of prostaglandins, which explains the drug's antipyretic (fever-reducing) and analgesic (pain-reducing) properties.

Another group of substances involved in acute inflammation is leukotrienes. The primary sources for these molecules are leukocytes, and some leukotrienes are found in mast cells. This group promotes vascular leakage but not chemotaxis. They also cause vasoconstriction (a decrease in the diameter of blood vessels) and bronchoconstriction (a decrease in the diameter of air passageways in the

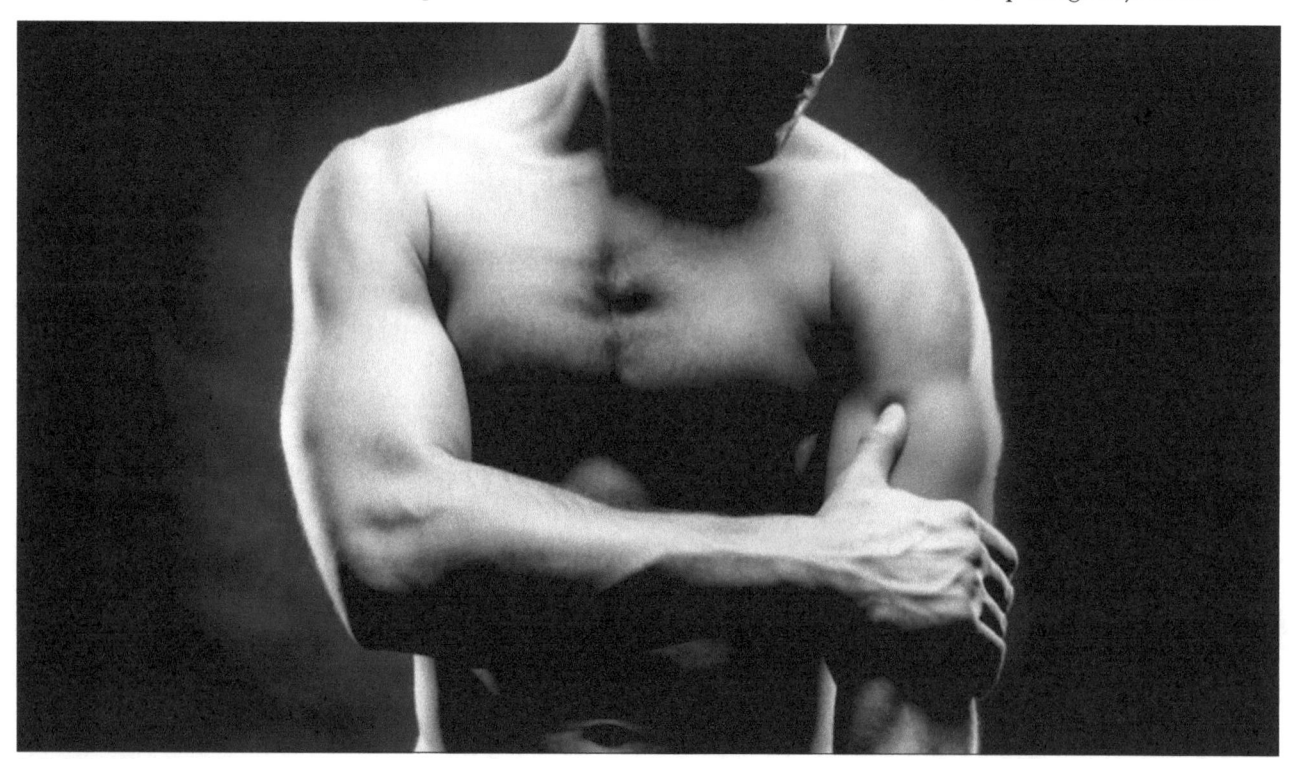

Inflammation occurs when tissues are injured by trauma, bacteria, toxins, or other causes. Photo via iStock/Staras. [Used under license.]

lungs). The effect of these leukotrienes is to slow blood flow and restrict air intake and outflow. A different type of leukotriene is found only in leukocytes. This type enhances chemotaxis but does not contribute to vascular leakage. In addition, leukotrienes cause white blood cells to stick to damaged tissues, speeding the removal of bacteria and promoting healing.

Other chemical substances are known to be involved with inflammation: platelet-activating factor, tumor necrosis factor, interleukin-1, cationic (positively charged) proteins, neutral proteases (enzymes that break down proteins), and oxygen metabolites (molecules resulting from reactions with oxygen). The sources of these are generally leukocytes, although some are derived from macrophages. They reinforce the effects of prostaglandins and leukotrienes.

There are four different outcomes for acute inflammation. There may be a complete resolution in which the injured site is restored to normal; this outcome usually follows a mild injury or limited trauma where there has been only minor tissue destruction. Healing with scarring may occur, in which injured tissue is replaced with scar tissue rich in collagen, giving it strength but at the cost of normal function; this outcome follows more severe injury or extensive destruction of tissue. There may be the formation of an abscess, characterized by pus, which follows injuries that become infected with pyogenic (pus-forming) organisms. The fourth outcome is chronic inflammation.

Chronic inflammation. Acute inflammation may be followed by chronic inflammation. This reaction occurs when the organism, factor, or agent responsible for the acute inflammation is not removed or when the normal healing processes fail to occur. Repeated episodes of acute inflammation may also lead to chronic inflammation. The stages of acute inflammation seem to remain for long periods. In addition, chronic inflammation may begin insidiously, such as with a low-grade infection or other processes that do not display the usual signs of acute inflammation; tuberculosis, rheumatoid arthritis, and chronic lung disease are examples of this third alternative.

Chronic inflammation typically occurs in one of the following conditions: prolonged exposure to potentially toxic substances such as asbestos, coal dust, and silica that are nondegradable; immune reactions against one's tissue (autoimmune diseases such as lupus and rheumatoid arthritis); and persistent infection by an organism that is either resistant to drug therapy or insufficiently toxic to cause an immune reaction (such as viruses, tuberculosis, and leprosy). The characteristics of chronic inflammation are similar to those of acute inflammation but are less dramatic and more protracted.

—*L. Fleming Fallon Jr.*

Further Reading

Challem, Jack. *The Inflammation Syndrome: Your Nutritional Plan for Great Health, Weight Loss, and Pain-Free Living.* Rev. ed., Wiley-Blackwell, 2010.

Dartt, Darlene A. *Immunology, Inflammation and Diseases of the Eye.* Academic Press, 2011.

Gallin, John I., and Ralph Snyderman, editors. *Inflammation: Basic Principles and Clinical Correlates.* 3rd ed., Raven Press, 1999.

Górski, Andrzej, Hubert Krotkiewski, and Michal Zimecki, editors. *Inflammation.* Kluwer, 2001.

Guha, Sushovan, et al. *Inflammation, Lifestyle, and Chronic Disease: The Silent Link.* CRC Press, 2012.

Kumar, Vinay, et al., editors. *Robbins and Cotran: Pathologic Basis of Disease.* 8th ed., Saunders/Elsevier, 2010.

McPherson, R. "Inflammation and Coronary Artery Disease: Insights from Genetic Studies." *The Canadian Journal of Cardiology*, vol. 28, no. 6, 2012, pp. 662-66.

Meggs, William Joel, and Carol Svec. *The Inflammation Cure.* Contemporary Books, 2004.

Preddy, Victor R., and Ronald R. Watson. *Bioactive Food as Interventions and Related Inflammatory Diseases.* Elsevier/Academic Press, 2013.

Yian, Gu, and Nikolas Scarmeas. "Dietary Inflammation Factor Rating System and Risk of Alzheimer Disease in Elder." *Alzheimer Disease and Associated Disorders*, vol. 25, no. 2, 2011, pp. 149-54.

Iron-Deficiency Anemia

Category: Condition
Specialties and related fields: Dietetics, hematology, nutrition, sports medicine
Definition: a type of anemia that develops if you do not have enough iron in your body

KEY TERMS

anemia: a condition in which the blood doesn't have enough healthy red blood cells

anisocytosis: a condition in which red blood cells are unequal in size

bone marrow: a soft fatty substance in the cavities of bones where blood cells are produced

duodenum: the first part of the small intestine; it is located between the stomach and the middle part of the small intestine, or jejunum

erythropoiesis: a tightly regulated, complex process originating in the bone marrow from a multipotent stem cell and terminating in a mature, enucleated erythrocyte.

hematopoiesis: the formation of blood cellular components

hemoglobin: a protein inside red blood cells that carries oxygen from the lungs to tissues and organs in the body and carries carbon dioxide back to the lungs

microcytosis: a condition in which red blood cell size smaller than the normal range

mucosa: the moist, inner lining of some organs and body cavities (such as the nose, mouth, lungs, and stomach

ERYTHROCYTE PRODUCTION

Anemia is a physical condition characterized by red blood cell deficiencies. Red blood cell production is a multistep process called "erythropoiesis." Erythropoiesis is a subprocess of the larger process of hematopoiesis, how all blood cells are made from hematopoietic stem cells in the bone marrow.

Hematopoiesis occurs in the bone marrow, predominantly in the pelvis, ribs, and sternum. Bone marrow resides inside the bone and contains various cell types. One bone marrow cell type is the hematopoietic stem cells (HSCs). Stem cells can divide throughout their lifetime, and their progeny can differentiate into various cell types. HSCs divide, and one cell remains an HSC, but the daughter cell becomes a progenitor of myeloid cells (erythrocytes, megakaryocytes, basophils, macrophages, eosinophils, or neutrophils) or lymphoid cells (B- and T-lymphocytes or natural killer cells). This progenitor cell responds to available signals to become one blood cell type or another. These signals are cytokines, growth factors, or cell adhesion events.

During infections, endothelial cells that line blood vessels and macrophages, T-lymphocytes, and natural killer cells secrete glycoproteins called granulocyte-macrophage colony-stimulating factor (GM-CSF) or granulocyte colony-stimulating factor (G-CSF). Granulocyte-macrophage colony-stimulating factor activates HSC daughter cells to divide and differentiate into monocytes, neutrophils, eosinophils, and basophils. This growth factor hastens the maturation of these white blood cells. Granulocyte colony-stimulating factor specifically induces neutrophil maturation.

Platelets bud from megakaryocytes in the bone marrow and are released into the bloodstream. Thrombopoietin, a growth factor made by the liver and kidneys, stimulates megakaryocyte differentiation and accelerates platelet production.

The cytokine erythropoietin is synthesized by the kidneys and, to a lesser extent, the liver. Erythropoietin drives HSC daughter cells to become erythrocytes or red blood cells. Red blood cells (RBCs) begin as proerythroblasts with large nuclei and many ribosomes. The proerythroblast becomes a basophilic erythroblast when the nucleus shrinks, and the cytoplasm contains increased numbers of ribosomes producing the protein hemoglobin. The next stage is the polychromatic erythroblast. This stage is the last precursor capable of mitosis. This precursor has a very gray cytoplasm because of the presence of hemoglobin.

The normoblast stage is the first nonmitotic precursor of erythropoiesis. Normoblasts have a small, dense nucleus. The next stage is the reticulocyte stage, when the nucleus is extruded. A reticular network of ribosomes in the cytoplasm gives the cell a stippled appearance in the microscope. Reticulocytes can carry oxygen and are gradually released into the bloodstream. In adults, 0.5 to 2.0 percent and in infants 2 to 6 percent of their RBCs are reticulocytes. Once all the ribosomes are cleared from the cytoplasm, the cell is a mature erythrocyte.

Red blood cells are packed with the protein hemoglobin. Hemoglobin contains four polypeptide chains, and four flat molecules called "hemes" with an iron ion at their center. Heme synthesis begins by combining a Krebs cycle intermediate known as succinyl-coenzyme with the amino acid glycine to make 5-aminolevulinic acid (ALA). The enzyme catalyzing this reaction, ALA synthase, uses a pyridoxal phosphate coenzyme. Pyridoxal phosphate is made from dietary vitamin B_6. Dietary vitamin B_6 deficiencies can cause hemoglobin deficiencies and anemia.

Hemoglobin production also requires lots of iron. Insufficient bodily iron decreases hemoglobin synthesis, causing iron-deficiency anemia (IDA). Iron-deficiency anemia is the most common type of anemia worldwide.

Red blood cells use their iron-laden hemoglobin molecules to ferry molecular oxygen to tissues and cells. Oxygen is the terminal electron acceptor for the electron transport chains in our cells through which cells make most of their adenosine triphosphate (ATP). Without oxygen, cells become anoxic and may die.

Red blood cells usually live 120 days. When they die, their iron is recycled, and their heme is degraded to bilirubin. Bilirubin is processed and excreted by the liver, derivatized in the intestines, and excreted by the kidneys. We lose about 1 milligram (mg) of iron every day through sweat, sloughed skin cells, and lost gastrointestinal cells excreted in feces. Daily iron intake averages about 10 to 20 mg, and people absorb about ten percent of it (1 to 2 mg).

IRON PHYSIOLOGY

Human diets consume two forms of iron. Iron bound to heme (heme iron) that comes from meat and nonheme iron found in plant-based foods like beans and spinach. Heme iron is in the Fe^{+2} or ferrous state, and heme-free iron is in the ferric or Fe^{+3} state.

When iron-containing food is digested in the gastrointestinal tract, its iron is released. Heme iron is directly absorbed by duodenal mucosal cells. These cells degrade the heme and free the Fe^{+2} iron. Nonheme ferric iron is reduced to ferrous iron by ferrireductase enzymes in the duodenum. Stomach acid activates ferrireductase (Dcytb) with the help of ascorbic acid (vitamin C). The iron transporter DMT-1 transports Fe^{+2} into duodenal mucosal cells where a protein, ferritin, binds it. Ferritin temporarily stores the iron until the body needs it.

When the body needs iron, the enzyme hephaestin converts Fe^{+2} to Fe^{+3}. The iron transport protein transferrin binds ferric iron and ferries it to cells that need it. Transferrin binds to transferrin receptors, and target cells use receptor-mediated endocytosis to engulf the transferrin and its iron. Cells can store excess iron in ferritin if needed.

CAUSES AND SYMPTOMS

Iron-deficiency anemia results from decreased dietary iron intake, decreased iron absorption, decreased iron demand, or decreased iron loss. The most common cause of IDA is decreased iron intake, particularly in infants, since breast milk is low in iron. Vegetarians who eat nonheme iron sources, which are more difficult to absorb, also are at higher risk of IDA.

Iron-deficiency anemia, due to decreased iron absorption, may result from diminished stomach acid production. People who have had part of their stomach surgically removed (gastrectomy) or take proton pump inhibitors (e.g., omeprazole, lansoprazole, rabeprazole, esomeprazole, pantoprazole, and others) may suffer from IDA due to poor iron absorption. Alternatively, inflammatory bowel diseases such as Crohn disease or celiac disease can damage duodenal cells, inhibiting iron absorption.

Increased iron demand usually occurs in rapidly growing children and adolescents who require more iron to make more hemoglobin. Pregnancy also increases iron demand since the growing fetus requires more iron from the mother's body.

Increased iron loss commonly occurs in those with slow bleeds. Older individuals with colon cancer may have black, tarry stools that result from cancers of the right, ascending colon that routinely bleed. Iron-deficiency anemia is one of the first symptoms of colon cancer. Women with frequent or heavy menstrual cycles or those with bleeding gastric ulcers may also suffer from IDA. *Helicobacter pylori* infections of the stomach cause gastric ulcers and gastrointestinal bleeding. *H. pylori* can sequester iron from various bodily sources, depriving the body of iron. Hookworm infections in developing countries are another source of constant blood loss that causes IDA.

Iron-deficiency anemia prevents normal hemoglobin production. Insufficient hemoglobin levels cause the bone marrow to make smaller (microcytic) RBCs. These microcytic RBCs also have a pale look, making them hypochromic. Consequently, IDA causes microcytic and hypochromic anemia.

Microcytic, hypochromic RBCs poorly transport oxygen to tissues, starving the tissues of oxygen and causing hypoxia. Hypoxia generates signals to the bone marrow to increase RBC production. The bone

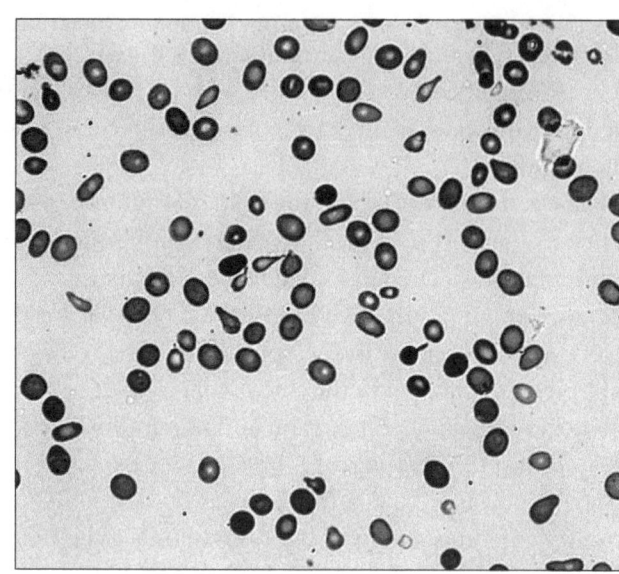

Figure 1. Human red blood cells showing poikilocytosis. Photo by Dr. Graham Beards, via Wikimedia Commons

marrow starts to make poorly formed RBCs, like a bakery with too little time to make too many biscuits. The bone marrow produces RBCs of various shapes (poikilocytosis) and sizes (anisocytosis; Fig. 1).

Iron-deficiency anemia—induced anoxia also adversely affects ATP production. The most heavily affected are fast-growing cells found in hair, finger, and toenails. Thin, fragile hair with seemingly inexplicable alopecia (hair loss) and brittle nails that crack and grow slowly are signs of IDA. Symptoms include pale skin (pallor), racing, irregular heartbeat (palpitations), shortness of breath (dyspnea), and a lack of stamina (easy fatiguability). Some with IDA may have an appetite for nonfood items like dirt, paper, or clay (pica). Iron-deficiency anemia can also cause spooning of the fingernails (koilonychia; Fig. 2).

Other diseases can cause IDA secondarily. Plummer-Vinson syndrome, a disease with no known cause, produces a triad of symptoms, including anemia, difficulty swallowing, and growths at the back of the throat (esophageal web). This condition also causes tongue inflammation (glossitis) and damage to the esophageal epithelium and mucosae.

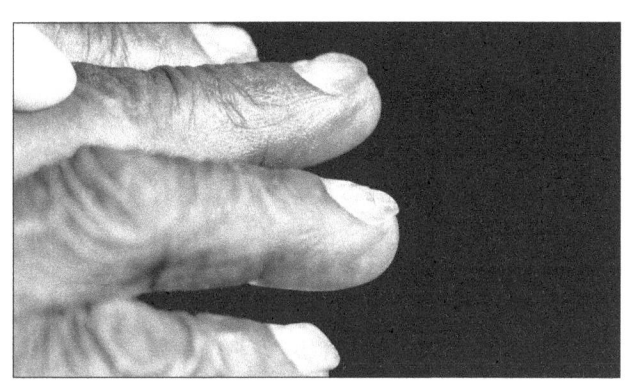

Figure 2. Koilonychia in an IDA patient. Photo by CHeitz, via Wikimedia Commons.

Plummer-Vinson syndrome increases the risk of pharyngeal or esophageal carcinoma.

TREATMENT AND THERAPY

Anemia diagnosis requires several blood tests. The most important is a complete blood count (CBC). Iron-deficiency anemia shows abnormally low hemoglobin levels that are < 13.5 g/dL in males and < 12.0 g/dL in females. The mean corpuscular volume (MCV) decreases since the RBCs are microcytic.

Other blood tests should measure iron, ferritin, and total iron-binding capacity (TIBC), which measures unbound transferrin in blood. Serum iron and ferritin levels are low in IDA patients, but the TIBC is higher than normal levels (Table 1).

Red blood cell size distribution also shows abnormally wide variability. The RBC distribution width or RDW measures the range of RBC sizes. Normal. Red blood cells have a small size variation range, and a normal RDW is 12 to 15 percent. However, an RDW of over ninety percent in IDA is not uncommon.

A blood smear of freshly drawn blood viewed with brightfield microscopy shows microcytic RBCs with anisocytosis.

Iron-deficiency anemia treatment requires oral or parenteral iron supplements. Ferrous sulfate is the most common oral iron supplement. This compound comes as a powder that is mixed with beverages and quaffed. Taking ferrous sulfate with acidic drinks like orange juice or soda increases its absorption. Ferrous sulfate heavily stains the teeth and gums. Therefore, drinking it through a straw and washing your mouth can avert this unpleasant side effect. Other oral iron formulations include ferrous gluconate and ferrous fumarate. People should take 2 to 5 mg of iron per kilogram of body weight daily. Patients should take all oral iron supplements on an empty stomach since food decreases iron absorption.

Health-care providers should use oral iron supplements with caution in people with peptic ulcer disease, regional enteritis, ulcerative colitis, and severe liver disease. Administering iron with antacids or the antibiotic tetracycline reduces iron absorption. Suppose a patient must take both drugs. Then they should separate their administration by at least two hours. Pregnancy increases iron absorption but also increases the incidence of gastrointestinal complications. Finally, giving iron supplements with dairy products can interfere with iron absorption.

If IDA individuals cannot take oral iron supplements, then the drug of choice is intravenous iron supplements. Four different intravenous iron supplements exist, including iron dextran, ferumoxytol, iron sucrose, and sodium iron gluconate complex (SFGC).

Iron dextran is contraindicated in IDA patients on dialysis. Some patients also have severe allergic reactions to the dextran component of iron dextran. Allergies to other intravenous iron supplements are

TABLE 1 – NORMAL LABORATORY IRON BLOOD TEST RESULTS

Blood Iron Levels	Blood Ferritin Levels	TIBC
60–170 mcg/dL, or 10.74–30.43 micromol/L	Male: 12–300 ng/mL Female: 12–150 ng/mL	240–450 mcg/dL, or 42.96–80.55 micromol/L

rare. When using iron dextran, health-care providers should give a test dose first. If that test dose is well tolerated, the health-care providers should prepare life-support equipment first, then administer the iron dextran while keeping injectable epinephrine ready.

Ferumoxytol (Feraheme) is limited to those with chronic kidney disease, even if they are on dialysis or receiving erythropoietin. Patients receive two ferumoxytol doses over three to eight days.

Iron-deficiency anemia patients receive three to ten doses of iron sucrose over several weeks. This drug is administered to patients with chronic kidney disease regardless of their dialysis status. Sodium iron gluconate complex has the same dosing schedule as iron sucrose. It is used in IDA patients undergoing long-term hemodialysis.

The common adverse effect of oral iron supplementation is gastrointestinal distress (nausea, constipation, heartburn) with oral formulations. This unfortunate side effect may resolve with continued use of the supplements. Oral iron supplements are usually taken on an empty stomach, but should the patient find the gastric disturbance intolerable, administer them with food and acidic drinks (preferable orange juice). Primary care providers should monitor the patient's bowel pattern and intervene as needed.

Other complications of intravenous iron supplements include low blood pressure (hypotension). Health-care providers should monitor all vital signs while administering intravenous iron. In children, fatal iron toxicity can occur if they consume 2 to 10 grams (gm) of iron. Iron toxicity causes severe gastrointestinal symptoms, shock, acidosis, and liver and heart failure. To treat this, providers should give the iron-chelating agent deferoxamine. No one should even receive oral and parenteral iron supplements simultaneously.

All IDA patients should increase their water and fiber intake and maintain an exercise program to counter the constipation effects of iron. Patients should consume iron-rich foods, including liver, egg yolks, muscle meats, yeast, grains, and green leafy vegetables.

If iron supplements work, the patient's reticulocyte count should increase at least one week after beginning iron therapy. The patient's hemoglobin level should increase by 2 g/dL one month after beginning therapy. Finally, their fatigue and pallor should disappear, and the patient should show increased energy levels.

Severe IDA cases that resist treatment with iron supplements may require a blood transfusion.

Iron toxicity is treated with iron chelators. These include deferoxamine (Desferal), administered subcutaneously, and deferasirox (Exjade® or Jadenu®). Deferasirox is a once-daily oral chelator that comes as a dispersible or film-coated tablet.

PERSPECTIVE AND PROSPECTS

The German physiologist Karl Vierordt and his student H. Welcher discovered IDA in 1852. Vierordt pioneered techniques for determining erythrocyte numbers in blood and invented the precursor to the blood pressure cuff. Vierordt's discoveries remained dormant until 1949 when C. A. Finch and his colleagues observed cultured reticulocytes incorporated iron from blood plasma to make hemoglobin. These observations established the importance of iron for hemoglobin synthesis. Twenty years later (1969), Evan Morgan and his colleagues demonstrated the role of transferrin in bringing iron to cells. Morgan observed that cells internalized the bound transferrin and made one of the first observations of the internalization of a membrane protein. Ten years after Morgan's blockbuster discovery (1979), T. H. Bothwell, with C. A. Finch and others, published a monograph on iron physiology in the human body. This work shows that iron metabolism was well understood at this time.

In 1990, the Nobel Committee awarded E. Donnall Thomas the Nobel Prize in Medicine for his discoveries about bone marrow transplantation. A coauthor with C. A. Finch on his pioneering 1949 paper, Thomas earned his medical degree at Harvard University in 1946. Thomas showed that providing new bone marrow cells from healthy donors to leukemia patients through transplants saved their lives.

Work on iron and RBC production provided new dietary recommendations concerning iron. Consequently, the worldwide anemia prevalence decreased from 40.2 percent to 32.9 percent between 1990 and 2010.

Several studies have established that young female athletes are at higher risk for IDA than nonathletes. Male athletes also may suffer from IDA, but their risk remains lower than women's. Coaches, athletic trainers, physical therapists, and sports physicians who train and watch over female athletes should remain vigilant for IDA signs and symptoms. A review of iron supplementation studies by the Cochrane Reviews concluded that iron supplementation effectively reduces anemia incidence in young women. Therefore, athletic programs should provide athletes with regular nutritional advice and iron-based supplements if necessary. Also, any athlete at risk for iron deficiency should perform non-weight-bearing, low-intensity sports to avoid inducing hemolysis that leads to IDA.

—*Michael A. Buratovich*

Further Reading

Garrison, Cheryl. *The Iron Disorders Institute Guide to Anemia: Understanding the Causes, Symptoms, and Healing of Iron Deficiency and Other Anemias.* 2nd ed., Cumberland House, 2009.

"Iron-Deficiency Anemia." *American Society of Hematology,* 2022, www.hematology.org/education/patients/anemia/iron-deficiency.

"Iron-Deficiency Anemia." *Mayo Clinic,* 4 Jan. 2022, www.mayoclinic.org/diseases-conditions/iron-deficiency-anemia/symptoms-causes/syc-20355034.

Low, Michael Sze Yuan, et al. "Daily Iron Supplementation for Improving Anaemia, Iron Status and Health in Menstruating Women." *The Cochrane Database of Systematic Reviews,* vol. 4, CD009747, 2016, doi:10.1002/14651858.CD009747.pub2.

Ponorac, Nenad, et al. "Professional Female Athletes Are at a Heightened Risk of Iron-Deficient Erythropoiesis Compared with Nonathletes." *International Journal of Sport Nutrition and Exercise Metabolism,* vol. 30, no. 1, 2020, pp. 48-53, doi:10.1123/ijsnem.2019-0193.

Sheftel, Alex D., et al. "The Long History of Iron in the Universe and in Health and Disease." *Biochimica et Biophysica Acta,* vol. 1820, no. 3, 2012, pp. 161-87, doi:10.1016/j.bbagen.2011.08.002.

Thomas, E. Donnall. "Facts." *Nobel Prize Outreach AB 2022,* NobelPrize.org, 24 June 2022, www.nobelprize.org/prizes/medicine/1990/thomas/facts/.

Lactate Threshold

Category: Physical training

Specialties and related fields: Biochemistry, exercise science, physical fitness, strength and conditioning

Definition: the point during exercise when the human body begins to make more lactate, or lactic acid, than it can simultaneously break down

KEY TERMS

aerobic: metabolic processes that utilize oxygen

anaerobic: metabolic processes that occur in the absence of oxygen

lactate: an organic acid the body forms when it breaks down carbohydrates to use for energy, while oxygen levels are low

metabolism: the sum of biochemical reactions that occur in the human body's cells. These reactions include anabolic reactions, energy-demanding reactions that build larger, more complex molecules from smaller, simpler precursors, and catabolic reactions that yield energy by degrading larger, reduced molecules into smaller, more oxidized ones

INTRODUCTION

The lactate threshold is the point at which the human body begins to make more lactate or lactic acid than it can simultaneously break down. The body creates lactate mainly during intense exercise when the body requires large amounts of oxygen. Lactate can build up in the body and cause several side effects, including burning muscles. Understanding the lactate threshold is important for athletes. Athletes who exercise just below their lactate thresholds can avoid the sore muscles common to lactic acid buildup. Exercising just below this level can also help athletes' bodies take in more oxygen. A person's lactate threshold depends on more than just exercise. Age, weight, body chemistry, and other factors affect a person's lactate threshold. Furthermore, people with certain health conditions will have different lactate thresholds.

BACKGROUND

Intense exercise can be very beneficial for the human body as it increases the heart rate and the amount of oxygen in the blood. This increased oxygen and increased body temperature can also cause many different chemical reactions in the body. The chemical reactions that take place in the body are affected by numerous variables. For example, a person's age, size, sex, and blood type can all affect chemical reactions in the body.

Some chemical changes take place in people's blood. When people exercise, the body needs to find ways to get energy quickly. The human body com-

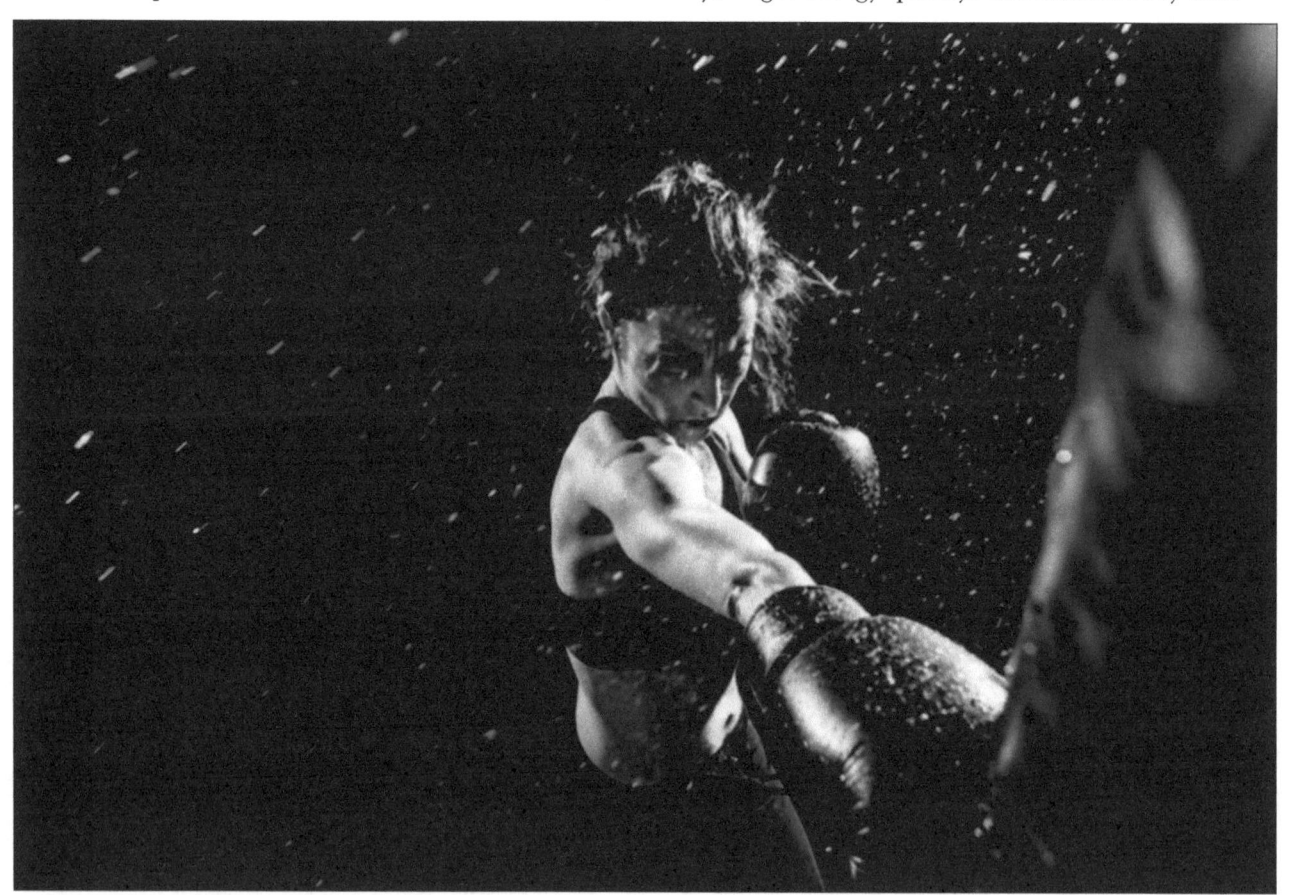

An individual's lactate threshold defines the upper limits of their sustainable training efforts. Photo via iStock/sanjeri. [Used under license.]

pletes two functions to produce energy: aerobic and anaerobic respiration. The body breaks down glucose to make energy through aerobic respiration. This process requires oxygen. However, when a person exercises at a high intensity, the body does not bring in enough oxygen to get all its energy from aerobic respiration. The body can also get energy through anaerobic respiration. This process creates energy and does not require oxygen.

When the body does not have enough oxygen, one of the waste products of anaerobic respiration is lactate or lactic acid. Although anaerobic respiration is useful because it gives the body energy during intense workouts, the lactic acid can build up in the body, causing negative side effects. Once a person reaches the point in exercise where the body no longer has enough oxygen to break down the lactic acid, and the lactic acid begins to build up, that person has reached the lactate threshold.

OVERVIEW

As people increase the intensity of their workouts, their bodies' lactic acid output also increases. When the body is ridding the body of lactic acid faster than it produces the acid, the body has not met the lactic threshold. A person's lactate threshold is the point when lactate begins to build up in the body, causing lactic acidosis. Lactic acidosis occurs when people surpass the lactate threshold and have lactate in their system. Lactic acidosis can cause side effects for some people. For example, some people experience stomachache, nausea, and rapid breathing. Since lactic acid is acidic, it can cause a burning sensation in the muscles and make them sore for days. The effects of lactic acidosis are generally temporary. They will usually go away after a period of rest. However, the symptoms can be unpleasant when a person experiences them. If the symptoms persist, the person should see a medical professional.

When a person feels the symptoms of lactic acidosis, that person should begin to decelerate their exercise. However, it is not generally recommended to stop intense exercise abruptly. Instead, a person can begin to slow the physical activity and eventually stop the exercise altogether. People who experience lactic acidosis should rest and give their bodies time to recuperate before exercising again. People who experience lactic acidosis should also drink plenty of water. Although intense exercise is among the most common causes of the body reaching the lactate threshold, it is not the only cause. Medical disorders, such as cancer, seizures, shock, and sepsis, can also cause lactic acidosis.

Medical professionals and scientists can determine the lactate threshold through medical testing. To test a person's lactate threshold, a researcher will have the person perform vigorous physical activity. Then, the research will collect blood samples to measure the amount of lactate in the blood. When the body begins accumulating lactate, the researchers know a person has exceeded the lactate threshold. Researchers measure lactate threshold to understand more about intense exercise and body function. They also measure the lactate threshold to help individual athletes understand their lactate thresholds. Athletes who know their lactate thresholds can measure the intensity of a workout and understand what level of intensity is as high as it can be without passing the threshold. That means the athlete can work out as much as possible without getting the buildup of lactate in the muscles that causes discomfort.

Athletes are interested in their lactate threshold since it can indicate their ideal level of exercise intensity. If athletes exercised lower than their lactate threshold, they would not be working as hard as they could; however, if they worked at higher than their lactate threshold, they would experience lactic acidosis, which would hurt their performance in the end. Athletes who train just at their lactate threshold can increase their lactate threshold. When athletes work out, they increase their bodies' ability to take in oxygen. As a person's body takes in more oxygen, the body can rid itself of more lactic acid. For this and other reasons, most athletes aim to increase the amount of oxygen their bodies can bring in.

Some athletes use interval training to increase their lactate threshold. In interval training, a person performs intervals of extremely intense physical exercise and intervals of much less intense exercise. If athletes feel that the intensity at which they are excising is too easy, they might be tempted to increase the intensity; however, their bodies will begin to produce excess lactate if they increase the intensity past the lactate threshold. Instead, athletes can increase the duration of their workouts so they can fully exhaust themselves without ever producing an overabundance of lactate and experience the negative side effects that lactate buildup can cause.

—Elizabeth Mohn

Further Reading

Blahd, William. "Lactic Acidosis and Exercise: What You Need to Know." *WebMD*, 14 July 2017, www.webmd.com/fitness-exercise/guide/exercise-and-lactic-acidosis#1. Accessed 11 June 2019.

Blessing, Jill. "The Chemical Reaction That Takes Place in the Body after Exercise." *Live Strong*, www.livestrong.com/article/375841-the-chemical-reaction-that-takes-place-in-the-body-after-exercise/. Accessed 11 June 2019.

Ghosh, Asok Kumar. "Anaerobic Threshold: Its Concept and Role in Endurance Sport." *US National Library of Medicine*, 2004, www.ncbi.nlm.nih.gov/pmc/articles/PMC3438148/. Accessed 11 June 2019.

Hyman, Lindsay. "The Performance Benefits of Lactate Threshold Testing and Training." *CTS*, trainright.com/the-performance-benefits-of-lactate-threshold-testing-and-training/. Accessed 11 June 2019.

Kravitz, Len, and Lance Dalleck. "Lactate Threshold Training." *University of New Mexico*, www.unm.edu/~lkravitz/Article%20folder/lactatethreshold.html. Accessed 11 June 2019.

"Lactate Threshold 101." *Bicycling*, 30 Apr. 2010, www.bicycling.com/training/a20017067/lactate-threshold-101/. Accessed 12 June 2019.

"Lactate Threshold Testing." *Exercise Physiology Core Laboratory*. University of Virginia Health System, med.virginia.edu/exercise-physiology-core-laboratory/fitness-assessment-for-community-members/lactate-threshold-testing/. Accessed 12 June 2019.

Quinn, Elizabeth. "Lactate Threshold Training for Athletes." *VeryWell Fit*, 19 Nov. 2018, www.verywellfit.com/lactate-threshold-training-3120092. Accessed 11 June 2019.

Sparacino, Alyssa. "How to Improve Your Lactate Threshold." *Shape*, 4 Apr. 2019, www.shape.com/fitness/tips/how-improve-lactate-threshold-workouts. Accessed 12 June 2019.

Metabolism

Category: Biology

Specialties and related fields: Biochemistry, cytology, exercise physiology, gastroenterology, nutrition, pharmacology, physiology

Definition: the processes by which the substance of plants and animals incidental to life is built up and broken down

KEY TERMS

adipose tissue: tissue that stores fat; occurs in humans beneath the skin, usually in the abdomen or in the buttocks

anabolism: the metabolic activity through which complex substances are synthesized from simpler substances

basal metabolic rate (BMR): the standardized measure of metabolism in warm-blooded organisms

beta-oxidation: the catabolic process by which fatty acid molecules are broken down

calorie: a measurement of heat, particularly in measuring the value of foods for producing energy and heat in an organism

catabolism: the complete breaking down of molecules by an organism to obtain chemical building blocks and capture and store energy *essential nutrients*: molecules that an organism needs for survival but cannot manufacture itself

glycolysis: the breakdown of glucose by enzymes, releasing energy and pyruvic acid

ketogenesis: the biochemical process through which organisms produce ketone bodies by breaking down fatty acids and ketogenic amino acids

Krebs cycle: the sequence of reactions by which most living cells generate energy during aerobic respiration. It takes place in the mitochondria, consuming oxygen, producing carbon dioxide and water as waste products, and converting adenosine diphosphate (ADP) to energy-rich adenosine triphosphate (ATP)

mitochondria: an organelle found in large numbers in most cells, in which the biochemical processes of respiration and energy production occur; it has a double membrane, the inner layer being folded inward to form layers (cristae)

oxidative phosphorylation: the metabolic pathway in which cells use enzymes to oxidize nutrients, thereby releasing chemical energy to produce adenosine triphosphate

standard metabolic rate (SMR): the standardized measure of metabolism in cold-blooded organisms

storage compounds: areas in the body that store nutrients not immediately required by an organism

STRUCTURE AND FUNCTIONS

Metabolism is an ongoing process in living organisms. It is fundamentally concerned with the chemistry of life. An organism's metabolic rate is the rate at which it consumes the energy it derives from the nutrients that sustain it. Organisms consume energy by converting chemical energy to heat and external work; most of the latter is converted to heat as external work, such as walking or moving, overcomes friction. Therefore, a workable measure of metabolic rate is the rate at which an organism produces heat. The food that organisms ingest is measured in calories, each calorie being the quantity of energy required to raise the temperature of one kilogram of water molecule one degree Celsius.

Metabolism consists of two essential underlying processes, anabolism, and catabolism. Anabolism is the energy-demanding process of synthesizing biological molecules from simpler precursors. Catabolism is the degradation of larger food molecules to harvest the energy stored in their chemical bonds.

In vertebrates, the food ingested is masticated by the teeth and mixed with digestive enzymes in the mouth. The salivary glands produce alpha-amylase enzymes that degrade starch, a plant-based glucose polymer, to maltose (Fig. 1).

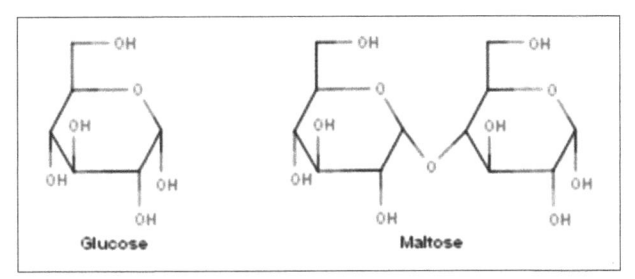

Figure 1. Glucose and maltose. Brush-border enzymes like maltase hydrolyze maltose to glucose. Image by M. Buratovich.

Swallowing the food bolus brings it to the stomach. The stomach secretes hydrochloride acid and the proteolytic enzyme pepsin. Acid denatures molecules and makes them easier to degrade. Pepsin is an acid-stable protease that clips proteins into small oligopeptides. After passing from the stomach to the small intestine, a cocktail of pancreatic enzymes degrades complex carbohydrates, proteins, and fats to simpler precursors. Bile salts made by the liver and stored in the gall bladder solubilize dietary fats, facilitating their degradation. Pancreatic bicarbonate neutralizes acid from the stomach to prevent it from eroding the mucosal lining of the small intestine.

Protein degradation yields amino acids, which are absorbed by the mucosal epithelium. These mucosal cells secrete the food-derived molecules into the bloodstream. Another enzyme, pancreatic amylase, degrades starch to maltose, maltotriose, and small, branched oligosaccharides called "limit dextrins." These smaller molecules pass through the intestinal mucosal cells into the bloodstream. Intestinal lipases and bile salts degrade fats and other lipids to free fatty acids and glycerol. The small intestinal mucosal cells absorb free fatty acids and glycerol and use them to resynthesize fats. Fatty acids are poorly soluble in the bloodstream, and dietary fats and cholesterol are assembled into chylomicron particles. Chylomicrons are too large to be secreted into the bloodstream. Instead, intestinal enterocytes release them into the lymphatic system. After sojourning in the lymphatic system, chylomicrons pass into the bloodstream. They are removed from the circulation by the liver.

Organisms typically cannot digest all the types of nutrients they ingest. Most vertebrates, for example, cannot digest cellulose, the major carbohydrate component of most plants. This material, therefore, passes through the digestive system and is excreted. Fiber passes through the digestive tract essentially undigested. Still, it keeps the colon clear and prevents colon cancer over the long term.

A remarkably complex biochemical process occurs when the circulatory system delivers its absorbed sugars, lipids, and amino acids to the parts of the body where they are needed to build new cells and repair existing cells. Sometimes, this process requires the conversion of sugar molecules to fat molecules or amino acids. For a cell to construct a protein, it must use its available pools of amino acids for protein synthesis, a highly complex process. Human cells can synthesize twelve of the twenty-one required amino acids. Since cells can synthesize these "nonessential" amino acids, they do not need to come from the diet. Nine other amino acids must come from the diet since human cells lack the biosynthetic pathways to construct these so-called essential amino acids. Because green plants can synthesize all twenty forms of amino acids, they are a major and ready source of the essential nutrients required to sustain life. The table below lists the nonessential and essential amino acids (Table 1).

TABLE 1

Nonessential amino acids	Essential amino acids
Alaine	Histidine
Arginine	Isoleucine
Aspartate	Leucine
Asparagine	Lysine
Cysteine	Methionine
Glutamate	Phenylalanine
Glutamine	Threonine
Glycine	Tryptophan
Histidine	Valine
Proline	
Serine	
Tyrosine	

Any molecules organisms need to survive but cannot manufacture are obtained through ingestion and digestion. Such molecules are essential nutrients. For example, there are three essential fatty acids that human cells cannot synthesize. People must acquire them from their diets. The three essential fatty acids are alpha-linolenic acid (ALA), eicosapentaenoic acid (EPA), and docosahexaenoic acid (DHA). Plant oils like flaxseed, soybean, and canola oil contain ALA. Fish and other seafood provide good sources of DHA and EPA. The structures of the essential fatty acids are shown below (Fig. 2).

Also, neither humans nor chickens can synthesize valine, an essential amino acid. However, chickens obtain valine by eating valine-rich grain. Humans eat chickens through which they obtain valine. This amino acid is also available to humans through the green vegetables they eat.

The food that organisms ingest provides the necessary building blocks for synthesizing membranes, enzymes, and other parts of cells and provides energy. Suppose the quantity of ingested nutrients exceeds the body's requirements for synthesis and energy production. In that case, they are stored within

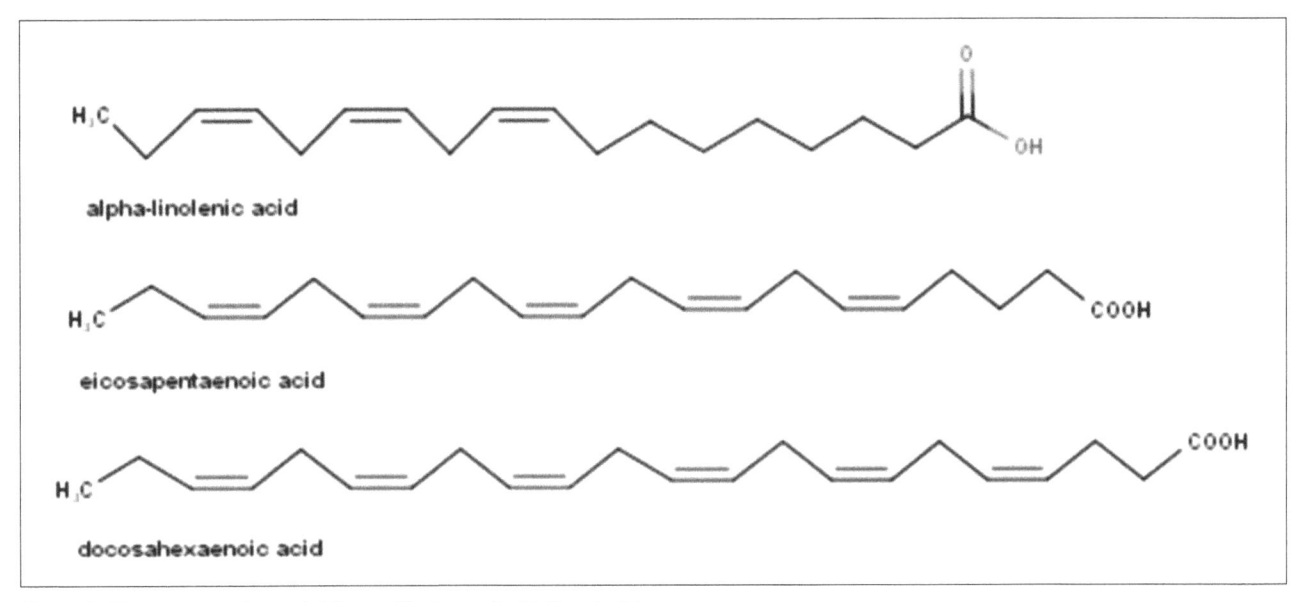

Figure 2. The structure of essential fatty acids. Image by M. Buratovich.

the organism. The excess is stored in the form of lipids. In humans, such excesses are stored around the abdomen and buttocks, where they can accumulate in considerable quantity.

Suppose a human's food supply is severely reduced or completely cut off. In that case, the body draws on these reserves, using the stored fat until it is completely depleted. Afterward, nutrients, mostly proteins, are drawn from muscle mass, the sudden reduction of which can quickly eventuate in death.

The survival of organisms is usually dependent upon the work that they perform. Energy to carry out work is derived through splitting the chemical bonds of adenosine triphosphate (ATP). A highly sophisticated biochemical process called "cellular respiration" transfers energy from the chemical bonds of nutrient molecules to those of ATP.

Almost every cell in the body has the enzymes and cellular equipment to carry out aerobic catabolism and manufacture its ATP. There are two ways to synthesize ATP in cells, substrate-level phosphorylation and oxidative phosphorylation (also known as cellular respiration). Substrate-level phosphorylation (SLP) transfers the energy of a high-energy phosphate group to adenosine diphosphate to make ATP. Oxidative phosphorylation in the human body requires molecular oxygen (O_2) as a terminal electron acceptor. It also requires reduced niacin or riboflavin-based electron carriers, an intact biological membrane, and several membrane-embedded electron carriers. Oxygen, carried through the blood, is the essential ingredient in aerobic catabolism, which results in the oxidization and degradation of nutrient molecules into small molecules composed largely of carbon dioxide and water. In this process, energy is released, some of it lost as heat, and some of it conserved in the bonds of ATP.

The main biochemical pathway that degrades food-based molecules is glycolysis. Glycolysis is a stepwise, consecutive set of enzyme-catalyzed reactions that begin with the six-carbon compound glucose and degrade it to two three-carbon molecules, pyruvate. Glycolysis produces two net ATP molecules per glucose and two reduced electron carriers (Fig. 3).

Pyruvate, the end-product of glycolysis, is transported from the cell cytoplasm into an organelle called the "mitochondrion." The pyruvate

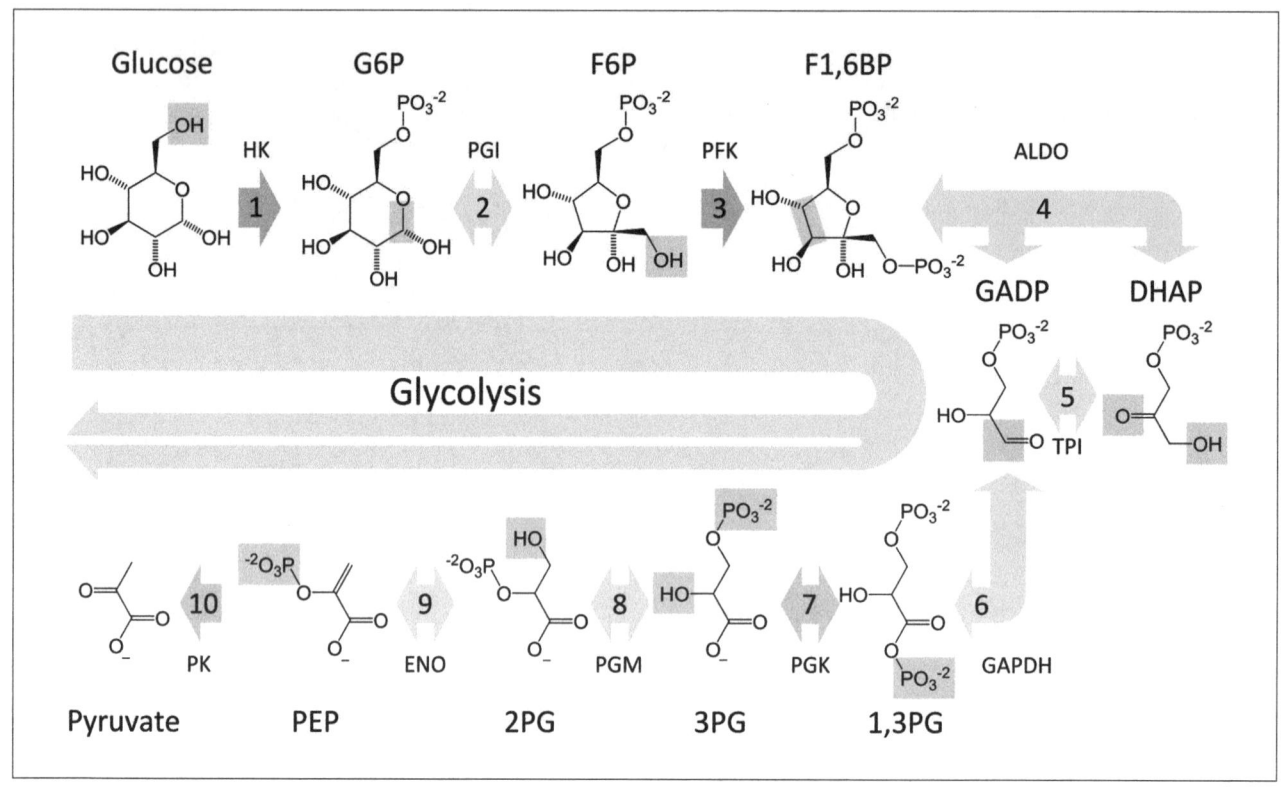

Figure 3. The metabolic pathway of glycolysis converts glucose to pyruvate via a series of intermediate metabolites. A different enzyme catalyzes each chemical modification. Steps 1 and 3 consume ATP, and steps 7 and 10 produce ATP. Since steps 6–10 occur twice per glucose molecule, this leads to a net production of ATP. Image by Thomas Shafee, via Wikimedia Commons.

dehydrogenase enzyme complex oxidizes pyruvate to acetic acid within the mitochondrion. The acetic acid is connected to a carrier molecule called "coenzyme A" to form acetyl-coenzyme A (Fig. 4). This reaction generates one carbon dioxide molecule and one reduced electron carrier (NADH). This reaction requires several coenzymes, including lipoate, FAD (flavin adenine dinucleotide), and thiamine.

Acetyl-coenzyme A remains in the mitochondrion and feeds a cyclical pathway called the "Krebs cycle." The metabolite oxaloacetate condenses with acetyl-coenzyme A to form citric acid. For this reason, the Krebs cycle is called the "citric acid" or "tricarboxylic acid" cycle. Citric acid undergoes several oxidation reactions that completely oxidize the acetate to carbon dioxide and regenerate oxaloacetate to perpetuate this biochemical pathway (Fig. 5).

Glycolysis, the pyruvate decarboxylase reaction, and the Krebs cycle generate many reduced electron carriers, NADH and $FADH_2$. These reduced molecules are fed into the electron transport chain embedded in the inner mitochondrial membrane. These electrons move through the electron transport chain to molecular oxygen, reducing it to water. As the electrons move through the electron transport chain, the carriers pump hydrogen ions (H^+) to the opposite side of the inner mitochondrial membrane. This hydrogen ion surfeit on the opposite side of the membrane and creates a charge and concentration disparity across the membrane that provides an energy source. The mitochondrion returns the hydrogen ions into the mitochondrion with an enzyme called ATP synthase (ATPase). ATPase has a channel through which the hydrogen ions move through the membrane. While passing through the ATPase, the enzyme utilizes the energy expended by this transfer to synthesize ATP from ADP and inorganic phosphate (PO_4^{-3}). This process, whereby the cell uses an ATP synthase driven by a hydrogen ion concentration gradient across a membrane to make ATP, is called "oxidative phosphorylation" or cellular respiration.

Amino acids are absorbed into the bloodstream and taken to the liver. Liver cells remove the amine (NH_2-) group from dietary amino acids to form alpha-keto acids. Enzymes called "transaminases" catalyze amino acid deamination reactions. Transaminases use the coenzyme pyridoxal phosphate, derived from dietary vitamins B_6.

Deamination reactions generate ammonium (NH_4^+), which is poisonous to cells. Liver cells use a cyclic pathway called the "urea cycle" to convert ammonium into urea, a vastly more innocuous molecule than ammonium. The kidney excretes urea in the urine.

Cells feed alpha-keto acids made by amino acid deamination into glycolysis or the Krebs cycle. The exception is the amino acid glycine. Glycine is directly oxidized in mitochondria by the glycine cleavage system. The electron transport chain oxidizes any reduced electron carriers made from amino acid oxidation to produce water and make ATP.

Chylomicrons, made by small intestinal mucosal cells, transport dietary fats to the liver. Liver cells use lipase to hydrolyze fats into glycerol and free fatty acids. Glycerol is oxidized by glycolysis. Fatty acids are transported into mitochondria, where they undergo oxidation by beta-oxidation to acetyl-coenzyme A. Acetyl-coenzyme A molecules enter the Krebs cycle for complete oxidation to carbon dioxide, water, and ATP.

Some organs such as the liver, kidneys, skeletal and cardiac muscles preferentially utilize fatty acids to spare glucose for the brain. The brain gains its energy almost exclusively through glucose oxidation.

During starvation, glucagon levels soar, and insulin levels drop. Glucagon stimulates fat degradation and the release of fatty acids, the degradation of liver glycogen and release of sugar into the bloodstream, and the synthesis of "ketone bodies." Ketone bodies are made from fatty acids and some amino acids. Ketogenic amino acids include leucine, lysine, phenylalanine, isoleucine, threonine, tryptophan and tyrosine. Beta-oxidation degrades fatty acids to acetyl-coenzyme A. Ketone body synthesis, or ketogenesis, begins with attaching two acetyl-coenzyme A molecules to make acetoacetyl-coenzyme A in mitochondria. The enzyme acetyl-coenzyme A acyl

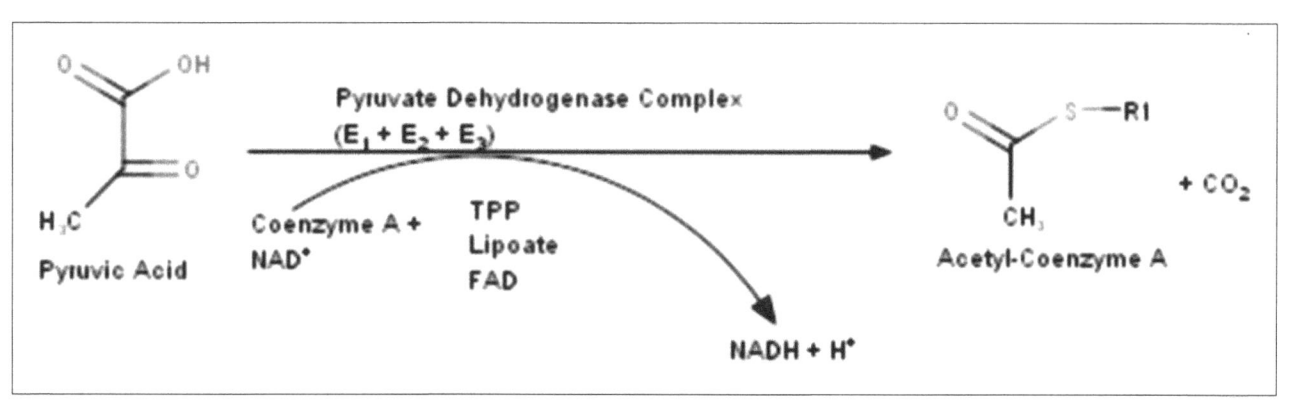

Figure 4. The pyruvate dehydrogenase complex catalyzes, through five sequential reactions, the oxidative decarboxylation of pyruvate, an α-keto acid, to form a carbon dioxide molecule (CO_2) and the acetyl group of acetyl-coenzyme A or acetyl-CoA, with the release of two electrons, carried by NAD. Image by M. Buratovich.

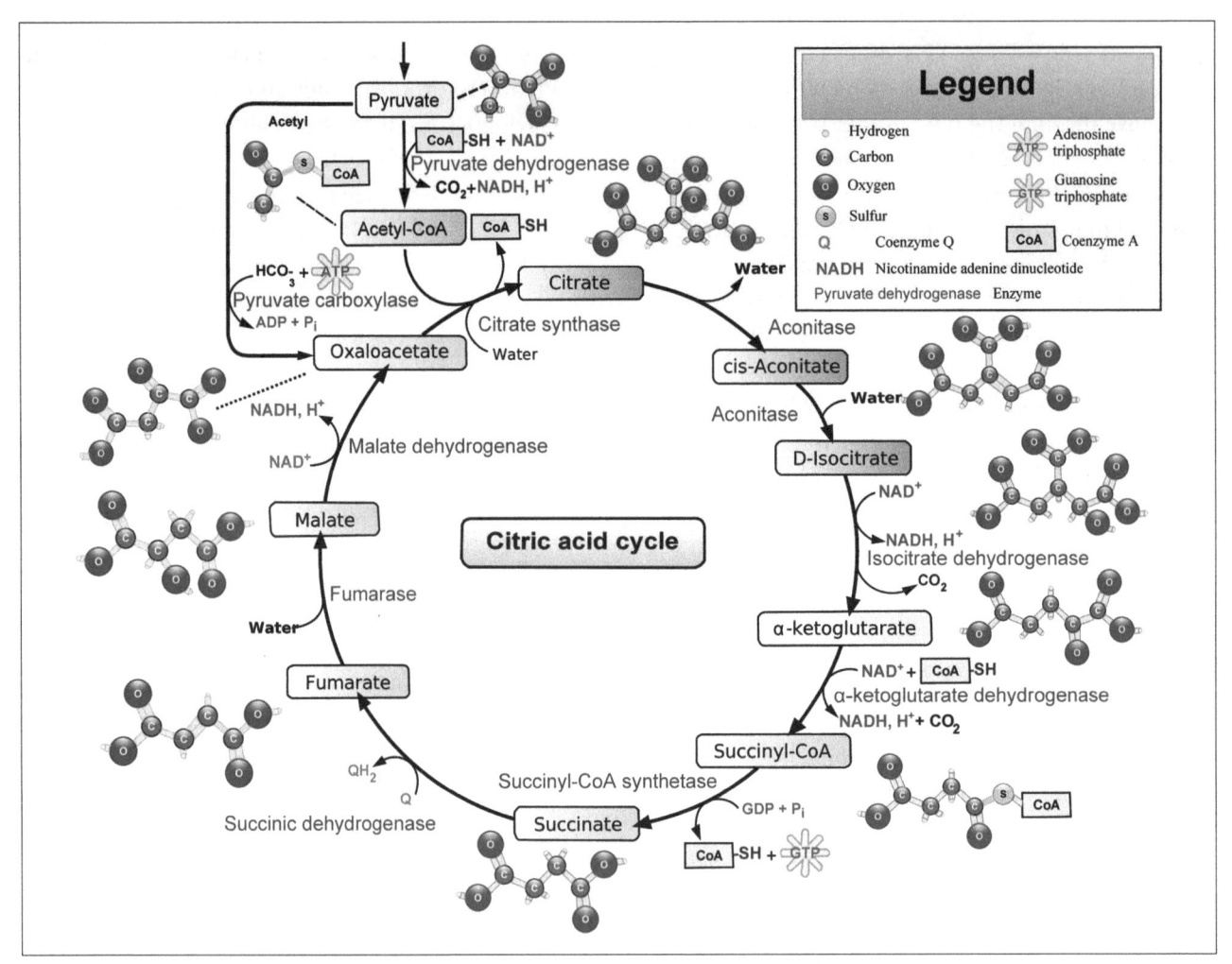

Figure 5. Citric acid overview cycle. Image by Narayanese, YassineMrabet, TotoBaggins, via Wikimedia Commons.

transferase (ACAT) catalyzes this reaction. The next step combines another acetyl-coenzyme A with acetoacetyl-coenzyme A to make 3-hydroxy-3-methylglutaryl coenzyme A or HMG-coenzyme A. This reaction is catalyzed by HMG-CoA synthase and is the rate-limiting or slowest step of ketone synthesis. The next step is catalyzed by HMG-coenzyme A lyase, which degrades HMG-coenzyme A to acetoacetate and acetyl-coenzyme A. Acetoacetate is the first ketone body made during ketogenesis. Beta-hydroxybutyrate dehydrogenase uses NADH to reduce acetoacetate to make beta-hydroxybutyrate, the second ketone body.

Acetoacetate and beta-hydroxybutyrate are organic acids that cause metabolic acidosis when they accumulate in the bloodstream. Acetoacetate enters the blood, and some of it spontaneously degrades to acetone, the third ketone body. Acetone is a volatile organic compound exhaled from the lungs. It causes the fruity smell of the breath of people with diabetes. Ketone body excretion by the kidneys causes excessive water and electrolyte loss, leading to dehydration and electrolyte abnormalities. Ketogenesis is carefully controlled during starvation, but in people with diabetes, abnormally high glucagon levels cause run-away ketogenesis.

Beta-hydroxybutyrate and acetoacetate enter the bloodstream and diffuse into peripheral tissues, including the brain, skeletal muscle, and the kidneys. Ketone bodies are metabolized in mitochondria. Red blood cells do not have mitochondria and, therefore, cannot use ketone bodies. Cells use the enzyme thiophorase to make acetyl-coenzyme A from acetoacetate. Acetyl-coenzyme A runs the Krebs cycle in cells to help them make enough energy to survive. The liver lacks thiophorase and cannot utilize ketone bodies. Thus, the liver makes ketone bodies for other organs but cannot use them for energy.

During anaerobic glycolysis, cells exclusively use glycolysis to produce ATP without oxygen. Pyruvate, under anaerobic conditions, does not enter mitochondria but is reduced to lactic acid by the enzyme lactate dehydrogenase. Heavily exercising muscle uses lactic acid fermentation to produce ATP when its intense activity cannot keep up with oxygen delivery by the circulatory system. Under anaerobic conditions, skeletal muscle primarily uses glucose from the bloodstream or its glycogen stores to produce lactic acid. Lactic acid is released into the bloodstream after exercise and is metabolized by the liver and either converted to glucose or oxidized aerobically by the renal cortex of the kidneys to release additional energy. The body does not excrete lactic acid.

Anabolic reactions expend ATP to synthesize proteins, complex carbohydrates, fats and other lipids, and nucleic acids from simpler precursors. Amino acids are made from glycolytic and Krebs cycle metabolites. For example, the amino acid, aspartic acid is made from oxaloacetate, and asparagine is made from aspartate. Glutamate is made from the Krebs cycle intermediate alpha-ketoglutarate, and glutamine is made from glutamate. Enzymes called transfer ribonucleic acid (tRNA) aminoacyl synthetases attach each amino acid to their cognate tRNAs. Amino acid-tRNA adducts are polymerized into proteins on the surface of ribosomes during protein synthesis.

Glucose is made in the liver by gluconeogenesis. This biochemical pathway largely runs the reactions of glycolysis in reverse, except for three bypass reactions. Glucose is made from alpha-keto acids and other small molecules that are converted to oxaloacetate, the starting molecule for gluconeogenesis. Humans and other animals, unlike plants, cannot make sugar from fat. The hormone glucagon stimulates gluconeogenesis and glycogen degradation in the liver. Conversely, insulin inhibits gluconeogenesis and promotes glucose uptake, glycogen synthesis, and glycolysis.

Complex carbohydrates are synthesized one sugar at a time. Glucose or other monosaccharides are activated by reacting them with uridine triphosphate (UTP) to form sugar-uridine diphosphate adducts. Sugar transferases link these UDP-sugar substrates into the growing polysaccharide chain one at a time. Sugar transferases also attach sugars to proteins to form glycoproteins and lipids to form glycolipids. Some complex carbohydrates, such as "N-linked" (asparagine) oligosaccharides, are pre-made and attached to proteins.

Lipids are made from acetyl-coenzyme A molecules that are carboxylated to make malonyl-coenzyme A. The enzyme acetyl-coenzyme A carboxylase (ACC) catalyzes this reaction. This enzyme is activated by insulin and inhibited by glucagon. Cholesterol is also made by polymerization of acetyl-coenzyme A. The key enzyme in cholesterol biosynthesis is beta-hydroxyl-beta-methylglutaryl-coenzyme A (HMG-CoA) reductase which makes mevalonic acid. Mevalonic acid is converted into activated isoprene units linked together to form lanosterol and cholesterol. The hormone insulin also activates cholesterol biosynthesis.

Nucleic acids are made from glucose and other precursors. The pentose phosphate pathway synthesizes ribose-5 phosphate from glucose. Pyrimidine bases are made from the amino acid aspartate, ammonium, and carbon dioxide. Pyrimidines are linked to ribose after their synthesis. Purine bases are made while attached to ribose and utilize the amino acids glutamine, aspartate, glycine, and the cofactor tetrahydrofolate. These biosynthetic pathways represent *de novo* or synthesis of nucleotides from scratch. However, salvage pathways synthesize nucleotides from recycled bases. All nucleotides are made as ribonucleotides. The enzyme ribonucleotide reductase converts ribonucleotides into deoxyribonucleotides for DNA synthesis. The enzyme RNA polymerase and DNA polymerase use the triphosphorylated forms of nucleotides to synthesize RNA and DNA. Some anticancer drugs, the antimetabolites, inhibit nucleotide synthesis to halt the growth of fast-growing cancer cells. Azathioprine's metabolites inhibit phosphoribosyl pyrophosphate (PRPP) synthetase, the enzyme that converts PRPP to inosine monophosphate (IMP). Inosine monophosphate can be converted to AMP or GMP.

As vertebrates age, their metabolic rate often decreases. In humans, a decreased metabolic rate, reduced activity in old age, and a failure to reduce caloric intake can result in substantial weight gain. Therefore, as humans age, their physicians usually encourage them to engage in physical activity and reduce the overall number of calories consumed. Physical activity generally helps sustain the basal metabolism at levels higher than those found among the sedentary.

DISORDERS AND DISEASES

All metabolic disorders stem from genetic or environmental origins or interactions between the two. For example, a person with a predisposition for diabetes, an inherited genetic disorder, may exacerbate this predisposition by indulging in a diet high in fats and carbohydrates, overindulging in alcoholic beverages, and engaging in little physical activity.

Environmental factors such as diet and exercise can hasten the onset of certain diseases. People at higher risk for diabetes, heart disease, or liver failure who control their diet and alcohol consumption and who make strenuous exercise a regular part of their daily activity may forestall the onset of the disease, possibly keeping it at bay for their entire lifetimes.

Significant advances were first made in the 1960s in tracing the genetic origins of diseases. The discovery that DNA, the molecular basis of heredity, was a major biochemical discovery has led to vastly increased insights into heredity and metabolic disorders of genetic origin, certainly the overwhelming majority of all such disorders. Among the many inherited metabolic disorders are diabetes, arthritis, gout, phenylketonuria (PKU), Tay-Sachs disease, Niemann-Pick disease, and hemochromatosis.

Genetic metabolic diseases result from loss-of-function mutations in genes that encode enzymes that catalyze the synthesis of essential biomolecules or enzymes that degrade biomolecules. For example, maple syrup urine disease occurs in approximately 1 in 86,800 to 185,000 live births. This genetic disease prevents the body from breaking down branched-chain amino acids. These amino acids and their metabolites buildup in the body cross the blood-brain barrier and interfere with normal brain function. Maple syrup urine disease is due to mutations in the genes that encode the branched-chain alpha-keto acid dehydrogenase (BCKD) components. Without functional BCKD, branched-chain alpha-keto acids accumulate and cause branched-chain ketoacidosis. Isoleucine spontaneously converts to alloisoleucine, and isoleucine and alloisoleucine react to form sotolone. This aromatic molecule gives maple syrup and caramel their sweet smell.

A second example is pyruvate decarboxylase deficiency. People with this genetic disease cannot oxidize pyruvate in their mitochondria and make lactic acid by default. The flood of lactic acid into the blood causes lactic acidosis and neurological manifestations.

Dietary deficiencies can deplete stores of essential coenzymes. Without such coenzymes, specific reactions cease, and whole metabolic pathways grind to a halt. For example, thiamine deficiencies prevent pyruvate metabolism to acetyl-coenzyme A. Dietary thiamine deficiencies cause a nutritional disease called "beriberi," which causes encephalopathy since the brain heavily depends on glucose catabolism. Chronic alcoholism also robs the body of thiamine. Alcohol prevents the conversion of thiamine into its active form (thiamine pyrophosphate), inhibits thiamine absorption by the small intestine, and interferes with thiamine storage in the liver. The resulting alcohol-induced thiamine deficiency causes Wernicke-Korsakoff syndrome. It adversely affects movement and balance, facial and eye movements, heart rate, and breathing.

Another example is vitamin B_6 deficiency. Vitamin B_6 participates in transamination reactions, heme, and neurotransmitter syntheses. Consequently, vitamin B_6 deficiencies cause neurological symptoms (seizures and peripheral neuropathy) and sideroblastic anemia. People with liver or kidney dysfunction can suffer from vitamin B_6 deficiencies, as can those on oral contraceptives or the antituberculosis drug isoniazid.

Genetic manipulation in utero can alter some metabolic disorders, bypassing or modifying faulty or abnormal genes. Perinatologists can detect several abnormalities in fetuses by analyzing the amniotic fluid surrounding them in the womb. This process, known as "amniocentesis," can identify more than twenty inherited metabolic disorders before an infant is born. The genes of a person with a predisposition for a metabolic defect usually do not carry the information required for synthesizing a particular protein, usually an enzyme. This deficiency inhibits catalytic activity and blocks a metabolic pathway, resulting in a genetic abnormality.

In a minority of cases, the protein serves a role in transport or acts as a cell-surface receptor. Whatever protein's role serves, a delicate balance exists within the cells. When this balance is disturbed, metabolic problems ensue. For example, a gene may be responsible for producing an enzyme that converts one substance to another substance. If this gene is defective, the enzyme derived from it may be deficient and fail to carry out the conversion or do so slowly as to result in an inefficient conversion. While the first substance, a protein, accumulates in the cell, causing a surplus, it will be in short supply in the cell involved in the conversion, resulting in a deficiency. The surplus or the shortage may eventuate in a metabolic disorder, the genetic disbalance often revealing itself in overt symptoms.

Evidence of metabolic disorders can occur at any time in a person's life. They sometimes are detectable prenatally, but they may occur in early childhood, adolescence, adult life, or old age. In some cases, the onset of a serious metabolic disorder will be followed quickly by death. Many people suffering from such disorders live long, active, full lives, many exceeding the average life span. Some metabolic disorders, such as diabetes, are manageable over long periods through diet and medication.

Some types of metabolic disorders can be treated successfully with massive doses of vitamins. At least twenty fairly common disorders respond favorably to such treatment. For example, Wilson disease, which results in excessive amounts of copper accumulated in the tissues, is treated successfully with D-penicillamine. This compound removes copper from the tissues and deposits it into the urinary system for excretion as urine.

Certain nutrients trigger metabolic disorders in some organisms. The avoidance of these nutrients can prevent the triggering of the disorder permanently. Also, where the disorder results from an inability to synthesize the end product of a biochemical pathway, the disorder may be forestalled by replacing the end product.

PERSPECTIVE AND PROSPECTS
Metabolism was scarcely understood until the 1770s when Joseph Priestley discovered oxygen and set other researchers on the path to understanding its role in the biochemical aspects of all life. In the next decade, Antoine-Laurent Lavoisier and Adair Crawford were the first researchers to measure the heat produced by animals and to suggest convincingly that animal catabolism is a form of combustion.

These early, tentative steps toward understanding how organisms derive energy and how they expend it led to further research that, in 1828, resulted in Friedrich Wohler's synthesis of an organic compound, urea, from inorganic substances, demonstrating that the compounds that living organisms produce can be converted from inorganic to organic through metabolism.

It was not until 1842 that Justus von Liebig did not categorize foods as falling into three essential types: carbohydrates, lipids, and proteins. He measured the caloric values of nutrients and advanced considerably what was known about nutrition and its role in metabolism. At about the same time, Julius Robert von Mayer and James Joule discovered that motion, heat, and electricity are all forms of the same thing, energy. It was not until the 1890s that Max Rubner and Wilbur Atwater demonstrated conclusively through empirical data that animals release energy according to thermodynamic and biochemical principles established through studies of inanimate systems.

Landmark discoveries about metabolism proceeded into the twentieth century. In 1907, Walter Fletcher and Frederick Gowland Hopkins discovered that lactic acid results when glucose is subjected to the anaerobic contraction of muscles. Five years later, Hopkins discovered substances now recognized as vitamins, invented in 1912 by Casimir Funk. Ten years later, Frederick Banting and others pinpointed insulin as a substance that could be synthesized and used to reduce human blood sugar levels, making diabetes a manageable rather than fatal disorder.

Advances in protein chemistry led to the realization that metabolic disorders result from faulty proteins that result from abnormal genes. A turning point in understanding metabolism and especially metabolic disorders came in 1926 when James B. Sumner purified the first enzyme, showing it to be a protein. In 1941, Fritz Lipmann established the central role of ATP as a carrier of energy in living organisms. The following year, Rudolf Schoenheimer demonstrated that the adult body's chemical constituents are in constant flux, suggesting that normal, healthy organisms are constantly renewing themselves.

As one surveys the future in terms of the rapidly increasing knowledge of metabolism and genetics, it is clear that genetic engineering offers daunting biological challenges. Obstetricians can detect congenital disabilities well before birth. Amniocentesis can reveal abnormalities such as metabolic disorders by the second trimester of pregnancy. It is now within the capability of genetic engineering to predetermine the sex of a fetus and to control matters of gender.

The capabilities that currently lie within reach pose substantial ethical problems and challenges. For example, suppose a fetus clearly shows evidence of being afflicted with a metabolic disorder. What use should be made of this information? Some parents would elect to terminate the pregnancy, given the challenges of raising such a child.

—*Michael A. Buratovich*

Further Reading
Appleton Amber, et al. *Metabolism and Nutrition.* Mosby/Elsevier, 2013.

Barasi, Mary E. *Human Nutrition: A Health Perspective*. 2nd ed., Oxford UP, 2003.

Becker, Kenneth L., et al., editors. *Principles and Practice of Endocrinology and Metabolism*. 3rd ed., Lippincott Williams and Wilkins, 2001.

Devlin, Thomas M., editor. *Textbook of Biochemistry: With Clinical Correlations*. 7th ed., Wiley-Liss, 2011.

Edwards, Christopher R., and Dennis W. Lincoln, editors. *Recent Advances in Endocrinology and Metabolism*. 4th ed., Churchill Livingstone, 1992.

Feek, Colin, and Christopher Edwards. *Endocrine and Metabolic Disease*. Springer, 1988.

Gropper, Sareen S., and Jack L. Smith. *Advanced Nutrition and Human Metabolism*. 6th ed., Cengage Learning, 2013.

Hoffmann, Georg F., et al. *Inherited Metabolic Diseases*. Lippincott Williams & Wilkins, 2002.

Isaacs, Scott, and Neil Shulman. *The Hormonal Balance: Understanding Hormones, Weight, and Your Metabolism*. Bull, 2007.

Karsenty, Gerard. *Translational Endocrinology of Bone: Reproduction, Metabolism, and the Central Nervous System*. Elsevier/Academic, 2013.

Kronenberg, Henry M., et al., editors. *Williams Textbook of Endocrinology*. 12th ed., Saunders/Elsevier, 2011.

Lieberman, Michael A., and Alisa Peet. *Marks' Basic and Medical Biochemistry*. 6th ed., Lippincott Williams & Wilkins, 2022.

Thompson, Janice, et al. *The Science of Nutrition*. 5th ed., Pearson, 2019.

Motor Control

Category: Physiology

Specialties and related fields: Emergency medicine, neurology, neurosurgery, occupational therapy, physical therapy

Definition: the regulation of movement in organisms that possess a nervous system

KEY TERMS

motor nerve: a nerve carrying impulses from the brain or spinal cord to a muscle or gland

nervous system: a highly complex part of an animal that coordinates its actions and sensory information by transmitting signals to and from different parts of its body

synapse: microscopic gaps that separate the terminal buttons of one neuron from receptors (usually located on the dendrites) of another neuron; when neurons communicate, they release chemicals that must travel across this gap to stimulate the postsynaptic receptors.

INTRODUCTION

Motor control is a person's ability to carry out voluntary movements. Motor control is also defined as the acquisition and development of distinct motor skills. It is important to note that motor control specifically refers to voluntary muscle movements and not to involuntary movements, such as shivering or flinching, which are controlled through different physiological systems. There are two types of motor control: gross motor control and fine motor control. Gross motor control refers to a person's ability to move a large muscle group or specific body part. Waving one's arm is an example of gross motor control. Fine motor control refers to a person's ability to execute more precise movements. Examples of fine motor control are the ability to write by hand and manipulate a pair of scissors. All motor control is made possible regardless of type through integrated cooperation among the muscles, bones, and central nervous system.

BACKGROUND

Motor control is primarily made possible by the nervous system. The nervous system is one of the body's most important organ systems. It is divided into two components: the central nervous system (CNS) and the peripheral nervous system (PNS). The CNS includes the brain and spinal cord, while the PNS consists of the nerves and ganglia that connect the CNS to the rest of the body. The PNS is further subdivided into the somatic motor system (SMS) and the autonomic motor system (AMS). The SMS branch of the PNS carries nerve impulses to the skeletal muscles that a person directly controls. Meanwhile, the AMS branch carries nerve impulses to muscles such as the heart that a person cannot directly control. The SMS is, therefore, the relevant branch of the PNS in terms of motor control.

The brain and spinal cord coordinate all forms of voluntary movement. This includes the planning, preparation, and execution of motor movements. The brain and spinal cord also play a key role in developing motor skills. One of the most important elements of the CNS's ability to coordinate motor movements is the neuronal structure found within the spinal cord. This unique structure is composed of neurons. Neurons are unique cells that transmit nerve impulses through the nervous system. The neuronal structure in the spinal cord is made up of special neurons called "motor neurons." Motor neurons are nerve cells forming part of the pathway along which nerve impulses travel from the CNS to other body parts. Motor neurons in the spinal cord synapse, or come together, with neurons connected to pathways in the brain and transmit information between the brain and various muscles throughout the body. By facilitating the exchange of information between the brain and muscles, motor neurons effectively make voluntary movements possible. This means that the SMS is the nervous system compo-

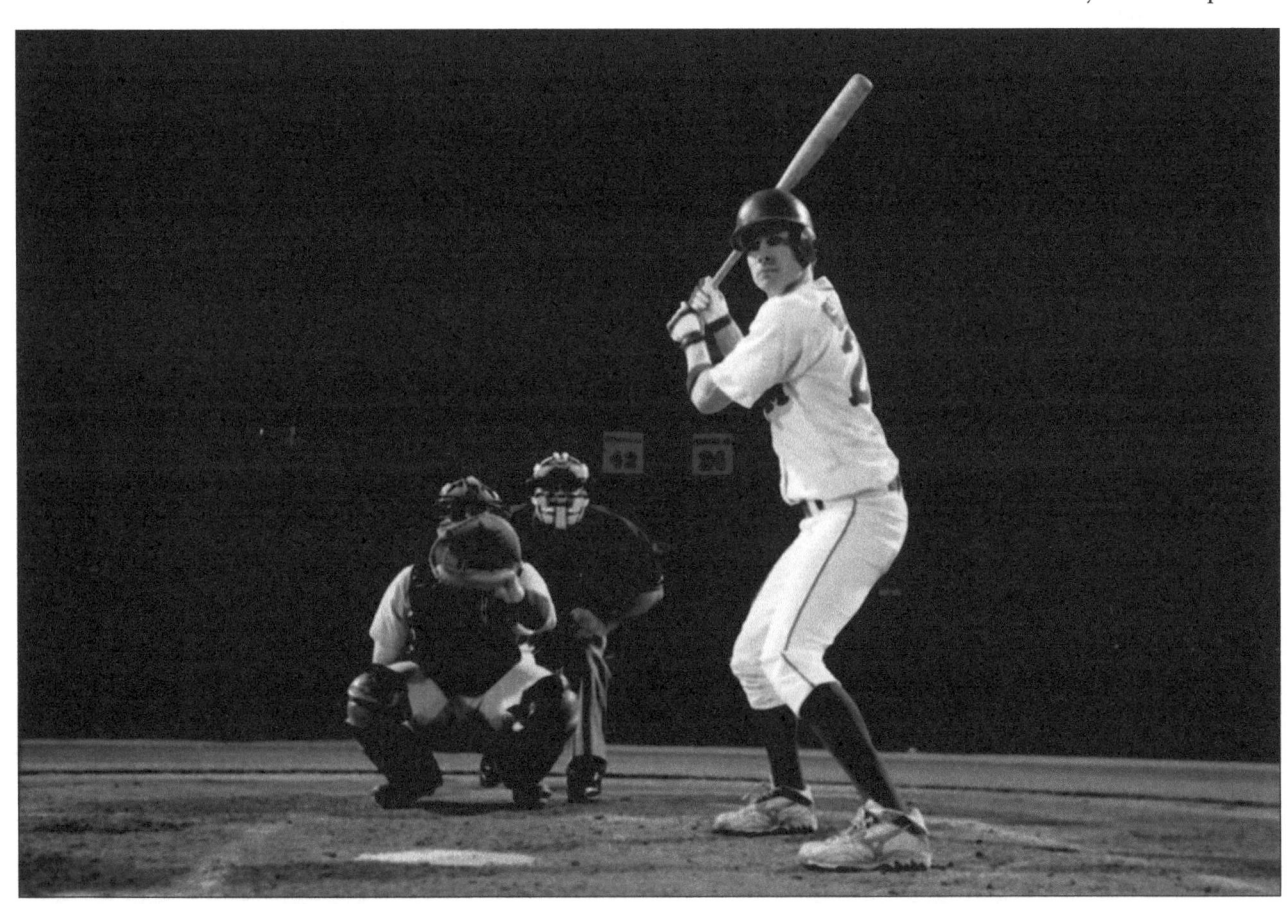

Motor skills are tasks that require voluntary control over movements of the joints and body segments to achieve a goal, e.g., hitting a baseball with a bat. Photo via iStock/Donald Miralle. [Used under license.]

nent that provides the underlying functionality essential to motor control. It also means that the SMS is a critical factor in the initial development of basic motor control during the early stages of life.

OVERVIEW

Motor control refers to a person's ability to control the movements of their body. There are two types of motor control: gross motor control and fine motor control. Gross motor control is the ability to make large general movements like moving one's arm or turning one's head. Executing the kinds of movements associated with gross motor control requires coordination among muscles, bones, and nerves. The acquisition of gross motor control is a significant developmental milestone in infants that typically precedes the acquisition of fine motor control. Fine motor control is the more precise coordination of muscles, bones, and nerves to carry out smaller, more exact movements. Writing by hand and picking up an object with the index finger and thumb are examples of fine motor control. The degree of fine motor control exhibited by a child is often used to estimate developmental age. Children develop fine motor control gradually over time as they learn and practice specific skills. To properly develop fine motor control, a child must have adequate awareness and planning, coordination, muscular strength, and normal sensation. Many simple motor control tasks can only be completed if the nervous system develops and functions correctly.

Two concepts that go hand-in-hand with motor control are motor planning and motor coordination. Motor planning refers to a person's ability to organize their body's actions to complete a given task. A motor plan for a particular task would include all the steps required to complete that task organized in the correct order. For example, the task of throwing a football to a friend would include steps for lifting the football, gripping it properly, aiming at the target, and propelling the football with the appropriate amount of force. People who experience difficulty with motor planning are said to have a medical condition known as "dyspraxia." Children with dyspraxia typically have normal strength and muscle tone. Still, they lack the planning ability and coordination to use their muscles appropriately. Motor coordination refers to a person's ability to use multiple body parts to complete a task. To ride a bicycle, for example, one must use their arms and hands to steer while simultaneously using their legs and feet to pedal. Riding a bicycle also requires a person to have adequate bilateral coordination, which is the ability to use both sides of the body simultaneously.

Acquiring gross and fine motor control is one of the most important aspects of childhood development. Learning basic motor control skills is a key part of childhood growth and a foundational element of early independence. Motor control develops over time through the course of three distinct stages of learning. The three phases of motor learning include the cognitive, associative, and autonomous stages. In the cognitive stage, movements are generally slow, inconsistent, and inefficient. Also, during this stage, a great deal of attention is required to understand what body part or parts must move to complete a particular task. Often, most of the resulting movement is consciously controlled. In the associative stage, movements typically become more fluid, reliable, and efficient. This stage also sees changes in how movements are controlled. While some movements are still consciously controlled, others become automatic. During the autonomous stage, movements are accurate, consistent, and efficient. Movements are also predominantly automatic at the autonomous stage.

There are a variety of medical conditions that can impair motor control in one way or another. These conditions are generally grouped into three broad categories: spinal cord disorders, cortical disorders, and subcortical disorders. Spinal cord disorders are conditions that specifically affect the spinal cord and disrupt the exchange of information between the brain and the rest of the body. The most common spinal cord disorders are those directly resulting from physical injury. Nerve injuries can take a long time to heal. Some nerve injuries can even be permanent. When a nerve is injured and can no longer relay the messages that tell muscles to move, paralysis may result. This can be especially problematic in the case of spinal cord injuries. Severe spinal cord injuries can lead to complete paralysis of the limbs or trunk. In many instances, such injuries are irreversible, meaning that the resulting paralysis is permanent. As a result, spinal cord injuries can seriously or even completely disrupt motor control. There are also several spinal cord conditions not related to physical injury that can disrupt motor control. These include myasthenia gravis, multiple sclerosis (MS), and motor neuron disease. Myasthenia gravis is a condition tied to a neurotransmitter called acetylcholine (ACh), released from motor neurons in the spinal cord. While ACh is released normally in people with myasthenia gravis, an autoimmune response against ACh receptors causes a stark reduction in the number of ACh receptor cells on muscles. This ACh receptor reduction can lead to muscle weakness or fatigue and a decline in motor control. MS is a condition in which a reduction in the fatty insulation found in neurons leads to a disruption in the flow of information within the brain and between the brain and the rest of the body. Motor neuron disease involves the death of motor neurons in the spinal cord. Cortical disorders are conditions that occur within the brain's cerebral cortex. Some examples include hemiplegia, cerebral palsy, and apraxia. Hemiplegia is a form of brain damage caused by a loss of blood supply due to an aneurysm, hemorrhage, or blood clot. Cerebral palsy arises from fetal trauma or trauma suffered during birth. Apraxia is a form of brain damage that occurs when damage to a certain part of the brain leaves a person unable to perform a particular action. All of these conditions can adversely affect motor control. Subcortical disorders affect the brain's basal ganglia, a group of structures located just below the cerebral cortex. Subcortical disorders progress slowly and lead to a gradual loss of motor control. These conditions arise from damage, diseases, or disorders that affect either parts of the basal ganglia or the pathways between the basal ganglia and the cerebral cortex and thalamus. Common subcortical disorders include Parkinson's, Huntington's, and Tourette syndrome.

—*Jack Lasky*

Further Reading

"Fine Motor Control." *MedlinePlus*, n.d., medlineplus.gov/ency/article/002364.htm. Accessed 8 Jan. 2019.

"Gross Motor Control." *MedlinePlus*, n.d., medlineplus.gov/ency/article/002368.htm. Accessed 8 Jan. 2019.

Holecko, Catherine. "Motor Planning, Control, and Coordination." *VeryWell Family*, 26 Oct. 2018, www.verywellfamily.com/what-is-motor-planning-1256903. Accessed 8 Jan. 2019.

Logsdon, Ann. "Learn about Gross Motor Skills Development." *VeryWell Family*, 30 Aug. 2017, www.verywellfamily.com/what-are-gross-motor-skills-2162137. Accessed 8 Jan. 2019.

"Motor Control and Learning." *Physiopedia*, n.d., www.physio-pedia.com/Motor_Control_and_Learning. Accessed 8 Jan. 2019.

"Motor Control and Movement Disorders." *AllPsychologyCareers*, n.d., www.allpsychologycareers.com/topics/motor-control.htmltest. Accessed 8 Jan. 2019.

"Motor Control & Motor Learning." *Trek Education*, n.d., exercise.trekeducation.org/motor-learning. Accessed 8 Jan. 2019.

"Motor Skills." *Pathways*, pathways.org/topics-of-development/motor-skills-2. Accessed 8 Jan. 2019.

Motor Skill Development

Category: Development
Specialties and related fields: Exercise physiology, genetics, neonatology, neurology, orthopedics, pathology, pediatrics, perinatology, physical therapy, psychology, sports medicine
Definition: the process of change in motor behavior with advancing age and the numerous physiological and psychological processes that underlie these changes, which describe the adjustments in posture, movement, and skillful manipulation of objects achieved through the coordination of several neurologic control structures

KEY TERMS

central nervous system: the brain and spinal cord, which process incoming information from the peripheral nervous system and form the main network of coordination and control in advanced organisms

motor control: the nature and cause of movement, which focuses on stability and movement of the body, and the manipulation of objects, which is achieved through the coordination of many structures organized both hierarchically and in a parallel manner

motor learning: the acquisition and modification of movement as a result of practice and experience, which leads to relatively permanent intrinsic changes in the ability to perform skilled activities; not directly measurable but inferred from measures of motor performance

motor performance: the directly measurable extent to which the objective of a motor task is met, the scientific study of which originated as a branch of experimental psychology

motor skills: skills in which both movement and the outcome of actions are emphasized

peripheral nervous system: the system of nerves that link the central nervous system to the rest of the body; consists of twelve pairs of cranial nerves, thirty-one pairs of spinal nerves, and the autonomic nervous system

skeletal muscle: striated muscle that contracts voluntarily and involuntarily to carry out the functions of body support, posture, and locomotion

somatosensory system: the system by which muscle, joint, and cutaneous sensory receptors contribute to the perception and control of movement through ascending pathways

PHYSICAL AND PSYCHOLOGICAL FACTORS

Motor skill development, the process of change in motor behavior with increasing age, focuses on adjustments in posture, movement, and the skillful manipulation of objects. Early researchers attributed all developmental changes to modifications occurring within the central nervous system, with increasing motor abilities reflecting increasing neural maturation. Modern researchers have determined that the central nervous system works in combination with other body systems (such as the musculoskeletal, cardiovascular, and respiratory systems) and the environment to influence motor development, with all systems interacting in an extremely complex fashion as the individual ages.

Prenatal development of motor behavior occurs approximately seven weeks after conception and birth, as was first determined during the 1970s using technology to visualize the fetus in utero. Following approximately eight weeks of gestation, the fetus can exert reflex, reaction, and active, spontaneous movement. It is currently believed that the ability to self-initiate movements within the womb is an integral part of development compared to the traditional view that the fetus is passive and reflexive.

Infancy, the period from birth until the child can stand and walk, lasts approximately twelve months. The neonate begins life essentially helpless against the force of gravity and gradually develops the ability to align body segments with respect to other body segments and the environment. The Bayley Scales of Infant Development measure the following milestones of motor skill development for the first year of life (with the average age of accomplishment listed in parentheses): erect and steady head holding (0.8 months), side to back turning (1.8 months), supported sitting (2.3 months), back to side turning (4.4 months), momentary independent sitting (5.3 months), rolling from back to stomach (6.4 months), steady independent sitting (6.6 months), early supported stepping movements (7.4 months), arm pull to standing position (8.1 months), assisted walking (9.6 months), independent standing (11.0 months), and independent walking (11.7 months). The transition from helplessness to physical independence during the first twelve months creates many changes for growing children and their caregivers. New areas of exploration open up for the baby as greater body control is gained, the force of gravity is conquered, and less dependence on holding and carrying by caregivers is required.

During the first three months after birth, the infant's motor skill development focuses on getting the head aligned from the predominating flexion posture. Flexor tone, the tendency to maintain a flexed posture and rebound back into flexion when the limbs are extended and released, probably results from a combination of the elasticity of soft tissues confined to a flexed position while in the womb and central nervous system activity. As antigravity activity progresses, the infant develops the ability to lift the head. Movements during this period involve brief periods of stretching, kicking, and thrusting of the limbs, in addition to turning and twisting of the trunk and head. Infants tend to be the most active before feeding and quieter and sleepier after feeding.

Great strides mark the third to sixth months after birth in overcoming the force of gravity by flexion and extension movements. The infant becomes more competent in head control with respect to symmetry and midline orientation with the rest of the body, can sit independently for brief periods, and can push up onto hands and knees. These major milestones enable considerably more independence and permit a greater ability to interact with the rest of the world.

The infant constantly moves and explores the surrounding environment during the sixth to ninth months after birth. As nine months approach, most babies can pull themselves into a standing position using a support such as furniture. The child expends a great deal of energy to stand and often bounces up and down once standing is achieved. The up-and-down bouncing eventually leads to shifting body weight from side to side and taking first steps, with a caregiver assisting alongside the furniture; this is often called "cruising".

The ninth to twelfth months involve forward creeping on hands and knees. This locomotor pattern requires more complicated alternating movements of the opposite arms and legs. Some infants prefer creeping even after they can walk independently, and many prefer plantigrade creeping (on extended arms and legs) to walking. The ease with which the child moves from sitting to creeping, kneeling or standing is greatly improved. Balance is developed to the point where the child can pivot around in circles while sitting, using the hands and feet for propulsion. The child begins to move efficiently from standing to floor sitting and can initiate rolling from the supine position using flexed legs. Unsupported sitting is accomplished with ease, and weight while sitting can be transferred easily from buttocks to hands.

The early childhood period lasts from infancy until about six years. It involves the child attaining new skills but not necessarily new patterns of movement, with the learning patterns acquired during the first year of life being used in more meaningful activities.

The locomotor pattern of walking is refined, and new motor skills that require increased balance and control of force—such as running, hopping, jumping, and skipping—are mastered.

Running is usually begun between years two and four, as the child learns to master the flight phase and the anticipatory strategies necessary when there is temporarily no body contact with the ground. It is not until age five or six that control during running with respect to starting, stopping, and changing directions are effectively mastered. Jumping develops at about age 2.5, as the ability and confidence to land after jumping from a height such as a stair is achieved. The ability to jump to reach an overhead object emerges, with early jumpers revealing a shallow preparatory crouch that progresses to a deeper crouch. Hopping, an extension of the ability to balance while standing on one leg, begins at about age 2.5. Still, it is not performed well until about age six, when a series of about ten hops can be performed consecutively and are incorporated into games such as hopscotch. Skipping, a step and a hop on one leg followed by a step and hop of the other leg is generally not achieved until about six years, with the opportunity and encouragement for practice being a primary determining factor, as with other locomotor skills.

Throwing is typically acquired during the first year, but advanced throwing, striking (such as with a plastic baseball and bat), kicking (such as with a soccer ball), and catching are not developed until early childhood. Catching develops at approximately age three, with the child initially holding the arms in front of the body and later making anticipatory adjustments to account for the thrown object's direction, speed, and size. Kicking, which requires balancing on one foot while transferring force to an object with the other foot, begins with a little preparatory backswing and eventually develops to involve the knee, hip, and lean of the trunk at about age six.

Fine motor manipulation skills in the upper extremity that are important to normal activities of daily living such as feeding, dressing, grooming, and handwriting, are greatly improved in early childhood. The key components include locating a target, which requires the coordination of eye-head movement; reaching, which requires the transportation of the hand and arm in space; and manipulation, which includes grip formation, grasp, and release.

During later childhood (the period from seven to about eleven years), adolescence, and adult life throughout the remainder of the life span, changes in movement are influenced predominantly by age. Adolescence begins with the onset of the physical changes of puberty, at approximately eleven to twelve years of age in girls and twelve to thirteen years of age in boys, and ends when physical growth is curtailed. Most authorities believe that the growth spurt of adolescence leads to the emergence of new patterns of movement within the skills that have already been acquired. Most adolescents have strong drives to develop self-esteem and become socially acceptable with their peers in school and various recreational activities. Cooperation and competition become strong components of motor skill development, stabilizing many skills before adolescence and preferences for various sports activities emerge. Boys typically demonstrate increased speed and strength compared to girls, despite recent dramatic changes in opportunities for girls in recreational and competitive sports activities. Even though age-related changes in motor behavior continue throughout adulthood, the physical skills that permit independence are primarily acquired during the first year of life.

Psychological factors influencing motor skill development include attention level, stimulus-response compatibility, arousal level, and motivation. The level of attention when attempting a motor task is critical, with humans displaying a relatively fixed capacity for concentration during different stages of development. Stimulus identification, response selection, and response programming stages—whereby an individual remembers or determines how to perform a task—affect skill development because the central nervous system takes longer to synthesize and respond to more complex skills. Also important are stimulus-response compatibility—the better the stimulus matches the response, the shorter the reaction time—and arousal, which is described as an "inverted U" by the Yerkes-Dodson model. The inverted U hypothesis implies an optimal level of psychological arousal to learn or perform a motor skill efficiently, with performance declining when the arousal level at a given moment is too great or too small. At a low level of arousal, the scope of perception is broad, and all stimuli (including irrelevant information) are processed. As arousal level increases, perception narrows so that when the optimal level of arousal is reached, and attention is sufficiently focused, concentration on only the stimuli relevant to successful skill learning and performance is enabled. Suppose arousal level surpasses this optimal level, and perception narrows to the point of tunnel vision. In that case, some relevant stimuli are missed, and learning and skill performance are reduced. The influence of personal motivation during motor skill development encompasses the child's perceived relevance of the activity and the child's individual ability to recognize the goal of the activity and desire to achieve it.

Three main factors that affect motor skill development in early and later childhood include feedback, amount of practice, and practice conditions. Feedback can be intrinsic, arising from the somatosensory system and senses such as vision and hearing, as information is gathered about a movement and its consequences rather than the actual achievement of the goal. In pathological conditions such as cerebral palsy, intrinsic feedback is often greatly impaired. Feedback can also be extrinsic and is often divided by researchers into the knowledge of results, or information about the movement's success in accomplishing the goal that is available after the skill is completed, and knowledge of performance, or information about skill performance technique or strategy. Knowledge of results provides information about errors as well as successes. True learning occurs through trial and error, with the nervous system detecting and correcting inappropriate or inefficient movements.

DISORDERS AND EFFECTS

Physical therapists, psychologists, teachers, and other professionals who work with pediatric patients often plan their treatment interventions and instructional lessons based on the normal age-related progression of motor skill development. Motor skill development is often significantly decreased due to neurological impairment; however, the child's resulting movement patterns reveal primary impairments such as inadequate muscle activation, secondary impairments such as contractures, and compensatory strategies adopted to overcome the impairment and achieve mobility. The categories for impairments that impact motor development can generally be divided into musculoskeletal, neuromuscular, sensory, perceptual, and cognitive.

Damage to various nervous system structures somewhat predictably reduces the motor control of movement via positive symptoms (the presence of abnormal behavior) and negative symptoms (the loss of normal behavior). Positive symptoms include the presence of exaggerated reflexes and abnormalities of muscle tone. Negative symptoms include the loss of muscular strength and the inappropriate selection of muscles during task performance. The broad spectrum of muscle tone abnormalities ranges from flaccidity to rigidity, with muscle spasticity defined as the velocity-dependent increase in tonic stretch reflexes (also called "muscle tone"), with exaggerated tendon jerks resulting from changes in the threshold of the stretch reflex.

Secondary effects of central nervous system lesions are not directly caused by the lesions themselves but develop as a consequence of the lesions. For example, children with cerebral palsy often exhibit the primary problem of spasticity in muscles of the lower extremities, which causes the secondary problem of muscular and tendon tightness in the ankles, knees, and hips. The secondary problem of a limited range of motion in these important areas for movement often impairs motor skills more than the primary problem of spasticity, with the resulting movement strategies reflecting the growing child's best attempt to compensate.

Another common compensatory strategy in children with a motor development dysfunction involves standing with the knee hyperextended because of an inability to generate enough muscular force to keep the knee from collapsing. Standing with the knee in hyperextension keeps the line of gravity in front of the knee joint. Contractures of joints are frequent consequences of disordered postural and movement patterns. For example, a habitual crouched sitting posture results in chronic shortening of the hamstring, calf, and hip flexor muscles, and a backward-tipped pelvis accommodates the shortened hamstrings. Chronic shortening of the calf muscles often results in toe walking (in which the heel does not strike the ground) and a reduced walking speed and stride length because of decreased balance and leg muscle strength. Changes in the availability of sensory information and cognitive factors such as fear of falling and inattention may also contribute strongly to motor skill development in some pediatric patients.

PERSPECTIVE AND PROSPECTS

Interest in the scientific study of motor development was greatly enhanced by Myrtle B. McGraw's *The Neuromuscular Maturation of the Human Infant* (1945). It described four stages of neural maturation: a period in which reflexes govern movement as a result of the dominance of lower centers within the central nervous system; a period in which reflex expression declines as a result of maturation of the cerebral cortex, and the inhibitory effect of the cortex over lower centers; a period in which an increase in the voluntary quality of activity as a result of increased cortical control produces deliberate or voluntary movement; and a period in which integrative activity of the neural centers takes place, as shown by smooth and coordinated movements.

Arnold Gesell then used cinematography to conduct extensive observations of infants during various stages of growth. He described the maturation of infants based on four behavior categories: motor behavior, adaptive behavior, language development, and personal-social development. Gesell identified six principles of development. The principle of motor priority and fore-reference states that the neuromotor system is laid down before it is voluntarily utilized. The principle of developmental direction states that development proceeds in head-to-foot and proximal-to-distal directions. The principle of reciprocal interweaving states that opposing movements such as extension and flexion show a temporary dominance over one another until they become integrated into mature motor patterns. The principle of functional asymmetry states that humans have a preferred hand, a dominant eye, and a lead foot. This unilateral dominance is subject to change during development. The principle of self-regulation states that periods of stability and instability culminate into more stable responses as maturity proceeds. The principle of optimal realization states that the human action system has strong growth potential toward normal development if environmental and cultural conditions are favorable and compensatory. Regeneration mechanisms come into play when damage occurs to facilitate the maximum possible growth.

Esther Thelen suggested the dynamic systems theory. This theory argues that the maturing nervous system interacts with other biomechanical, psychological, and social environment factors to create a dimensional system whereby behavior represents a compression of the degrees of freedom.

A more refined systems theory of motor control developed by Anne Shumway-Cook and Marjorie Woollacott claims that the three main factors that interact in the development of efficient locomotion are progression (ability to generate rhythmic muscular patterns to move the body in the desired direction), stability (the control of balance), and adaptation (the ability to adapt to changing task and environmental requirements). These three factors generally appear sequentially, with muscular patterns appearing first, followed by equilibrium control, and finally adaptive capabilities. Although research on the emergence of human motor skills has primarily concentrated on the developmental milestones of infants and children, it appears that important changes in motor behavior continue throughout the human life span.

—Daniel G. Graetzer

Further Reading

Berk, Laura E. *Child Development*. 9th ed., Pearson/Allyn & Bacon, 2013.
Feldman, Robert S. *Development Across the Life Span*. 6th ed., Pearson/Prentice Hall, 2011.
Haywood, Kathleen, et al. *Advanced Analysis of Motor Development*. Human Kinetics, 2012.
Kail, Robert V., and John C. Cavanaugh. *Human Development: A Life-Span View*. 6th ed., Wadsworth Cengage Learning, 2013.
Kalverboer, Alex F., et al., editors. *Motor Development in Early and Later Childhood: Longitudinal Approaches*. Cambridge UP, 1993.
Ludlow, Ruth, and Mike Phillips. *The Little Book of Gross Motor Skills*. Featherstone Education, 2012.
Nathanson, Laura Walther. *The Portable Pediatrician: A Practicing Pediatrician's Guide to Your Child's Growth, Development, Health, and Behavior from Birth to Age Five*. 2nd ed., HarperCollins, 2002.
Newell, K. M. "Motor Skill Acquisition." *Annual Review of Psychology*, vol. 42, 1991, pp. 213-37.
Shumway-Cook, Anne, and Marjorie Woollacott. *Motor Control: Translating Research into Clinical Practice*. 4th ed., Philadelphia: Lippincott Williams & Wilkins, 2012.
Sugden, David, and Michael G. Wade. *Typical and Atypical Motor Development*. Mac Keith Press, 2013.
Thelen, Esther, and Linda B. Smith. *A Dynamic Systems Approach to the Development of Cognition and Action*. 5th ed., MIT Press, 2002.

NEUROPLASTICITY

Category: Rehabilitation
Specialties and related fields: Neurology, occupational therapy, physical therapy, physical medicine and rehabilitation, psychology, sports medicine
Definition: the ability of the brain to form and reorganize synaptic connections, especially in response to learning or experience or following injury

KEY TERMS

axons: the long threadlike part of a nerve cell along which impulses are conducted from the cell body to other cells
dendrites: branched extensions of nerve cells that propagate the electrochemical stimulation received from other neural cells to the cell body, or soma or the neuron from which the dendrites project
neurons: a specialized, impulse-conducting cell that is the functional unit of the nervous system, consisting of the cell body and its processes, the axon and dendrites

INTRODUCTION

Neuroplasticity is the ability of the human brain to "rewire" itself by establishing new neural connections in response to injury, developmental or environmental changes, or changes in sensory input. The brain is a complex organ responsible for mental functions such as memory and emotions; it also controls the central nervous system and provides operating instructions to other organs in the body. It is divided into several sections, each responsible for a specific function. Scientists have discovered that the brain can adapt to changes by physically altering its structure to reorganize these functions. This "plastic" capability of the brain can compensate for injuries and illness by rerouting tasks normally assigned to one section of the brain to another. It can also help maintain and strengthen healthy brains by developing new skills and improving memory.

BACKGROUND

The average human brain weighs about three pounds and makes up about 2 percent of a person's body weight. Compared to other vertebrates, humans have the largest brains relative to their body size. The brain is one of the most vital organs in the body, acting as both a source of mental activity and the command center for operating the body's other organs and systems. The brain does this through a network of billions of nerve cells called "neurons." Neurons communicate by transmitting electrical and chemical signals containing specific information or instructions the body needs to function. The parts of the neuron that transmit these messages are nerve fibers called "axons" and "dendrites." Axons transmit electrical impulses away from the neuron, and dendrites act as receivers for the impulses. The brain and central nervous system contain trillions of connections that send or receive information along a specific neural pathway or network.

Neurons go about their tasks in a brain divided into several sections, each responsible for a specific function in the body. The cerebrum, the largest and outermost section of the brain, is separated into two hemispheres and contains the cerebral cortex, the area responsible for complex thought. The cerebral cortex is divided into four lobes, each of which manages its own tasks such as visual processing, memory,

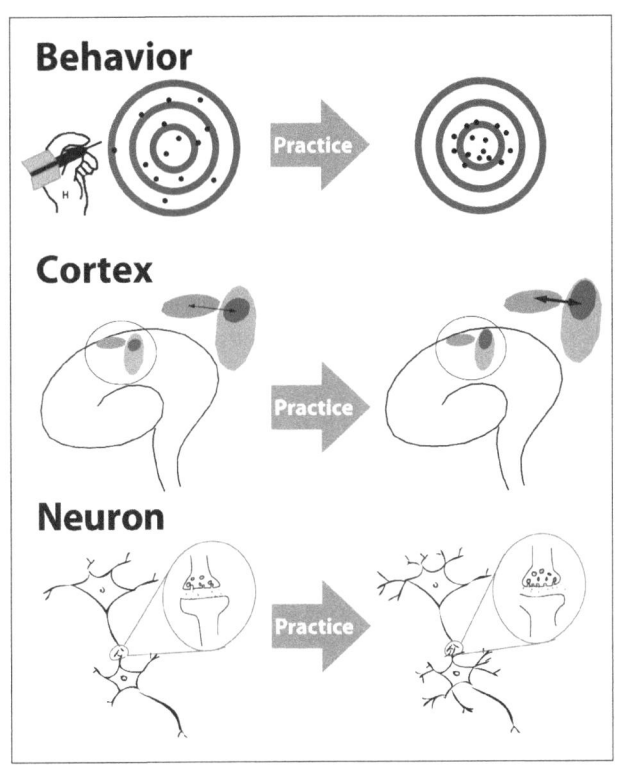

Schematic illustration of brain plasticity after skill practice. Image by Bokkyu Kim at English Wikipedia, via Wikimedia Commons.

language, sensory perception, and emotion. The two hemispheres of the brain control functions on the opposite side of the body; for instance, the left area controls the right side of the body, and the right area controls the left. Other, deeper sections of the brain control basic tasks such as hunger, sleep, balance, and heart and lung functions.

OVERVIEW

The idea that the neural connections in the human brain develop over time is a concept that dates back to the nineteenth century. Researchers, however, thought that these changes occurred only in early childhood. The adult brain's connections were believed to have been fully formed and locked into place. In the early twentieth century, pioneering neuroscientist Santiago Ramón y Cajal suggested some "neuronal plasticity" was possible in adults. Still, his ideas were often disputed by other scientists. In the 1960s, technological advances such as magnetic resonance imaging (MRI) and electron microscopy allowed researchers to observe the brain in more detail. They discovered that neural pathways did continue to evolve into adulthood, and the process continued through a person's lifetime.

As the field was called, research into neuroplasticity increased in the late twentieth century, leading scientists to reexamine previous notions about the brain. It had long been accepted that injured or damaged nerve cells could not be regenerated; however, scientists found that undamaged axons could regrow nerve endings to repair a damaged neural pathway. Axons could also grow nerve endings to reestablish connections with undamaged neurons, bypassing the injured section of the brain and rerouting the transmission of electrochemical information. For example, a person who suffered an injury to the language center in the brain's left hemisphere may have language functions taken over by the right hemisphere. The process's effectiveness depends on the injury's severity and can be aided with rehabilitation. Neuroplasticity may have negative effects, such as a deaf person developing a constant ringing in the ears. This ringing signifies that the body is trying to rewire the brain to compensate for the lack of sound. It is also responsible for the phantom limb phenomenon, in which amputees feel pain or sensation in an arm or leg that has been removed.

Neuroplasticity can also play a role in improving the function of healthy brains through mental stimulation and brain workouts. Human cognitive ability tends to peak between the ages of twenty and thirty. As people get older, memory, attention, and learning skills decline. However, the brain's "plastic" capabilities do not deteriorate with age. People can stimulate neuron growth and improve brain function by performing specific mental exercises focusing on sensory input, movement, and cognitive patterns. These tests may include identifying different colored objects from only a brief glimpse, recognizing whether a sound is increasing or decreasing in frequency, or finding a pattern in a sequence of symbols. Researchers have also found that simple activities such as physical activity, learning a skill, or interacting in new social situations positively affect mental ability.

Brains stimulated by mental exercises tend to be more alert and motivated, two conditions that can increase the production of neurochemicals that facilitate neuron growth. Practicing the exercise and focusing on the task increase its effectiveness; distractions and irrelevant mental clutter can slow or impair the process. While initial progress is sometimes temporary, the brain can remember positive results and build upon them to make more lasting changes. In time, enhancing certain brain connections can also diminish activity in others, reducing distractions and increasing the ability to focus.

—*Richard Sheposh*

Further Reading
Costandi, Moheb. *Neuroplasticity*. MIT Press, 2016.
Doidge, Norman. *The Brain's Way of Healing: Remarkable Discoveries and Recoveries from the Frontiers of Neuroplasticity*. Penguin Books, 2015.
Fuchs, Eberhard, and Gabriele Flügge. "Adult Neuroplasticity: More than 40 Years of Research." *Neural Plasticity*, vol. 2014, 4 May 2014, www.hindawi.com/journals/np/2014/541870/. Accessed 11 Jan. 2017.
Hampton, Debbie. "Neuroplasticity: The 10 Fundamentals of Rewiring Your Brain." *Reset.me*, 28 Oct. 2015, reset.me/story/neuroplasticity-the-10-fundamentals-of-rewiring-your-brain/. Accessed 11 Jan. 2017.
Lewis, Tanya. "Human Brain: Facts, Functions & Anatomy." *Live Science*, 25 Mar. 2016, www.livescience.com/29365-human-brain.html. Accessed 11 Jan. 2017.
Liou, Stephanie. "Neuroplasticity." *Huntington's Outreach Project for Education at Stanford*, web.stanford.edu/group/hopes/cgi-bin/hopes_test/neuroplasticity/. Accessed 11 Jan. 2017.

Medeiros, João. "Game Your Brain: The New Benefits of Neuroplasticity." *Wired*, 16 May 2014, www.wired.co.uk/article/game-your-brain. Accessed 11 Jan. 2017.

Perlmutter, David. "Making New Connections: The Gift of Neuroplasticity." *Integrative Practitioner*, 19 Apr. 2010, www.integrativepractitioner.com/topics/brain-health/making-new-connections-the-gift-of-neuroplasticity/. Accessed 11 Jan. 2017.

Osmosis

Category: Physiology
Specialties and related fields: Biochemistry, genetics, molecular biology, physiology
Definition: a process by which molecules of a solvent tend to pass through a semipermeable membrane from a less concentrated solution into a more concentrated one, thus equalizing the concentrations on each side of the membrane

KEY TERMS

concentration gradient: the gradual change in the concentration of solutes in a solution across a specific distance

diffusion: the process by which different particles, such as atoms and molecules, gradually become intermingled due to random motion caused by thermal energy

equilibrium: the state that exists when the forward activity is exactly equal to the reverse activity of that process

hypertonic: describes a solution with a greater concentration of solutes than the solution to which it is being compared; in biology, a solution with a greater solute concentration than the cytoplasm of a cell

hypotonic: describes a solution with a lower concentration of solutes than the solution to which it is being compared; in biology, a solution with a lower solute concentration than the cytoplasm of a cell

isotonic: describes a solution with the same concentration of solutes as the solution to which it is being compared; in biology, a solution with the same solute concentration as the cytoplasm

osmotic pressure: the pressure that would have to be applied to a solution to prevent the flow of solvent through a semipermeable membrane

reverse osmosis: the application of pressure to a solution to overcome the osmotic pressure of a semipermeable membrane and force water to pass through it in the direction opposite to normal osmotic flow

semipermeable membrane: a membrane that allows the passage of a material, such as water or another solvent, from one side to the other while preventing the passage of other materials, such as dissolved salts or another solute

solute: any material dissolved in a liquid or fluid medium, usually water

solvent: any fluid, most commonly water, that dissolves other materials

VISUALIZING THE CONCEPT OF OSMOSIS

Osmosis is the process by which molecules of a solvent pass through a semipermeable membrane that separates two solutions with differing concentrations of solute. The solvent moves from the solution with the lower concentration (the hypotonic solution) toward the one with the higher concentration (the hypertonic solution). The process will continue until the concentrations of both solutions are equal, and equilibrium is achieved.

A semipermeable membrane is necessary for osmosis to occur. Such a membrane acts as a porous barrier that will allow the passage of solvent molecules but not dissolved materials, such as various mineral salts. Water molecules, though polar, are electrically neutral and very small. When salts such as sodium chloride are dissolved in water, they dissociate into ions, which are electrically charged and significantly larger than the surrounding water mol-

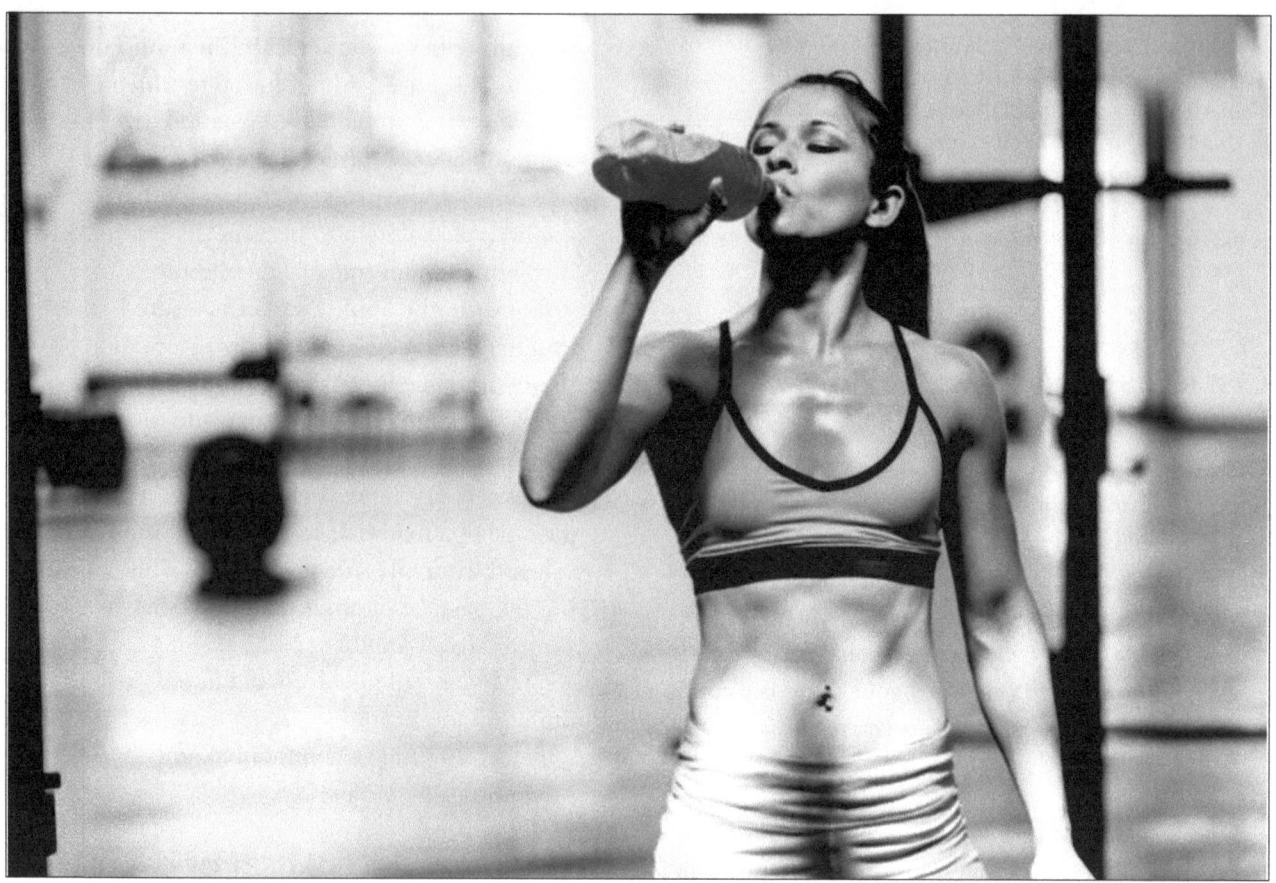

When an athlete drinks a sports drink, water diffuses into cells by osmosis, leading to rapid rehydration. Photo via iStock/mihailomilovanovic. [Used under license.]

ecules. A porous membrane with pores big enough to allow electrically neutral water molecules to pass through, but not the larger electrically charged dissolved ions, is said to be semipermeable. Other types of dissolved materials, such as various sugars and proteins, are too large to pass through the membrane's pores and so are subject to the process of osmosis as well. The presence of a semipermeable membrane can produce an osmotic system. In an osmotic system, the hypotonic solution is confined to one side of the membrane, and the hypertonic solution is contained on the other side. Osmosis occurs spontaneously and continues until the two solutions become isotonic, meaning that both solutions have the same concentration of solutes.

DIFFUSION AND OSMOTIC PRESSURE

Diffusion can be demonstrated simply by adding a few drops of food coloring to a container of water, being careful not to mix them, and then letting the water stand undisturbed. At first, the food coloring will remain where it was placed. Still, over time it will become evenly distributed throughout the water. The water molecules are in constant motion. As they continually bump into the food coloring molecules, they eventually spread them throughout so that the two become mixed. During this process, the distribution of the food coloring in the water follows a concentration gradient, which is the difference in concentration of a solute when the concentration is not constant throughout the solution. Once the food coloring is evenly distributed, the result of this mixing is the same as if the solution had been stirred or agitated, but it requires a much longer time.

Diffusion is the mechanism that drives water molecules through the pores of a semipermeable membrane. Once they are through the membrane, the water molecules interact with the dissolved salts in that solution and remain. The process is reversible, so some water molecules are driven through the membrane in the opposite direction simultaneously. However, the difference in concentration ensures that the net flow of water molecules is toward the hypertonic solution until equilibrium is achieved.

Osmosis can be prevented by applying pressure to the hypertonic solution. The amount of pressure that must be applied to stop osmosis is termed the membrane's osmotic pressure, and it depends on the temperature and the difference in concentration between the two solutions. Osmotic pressure was first described by Jean-Antoine Nollet (1700-1770), also known as Abbé Nollet, in 1748 and first measured directly by Jacobus Henricus van't Hoff (1852-1911) in 1877. The osmotic pressure is given the symbol ϖ and, in the case of an ideal solution, is defined by the van't Hoff equation as:

$$\varpi = RT(C_B - C_A)$$

where T is the temperature in kelvins and C is the concentration in moles per liter (mol/L), or molars (M). R is the gas constant, 8.314 J K^{-1} mol^{-1}. An ideal solution is a solution in which the molecules of solute and solvent interact with each other in the same way they interact with themselves. If the solution is not ideal, then an osmotic coefficient must be included in the equation.

By applying pressure above the osmotic pressure, the process can be driven in reverse. Reverse osmosis forces water molecules to pass through a semipermeable membrane from the hypertonic solution into the hypotonic solution. Through this process, salt-free potable water can be produced from salty seawater or other nonpotable sources.

A DEMONSTRATION OF OSMOSIS

The process of osmosis and osmotic pressure can be readily demonstrated and observed. The essential feature of the demonstration is that two solutions are separated by a semipermeable membrane and cannot mix. This can be done by using the membrane as a partition to separate one half of the inside of a beaker from the other half. The solution on one side of the membrane is a salt solution in water, while on the other is just plain water. As osmosis takes place, the level of the saltwater solution will increase as the level of the unadulterated water decreases. The rate at which the levels change depends on the area of the membrane that is exposed to both solutions.

As water molecules pass through the membrane, the concentration of dissolved salt in the hypertonic solution decreases, and the concentration in the hypotonic solution increases. The same effect will be observed if both solutions contain dissolved salt but in different amounts. Still, it will cease when the concentrations of the two solutions become equal. When the two solutions become isotonic at the equilibrium point, water molecules pass through the membrane in both directions at the same rate.

OSMOSIS IN BIOLOGICAL SYSTEMS

Cell membranes function as semipermeable membranes in living systems, allowing water, oxygen, carbon dioxide, sugars, enzymes, ions, hormones, metabolites, and various other cellular components to pass through as necessary. Living systems use a complex mechanism of osmoregulation that actively brings water into the cells to replace water lost through osmosis to maintain the proper amount of water in cells and prevent dehydration. Anything that interferes with this mechanism, such as the consumption of alcohol, use of drugs, smoking, or lack of sufficient water in the diet, adversely affects the system's viability. Hangovers, for example, are partly the result of dehydration of cell fluids as alcohol is metabolized and often persists until the osmotic balance of the cells is restored.

—Richard M. Renneboog

Further Reading

Cooke, David, editor. *Microbiology: Concepts and Applications*. Callisto Reference, 2018.

Costanzo, Linda S. *Physiology: Cases and Problems*. 4th ed., Lippincott, 2012.

Kucera, Jane. *Reverse Osmosis: Design, Processes, and Applications for Engineers*. Wiley, 2010.

Lafferty, Peter, and Julian Rowe, editors. *The Hutchinson Dictionary of Science*. 2nd ed., Helicon, 1998.

Lodish, Harvey, et al. *Molecular Cell Biology*. 9th ed., W. H. Freeman, 2021.

Urry, Lisa A., et al. *Campbell Biology*. 12th ed., Cummings, 2020.

OSTEOARTHRITIS

Category: Disease/Disorder

Specialties and related fields: Exercise physiology, occupational therapy, orthopedics, physical therapy, podiatry

Definition: a degenerative joint disease that results from the wearing away of the cartilage of bones, causing inflammation, swelling, and pain in affected joints and eventually causing joint stiffness and limitation of movement, misalignment, and knob-like bone growths in the hands

KEY TERMS

Bouchard's nodes: osteophytes or bony spurs that develop as a result of the destruction of joint cartilage in proximal interphalangeal joints

cartilage: a smooth material covering the ends of bone joints that cushions the bone, allowing the joint to move easily

collagen: a fibrous protein substance in connective tissue, bone, tendons, and cartilage

crepitus: the scraping or grinding sound heard or felt when bone rubs over bone in joint spaces

degenerative: marked by progression to a state below what is considered normal or desirable

distal: away from the point of origin

distal interphalangeal joints: the distal joints of the fingers

Herberden's nodes: osteophytes or bony spurs that develop as a result of the destruction of joint cartilage in distal interphalangeal joints

inflammatory: irritation that causes swelling, heat, and discomfort

joints: the junctions at the ends of bones that allow for movement

proximal: toward the point of origin

proximal interphalangeal joints: the proximal joints in the fingers

synovial fluid: fluid contained in the synovium of joint margins that reduces friction during movement of the joints

synovium: fluid-filled sacs in joint margins

CAUSES AND SYMPTOMS

There are several causes of osteoarthritis (OA), including traumatic injuries, joint overuse or repetitive movement of a joint, obesity, and genetic or metabolic diseases. The most commonly affected joints are the hands, hips, knees, and spine. An inherited genetic defect in collagen production leads to defective cartilage and more rapid joint deterioration. OA in the hands or hips may be hereditary. Osteoarthritis in the knees is linked to excess weight. X-rays of more than half the population over sixty-five would show OA in at least one joint.

Cartilage containing synovial fluid and elastic tissue reduces friction as joints move. Osteoarthritis develops when the cartilage wears away, and bone rubs against bone. The most prominent symptom of OA is joint pain. Other symptoms include morning stiffness or stiffness after long periods of immobility. Early in the disease, individuals may experience joint pain after strenuous exercise. As the disease progresses, joints stiffen, and diminished joint mobility is experienced even with slight activity. As joint mobility decreases, the muscles surrounding the joint weaken, thereby increasing the likelihood of further injury to the joint. As the cartilage wears away, crepitus can often be heard as the bone moves against bone. The development of Herberden's nodes on the distal interphalangeal joints and Bouchard's nodes on the proximal interphalangeal joints of the hands is not uncommon.

Confirmation of OA is based on a history of joint pain and physical findings that indicate arthritic joint changes. An X-ray shows a loss of joint space, osteophytes, bone cysts, and sclerosis of subchondral bone. Sometimes, a computed tomography (CT) scan or magnetic resonance imaging (MRI) may help confirm the presence of OA.

TREATMENT AND THERAPY

The goal of treatment for OA is to preserve physical function and reduce pain. Education, physical therapy, and occupational therapy are instrumental in maintaining independence and improving muscle strength around affected joints. Pacing activities to avoid overexertion of the affected joints is an effective means to prevent further pain and injury. Heat therapies such as warm soaks, paraffin, and mud treatments may help lessen the discomfort in tender joints. Moderate exercise such as walking, swimming, strength training, and stretching may help maintain mobility in arthritic joints and improve posture and balance. Relaxation techniques, stress reduction activities, and biofeedback may also be helpful.

Topical analgesic ointments may help to reduce joint swelling and pain. Acetaminophen is very effective for controlling OA pain. However, people taking blood-thinning medicines, having liver disease, or consuming large amounts of alcohol should use acetaminophen with caution. Nonsteroidal anti-inflammatory drugs (NSAIDs) such as ibuprofen and naproxen are also effective for pain relief. Still, they may cause gastrointestinal bleeding, kidney damage, and increased heart attack and stroke risk. COX-2 selective inhibitors are the most recently introduced NSAIDs. This class of drugs selectively blocks the enzyme COX-2, thus controlling the production of prostaglandins. These natural chemicals contribute to body inflammation and cause the pain and swelling of arthritis. Since they do not block the COX-1 enzyme cyclooxygenase-1, which is present in the stomach and inflammation sites, the natural mucous linings of the stomach and intestine are protected, thereby reducing the incidence of upset, ulceration, or bleeding. This feature of blocking COX-2 but not COX-1 makes these drugs unique among traditional NSAIDs. COX-2 selective inhibitors include Celebrex (celecoxib). Two other COX-2-specific inhibitors, Vioxx (rofecoxib) and Bextra (valdecoxib), were withdrawn from the market because they increased the risks of heart attacks and strokes. Other COX-2 inhibitors sold outside the United States include Prexige (lumiracoxib) and Arcoxia (etoricoxib). Any

---

INFORMATION ON OSTEOARTHRITIS

Causes: Traumatic injuries, joint overuse, obesity, genetic or metabolic diseases

Symptoms: Joint pain (commonly in hands, hips, knees, spine); stiffness in the morning or after long periods of immobility; development of nodes

Duration: Chronic and progressive

Treatments: Occupational therapy; physical therapy; moderate exercise; heat therapy (warm soaks, paraffin, mud treatments); pain medications such as topical analgesic ointments, acetaminophen, NSAIDs (ibuprofen, naproxen); COX-2 inhibitors; glucosamine; chondroitin; injections of cortisone or hyaluronic acid; surgery in severe cases.

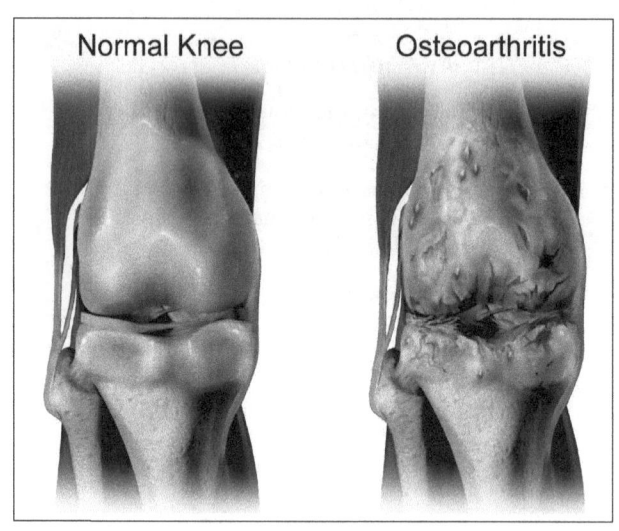

Image by Bruce Blaus, via Wikimedia Commons.

medication used to treat OA should be taken under the direction of a health-care provider.

Glucosamine and chondroitin naturally occur in the body. Both have been promoted for the treatment of OA. Glucosamine may promote the formation and repair of cartilage. In contrast, chondroitin may promote water retention and elasticity in cartilage and prevent cartilage breakdown. However, recent studies indicate that taking glucosamine for arthritis may increase a patient's risk of developing glaucoma.

When interventions to relieve symptoms of OA no longer work, an orthopedic surgeon may inject cortisone or hyaluronic acid into joint spaces such as the knee. Hyaluronic acid replaces the synovial fluid that a joint has lost to maintain knee movement without pain. Orthopedic physicians may inject cortisone into affected joint spaces to temporarily relieve joint pain. Surgical intervention to trim torn and damaged cartilage from joint spaces, replace severely damaged joints partially or totally in the knees and hips, or fuse bones together are effective treatments in OA's most severe, debilitating stages. Realignment of a joint (osteotomy) is another possible procedure.

PERSPECTIVE AND PROSPECTS

Arthritis comprises more than one hundred diseases and conditions and is the major cause of disability in the United States. Almost 27 million people in the United States have OA, the most common form of arthritis. Osteoarthritis incidence increases with age but can affect individuals as young as eighteen. OA is three times more common among women, although before forty-five years of age, it is more common in men. Costs for treatment of arthritis in the United States exceed $128 billion annually. There is no cure for OA, but a healthy diet, regular exercise, and weight control are measures that can slow its progress.

—Sharon W. Stark, Victoria Price

Further Reading

Ali, Naheed. *Arthritis and You: A Comprehensive Digest for Patients and Caregivers*. Rowman and Littlefield, 2013.
Brower, Anne C. *Arthritis in Black and White*. Elsevier Saunders, 2012.
Fox, Barry, and Nadine Taylor. *Arthritis for Dummies*. 3rd ed., For Dummies, 2022.
Ive, Frances. *One Step Ahead of Osteoarthritis*. Hammersmith Health Books, 2019.
Lane, Nancy E., and Daniel J. Wallace. *All About Osteoarthritis: The Definitive Resource for Arthritis Patients and Their Families*. Oxford UP, 2002.
Peterson, Lynne. *Mayo Clinic Guide to Arthritis: Managing Joint Pain for an Active Life*. Mayo Clinic Press, 2020.
Shlotzhauer, Tammi L. *Living with Rheumatoid Arthritis*. 3rd ed., Johns Hopkins UP, 2014.

PAIN

Category: Disease/Disorder
Specialties and related fields: Most, especially anesthesiology, general surgery, genetics, internal medicine, neurology, oncology, physical therapy, psychiatry, rheumatology, sports medicine

Definition: an unpleasant, subjective experience of physical or mental suffering, a symptom of a real or potential underlying cause, condition, or injury

KEY TERMS

acute pain: sudden, extreme pain that is short-term; serves as a warning of damage or disease

analgesic: a drug or medication that alleviates pain by blocking pain receptors

chronic pain: a deeper, aching pain that comes on slowly and lasts longer than the normal course for a specific injury or condition; it may be constant or intermittent

cutaneous pain: caused by injuries to the skin or superficial tissues; brief and localized

endorphins: brain chemicals released by the body that act as natural painkillers

nociception: the process of transmitting pain messages to the brain through the spinal cord by sensitive nerve endings in skin and tissues

referred pain: pain experienced at a site other than the site of origin

substance P: a peptide found in nerve cells in the body, which serves as a chemical messenger (neurotransmitter) that carries pain messages along pathways to the brain

visceral pain: throbbing or aching pain that originates in the deeper body tissues and organs; of longer duration than cutaneous pain

CAUSES AND SYMPTOMS

Not all causes of pain are known or understood, but some basic causes of the most commonly reported pain include inflammation, as in arthritis, rheumatism, and infection; work-related and sports-related injuries; stress and tension; nerve pain, as from shingles, diabetic neuropathy, and sciatica; and pain related to such diseases as osteoporosis and cancer.

People have similar pain thresholds but different levels of pain tolerance or how much pain they can bear. One congenital anomaly inhibits or eliminates

> ### INFORMATION ON PAIN
>
> **Causes**: Infection, trauma, disease
>
> **Symptoms**: Sensation may range from mild to severe
>
> **Duration**: Acute to chronic
>
> **Treatments**: Wide-ranging; may include drug therapy, surgery, physical therapy, alternative medicine

the perception of pain. Pain tolerance is therefore subjective and can be influenced by socioeconomic status, cultural background, and socialization, with disparities noted in who suffers pain, what type of pain a person suffers, and how the individual perceives pain.

Physiological pain is the body's response associated with tissue damage or inflammation or as a warning system to alert the body to potential physical harm. The most commonly reported types of pain are the lower back, severe or migraine headaches, and joint pain, particularly in the knees. Although pain may be produced without a defined stimulus, such as with emotional or psychological pain, physiological pain is transmitted through stimulation of nerve pathways, a process called "nociception." Nociceptors are free, sensitive nerve endings outside the spinal column; they are found in skin and internal surfaces, such as on the joints. Nociceptors, when stimulated, send signals through sensory neurons to the posterior horn of the spinal cord that are then transmitted to other nerve fibers, which travel upward through the brain stem to the thalamus, the gateway to conscious action in the brain. There, information is coordinated, localized, and sent to the cerebral cortex, where a conscious reaction to the stimulus is produced.

Pain is said to be referred when it is experienced at a location other than its site of origin. Referred pain occurs when nerve fibers carrying pain messages enter the spinal cord at the same place as other nerve fibers from other body parts using the same pathways. The other nerve fibers may become stimulated and result in painful perceptions in healthy areas of the body, such as referred pain from the heart to the neck, arm, and stomach.

Among theories of pain transmission, Ronald Malzack and Patrick Wall's Gate Control theory helps explain the differing degrees of pain that people may suffer. It is related to the amount of substance P, a peptide found in nerve cells throughout the body, that reaches the brain. The transmission of neurons is generally very rapid, as touching a hot stove produces immediate action to protect the body from damage. However, messages carried by substance P travel more slowly since they must pass through a special gateway in the spinal cord. At the same time, pain signals also prompt the brain to release chemical endorphins, the body's natural painkillers, which must descend through the same gate. Thus, there is some competition for passage. The fewer available receptors for substance P once it arrives in the brain, the lower the pain perception. With healing, the gate closes, but when chronic pain occurs, it remains open even after healing or without an identified underlying cause.

The two basic types of pain are acute and chronic. Acute pain comes on suddenly and, although extreme, is generally brief. Acute pain warns the body about damage or disease, is localized, and is more easily treated. Chronic pain, however, occurs daily and lasts longer than would be common for a specific injury. It no longer serves to warn and is much more difficult to treat, although

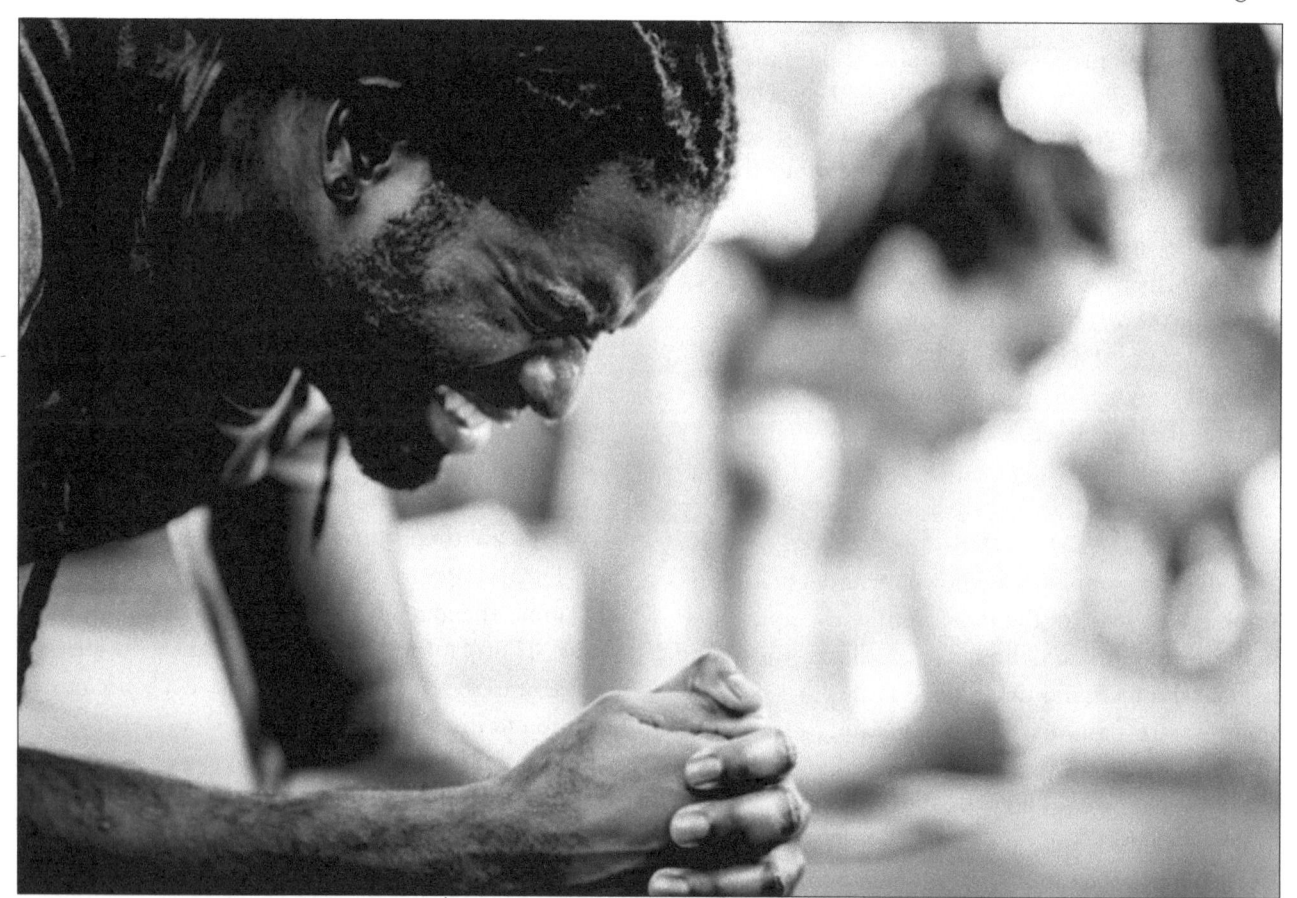

Painful sports-related injuries include sprains, strains, fractures, dislocations, and knee injuries. Photo via iStock/skynesher. [Used under license.]

most sufferers can be helped. Chronic pain may last beyond the resolution of an underlying cause or grow out of an acute condition. In this case, it may become a learned response that no longer has a purpose but continues to hurt. Chronic pain may also occur without apparent cause, creating disability, depression, and suffering.

Pain may be medically classified as either superficial or deep. Superficial pain also called "fast or cutaneous pain," is carried by nerve fibers on the skin and outer linings of the organs. These nerve fibers are plentiful in the intestines, cornea, and nose, for example, and pain messages are quickly delivered to the brain, such as when one is cut or burned. Also termed somatic pain, it is experienced as intense or burning. Kidney stones or acid reflux from the stomach may create waves of this burning pain. Deep pain, on the other hand, also referred to as slow or visceral pain, comes from nerve fibers located in muscles, bones, and tissues of the internal organs. It travels more slowly, taking longer to reach the brain. It may be experienced as dull aching or throbbing pain. The two types of pain may also occur at the same time.

TREATMENT AND THERAPY

The major treatment for pain in the United States has been analgesic medications or drug therapy. Sufferers spend over an estimated $18 billion annually for relief from prescription and over-the-counter medications. There are no standard guidelines for analgesics since the degree of relief varies from patient to patient. These medications are classified as narcotics, such as morphine or opium-based addictive drugs, and nonnarcotic, such as aspirin, ibuprofen, and acetaminophen. Since patients respond differently, and many analgesics can carry significant side effects with cardiovascular, renal, and gastrointestinal toxicity, the lowest dose of the preferred medication is usually recommended to start. Painkillers must also often be administered with other medications directed to the underlying cause of the pain and must therefore be compatible.

One subcategory of nonnarcotic analgesics comprises nonsteroidal anti-inflammatory drugs (NSAIDs). Another alternative, acetaminophen, addresses pain but does not affect inflammation. Another nonnarcotic class of drugs, known as "COX-2 inhibitors," suppresses the COX-2 enzyme, which triggers inflammation. Although these drugs are seemingly well-tolerated and effective, many endanger the heart, and several were withdrawn from the market.

Narcotic analgesics are the most effective, but long-term use can create dependency. These drugs are stringently protected in the United States by state and federal laws. Doctors have therefore been hesitant to use them for severe chronic pain, even in patients dying from cancer or other painful diseases, when other medications are not working. This situation appears to be changing.

Nondrug therapies include such techniques as transcutaneous electrical nerve stimulation (TENS), massage therapy, neurosurgery, physical therapy and exercise, and mind-body therapies such as guided imagery, meditation, relaxation, and hypnosis. These therapies attempt to alleviate chronic pain in various ways by stimulating blood circulation, blocking nerve pain messengers, and enlisting the help of the brain, where pain messages are processed.

A combination of biomedical and nonbiomedical therapies also utilizes several alternative therapies for pain. Acupuncture and acupressure, the foundation of Chinese medicine, are thought to stimulate blood circulation and possibly the autonomic nervous system by inserting very fine needles at crucial points in the body. Herbal medicine uses substances derived from plants with therapeutic or pharmacologic properties and benefits. Many of today's medicines have ingredients that originated in plants and can be synthesized in the laboratory. Guided imagery, aromatherapy, creative arts therapy, magnet therapy, and therapeutic touch are often used as adjuncts to dealing with pain, but most have not been proven. Like analgesics, these therapies address the control and management of pain rather than offering a cure.

Although many of these complementary therapies are not biomedically sanctioned or recognized, many chronic pain sufferers try some form of complementary medicine. Little or no research has been done on many of these therapies. Still, their popularity relates to chronic pain being closely connected with the brain, affecting emotions, attitudes, and psychological stability, which are not addressed by conventional medicine and treatment. Some of these therapies may work through the placebo effect, meaning that if one expects the therapy to alleviate pain, it will. Some approaches are backed by positive evidence, while others have no effect. Very little evidence exists about how or why many of these therapies are successful, but combination therapies are vital in alleviating pain; however, they may work.

PERSPECTIVE AND PROSPECTS
The development of pain medicine and clinics devoted solely to the study and alleviation of pain is fairly recent. Since pain was traditionally seen as a symptom rather than a disease or condition in itself, the medical profession has generally focused on treating the cause, considering it purely a diagnostic tool. However, the discovery and development of anesthetics for surgical procedures in the mid-nineteenth century was a huge advance in medical care and treatment and was a precondition for the later development of pain medicine. Anesthesiologists not only had to address traumatic and postoperative pain but also worked to refine techniques and developed expertise in management relating to other types of pain.

Anesthesiology progressed rapidly during World War II, with improved nerve blocking and analgesic use. Anesthesiologist John Bonica contributed significantly to this development of pain medicine. He was faced with extreme, intractable, complex, and phantom limb pain (the sensation of pain felt in a limb no longer there) in the injured during wartime and lacked knowledge or methods to treat them. As pain persisted and physiological causes could not be identified, it became necessary to look elsewhere for the source of the pain. It became obvious that numerous specialists, including psychologists and psychiatrists, needed to consult and discuss their varied findings and opinions.

As defined by the American Academy of Pain Medicine, the specialty concerns the study, prevention, evaluation, treatment, and rehabilitation of people in pain. Practitioners of pain medicine mostly come from other medical fields most closely related to pain, such as neurology, anesthesiology, and rehabilitation. Many are certified as pain specialists through the American Board of Anesthesiology. While some pain clinics focus on specific types of pain, such as bone and joint, others address a broader spectrum of suffering and tend to use various methods and treatments, including alternative therapies, to find whatever works. Some pain cannot be eliminated but can be minimized or controlled to allow the patient to function.

The need to study and understand the causes and alleviation of pain have become more urgent. According to the National Center for Health Statistics, one in four adults in the United States reported suffering pain lasting for at least twenty-four hours during the previous month. One in ten reported pain lasting a year or more. Pain is usually seen as a result of another physical condition. Still, considering the costs that accompany pain and resulting disability in dollars and loss of individual function reflected in absenteeism in the workplace, pain places an increasing burden on the

American health-care system. The general cost of pain and pain-related items is estimated to top $100 billion annually.

Research is being conducted into the origins and mechanics of pain to identify new and more effective therapies. A study funded by the National Institutes of Health found that the perception of pain (the extent to which one feels pain) is inherited through a gene with a specific variant. This gene variant affects sensitivity to acute pain and the risk of developing chronic pain. Other genes may also play a role. This study opens up pathways for developing new treatments and approaches to pain.

Such professional organizations as the American Academy of Pain Medicine, the American Pain Foundation, the American Pain Society, and the International Association for the Study of Pain represent only a few of the growing number of resources for studying pain and pain management. Alternative approaches are represented through organizations for specific therapies and the National Center for Complementary and Alternative Medicine.

—Martha Oehmke Loustaunau

Further Reading

Ballantyne, Jane C., et al., editors. *Bonica's Management of Pain*. 5th ed., Lippincott Williams & Wilkins, 2018.

Baszanger, Isabelle. *Inventing Pain Medicine: From the Laboratory to the Clinic*. Rutgers UP, 1998.

Bellenir, Karen, editor. *Pain Sourcebook: Basic Consumer Health Information About Specific Forms of Acute and Chronic Pain*. 2nd ed., Omnigraphics, 2002.

Coakley, Sarah, and Kay Kaufman Shelemay, editors. *Pain and Its Transformations: The Interface of Biology and Culture*. Harvard UP, 2008.

Vertosick, Frank T., Jr. *Why We Hurt: The Natural History of Pain*. Harcourt, 2000.

Waldman, Steven D. *Atlas of Uncommon Pain Syndromes*. Elsevier, 2014.

Wall, Patrick David. *Pain: The Science of Suffering*. Columbia UP, 2013.

STEROIDS

Category: Treatment
Specialties and related fields: Biochemistry, biotechnology, endocrinology, immunology, pharmacology substance use, treatment, and therapy
Definition: a class of natural or synthetic organic compounds characterized by a molecular structure of seventeen carbon atoms arranged in four rings that comprise the "steroid nucleus"

KEY TERMS

anabolic steroid: a synthetic steroid hormone that resembles testosterone and promotes muscle growth; used medicinally to treat some forms of weight loss and illegally by some athletes and others to enhance physical performance

bile acids: steroid acids, synthesized in the liver, found predominantly in the bile of mammals and other vertebrates, conjugated with taurine or glycine residues to give anions

chylomicrons: lipoprotein particles that consist of triglycerides, phospholipids, cholesterol, and proteins and transport dietary lipids from the intestines to other locations in the body

endocrine glands: glands that release hormones directly into the bloodstream

gonads: a collective term referring to the testes and ovaries

hormone: a class of signaling molecules in multicellular organisms that are transported to distant organs to regulate physiology and behavior

semisynthetic: about compounds that are obtained by altering or augmenting the molecular structure of a compound obtained from a natural source

synthetic: about compounds that are produced entirely by synthesis reactions carried out in the laboratory from simple starting materials

very low-density lipoproteins: one of the major groups of lipoproteins that enable fats and cholesterol to move within the water-based solution of the bloodstream

STRUCTURE AND FUNCTIONS

Steroids are a group of organic compounds distinguished by a unique molecular arrangement of seventeen carbon atoms conjoined in four adjacent rings. These four rings are referred to as the steroid nucleus and are common to all steroid compounds (Fig. 1). Three of these rings are hexagonal six-carbon rings arranged in a bent-line fashion to form a phenanthrene group. The fourth group or ring contains only five carbon atoms. Steroids vary with the nature of the attached groups, the position of a given attached group, or some alteration to the configuration of the steroid nucleus. Small chemical differences in the structure of steroids can reflect great differences in specific biological effects. Steroids are included in the lipid category of biological molecules because they are nonpolar and insoluble in water.

Any steroid that contains a hydroxyl group (-OH) is called a "sterol." This term comes from a Greek word meaning "solid." Sterols were so named because they were among the earliest compounds found to be solid at room temperature. Once chemical structures were determined, other compounds with similar structures were named steroids, which means "sterol-like." The suffix *-oid* comes from Greek and means "similar to."

Chemists have isolated hundreds of steroids from plants and animals; additionally, thousands have been manufactured by chemically modifying natural steroids or synthesizing the entire molecule. Cholesterol is the parent, or precursor compound, for bile acids and the biologically important steroids to the body.

The metabolic precursor for steroids is acetic acid. Various enzymes catalyze the polymerization of acetic acid and the transformation of those polymers into several other compounds, ultimately synthesizing cholesterol. The rate-limiting step of cholesterol biosynthesis is the reduction of 3-hydroxy-3-methylglutaryl-coenzyme A to mevalonic acid. The enzyme catalyzing this step, 3-hydroxy-3-methylglutaryl-coenzyme A (HMG-CoA reductase), is the most heavily regulated in this pathway. Statins, a class of medications that low serum cholesterol levels, also target this enzyme.

Cholesterol is the most common steroid in the human body, as it is a structural component of cellular membranes. The prefix *chole-* came from the Greek word for liver bile, a digestive fluid manufactured by the liver and secreted into the intestines. The name is appropriate since the bile contains a considerable amount of cholesterol.

Liver cells (hepatocytes) synthesize bile from cholesterol. Hepatocytes use the enzyme 7-alpha-hydroxylase to convert cholesterol into two primary bile acids, cholic acid, and chenodeoxycholic acid. The liver conjugates the amino acids glycine or taurine to the primary bile acids to form taurocholic

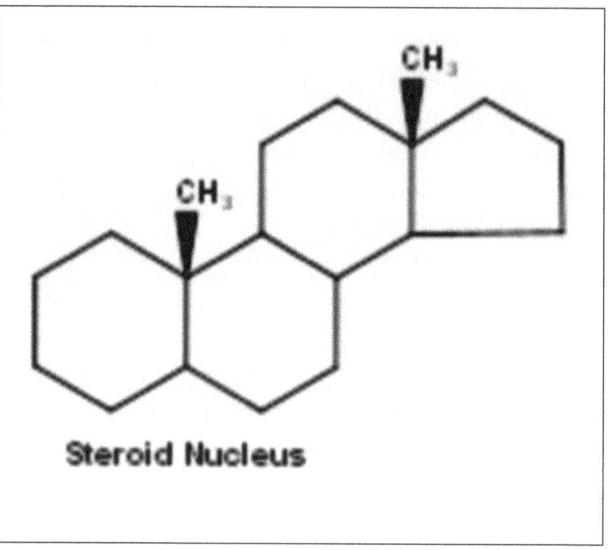

Figure 1. Four-ring steroid nucleus. All steroids, natural or synthetic, have molecular structures derived from the basic one shown above. Image by M. Buratovich.

acid, glycocholic acid, taurodeoxycholic acid, and glycodeoxycholic acid. These bile acids are the main components of bile.

In the intestines, resident microorganisms dehydroxylate (remove a hydroxyl [-OH] group) the primary bile acids and remove their taurine and glycine groups. These reactions generate secondary bile acids, deoxycholic acid, and lithocholic acid.

Bile is stored and concentrated in the gallbladder. Cholesterol is not very soluble; if it accumulates in great enough quantities, it forms small crystals in the bile. These crystals may aggregate to form larger particles that can block the narrow duct that leads from the gallbladder to the intestines. These aggregations of particles are called "gallstones" and are composed of almost pure cholesterol. The blockage can result in a buildup of pressure and cause much pain. Often, surgery is required to remove the obstruction.

Thirty minutes or so after eating, digested food, known as "chyme," enters the duodenum, the first part of the small intestine. The innermost cell layer of the duodenum, the mucosae, contains special cells called "I-cells" that detect the chyme and secrete a peptide hormone, cholecystokinin (CCK). CCK moves through the bloodstream and stimulates the gall bladder to contract and squirt the bile into the common bile duct. Cholecystokinin also relaxes the muscular valve (sphincter of Oddi) that is the door between the common bile duct and the duodenum. Bile flows into the duodenum to mix with the chyme.

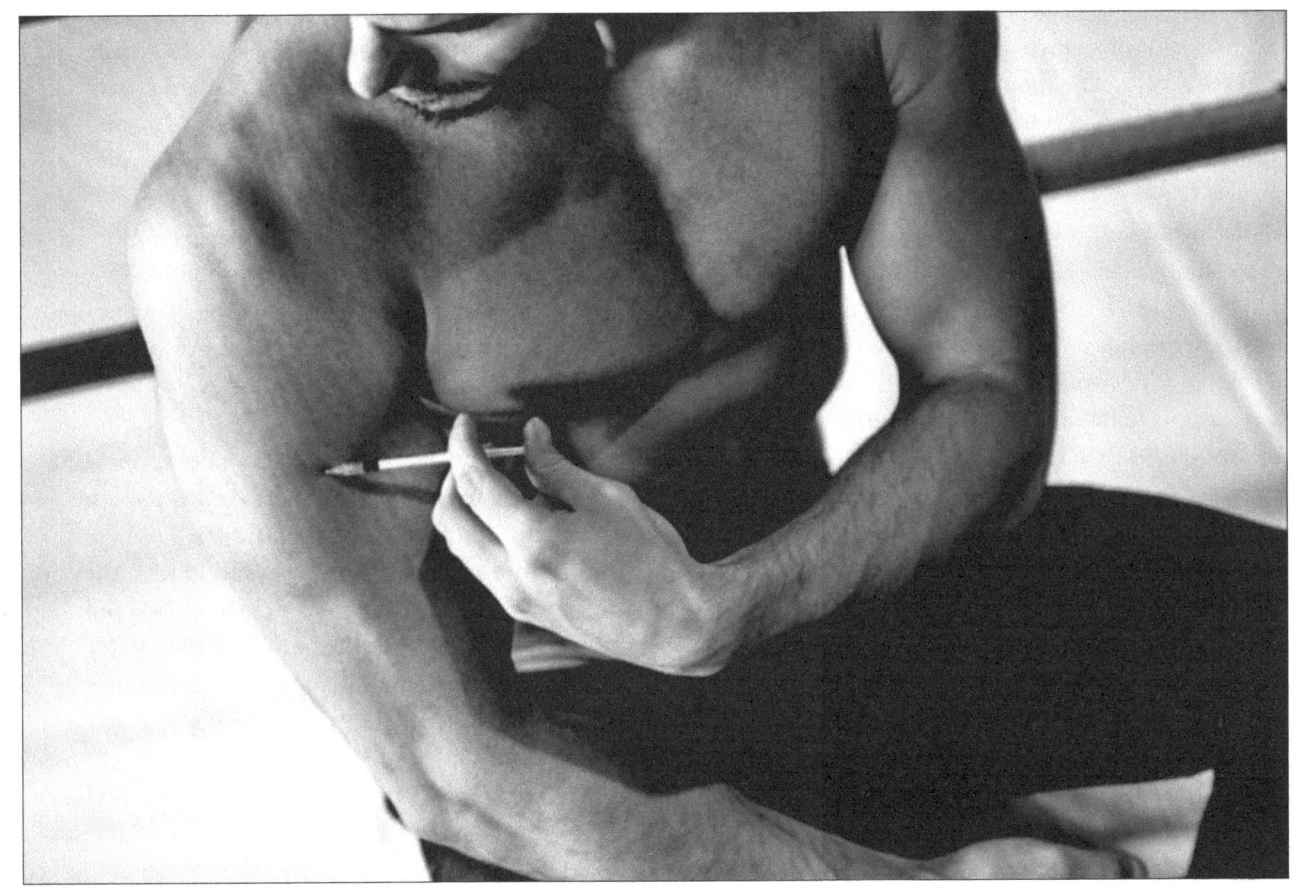

Using performance-enhancing steroids can have serious long-term health effects. Photo via iStock/GeorgeRudy. [Used under license.]

Bile salts have a water-loving side and a water-hating side (amphipathic). This unique property causes bile salts to self-assemble into tiny, bubble-like structures called "micelles" in water. Fats insert themselves into these micelles, providing a large surface for lipase enzymes to bind and degrade fats.

Cholesterol is also important because it is the precursor or parent molecule for the steroid hormones produced by the gonads and the adrenal cortex. Cholesterol is delivered to cells by very low-density lipoproteins (VLDLs). Pancreatic lipases degrade dietary fat in the duodenum (first part of the small intestine) to free fatty acids, glycerol, and monoglycerides. Duodenal mucosal cells absorb these molecules and use them to re-synthesize fats. A transport protein called Neimann-Pick-like Protein-1 (NPCL-1) in the apical membrane of duodenal mucosal cells moves dietary cholesterol into the duodenal cells. The mucosal cells use the enzyme acyl-coenzyme A acyl transferase (ACAT) to attach a fatty acid to the hydroxyl group of cholesterol to form a "cholesterol ester." The mucosal cells use cholesterol esters and fats to construct a macromolecular assemblage called a "chylomicron." This particle has a shell of phospholipids surrounding a core of fats and cholesterol esters. Free cholesterol molecules and special proteins called "apolipoproteins" are embedded in the phospholipid shell. Apolipoproteins are structurally complex molecules, with one side facing the aqueous environment and another facing the water-hating chylomicron interior. Chylomicrons have several apolipoproteins on their surfaces. The most important structural apolipoprotein is apoB48 and other apolipoproteins aid chylomicron function.

Chylomicrons are too large to enter the bloodstream after the mucosal cell releases them from their basal surfaces. Instead, chylomicrons enter the lymphatic vessels and sojourn through the lymph system for a time. Eventually, the lymph feeds into the bloodstream through the thoracic duct. The liver removes chylomicrons from the circulation and uses its fats and cholesterol to construct a different lipoprotein called a VLDL. Once released from the liver, VLDLs move through the bloodstream, delivering cholesterol and fats to various tissues.

The gonads, a collective term referring to the testes and ovaries, use cholesterol, delivered to them by serum VLDLs, to synthesize the sex steroids. Sex steroids include estradiol and progesterone from the ovaries and testosterone from the testes. The adrenal cortex secretes corticosteroids, including cortisol, aldosterone, and other steroid compounds. Some steroid hormones are specialized in their function and do not produce general effects on metabolism. Sex hormones influence reproduction by acting on sexual organs to stimulate their development and function, influencing sexual behavior, and stimulating the development of secondary sex characteristics. Some of the steroids secreted by the adrenal cortex have more general effects on the metabolism of carbohydrates and proteins in many tissues.

Steroid hormones bind to specific receptors in the cytoplasm of responsive tissues. Since these hormones are lipid-soluble, they pass readily through cell membranes, mostly composed of phospholipids. Inside the cytoplasm, a steroid receptor protein receptor binds to the hormone. The hormone-receptor complex translocates to the nucleus. In the nucleus, the activated steroid receptor complex binds to specific deoxyribonucleic acid (DNA) sequences called steroid response elements (SREs). When steroid/steroid receptor complexes bind SREs, they create binding sites for ribonucleic acid (RNA) polymerase and general transcription factors. RNA polymerase transcribes the gene to make a messenger RNA (mRNA). The mRNA goes to the cytoplasm, where it is translated into protein by ribosomes. Activation of gene expression induces the synthesis of production of target proteins that are either used by the cell or secreted elsewhere.

CATEGORIES OF STEROID HORMONES

The adrenal glands are atop the kidneys, covered by a thick connective tissue capsule. The adrenal gland has two regions, an outer cortex and an inner medulla. The cortex has three layers, an outermost zona glomerulosa, an inner zona fasciculata, and the innermost zona reticularis. The zona glomerulosa secretes mineralocorticoids, the middle zona fasciculata produces glucocorticoids, and the zona reticularis makes sex steroids.

The steroid hormones of the adrenal cortex have separate actions and sites of action. Aldosterone is the principal mineralocorticoid and plays an important role in regulating sodium and potassium body levels. Cortisol, the major glucocorticoid, regulates carbohydrate metabolism. Adrenal androgens are also produced but have only weak activity and play a minor physiological role under most conditions. All adrenal steroids are derived from cholesterol.

The hypothalamus-pituitary axis controls adrenal hormone production. The hypothalamus lies at the base of the brain above the pituitary gland. The hypothalamus releases a small peptide hormone, corticotropin-releasing hormone (CRH). CRH is released into the bloodstream and flows directly to the pituitary gland. The pituitary contains cells called "corticotrophs" that respond to CRH by releasing the protein hormone adrenocorticotrophic hormone (ACTH) into the bloodstream. Adrenocorticotrophic hormone travels to the adrenal glands and binds to receptors embedded in the membranes of adrenal gland cortex cells, inducing adrenal cortex cells to take up cholesterol and convert it to pregnenolone in their mitochondria. The enzyme cholesterol desmolase catalyzes this reaction which ACTH also induces. Increased cortisol blood levels inhibit ACTH and CRH secretion by the anterior pituitary and hypothalamus.

Mineralocorticoids. Mineralocorticoids are adrenal steroids that regulate potassium and sodium levels in the body. They are synthesized in the zona glomerulosa of the adrenal cortex. Only the zona glomerulosa cells have the enzyme aldosterone synthase, which makes aldosterone, the main mineralocorticoid, from other corticosterone. The peptide signaling molecule angiotensin II induces aldosterone synthase expression.

Mineralocorticoids affect the distal tubules of the kidney by stimulating the excretion of potassium and sodium reabsorption. Their net effect is to increase the volume of body fluids. The adrenal cortex secretes aldosterone at about 0.1 milligrams per day.

Glucocorticoids. Glucocorticoids are the adrenal steroids made in the zona fasciculata. These hormones regulate glucose metabolism. In humans, cortisol is responsible for most of the glucocorticoid activity. It is secreted by the adrenal cortex at about 20 milligrams per day and metabolically affects tissues throughout the body. Cortisol is regulated by the central nervous system and the body's permissive or stimulatory messenger molecules. Generally, glucocorticoids stimulate glucose production and enhance the use of fat and protein as energy sources. Glucocorticoids are not stored but released as they are made. The adrenal gland secretes cortisol in pulses and peaks in the early morning, around 6 AM.

Androgens. Androgens are steroid hormones secreted primarily by the testes, adrenal glands, and ovaries. The innermost layer of the adrenal cortex, the zona reticularis, receives steroid metabolites, 17-alpha-hydroxypregnenolone and 17-alpha-hydroxyprogesterone, from the zona fasciculata. The zona reticularis cells use the enzyme 17,20 lyase to convert 17-alpha-hydroxypregnenolone into dehydroepiandrosterone (DHEA) and 17-alpha-hydroxyprogesterone into androstenedione. Dehydroepiandrosterone and androstenedione are interchangeable since the enzyme 3-beta-hydroxysteroid dehydrogenase readily converts one into the other. Androstenedione and DHEA are precursors of testosterone. Testosterone is converted to estrogen by the enzyme aromatase. The testosterone and estrogen made by the adrenal cortex are rather small compared to the testosterone made by the testes and estrogen synthesized by the ovaries. The small amount of testosterone made by the female adrenal cortex influences secondary sex characteristic development like underarm and pubic hair.

Testosterone is the principal androgen secreted by the testes; it regulates the development and function of male sex accessory organs. Increased testosterone secretion during puberty is required for seminal vesicle and prostate growth. Removal of androgens by castration results in these organs undergoing atrophy.

Androgens promote protein synthesis or anabolic activity in skeletal muscle, bone, and kidneys. They stimulate the growth of the larynx and cause the lowering of the voice. They increase hemoglobin synthesis, which is higher in males than females, and affect bone growth by causing the conversion of cartilage to bone. As a class of compounds, androgens are reasonably safe since they have limited and relatively predictable side effects. In human males, testosterone is synthesized by the testes at the rate of about 8 milligrams per day.

Estrogens and progesterone. Estrogens and progesterone are primarily produced in the ovaries of nonpregnant adult women. The ovary contains ovarian follicles comprised of an oocyte (egg) surrounded by an inner layer of granulosa cells and an outer layer of thecal cells. Serum VLDLs deliver cholesterol to thecal cells (granulosa cells are too far from the blood supply). Thecal cells use the enzyme cholesterol desmolase to convert cholesterol to pregnenolone. Most of the pregnenolone is converted into androstenedione. Androstenedione diffuses to the granulosa cells. Granulosa cells use two enzymes, 17-beta-hydroxysteroid dehydrogenase to convert androstenedione to testosterone and aromatase to convert testosterone to 17-beta-estradiol. Aromatase is induced by the hormone follicle-stimulating hormone (FSH) secreted by the anterior lobe of the pituitary gland. During the luteal phase of the menstrual cycle (after ovulation), low FSH levels decrease aromatase levels, and granulosa cells convert pregnenolone into progesterone. Consequently, before ovulation, the ovaries make more estrogen than progesterone, and after ovulation, they make more progesterone than estrogen.

During pregnancy, the placenta is the major estrogen and progesterone production site. Smaller estrogen synthesis involves the liver, kidney, skeletal muscle, and testes. Progesterone and estrogen are released into the bloodstream and bound by plasma proteins like albumin, sex-binding hormone globulin (SBHG), and transcortin. These hormones are transported throughout the body and have systemic effects. The systemic effects of estrogen and progesterone begin at puberty. Estrogen and progesterone drive the maturation of the female reproductive system, including the fallopian tubes, uterus, cervix, and vagina. Estrogen stimulates secondary sexual characteristics, such as fat distribution on the hips, thighs, and buttocks, hip widening, and breast growth. Estrogen also increases bone density and blood vessel flexibility and lowers low-density lipoprotein levels. Progesterone increases skin elasticity and improves bone health.

USES AND COMPLICATIONS

When cortisone was initially discovered, it was labeled a "wonder drug" and thought to possess overall effectiveness in many areas of medicine. Although these expectations have not been realized, various steroids are effective in medical practice and treatment. Steroids are commonly prescribed for those persons whose bodies cannot produce specific steroid hormones in adequate quantities. Steroids are effective anti-inflammatory agents, reducing inflammatory reactions in various body tissues. They are also prescribed for patients who have undergone organ transplantation or have highly sensitive allergies because they inhibit the immune system's responsiveness.

The primary therapeutic use of androgens is for testicular deficiency. Fluoxymesterone and methyltestosterone are two oral testosterone, and testosterone esters like testosterone cypionate are long-acting testosterones injected intramuscularly. These drugs effectively replace testosterone in males with hypogonadism with low testosterone levels that cause delayed puberty. In these cases, supplemental doses of androgens are given to stimulate and enhance the development of sexual and accessory sex characteristics. Androgens are also effective in treating some anemias when persons have reduced levels of red blood cells. Androgens are used to treat osteoporosis, a decrease in bone or skeletal mass. Androgens are given to women in breast cancer treatment and are effective about 20 percent of the time. They treat the abnormal growth of endometrial tissue in the peritoneal cavity of women, a disease called "endometriosis," and are effective in that role.

Steroids also have anabolic activities that are manifested by stimulating increases in protein production, enhancing the uptake of amino acids into cells, and inhibiting the glucocorticoids from breaking down proteins. They influence embryonic development, especially the differentiation of the central nervous system and the male reproductive tract. The excitatory function of androgens occurs at puberty, during which the reproductive organs are activated to produce sex cells. Androgens also maintain the body's sexual characteristics in the adult. Thus, in cases of androgen deficiency, there is a regression of male sexual behavior, libido, and reproductive function; this regression is reversible with treatment.

Anabolic steroids are synthetic androgens with chemical modifications that increase their anabolic activity. Nandrolone and oxandrolone are two anabolic steroids that treat aplastic anemia, a condition caused by the bone marrow no longer producing enough red blood cells. Unfortunately, these drugs and testosterone derivatives are abused because of their anabolic effects. Athletes and bodybuilders searching for accelerated muscle building or physical definition are two groups in which such abuse has been seen. One complication is that the stimulatory effects of anabolic steroids reinforce their abuse, making them addictive. Frequent users of anabolic steroids should be aware of conditions such as dependence, withdrawal, and other problematic side effects of heavy steroid use. Such effects may include increased periods of sleep disturbance, paranoia, anger and agitation, mood swings or instability of mood, violence or other impulsive behavior, and concentration and memory disturbance. Physical problems may include severe acne, jaundice, excess water retention, decreased sperm count, high cholesterol, liver problems, and difficulty controlling blood sugar.

The condition known as "Addison's disease" is caused by a failure of the adrenal gland to secrete adequate amounts of both glucocorticoids and mineralocorticoids. Adrenal insufficiency can be primary, secondary, or tertiary—primary adrenal insufficiency results from problems with the adrenal cortex. Autoimmune diseases of the adrenal glands or disseminated tuberculosis, human immunodeficiency virus (HIV), or fungal infections are causes of primary adrenal insufficiency. Pituitary gland abnormalities cause secondary adrenal insufficiency. Pituitary gland tumors or other conditions prevent it from secreting ACTH. Tertiary adrenal gland insufficiencies result from hypothalamic dysfunction that prevent CRH secretion. The symptoms of this disease are imbalances in body levels of sodium and potassium, dehydration, reduced blood pressure, rapid weight loss, and generalized weakness. People with primary adrenal insufficiency may also show hyperpigmentation inside the mouth, creases of the palm, and knuckles. Decreased cortisol production increases ACTH production. ACTH is made from a larger precursor that produces melanocyte-stimulating hormone (MSH). Melanocyte-stimulating hormone increases pigment concentration in some body areas. A person with Addison's disease will die if not treated with fludrocortisone and hydrocortisone because of severe electrolyte imbalance and dehydration.

Another disorder, Cushing's syndrome, results when the adrenal gland secretes corticosteroids in excessive quantities. Symptoms include high blood pressure, protein and carbohydrate metabolism alterations, high blood sugar concentrations, and muscular weakness. A tumor often causes this syndrome in the adrenal gland that promotes the secretion of corticosteroids. Surgical intervention is often used to remove the portion of the malfunctioning gland. Symptoms similar to those seen in Cushing's syndrome are found in people with inflammatory diseases who receive lengthy treatments with corticosteroids to reduce the inflammation.

Adrenogenital syndrome results from excessive sex steroids, and adrenal gland hyperactivity is usually the main cause. Androgen is the major sex steroid involved in this clinical condition, which causes premature puberty and enlarged genital sex organs in young children. Other characteristics are increased body and facial hair and deepening of the voice.

Synthetic estrogens like ethinyl estradiol and mestranol treat primary hypogonadism in young girls that results from low estrogen levels. These synthetic estrogens come as vaginal creams, transdermal patches, and intramuscular injections.

The most frequent use of estrogens is for oral contraceptives or birth control pills. This method is convenient, reversible, and relatively inexpensive; its use is worldwide and includes approximately 16 percent of American women of childbearing age and 25 percent of all contraceptive users. Most oral contraceptives combine estrogen ethinyl estradiol and a synthetic progestin or consist of a synthetic progestin alone (minipills). Combination oral contraceptives come as monophasic or multiphasic oral contraceptive pills (OCPs). Monophasic OCPs contain a fixed dose of estrogen and progestin in every pill. Multiphasic OCPs vary the dose of one or both hormones throughout the twenty-eight-day cycle. Traditional preparations contain twenty-one active pills and seven placebos. The traditional formulation results in thirteen withdrawal bleeds per year. Other regimens have few hormone-free days (two to four placebo or iron tablets per twenty-day cycle) or continuous (also called extended) cycles with fewer withdrawal bleeds per year. Continuous OCPs effectively treat women with dysmenorrhea, premenstrual syndrome, or premenstrual dysphoric disorder. Progestin-only pills, minipills, contain norethindrone. Women take minipills continuously without a break. Breastfeeding women and those who do not tolerate estrogen usually take minipills. These steroids inhibit the release of gonadotropic hormones by the pituitary gland's anterior lobe, which normally stimulates ovulation. Hormones were also once the primary treatment for menopausal symptoms. However, the Women's Health Initiative Study showed that while hormone therapy had some benefits, it also increased the risk for blood clots, breast cancer, heart attacks, and strokes.

Antiandrogens are substances that prevent or depress the action of androgens, or testosterone, on the body. Flutamide competitively inhibits the androgen receptor. This drug treats prostate cancer since this cancer depends on androgens for survival in the early course of the disease. Flutamide causes breast enlargement (gynecomastia), sexual dysfunction, and vomiting. Spironolactone is a diuretic that also inhibits the androgen receptor. It treats excessive hair growth (hirsutism) caused by polycystic ovary disease. In men, spironolactone treats male pattern baldness. This drug causes gynecomastia in men, and women who take this drug stop having periods.

For nonmetastatic castration-resistant prostate cancer, the US Food and Drug Administration (FDA) has approved three different androgen receptor inhibitors, darolutamide (Nubeqa), apalutamide (Erleada), and enzalutamide (Xtandi).

The prostate depends on dihydrotestosterone for androgenic stimulation. 5-alpha reductase inhibitors prevent the conversion of testosterone to dihydrotestosterone. 5-alpha reductase inhibitors like finasteride and dutasteride treat benign prostatic hyperplasia and hair loss in men. These drugs cause gynecomastia, infertility, and sexual dysfunction, but not as frequently as other antiandrogens.

Antiandrogens are valuable for managing patients whose bodies are producing abnormally high levels of androgens, who are undergoing premature puberty, or who are affected with acne, hirsutism (excessive hairiness, especially in women), and certain tumors or neoplasms. Potentially, these drugs can be utilized to cause sterility in males.

Treatment of abnormal growths, malignant cancers, or benign tumors in the male prostate gland has frequently used natural or synthetic steroids. Natural body androgens stimulate the growth of the prostate gland in males and enhance the proliferation of many prostate cancers. Estradiol, a form of the female sex steroid estrogen, is used to control the advancement of prostate carcinoma in some males and can induce remission in 50 to 80 percent of the cases of prostate tumors. Estrogens exert their effect by interfering with androgen production or inhibiting androgen-responsive tissues' function. Thus, in some cases, estrogens inhibit abnormal cellular growth. A manufactured synthetic drug, cyproterone acetate, is also used to treat benign prostatic enlargement in men. Cyproterone acetate is very effective in treating prostate cancers and tumors. It does not have the feminizing side effects of the estrogens; however, it does cause inhibition of sperm production and loss of sexual drive.

PERSPECTIVE AND PROSPECTS

The use of steroids as therapeutic agents began in the early 1930s. At that time, Philip Showalter Hench, who was working in the Mayo Clinic, noticed that the symptoms of arthritic women were alleviated when they became pregnant. He suggested that increased secretions from the adrenal cortex might be the responsible agents. Later, clinical trials were conducted to test the role of corticosteroids in treating acute arthritis. With the use of adequate dosages, the clinical response was impressive. The 1950 Nobel Prize in Physiology or Medicine was awarded to Hench and his coworkers to find that cortisone was effective in treating arthritis.

Pharmaceutical firms have manufactured numerous steroid derivatives, all of which have different effectiveness levels as glucocorticoids, mineralocorticoids, or sex steroids. Organic chemists synthesize adrenal steroid analogs to create compounds that produce heightened biological effects with minimal or no side effects. Consequently, hundreds of different steroids are available. Most of these are characterized according to their biological effectiveness, such as reducing inflammation or inhibiting the immune system. When determining a course of treatment, a physician chooses a particular steroid that enhances desired effects and has minimal effects in related areas. The skin very poorly absorbs some pharmaceutical derivatives of adrenal steroids. These derivatives are especially useful to apply to the skin when a maximal local effect is desired without a generalized effect on other body regions.

However, steroids can also have negative and sometimes dangerous effects on the body, whether ingested (cholesterol) or injected (anabolic steroids). Evidence indicates that high blood cholesterol levels are associated with an increased risk of atherosclerosis, a clinical condition in which localized plaques (or atheromas) build up in the walls of arteries, reducing blood flow. Atheromas serve as locations for blood clot formation, further blocking the blood supply to a vital organ such as the heart, brain, or lung. High blood cholesterol may result from a diet rich in cholesterol and saturated fat or an inherited condition (familial hypercholesterolemia) in which affected individuals have extremely high cholesterol concentrations regardless of their diet. In the latter case, affected persons usually suffer heart attacks during childhood.

Cholesterol is found in foods prepared from animal products. Cholesterol-rich foods include most meats, eggs, and dairy products such as cheese, cream, and butter. Humans readily absorb cholesterol from dietary sources. Most Western diets contain 400 to 600 milligrams of cholesterol per day. About 75 percent is readily absorbed into the bloodstream from the dietary tract. Cholesterol is carried to the arteries by proteins in the blood plasma called low-density lipoproteins (LDLs). A given cell may engulf the LDLs and use the cholesterol for different purposes. The LDLs in a given location may stimulate other cells to secrete growth factors that either begin or contribute to atheroma development. Thus, the risk of atherosclerosis is greatly increased. Most people can significantly lower their blood cholesterol levels through controlled exercise and diet. Since saturated fat raises blood cholesterol levels, many health experts recommend limiting their intake of foods such as fatty meat, egg yolk, and liver. Fat should contribute less than 30 percent to the total calories, though others have challenged this assumption.

The use and abuse of anabolic steroids to increase muscle mass and strength is widespread in amateur and professional sports. Although those promoting steroid use claim increases in muscle mass, strength, and endurance, controlled clinical trials show minimal enhancement of muscle mass and strength. Testosterone may also enhance training efforts by promoting aggressive behavior. The use of these compounds poses ethical questions. It increases the risk of serious toxicity because of the extremely high doses administered, often as much as one hundred times the usual therapeutic dosages.

—Michael A. Buratovich

Further Reading

"Anabolic Steroid (Oral Route, Parenteral Route)." *Mayo Clinic*, 1 Feb 2022, www.mayoclinic.org/drugs-supplements/anabolic-steroid-oral-route-parenteral-route/description/drg-20069323. Accessed 18 Jun. 2022.

"Anabolic Steroids." *MedlinePlus*, 2 June 2021, medlineplus.gov/anabolicsteroids.html. Accessed 18 June 2022.

Craig, Charles R., and Robert E. Stitzel, editors. *Modern Pharmacology with Clinical Applications*. 6th ed., Lippincott, 2004.

Guyton, Arthur C., and John E. Hall. *Human Physiology and Mechanisms of Disease*. 6th ed., W. B. Saunders, 1997.

Henry, Helen L., and Anthony W. Norman, editors. *Encyclopedia of Hormones*. 3 vols. Academic Press, 2003.

Melmed, Schlomo, et al., editors. *Williams Textbook of Endocrinology*. 14th ed., Elsevier, 2019.

Montgomery, Rex, et al. *Biochemistry: A Case-Oriented Approach*. 6th ed., Mosby, 1996.

"Steroids." *MedlinePlus*, 16 Mar. 2016, medlineplus.gov/steroids.html. Accessed 18 Jun. 2022.

Tortora, Gerard J., and Bryan Derrickson. *Principles of Anatomy and Physiology*. 16th ed., John Wiley and Sons, 2020.

Zelman, Mark, et al. *Human Diseases: A Systemic Approach*. 8th ed., Pearson, 2014.

Exercise Training

"Fitness is attained one exercise session at a time."

—Tom Miles, *A Year for Change*

Most people go to a gym and start bench pressing or running several miles if they want to start exercising. Is there a better way to go about it? As this section shows, the answer is yes. The risk of injuries, tiredness, and even sickness is elevated if beginning or returning to an exercise regimen too quickly, not to mention the demoralizing effects of unrealistic expectations. Exercise, if done regularly, can have long-lasting good effects on strength, fitness, weight, balance, and energy levels. A few approaches outlined in this segment include: aerobics, cross training, HITT training, stretching, and weight training.

Aerobics

Category: Biology
Specialties and related fields: Exercise physiology, sports medicine

KEY TERMS

aerobic exercise: any type of cardiovascular conditioning that increases the heart rate
cardiovascular: activities or conditions that affect the heart and blood vessels
exercise: activity requiring physical effort, carried out to sustain or improve health and fitness
metabolism: the biochemical processes in our bodies by which it degrades food, converts it to energy, and uses that energy to carry out the processes of life

BRIEF HISTORY

Aerobics, from the Greek words for air and life, is a term from the field of biology. It refers to sustained moderate physical activity during a specific period that requires an additional effort from the cardiovascular system—that is, the heart and lungs—to increase oxygen transport to the muscles. Aerobic exercise is aimed at improving cardiovascular conditioning and lung function. Since its early days as a dance and exercise routine, aerobics has fueled a multibillion-dollar industry and become a vital part of American culture.

In biology, the word "aerobic" describes organisms that need oxygen to live. Aerobics exercises then stimulate breathing are designed to improve how the body oxygenates. Aerobics is an exercise discipline that began in the postwar years of the twentieth century, when a medical doctor and former military officer, Kenneth H. Cooper, authored the book *Aerobics* (1968). Cooper was already a respected exercise expert because of his studies in the military. He worked not only to improve the physical condition of American soldiers but also to identify their limitations.

Cooper soon became known beyond military circles. He expanded his research to understand better the benefits of intense physical activity called "cardiovascular workout." His research explored not only physical benefits but also mental benefits. He continued to publish books on his findings. Still, it wasn't until 1982 that he could put into practice the overall techniques described in his work. In the beginning, however, aerobics lacked widespread acceptance. Some of the obstacles it faced to becoming universally popular were the lack of adequate spaces to practice it and the monotony of repetitive exercise.

Cooper's first book has sold about 30 million copies worldwide. Nevertheless, the books and workout videos produced by actor Jane Fonda turned aerobics into an unprecedented mass phenomenon. By the 1990s, advances in biomechanics and physiology brought radical changes to the field of aerobics. These studies reduced the incidence of injuries incurred during aerobic exercise and helped increase the benefits to the body.

Aerobics is the most practiced exercise worldwide. The addition of music, dance elements, and attractive gear made aerobic exercise more appealing and played a fundamental role in its widespread popularity. Aerobics instructors added other cardiovascular exercises, including boxing, martial arts, water exercises, and bicycling. Technology expanded apace, and gadgets meant to measure factors such as cardiovascular workout and calorie loss entered the market.

OVERVIEW

What made aerobics different from other exercise routines, such as calisthenics, is the link to dance music. This novelty and the fact that it is usually practiced in groups increased its popularity. Eventually, aerobics became a common household experience, as routines recorded on videocassettes by ex-

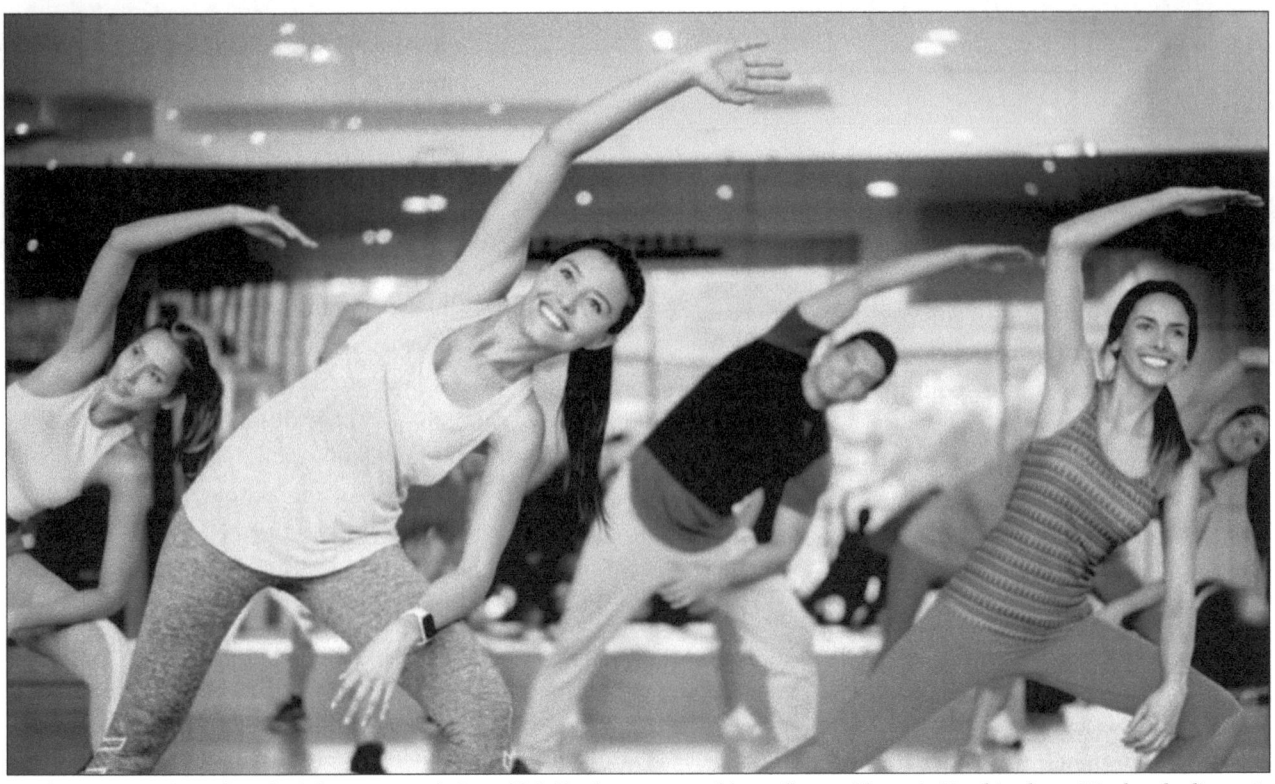

Aerobic exercise reduces the risk of obesity, type-2 diabetes, high blood pressure, and heart disease. Photo via iStock/andresr. [Used under license.]

perts and celebrities, especially Jane Fonda and Richard Simmons, could be played at home. In time, fitness programs became incorporated into many workplaces.

Another reason for the popularity of aerobics is that practically everybody can practice it without being an athlete. A typical aerobics routine consists of warming and stretching exercises for about twenty to thirty minutes to raise the cardiac rate to its target level. Exercise intensity then decreases. The appropriate level depends upon age and health conditions. Some exercise programs include a strength sequence for body-sculpting purposes. Merging aerobics with elements of other dance forms or sports has become commonplace, producing jazzercise, Zumba, spinning, kickboxing, and many others.

Many social forces came together that helped spread the popularity of fitness by way of aerobic exercise. These social forces included science, such as the studies on the health benefits of fitness, government incentives, commercial interests, and national culture. In the United States, the cultivation of health and fitness has long been a cultural factor. Experts and popular periodicals have touted the benefits of a healthy lifestyle since the nineteenth century. Nevertheless, before World War II, to be overly concerned with physical prowess and health was considered strange.

Decades before the success of aerobics, trailblazer Jane Fonda, strongman Charles Atlas (1892-1972), and exercise guru Jack LaLanne (1914-2011) ran extremely successful marketing campaigns touting the benefits of proper nutrition and exercise. In 1956, President Dwight Eisenhower created the President's Council on Youth Fitness, with the main objective of raising public awareness. It developed a plan of action and a nationwide pilot program that studied the fitness level of more than eight thousand children between the ages of five and twelve. In 1965, under President Lyndon B. Johnson, another nationwide fitness study took place with children ages ten to seventeen years of age.

These government studies highlighted a concern, specific to the Cold War period, with the health and fitness of the young. They heralded the eventual popularity of aerobics and other new fitness sports, such as jogging, which became a craze in the 1970s. Jogging, however, is a mostly solitary sport. In the 1980s, a preference for the shared experience of health clubs and gyms prevailed.

In the second decade of the twenty-first century, the revenues from the health and fitness industry reached about $33 billion a year, with continued expectations for growth. Approximately 45 million Americans spend money on exercise technology and gear, club memberships, and various other products related to fitness. The expense and other social factors associated with exercise programs have been cited as causes for exclusion. According to many social scientists, fitness has become a vital part of American identity, raising questions about who gets left behind from participation in it and why. The fact that many cannot afford gym memberships and gear suggests a link between fitness and issues of social class.

—*Trudy Mercadal, Geraldine Marrocco*

Further Reading

Bishop, Jan Galen. *Fitness through Aerobics*. Cummings, 2013.
Black, Jonathan. *Making the American Body: The Remarkable Saga of the Men and Women Whose Feats, Feuds, and Passions Shaped Fitness History*. U of Nebraska P, 2013.
Cooper, Kenneth H. *Aerobics Program for Total Well-Being: Exercise, Diet and Emotional Balance*. Bantam, 2013.
———. *Regaining the Power of Youth at Any Age: Startling New Evidence from the Doctor Who Brought Us Aerobics, Controlling Cholesterol, and the Antioxidant Revolution*. Nelson, 2005.
Ehrman, Jonathan, et al. *Clinical Exercise Physiology*. 3rd ed., Human Kinetics, 2013.
Malcolm, Dominic. *The Sage Dictionary of Sports Studies*. Sage, 2008.
McKenzie, Shelley. *Getting Physical: The Rise of Fitness Culture in America*. UP of Kansas, 2013.
Zoumbaris, Sharon K., editor. *Encyclopedia of Wellness*. Greenwood, 2012.

Autogenic Training

Category: Therapy or technique
Also known as: Autosuggestion, hypnosis, relaxation
Definition: a method of self-control therapy that teaches a person to use specific phrases to enter a state of deep relaxation and achieve healing

KEY TERMS

autosuggestion: the hypnotic or subconscious adoption of an idea that one has originated oneself, sometimes by repeating verbal statements to oneself to change behavior
selective awareness: the process of directing our awareness to relevant stimuli while ignoring other stimuli in the environment
self-hypnosis: putting oneself in a highly suggestive state to focus, motivate, become more self-aware, and make the best use of innate skills
trigger: an event or situation that can induce certain mental states to occur

OVERVIEW

Autogenic ("generated from within") training, or AT, is one of the oldest biobehavioral methods used in clinical psychology and stress management. Developed in the 1920s by Johannes H. Schultz as a self-hypnotic procedure, it drew on the observation that persons often reported a sensation of heaviness (muscle relaxation) and warmth (vascular dilation) in their limbs under hypnosis.

A firm believer in the self-regulatory capacities of the human body, Schultz considered that hypnosis occurred not only because the patient allowed it but also because they induced it. Consequently, Schultz looked for an autogenic "trigger," or formula, that he could use to enter this state. Ultimately, he perfected a series of simple mental exercises that allow the mind to calm itself by turning off the body's stress responses.

The technique uses autosuggestion to establish a new mind/body balance through changes in the autonomic nervous system. Unlike progressive muscular relaxation and biofeedback, AT does not involve a conscious attempt to relax the muscles or control physiological functions. Rather, through passive self-suggestion ("observing" concentration and nonforcing), the person tries to render specific body regions warm and heavy. The training process involves focusing on and subvocally repeating one of six basic autogenic phrases, or orientations, several minutes each day for one week or more. These phrases (with many possible variations) are "My arms and legs are heavy," "My arms and legs are warm," "My heartbeat is calm and regular," "My lungs are breathing for me," "My abdomen is warm," and "My forehead is cool." The practitioner can change the words without altering the method's effectiveness to suit the practitioner's mind and circumstances. Within months of training, achieving a state of deep relaxation and beneficial physiological changes will take only seconds.

MECHANISM OF ACTION

The AT verbal suggestions represent self-hypnosis, which is very powerful in inducing deep relaxation. Autogenic training uses selective awareness (SA),

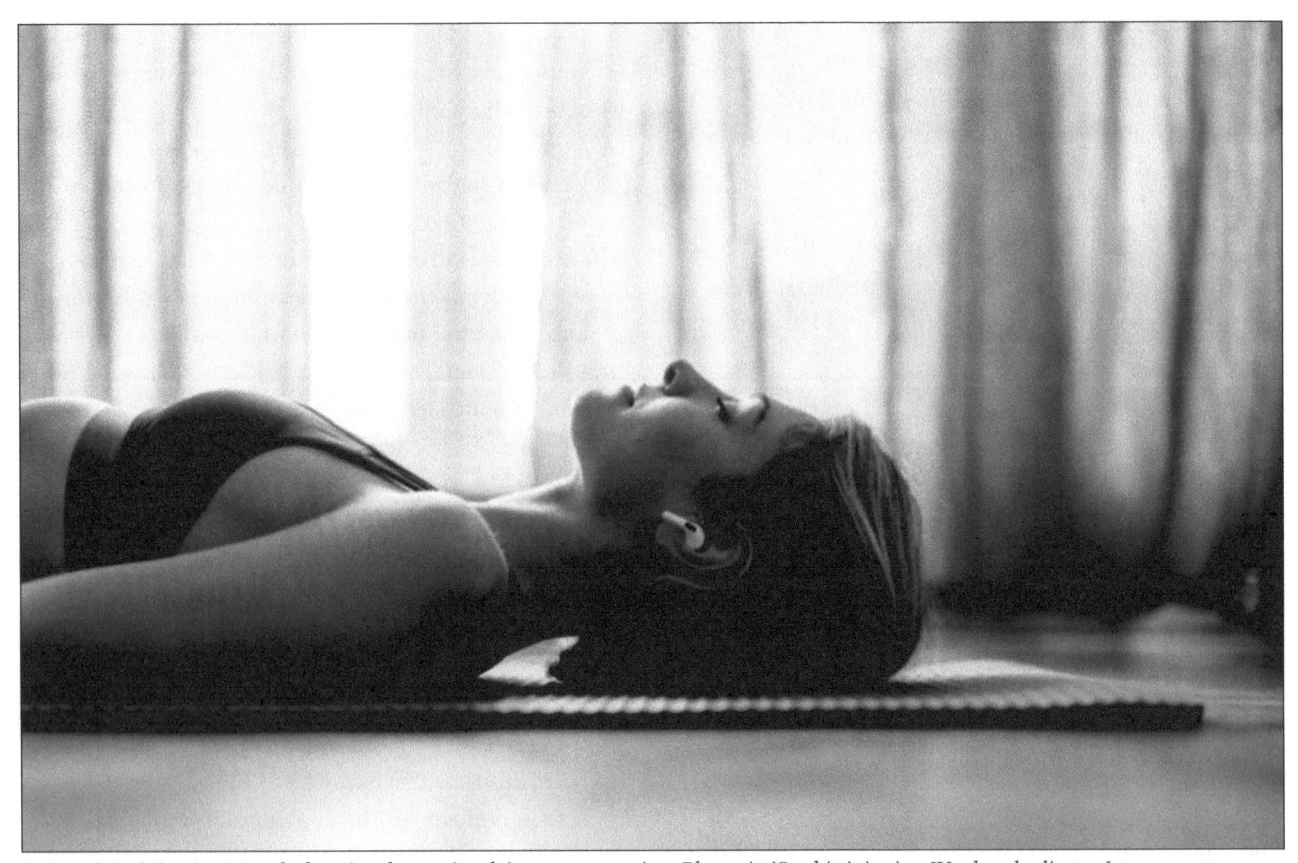

Autogenic training is a type of relaxation therapy involving autosuggestion. Photo via iStock/miniseries. [Used under license.]

which represents the receptivity of the conscious mind to receive and acknowledge specific thoughts. Under SA circumstances, the censorship exerted by the ego should be eradicated, and thoughts should be allowed to travel freely from the conscious to the unconscious realm. The absence of censorship can dramatically improve the mind's ability to influence physiological processes as desired. In this receptive state, pain sensations are also significantly reduced.

Worldwide, abundant anecdotal reports of persons accomplishing daunting physical tasks while severely injured bear witness to the power of this phenomenon. Still insufficiently understood, the interplay between conscious and unconscious can nevertheless play important roles in maintaining physiological and psychological homeostasis. The method appears to exert a balancing effect upon the two branches of the autonomic nervous system (sympathetic and parasympathetic, fight-or-flight and rest-and-digest, respectively).

During AT sessions, sudden physical and emotional reactions, such as numbness, muscle twitching, or tears, may result from the release of unconscious thoughts. The manifestation, considered normal and even beneficial, is called "autogenic discharge."

USES AND APPLICATIONS

Autogenic training is most used to reduce anxiety, fatigue, chronic pain, and stress. The sensations of warmth and heaviness can induce sleep, thus rendering the method useful in persons with insomnia.

Other proposed uses for the method include constipation and diarrhea, gastritis, ulcers, headaches, high blood pressure, hyperventilation, asthma, irregular and rapid heartbeat, and Raynaud's phenomenon (episodic vasospasm of fingers and toes). Evidence suggests that AT may enhance mental well-being and clinical outcome in persons with Meniere's disease (an inner-ear disorder that affects hearing and balance).

SCIENTIFIC EVIDENCE

Thousands of studies have been conducted on AT's effects and clinical applications, both in Europe since the introduction of the method and in the United States beginning in the 1980s. A wealth of data remains in languages other than English.

Ample experimental support exists for the hypothesis that AT affects sympathetic tone and even parasympathetic function (increased cardiac parasympathetic tone, with beneficial results). There is considerable difficulty in standardizing the technique, selecting participants, and measuring outcomes, so rigorous clinical studies are notoriously difficult to perform. Many studies have serious methodological flaws. Nevertheless, randomized-controlled trials have been conducted, with significant results indicating AT effectiveness in reducing anxiety and chronic pain, improving the symptoms of migraine headaches and alleviating the symptoms of irritable bowel syndrome and other conditions.

CHOOSING A PRACTITIONER

Autogenic training is more popular in Europe and Japan than in North America. The British Autogenic Society offers therapist training courses and maintains a directory of practitioners in the United Kingdom and abroad. These practitioners have various backgrounds and may be doctors, nurses, psychotherapists, psychologists, complementary therapists, social workers, or teachers. Interested persons can learn the technique from numerous books, websites, or, preferably, AT therapists. A specialist can confirm the quality of the practice, monitor progress, provide feedback, and implement variations from the standard.

SAFETY ISSUES

Autogenic training is generally safe and can be used by most people, except children younger than school age and persons with severe psychiatric disorders. However, before implementing the technique, persons should undergo a physical examination and discuss potential effects with a health-care practitioner. It has been suggested that rapid autonomic rebounds can lead to dizziness, disorientation, anxiety, panic, and even hallucinations. Finally, persons with cardiovascular diseases, diabetes, or other severe disorders should only use AT under medical supervision.

—*Mihaela Avramut*

Further Reading

Edlin, Gordon, and Eric Golanty. *Health and Wellness*. 10th ed., Jones and Bartlett, 2010.

Linden, Wolfgang. "The Autogenic Training Method of J. H. Schultz." *Principles and Practice of Stress Management*, edited by Paul M. Lehrer and Robert L. Woolfolk, 4th ed., Guilford Press, 2021, pp. 527-52.

Seaward, Brian L. *Managing Stress: Principles and Strategies for Health and Well-Being*. 6th ed., Jones and Bartlett, 2009.

"Welcome to the British Autogenic Society." *British Autogenic Society*, 2022, britishautogenicsociety.uk/. Accessed 28 May 2022.

Blood Flow Restriction (BFR) Training

Category: Training

Specialties and related fields: Athletic training, physical therapy

Definition: a tissue category composed of adipose (fat), blood, bone, cartilage, ligaments, and tendons; the function of connective tissue is to connect, support, bind, protect, and store materials

KEY TERMS

blood clots: an important process that prevents excessive bleeding when a blood vessel is injured

Kaatsu training: a patented exercise method developed by Dr. Yoshiaki Sato that is based on blood flow moderation exercise involving compression of the vasculature proximal to the exercising muscles

INTRODUCTION

Blood flow restriction (BFR) training is used to increase muscle size and strength. It is employed by physical therapists as well as bodybuilders and athletes. It is also known as "occlusion therapy." It involves using some form of compression device wrapped around the upper portion of a limb to restrict blood flow. The controlled restriction of blood flow causes changes in the muscle cells. Proponents say these changes promote rapid growth in the muscle cells, allowing faster healing for injured limbs and increasing the strength and performance of healthy limbs. However, the practice risks cutting off too much blood flow or causing blood clots. Athletes should do it under the supervision of a physical therapist or another trained professional.

OVERVIEW

Blood flow restriction training is also known as "Kaatsu training." This name was given by the person generally credited with developing the method, Yoshiaki Sato. While maintaining a kneeling position for a long period during a Buddhist prayer service in 1966, Sato noticed that the muscles in his leg swelled much like they did while he exercised.

After years of experimentation that sent him to the emergency room at least once with a blood clot, Sato developed a technique for using a compression device around his limbs that increased the effects of exercise. He called this Kaatsu training. The technique has been popular in Japan for years and eventually spread worldwide.

Blood flow restriction training involves using a compression device similar to a blood pressure cuff applied to the upper portion of an arm or leg before exercise. Specially made devices exist for this purpose, but some use compression bandages or tourniquets wrapped around the limb. The device or band is applied so that the blood carried by arteries deeper in the limb can get into the arm or leg, but the blood in the veins, which are closer to the surface, cannot flow back to the heart. In most cases, BFR training aims to restrict about 50 to 80 percent of the blood flow to the limb.

The person then engages in exercise with the device in place. This forces blood to fill blood vessels and muscles that proponents of the technique claim tricks the brain into believing the body is exercising harder than it is. This technique increases lactic acid production, the substance that makes muscles burn when a person uses them strenuously. Lactic acid breaks down muscle fibers, so new ones are made. The technique also increases other hormones and chemicals related to muscle growth. Therefore, proponents claim that BFR training promotes a fast buildup of new muscle, which is beneficial to both patients recovering from an illness or injury and those who are building muscle for athletic purposes.

Medical experts caution against using the technique without the supervision of a trained expert. They point to the risk of blood clots and damage to the limb. They also note that additional studies need to be performed to determine what effect altering blood flow in this way will have on the heart.

—Janine Ungvarsky

Further Reading

Anderson, Jon R. "Kaatsu Training Is Blowing Fitness Researchers' Mind." *Military Times*, 6 Feb. 2015, www.militarytimes.com/2015/02/06/kaatsu-training-is-blowing-fitness-researchers-minds/. Accessed 22 Oct. 2018.

"Blood Flow Restriction Training." *American Physical Therapy Association*, www.apta.org/PatientCare/BloodFlowRestrictionTraining/. Accessed 22 Oct. 2018.

Gaddour, B. J. "The Fastest Way to Make Your Muscles Grow." *Men's Health*, 21 Dec. 2016, www.menshealth.com/fitness/a19534758/blood-flow-restriction-to-build-muscle/. Accessed 22 Oct. 2018.

Matthews, Mike. "Does Blood Flow Restriction (Occlusion) Training Really Work?" *Legion Athletics*, legionathletics.com/blood-flow-restriction-occlusion-training/. Accessed 22 Oct. 2018.

Mazzone, Nicholas. "Blood Flow Restriction Training: What Is It and Will It Work for My Patients?" *New Grad Physical Therapy*, 8 May 2017, newgradphysicaltherapy.com/blood-flow-restriction-training/. Accessed 22 Oct. 2018.

Sato, Y. "The History and Future of KAATSU Training." *International Journal of Kaatsu*, 2005, www.kaatsu-global.com/Assets/Files/Presentations/The_history_and_future_of_KAATSU_Training.pdf. Accessed 22 Oct. 2018.

Spranger, Marty D., et al. "Blood Flow Restriction Training and the Exercise Pressor Reflex: A Call for Concern." *American Journal of Physiology—Heart and Circulatory Physiology*, Nov. 2015, www.physiology.org/doi/full/10.1152/ajpheart.00208.2015. Accessed 22 Oct. 2018.

Wilson, Jacob. "Your Complete Guide to Blood Flow Restriction Training." *Body Building*, 27 July 2018, www.bodybuilding.com/content/your-complete-guide-to-blood-flow-restriction-training.html. Accessed 22 Oct. 2018.

CROSS-TRAINING

Category: Training

Specialties and related fields: Athletic training, exercise science, strength and conditioning

Definition: an athletic training method that combines different types of exercise to reduce injury risk and increase strength in little-used muscles

KEY TERMS

exercise routine: physical exertion to improve one's fitness for athletic competition, ability, or performance that consists of regularly doing a series of things in a fixed order

repetitive strain injury: injuries to muscles, nerves, ligaments, and tendons caused by improper technique or overuse that most commonly affect the elderly

INTRODUCTION

In general terms, cross-training can refer to routinely practicing more than one subject, professional endeavor, or sport to improve one's overall performance. The term is most commonly applied to the field of sports. It refers to a training or exercise program designed to help an athlete's overall performance in their main sport (e.g., bicycling, running, or swimming) while reducing the risk of injury caused by the repetitive movements or motions associated with the sport. Cross-training gained popularity in the early 1980s and has since become an accepted training approach. Athletic coaches, trainers, and medical professionals recommend it to help athletes improve their overall health, physical fitness, and athletic ability and performance.

OVERVIEW

Cross-training has a long history; the first Olympic athletes routinely cross-trained by varying their exercise routines to include running, weight training, and wrestling (typically with animals) to improve their overall endurance, strength, and performance in the games. These ancient cross-training programs, referred to as the tetrad, outlined the Olympians' exercise routines over four days, with each day of the cycle focused on a different activity.

Today, cross-training in modern sports training has become an accepted practice by athletic trainers, coaches, medical professionals, and athletes to help athletes avoid injuries caused by repetitive movements and increase an athlete's overall performance and health. Commonly used in training programs for competitive runners, cyclists, and swimmers, cross-training helps these athletes avoid common injuries caused by repetitive motions that come with these sports (e.g., knee and shoulder injuries). However, noncompetitive athletes and sports enthusiasts also practice cross-training because these programs tout various other benefits, including reducing boredom with a training program, helping the body adapt to new activities, and allowing certain groups of muscles to rest. In contrast, other muscles are strengthened, improving a person's overall recovery

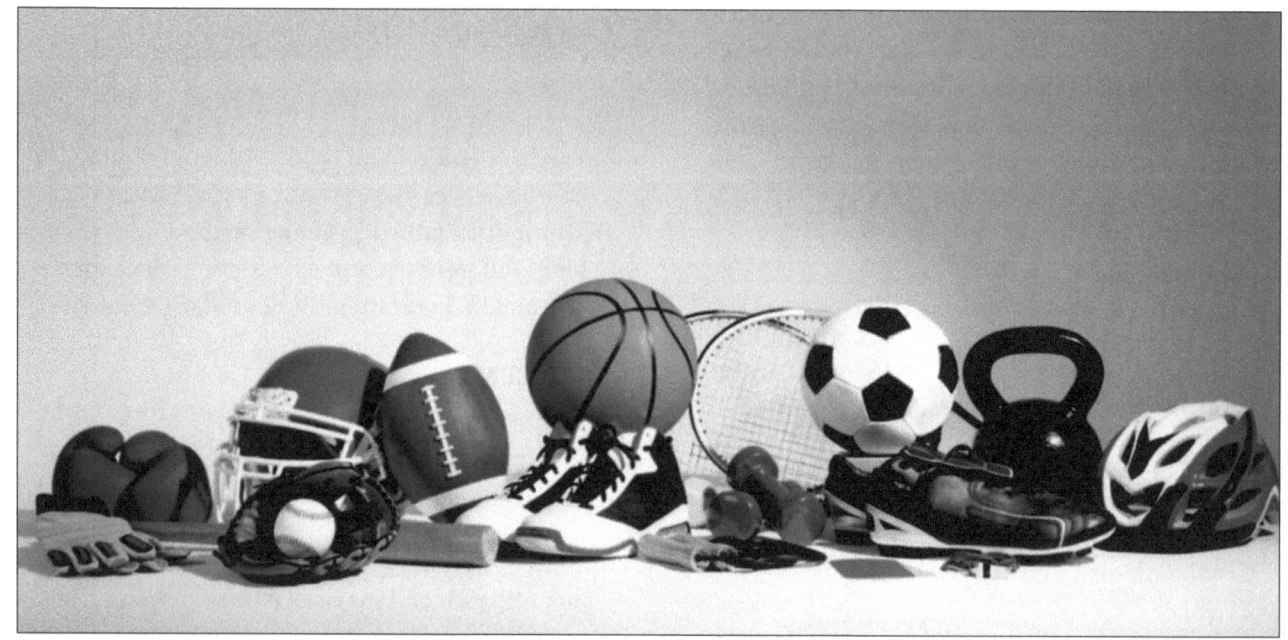

Athletes cross-train, or engage in sports other than their usual sport, to improve overall performance. Photo via iStock/AndreyPopov. [Used under license.]

time. Additional benefits of cross-training referenced by sports experts and medical professionals include building stamina, aerobic and flexibility capacity, and muscle strength.

The risk of repetitive strain injuries caused by overuse is reduced when an athlete's exercise routine alternately works various muscle groups and joints. The exercise variation takes place either daily or weekly. Typical variations include rotating the time a person spends practicing the main activity with other exercises that focus on weight and strength training.

A person does not have to be a competitive athlete to benefit from a cross-training program. Many people who routinely exercise vary their routines and techniques as a normal part of their exercise regimen. This variation can reduce boredom and increase overall motivation for engaging in a routine exercise program.

—L. L. Lundin

Further Reading

Anderson, Marcia K. *Foundations of Athletic Training: Prevention, Assessment, and Management*. Philadelphia: Lippincott Williams & Wilkins, 2012.

"Cross-training for Fun and Fitness." *American Council on Exercise (ACE)*, 2013, acewebcontent.azureedge.net/assets/education-resources/lifestyle/fitfacts/pdfs/fitfacts/itemid_2547.pdf.

Ellis, Marie. "Heart Benefits Linked to Marathon Training, Researchers Say." *Medical News Today*, 28 Mar. 2014, www.medicalnewstoday.com/articles/274749.php.

Joubert, Dustin P., Gary L. Oden, and Brent C. Estes. "The Effects of Elliptical Cross Training on VO_2max in Recently Trained Runners." *International Journal of Exercise Science*, vol. 4 no. 1, 2011, pp. 4-12.

Kisner, Carol, and Lynn Allen Colby. *Therapeutic Exercise: Foundations and Techniques*. 5th ed., Philadelphia: Davis, 2007.

Kolata, Gina. "Perks of Cross-Training May End Before Finish Line." *New York Times*, 15 Aug. 2011, www.nytimes.com/2011/08/16/health/16best.html.

Millet, G. P., et al. "Modeling the Transfers of Training Effects on Performance in Elite Triathletes." *International Journal of Sports Medicine*, vol. 1, 2002, pp. 55-63.

Starkey, Chad, editor. *Athletic Training and Sports Medicine: An Integrated Approach*. American Academy of Orthopaedic Surgeons, 2013.

Endurance Training

Category: Training

Specialties and related fields: Exercise science, personal training

Definition: exercising to train the aerobic system as opposed to the anaerobic system to increase endurance

KEY TERMS

adventure races: a multidisciplinary team sport involving navigation over an unmarked wilderness course with races extending anywhere from two hours up to two weeks in length

endurance: denoting or relating to a race or other sporting event that takes place over a long distance or otherwise demands great physical stamina

triathlon: an athletic contest consisting of three different events, typically swimming, cycling, and long-distance running

INTRODUCTION

Endurance training involves any exercise program that helps to improve aerobic capacity and the health of the cardiovascular system. It is one of the four main types of exercise, including balance, flexibility, and strength. Endurance training sometimes is referred to as aerobic exercise because it involves activities that raise the heart rate and increase breathing for a sustained period. These exercises help the body's heart, lungs, and circulatory system work more efficiently by increasing the amount of oxygen the body can utilize during intense exercise over time. Such conditioning can improve various health issues, including conditions related to heart disease and obesity.

REASONS FOR ENDURANCE TRAINING
There are many reasons why a person might choose endurance training. First, endurance training is one of the best ways to increase a person's overall health and fitness. Additionally, endurance training can help reduce the risk of certain diseases and help people manage many health conditions. This type of training also may help reduce the risk of heart disease, stroke, cancer, and obesity.

Doctors often prescribe endurance training to help patients deal with various conditions such as multiple sclerosis (MS), diabetes, arthritis, and chronic obstructive pulmonary disease (COPD). They also may recommend endurance exercises to help patients recover from heart attacks or strokes because regular aerobic exercise can help prevent the likelihood of another traumatic cardiovascular event.

Endurance training burns fat. It can help a person lose weight or maintain healthy body weight. Endurance training and other aerobic exercises also release endorphins, chemicals in the body that boost good feelings. Exercise-induced endorphin release can help people deal with certain mental health conditions, including stress, depression, and anxiety. Some studies even show that endurance training may help reduce the risk of developing Alzheimer's disease later in life.

TYPES OF ENDURANCE EXERCISES
There are many types of endurance exercises. Some endurance exercises include running, jogging, and brisk walking sports such as soccer, skiing, tennis, basketball, biking, swimming, dancing, rowing, skating, jumping rope, stair climbing, cross-training on elliptical trainers, stationary bicycles, and ski machines. All these exercises work the larger muscle groups in the body and increase heart rate.

RECOMMENDATIONS
Experts recommend that people consult their doctors before beginning endurance training to rule out any potential health risks. Endurance training can be beneficial for people of all ages and fitness backgrounds. Because there are so many endurance exercises, individuals can choose a workout that fits their specific needs and lifestyle.

Endurance training is a great way for people to meet their weekly fitness recommendations. Specific recommendations for how often someone should engage in aerobic exercise depend on the person's goals. The government recommends that adults engage in at least thirty minutes of moderate-intensity

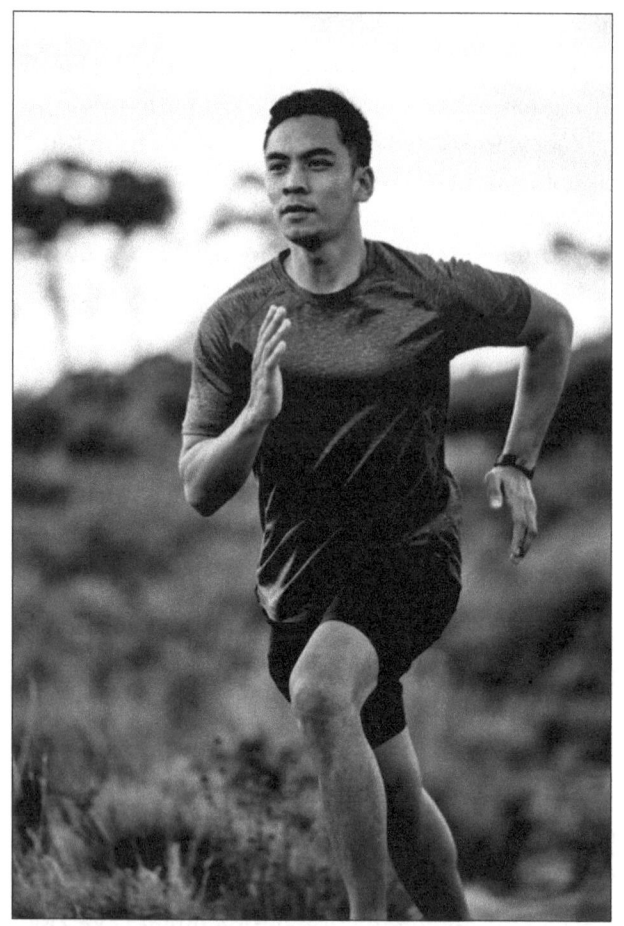

Photo via iStock/PeopleImages. [Used under licnense.]

exercise on most days of the week to help reduce the risk of chronic diseases. Adults should perform moderate to vigorous-intensity exercises for sixty minutes on most days of the week to avoid weight gain. People hoping to lose weight need to perform sixty to ninety minutes of moderate-intensity exercise on most days of the week. Experts caution people who are new to endurance training not to begin a high-intensity program right away. People often need to build up their endurance over time, so it is recommended that beginners start slow and work their way up to more strenuous workouts.

Individuals should warm up before starting an endurance training exercise. Warm-ups loosen the muscles and help prevent injury during exercise. These warm-up activities can include walking, jumping jacks, or stretching. Additionally, athletes should follow each exercise with a cooldown period that helps bring the heart rate back down. Cooldown activities may include stretching or walking.

ENDURANCE COMPETITIONS

Some athletes specifically train for different endurance competitions. One of the most well-known endurance sports is the marathon, a running race of 26.2 miles (42.2 kilometers). There also are ultramarathons. These events are longer than regular marathons, but there is no standard distance for an ultramarathon. They can range anywhere from 31.1 to 100 miles (50.1 to 160.9 kilometers). Another famous endurance competition is the triathlon. A triathlon involves three events: swimming, biking, and running. There are different levels of triathlons. The Olympic level includes a 1,500-meter (1,640-yard) swim, a 24.8-mile (40-kilometer) bike race, and a 6.2-mile (10-kilometer) run. A sprint-level triathlon is any triathlon that is shorter than the Olympic-level triathlon. The other common level is the Ironman triathlon. This competition includes a 2.4-mile (3.9-kilometer) swim, a 112-mile (180.2-kilometer) bike race, and a 26.2-mile (42.2-kilometer) run.

There also are endurance competitions called "adventure races," during which participants must reach a series of checkpoints by a designated time. These events usually include at least two endurance activities, running, swimming or hiking, and kayaking. They can take place in various terrains, including a desert or a forest. Some of these races last several hours, while others last for days. Most races

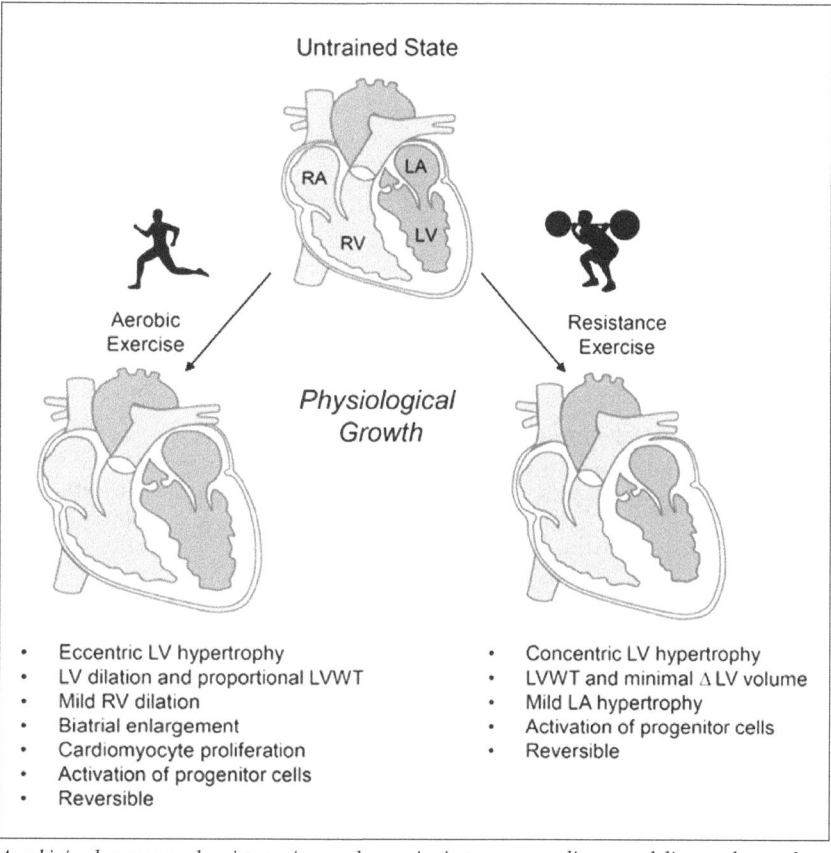

Aerobic/endurance and resistance/strength exercise impact on cardiac remodeling and growth. Image by Kyle Fulghum and Bradford G. Hill, via Wikimedia Commons.

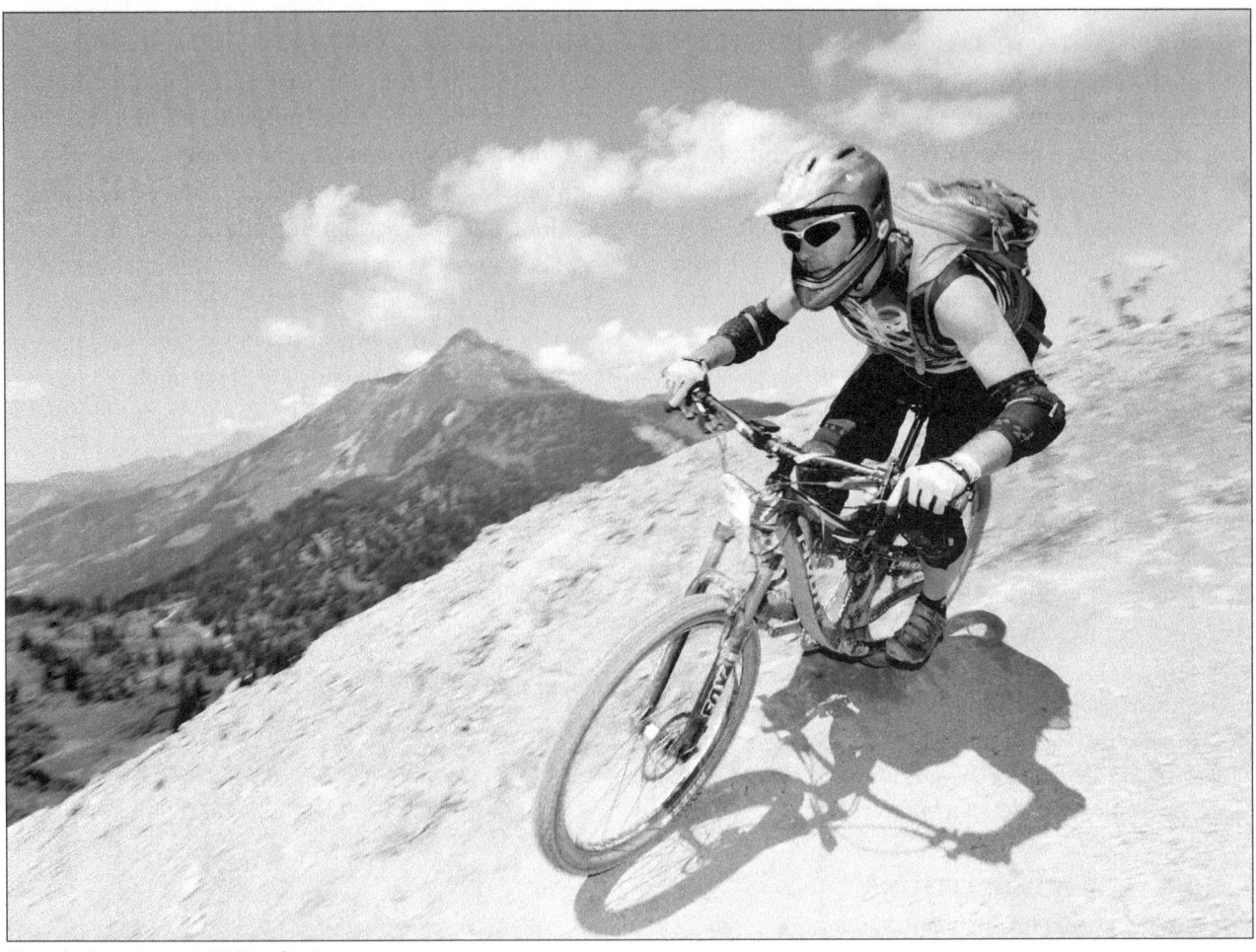

Photo by Jussarian, via Wikimedia Commons.

feature teams of individuals, but some competitions are solo events. Adventure races are considered some of the toughest endurance competitions. Experts recommend that novice athletes forego participating in these activities because competitors must be in excellent physical condition to complete an adventure race.

—*Rebecca Zukauskas*

Further Reading

Breene, Sophia. "13 Mental Health Benefits of Exercise." *Huffington Post*. TheHuffingtonPost.com, 27 Mar. 2013, www.huffingtonpost.com/2013/03/27/mental-health-benefits-exercise_n_2956099.html.

"Endurance Exercise (Aerobic)." *American Heart Association*, 24 Mar. 2015, www.heart.org/HEARTORG/HealthyLiving/PhysicalActivity/FitnessBasics/Endurance-Exercise-Aerobic_UCM_464004_Article.jsp#.VtSlGubl9pA.

Hill, Z. B. *Endurance and Cardio Training*. Mason Crest, 2015.

Kenney, W. Larry, et al. *Physiology of Sport and Exercise*. 6th ed., Human Kinetics, 2015.

Mihalka, Matthew. "Pushing the Limits: Ultramarathons, Ironman, and the Modern Athlete." *American History through American Sports: From Colonial Lacrosse to Extreme Sports,* edited by Danielle Sarver Coombs and Bob Batchelor, vol. 3, Praeger, 2013, pp. 279-93.

Ergogenic Aids

Category: Biology
Specialties and related fields: Biochemistry, endocrinology, ethics, exercise physiology, family medicine, hematology, internal medicine, nephrology, orthopedics, pharmacology, psychology, sports medicine, toxicology
Definition: substances used by athletes to gain an advantage; most of these substances are illegal and unethical within competitive sports

KEY TERMS

anabolic-androgenic steroids (AAS): natural androgens like testosterone as well as synthetic androgens that are structurally related and have similar effects to testosterone

androstenedione: a naturally occurring steroid hormone, also available as a dietary supplement, believed to increase serum testosterone levels.

creatine: a compound formed in protein metabolism and present in much living tissue; it is involved in the supply of energy for muscular contraction

growth hormone (GH): a peptide hormone that stimulates growth, cell reproduction, and cell regeneration

INTRODUCTION

In the history of sport, athletes have attempted to find a competitive advantage through advanced techniques in training, nutrition, and even ergogenic aids, such as nutritional supplements and pharmacological aids. The use of these substances—such as anabolic-androgenic steroids (AAS), testosterone precursors (such as androstenedione), and nonsteroidal aids such as human growth hormone (GH) and creatine-have become increasingly popular in recent years, even without specific scientific data supporting their efficacy and safety.

The population using such performance-enhancing drugs ranges from collegiate to professional athletes to adolescents and high school students. Recent meta-analyses estimate that 3 to 12 percent of adolescent boys have used an anabolic steroid at least once, and 28 percent of collegiate athletes admit to taking creatine. Other studies have suggested that the number may be closer to 41 percent.

Though such ergogenic aids are thought to improve strength, endurance, agility, and overall performance, most athletic improvement is anecdotal at best. Scientific evidence supporting these ideas is scarce and incomplete. Even with aids that may improve strength and performance, the safety of these substances has been seriously questioned, such as with the use of AAS, GH, and ephedra.

TYPES OF ERGOGENIC AIDS

Anabolic-androgenic steroids as ergogenic aids in sports are chemical compounds that resemble the structure of testosterone. This naturally occurring male sex hormone affects muscle growth and strength. "Anabolic" refers to the growth of cells, and "androgenic" refers to the stimulation of the growth of male sex organs and masculine sex characteristics. Anabolic-androgenic steroids bind to cells that are used for muscle repair and that can transform into muscle fibers.

Anabolic-androgenic steroids have been one of the most studied ergogenic aids. Yet, many of its mechanisms and adverse effects are still not well understood. Studies have shown that increased doses of testosterone can decrease total body adipose tissue in the body and increase strength and fat-free mass. Adverse effects of AAS use include hypothalamic-pituitary dysfunction, gynecomastia, severe acne, infection because of sharing needles, aggressive and depressive behavior, and a possible association with premature death.

Androstenedione (andro) is a testosterone precursor produced by the adrenal glands and gonads. Its ergogenic effect occurs after it is converted to testosterone in the testes and other tissues. The body can also convert it to estrone and estradiol, which are steroid compounds that are primary female sex hormones (found in both men and women). Testosterone synthesis is regulated by the concentration of testosterone precursors in the body. Theoretically, an increase in androstenedione would increase testosterone production and thus can increase protein synthesis, lean body mass, and strength.

Older studies showed that andro supplementation results in increased serum testosterone levels. However, more recent studies have shown that andro supplementation fails to directly improve lean body mass, muscular strength, or serum testosterone levels. Possible side effects of andro use are suppressed testosterone production, liver dysfunction, cardiovascular disease, testicular atrophy, baldness, acne, and aggressive behavior.

Like androstenedione, dehydroepiandrosterone (DHEA) is a precursor of testosterone and is also formed in the adrenal glands and gonads. Dehydroepiandrosterone is the most abundant steroid hormone in circulation. It is a precursor to androstenedione and other testosterone precursors (such as androstenediol). Studies of DHEA supplementation have not been shown to increase lean body mass, strength, or testosterone levels. Possible side effects are similar to andro and AAS use.

Human GH is a metabolic hormone secreted into the blood by cells found in the anterior pituitary gland. After its secretion, GH stimulates the production of insulin-like growth factor (IGF)-1 in the liver. These hormones stimulate bone growth, protein synthesis, and the conversion of fat to energy. Athletes have been attracted to GH because of such theoretical benefits and the limited techniques for detecting GH in the urine. Growth hormone levels vary in individuals of different ages, sex, and activity and can vary throughout the day, so no reliable benchmark is available to determine if illicit use has occurred.

Scientific studies have been unable to show that GH leads to increased muscle strength and exercise performance or changes in protein synthesis. Because of ethical limitations, it is difficult to study the effect of larger doses of GH on healthy individuals. Adverse effects of GH use include cosmetic damage, joint pain, muscle weakness, fluid retention, impaired glucose regulation (which may lead to diabetes mellitus), cardiomyopathy, hyperlipidemia, and possibly death.

Erythropoietin (EPO) is a hormone secreted by the kidneys that signals to hematopoietic stem cells in the bone marrow. Erythropoietin increases the oxygen-carrying capacity of blood and, as a result, aids in endurance and aerobic respiration. The appeal of EPO among athletes is this endurance-enhancing effect. As a result, many users are skiers, cyclists, and other athletes who require high endurance levels. Early use of EPO as an ergogenic aid, termed "blood doping," came in the form of autologous blood transfusions. Athletes would harvest their red blood cells and reintroduce them into their systems before events. A synthetic form of EPO, recombinant human erythropoietin (r-HuEPO), became available in 1988.

Scientific studies have shown that EPO and r-HuEPO treatments increase certain blood concentrations and can aid in endurance. However, EPO may also have serious and dangerous side effects, such as hypertension, seizures, thromboembolic events, and possibly death.

Creatine monohydrate is an amine synthesized in the kidneys, pancreas, and liver. Athletes can also obtain it through a diet of meat and fish. Approximately 90 to 95 percent of creatine in the body is found in skeletal muscle. Creatine is converted to creatine phosphate (PCr), an important limiting factor in adenosine triphosphate (ATP) resynthesis, which plays a significant role in energy reserves within the body. Theoretically, an increase of PCr in the body would increase the regeneration of ATP, increasing sustained maximal energy production for short-term exercise. Increased ATP synthesis could lead to increased intensity and repetition frequency, thus possibly increasing skeletal muscle mass.

In 2002, A. M. Bohn and colleagues argued in an article in *Current Sports Medicine Reports* that there are "no studies demonstrating benefit with the relatively indiscriminant use of variable amounts of creatine by large numbers of athletes on a specific team." Nevertheless, creatine has been shown to enhance performance in small populations of athletes in various sports. Creatine's possible adverse effects include muscle cramping, dehydration, gastrointestinal distress, weight gain, increased risk of muscle tears, inhibited insulin and creatine production, renal damage, and possibly nephropathy.

Stimulants are drugs that increase nervous system activity. Examples of stimulants commonly used as ergogenic aids include the class of drugs called "amphetamines" and specific chemical compounds such as caffeine and ephedrine. The use of caffeine improves exercise time to exhaustion and may significantly increase intestinal glucose absorption. It has been suggested that caffeine increases fat utilization for energy and delays glycogen depletion (the stored form of glucose). As a result, caffeine and other stimulants are popular ergogenic aids for extended aerobic activity.

Caffeine in small doses has been shown to increase performance. Caffeine's possible adverse effects may include anxiety, dependency, withdrawal, and possibly a diuretic effect (dehydration). Ephedrine may have similar adverse effects. Other stimulants, such as amphetamines or cocaine, have more serious and detrimental effects.

PERSPECTIVE AND PROSPECTS

The use of ergogenic aids in the history of sport has progressively moved from primitive aids to more sophisticated performance enhancers. Crude natural concoctions and stimulants have paved the way for complex pharmacological agents (such as erythropoietin) and designer anabolic steroids (tetrahydrogestrinone). Athletes and trainers have utilized any means to gain a competitive edge, even if that results in damage to health and even a risk of death.

The biggest problem stemming from such aids is the difficulty in detecting them. Consider the recent media attention given to ergogenic aids and their popularity in the 2007 Mitchell Report. This independent congressional investigation examined the use of performance-enhancing drugs in Major League Baseball. Other examples include the 2012 discoveries of abuse by high-profile cyclists and athletes at the Summer Olympics held in London. This media attention has also shown the difficulties among investigators, such as the International Olympic Committee, the World Anti-Doping Agency, and the United States Anti-Doping Agency, in detecting new designer steroids and new ergogenic aids among elite athletes.

—*Julien M. Cobert, Jeffrey R. Bytomski*

Further Reading

"Anabolic Steroids." *MedlinePlus*, 2 June 2021, medlineplus.gov/anabolicsteroids.html.

Bohn, Amy Miller, Stephanie Betts, and Thomas L. Schwenk. "Creatine and Other Nonsteroidal Strength-Enhancing Aids." *Current Sports Medicine Reports*, vol. 1, no. 4, 2002, pp. 239-45.

Foster, Zoë J., and Jeffrey A. Housner. "Anabolic-Androgenic Steroids and Testosterone Precursors: Ergogenic Aids and Sport." *Current Sports Medicine Reports*, vol. 3, no. 4, 2004, pp. 234-41.

Graham, T. E. "Caffeine and Exercise: Metabolism, Endurance, and Performance." *Sports Medicine*, vol. 31, no. 11, 2001, pp. 785-807.

Juhn, Mark S. "Ergogenic Aids in Aerobic Activity." *Current Sports Medicine Reports*, vol. 1, no. 4, 2002, pp. 233-38.

Krans, Brian. "Performance Enhancers: The Safe and the Deadly." *Healthline*, 5 Feb. 2021, www.healthline.com/health/performance-enhancers-safe-deadly.

"Performance-Enhancing Drugs: Know the Risks." *Mayo Clinic*, 4 Dec. 2020, www.mayoclinic.org/healthy-lifestyle/fitness/in-depth/performance-enhancing-drugs/art-20046134.

Powers, Michael E. "The Safety and Efficacy of Anabolic Steroid Precursors: What Is the Scientific Evidence?" *Journal of Athletic Training*, vol. 37, no. 3, 2002, pp. 300-305.

Shekelle, Paul G., et al. "Efficacy and Safety of Ephedra and Ephedrine for Weight Loss and Athletic Performance: A Meta-analysis." *Journal of the American Medical Association*, vol. 289, no. 12, 2003, pp. 1537-45.

Sotas, Pierre-Edouard, et al. "Prevalence of Blood Doping in Samples Collected from Elite Track and Field Athletes." *Clinical Chemistry*, vol. 57, no. 5, 2011, pp. 762-69.

Stacy, Jason J., Thomas R. Terrell, and Thomas D. Armsey. "Ergogenic Aids: Human Growth Hormone." *Current Sports Medicine Reports*, vol. 3, no. 4, 2004, pp. 229-33.

Yesalis, C. E., and M. S. Bahrke. "Doping Among Adolescent Athletes." *Baillieres Best Practice and Research in Clinical Endocrinology and Metabolism*, vol. 14, no. 1, 2000, pp. 25-35.

High-Intensity Interval Training (HIIT)

Category: Exercise training
Specialties and related fields: Personal training, strength and conditioning
Definition: a form of exercise in which short periods of extremely demanding physical activity are alternated with less intense recovery periods

KEY TERMS

intensity: the difficulty of an exercise, typically based on the amount of weight you lift

fitness training: regular, structured activity designed to promote health in human beings

INTRODUCTION

High-intensity interval training (HIIT)—also known as high-intensity intermittent exercise (HIIE) or sprint interval training (SIT)—is a type of exercise regimen used by many athletes. The exercise regimen usually begins with a warm-up period, in which a person conditions their body for a high-intensity workout. The person does several repetitions of the exercise in quick succession and then switches to a medium-intensity version of the exercise, followed by a cool-down period. The medium-intensity version of the exercise is usually performed at around 50 percent intensity. It is meant to let the muscles relax while still benefiting from the exercise.

The number of repetitions in HIIT can vary from exercise to exercise or training regimen to training regimen. Still, no real formula exists regarding how exactly a HIIT regimen needs to be performed for maximum health benefits. However, it is generally advised to do no more than three repetitions or twenty seconds of intense exercise in a row, as exceeding this limit is considered debilitating to the human body. Through HIIT, the body is meant to give an all-out effort for a short but intense burst. Athletic training aims to keep the body's heart rate up consistently so that the body can burn the maximum amount of fat in the shortest time.

BACKGROUND

Dr. Woldemar Gerschler initially developed interval training in the late 1930s. At the time, Gerschler was working as head coach of Dresdner SC, a major German sports club in the time before World War II. Gerschler attempted to base his training methods on physiological and psychological conditioning, although he was trained more in the psychological. To perfect the technique, Gerschler recruited noted cardiologist Dr. Herbert Reindell. Between 1935 and 1940, the two experimented on more than three thousand subjects whose precise heart rate they monitored over twenty-one days of training. In their experiments, Gerschler and Reindell found great performance improvements over this period and that the heart volume increased by over one-fifth.

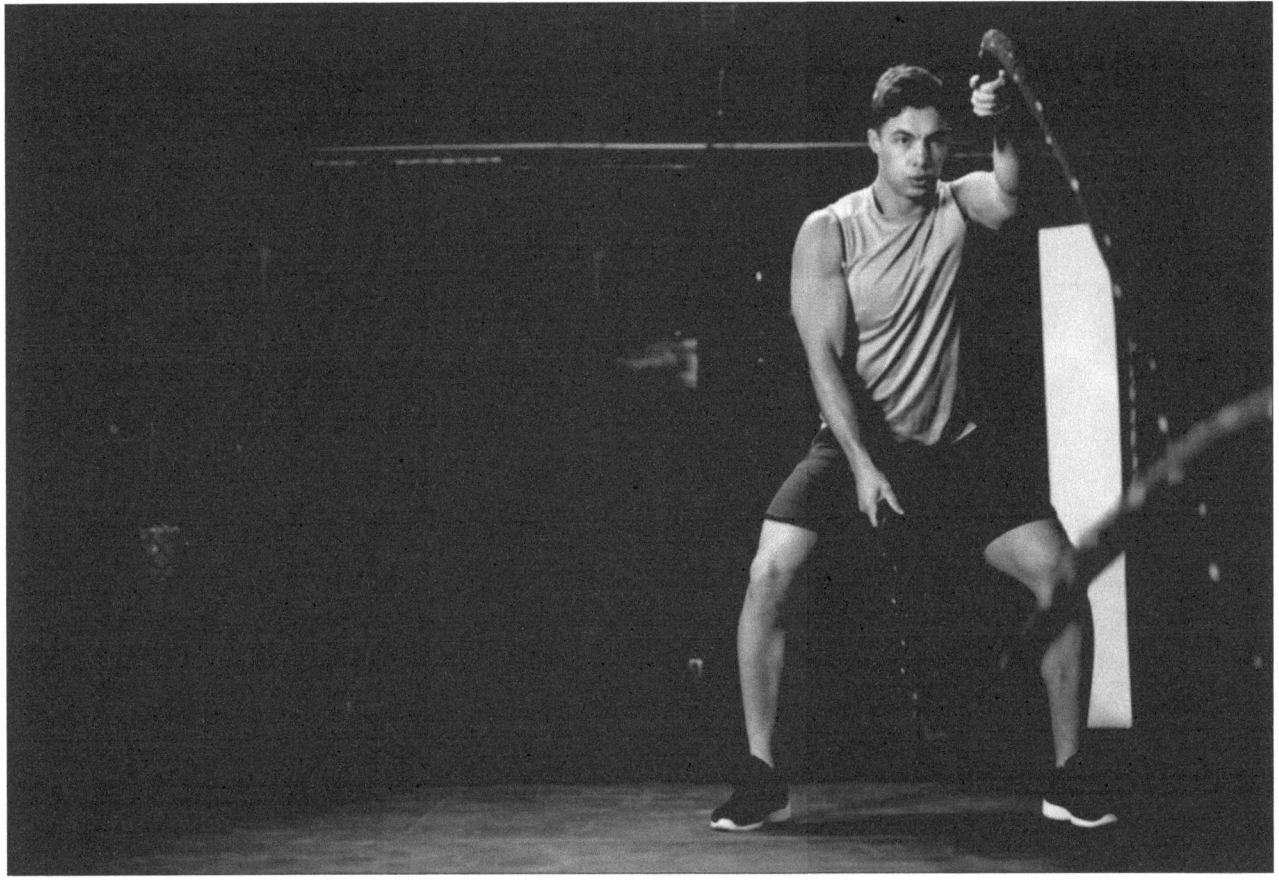

HITT training incorporates short periods of intense exercise. Photo via iStock/PeopleImages. [Used under license.]

The experiments by Gerschler and Reindell helped the two doctors develop the technique known as "interval training," where athletes would run short distances or lift weights for a relatively short period at full capacity, followed by a short recovery period. The original form of interval training was based on the idea that the body's blood volume is constant and that the effect gained from training at maximum capacity for a short time will come when the heart rate decreases due to the increased quantity of blood that is pumped during training.

Gerschler used this technique in his coaching after World War II. Coached using Gerschler's interval training technique, athlete Josy Barthel became the surprise winner of the men's 1500-meter race at the 1952 Summer Olympics. This success story brought widespread attention to the technique, and Gerschler later coached Roger Moens in this technique to win the silver medal in the 800-meter race at the 1960 Summer Olympics.

NEW INTERVAL TRAINING
Others later refined Gerschler's technique. Individuals such as athletic coach Peter Coe, Professor Izumi Tabata, and Professor Martin Gibala made vast improvements to the technique. Each of these individuals came up with their regimens based on interval training, which culminated in the formation of modern HIIE.

In 1996, Tabata published his study on the effects of HITT in conjunction with the National Institute of Fitness and Sports in Kanoya, Japan. In this study, Tabata followed training methods used by Japanese speed skaters. He broke athletes participating in the study into two groups and monitored them over six days. During the study, Tabata had one group engage in moderate-intensity exercise for one hour on an exercise bicycle; the other group trained using the method he saw Japanese speed skaters using: a ten-minute warm-up and four minutes of intense exercise and rest at a 2:1 ratio, with eight total intervals taking place. Tabata noted in the study that only the second group received a noted increase in anaerobic capacity.

In February 2012, Jamie Timmons, a professor of systems biology at the University of Loughborough, further refined the technique and debuted his take on HIIE on the BBC program Horizon, putting BBC science journalist and television host Michael Mosley through a rigorous exercise regimen that he designed. The three-minute HIIE program was effective with just six repetitions a week, with forty seconds of the regimen being done at maximum speed. Timmons has demonstrated that his approach can improve insulin sensitivity in just two weeks and can help prevent type 2 diabetes, obesity, and cardiovascular disease, among other conditions.

High-intensity interval training is widely used in personal training, as it is a great technique to burn fat without promoting muscle loss. In athletics, HIIT is often used by sprinters and swimmers looking to gain stamina without losing speed or precision. In general, the technique is used by those looking for a quick but intense workout that fits into their lifestyle.

—*Daniel Horowitz*

Further Reading

Little, Jonathan P., et al. "A Practical Model of Low-Volume High-Intensity Interval Training Induces Mitochondrial Biogenesis in Human Skeletal Muscle: Potential Mechanisms." *Journal of Physiology*, vol. 588, no. 6, 2010, pp. 1011-22.

Laursen, Paul B., and David G. Jenkins. "The Scientific Basis for High-Intensity Interval Training: Optimizing Training Programs and Maximizing Performance in Highly Trained Endurance Athletes." *Sports Medicine*, vol. 32, no. 1, 2002, pp. 53-73.

Mosley, Michael, and Peta Bee. "A Few Workouts and Tips." *Fast Exercise*. Author, n.d. Accessed 24 Aug. 2016.

Reynolds, Gretchen. "One Minute of All-Out Exercise May Have Benefits of 45 Minutes of Moderate Exertion." *New York Times*, 27 Apr. 2016.

Tabata, I., et al. "Effects of Moderate-Intensity Endurance and High-Intensity Intermittent Training on Anaerobic Capacity and VO2max." *Medicine and Science in Sports and Exercise* vol. 28, no. 10, 1996, pp. 1327-30.

PROGRESSIVE MUSCLE RELAXATION

Category: Therapy or technique; Physiotherapy

Specialties and related fields: Occupational therapy. pain medicine, physical therapy, psychology, therapeutic massage

Definition: a nonpharmacological method of deep muscle relaxation, based on the premise that muscle tension is the body's psychological response to anxiety-provoking thoughts and that muscle relaxation blocks anxiety

KEY TERMS

autonomic nervous system: the part of the nervous system responsible for the control of the bodily functions not consciously directed, such as breathing, the heartbeat, and digestive processes

behavioral medicine: an interdisciplinary field of research and practice that focuses on how people's thoughts and behavior affect their health

vasodilation: the dilatation of blood vessels, which decreases blood pressure

OVERVIEW

The positive effects of relaxation and the contributory influences of prolonged stress and tension on illness have long been recognized. Progressive muscle relaxation (PMR) is a technique aimed at reducing the somatic (bodily) consequences of stress, such as muscle tension, by lowering physiologic arousal and, thereby, inducing relaxation.

RELAXATION TECHNIQUES

Relaxation techniques include several practices, such as PMR, guided imagery, biofeedback, self-hypnosis, and deep breathing exercises. The goal is similar in all: consciously producing the body's natural relaxation response, characterized by slower breathing, lower blood pressure, and a feeling of calm and well-being.

Relaxation is more than a state of mind; it physically changes how the body functions. Using relaxation techniques to produce the relaxation response may counteract the effects of long-term stress, which may contribute to or worsen a range of health problems, including depression, digestive disorders, headaches, high blood pressure, and insomnia.

When a person is under stress, the body releases hormones that produce the fight-or-flight response: Heart rate and breathing rate go up, and blood vessels narrow (restricting blood flow). This response allows energy to flow to body parts, such as the muscles and the heart, that need to take action. However useful this response may be in the short-term, evidence shows that emotional or physical damage can occur when the body remains in a stress state for a long time. Long-term or chronic stress (lasting months or years) may reduce the body's ability to fight illness and lead to or worsen certain health conditions. Chronic stress may lead to high blood pressure, headaches, stomachache, and other symptoms. Stress may worsen certain conditions, such as asthma. Stress is also linked to depression, anxiety, and other mental illnesses.

In contrast to the stress response, the relaxation response slows the heart rate, lowers blood pressure, and decreases oxygen consumption and levels of stress hormones. Because relaxation is the opposite of stress, the theory is that voluntarily creating the relaxation response through traditional relaxation techniques could counteract the negative effects of stress.

Commonly used models of progressive relaxation are based on the principles identified by American psychiatrist Edmund Jacobson in the 1930s. The basic technique developed by Jacobson involves alternately tensing and relaxing major muscle groups of the body while concurrently focusing on sensations associated with the tensing and relaxing.

Regardless of the reasons for its application, current PMR methods begin with a rationale for its use. The fundamental premise is that muscle tension, even when not overtly perceived, causes anxiety (and often pain, discomfort, and agitation) and that a significant reduction in associated symptoms will result if tense muscles are relaxed.

Participants learning PMR are requested to loosen tight clothing and sit in a comfortable chair in a quiet setting, relatively free from distraction. A trained therapist then instructs and demonstrates how to isolate, tense, and relax muscles and systematically guides the person through the different muscle groups in a fixed order.

During the "tensing" phase of the procedure, the person is directed to constrict the identified muscle as tightly as possible while keeping other muscle groups loose and relaxed. Attention is directed to the sensations associated with tensing, such as tightness and discomfort. The tensing phase lasts approximately ten seconds and is followed by the "relaxing" or "releasing" phase, wherein muscle tension is "let go," and muscles are allowed to become limp. The participant then focuses on the tension and discomfort draining from the muscle and takes notice of the contrast between the warmth and comfort of relaxed muscles and the discomfort of tensed muscles.

After about ten to fifteen seconds of relaxing, the sequence is repeated with another muscle group. A typical sequence of muscle groups addressed in the technique is the following: hands, biceps and triceps, shoulders, chest, neck, mouth and lips, eyes, forehead, scalp, back, stomach, thighs, calves, feet, and toes. After completing the tensing and releasing phases, participants take an "inventory" of their muscle groups and relax those with remaining tension. The procedure takes about twenty to thirty minutes to complete.

During the procedure, participants are encouraged to avoid blocking thoughts that might intrude upon their consciousness and either allow these thoughts to flow through their mind or shift their focus toward breathing if they find themselves distracted. For a period following the exercise, participants may engage in slow, steady, and even breathing to enhance the relaxation response. They may also repeat a calming word or phrase such as "relax," "release," or "let go" each time they exhale so that the word or phrase becomes a cue for promoting relaxation, a practice known as "cue-controlled relaxation".

Nonguided practice sessions are encouraged to further enhance skills, with the goal of the person being able to achieve a highly relaxed state without guidance. Two or three guided relaxation sessions are typically conducted to develop basic proficiency with the exercise. Common variations to the procedure include abbreviated protocols such as "release only" methods, whereby the tensing phase is eliminated, or emphasis is directed at specific muscle groups that are identified as particularly key in inducing overall relaxation. Audiotapes of the relaxation procedure may also be used to develop relaxation skills.

MECHANISM OF ACTION
Progressive muscle relaxation has been found to affect the autonomic nervous system, which, among other functions, regulates how the body reacts to changes in the environment. These effects include decreases in heart rate, blood pressure, muscle tension, and general arousal. Vasodilation of blood vessels also occurs, causing increased blood flow throughout the body, most noticeably in the extremities. These responses are the opposite of those produced by anxiety and lead to subjective feelings of warmth, comfort, and calmness.

USES AND APPLICATIONS
Progressive muscle relaxation has a long history in psychiatry, psychology, and behavioral medicine. The procedure has been employed as a stand-alone therapy and a component of multifaceted protocols treating psychiatric and medical illnesses. The procedure is commonly used in nonmedical settings to promote overall wellness and healthy adaptation to life stressors.

SCIENTIFIC EVIDENCE
A large body of research has demonstrated that PMR effectively reduces symptoms stemming from various medical and psychiatric conditions. A double-blind, placebo-controlled study in 2005 examined the technique as applied in a medical setting. The study showed that asthmatic female adolescents' lung function, heart rate, and blood pressure improved after learning and employing PMR. Another double-blind, placebo-controlled study in 2009 examined the technique's psychiatric application. The study found that PMR improved anxiety symptoms in hospitalized adults with schizophrenia.

CHOOSING A PRACTITIONER
Trained and licensed mental health or medical professionals should be consulted for persons seeking PMR treatment for psychiatric, psychological, or medical conditions. For nonmedical applications, trained nonprofessionals and audiotapes are usually appropriate.

SAFETY ISSUES

Before participating in PMR, interested persons should consult a physician or other health-care provider.

—Paul F. Bell

Further Reading

Corbett, Christina, et al. "A Randomised Comparison of Two 'Stress Control' Programmes: Progressive Muscle Relaxation versus Mindfulness Body Scan." *Mental Health & Prevention*, vol. 15, 2019, p. 200163, doi:10.1016/j.mph.2019.200163.

Cuncic, Arlin. "Chill Out: How to Use Progressive Muscle Relaxation to Quell Anxiety." *Verywell Mind*, 13 July 2019, www.verywellmind.com/how-do-i-practice-progressive-muscle-relaxation-3024400.

Dunford, Emma, and Miles Thompson. "Relaxation and Mindfulness in Pain: A Review." *Reviews in Pain*, vol. 4, no. 1, 2010, pp. 18-22, doi:10.1177/204946371000400105.

Pangotra, Aditi, et al. "Effectiveness of Progressive Muscle Relaxation, Biofeedback and L-Theanine in Patients Suffering from Anxiety Disorder." *Journal of Psychosocial Research*, vol. 13, no. 1, 2018, pp. 219-28, doi:10.32381/jpr.2018.13.01.21.

Selva, Joaquin. "Progressive Muscle Relaxation (PMR): A Positive Psychology Guide." *PositivePsychology.com*, 4 July 2019, positivepsychology.com/progressive-muscle-relaxation-pmr/.

Smith, Karen E., and Greg J. Norman. "Brief Relaxation Training Is Not Sufficient to Alter Tolerance to Experimental Pain in Novices." *PLOS One*, vol. 12, no. 5, 2017, doi:10.1371/journal.pone.0177228.

Static Stretching

Category: Conditioning

Specialties and related fields: Athletic training, occupational therapy, orthopedics, physical therapy, strength and conditioning

Definition: stretching a muscle to near its furthest point and then holding that position for at least fifteen or twenty seconds

KEY TERMS

agonist muscle: the muscle contracting during an activity

antagonist muscle: the muscle relaxing or lengthening during an activity

ligament: a membranous fold that supports an organ and keeps it in position.

tendon: a flexible but inelastic cord of strong fibrous collagen tissue attaching a muscle to a bone

INTRODUCTION

Static stretching is used to stretch muscles while the body is stationary. This method stretches the muscle to a point beyond its normal limit and then holds it there for about thirty seconds. Some advocate static stretching before more strenuous exercise to warm and loosen the muscles. However, other research has indicated that static stretching should be employed after vigorous exercise to help lengthen the muscles and increase flexibility or range of motion around a joint. This research also states that other stretching methods, such as dynamic stretching, should be used before activity since dynamic stretching helps to increase heat and blood flow to the muscles.

OVERVIEW

To perform a static stretch, individuals move their bodies into a position that will enable a muscle or group of muscles to be stretched using tension or tightness. The muscle or muscles that will be stretched are called the "agonists," while the opposing muscles are called the "antagonists." After positioning the body in a specific way to increase the tension on the agonist, the individual holds this position without moving for a few seconds. During this time, individuals should take slow, deep breaths. They should remain still and not bounce when performing static stretches. They should concentrate on holding the position rather than on the stretch itself. The stretch can be repeated several times. A common example of a static stretch is bending over to touch one's toes.

Static stretching has several advantages in addition to lengthening muscles and increasing flexibility. It can help relax the body both physically and mentally. Stress increases tension in muscles, and stretching helps reduce this tension. In addition, the deep breaths one takes during stretching can help relieve stress. Tight muscles can affect joints and lead to muscular imbalances. Tight muscles put individuals at risk for injuries. Static stretching loosens muscles to improve balance and decrease the risk of injury.

TYPES OF STATIC STRETCHING

Two types of static stretching exist: passive and active. A person performing passive static stretching does not have to exert any effort. For example, if people perform leg lift stretches passively, they would lift one of their legs into the air and place their leg on something such as a chair or have another person hold it in place for the duration of the stretch. Doing this stretches the leg and hip muscles, but it does not require other muscles to work to hold the leg up in the air.

Passive static stretching is used to work the muscles of people who cannot move independently, such as those who are disabled, paralyzed, or in a coma. It is also employed by those who are not very strong to strengthen the muscles and keep them moving. Some researchers claim that passive static stretching is more effective for readying muscles for exercise than other forms of stretching.

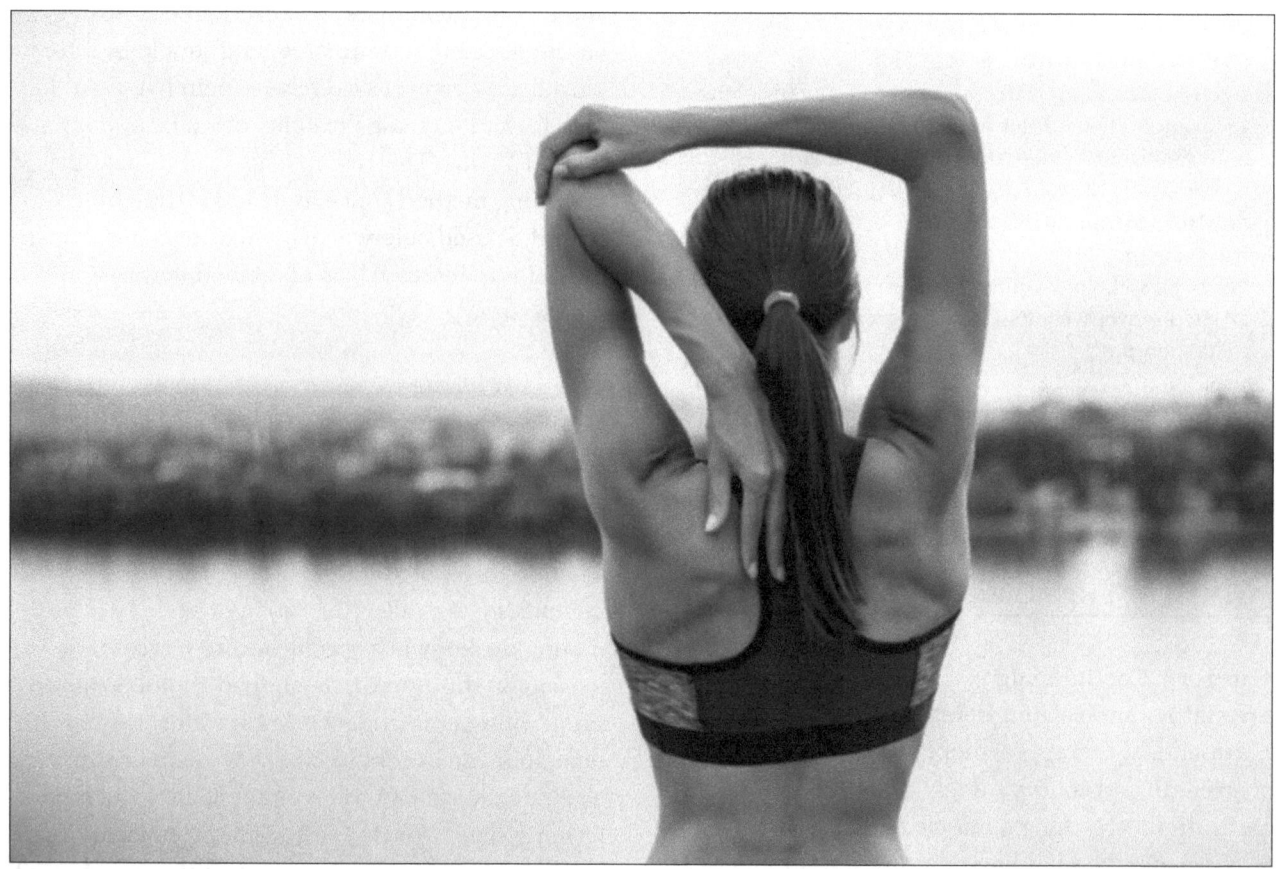

Static stretching involves standing, sitting, or lying still and holding a single position for about 45 seconds. Photo via iStock/LittleBee80. [Used under license.]

Active stretches are typically more difficult to perform than passive stretches, so they are usually only held for a few seconds. On the other hand, a person who performs active static stretching has to put forth work. For example, for the same leg lift stretch using active stretching, individuals raise their legs but do not use anything to prop their legs up; they instead use other muscles in the body to hold their legs up without assistance.

Static stretches are similar to some yoga moves, but many of them are much easier to perform. More people perform active stretches because nothing but the body is needed to perform these types of stretches. Examples of active static stretches include lifting the arms in the air and holding them there or performing a lunge and staying in that position. People of all activity levels can perform active static stretching. It is a good activity for individuals new to exercise and those who are mostly sedentary (not active).

DYNAMIC STRETCHING

Dynamic stretching is a type of stretching that uses movement to stretch muscles. Dynamic stretching differs from static stretching because static stretching holds muscles still during the stretch. Athletes like baseball players and runners typically use dynamic stretches to prepare their muscles for sudden movements, prevent strain, and increase flexibility. Dynamic stretches raise the body temperature to warm up the muscles and prepare them for swift movements.

These types of stretches are generally employed before workouts or competitions. The stretches can be tailored to correspond with specific sports played. This helps the body become used to particular movements to prevent injury. An example of a dynamic stretch used by a sprinter is raising alternate knees as high as possible while walking in place. This readies muscles in the legs and back for sprinting. An example typically used by baseball players is swinging the arms next to the body in circles. This exercise stretches muscles in the arms, shoulders, and lower back to prepare baseball players to throw the ball and swing the bat during games.

—*Angela Harmon*

Further Reading

Boelcke, Allison. "What Is Dynamic Stretching?" *Wise Geek*. Conjecture Corporation, 20 Mar. 2015, www.wisegeekhealth.com/what-is-dynamic-stretching.htm. Accessed 24 Mar. 2015.

Ellis-Christensen, Tricia. "What Is Static Stretching?" *Wise Geek*. Conjecture Corporation, 23 Mar. 2015, www.wisegeekhealth.com/what-is-static-stretching.htm. Accessed 24 Mar. 2015.

Moore, Heather. "Static vs. Dynamic Stretching." *Philly.com*. Interstate General Media, LLC., 28 Jan. 2014, www.philly.com/philly/blogs/sportsdoc/Static-vs-dynamic-stretching.html?c=r. Accessed 24 Mar. 2015.

Reynolds, Gretchen. "Stretching: The Truth." *Play Magazine*. The New York Times Company, 31 Oct. 2008, www.nytimes.com/2008/11/02/sports/playmagazine/112pewarm.html. Accessed 24 Mar. 2015.

St. Laurent, Christine. "Static Stretching Advantages." *Livestrong.com*. Demand Media, Inc., 20 Oct. 2013, www.livestrong.com/article/437963-static-stretching-advantages/. Accessed 24 Mar. 2015.

Walker, Brad. *The Anatomy of Stretching*. North Atlantic Books, 2007.

STRETCHING

Category: Conditioning

Specialties and related fields: Athletic training, occupational therapy, orthopedics, physical therapy, strength and conditioning

Definition: stretching a muscle to near its furthest point and then holding that position for at least 15 or 20 seconds

KEY TERMS

agonist muscle: the muscle contracting during an activity

antagonist muscle: the muscle relaxing or lengthening during an activity

ligament: a membranous fold that supports an organ and keeps it in position

tendon: a flexible but inelastic cord of strong fibrous collagen tissue attaching a muscle to a bone

INTRODUCTION

Stretching, as it relates to physical fitness, is the process of positioning the body's limbs in ways that will lengthen the muscles and surrounding soft tissue. Stretching builds muscle elasticity and tone, as well as creates better flexibility. Stretching also increases a person's range of motion, improves circulation, relieves muscle soreness, and reduces overall fatigue. The two basic types of stretching are static stretching and dynamic stretching. Proper technique is an important component of stretching. Incorrect stretching can lead to injury.

UNDERSTANDING STRETCHING

When the body is stretching, several things take place deep in the muscles and soft tissue. A muscle contains thousands of tiny string-like cells called "muscle fibers." Muscle fibers are situated close together within a muscle and are usually very long. Muscle fibers are composed of thousands of even smaller threads called "myofibrils," which allow muscles to lengthen, relax, and contract. Within the myofibrils are millions of minuscule bands called "sarcomeres," which are made up of overlapping strands of protein-laden myofilaments. Stretching a muscle lengthens and narrows the muscle fibers and their smaller components. When a muscle is lengthened during stretching, the connective tissue and sheath of the muscle tendons elongate. As the body gets used to stretching, the

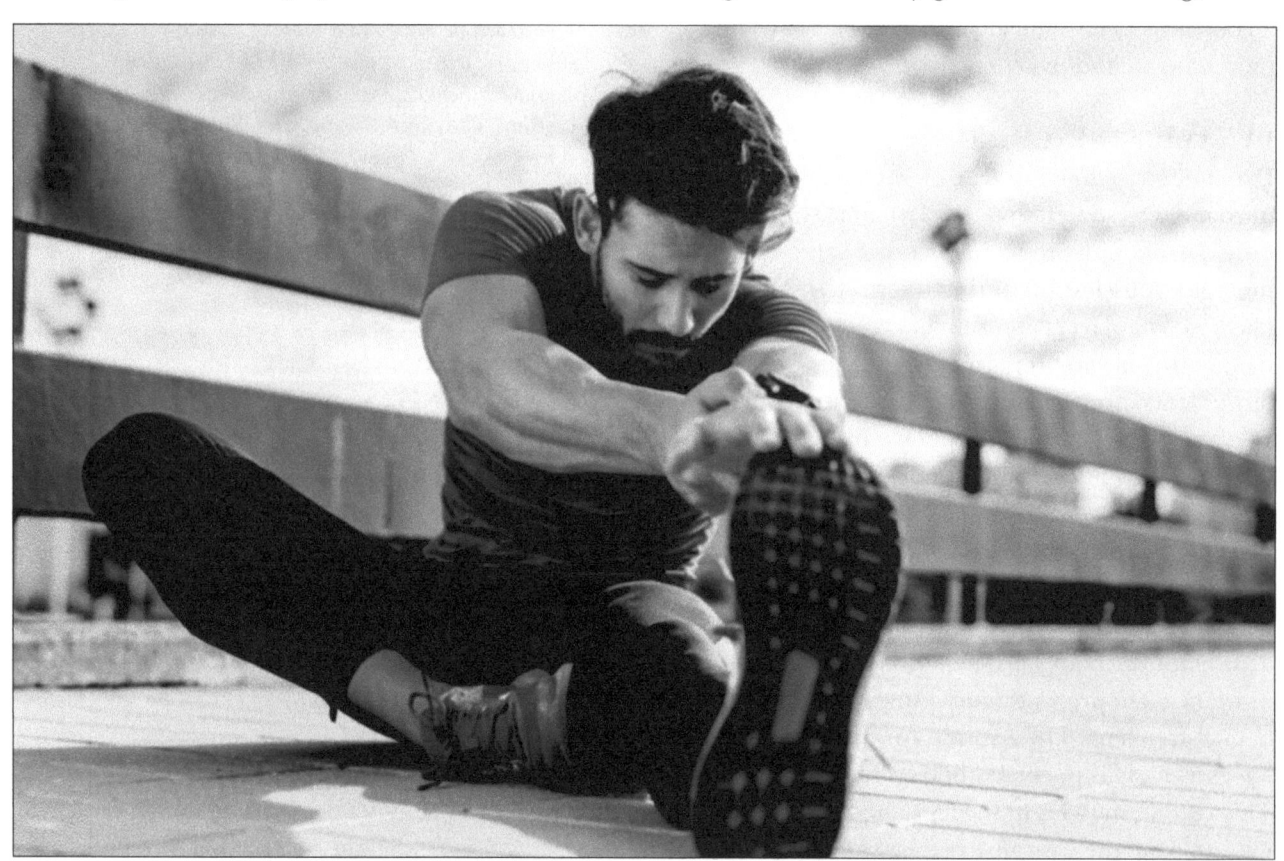

Photo via iStock/Ivanko_Brnjakovic. [Used under license.]

surrounding ligaments, tendons, connective tissue, skin, and scar tissue begin to adapt to the movement. Continual stretching over long periods leads to many benefits.

THE BENEFITS OF STRETCHING

Stretching improves a person's overall athletic ability. Stretching the muscles leads to greater flexibility, allowing for a greater range of motion. The activity improves the range of motion by reducing muscle tension in the stretched part of the body. Improved range of movement allows the limbs to move farther apart without the muscles or tendons becoming damaged. Consistent stretching after athletic activity reduces an athlete's risk of injury.

Besides reducing the risk of injury, stretching also eases postexertion muscle soreness. Soreness occurs after strenuous exercise and results from microtears in the muscle fibers, blood pooling in the legs, and waste accumulation, such as lactic acid buildup. Lengthening the muscle fibers during a stretch increases blood circulation and helps eliminate waste products. Stretching after a workout also reduces bodily fatigue, which can diminish future physical and mental performance. Fatigue creates greater muscle tension and forces the body to work harder during physical activity. Greater flexibility relieves muscle pressure, and the body requires less effort from the working muscles.

A person can learn many things about the body by performing frequent stretches, leading to greater relaxation and stress relief. Regular stretching also corrects posture and strengthens physical coordination. Better circulation also leads to increased energy.

TYPES OF STRETCHES

Stretching falls into two basic categories: static stretching and dynamic stretching. Static stretches are done without other types of movement. A static stretch involves a person getting into a stretch and remaining there for a given time. The position of the stretch is meant to place gradual tension on the muscle as it is stretched. Static stretching is recommended for beginners and people who are not very active. Other static stretches include passive stretching, active stretching, and isometric stretching. Passive stretching involves another person or apparatus moving a limb to create a stretch. Active stretching is using muscle strength to generate a stretch in a specific area. Raising the leg high in the air and keeping it there without external assistance is an example of an active stretch. Isometric stretches are passive stretches that lengthen muscles for extended amounts of time with great intensity.

Dynamic stretches involve stretching and movement. While stretching a specific body part, a person also swings or bounces the body part to extend its range of motion. The force of the bouncing or swinging creates greater flexibility in the limb. Dynamic stretches can also work to strengthen muscles. Resistance stretching and loaded stretching contract and elongate a muscle simultaneously. The muscle is stretched through its full range of motion while contracted, increasing strength. Due to the demands dynamic stretching places on the musculoskeletal system, this type of stretching is most beneficial to regularly active people.

STRETCHING SAFELY

Stretching can do serious damage to the body if performed incorrectly. Individuals should listen to their bodies when stretching. Any movement that causes pain or discomfort should be avoided. A person should never stretch an injured body area until the area has recovered or a physician has cleared the individual to perform the activity. Warming up is also very important before stretching. Stretching cold muscles can lead to muscle damage. Body heat loosens muscles, making them more pliable for stretching. Warm-ups also increase blood flow and release oxygen into a person's system, nourishing the muscles. Comprehensive stretching of all major muscle groups in the body is an important part of physical activity. Expert opinion varies regarding whether stretching before exercise is beneficial. Still, most agree that stretching after a workout is crucial to muscle recovery.

—*Cait Caffrey*

Further Reading

Reynolds, Gretchen. "Stretching: The Truth." *Play Magazine*, 31 Oct. 2008, www.nytimes.com/2008/11/02/sports/playmagazine/112pewarm.html.

Roberts, Melanie, and Stephanie Kaiser. "The Different Types of Stretching." *Idiot's Guides: Stretching*. Alpha Books, 2013.

"Stretching: Focus on Flexibility." *Mayo Clinic*, 23 Mar. 2015, www.mayoclinic.org/healthy-living/fitness/in-depth/stretching/art-20047931.

Walker, Brad. *The Anatomy of Stretching*. Atlantic Books, 2007.

STRESS REDUCTION

Category: Treatment

Specialties and related fields: Alternative medicine, environmental health, immunology, occupational health, preventive medicine, psychiatry, psychology

Definition: a set of procedures to decrease bodily and mental tension by increasing rest and coping skills

KEY TERMS

palliative treatments: therapies that reduce symptoms without completely eradicating a disorder

psychotherapy: treatment using the mind to remedy problems related to disordered behavior or thinking, emotional problems, or disease

stress: physical, environmental, or psychological strain experienced by an individual that requires adjustment

INDICATIONS AND PROCEDURES

Stress can exacerbate difficulties in daily functioning, slow recovery from mental or physical problems, and impede immunological functioning. Stress reduction techniques represent a cluster of procedures that aim to reduce bodily and emotional tension: drug and physical therapies, exercise, biofeedback training, meditation, hypnosis, psychotherapy, relaxation training, and stress inoculation therapy.

The drugs used in stress reduction are designed to provide overall bodily relaxation, induce rest, or decrease the anxious thinking that exacerbates stressful experiences. Examples of such drugs include sedatives, tranquilizers, benzodiazepines, antihistamines, beta-blockers, and barbiturates. Similarly, physical therapies and exercise are recommended for these purposes. Baths (hydrotherapy), massages, and moderate exercise can also be part of a stress reduction program.

Psychotherapy is a common treatment for stress implemented by psychiatrists, psychologists, social workers, psychiatric nurses, and counselors. Not only does it help individuals to sort out their problems mentally, but it is also an effective stress management strategy. When individuals analyze their lifestyles and life events, stress-inducing behaviors and life patterns can be explored and targeted for modification.

Biofeedback, meditation, hypnosis, and relaxation training focus on inducing relaxation or altered consciousness by shifting a person's attention. Biofeedback uses monitoring devices attached to the body to provide visual or aural feedback to the trainee. Such devices include the electromyograph (EMG), which measures muscle tension, and the psychogalvanometer, which measures galvanic skin response (GSR). An EMG involves placing sensors on various muscle groups to record muscular electrical potentials. Galvanic skin response also relies on sensors, which record bodily responses caused by sweat gland activity and emotional arousal. The feedback from such devices allows trainees to learn to control certain bodily processes (e.g., muscle tension, brain waves, heart rate, temperature, and blood pressure). Biofeedback training treats headaches, temporomandibular joint (TMJ) syndrome, high blood pressure, and tics. It can also facilitate neuromuscular responses in stroke patients.

Meditation is a focused thinking exercise involving a quiet setting and the repetition of a word or phrase called a "mantra." By blocking distracting thoughts and refocusing attention, meditation reduces anxious thinking. It is useful for mild anxiety, minor concentration difficulties, and daily relaxation.

Hypnosis involves using suggestion, concentrated attention, or drugs to induce a sleeplike state or trance. Hypnosis can be induced by a hypnotist or via self-hypnosis. Hypnotic states are characterized by increased suggestibility, recall of forgotten events, decreased pain sensitivity and increased vasomotor control. The ability to be hypnotized varies from person to person based on susceptibility to suggestion and psychological needs. Hypnosis is a brief therapy targeting problems such as insomnia, pain, panic, and sexual dysfunction. In addition, hypnosis is sometimes used when drugs are contraindicated for anesthetic use, particularly for dental procedures.

Relaxation training involves three primary methods: autogenic training, which involves head, heart, and abdominal exercises; progressive relaxation, which involves becoming aware of tension in the various muscle groups by relaxing one group at a time in a specific order; and breathing exercises. Relaxation training is best learned when a therapist trains an individual in person and the exercises are practiced independently. Relaxation can be practiced several times daily and in response to stressful events. High blood pressure, ulcers, insomnia, asthma, drug and alcohol problems, spastic colitis, tachycardia (rapid heartbeat), pain management, and moderate-to-severe anxiety disorders are treated with relaxation training.

Stress inoculation therapy is a specific type of psychotherapy involving techniques that alter patterns of thinking and acting. It is useful for treating anxiety disorders related to stress. It comprises three steps: education about stress and fear reactions, rehearsal of coping behaviors, and application of coping behaviors in stress-provoking situations.

USES AND COMPLICATIONS

Individuals should not apply stress reduction procedures without proper consultation; medical conditions that might be causing symptoms should be assessed or ruled out first. Biofeedback training for headaches, for example, would be unwarranted until other, more serious causes of headaches had been eliminated from consideration. Similarly, exercise, drug, and physical therapies could worsen conditions such as high blood pressure, alcohol and drug problems, and chronic pain if applied incorrectly. For example, where stress or pain is chronic, drug therapies might encourage the development of drug dependence.

Training via self-help materials alone or by an unskilled provider may provide no benefit or create difficulties. Instead, skilled providers should administer these procedures. Poor training could result in frustration, hypervigilance, heightened anxiety, depression, or pain caused by overattention to symptoms or conflicts. Some individuals are prone to these effects even with good training. Therefore, ongoing assessment is necessary. Finally, interpretation of any memories provoked by hypnosis should be approached with caution because of the suggestibility characteristic of hypnotic states.

PERSPECTIVE AND PROSPECTS

Stress reduction techniques evolved from ancient meditation practices and simpler pain management methods predating the development of modern anesthetics. These techniques' palliative and preventive effects have given these procedures a sure hold in future medical practice. In contrast, employee benefits such as decreased absenteeism and increased feelings of wellness have secured these strategies in the workplace. The expanded use of stress reduction procedures in prenatal care and with the elderly is likely.

—*Nancy A. Piotrowski*

Further Reading

Davis, Martha, et al. *The Relaxation and Stress Reduction Workbook*. 5th ed., New Harbinger, 2000.

Humphrey, James H. *Stress Among Older Adults: Understanding and Coping*. Charles C Thomas, 1992.

Manning, George, et al. *Stress: Living and Working in a Changing World*. Whole Person Associates, 1999.

Newton, Tim, et al. *Managing Stress: Emotion and Power at Work*. Sage, 1996.

Pelletier, Kenneth. *The Best Alternative Medicine*. Fireside, 2002.

Schafer, Walt, and Sharrie A. Herbold. *Stress Management for Wellness*. 4th ed., Thomson/Wadsworth, 2000.

Seaward, Brian Luke. *Managing Stress: Principles and Strategies for Health and Well-Being*. 6th ed., Jones and Bartlett, 2009.

Weight Training

Category: Conditioning

Specialties and related fields: Athletic training, personal training, physical therapy, strength and conditioning

Definition: also called "strength training," it is a type of physical activity that refers to lifting weights (dumbbells) or using resistance (weight-bearing) machines to stress the muscles, causing them to get stronger

KEY TERMS

muscle fitness: having muscles that can lift heavier objects or muscles that will work longer before becoming exhausted

muscles: a band or bundle of fibrous tissue in a human or animal body that can contract, move in, or maintain the position of parts of the body.

resistance training: the performance of physical exercises that are designed to improve strength and endurance, often associated with the lifting of weights

workout: a session of vigorous physical exercise or training

INTRODUCTION

Weight training has many benefits for the body. It strengthens the bones and muscles, increases a person's strength, wards off diseases, helps people lose and maintain weight, and improves their overall health.

Many people—women especially—mistakenly believe that lifting weights will cause them to become bulky. This is not true since women do not have high testosterone levels, allowing men to add bulky muscles to their bodies. However, weight training can cause injury if a person does not follow proper lifting techniques.

GETTING STARTED

Before individuals begin any weight training routine, they should visit their doctor to ensure they are healthy enough to participate in the exercise. A doctor can assess a person's overall health to determine if there will be any risks associated with lifting weights. Anyone seeking the begin a weightlifting program should address the following health concerns with a doctor:

- Does the person have heart trouble, diabetes, or asthma conditions?
- Does physical activity cause chest pain or pain in the neck, shoulder, or arm?
- Does the person suffer from faintness or dizzy spells?
- Does physical activity cause the person to become winded or have trouble catching their breath?

- Are weight-bearing exercises difficult because of bone or joint problems, such as arthritis?
- Is the person over the age of forty?
- Is the person inactive?
- Does the person have health problems that might be impacted or made worse by lifting weights?

PROPER TECHNIQUE

Once individuals have determined that they are healthy enough to begin weight training, they should learn proper techniques. If people improperly lift weights, they can risk injuries, such as sprains, strains, and fractures. These can lead to more serious issues if they are left untreated.

Individuals new to weightlifting should work with a trainer at a fitness facility to learn how to use the machines and the proper ways to lift weights. People who do not belong to a fitness center can use other resources such as online tutorials and books to learn proper techniques.

Before a workout, a person should gently warm their muscles since cold muscles are more prone to injuries. A person can walk briskly or perform another aerobic activity such as jumping jacks for five to ten minutes to prepare the body for exercise.

Beginners should not lift weights that are too heavy. A few pounds are typically fine for beginners as the body's muscles, tendons, and ligaments quickly get used to weight training. A person will be able to

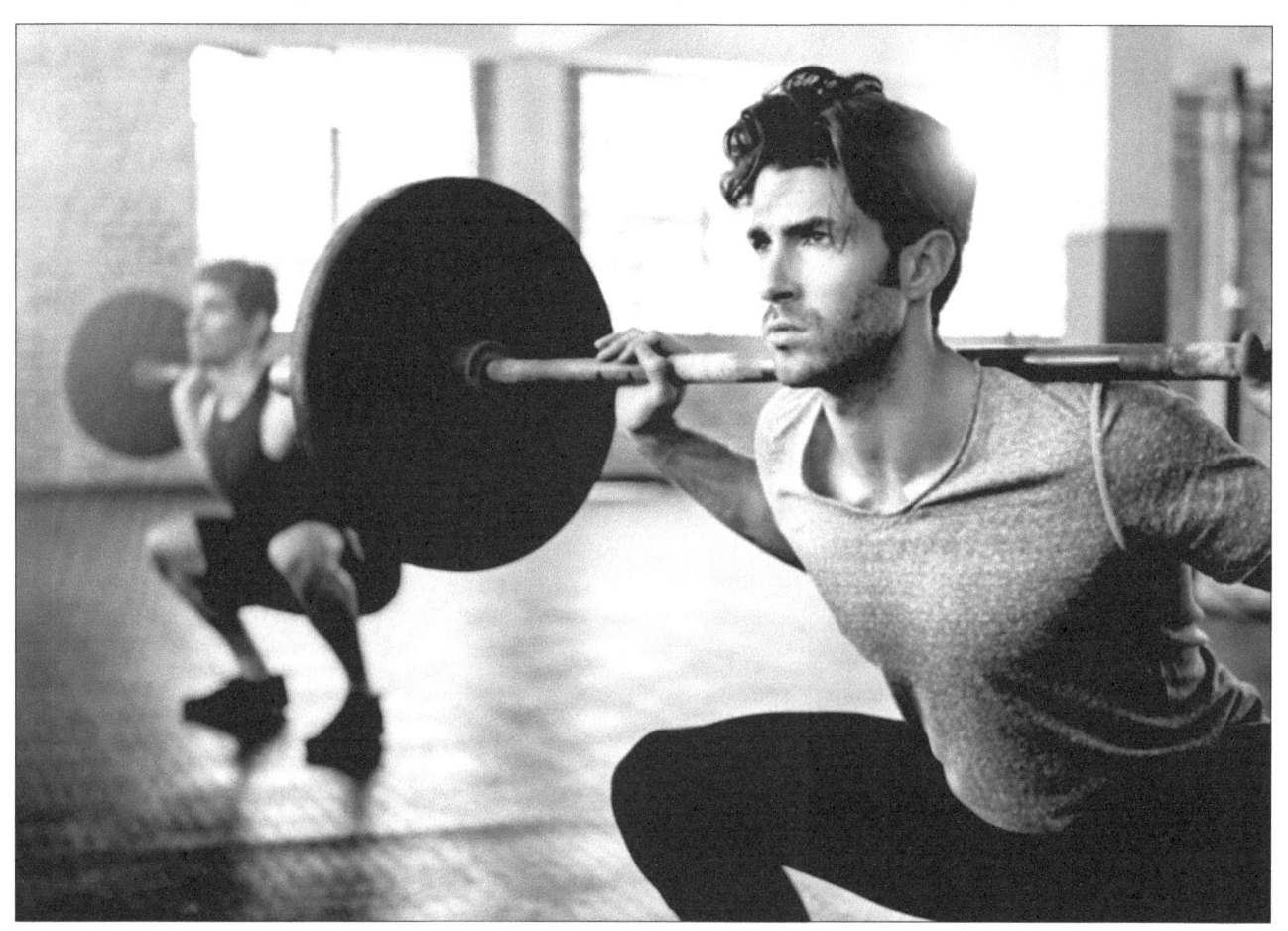

Weight training can increase metabolism and assist in weight loss. Photo via iStock/gradyreese. [Used under license.]

lift heavier weights as time progresses. The proper weight to lift allows a person to tire their muscles after about ten to fifteen repetitions. The last repetition should be difficult for the person to complete. There is no correct number of repetitions or sets for each person. It is up to the individual. A good rule of thumb is about three sets of twelve repetitions per exercise with thirty to ninety seconds of rest time between sets. Once a person can easily complete twelve repetitions per set, the person can gradually increase the weight. The right weight makes the last repetition difficult for the person to complete.

Individuals should practice good posture when lifting weights. They should start with their shoulders back and chest out in seated or standing positions. They also should keep their abdominal muscles tight.

Muscles need time to recover and repair themselves; therefore, individuals should rest for about a full day before exercising the same muscle group. Consequently, people should not work their leg muscles two days in a row. Instead, they should focus on arms one day, shoulders and back the next day, legs on the third day, and repeat. Individuals should rest a day or two between lifting weights to ensure the muscles have adequate time to repair.

BENEFITS
Individuals should aim to weight train for at least twenty to thirty minutes, two to three days a week. They should also perform cardiovascular exercises such as running or walking and eat a healthy diet for optimum health.

Weight training not only strengthens muscles but also increases bone density. It helps to reduce the risk of breaks and fractures. Lifting weights improves balance and reverses age-related muscle loss. It helps to ease anxiety and improve mood. It also helps a person sleep better.

Weight training improves a person's appearance and can help a person lose more weight than doing cardiovascular exercise alone. Research has shown that lifting weights provides a person with a metabolic spike that helps the body burn more calories after the workout because the body is working to repair the muscles. In addition, weight training helps a person improve their performance in other activities such as running or biking.

—*Angela Harmon*

Further Reading

"Best Beginner Weight-Training Guide with Easy-to-Follow Workout!" *Bodybuilding.com*, 8 Sept. 2015, www.bodybuilding.com/fun/beginner_weight_training.htm.

Klein, Sarah. "13 Reasons to Start Lifting Weights." *Huffington Post*, 12 Jan. 2015, www.huffingtonpost.com/2015/01/12/benefits-of-lifting-weights_n_6432632.html.

Plosser, Liz. "A WH Fitness Face Off." *Women'sHealth*, 2 Aug. 2007, www.womenshealthmag.com/fitness/cardio-vs-strength-training-workouts.

Sinkler, Jen. "4 Myths about Strength-Training Busted!" *Women'sHealth*, 24 Dec. 2013, www.womenshealthmag.com/fitness/strenght-training-myths.

"Weight Training: Improve Your Muscular Fitness." *Mayo Clinic*, 14 Aug. 2015, www.mayoclinic.org/healthy-lifestyle/fitness/in-depth/weight-training/art-20047116.

Nutrition and Supplements

If you are what you eat, then your workouts depend on what you eat. Americans spend huge sums of money on dietary supplements, even though the evidence that these supplements augment health or athletic prowess is wanting. Look here to see what to eat and how to best invest in your health. Diet plays a major role in providing energy for training, regulating metabolism, and providing nutrients to maintain and repair tissue. It also affects energy levels and focus. Topics explained in this section include: sports energy drinks, glucosamine, carbohydrates, essential nutrients, and creatine.

Amino Acids

Category: Biochemistry, organic chemistry
Specialties and related fields: Biochemistry, microbiology, nutrition
Definition: simple organic compounds that contain a carboxyl (-COOH) and an amino ($-NH_2$) group that are the building blocks of proteins

KEY TERMS

amino group: a functional group containing a nitrogen atom bonded to two hydrogen atoms ($-NH_2$)

carboxyl group: a functional group containing a carbon atom double-bonded to an oxygen atom and single-bonded to a hydroxyl group (-OH); has the formula CO_2H, typically written -COOH

catalyst: a chemical species that initiates or speeds up a chemical reaction but is not consumed in the reaction

peptide bond: a covalent bond that links the carboxyl group of one amino acid to the amine group of another, enabling the formation of proteins and other polypeptides

protein: a biological polymer consisting of one or more long chains of amino acids linked by peptide bonds in a sequence specified by an organism's deoxyribonucleic acid (DNA)

THE NATURE OF AMINO ACIDS

An amino acid is any compound whose molecular structure contains both an amino group and a carboxyl group, also called a "carboxylic acid group"—hence, the term "amino acid." However, the term refers to the specific group of amino acids that compose those proteins encoded by the deoxyribonucleic acid (DNA) molecule. These twenty (or sometimes twenty-three, depending on how they are classified) amino acids are called "proteinogenic amino acids," which means they are the main amino acids used to create proteins, enzymes, and other biomolecules. The three disputed amino acids are selenocysteine and pyrrolysine, which are not directly coded for in the genetic code but rather synthesized by other means and incorporated later, and N-formylmethionine, which initiates protein synthesis in some prokaryotes but is typically removed afterward. Selenocysteine is the only one of the three found in eukaryotes.

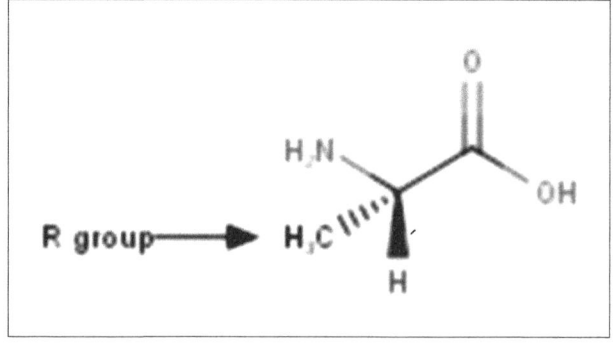

The chemical structure of the amino acid alanine. The R group in alanine is a "methyl" or $-CH_3$ group. Each amino has a unique R group, but the molecular skeleton remains the same for all amino acids, except for proline, whose R group forms a ring with the "amino" or $-NH2$ group. Image by M. Buratovich.

Of the standard twenty proteinogenic amino acids, nine are deemed "essential" because they are not synthesized in human metabolism but must be acquired through diet. Humans' nine essential amino acids include histidine, isoleucine, leucine, lysine, methionine, phenylalanine, threonine, tryptophan, and valine. Chemically, all proteinogenic amino acids are α-amino acids," meaning that their amino and carboxyl groups are bonded to the same carbon atom, known as the α-carbon (alpha carbon). This same carbon atom is also bonded to a hydrogen atom. The fourth atom or group bonded to the α-carbon, the so-called R group, determines the identity and chemical characteristics of the amino acid.

Chemically, amino acids have unique properties due to a basic amino or $-NH_2$ group and an acidic, carboxylic acid or COOH, group in the same molecule. An amino group is a basic group because it removes hydrogen ions (H⁺) from the solution. The -NH₂ binds the H⁺ ion from the solution to become a charge -NH₃⁺ group. The carboxylic acid, -COOH, group is an acidic group because it donates or releases hydrogen ions into the solution. Consequently, the -COOH group releases its hydrogen to become a negatively-charged -COO⁻ group, plus an H⁺ ion, released into the solution. A "zwitterion" is a state in which the amino acid is electrically neutral since a positive and a negative charge co-exist in separate parts of the molecule simultaneously.

In addition, each amino acid has a unique isoelectric point, which is the specific degree of acidity or basicity (pH) called its "isoelectric point" (pI), at which the amino acid has no net electrical charge. These particular characteristics are responsible for most, if not all, of the behavior of amino acids and the much larger compounds they form, such as proteins and enzymes. The names of all the amino acids, their single-letter symbol, and the codons that encode them are listed in the table on the following page.

FORMATION OF PROTEINS AND ENZYMES

The structures of all proteins are determined by the sequence of amino acids encoded in the DNA mole-

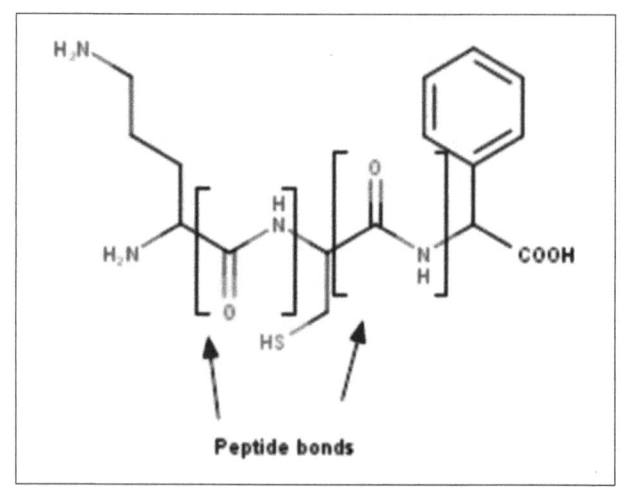

A peptide bond is the standard amide structure that forms between a carboxylic acid and an amine. Image by M. Buratovich

Zwiterrion state, in which the amino acid is electrically neutral. Image by M. Buratovich

cule. Most proteins and enzymes contain far more than just twenty amino acids. With just one of the twenty standard amino acids, there are thousands of trillions of possible ways to arrange them in a "polypeptide chain."

The synthesis of polypeptides and their formation into proteins is rapid, taking as little as six minutes, according to various tracer studies using radioactively labeled amino acids. The process begins with transcription, during which specific enzymes called ribonucleic acid (RNA) polymerases locally unwind the double-stranded structure of a DNA molecule and synthesize RNA copies of the DNA sequence. Each RNA molecule made from the DNA template used to synthesize proteins, so-called messenger RNAs (mRNAs), carry linear, consecutive, three-nucleotide sequences called "codons."

During the next step, translation, RNA-protein complexes called "ribosomes" bind the mRNA and translate the nucleotide sequence, originally from DNA, into a protein with a specific amino acid sequence. Ribosomes are macromolecular complexes of ribosomal RNA (rRNA) and ribosomal proteins. Translation links specific amino acids together in a specific order according to the sequence specified by the mRNA. Translation occurs in four steps: (1) activation of the amino acids; (2) initiation of the ribosome/mRNA complex; (3) elongation of the protein chain; and (4) termination when the ribosome encounters one of three stop codons that do not encode for an amino acid.

Amino acid activation culminates in the conjugation of each amino acid to a specific transfer RNA. The enzymes that catalyze activation, aminoacyl tRNA synthetases, specifically recognize each amino acid and its cognate tRNA and, in an energy-demanding reaction, link the amino acid to the 3' terminus of the tRNA.

Initiation requires the small ribosomal subunit (30S in prokaryotes and 40S in eukaryotes), the mRNA, the initiator tRNA, charged with methionine in eukaryotes, and N-formylmethionine in some prokaryotes, and special proteins called "initiation factors." These complexes position the mRNA on the ribosomal subunit and ready it for elongation. Once the start codon, AUG, is properly set on the ribosomal subunit, the large ribosomal subunit (50S in prokaryotes and 60S in eukaryotes) binds to the small ribosomal subunit, and elongation begins. Elongation requires proteins called "elongation factors" that ferry the tRNAs charged with their cognate amino acids to the ribosome. When the two appropriate amino acids are set next to each other, the large ribosomal RNA in the large ribosomal subunit catalyzes the formation of a peptide bond between the two amino acids. A peptide bond is just the stan-

Amino Acid	Single Letter Symbol	mRNA Codons that Encode Each Amino Acid
Alanine	A	GCA, GCC, GCG, GCU
Arginine	R	AGA, AGG, CGA, CGG, CGC, CGU
Asparagine	N	AAC, AAU
Aspartic acid	D	GAC, GAU
Cysteine	C	UGC, UGU
Glutamic acid	E	GAA, GAG
Glutamine	Q	CAG, CAA
Glycine	G	GGA, GGC, GGG, GGU
Histidine	H	CAC, CAU
Isoleucine	I	AUA, AUC, AUU
Leucine	L	CUA, CUC, CUG, CUU, UUA, UUG
Lysine	K	AAA, AAG
Methionine	M	AUG
Phenylalanine	F	UUU, UUC
Proline	P	CCA, CCC, CCG, CCU
Serine	S	AGC, AGU, UCA, UCG, UCC, UCU
Threonine	T	ACA, ACG, ACC, ACU
Tryptophan	W	UGG
Tyrosine	Y	UAC, UAU
Valine	V	GUA, GUG, GUC, GUU
Start codon	M	AUG
Stop codons	-	UUA, UGA, UAG

dard amide structure that forms between a carboxylic acid and an amine. The term refers specifically to an amide bond formed between amino acids in a polypeptide.

The ribosome reads the mRNA one codon at a time. Translation terminates once the ribosome encounters UAA, UAG, or UGA codons. There are no tRNAs that recognize these three "stop codons." Therefore, special proteins called "release factors" bind to the ribosome, liberate the nascent polypeptide chain from the ribosome and dissociate the small and large ribosomal subunit.

TRANSLATING THE GENETIC CODE INTO PROTEINS

The DNA and RNA molecules use only four different nucleotide bases to specify the entire genetic code. Yet, the number of possible three-nucleotide codons formed from these is more than sufficient to differentiate the twenty standard amino acids. The system is redundant, with several different codons signifying the same amino acid. Specific nucleotide sequences also designate the starting and ending points of a particular sequence of amino acids and hence the protein structure that derives from that sequence. Deoxyribonucleic acid was first identified in the late 1860s by Swiss chemist Friedrich Miescher. Still, it was not thought to be related to genetic information until Oswald Avery and colleagues established its connection in 1943. Subsequent research eventually revealed the structure and function of DNA and RNA. By preparing synthetic sequences of mRNA codons, researchers determined which codons encoded for each specific amino acid in transcription and translation. The code is translated in the accompanying chart.

Interestingly, the same codon, AUG, indicates both methionine and the start sequence, while the three stop codons are unique. The context in which the AUG codon appears determines whether it functions as a start codon or the codon for methionine.

AMINO ACIDS AND PROTEINS

The sequence of amino acids in a protein molecule defines its primary structure. Since each amino acid group has a specific geometry dictated by molecular structure and bond formation rules, no polypeptide chain or protein can be just a linear molecule. The angles of the bonds at each atom create all sorts of twists and turns along the entire length of the polypeptide molecule, moving the various functional groups on each amino acid into positions that allow them to interact with each other. Some protein segments form larger, local structures, such as spirals (alpha-helices) or flattened sheets (beta sheets). These constitute the secondary structure of the protein. A third or tertiary structure results from packaging various secondary structures into three-dimensional structures that give the protein its characteristic and unique shape. Tertiary structures often require the interaction of the various amino acid functional groups as they form bonds due to their proximity. For example, positively charged amino acids like arginine or lysine may form ionic bonds with nearby negatively charged amino acids like aspartate or glutamate. Alternatively, the amino acid cysteine, which contains a sulfhydryl functional group (-SH), can form disulfide bonds (-S-S-) with adjacent cysteine residues to reinforce or drive the protein into particular tertiary structures. Disulfide bonds are formed by enzymes called "protein disulfide isomerases." Protein disulfide isomerases are restricted to the endoplasmic reticulum in eukaryotes and the periplasm in prokaryotes. A fourth, or quaternary, structure results when two or more protein subunits combine to form a larger, functional complex.

—*Richard M. Renneboog, Michael A. Buratovich,*

Further Reading
Berg, Jeremy M., et al. *Biochemistry*. 9th ed., W.H. Freeman, 2019.

Klein, David R. *Organic Chemistry and a Second Language*. 5th ed., Wiley, 2019.

Lodish, Harvey, et al. *Molecular Cell Biology*. 9th ed., W.H. Freeman, 2021.

Nelson, David L., and Michael M. Cox. *Lehninger Principles of Biochemistry*. 8th ed., W.H. Freeman, 2021.

Winter, Arthur. *Organic Chemistry for Dummies*. 2nd ed., For Dummies, 2016.

ANTI-INFLAMMATORY DIET

Category: Therapy or technique

Also known as: Diet-based therapy, nutritional medicine

Specialties and related fields: Dietetics, nutrition, rheumatology

Definition: therapy that uses food with anti-inflammatory activities to treat and prevent chronic degenerative diseases

KEY TERMS

cytokines: any of a class of immunoregulatory proteins (such as interleukin or interferon) that are secreted by cells, especially of the immune system

eicosanoids: any of a class of compounds (such as the prostaglandins) derived from polyunsaturated fatty acids (such as arachidonic acid) and involved in cellular activity

inflammation: a local response to cellular injury that is marked by capillary dilatation, leukocytic infiltration, redness, heat, and pain and that serves as a mechanism initiating the elimination of harmful agents and damaged tissue

interleukins: any of various cytokines of low molecular weight that are produced by lymphocytes, macrophages, and monocytes and that function especially in the regulation of the immune system and especially cell-mediated immunity

omega-3 fatty acids: being or composed of polyunsaturated fatty acids that have the final double bond in the hydrocarbon chain between the third and fourth carbon atoms from the end of the molecule opposite that of the carboxyl group and that are found especially in fish, fish oils, green leafy vegetables, and some nuts and vegetable oils

OVERVIEW

Numerous evidence-based research studies in the twenty-first century support the use of anti-inflammatory diets to treat and prevent chronic degenerative diseases. These studies examined dietary properties that included raw versus processed, organic versus commercially grown, and natural versus genetically modified. The studies also looked at the dietary effects of herbs and spices, fruits and vegetables, nuts and seeds, grains and legumes, minerals and vitamins, and phytochemicals and polyunsaturated fatty acids such as omega-3 fatty acids.

MECHANISM OF ACTION

Few direct or indirect pathways (based on the specific inflammatory biomarkers) explain how the anti-inflammatory diet works. The eicosanoid-related anti-inflammatory pathway is typical for foods with high omega-3 fatty acid content. This pathway decreases levels of arachidonic acid and inflammatory mediators such as cytokines, related prostaglandins, and related metabolites. This process also decreases the activities of inflammatory cells in the immune system.

Food with active phytochemicals (resveratrol and epigallocatechin gallate) works through an inhibitory effect on nuclear transcription (for example, nuclear transcription factor) and a signaling process.

THERAPEUTIC USES

Based on recent research studies, the anti-inflammatory diet could be used to treat chronic degenerative diseases with chronic inflammation as a common denominator. These diseases include diabetes, cardio-

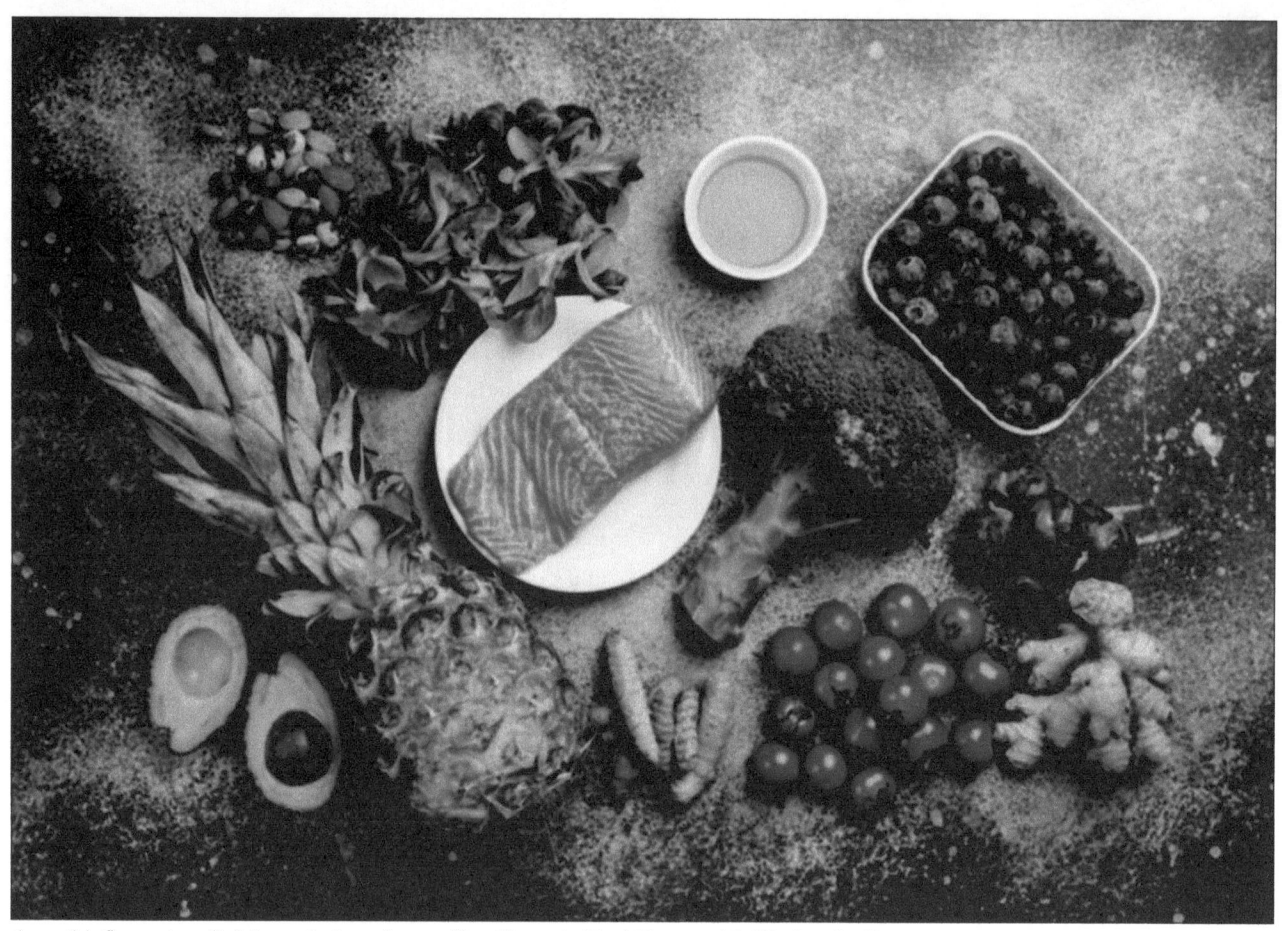

An anti-inflammatory died favors fruits and vegetables. Photo via iStock/thesomegirl. [Used under license.]

vascular diseases, obesity, certain cancers, arthritis, osteoporosis, and other immune system disorders.

SCIENTIFIC EVIDENCE

Evidence-based research shows that an anti-inflammatory diet is beneficial in treating many chronic degenerative disease conditions. A 2003 double-blind, crossover study included sixty-eight persons diagnosed with rheumatoid arthritis. Participants were divided into two groups for eight months of observation. One group was on a regular Western diet. The other group was on an anti-inflammatory diet with specific regulations on arachidonic acid (low intake). Both groups received placebo or fish oil capsules for three months. Persons on the anti-inflammatory diet, but not those on the typical Western diet, showed improvements in tender and swollen joints and even greater improvements when added to fish oil. The basic anti-inflammatory diet can augment the beneficial effects of any single, added anti-inflammatory food component.

In a 2010 double-blind, placebo-controlled, crossover study with a treatment period of five weeks, thirty-six healthy overweight persons received what was called an anti-inflammatory dietary mix (AIDM), which included green tea extract, resveratrol (grape extract), vitamin C, vitamin E (alpha-tocopherol), tomato extract, and omega-3 fatty acids. All these food components are described as an anti-inflammatory by human and animal research studies. Serum and urine inflammatory biomarkers were measured. The AIDM decreased inflammation and oxidative stress (a marker for risk of inflammation) and changes in lipid metabolism (with a decrease in triglycerides and with an improvement of endothelial function).

In a 2010 single-blind, randomized study, thirty-five persons diagnosed with obesity and metabolic syndrome were put on either an anti-inflammatory diet (green tea or green tea extract) or no diet for eight weeks. The group on green tea beverages or green tea extract showed lower levels of interleukin (one of the biomarkers for inflammation).

SAFETY ISSUES
No adverse side effects have been reported with the anti-inflammatory diet. Beneficial changes in bowel habits can occur in the beginning, however.

—Zuzana Bic

Further Reading
Fletcher, Jenna. *Anti-Inflammatory Diet: What to Know*. Medical News Today, MediLexicon International, 3 Jan. 2020, www.medicalnewstoday.com/articles/320233. Accessed 26 May 2022.
"Foods That Fight Inflammation." *Harvard Health Publishing*, 7 Nov. 2018, www.health.harvard.edu/staying-healthy/foods-that-fight-inflammation. Accessed 26 May 2022.
"How an Anti-Inflammatory Diet Can Relieve Pain as You Age." *Health Essentials from Cleveland Clinic*, 7 Oct. 2019, health.clevelandclinic.org/anti-inflammatory-diet-can-relieve-pain-age/. Accessed 26 May 2022.
"How to Use Food to Help Your Body Fight Inflammation." *Mayo Clinic*, 13 Aug. 2019, www.mayoclinic.org/healthy-lifestyle/nutrition-and-healthy-eating/in-depth/how-to-use-food-to-help-your-body-fight-inflammation/art-20457586. Accessed 26 May 2022.
Spritzler, Franziska. "The 13 Most Anti-Inflammatory Foods You Can Eat." *Healthline*, 19 Dec. 2019, www.healthline.com/nutrition/13-anti-inflammatory-foods. Accessed 26 May 2022.

BIOTIN

Category: Herbs and supplements
Also known as: Related term: Biocytin (brewer's yeast biotin complex)
Specialties and related fields: Biochemistry, dietetics, nutrition
Definition: natural substance used as a supplement to treat specific health condition

KEY TERMS
B vitamins: a class of water-soluble vitamins that play important roles in cell metabolism and synthesis of red blood cells and tend to coexist in the same foods
dietary supplement: a manufactured product that, when consumed, provides nutrients above the recommended daily requirements
enzymes: molecules, usually proteins, produced by living organisms that act as a catalyst to accelerate the rate of specific biochemical reactions

OVERVIEW
Biotin is a water-soluble B vitamin that plays an important role in metabolizing the energy humans obtain from food. Biotin assists four essential enzymes that break down fats, carbohydrates, and proteins.

Biotin deficiency is rare, except, possibly, among pregnant women. All proposed therapeutic uses of biotin supplements are highly speculative.

REQUIREMENTS AND SOURCES
Although biotin is a necessary nutrient, humans usually get enough from bacteria living in the digestive tract. Severe biotin deficiency has been seen in people who frequently eat large quantities of raw egg whites. Raw egg whites contain a protein that blocks the absorption of biotin. Cooked egg whites do not present this problem.

The official US and Canadian recommendations for daily intake of biotin are as follows: for infants, zero to five months, five micrograms (mcg); six to eleven months, six mcg; for children, one to three years, eight mcg; four to eight years, 12 mcg; and nine to thirteen years, 20 mcg; for teenagers, fourteen to eighteen years, 25 mcg; and for adults nineteen years and older, 30 mcg. The recommended intake for pregnant women is 30 mcg, and for nursing women, 35 mcg. Good dietary sources of biotin include brewer's yeast, nutritional (torula) yeast, whole grains, nuts, egg yolks, sardines, legumes, liver, cauliflower, bananas, and mushrooms.

There is some evidence that slight biotin deficiency may occur during normal pregnancy. For this reason, pregnant women are advised to take a prenatal vitamin that contains the recommended amount of biotin.

Common Synonyms for Biotin	
Beta-biotin	Beta-biotin
Bioepiderm	Bioepiderm
Bios II	Bios II
Biotina	Biotina
Biotine	Biotine
Biotinum	D-biotin
Coenzyme R	

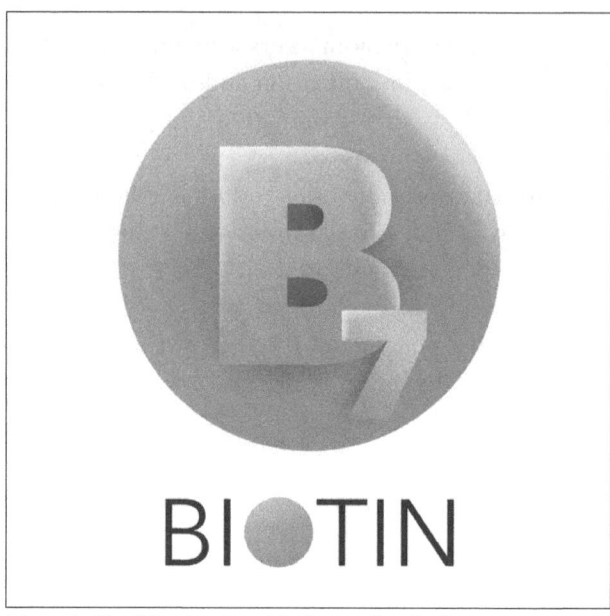

Photo via iStock/Dmitry Kovalchuk. [Used under license.]

THERAPEUTIC DOSAGES

For people with diabetes, the usual recommended dosage of biotin is 7,000 to 15,000 mcg daily. For treating "cradle cap" (a scaly head rash often found in infants), the usual dosage of biotin is 6,000 mcg daily, given to the nursing mother (not the child). A lower dosage of 3,000 mcg daily is used to treat brittle fingernails and toenails.

There are indirect indications that individuals taking antiseizure medications might benefit from biotin supplementation at nutritional doses. However, it has been suggested that people take biotin at least two hours before or after the medication dose to avoid potential interference with the medication's absorption. In addition, people should avoid excessive biotin supplementation (above nutritional needs) because it might interfere with seizure control. All these proposed interactions are quite speculative. Even if they do exist, they may not be important enough to make a difference in real life.

THERAPEUTIC USES

All the proposed uses of biotin discussed here are speculative and based on incomplete evidence. Preliminary research suggests that supplemental biotin might help reduce blood sugar levels in people with either type 1 (childhood-onset) or type 2 (adult-onset) diabetes and possibly reduce the symptoms of diabetic neuropathy.

SCIENTIFIC EVIDENCE

No double-blind, placebo-controlled studies have been reported on these potential uses of biotin. Two double-blind studies have found benefits for diabetes with a mixture of biotin and chromium; however, it is not clear how much the biotin in this combination contributed.

Weak evidence, too weak to rely upon, has been used to support the theory that biotin supplements are helpful for brittle nails. Based on virtually no evidence, biotin has been proposed for treating cradle cap in infants.

SAFETY ISSUES
Biotin appears to be quite safe. However, maximum safe dosages for young children, pregnant or nursing women, or those with severe liver or kidney disease have not been established.

IMPORTANT INTERACTIONS
Persons taking anticonvulsant medications may need extra biotin. Still, they should not take more than the dosage recommendations listed in the Requirements and Sources section. In addition, one should take the vitamin two to three hours apart from the medication.

—*EBSCO CAM Review Board*

Further Reading

"Biotin: Fact Sheet for Health Professionals." *NIH Office of Dietary Supplements*. US Department of Health and Human Services, 10 Jan. 2022, ods.od.nih.gov/factsheets/Biotin-HealthProfessional/. Accessed 28 May 2022.

Lipner, Shari R. "Rethinking Biotin Therapy for Hair, Nail, and Skin Disorders." *Journal of the American Academy of Dermatology*, vol. 78, no. 6, 2018, pp. 1236-38.

Mock, Donald M. "Biotin: From Nutrition to Therapeutics." *The Journal of Nutrition*, vol. 147, no. 8, 2017, pp. 1487-92.

Patel, Deepa P., et al. "A Review of the Use of Biotin for Hair Loss." *Skin Appendage Disorders*, vol. 3, no. 3, 2017, pp. 166-69.

BRANCHED-CHAIN AMINO ACIDS

Category: Herbs and supplements
Specialties and related fields: Athletic training, biochemistry, body building, dietetics, nutrition
Definition: natural substance of the human body used as a supplement to treat specific health conditions

KEY TERMS

amyotrophic lateral sclerosis: a nervous system disease that weakens muscles and impacts physical function

isoleucine: an essential hydrophobic amino acid that is one of three branch-chain amino acids and a constituent of most proteins; it is an essential nutrient in the diet of vertebrates

leucine: a hydrophobic amino acid that is one of three branch-chain amino acids and a constituent of most proteins; it is an essential nutrient in the diet of vertebrates

valine: a hydrophobic α-amino acid used in the biosynthesis of proteins that is a member of the branch chain amino acids; in humans, valine must be obtained from the diet

OVERVIEW

Branched-chain amino acids (BCAAs) are naturally occurring molecules (leucine, isoleucine, and valine) that the body uses to build proteins. The term "branched-chain" refers to the molecular structure of these particular amino acids. Muscles have a particularly high content of BCAAs. For reasons that are not entirely clear, BCAA supplements may improve appetite in cancer patients and slow the progression of amyotrophic lateral sclerosis (ALS, or Lou Gehrig's disease, a condition that leads to degeneration of nerves, atrophy of the muscles, and eventual death). Branched-chain amino acids have also been proposed as a supplement to boost athletic performance.

REQUIREMENTS AND SOURCES
Dietary protein usually provides all the BCAAs needed. However, physical stress and injury can increase a person's need for BCAAs to repair muscle damage, so that supplementation may be helpful.

Branched-chain amino acids are present in all protein-containing foods, but red meat and dairy products are the best sources. Chicken, fish, and eggs are excellent sources as well. Whey protein and egg protein supplements are another way to ensure that a person gets enough BCAAs. Supplements may contain all three BCAAs together or individual BCAAs. The typical dosage of BCAAs is 1 to 5 grams (g) daily.

THERAPEUTIC USES
Preliminary evidence suggests that BCAAs may improve appetite in people undergoing treatment for cancer. There is also some evidence that BCAA supplements may reduce symptoms of amyotrophic lateral sclerosis (ALS, or Lou Gehrig's disease); however, not all studies have had positive results.

Preliminary evidence from a series of small studies suggests that BCAAs might decrease symptoms of tardive dyskinesia, a movement disorder caused by long-term usage of antipsychotic drugs. Branched-chain amino acids have also shown a bit of promise for enhancing recovery from traumatic brain injury.

Because of how they are metabolized in the body, BCAAs might be helpful for individuals with severe liver disease (such as cirrhosis). Branched-chain amino acids have also been tried to aid muscle recovery after bed rest following surgery.

Although there is little supportive evidence on balance, current research does not indicate that BCAAs effectively enhance sports performance. One preliminary study suggests that BCAAs might aid recovery from long-distance running. Branched-chain amino acids have also as yet failed to prove effective for muscular dystrophy.

SCIENTIFIC EVIDENCE
Appetite in cancer patients. A double-blind study tested BCAAs on twenty-eight people with cancer who had lost their appetites because of the disease itself or its treatment. Appetite improved in 55 percent of those taking BCAAs (4.8 g daily) compared with only 16 percent of those taking a placebo.

Amyotrophic lateral sclerosis (ALS) (also known as Lou Gehrig's disease). A small double-blind study found that BCAAs might help protect muscle strength in people with Lou Gehrig's disease. Eighteen individuals were given either BCAAs (taken four times daily between meals) or a placebo and followed for one year. The results showed that people taking BCAAs declined much more slowly than those receiving a placebo. Five of nine participants lost their ability to walk in the placebo group, two died, and another required a respirator. Only one of the nine participants receiving BCAAs became unable to walk during the study period. This study is too small to provide conclusive evidence, but it does suggest that BCAAs might be helpful for this disease. However, other studies found no effect. One found a slight increase in deaths during the study period among those treated with BCAAs compared with those treated with a placebo.

Muscular dystrophy. One double-blind, placebo-controlled study found leucine (one of the amino acids in BCAAs) ineffective at the dose of 0.2 g per kilogram body weight (e.g., 15 g daily for a 75-kilogram woman) in ninety-six individuals with muscular dystrophy. Over one year, no differences were seen between the effects of leucine and a placebo.

SAFETY ISSUES

Branched-chain amino acids are believed to be safe; they are converted into other amino acids when taken in excess. However, like other amino acids, BCAAs may interfere with medications for Parkinson's disease. They may reduce the effectiveness of medications for Parkinson's disease (such as levodopa).

—*EBSCO CAM Review Board*

Further Reading

Fouré, Alexandre, and David Bendahan. "Is Branched-Chain Amino Acids Supplementation an Efficient Nutritional Strategy to Alleviate Skeletal Muscle Damage? A Systematic Review." *Nutrients*, vol. 9, no. 10, 2017, p. 1047.

Solon-Biet, Samantha M., et al. "Branched-Chain Amino Acids Impact Health and Lifespan Indirectly via Amino Acid Balance and Appetite Control." *Nature Metabolism*, vol. 1, no. 5, 2019, pp. 532-45.

Vandusseldorp, Trisha, et al. "Effect of Branched-Chain Amino Acid Supplementation on Recovery Following Acute Eccentric Exercise." *Nutrients*, vol. 10, no. 10, 2018, p. 1389.

Wolfe, Robert R. "Branched-Chain Amino Acids and Muscle Protein Synthesis in Humans: Myth or Reality?" *Journal of the International Society of Sports Nutrition*, vol. 14, no. 1, 2017, doi.org/10.1186/s12970-017-0184-.

Zhang, Zhen-Yu, et al. "Branched-Chain Amino Acids as Critical Switches in Health and Disease." *Hypertension*, vol. 72, no. 5, 2018, pp. 1012-22.

CARBOHYDRATES

Category: Biology
Also known as: Sugars, saccharides
Specialties and related fields: Biochemistry, endocrinology, nutrition
Definition: organic compounds consisting of carbon, hydrogen, and oxygen, in which hydrogen and oxygen are in a 2:1 ratio; the simplest carbohydrates (monosaccharides) contain an aldehyde or a ketone functional group and usually one hydroxyl group per carbon atom

KEY TERMS

alpha-amylase: an enzyme that hydrolyses alpha-linked polysaccharides, such as starch and glycogen, yielding shorter sugar chains

monosaccharide: any of the class of sugars such as glucose that cannot be hydrolyzed to give a simpler sugar

polysaccharide: a carbohydrate whose molecules consist of many sugar molecules bonded together

starch: a glucose polymer consisting of numerous glucose units joined by glycosidic bonds and is the major storage carbohydrate in plants and photosynthetic bacteria

DIGESTION AND ABSORPTION

Dietary carbohydrates include monosaccharides, such as glucose, fructose, and lactose; disaccharides (two monosaccharides linked together), sucrose, and lactose; and polysaccharides (many monosaccharides linked together in polymers), such as starches and fiber.

Starches are first broken down in the mouth by salivary alpha-amylase and then in the small intestine by alpha-amylases of salivary and pancreatic origin. The resulting simpler sugars are further digested by enzymes linked to the small intestine's inner lining: maltase, sucrase, and trehalase, which yield absorbable monosaccharides. These sugars cross the cells lining the small intestine via specialized molecular transport mechanisms and then diffuse into the intestinal capillaries and reach the bloodstream.

METABOLISM

In the body, the main role of carbohydrates is energy production and storage. Carbohydrates can also be joined to proteins (glycoproteins, for cell-cell

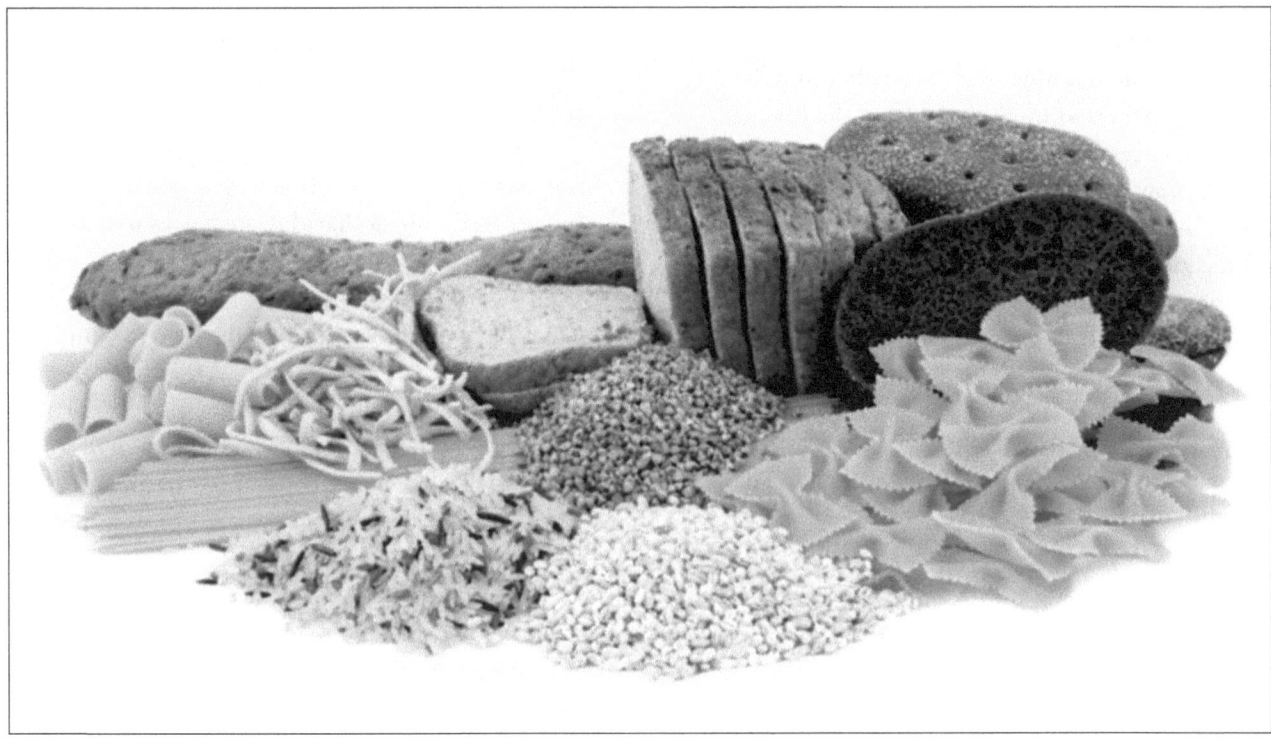

Carbohydrates are important for maximum energy, speed, and stamina. Photo via iStock/EvgeniaSh. [Used under license.]

interactions) or fatty acids (glycolipids, which provide energy and markers for cellular recognition).

The body converts most digestible carbohydrates into glucose, a universal energy source for cells. Glucose is maintained at a constant level in the blood by the interplay of insulin, glucagon, and other hormones. Excess glucose is stored as glycogen (glycogenesis), which can be broken down (glycogenolysis) when energy is needed.

Carbohydrate-related diseases are often genetic, linked to inborn errors in enzymes or cellular transporters. Examples are galactosemia, glycogen storage diseases, and lactose intolerance. Diabetes mellitus is a metabolic disorder characterized by excessive blood glucose. Type 1 diabetes is caused by insulin deficiency; type 2 can result from insulin resistance, impaired insulin secretion, and increased glucose production.

According to current recommendations, carbohydrates, preferably starches and natural sugars, should represent 40 to 60 percent of total calorie intake. Refined simple sugars provide calories but very little nutrition, and their intake should therefore be limited.

PERSPECTIVE AND PROSPECTS

Food availability in developed countries has reached unprecedented levels. The per capita consumption of carbohydrates, particularly refined sugars, increased dramatically in the late twentieth and early twenty-first centuries. Since the 1990s, the incidence of obesity has been climbing steadily. It so has the incidence of diabetes and related health problems. Current research in nutrition and carbohydrate metabolism addresses the problem, which has reached epidemic proportions. Great progress is being made in dietary manipulations and drug development.

—*Donatella M. Casirola*

Further Reading

"Carbohydrate Choice Lists." *Centers for Disease Control and Prevention*, 10 Aug. 2021, www.cdc.gov/diabetes/managing/eat-well/diabetes-and-carbs/carbohydrate-choice-lists.html. Accessed 2 Jun. 2022.

"Carbohydrates." *MedlinePlus*, 17 Jan. 2022, medlineplus.gov/carbohydrates.html. Accessed 2 Jun. 2022.

"Carbohydrates: How Carbs Fit into a Healthy Diet." *Mayo Clinic*, 22 Mar. 2022, www.mayoclinic.org/healthy-lifestyle/nutrition-and-healthy-eating/in-depth/carbohydrates/art-20045705. Accessed 2 Jun. 2022.

Fox, Stuart, and Krista Rompolski. *Human Physiology*. 16th ed., McGraw-Hill, 2021.

McGraw-Hill Encyclopedia of Science and Technology. 11th ed., McGraw-Hill, 2012.

Stanhope, K. L., and P. J. Havel. "Fructose Consumption: Considerations for Future Research on Its Effects on Adipose Distribution, Lipid Metabolism, and Insulin Sensitivity in Humans." *Journal of Nutrition*, vol. 139, no. 6, 2009, pp. 1236S-41S.

CETYLATED FATTY ACIDS

Category: Herbs and supplements
Specialties and related fields: Alternative medicine, dietetics, nutrition
Definition: fatty acids esterified to cetyl alcohol (1-hexadecanol)

KEY TERMS

cetyl alcohol: C-16 fatty alcohol with the formula CH(CH)OH

ester: an organic compound formed by reacting a carboxylic acid with an alcohol with the elimination of a water molecule. Many naturally occurring fats and essential oils are esters of fatty acids; they are among the most fragrant organic molecules

OVERVIEW

In 2004, a special mixture of fats called "cetylated fatty acids" began to be widely marketed as a treatment for osteoarthritis. Although the claims associated with this product appear to exceed what has been proven, it is fair to say that cetylated fatty acids have shown definite promise in preliminary trials.

REQUIREMENTS AND SOURCES

There is no dietary requirement for cetylated fatty acids.

THERAPEUTIC DOSAGES

Cetylated fatty acids are used both orally and as a topical cream. A typical oral dose of cetylated fatty acids is 1,000 to 2,000 milligrams daily. Cetylated fatty acid creams are applied twice to the affected area daily.

THERAPEUTIC USES

Three double-blind, placebo-controlled studies have found cetylated fatty acids helpful for osteoarthritis. Two involved a topical product, and one used an oral formulation.

In one study using a cream, forty people with osteoarthritis of the knee applied either cetylated fatty acids or a placebo to the affected joint. The results over thirty days showed greater improvements in range of motion and functional ability among people using the real cream than among those using the placebo cream. In another thirty-day study, also enrolling forty people with knee arthritis, the use of cetylated fatty acid cream improved postural stability, presumably because of decreased pain levels.

In addition, a sixty-eight-day double-blind, placebo-controlled study of sixty-four people with knee arthritis tested an oral cetylated fatty acid supplement (the supplement also contained lesser amounts of lecithin and fish oil). Participants in the treatment group experienced improvements in swelling, mobility, and pain level compared with those in the placebo group. Inexplicably, the study report does not discuss whether side effects occurred.

Although this is a promising body of research, it is far from definitive. Current advertising claims for cetylated fatty acids go far beyond the existing evidence. For example, several websites claim that cetylated fatty acids are more effective than glucosamine or chondroitin. However, no comparison studies have been performed upon which such a claim could be rationally based.

It is not known how cetylated fatty acids might help osteoarthritis. Proponents cite the known benefits of fish oil for rheumatoid arthritis. However, the fatty acids in fish oil are rather different from those in cetylated fatty acids. Also, the origin of rheumatoid arthritis is quite unlike that of osteoarthritis. Consequently, there is little relevance to these observations. Proponents also make specific claims, including that cetylated fatty acids reduce inflammation, protect cartilage from damage, lubricate cell membranes, and increase fluid in joints. However, none of these explanations have more than speculative scientific support. If cetylated fatty acids do help osteoarthritis, their mechanism is not known. Cetylated fatty acid creams have also been proposed for the treatment of psoriasis.

SAFETY ISSUES

Cetylated fatty acids appear to have a low level of toxicity, according to safety studies conducted by the primary manufacturer. However, maximum safe doses in young children, pregnant or nursing women, and people with severe liver or kidney disease have not been established.

—*EBSCO CAM Review Board*

Further Reading

"Cetylated Fatty Acids Help Osteoarthritis Joints." *Health24*, 19 Jan. 2017, www.health24.com/Medical/Arthritis/Managing-pain/Cetylated-fatty-acids-help-joints-20120721.

Hudita, Ariana, et al. "In Vitro Effects of Cetylated Fatty Acids Mixture from Celadrin on Chondrogenesis and Inflammation with Impact on Osteoarthritis." *Cartilage*, vol. 11, no. 1, 2018, pp. 88-97.

Wong, Cathy. "The Health Benefits of Cetyl Myristoleate." *Verywell Health*, 25 Nov. 2019, www.verywellhealth.com/the-benefits-of-cetyl-myristoleate-89434.

CREATINE

Category: Herbs and supplements
Specialties and related fields: Biochemistry, dietetics, nutrition, personal training, sports medicine
Definition: natural substance of the human body used as a supplement to treat specific health conditions and enhance sports performance enhancement

KEY TERMS

creatine kinase: an enzyme expressed by various tissues and cell types that catalyzes the conversion of creatine and uses adenosine triphosphate (ATP) to create phosphocreatine and adenosine diphosphate (ADP)

creatine phosphate: a compound in muscles that regenerates ATP from ADP

creatinine: a breakdown product of creatine phosphate from muscle and protein metabolism. It is released at a constant rate by the body

OVERVIEW

Creatine is a naturally occurring substance that plays an important role in producing energy in the body. The body converts it to phosphocreatine, a form of stored energy used by muscles.

Although the evidence for creatine is not definitive, it has the most evidence behind it among all the sports supplements. Numerous small double-blind studies suggest that it can increase athletic performance in sports that involve intense but short bursts of activity. The theory behind its use is that supplemental creatine can build up a reserve of phosphocreatine in the muscles to help them perform on demand. Supplemental creatine may also help the body make new phosphocreatine faster when used up by intense activity.

REQUIREMENTS AND SOURCES

Although some creatine exists in the daily diet, it is not an essential nutrient because the human body can make it from the amino acids L-arginine, glycine, and L-methionine. Provided enough animal protein (the principal source of these amino acids) is consumed, the body will make all the creatine needed for good health.

Meat (including chicken and fish) is creatine's most important dietary source and its amino acid building blocks. For this reason, vegetarian athletes may potentially benefit most from creatine supplementation.

THERAPEUTIC DOSAGES

A typical dosage schedule for bodybuilding and exercise enhancement starts with a loading dose of around 15 to 30 grams daily (divided into 2 or 3 separate doses) for three to four days, followed by 2 to 5 g daily. Some authorities recommend skipping the loading dose. (By comparison, humans typically get only about 1 g of creatine in their daily diet.)

Creatine's ability to enter muscle cells can be increased by combining it with glucose, fructose, or other simple carbohydrates; in addition, prior use of creatine might enhance the sports benefits of carbo-

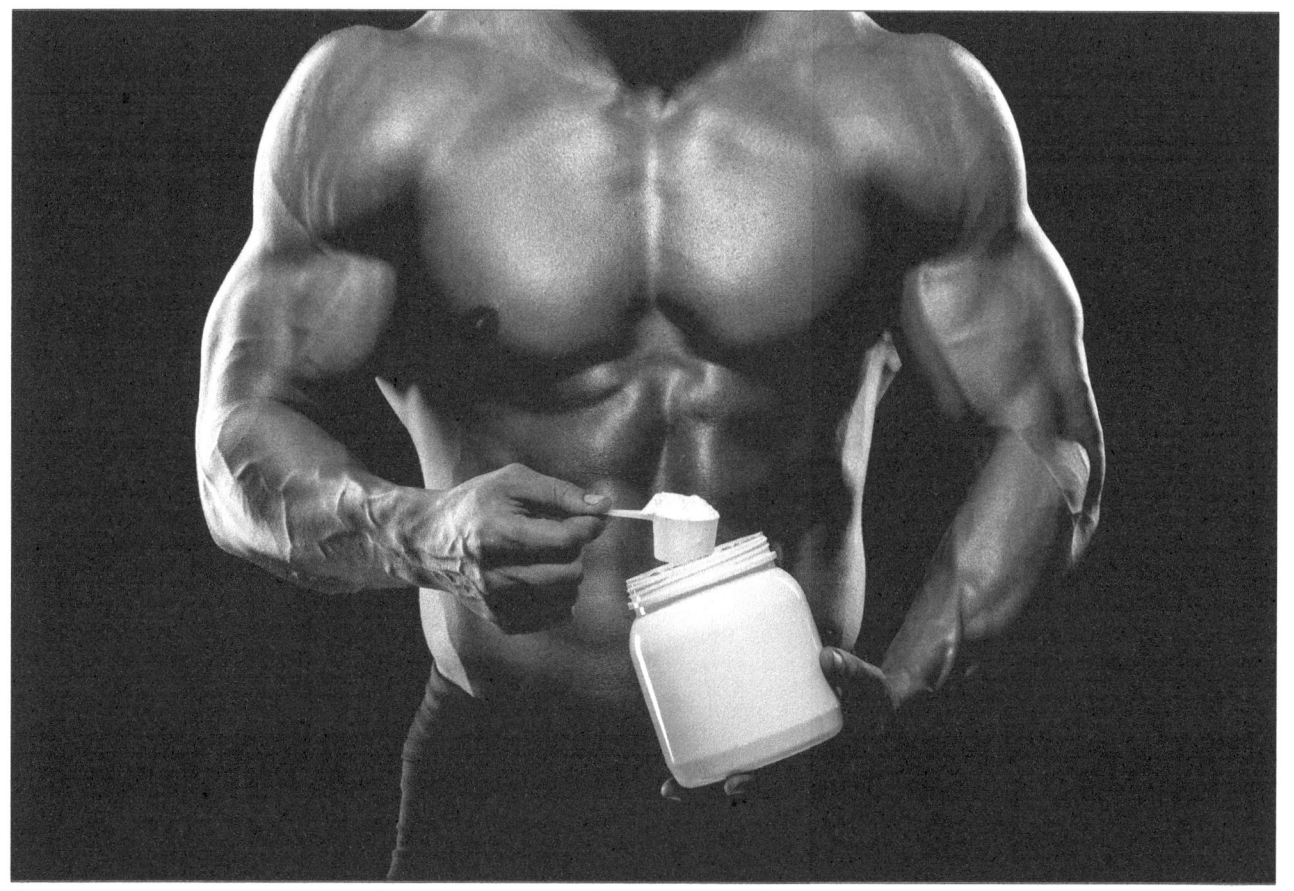

Creatine maintains a continuous supply of energy to working muscles. Photo via iStock/MRBIG_PHOTOGRAPHY. [Used under license.]

hydrate-loading. Caffeine may block the effects of creatine.

THERAPEUTIC USES
Creatine is one of the best-selling and best-documented supplements for enhancing athletic performance. Still, the scientific evidence that it works is far from complete. The best evidence points to potential benefits in forms of exercise that require repeated short-term bursts of high-intensity exercise; this has been seen more in artificial laboratory studies than in studies involving athletes during regular sports performance. It might also be helpful for resistance exercise (weight training), although not all studies have found benefits.

Creatine has also been proposed as an aid to promote weight loss and reduce the proportion of fat to muscle in the body. Still, there is little evidence that it is effective for this purpose. Preliminary evidence suggests that creatine supplements may be able to reduce levels of triglycerides in the blood. Triglycerides are fats related to cholesterol that also increase the risk of heart disease when elevated in the body. Creatine supplements might also help counter the loss of muscle strength that occurs when a limb is immobilized, such as following injury or surgery; however, not all results have been positive.

Studies, including small double-blind trials, inconsistently suggest that creatine might help reduce fatigue and increase strength in various illnesses where muscle weakness occurs, including chronic obstructive pulmonary disease (COPD), congestive heart failure, dermatomyositis, Huntington's disease, McArdle disease, mitochondrial illnesses, muscular dystrophy, and myotonic dystrophy.

One study claimed to find evidence that creatine supplements can reduce blood sugar levels. However, the results are somewhat questionable because dextrose (a form of sugar) was used as the placebo in this trial.

Evidence from animal and open human trials suggested that creatine improved strength and slowed the progression of amyotrophic lateral sclerosis (ALS). For this reason, many people with ALS tried it. However, these hopes were dashed in 2003 when a ten-month double-blind, placebo-controlled trial of 175 people with ALS was announced. The use of creatine at a dose of 10 g daily failed to benefit symptoms or disease progression. Negative results were also seen in subsequent, slightly smaller studies. Creatine also does not strengthen muscles in people with wrist weakness due to nerve injury.

Long-term use of corticosteroid drugs can slow a child's growth. One animal study suggests that supplemental creatine may help prevent this side effect. Creatine has also shown some promise for improving mental function, particularly after sleep deprivation. However, one small study showed no similar benefit in young adult subjects who were not sleep-deprived.

One study failed to find creatine helpful for maintaining muscle mass during treatment for colon cancer. Another study found little to no benefits in Parkinson's disease, and another failed to find any benefit in schizophrenia.

By 2020, several studies were conducted to analyze creatine supplementation's efficacy for reducing age-related muscle loss (sarcopenia). A meta-analysis in 2021 by dos Santos and colleagues showed that creatine supplementation reduces age-related sarcopenia. However, this same meta-analysis argued that the quality of the evidence was wanting, and larger, higher-quality studies were warranted.

SCIENTIFIC EVIDENCE
Exercise performance. Several small double-blind studies suggest that creatine can improve performance in exercises that involve repeated short bursts of high-intensity activity. For example, a double-blind study investigated creatine and swimming performance in eighteen men and fourteen women.

Compared with men taking a placebo, men taking the supplement had significant speed increases when doing six bouts of 50-meter swims starting at three-minute intervals. However, their speed did not improve when swimming ten sets of 25-yard lengths started at one-minute intervals. It may be that the shorter rest time between laps was not enough for the swimmers' bodies to resynthesize phosphocreatine.

None of the women enrolled in the study showed any improvement with the creatine supplement. The authors of this study noted that women normally have more creatine in their muscle tissue than men do, so perhaps creatine supplementation (at least at this level) is not beneficial to women as it appears to be for men. Further research is needed to understand this gender difference in response to creatine fully.

In another double-blind study, sixteen physical education students exercised ten times for six seconds on a stationary cycle, alternating with a thirty-second rest period. The results showed that individuals who took 20 g of creatine for six days were better able to maintain cycle speed. Similar results were seen in many other studies of repeated high-intensity exercise. According to some studies, isometric exercise capacity (pushing against a fixed resistance) also may improve with creatine. However, benefits are generally minimal in studies involving athletes engaged in normal sports rather than contrived laboratory tests.

In addition, two double-blind, placebo-controlled studies, each lasting twenty-eight days, provide some evidence that creatine and creatine plus beta hydroxymethyl butyrate (HMB) can increase lean muscle and bone mass. The first study enrolled fifty-two college football players during off-season training. The other followed forty athletes engaged in weight training.

However, studies of endurance or nonrepeated exercise have not shown benefits. Therefore, creatine probably will not help those running marathons or single sprints.

High triglycerides. A fifty-six-day double-blind, placebo-controlled study of thirty-four men and women found that creatine supplementation can reduce triglycerides in the blood by about 25 percent. Effects on other blood lipids such as total cholesterol were insignificant.

Congestive heart failure. Easy fatigability is one unpleasant symptom of congestive heart failure. Creatine supplementation has been used to treat this symptom, with some positive results. A double-blind study examined seventeen men with congestive heart failure given 20 g of creatine daily for ten days. Exercise capacity and muscle strength increased in the creatine-treated group. Similarly, a double-blind, placebo-controlled crossover study of twenty men with chronic heart failure improved muscle endurance. Treatment with 20 g of creatine for five days increased the amount of exercise they could complete before they reached exhaustion. These results were promising, but further study is needed.

SAFETY ISSUES

Creatine appears to be relatively safe. No significant side effects have been found with several days of a high dosage regimen followed by six weeks of a lower dosage. A study of one hundred football players found no adverse consequences during ten months to five years of creatine supplementation. However, medical professionals recommend that teens refrain from regularly using the supplement because studies have not determined the potential effect of creatine supplementation on development. It has often been observed that young adults do not follow dosage guidance. Contrary to early reports, creatine does not adversely affect the body's ability to exercise under hot conditions and might even be beneficial.

Dividing the dose may help avoid gastrointestinal side effects (diarrhea, stomach upset, and belching). In one study of fifty-nine male soccer players, administering two separate 5 g doses was associated with less diarrhea than a single 10 g dose.

However, there are some potential concerns with creatine. Because the kidneys metabolize it, fears have been expressed that creatine supplements could cause kidney injury. There are two worrisome case reports. However, evidence suggests that creatine is safe for people whose kidneys are healthy to begin with, and who do not take excessive doses. Furthermore, a one-year double-blind study of 175 people with amyotrophic lateral sclerosis found that the use of 10 g of creatine daily did not adversely affect kidney function. Nonetheless, prudence suggests that individuals with kidney disease, especially those on dialysis or people with conditions that could increase the risk of developing kidney disease, should avoid creatine supplements.

A small number of deaths have been reported in individuals taking creatine, but other causes were most likely responsible. Another concern is that creatine is metabolized to the toxic substance formaldehyde in the body. However, it is not clear whether the amount of formaldehyde produced in this way will cause any harm.

A few reports suggest that creatine could, at times, cause heart arrhythmias. It has also been suggested that oral creatine would increase urine levels of the carcinogen N-nitrososarcosine, but this does not seem to be the case. As with all supplements taken in very high doses, it is important to purchase a high-quality form of creatine because contaminants present in very low concentrations could conceivably build up and cause problems.

—*EBSCO CAM Review Board*

Further Reading

Astorino, T. A., et al. "Is Running Performance Enhanced with Creatine Serum Ingestion?" *Journal of Strength Conditioning Research*, vol. 19, 2005, pp. 730-34.

Bemben, M. G., et al. "Creatine Supplementation During Resistance Training in College Football Athletes." *Medicine and Science in Sports and Exercise*, vol. 33, 2001, pp. 1667-73.

Candow, Darren G., et al. "Variables Influencing the Effectiveness of Creatine Supplementation as a Therapeutic Intervention for Sarcopenia." *Frontiers in nutrition*, vol. 6, 2019, doi:10.3389/fnut.2019.00124. Accessed 25 June 2020.

Chilibeck, P. D., et al. "Effect of Creatine Ingestion After Exercise on Muscle Thickness in Males and Females." *Medicine and Science in Sports and Exercise*, vol. 36, 2004, pp. 1781-88.

Cramer, J. T., et al. "Effects of Creatine Supplementation and Three Days of Resistance Training on Muscle Strength, Power Output, and Neuromuscular Function." *Journal of Strength Conditioning Research*, vol. 21, 2007, pp. 668-77.

"Creatine." *MedlinePlus*, 26 Oct. 2021, medlineplus.gov/druginfo/natural/873.html.

Deacon, S. J., et al. "Randomized Controlled Trial of Dietary Creatine as an Adjunct Therapy to Physical Training in COPD." *American Journal of Respiratory and Critical Care Medicine*, vol. 178, 2008, pp. 133-39.

Eckerson, J. M., et al. "Effect of Creatine Phosphate Supplementation on Anaerobic Working Capacity and Body Weight After Two and Six Days of Loading in Men and Women." *Journal of Strength Conditioning Research*, vol. 19, 2005, pp. 756-63.

Kambis, K. W., and S. K. Pizzedaz. "Short-Term Creatine Supplementation Improves Maximum Quadriceps Contraction in Women." *International Journal of Sport Nutrition and Exercise Metabolism*, vol. 13, 2003, pp. 97-111.

Neighmond, Patti. "Is the Warning That Creatine's Not for Teens Getting Through?" *NPR*, 2 Jan. 2017, www.npr.org/sections/health-shots/2017/01/02/507478762/is-the-warning-that-creatines-not-for-teens-getting-through. Accessed 25 June 2020.

Pluim, B. M., et al. "The Effects of Creatine Supplementation on Selected Factors of Tennis Specific Training." *British Journal of Sports Medicine*, vol. 40, 2006, pp. 507-11.

Essential Nutrients

Category: Anatomy/Biology
Specialties and related fields: Dietetics, gastroenterology, nutrition
Definition: essential nutrients are those nutrients an organism cannot synthesize on its own or cannot produce in sufficient quantities; such an organism must obtain these essential nutrients from outside sources; if deprived of these essential nutrients, it cannot function properly and ultimately dies

KEY TERMS

carbohydrates: a large group of food-based organic compounds that contain hydrogen and oxygen in the same ratio as water

fats: an essential nutrient that mostly consists of triglycerides composed of three fatty acids esterified to a glycerol molecule

proteins: nitrogenous organic compounds composed of one or more long chains of amino acids

vitamin: any organic compound essential for normal growth and nutrition that cannot be synthesized by the body and is required in small dietary quantities

STRUCTURE AND FUNCTION

While specific essential nutrients vary from organism to organism, the human body requires six essential nutrients to maintain its health: water, proteins, carbohydrates, fats, vitamins, and minerals. A lack of one of these will cause a person to become ill due to malnutrition, and a severe deficiency can result in death. Because of this, it is important to understand the sources of essential nutrients to maintain good health.

In developed nations, adequate levels of essential nutrients are easily acquired through diet throughout the year. Potable water and reasonably priced sources of the macronutrients—fats, proteins, and carbohydrates—are readily available.

Fats are a significant energy source and can increase the body's absorption of fat-soluble vitamins. Fats in the form of oil, butter, and foods such as avocado, fish, and nuts are typically close at hand. Fats include the essential fatty acids: alpha-linolenic acid, an omega-3 fatty acid found in soy, rapeseed, and flax; and linolenic acid, an omega-6 fatty acid that can be found in a variety of vegetable oils.

Proteins are a vital component of all cells. They are made of chains of amino acids. They are found in relatively inexpensive and readily available foods such as eggs, nuts, meats, and soy protein. Of the twenty-one amino acids that make up proteins, nine are essential in human nutrition and cannot be synthesized.

Carbohydrates, the third class of macronutrients, are a vital energy source for the human body. People can obtain complex carbohydrates from cereals, bread, and pasta. In contrast, simple carbohydrates include a variety of sugars.

The essential micronutrients include vitamins and minerals. The thirteen essential vitamins are vitamin A, the eight B vitamins (thiamine, riboflavin, niacin, pantothenic acid, biotin, vitamin B_6, vitamin B_{12}, and folate), vitamin C, vitamin D, vitamin E, and vitamin K. Vitamins perform a variety of essential functions in the body. They are found in dark-colored fruits, dark leafy vegetables, egg yolks, fortified dairy products, whole grains, lentils, beans, fish, liver, and beef. Eating a varied diet is the best way to ensure one receives all the essential vitamins.

Minerals essential to human nutrition include sodium, potassium, calcium, magnesium, and iodine. Adequate sodium and potassium levels help maintain cell function and balance fluid volumes, while calcium is critical to bone health. Iodine is integral to the synthesis of thyroid hormone. Magnesium is critical for important physiological functions such as muscle contraction and relaxation, nerve function, vascular tone, and heart rhythm. It functions as a cofactor for over 300 enzyme-catalyzed reactions.

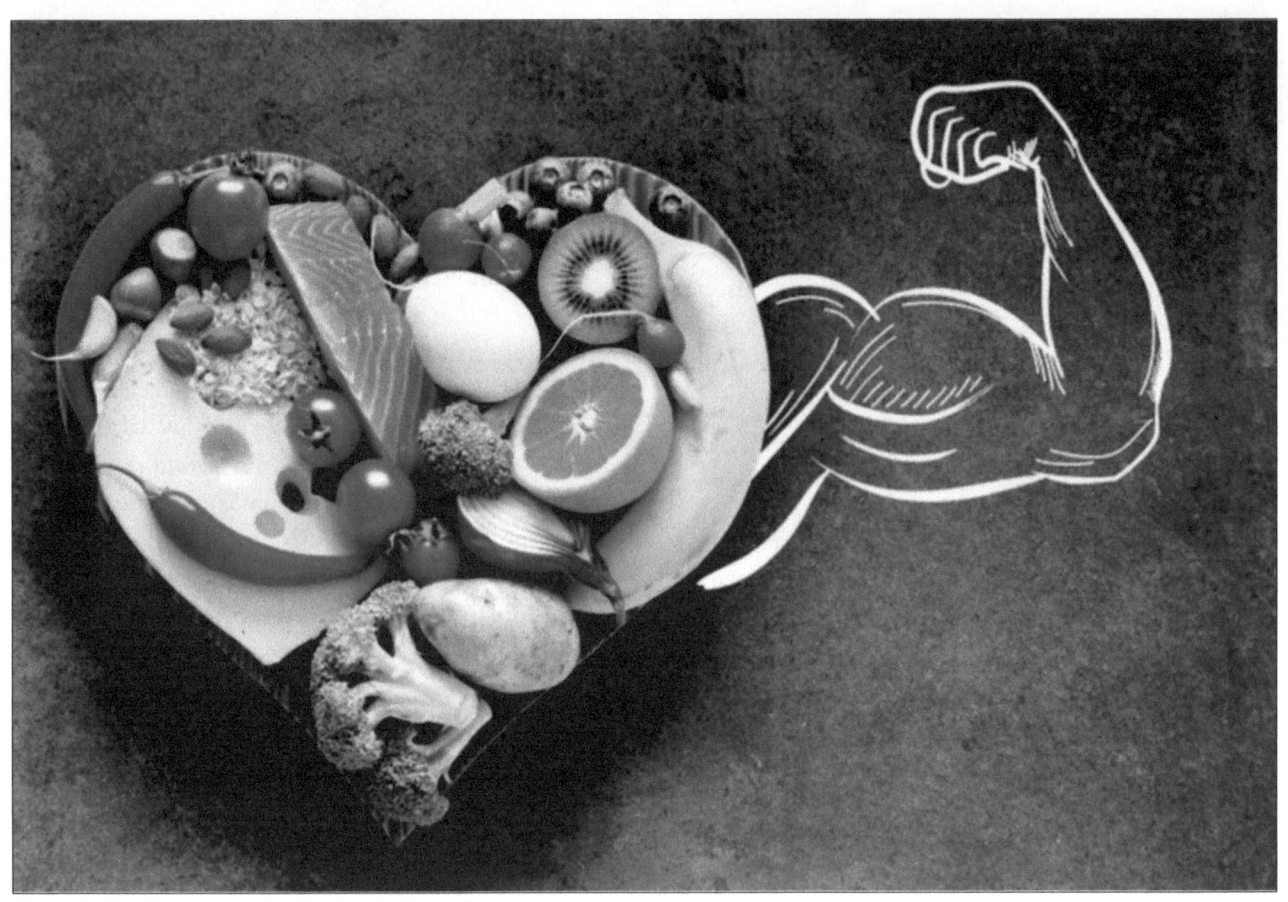

Photo via iStock/piotr_malczyk. [Used under license.]

Adequate supplies of foods containing essential nutrients effectively prevent several diseases attributed to nutritional deficiencies. All that is required is to eat a wide variety of foods or foods rich in the associated nutrients. Enriched foods and daily vitamins, for example, provide many essential nutrients. Many breakfast cereals and breads, as well as milk and salt, are enriched or fortified. However, it is important to check food labels to see what these foods have in the way of essential nutrients—and to seek sources for what is not included.

DISORDERS AND DISEASES

In some parts of the world, many people do not have access to the foods they require for a sufficient quantity of essential nutrients. When this is the case, people will be undernourished, which leads to various health problems and reduced resistance to illnesses. Adults who do not receive adequate nutrition are unlikely to have long life expectancies. Children who do not receive adequate nutrition will not reach their full physical or cognitive development potential. Infant mortality rates will also be high due to low birth weights and the effects of nutritional deficiencies; for example, folic acid deficiency is the principal cause of neural tube defects, a potentially fatal congenital disability.

Many conditions and some diseases result from a lack of essential nutrients. Insufficient quantities of iron, vitamin B6, or vitamin B_{12} result in anemia, which leads to extreme fatigue and weakness. While these are nearly unheard of in developed nations, they are serious ailments in developing nations. Some of the more well-known are rickets, beriberi, pellagra, scurvy, anemia, and goiter. Rickets results from a lack of vitamin D and causes bowed legs, weak bones, and dental deformities. Beriberi is due to insufficient thiamin intake and causes atypical muscle coordination and damage to the nerves, resulting in loss of feeling in the extremities and confusion. Pellagra results from insufficient niacin and causes dementia. Scurvy results from a lack of vitamin C and causes internal bleeding and severe problems with the teeth and gums. Goiter can arise from insufficient iodine; however, goiter due to iodine deficiency is rare in developed countries due to iodized salt. Symptoms of this disease include an enlarged thyroid gland and difficulties breathing. Each of these diseases can be prevented or reversed by adequate intake of essential nutrients.

The principal cause of nutritional deficiencies worldwide is poverty and limited access to a varied and healthy diet; however, fad diets, drug interactions, alcoholism, genetic abnormalities, or gastrointestinal problems can also lead to inadequate levels of essential nutrients in the body. The human body cannot synthesize these nutrients; without access to sources of these nutrients, people can't maintain good health. Whatever the cause of nutritional deficiencies, they take a significant toll on those affected and their countries and communities.

PERSPECTIVE AND PROSPECTS

Vegetarians (those who eat little or no meat) and vegans (those who neither eat nor use any animal products) are at risk for several deficiencies, including deficiencies in the essential amino acids lysine and methionine, riboflavin, calcium, and iron, and especially vitamin B_{12}, which is only present in animal products. Therefore, vegetarians and vegans should consider a vitamin B_{12} supplement. Vegetarian children not exposed to sunlight are at risk for vitamin D deficiencies. Since fruits and vegetables contain little zinc, and since a compound in whole grains called the "phytic acid" can sequester zinc and prevent its absorption, vegetarians and vegans can suffer from zinc deficiencies.

Women should ensure that their calcium intake is adequate to prevent osteoporosis. According to the National Academy of Sciences, the recommended calcium intake for women at risk for osteoporosis is 1,000 micrograms (mg) for women ages nineteen to fifty and 1,200 mg for those ages fifty to seventy. Regular consumption of dairy products can achieve such dietary calcium levels.

Vitamin D intake has generated some attention since many people who live and work indoors neither experience sufficient exposure to the sun (which helps the body synthesize vitamin D) nor get adequate quantities of vitamin D from food. Consumer Reports on Health in 2009 recommended a daily intake of 800-1,200 international units (IU) of vitamin D, and some people may benefit from a vitamin D supplement of 400-800 IU.

In 2015, the sale of dietary supplements in the US generated approximately $37 billion. Dietary supplements are recommended for very young children until they begin eating solid food and for people recovering from surgery or serious illness, pregnant women, and older adults who fail to eat properly. However, for the remaining population, dietary supplements are neither recommended nor necessary. High doses of vitamins above the Recommended Daily Allowance (RDA) do little good except waste money. While situations exist in which above-RDA dosages of vitamins can be beneficial, such vitamin dosages should be taken under medical supervision. The best way to get adequate vitamins and minerals is from foods in a balanced diet.

—*Gina Hagler, Michael A. Buratovich*

Further Reading

Barrett, Stephen, et al. *Consumer Health: A Guide to Intelligent Decisions*. 9th ed., McGraw-Hill Education, 2012.

Insel, Paul, et al. *Nutrition*. 6th ed., Jones, 2016.

Mann, Jim, and A. S. Truswell. *Essentials of Human Nutrition*. Oxford UP, 2012.

Nelms, Marcia, and Kathryn P. Sucher. *Nutrition Therapy and Pathophysiology*. 3rd ed., Brooks Cole, 2015.

Smolin, Lori A., and Mary B. Grosvenor. *Nutrition: Science and Applications*. 3rd ed., Wiley, 2013.

Thompson, Janice J., and Melinda Manore. *Nutrition: An Applied Approach*. 5th ed., Pearson, 2017.

"Vitamins and Minerals." *Centers for Disease Control and Prevention*, 11 Apr. 2022, www.cdc.gov/nutrition/infantandtoddlernutrition/vitamins-minerals/index.html. Accessed 8 June 2022.

Fatty Acid

Category: Biology
Specialties and related fields: Biochemistry, metabolism
Definition: carboxylic acids that contain long aliphatic hydrocarbon chains that serve as an energy source, structural compounds primarily in membranes, and precursors for other important biologically active compounds

KEY TERMS

α-linolenic acid (ALA): an essential fatty acid (EFA) from which EPA and DHA are synthesized

docosapentaenoic acid (DHA): an omega-3 fatty acid with 22 carbons and six carbon-carbon double bonds

eicosapentaenoic acid (EPA): an omega-3 fatty acid with 20 carbons and five carbon-carbon double bonds

essential fatty acid (EFA): a fatty acid that humans cannot synthesize

γ-linolenic acid (GLA): an essential fatty acid from which other fatty acids are synthesized

leukotriene: fatty acid-derived compounds that mediate inflammation and cause constriction of the bronchioles

nonsteroidal anti-inflammatory drugs (NSAIDs): compounds that inhibit the synthesis of prostaglandins and thromboxanes

omega-3 (ω-3 or n-3) fatty acid: unsaturated fatty acids with a carbon-carbon double bond, three carbons from the methyl end of the hydrocarbon chain

prostacyclin: a fatty acid-derived compound that inhibits platelet aggregation and blood clotting and acts as a vasodilator

prostaglandins: fatty acid-derived compounds that inhibit platelet aggregation and blood clotting, act as vasodilators, mediate inflammation and increase the perception of pain

saturated fatty acid: a fatty acid with no carbon-carbon double bonds

trans-fatty acid: a fatty acid with at least one carbon-carbon double bond where the hydrogens attached to the carbons that participate in the double bond are on opposite sides of the double bond

thromboxane: fatty acid-derived compounds that are vasodilators and promote platelet aggregation and blood clotting

unsaturated fatty acid: a fatty acid with at least one carbon-carbon double bond

STRUCTURE AND FUNCTIONS

A fatty acid is a carboxylic acid with a long aliphatic hydrocarbon chain. Fatty acids serve as cellular energy sources, cellular structural components, especially within membranes, and precursors for other important biological compounds such as the eicosanoids prostaglandins, thromboxanes, prostacyclins, and leukotrienes.

Naturally occurring fatty acids are usually found esterified to glycerol to form glycerides. Mono-, di- and triglycerides have one, two, and three fatty acids esterified to glycerol, respectively. Fatty acids found in nature usually have an even number of carbon atoms numbering as high as 24 or more. However, 16 and 18 are the most common. From shortest to longest, fatty acids are often grouped as short-chain fatty acids (with fewer than six carbon atoms, such as butyric acid, the fatty acid that provides the unpleasant smell of both human vomit and rancid dairy products), medium-chain fatty acids (with 6-12 carbons, often found as part of medium-chain triglycerides), long-chain fatty acids (13-21 carbons), or very-long-chain fatty acids (22 or more carbons). The carbon atoms are numbered from the carboxyl group (carbon 1) to the methyl (-CH3) end. Fatty acids are saturated if they have no carbon-carbon double bonds and unsaturated if they have no carbon-carbon double bonds.

Palmitic and stearic acids are examples of naturally-occurring 16-carbon and 18-carbon saturated fatty acids, respectively. Mono- and di-unsaturated fatty acids have one and two carbon-carbon double bonds, respectively. Palmitoleic and oleic acids are examples of naturally occurring 16-carbon and 18-carbon monounsaturated fatty acids. Polyunsaturated fatty acids have three or more carbon-carbon double bonds. Omega-3 (ω-3 or υ-3) fatty acids such as linolenic acid have a double bond three carbons from the noncarboxyl end of the amino acid (Omega is the last letter of the Greek alphabet). Double bonds can be either in the cis position, where the hydrogen atoms on either side of the double bond are on the same side of the hydrocarbon chain, or in the trans position, where the hydrogen atoms are on opposite sides of the chain. Trans fatty acids have at least one double bond. A cis double bond bends the hydrocarbon chain about 45 degrees. At room temperature, medium and long-chain saturated fatty acids such as those found in palm and coconut oil, which can contain up to 48 percent saturated fatty acids, are solid. In contrast, unsaturated fatty acids of the same length, such as those found in peanut, corn, and canola oils containing nearly 90 percent unsaturated fatty acids, are liquid.

Humans can catabolize all fatty acids normally consumed in the diet. The process, called "β-oxidation," occurs in the mitochondria of the liver and completely metabolizes the hydrocarbon chain to energy (ATP), carbon dioxide, and water. The carbon atoms derived from fatty acids cannot be used to synthesize glucose or other sugars. Most fatty acids required by humans can easily be synthesized from any two-carbon source. Such two-carbon sources are usually derived from glucose metabolism. Fatty acid synthesis occurs in the cytoplasm by a multi-subunit enzyme complex called "fatty acid synthase," whose main product is the 16-carbon saturated palmitic acid. Longer chains can be synthesized by adding two-carbon units to the carboxyl end of the fatty acid. Animals can place double bonds in the hydrocarbon chain, but not beyond carbon 9. Thus, α-linoleic acid, with double bonds at carbons 9 and 12, α-linolenic acid (ALA), double bonds at carbons 9, 12, and 15, and γ-linolenic acid (GLA) with double bonds at carbons 6, 9, and 12 are essential fatty acids (EFAs). People must acquire these fatty acids by consuming plants since plants can synthesize fatty acids that contain double bonds beyond carbon 9. Many longer-chain fatty acids required by humans can be synthesized from linolenic and linoleic acids via elongation and desaturation. Eicosapentaenoic acid (EPA), an omega-3 fatty acid with 20 carbons and five double bonds, and docosahexaenoic acid (DHA), a 22-carbon fatty acid with six double bonds, can be synthesized from linolenic acid and arachidonic acid (ARA), a 20-carbon nonessential fatty acid with four double bonds, but not fast enough and in quantities sufficient enough for fetuses and infants where DHA is utilized for retinal and neuronal development. Both EPA and DHA are found in marine food sources like phytoplankton, algae, and oily fish that have consumed phytoplankton and algae. Although human breast milk contains ARA, EPA, and DHA, the concentrations vary and largely depend on the mother's diet. ARA and DHA were first introduced into infant formula in Europe. They were introduced into infant formula in the United States in 2002.

Important biological compounds synthesized from fatty acid precursors are eicosanoids, including prostaglandins, thromboxanes, and leukotrienes. Prostaglandins inhibit platelet aggregation and blood clotting, act as vasodilators, mediate inflammation, and increase pain perception. Thromboxanes are vasodilators and promote platelet aggregation and blood clotting. Aspirin and other nonsteroidal anti-inflammatory drugs (NSAIDs) inhibit the synthesis of prostaglandins and thromboxanes and are often prescribed to prevent heart attacks and reduce inflammation and pain. Thromboxane receptor agonists can also inhibit the function of thromboxanes. Leukotrienes mediate inflammation and cause constriction of the bronchioles. Inhibitors of leukotriene receptors, such as montelukast (Singulair), are often prescribed to treat asthma.

Fatty acids are usually consumed as triglycerides emulsified by bile and digested in the small intestine by lipases that cleave the triglycerides into fatty acids, glycerides, and glycerol. The fatty acids, glycerides, and glycerol are absorbed into the intestinal mucosa. Short- and medium-chain fatty acids are transported via the blood bound to a blood protein called "albumin." Long-chain fatty acids are resynthesized into triglycerides in the intestinal mucosae and transported to the liver through the lymphatic system via lipoprotein particles called "chylomicrons." Fatty acids can immediately be used as an energy source or stored as triglycerides in various tissues. Several genetic diseases of fatty acid metabolism are known.

DISORDERS AND DISEASES

The most common disease of fatty acids is EFA deficiency which can lead to various symptoms, including inflammatory conditions such as arthritis, hypertension, immune disorders, mental disorders, eczema, atherosclerosis, and diabetes. Many of the symptoms of EFA deficiency can be improved with the administration or consumption of EFAs.

Several studies have concluded that a diet high in ω-3 fatty acids such as EPA and DHA derived from oily fish positively affect cardiovascular health by preventing stroke by reducing blood triglycerides, blood pressure, and blood clotting. EPA and DHA may compete with precursors to thromboxane synthesis and reduce the level of thromboxanes involved with blood clotting that may lead to stroke. However, large systematic literature reviews have failed to establish that dietary supplementation with fish oil significantly decreases the risk for death, cancer, stroke, or heart disease. More work remains to be done. EPA, DHA, and GLA can be converted to eicosanoid compounds that inhibit the inflammatory response and are modestly effective in treating rheumatoid arthritis.

—Charles Vigue, Bill Kte'pi

Further Reading

Abad-Jorge, Ana. "The Role of DHA and ARA in Infant Nutrition and Neurodevelopmental Outcomes." *Today's Dietitian*, vol. 10, no. 10, 2008, p. 66.

Ahmad, Moghis U., editor. *Fatty Acids: Chemistry, Synthesis, and Applications*. Academic Press and ACCS Press, 2017.

Lawrence, Glen D. *The Fats of Life: Essential Fatty Acids in Health and Disease*. Rutgers UP, 2010.

McColl. Janice. "An Introduction to Essential Fatty Acids in Health and Nutrition." *Bioriginal Food & Science Corporation*, 2017, www.bioriginal.com/page-articles/an-introduction-to-essential-fatty-acids-in-health-and-nutrition.

Ridgeway, Neale, and Roger McLeod, editors. *Biochemistry of Lipids, Lipoproteins, and Membranes*. Elsevier, 2015.

Today's Dietitian, www.todaysdietitian.com/newarchives/092208p66.shtml.

Valentine, Raymond C., and David L. Valentine. *Human Longevity: Omega-3 Fatty Acids, Bioenergetics, Molecular Biology, and Evolution*. CRC Press, 2015.

Watson, Ronald Ross, and Fabien De Meester, editors. *Handbook of Lipids in Human Function: Fatty Acids*. Academic Press and ACCS Press, 2015.

———. *Omega-3 Fatty Acids in Brain and Neurological Health*. Academic, 2014.

GLUCOSAMINE

Category: Herbs and supplements
Specialties and related fields: Alternative and complementary medicine, athletic training, orthopedics, personal trainer, sports medicine, strength, and conditioning
Definition: natural substance of the human body used as a supplement to treat osteoarthritis and related conditions

KEY TERMS

cartilage: the firm, whitish, flexible connective tissue found in various forms in the larynx and respiratory tract, in structures such as the external ear, and the articulating surfaces of joints; it is more widespread in the infant skeleton, replaced by bone during growth

chondrocytes: specialized cells that secrete cartilage matrix, eventually becoming embedded in it

osteoarthritis: degeneration of joint cartilage and the underlying bone, most common from middle age onward; it causes pain and stiffness, especially in the hip, knee, and thumb joints

OVERVIEW

Glucosamine, most commonly used in the form of glucosamine sulfate, is a simple molecule derived from glucose, the principal sugar found in the blood. In glucosamine, one oxygen atom in glucose is replaced by a nitrogen atom. The chemical term for this modified form of glucose is an amino sugar. Glucosamine is produced naturally in the body, where it is a key building block for making cartilage.

REQUIREMENTS AND SOURCES

There is no US Dietary Reference Intake for glucosamine. One's body makes all the glucosamine it needs from building blocks found in foods. Glucosamine is not usually obtained directly from food. Glucosamine supplements are derived from chitin, a substance found in the shells of shrimp, lobsters, and crabs.

THERAPEUTIC DOSAGES

Osteoarthritis is a disease in which cartilage in joints becomes stiffer and may wear away. Glucosamine is used to treat this condition. A typical dosage of glucosamine is 500 milligrams (mg) three times daily. A 1,500-mg dose taken once daily is another option.

Glucosamine is available in three forms: glucosamine sulfate, glucosamine hydrochloride, and N-acetyl glucosamine. All three forms are sold as tablets or capsules. There is some dispute over which form is best. One study provides some evidence that glucosamine hydrochloride and glucosamine sulfate are equally effective. Glucosamine is often sold in combination with chondroitin. It is not known whether this combination treatment is better than glucosamine alone. However, animal studies suggest that this may be the case.

THERAPEUTIC USES

Glucosamine is widely accepted as a treatment for osteoarthritis. However, the current evidence from

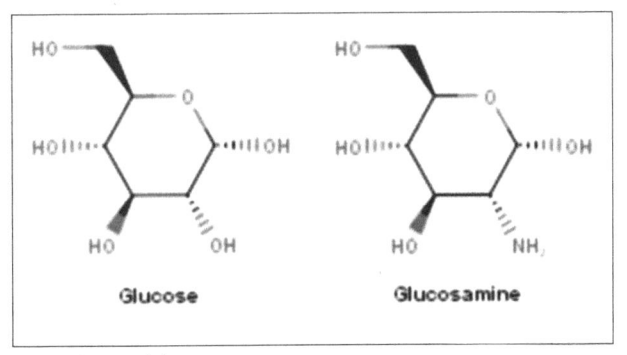

By M. Buratovich.

double-blind studies is highly inconsistent, with many of the most recent and best-designed studies failing to find significant benefits. According to the positive studies, glucosamine acts more slowly than conventional treatments, such as ibuprofen, but eventually produces approximately equivalent benefits. In addition, unlike conventional treatments, glucosamine might also help prevent progressive joint damage, thereby slowing the course of the disease. However, these potential benefits remain controversial in light of the most recent trials. Glucosamine has also shown some promise for osteochondritis of the knee, a cartilage disease related to osteoarthritis.

Some athletes use glucosamine in the (unproven) belief that it can prevent muscle and tendon injuries. It has also been suggested as a treatment for tendonitis. However, there is no meaningful scientific evidence to support these potential uses. Exercise can also produce short-term muscle soreness. In one study, glucosamine supplementation failed to prove effective in reducing this type of pain, increasing it. However, one study found somewhat inconsistent evidence hinting that glucosamine might aid recovery from acute knee injuries experienced by competitive athletes.

Glucosamine might also be helpful for rheumatoid arthritis, according to a double-blind, placebo-controlled study of fifty-one people. In this study, glucosamine at a dose of 1,500 mg daily significantly improved symptoms. However, it did not alter measures of inflammation as determined through blood tests.

SCIENTIFIC EVIDENCE
Relieving osteoarthritis symptoms. Inconsistent evidence suggests that glucosamine supplements might relieve pain and other symptoms of osteoarthritis. Two types of studies have been performed, those that compared glucosamine against placebo and those that compared it against standard medications.

In the placebo-controlled category, one of the best trials was a three-year, double-blind study of 212 people with knee osteoarthritis. Participants receiving glucosamine showed reduced symptoms compared with those receiving placebo. Benefits were also seen in other double-blind, placebo-controlled studies, enrolling more than a thousand people and ranging in length from four weeks to three years.

Other double-blind studies, enrolling more than four hundred people, compared glucosamine against ibuprofen. These studies found glucosamine and the drug equally effective. Furthermore, one of the placebo-controlled trials noted above (only reported in abstract form) also included people given the drug piroxicam and again found equivalent benefits.

However, most recent studies have been less promising. In four studies involving about five hundred people, glucosamine supplementation failed to improve symptoms significantly. The list goes on. In a study involving 222 participants with hip osteoarthritis, two years of treatment with glucosamine was no better than a placebo for pain, function, or X-ray findings. Another trial involving 147 women with osteoarthritis found glucosamine to be no more effective than home exercises over eighteen months.

In a double-blind trial, researchers evaluated the effects of stopping glucosamine after taking it for six months. This study enrolled 137 people with osteoarthritis of the knee and found that participants who stopped using glucosamine (and, unbeknownst to them, took a placebo instead) did no worse than people who stayed on glucosamine.

In another very large (1,583-participant) study, neither glucosamine (as glucosamine hydrochloride) nor glucosamine plus chondroitin was more effective than a placebo. Another trial failed to observe the benefits of glucosamine plus chondroitin. Finally, in a systematic review including ten randomized trials involving 3,803 patients with osteoarthritis of the hip or knee, researchers found that glucosamine alone or with chondroitin did not improve pain.

Most of the positive studies were funded by manufacturers of glucosamine products, and most of the studies performed by neutral researchers failed to find benefits.

Many popular glucosamine products combine this supplement with methylsulfonylmethane (MSM). One study published in India reported that both MSM and glucosamine improved arthritis symptoms compared with a placebo. MSM and glucosamine were even more effective than either supplement separately. However, India has not achieved a reputation for conducting reliable medical trials.

Slowing the course of osteoarthritis. Conventional treatments for osteoarthritis reduce the symptoms but do not slow the progress of the disease. Nonsteroidal anti-inflammatory drugs, such as indomethacin, might speed the progression of osteoarthritis by interfering with cartilage repair and promoting cartilage destruction (though the evidence for this is weak). In contrast, two studies reported that glucosamine might slow the progression of osteoarthritis.

LONG-TERM GLUCOSAMINE STUDY

New data from a long-term study of the dietary supplements glucosamine and chondroitin for treating knee osteoarthritis pain reveal that persons who took the supplements (alone or in combination) had outcomes similar to those experienced by persons who took celecoxib (Celebrex) or placebo pills. Earlier studies examined the effects of glucosamine and chondroitin on pain associated with knee osteoarthritis over a short duration—twenty-four weeks. This study, part of the Glucosamine/Chondroitin Arthritis Intervention Trial (GAIT), funded by the National Center for Complementary and Alternative Medicine and the National Institute of Arthritis and Musculoskeletal and Skin Diseases, was the first to assess the safety and effectiveness of the supplements over two years.

The study enrolled 662 GAIT participants with moderate-to-severe knee osteoarthritis who received either glucosamine (500 milligrams [mg] three times daily), chondroitin sulfate (400 mg three times daily), glucosamine and chondroitin sulfate combined (same doses), Celebrex (celecoxib; 200 mg once daily), or placebo. The study's primary outcome measure was a 20 percent reduction in pain scores (using the Western Ontario and McMaster Universities Osteoarthritis [WOMAC] pain scale).

All treatment groups experienced an improvement in pain and function over the two-year study period, with clinically detectable improvements seen as early as twenty-four weeks in all groups. However, none of the treatments was significantly better than the placebo. The odds of obtaining a 20 percent decline on the WOMAC scale when taking Celebrex were 1.2 times greater than that of obtaining this decline when taking a placebo. Likewise, the odds of obtaining a 20 percent decline for glucosamine alone, glucosamine and chondroitin sulfate combined, and chondroitin sulfate alone were 1.16, 0.83, and 0.69 times that for placebo, respectively. There were no statistically significant differences among the four treatment groups. Adverse reactions were mild and occurred among all treatment groups, and serious adverse events were rare.

The researchers noted that findings from their study provide important longer-term safety information on the use of glucosamine and chondroitin and the use of Celebrex, adding to the existing scientific literature on treatments people use for pain associated with osteoarthritis of the knee. Researchers also pointed out that their study data were obtained with dosages typically used to treat knee osteoarthritis.

A three-year, double-blind, placebo-controlled study of 212 people found indications that glucosamine may protect joints from further damage. Throughout the study, individuals given glucosamine showed some actual improvement in pain and mobility, while those given placeboes worsened steadily. Perhaps even more important, X-rays showed that glucosamine treatment prevented progressive damage to the knee joint. Another large, three-year study enrolling 202 people found similar results. Furthermore, a follow-up analysis, done five years after the conclusion of these two studies, found suggestive evidence that the use of glucosamine reduced the need for knee-replacement surgery.

Like the positive studies of glucosamine for reducing symptoms, all these studies were funded by a major glucosamine manufacturer.

Relieving knee pain due to osteochondritis. A twelve-week, double-blind, placebo-controlled study examined the effectiveness of glucosamine at 2,000 mg daily in fifty people with continuing knee pain, mostly caused by osteochondritis (damage to the articular cartilage of the knee) rather than osteoarthritis. The results were somewhat equivocal but indicated that glucosamine could improve symptoms. Some participants may have also had osteoarthritis, so the results of this study are a bit difficult to interpret.

SAFETY ISSUES

Glucosamine appears to be a generally safe treatment and has not been associated with significant side effects. A few case reports and animal studies raised concerns that glucosamine might raise blood sugar in people with diabetes. Still, subsequent studies have tended to lay these concerns to rest. Glucosamine does not appear to affect cholesterol levels either. There is one case report of an allergic reaction to a glucosamine/chondroitin product, causing exacerbation of asthma.

—*EBSCO CAM Review Board*

Further Reading

Arendt-Nielsen, L., et al. "A Double-Blind Randomized Placebo-Controlled Parallel Group Study Evaluating the Effects of Ibuprofen and Glucosamine Sulfate on Exercise-Induced Muscle Soreness." *Journal of Musculoskeletal Pain*, vol. 15, 2007, pp. 21-28.

Herrero-Beaumont, G., et al. "Glucosamine Sulfate in the Treatment of Knee Osteoarthritis Symptoms: A Randomized, Double-Blind, Placebo-Controlled Study Using Acetaminophen as a Side Comparator." *Arthritis and Rheumatism*, vol. 56, no. 2, 2007, pp. 555-67.

Kawasaki, T., et al. "Additive Effects of Glucosamine or Risedronate for the Treatment of Osteoarthritis of the Knee Combined with Home Exercise." *Journal of Bone and Mineral Metabolism*, vol. 26, 2008, pp. 279-87.

Ostojic, S. M., et al. "Glucosamine Administration in Athletes: Effects on Recovery of Acute Knee Injury." *Research in Sports Medicine*, vol. 15, 2007, pp. 113-24.

Rozendaal, R. M., et al. "Effect of Glucosamine Sulfate on Hip Osteoarthritis." *Annals of Internal Medicine*, vol. 148, 2008, pp. 268-77.

Usha, P. R., and M. U. Naidu. "Randomised, Double-Blind, Parallel, Placebo-Controlled Study of Oral Glucosamine, Methylsulfonylmethane, and Their Combination in Osteoarthritis." *Clinical Drug Investigation*, vol. 24, 2004, pp. 353-63.

IRON

Category: Supplements
Specialties and related fields: Dietetics, hematology, nutrition, obstetrics and gynecology, sports medicine
Related terms: Chelated iron, iron sulfate
Definition: natural substance of the human body used as a supplement to treat specific health conditions

KEY TERMS

anemia: a condition in which the body lacks enough healthy red blood cells to carry adequate oxygen to its tissues *ferritin*: a protein produced by mammalian cells that stores iron

hemoglobin: the iron-containing oxygen-transport metalloprotein in red blood cells of almost all vertebrates as well as the tissues of some invertebrates that carries oxygen from the respiratory organs to the rest of the body

iron-deficiency anemia: too few healthy red blood cells resulting from insufficient bodily iron levels

menstruation: the process in a woman of discharging blood and other materials from the lining of the uterus at intervals of about one lunar month from puberty until menopause, except during pregnancy

recommended daily allowance: average daily level of intake sufficient to meet the nutrient requirements of nearly all (97 to 98 percent) healthy people

INTRODUCTION

The element iron is essential to human life. As part of hemoglobin, the oxygen-carrying protein found in red blood cells, iron is integral in furnishing every cell in the body with oxygen. It also functions as a part of myoglobin, which helps muscle cells store oxygen. Without iron, the body could not make adenosine triphosphate (ATP, the body's primary energy source), produce deoxyribonucleic acid (DNA), or carry out many other critical processes.

Iron deficiency can lead to anemia, learning disabilities, impaired immune function, fatigue, and depression. However, individuals should not take iron supplements unless laboratory tests show they are genuinely deficient in iron.

REQUIREMENTS AND SOURCES

The official US recommendations (in milligrams [mg]) for daily intake of iron are as follows:

Infants to six months of age (0.27) and seven to twelve months (11); children one to three years (7) and four to eight years (10); males nine to thirteen years (8) and nineteen years and older (8); females nine to thirteen years (8), fourteen to eighteen years (15), nineteen to fifty years (18), and fifty years and older (9); pregnant women (27); and nursing women (9; 10 milligrams if age eighteen years or younger).

Iron deficiency is the most common nutrient deficiency in the world; worldwide, at least 700 million individuals have iron-deficiency anemia. Iron deficiency is widespread in the developing world, and it is prevalent in developed countries as well. Groups at high risk are children, teenage girls, menstruating women (especially those with excessively heavy menstruation, known as "menorrhagia"), pregnant women, and the elderly.

There are two major forms of iron: heme iron and non-heme iron. Heme iron is bound to the proteins hemoglobin or myoglobin, whereas non-heme iron is an inorganic compound. In chemistry, "organic" has a precise meaning that has nothing to do with farming. An organic compound contains carbon atoms. Thus, "inorganic iron" is an iron compound containing no carbon. Heme iron, obtained from red meats and fish, is easily absorbed by the body. Non-heme iron, usually derived from plants, is less easily absorbed.

Rich sources of heme iron include oysters, meat, poultry, and fish. The main sources of non-heme

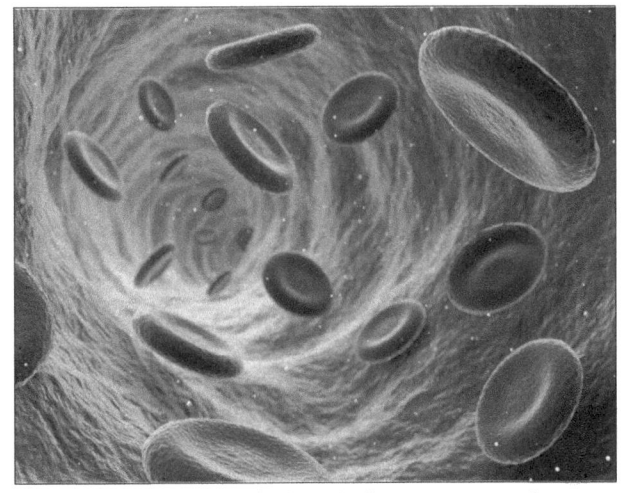

Iron is an important part of red blood cells. Image via iStock/ExperienceInteriors. [Used under license.]

iron are dried fruits, molasses, whole grains, legumes, leafy green vegetables, nuts, seeds, and kelp. Contrary to popular belief, no meaningful evidence exists that cooking in an iron skillet or pot provides a meaningful amount of iron supplementation.

Iron absorption may be affected by antibiotics in the quinolone (Floxin, Cipro) or tetracycline families, levodopa, methyldopa, carbidopa, penicillamine, thyroid hormone, captopril (and possibly other angiotensin-converting enzyme [ACE] inhibitors), calcium, soy, zinc, copper, manganese, or multivitamin/multimineral tablets. Conversely, iron may also inhibit the absorption of these drugs and supplements. In addition, drugs in the H2 blocker or proton pump inhibitor families may impair iron absorption.

THERAPEUTIC DOSAGES

The typical short-term therapeutic dosage to correct iron deficiency is 100 to 200 mg daily. Once the body's stores of iron reach normal levels, the patient should reduce this dose to the lowest level to maintain iron balance.

THERAPEUTIC USES

The most obvious use of iron supplements is to treat iron deficiency. Severe iron deficiency causes anemia, which in turn causes many symptoms. An iron deficiency that is too slight to cause anemia may also impair health. Several, though not all, double-blind trials suggest that mild iron deficiency might impair sports performance. In addition, a double-blind, placebo-controlled study of 144 women with unexplained fatigue who also had low or borderline-low levels of ferritin (a measure of stored iron) found that iron supplements enhanced energy and well-being. Another study found that iron supplements improved mental function in iron-deficient women. However, individuals should not take iron just because they feel tired; they should make sure to get tested to see whether they are indeed deficient. With iron, more is not better.

Excessively heavy menstruation (menorrhagia) can cause iron loss and may warrant iron supplements. Interestingly, a small double-blind trial found evidence that iron supplements might help reduce menstrual bleeding in women with menorrhagia who are also iron-deficient.

A study of seventy-one human-immunodeficiency-virus-positive (HIV-positive) children noted a high rate of iron deficiency. One observational study of 296 men with HIV infection linked a high iron intake to a decreased risk of acquired immunodeficiency syndrome (AIDS) six years later.

Individuals taking drugs in the ACE inhibitor family frequently develop a dry cough as a side effect. One study suggests that iron supplementation can alleviate this symptom. However, iron can interfere with ACE inhibitor absorption, so patients should take it at a different time of day.

Pregnant women commonly develop iron deficiency anemia. One study found evidence that a fairly low supplemental dose of iron (20 mg daily) is nearly as effective for treating anemia during pregnancy as 40 mg or even 80 mg daily and is less likely to cause gastrointestinal side effects. Iron supplements, however, can be hard on the stomach, thereby aggravating morning sickness.

Iron has been suggested as a treatment for attention deficit disorder. However, there is only preliminary evidence that it may be effective in hyperactive children with low iron levels, as indicated by ferritin levels.

Preliminary studies have linked low iron levels to restless legs syndrome. However, a small double-blind study found no benefit when researchers gave iron supplements to healthy people, that is, those who were not iron-deficient. In addition, one study tested whether supplemental iron could increase the saliva flow rate but failed to find benefits.

SCIENTIFIC EVIDENCE

Sports performance. A double-blind, placebo-controlled trial of forty-two women without anemia but with evidence of slightly low iron reserves found that iron supplements significantly enhanced sports performance. Participants were put on a daily aerobic training program for the last four weeks of this six-week trial. At the end of the trial, those receiving iron showed significantly greater gains in speed and endurance than those given placebo. In addition, a double-blind, placebo-controlled study of forty elite athletes without anemia but with mildly low iron stores found that twelve weeks of iron supplementation enhanced aerobic performance.

Benefits of iron supplementation were observed in other double-blind trials involving mild cases of low iron stores. However, other studies failed to find significant improvements, suggesting that the benefits of iron supplements for nonanemic, iron-deficient athletes are small at most.

Menorrhagia. One small double-blind study found good results using iron supplements to treat heavy menstruation. This study, performed in 1964, saw an improvement in 75 percent of the women who took iron, compared to 32.5 percent of those who took a placebo. Women who began with higher iron levels did not respond to treatment. These results suggest that supplementing with iron is a good idea only if an individual is deficient in it.

SAFETY ISSUES

Iron supplements commonly cause gastrointestinal upset, but when taken at recom-

IRON AND MENTAL FUNCTION

The element iron is essential to human life. Iron is an integral part of hemoglobin, the oxygen-carrying protein in red blood cells. Marked iron deficiency causes a reduction in red cell size and hemoglobin content known as "iron-deficiency anemia"; this, in turn, causes fatigue, depression, reduced immunity, impaired mental function, and many other symptoms. Iron-deficiency anemia, caused by malnutrition, is a common problem in developing countries, especially among children. In the United States, however, deficiency occurs most commonly in menstruating girls and women because of cyclical blood loss.

The famous "iron-poor blood" advertisements of the 1950s and 1960s popularized the notion that most women could benefit from iron supplements. However, this idea still lacks widespread acceptance. According to conventional medical wisdom, iron deficiency does not cause symptoms until it reaches the point of causing anemia. In addition, during the 1980s and 1990s, a theory was developed claiming that excess iron can increase the risk of heart disease and strokes. The value of iron supplements for women without iron-deficiency anemia is, therefore, quite controversial.

The situation has begun to change in recent years. The theory that excess iron is associated with increased heart attack has begun to lose ground. At the same time, a growing body of evidence suggests that marginal iron deficiency does indeed cause problems.

The human body stores iron in the form of ferritin. Evidence indicates that nonanemic women with low ferritin levels may feel somewhat tired and that iron supplementation might increase their energy and physical performance. Furthermore, a study published in 2007 suggests that iron supplements may improve mental function in nonanemic women with low ferritin. Thus, the "iron-poor blood" advertisements have been partially vindicated.

This study evaluated 149 women with varying levels of stored iron, ranging from adequate iron through mild deficiency to true iron-deficiency anemia. All participants were given either iron supplements or a placebo for sixteen weeks.

At the study's beginning, mental function tests showed a direct relationship between iron status and brain function. On average, participants with anemia performed poorly on these tests. In contrast, participants with mild iron deficiency performed in the middle, and those with adequate iron did the best. By the end of the study, performance improved markedly among those who showed an increase in iron stores. In other words, those who were deficient in iron (whether anemic or not) benefited more from iron supplements than from placebo. However, those who were not deficient did not show improvement.

One should not take iron supplements unless lab tests show that one is genuinely deficient. However, one should also check measures of iron storage (such as ferritin) because even mild iron deficiency may impair physical and mental function, though too mild to cause anemia.

—*Steven Bratman, MD*

mended dosages, serious adverse consequences are unlikely. However, excessive dosages of iron can be toxic, damaging the intestines and liver and possibly resulting in death. Iron poisoning in children is a common problem, so parents and grandparents should keep iron supplements out of the reach of children.

Mildly excessive levels of iron may be unhealthy for another reason: Iron acts as an oxidant (the opposite of an antioxidant), perhaps increasing the risk of cancer and heart disease (although this is controversial). Elevated levels of iron may also play a role in brain injury caused by stroke. In addition, excess iron appears to increase pregnancy complications. Suppose breast-fed infants who are not iron-deficient are given iron supplements. In that case, the effects may be negative rather than positive.

The simultaneous use of iron supplements and high-dose vitamin C can greatly increase iron absorption, possibly leading to excessive iron levels in the body. One study found that iron does not impair absorption of the drug methotrexate.

IMPORTANT INTERACTIONS

People who are taking antibiotics in the tetracycline or quinolone (Floxin, Cipro) families, levodopa, methyldopa, carbidopa, penicillamine, thyroid hormone, calcium, soy, zinc, copper, or manganese can avoid iron absorption problems by waiting at least two hours following their dose of medication or supplement before taking iron. Individuals who take drugs that reduce stomach acid, such as antacids, H_2 blockers, and proton pump inhibitors, may need extra iron.

Individuals taking iron simultaneously with high doses of vitamin C may be absorbing too much iron. For people taking ACE inhibitors, iron may reduce the coughing side effect; however, to avoid absorption problems, these individuals should wait at least two hours following their dose of medication before taking iron.

—*EBSCO CAM Review Board*

Further Reading

Binkoski, A. E., et al. "Iron Supplementation Does Not Affect the Susceptibility of LDL to Oxidative Modification in Women with Low Iron Status." *Journal of Nutrition*, vol. 134, 2004, pp. 99-103.

Dewey, K. G., et al. "Iron Supplementation Affects Growth and Morbidity of Breast-Fed Infants: Results of a Randomized Trial in Sweden and Honduras." *Journal of Nutrition*, vol. 132, 2002, pp. 3249-55.

Flink, H., et al. "Effect of Oral Iron Supplementation on Unstimulated Salivary Flow Rate." *Journal of Oral Pathology and Medicine*, vol. 35, 2006, pp. 540-47.

Hamilton, S. F., et al. "The Effect of Ingestion of Ferrous Sulfate on the Absorption of Oral Methotrexate in Patients with Rheumatoid Arthritis." *Journal of Rheumatology*, vol. 30, 2003, pp. 1948-50.

Konofal, E., et al. "Effects of Iron Supplementation on Attention Deficit Hyperactivity Disorder in Children." *Pediatric Neurology*, vol. 38, 2008, pp. 20-26.

Moriarty-Craige, S. E., et al. "Multivitamin-Mineral Supplementation Is Not as Efficacious as Is Iron Supplementation in Improving Hemoglobin Concentrations in Nonpregnant Anemic Women Living in Mexico." *American Journal of Clinical Nutrition*, vol. 80, 2004, pp. 1308-11.

Murray-Kolb, L. E., and J. L. Beard. "Iron Treatment Normalizes Cognitive Functioning in Young Women." *American Journal of Clinical Nutrition*, vol. 85, 2007, pp. 778-87.

Sankaranarayanan, S., et al. "Daily Iron Alone but Not in Combination with Multimicronutrients Increases Plasma Ferritin Concentrations in Indonesian Infants with Inflammation." *Journal of Nutrition*, vol. 134, 2004, pp. 1916-22.

Sharieff, W., et al. "Is Cooking Food in Iron Pots an Appropriate Solution for the Control of Anaemia in Developing Countries? A Randomised Clinical Trial in Benin." *Public Health Nutrition*, vol. 9, 2008, pp. 971-77.

Verdon, F., et al. "Iron Supplementation for Unexplained Fatigue in Non-anaemic Women." *British Medical Journal*, vol. 326, 2003, p. 1124.

Lecithin

Category: Herbs and supplements
Related terms: Egg lecithin, phosphatidylcholine in lecithin, soy lecithin
Definition: natural animal and plant substance used to treat specific health conditions

KEY TERMS

phosphatidylcholine: a class of phospholipids that incorporate choline as a headgroup and a major component of biological membranes; it is easily obtained from a variety of readily available sources, such as egg yolk or soybeans

ulcerative colitis: a chronic, inflammatory bowel disease that causes inflammation in the large intestine of the digestive tract

OVERVIEW

For decades, lecithin has been a popular treatment for high cholesterol, although there is little evidence that it works. More recently, lecithin has been proposed as a remedy for various psychological and neurological diseases, such as Tourette's syndrome, Alzheimer's disease, and bipolar disorder (earlier known as "manic depression)".

Lecithin contains phosphatidylcholine, which may be responsible for its medicinal effects. Phosphatidylcholine is a major part of the membranes surrounding human cells. However, when this substance is consumed, it is broken down into the nutrient choline rather than carried directly to cell membranes. Choline acts like folate, trimethylglycine, and SAMe (S-adenosylmethionine) to promote methylation. It is also used to make acetylcholine, a nerve chemical essential for proper brain function.

REQUIREMENTS AND SOURCES

Neither lecithin nor its ingredient phosphatidylcholine is an essential nutrient; however, choline has recently been recognized as essential. For use as a supplement or a food additive, lecithin is often manufactured from soy.

THERAPEUTIC DOSAGES

Standard lecithin contains about 10 to 20 percent phosphatidylcholine. However, European research has tended to use concentrated products containing 90 percent phosphatidylcholine in lecithin. The following dosages are based on that type of product. For psychological and neurological conditions, doses as high as 5 to 10 grams (g) taken three times daily have been used in studies. For liver disease, a typical dose is 350 to 500 milligrams (mg) taken three times daily; for high cholesterol, 500 to 900 mg taken three times daily has been tried.

THERAPEUTIC USES

For some time, lecithin/phosphatidylcholine was one of the most commonly recommended natural treatments for high cholesterol. However, this idea appears to rest entirely on studies of unacceptably low quality. The best-designed studies have failed to find any evidence of benefit. In Europe, phosphatidylcholine is also used to treat liver diseases, such as alcoholic fatty liver, alcoholic hepatitis, liver cirrhosis, and viral hepatitis. However, research into these potential uses remains preliminary and has yielded contradictory results.

Researchers have recently become interested in using phosphatidylcholine as a supportive treatment for severe ulcerative colitis. There may be insufficient phosphatidylcholine in the colon's mucus lining in persons with ulcerative colitis. Taking phosphatidylcholine may correct this deficiency.

In a small, double-blind, placebo-controlled study, sixty persons whose ulcerative colitis was poorly responsive to corticosteroids were randomized to receive either phosphatidylcholine (2 g per day) or a placebo for twelve weeks. One-half of the participants taking phosphatidylcholine showed a significant improvement in symptoms versus only

10 percent taking a placebo. Moreover, 80 percent taking phosphatidylcholine were able to discontinue their corticosteroids without disease flare-up, compared with 10 percent taking placebo.

Some evidence hints that phosphatidylcholine may reduce homocysteine levels, which in turn was thought likely to reduce heart disease risk. Because phosphatidylcholine plays a role in nerve function, it has also been suggested as a treatment for various psychological and neurological disorders, such as Alzheimer's disease, bipolar disorder, Parkinson's disease, Tourette's syndrome, and tardive dyskinesia (a late-developing side effect of drugs used for psychosis). However, the evidence that it works is limited to small studies with conflicting results.

SAFETY ISSUES

Lecithin is believed to be generally safe. However, some people taking high dosages (several grams daily) experience minor but annoying side effects, such as abdominal discomfort, diarrhea, and nausea. Maximum safe dosages for young children, pregnant or nursing women, and those with severe liver or kidney disease have not been determined.

—*EBSCO CAM Review Board*

Further Reading

Olthof, M. R., et al. "Choline Supplemented as Phosphatidylcholine Decreases Fasting and Postmethionine-Loading Plasma Homocysteine Concentrations in Healthy Men." *American Journal of Clinical Nutrition*, vol. 82, 2005, pp. 111-17.

Singh, N. K., and R. C. Prasad. "A Pilot Study of Polyunsaturated Phosphatidyl Choline in Fulminant and Subacute Hepatic Failure." *Journal of the Association of Physicians of India*, vol. 46, 1998, pp. 530-32.

Stremmel, W., et al. "Phosphatidylcholine for Steroid-Refractory Chronic Ulcerative Colitis." *Annals of Internal Medicine*, vol. 147, 2007, pp. 603-10.

Nicotinamide Adenine Dinucleotide (NAD)

Category: Herbs and supplements
Specialties and related fields: Alternative and complementary medicine, nutrition
Definition: natural substance of the human body used as a supplement to treat specific health conditions

KEY TERMS

nicotinamide: a compound that is the form in which nicotinic acid often occurs in nature

oxidation: a chemical process that removes electrons from molecules or atoms

reduction: a chemical reaction that adds electrons to molecules or atoms

OVERVIEW

Nicotinamide adenine dinucleotide (NAD) is an important cofactor or assistant that helps enzymes in their work throughout the body. Nicotinamide adenine dinucleotide particularly plays a role in the production of energy. It also participates in the production of L-dopa, which the body turns into the important neurotransmitter dopamine.

Based on these basic biochemical facts, NAD has been evaluated as a treatment for jet lag, Alzheimer's disease, Parkinson's disease, chronic fatigue syndrome, and depression, and as a sports supplement. However, only the first of these uses has any meaningful scientific evidence, and even that is highly preliminary.

REQUIREMENTS AND SOURCES

People do not get much NAD from their food. Healthy bodies make all the NAD they need, using vitamin B3 (niacin or nicotinamide) as a starting point. The highest concentration of NAD in animals is found in muscle tissues, which means that meat might be a good source, were it not that most of the NAD in meat is destroyed during processing, cooking, and digestion.

THERAPEUTIC DOSAGES

The typical dosage for supplemental NAD ranges from 5 to 50 milligrams (mg) daily, often taken sublingually (under the tongue). Stabilized NAD products are available.

THERAPEUTIC USES

Two small double-blind, placebo-controlled trials suggest that NAD may be useful for enhancing mental function under conditions of inadequate sleep, such as jet lag.

Supplemental NAD has also been proposed as a treatment for Alzheimer's, chronic fatigue syndrome, depression, and Parkinson's disease. Additionally, it has been tried as a sports performance enhancer. However, although a few studies have been performed to evaluate these potential uses, none were designed in such a way as to produce scientifically meaningful results.

SCIENTIFIC EVIDENCE

In a double-blind, placebo-controlled trial, thirty-five individuals taking an overnight flight across four time zones were given either 20 mg of NAD or a placebo sublingually (under the tongue) on the morning of arrival. Participants were twice given wakefulness and mental function tests: first at ninety minutes and then at five hours after landing. Individuals given NAD scored significantly better on these tests than those given a placebo.

The only supporting evidence comes from an unpublished double-blind, placebo-controlled, crossover study funded by the makers of an NAD product. In this study, twenty-five people were kept awake all night, and their cognitive function was tested the following day. People given NAD performed significantly better on various measures of mental function than those given placeboes. NAD did not, however, reduce daytime sleepiness or enhance mood.

SAFETY ISSUES

Nicotinamide adenine dinucleotide appears to be quite safe when taken at 5 mg daily or less. However, formal safety studies have not been completed. Safety in young children, pregnant or nursing women and those with severe liver or kidney disease has not been established.

—*EBSCO CAM Review Board*

Further Reading

Forsyth, L. M., et al. "Therapeutic Effects of Oral NADH on the Symptoms of Patients with Chronic Fatigue Syndrome." *Annals of Allergy, Asthma, and Immunology*, vol. 82, 1999, pp. 185-91.

Okabe, Keisuke, et al. "Oral Administration of Nicotinamide Mononucleotide Is Safe and Efficiently Increases Blood Nicotinamide Adenine Dinucleotide Levels in Healthy Subjects." *Frontiers in Nutrition*, vol. 9, 2022, 868640, doi:10.3389/fnut.2022.868640.

Radenkovic, Dina, et al. "Clinical Evidence for Targeting NAD Therapeutically." *Pharmaceuticals (Basel, Switzerland)*, vol. 13, no. 9, 2020, p. 247, doi:10.3390/ph13090247.

NUTRITION

Category: Biology

Specialties and related fields: Biochemistry, preventive medicine, public health

Definition: the science of food and beverage analysis, metabolism, physical needs for health, and disease prevention

KEY TERMS

calorie: a measure of the energy in food or of the energy used by the body *carbohydrate*: one of three macronutrients; foods that provide carbohydrates are starches, sugars, fruit, vegetables, and milk products

fat: one of three macronutrients; foods that provide fat are oils, margarine, butter, meat, and dairy

macronutrient: carbohydrate, protein, or fat

minerals: inorganic substances that are essential for body processes; the major minerals include calcium, phosphorus, magnesium, sodium, chloride, and potassium

protein: one of three macronutrients; foods that provide protein are meat and dairy, with smaller amounts of protein found in starches

vitamins: organic (carbon-containing) substances found in plants and animals that are essential for body processes; examples include vitamins A, C, and D, and the B vitamins

STRUCTURE AND FUNCTIONS

Nutrients are necessary for all aspects of living, including cellular metabolism, individual organ function, and multiple organ systems function. Breathing, moving, thinking, playing, and working all rely on the availability of nutrients. The study of nutrition has revolved around either healthy growth and development or nutrition concerning the prevention and treatment of disease. Periods of noticeable growth, such as pregnancy, infancy, childhood, and adolescence, are particular areas of study in nutrition because nutrient needs change during these periods.

The number of calories required to maintain a healthy weight during each life cycle stage depends upon the amount of energy expended. Because men generally have a larger body mass than women, they usually have a larger caloric requirement. Higher caloric requirements are found when body mass is relatively large, and energy output is relatively high, as seen in later adolescence and young adulthood.

Macronutrients. Carbohydrates are an important source of energy. The recommended intake range is 45 to 65 percent of the total caloric intake. Each gram of carbohydrate contributes four calories to the diet. Carbohydrates are found in starchy foods such as potatoes or corn, vegetables and fruits, and milk and yogurt. Carbohydrates are not found in meats or fats unless the food is a mixed dish, such as a hamburger casserole or a candy bar. Simple carbohydrates require little digestion, such as sucrose or sugar. Complex carbohydrates require more digestion, such as starches and fiber. General dietary guidelines suggest an increase in the higher fiber foods. The recommendation is to consume 25 to 35 grams of fiber daily; Americans generally consume 5 to 10 grams. In addition to fruits and vegetables, nuts and seeds, whole wheat bread, and cereal are high-fiber foods.

Dietary protein is required to supply essential amino acids so the body can synthesize new proteins such as enzymes, hormones, or structural proteins to build muscle. Meats (including pork, beef, chicken, or turkey), fish, eggs, and nuts contain substantial protein. Protein is also found in dairy products such as milk, cheese, and yogurt. Some protein can be found in most foods, including starches and vegetables, except those foods that are all fat, such as oil, or all simple carbohydrates, such as sugar. Each gram of protein contributes four calories to the diet. Protein requirements are closely related to caloric intake. With adequate or excess calories, protein is pared, meaning less can be consumed while still meeting all body demands for protein. In these cases, protein does not need to be used for energy. However, inadequate caloric intake requires higher protein levels to meet the body's needs. Some protein will also be converted to calories for energy needs. The recommended intake assumes that adequate calorie needs are consumed. Protein requirements may be higher than the recommended levels in cases of stress. Although both psychological and physical stress can increase protein requirements, physical stress (including surgery and burns) usually causes a more substantial increase in requirements.

Dietary fat is a risk factor in the development of atherosclerosis or heart disease. Because of this, dietary fat intake recommendations are restricted in total intake and type of fat ingested. Saturated fat is solid at room temperature and is derived from animals. Lard, shortening, and bacon fat are examples. Unsaturated fat can either have many unsaturated bonds (polyunsaturated) in the structure or one (monounsaturated). Polyunsaturated fat is liquid at room temperature and derived from plants such as corn or soybeans. Monounsaturated fat is derived from plants such as canola or olive oil. Whereas recommendations had previously specified levels of intake for both polyunsaturated and monounsaturated fats, current recommendations reflect only a limited total fat intake with a restriction on trans fats. Trans fat is unsaturated fat that has been partially hydrogenated. This process causes a liquid fat to become more solid and is sometimes desirable in baked products. Trans fats are linked to cardiovascular disease and should be limited. Foods that have higher values of trans fat should be labeled as such and are most often processed baked goods, such as cookies, cakes, or pies, or snack foods, such as chips. Regardless of the type of fat, each gram of fat contributes nine calories to the diet.

Minerals. The major minerals include calcium, phosphorus, magnesium, sodium, chloride, and potassium. These minerals are often called "electrolytes," meaning they can have a negative or positive charge, thus conducting electricity. In the body, these anions (negatively charged) and cations (positively charged) are important for the action potentials of cells, nerve conduction, and the excitation of muscles. The trace minerals are so-called because only very small amounts are needed daily. One of the most common trace minerals is iron. The minerals in a particular food often vary depending on the soil in which a plant is grown or the feed an animal consumes. Minerals are inorganic and cannot be destroyed with cooking or processing.

Calcium is required for normal growth and development of bone as well as nervous and muscular activity, enzyme regulation, and blood clotting. Poor calcium intake is associated with developing porous bones or osteoporosis. Food labels may designate a food as an excellent source (at least 200 milligrams of calcium) or a good source (100 to 199 milligrams of calcium).

Most phosphorus is in the bone as hydroxyapatite. However, phosphorus also occurs as phospholipids in most cell membranes. It is a component of nucleic acids—phosphorus functions as an acid-base buffer in enzymatic reactions and energy transfer. Phosphorus is found in nearly all foods, but good sources include meat, milk products, eggs, grains and legumes, and soft drinks.

Magnesium is essential for hundreds of enzymatic reactions and muscle contractions. About half of the body's magnesium is found in bone. Green leafy vegetables, fruits, grains, nuts, milk, meat, shellfish, and eggs are good sources of magnesium.

Potassium is found in many foods, including milk, meat, fruit, and vegetables. Together with sodium, potassium is involved in maintaining fluid balance. A diet high in sodium and low in potassium may be involved in developing high blood pressure or hypertension. The major source of sodium in the diet is salt, which is sodium chloride. Foods high in sodium include any food with visible salt (such as crackers and snack foods), pickled foods, processed foods such as lunch meat, canned soup, canned meat, and cured foods such as bacon and ham. A diet high in potassium and calcium and low in sodium is recommended to prevent hypertension.

Most of the body's iron is found in hemoglobin in red blood cells, which transport oxygen in the blood. Food sources of iron are either heme (from meat) or nonheme (from plant sources or iron-fortified foods). Very little iron is excreted from the body, with most of the iron from degraded hemoglobin being reabsorbed in the gastrointestinal tract. A deficiency of iron occurs gradually with chronic poor intake of iron-rich foods. Other causes of iron deficiency include excessive blood loss and malabsorption. Chronic iron deficiency will cause anemia.

Vitamins. Vitamin A food sources include both animal sources (retinoids) and plant sources (carotenoids). Good animal food sources of vitamin A include liver, egg yolks, milk fat, and fish oils. Carotenoids can be converted to retinol in the intestinal mucosa. They will then have the same metabolic role as retinoids from animal sources. The most common of these is beta carotene, but there are more than five hundred carotenoids. Vitamin A is required for optimal vision, with most of its effects found in maintaining night vision. Vitamin A also has a role in maintaining epithelial tissues, mucus production, and bone health. Vitamin A appears to have a role in fertility and maintaining immune function.

Vitamin C is an important antioxidant with the biochemical ability to neutralize free radicals. Free radicals are metabolites of oxygen used in the cell and are believed to promote aging and several chronic diseases. Good sources of vitamin C include citrus fruits, broccoli, kiwi, potatoes, strawberries, and tomatoes, as well as most other fruits and vegetables. Heat, alkalinity, and exposure to air will destroy vitamin C. Therefore, certain cooking, processing, and storage practices can greatly reduce the vitamin C content of food.

Another antioxidant is vitamin E. Vitamin E is a group of compounds, the most common of which is α-tocopherol. Good sources of vitamin E include vegetable oils, margarine, and nuts. Vitamin E is not destroyed by exposure to air, primarily because it is protected by dietary fat. Vitamin E can be destroyed by high temperatures, such as in frying.

Vitamin D food sources are very limited. While milk is fortified with vitamin D, other dairy products, such as cheese and yogurt, generally are not. Some new products are fortified with calcium and vitamin D, such as yogurt, margarine, and juice. Exposure of the skin to sunlight converts a pre-vitamin D compound to vitamin D_3 (cholecalciferol). Cholecalciferol will be hydroxylated in the liver and the kidney before it becomes active vitamin D. Vitamin D is required for calcium regulation and bone health. Still, emerging research areas suggest that vitamin D may also have a role in autoimmune diseases.

The B vitamins are water-soluble and include thiamin, niacin, riboflavin, pantothenic acid, vitamin B_6, biotin, folate, and vitamin B_{12}. As a group, the B vitamins are essential for the metabolism of macronutrients, cell growth, division, and all organ functions. The B vitamins are found in various foods, although vitamin B_{12} is primarily found in animal products. Once a concern for vegetarians, vitamin B_{12} is fortified in many kinds of cereal and nonmeat breakfast foods.

DISORDERS AND DISEASES

Most chronic diseases result from a complex interaction between genetics and environmental factors. Diet is an important environmental factor that is potentially modifiable, and it has received much attention in preventing chronic disease. Most chronic disease prevention or treatment includes a nutritional component. The most prevalent chronic diseases in the United States are cancer, cardiovascular disease, diabetes, obesity, and osteoporosis.

Cancer. Although overall rates are declining in the United States, cancer continues to be a major cause of mortality. Cancer generally involves three phases: initiation, promotion, and progression. During the initiation step, a genetic alteration may remain quiescent or continue through the second step of promotion. During promotion, cellular proliferation is stimulated, and the abnormal cells begin to grow without regulation. The third phase is progression, when the neoplastic cells become invasive and spread or metastasize to other body parts. Dietary components may be involved in initiating and promoting certain cancers and their inhibition. The dietary components that have been linked to the development of cancer include dietary fat, total calories, and alcohol, as well as salted, cured foods and molds that may grow in certain foods.

Antioxidants have been investigated as inhibitors of cancer. Fruits and vegetables are rich sources of antioxidants, and high fruit and vegetable intake has been linked to a lower incidence of certain cancers. The results of many studies, however, are inconclusive. Although a high intake of dietary fat and red meat has been associated with an increased risk of colon cancer, lower-fat diets have not proved to be an effective intervention in decreasing colon cancer incidence. Nevertheless, a diet high in fruits and vegetables, at least five servings each day, and lower in fat and alcohol is recommended as a preventive measure against cancer. Some of the benefits of high fruit and vegetable intake may be attributable to the fiber content of these foods. Higher fiber diets increase fecal bulk, diluting carcinogens that enter the gastrointestinal tract. By increasing intestinal motility, fiber also decreases the amount of time that fecal material is in the gastrointestinal tract, thereby limiting exposure of the mucosa to potential toxins.

Cardiovascular disease. Cardiovascular diseases are the leading cause of death in the United States. They include arrhythmias, congestive heart failure, and valvular diseases. Still, most of the morbidity and mortality are related to coronary heart disease or atherosclerosis. Hyperlipidemia is a risk factor for atherosclerosis, and dietary fat influences the level of blood lipids. According to the Center for Disease Control (CDC), the recommended fat intake is 25 to 35 percent of total calories per day. Of that dietary fat, less than 7 percent of total calories should be saturated fat, and less than 1 percent should be trans fat. Lower fat meats and dairy are recommended, as well as replacement of some meat with vegetable alternatives. Sources of trans fat should be limited. The effects of various levels of polyunsaturated and monounsaturated fats are debated. While limited cholesterol intake is recommended, cholesterol intake has had less effect on blood lipids than total fat and trans fat.

Eating fish, especially oily fish, is recommended as a source of omega-3 fatty acids, which are long-chain polyunsaturated fatty acids associated with a decreased risk of certain heart diseases. The two omega-3 fatty acids are eicosapentaenoic acid (EPA) and docosahexaenoic acid (DHA). Although fish may contain contaminants known to be hazardous to health, the benefits of eating it are believed to outweigh the risks for adults. Restricted intake may be recommended for children and pregnant women. Supplements of DHA and EPA are not recommended for the prevention of heart disease. However, they may be prescribed as treatment under a physician's supervision.

Higher intakes of fruits, vegetables, and whole grains are recommended to prevent heart disease. In addition to fiber, these foods may contain antioxidants or other bioactive compounds that are beneficial to health. In addition, these foods may displace other, higher-calorie foods from the diet, thus promoting a healthy weight. Limiting foods high in added sugars is recommended because of the association of these foods with weight gain and obesity. Obesity is a significant risk factor for cardiovascular disease, and achieving a healthy weight through diet and physical activity is important.

A healthy weight is also significant in the maintenance of optimal blood pressure. Because sodium intake is associated with increased blood pressure on average, limiting sodium intake is also recommended for heart health. Limited amounts of alcohol, if alcohol is consumed at all, is also included as a healthy lifestyle measure for the prevention of heart disease. Moderate alcohol intake is generally considered two drinks for men and one for women each day.

Foods being investigated concerning their role in the prevention of cardiovascular disease include soy and plant stanols. Supplements of antioxidants and fish oils for their DHA and EPA are generally not recommended. Still, foods containing these compounds may be beneficial.

Diabetes. The incidence of diabetes continues to grow in parallel to the incidence of obesity. Diabetes mellitus has been categorized as either type 1 diabetes (formerly known as insulin-dependent diabetes mellitus, IDDM) or type 2 diabetes (formerly known as non-insulin-dependent diabetes mellitus, NIDDM). Nutrition is an important component of both the prevention and treatment of diabetes, regardless of type.

Obesity enhances insulin resistance. Therefore, the main goal of type 2 diabetes management is to prevent or reduce obesity. Weight loss in obese persons with type 2 diabetes improves glycemic control and blood lipid profile. Because carbohydrates are the main determinant of postprandial plasma glucose, the number of carbohydrates and timing of foods eaten may need to be regulated. The total amount of carbohydrates in the diet or meal is more important than the type of carbohydrate, with certain exceptions. Liquid carbohydrates are more easily digested and absorbed than those from solid foods. Beverages such as milk and orange juice may cause a more rapid rise in blood glucose. Sucrose and sucrose-containing foods do not need to be eliminated. Still, these foods need to be included in the total carbohydrates and calories consumed for meal planning and coverage with medication. Restriction of sucrose and sucrose-containing foods usually relates to the restriction of total calories. The glycemic response to carbohydrates depends on many components, including the type of carbohydrate, the cooking or processing, prior food intake, other macronutrients in the food, and glycemic control of the individual. Because dietary modifications need to be individualized, people with diabetes should receive individualized medical nutrition therapy, preferably by a registered dietitian or certified diabetes educator.

Obesity. Obesity occurs when caloric intake exceeds the needs of the individual and is therefore stored in adipose tissue. Although normal weight varies with age, gender, and height, for each group, there are indicators of obesity. Usual indicators of obesity are based on the assumption that variations in weight at various heights are attributable to body fat and are often calculated as the body mass index (BMI). According to the CDC, a BMI between 25 and 30 is considered overweight, and above 30 is considered obese. The optimal macronutrient distribution to facilitate weight loss is not known. Without clear conclusions, higher and lower amounts of protein, fat, and carbohydrates have been investigated. Consuming fewer calories while increasing the number of calories used through physical activity remains the cornerstone of obesity prevention and treatment.

Osteoporosis. As with other chronic diseases, the incidence of osteoporosis continues to rise. Osteoporosis is asymptomatic until the condition produces deformity or contributes to fractures. While genetics play an important role in the development of osteoporosis, modifying risk factors include diet and physical activity. Optimal calcium levels are beneficial in maintaining high bone mineral density, which is critical in preventing osteoporosis. Most calcium is obtained from dairy products, although grain-based foods and juices are increasingly being fortified with calcium. Vitamin D plays a critical role in regulating calcium balance. Therefore, adequate vitamin D status is important in preventing osteoporosis. Vitamin D deficiency can contribute to osteoporosis in older individuals secondary to poor skin synthesis, lower hydroxylation of vitamin D in the kidneys, and inadequate nutritional intake. As with calcium, more food products are being fortified with vitamin D, increasing awareness of osteoporosis.

PERSPECTIVE AND PROSPECTS

Although the science of nutrition began as a branch of biochemistry, early discoveries of the health properties of food date to the eighteenth century and the discovery that limes could prevent the painful bleeding disorder scurvy. Since then, the knowledge of nutrition has progressed beyond identifying deficiency diseases to understanding and appreciating the complexity of nutrition in optimal health. In addition to further investigations into macronutrients, vitamins, and minerals, many bioactive substances in foods are being identified, such as bioflavonoids and probiotics. The interactions of these and more traditional nutrients are being investigated as potential modifiers of chronic disease and promoters of longevity.

—*Karen Chapman-Novakofski*

Further Reading

American Diabetes Association. *American Diabetes Association Complete Guide to Diabetes*. 4th Rev. ed., Bantam Books, 2006.

"Defining Adult Overweight and Obesity." *Overweight and Obesity, Centers for Disease Control*, 3 June 2022, www.cdc.gov/obesity/basics/adult-defining.html. Accessed 13 June 2022.

"Dietary Fats." *American Heart Association*, 1 Nov. 2021, www.heart.org/en/healthy-living/healthy-eating/eat-smart/fats/dietary-fats. Accessed 13 June 2022.

Duyff, Roberta Larson. *American Dietetic Association Complete Food and Nutrition Guide*. 3rd ed., John Wiley & Sons, 2007.

"Healthy Eating: Vitamins and Minerals for Older Adults." *National Institute on Aging*. National Institutes of Health, 2 Jan. 2021, www.nia.nih.gov/health/vitamins-and-minerals-older-adults. Accessed 13 June 2022.

Lichtenstein, Alice H., et al. "Diet and Lifestyle Recommendations Revision 2006: A Scientific Statement from the American Heart Association Nutrition Committee." *Circulation*, vol. 114, no. 1, 2006, pp. 82-96.

US Department of Health and Human Services and US Department of Agriculture. *Dietary Guidelines for Americans 2005*. 6th ed., Government Printing Office, 2005.

PROTEIN

Category: Biology
Specialties and related fields: Biochemistry, dietetics, nutrition
Definition: an important dietary nutrient with many essential functions in the body

KEY TERMS

essential amino acids: amino acids that cannot be synthesized by an organism and must come from diet
complete protein: proteins that provide all eight essential amino acids
incomplete protein: proteins that are missing at least one essential amino acid
kwashiorkor: a disease caused by severe protein deficiency; symptoms include apathy, diarrhea, inactivity, failure to grow, fatty liver, and edema

STRUCTURE AND FUNCTIONS

Proteins are composed of twenty-two different amino acids in various combinations joined together in a chain. The human body can synthesize thirteen amino acids, known as "nonessential amino acids." In contrast, the other nine, known as "essential amino acids," must be provided by the diet. Proteins from dietary sources are considered complete or incomplete based on their amino acid content. Complete proteins provide all eight essential amino acids. In contrast, incomplete proteins have low amounts or are missing at least one essential amino acid. Only fish, meat, poultry, eggs, cheese, and other foods from animal sources contain complete proteins. Peanuts, soy, nuts, seeds, green peas, legumes, and some grains provide the richest plant proteins. Omnivores typically eat a sufficient variety of foods to consume essential amino acids. Vegetarians ensure sufficient amino acid intake by consuming a variety of plant proteins.

Every cell in the body contains protein. Proteins are essential for cell structure and function and comprise major components of skin, tissues, muscles, and internal organs. Dietary protein, one of three nutrients used for energy, is required for building, maintaining, and repairing body tissue. Growth and development during childhood, adolescence, and pregnancy depend on proteins. Proteins participate in all cellular functions, acting as enzyme catalysts and transporting and storing molecules. They also provide mechanical support and immune protection, generate movement, transmit nerve impulses, and control growth and differentiation. Important classes of proteins include enzymes, hormones, and antibodies.

DISORDERS AND DISEASES

Protein deficiency is relatively rare in developed countries, although poverty can prevent adequate protein consumption. Protein deficiency can result from stringent weight-loss diets or in older adults. Severe protein deficiency is fatal. In developing countries, protein deficiency causes the disease known as "kwashiorkor," which includes symptoms such as apathy, diarrhea, inactivity, failure to grow, fatty liver, and edema. Since the body cannot store protein, too much protein can also be harmful, with a high-protein diet potentially leading to high cholesterol or other diseases and possible effects on kidney function. Excess protein may also result in immune system hyperactivity, liver dysfunction, bone loss, and obesity. Proteins contribute to food allergies, with many people allergic to proteins in milk (casein), wheat (gluten), or proteins found in peanut, shellfish, or other kinds of seafood.

PERSPECTIVE AND PROSPECTS

A nutritionally balanced diet provides adequate protein. The average diet in the United States includes nearly twice the amount of protein required to maintain a healthy body. Although it was once believed that vegetarians needed to combine proteins by consuming all amino acids in the same meal, it is now realized that the benefits of protein combining can be achieved over a longer period. In May 2013, the New York University Fertility Center published a study showing that women undergoing fertility treatment increased their chances of conception by increasing the amount of protein in their diets.

—*C. J. Walsh*

Further Reading

"Dietary Proteins." *MedlinePlus*, 25 Mar. 2015, medlineplus.gov/dietaryproteins.html.

Duyff, Roberta Larson. *American Dietetic Association Complete Food and Nutrition Guide*. John Wiley & Sons, 2006.

Marshall, Keri. *User's Guide to Protein and Amino Acids*. Basic Health Publications, 2005.

Norton, Amy, "Can High-Protein, Low-Carb Diet Boost Fertility Treatment?" *MedicalXpress*, 6 May 2013, medicalxpress.com/news/2013-05-high-protein-low-carb-diet-boost-fertility.html.

"Protein in Diet." *MedlinePlus*, n.d., medlineplus.gov/ency/article/002467.htm.

Shils, Maurice E., et al. *Modern Nutrition in Health and Disease*. 10th ed., Lippincott Williams & Wilkins, 2005.

Sports and Energy Drinks

Category: Nutrition
Specialties and related fields: Dietetics, nutrition
Definition: functional beverages whose stated purpose is to help athletes replace water, electrolytes, and energy before, during, and especially after training or competition

KEY TERMS

dehydration: loss of body fluid caused by illness, sweating, or inadequate intake

electrolytes: minerals in your blood and other body fluids that carry an electric charge

hydration: drinking water to replace bodily water lost through perspiration after intense exercise

INTRODUCTION

Despite the lack of scientific evidence, young athletes were advised by well-meaning but uninformed adults to avoid consuming too much water so they wouldn't become "logy," a vague term describing a condition akin to a slowness of reaction in sports that demanded a rapid response. Through the 1970s, marathon runners were cautioned about consuming too much water before and during races. At the same time, football players training in hot and humid climates had their water intake restricted to prevent any deterioration in their efforts. This misunderstanding was not only contrary to the athlete's needs. Still, it resulted in serious damage from heat stroke and, in some cases, the death of athletes who needed a replenishment for the electrolytes expended during exertion.

By the mid-1970s, it had become apparent to researchers in the growing field of exercise physiology that it was necessary to seriously consider the loss of vital fluids during prolonged periods of intense exercise, and this was especially important for young athletes less attuned to the signals of distress than adults with more experience in demanding conditions. The US Department of Health and Human Services recommended in 2008 that "young people need at least sixty minutes of physical activity daily" since "positive experiences with physical activity at a young age help lay the basis for being regularly active throughout life." This recommendation resulted from studies indicating that the rate of obesity in adolescents ages twelve to nineteen increased from 5 to 17.5 percent from 1980 to 2006. To ensure safe participation in a vigorous aerobic and bone-strengthening activity, researchers began experimenting with drinks designed to replace the electrolytes lost during prolonged physical activity, beginning with the pioneering studies conducted by scientists at the University of Florida College of Medicine who tested ten football players in 1965. Although the results were not completely conclusive, the Florida "Gators" victory in the Sugar Bowl in 1967 led to the marketing of a drink containing water, sodium, potassium, phosphate, lemon juice, and sugar initially called "Gator-Aid," and then designated *Gatorade*, the first and still most widely dispensed sports drink. The brand was hugely boosted when it was named the National Football League's "Official Drink" in 1967.

A MASS MARKETING MODEL

For almost a decade, Gatorade was the sole sports drink available. It was marketed primarily in its original formula, with fructose becoming the basic sweetener. As other sports drinks began to enter the market, Gatorade added a fruit punch in 1983 to the original lemon-lime and orange flavors, followed by watermelon and strawberry-kiwi in the 1990s. In 2004, an endurance formula containing more sodium and potassium was added to the line, a part of a trend to designate a particular product for a more specific event. Michael Jordan was engaged to endorse *Gatorade* in an ad campaign using the slogan "Be Like Mike" in 1991, and Tiger Woods was involved in promoting "Tiger Ade" before his loss of prestige. In addition, athletes like Peyton Manning took part in fitness tests of the product's capabilities, lending the imprimatur of their professional commitment to the brand. When Harry Carson and Jim Burt of the NFL's football Giants poured a container of Gatorade over their coach Bill Parcells to celebrate an important victory in 1985, a ritual was established, which has been continued with other liquids throughout the sports world since that time.

CONTENDING FOR MARKET SHARES

The market dominance of Gatorade was inevitably challenged by other brands as the consumption of sports drinks became standard practice for athletes at every level of competitive capability. For long-distance runners, the steady reduction in the world marathon "record" or fastest time was attributed to the widespread use of individual liquid preparations. At the same time, the "running boom" inspired by Frank Shorter's two Olympic medals in 1972 (gold) and 1976 (silver, a loss to a chemically assisted East German) vastly increased the numbers of recreational runners ready to follow trends in improved human performance. While Gatorade continued to increase revenue for the Van Camp and Pepsico corporations that distributed it in and beyond the United States, other drinks such as Powerade, developed by Coca-Cola, assumed about 21 percent of the market share by 2010 to Gatorade's 75 percent. Lesser-known brands like 10-K Thirst Quencher, bottled in the United States but owned by Suntory of Japan, and Staminade—developed in Australia in the late 1980s; and Accelearade, a protein-infused drink developed in the United Kingdom—entered an expanding market.

NEGATIVE EFFECTS OF LIQUID SUPPLEMENTS

The professional athletes featured in the marketing campaigns were expending energy at such a high level that the caloric contents of sports drinks didn't adversely affect their nutritional intake. For the participants of the recreational sport, especially those in the adolescent and mature adult cohort, the heavy dose of carbohydrates distorted a balanced diet and, especially for adolescents, resulted in significant weight gains. A 32-ounce bottle of Gatorade contains 53 grams of sugar, more than the suggested daily intake. Numerous exercise physiologists have determined that water without any additional ingredients will be sufficient for most athletes, with sports drinks appropriate for extreme conditions of temperature and humidity or prolonged activity of durations beyond an hour, such as marathons, ultramarathons, and full triathlons. As David Neiman, a leading researcher in the field, advises:

Thirst can lag behind actual body needs. So before, during, and after the exercise bout, one should drink plenty of fluids. A plan recommended by some sports-medicine experts is to drink 2 cups of water immediately before the exercise, 1 cup every 15 minutes during the exercise session, and then two more cups after the session.

While Neiman and other experts stress the importance of water as a necessity, Neiman observes that "a wide variety of sports drinks are available" and lists three reasons for using these drinks:
- To avoid dehydration
- To counter the loss of electrolytes
- To oppose the loss of body carbohydrate stores

Neiman notes that the electrolyte content of sweat is relatively low, and "most studies have shown such losses are rarely significant for properly nourished and acclimatized people."

Nonetheless, the marketing forces have so strongly encouraged the consumption of sports drinks that Neiman and colleagues have commented that "Extensive reviews of the literature have failed to find any convincing support for the role of supplementation in enhancing performance, hastening recovery or decreasing injury in healthy, well-adjusted adults undergoing athletic training." This caution is concentrated on vitamin and mineral supplements and applies to sports drinks.

ENERGY DRINKS

Sports drinks are designed as replacements; energy drinks are designed as stimulants. The concern about the negative effects of energy drinks and gels is less specific and more a matter of conjecture than the detailed studies of sports drinks. Still, there is sufficient evidence to indicate that casual consumption of beverages like Red Bull, Rock Star, Monster, and other popular brands can have the potential to damage healthy people and may pose a serious risk for people with some easily identifiable physiological characteristics. For instance, enamel demineralization may occur in younger consumers. Because there aren't regulations limiting the amounts of prime ingredients like caffeine, an awareness of the amount of each substance is valuable in deciding how frequently a product might be used. The December 2012 issue of *Consumer Reports* has a chart listing the primary ingredients in 28 energy products. The caffeine quotient in each sample ranges from 75 to more than 200 milligrams per serving. As a point of comparison, there are 34 milligrams of caffeine in standard servings of Coke and 55 milligrams in Mountain Dew.

Another important aspect concerning components is the specific substance that gives the product its characteristic effect or taste. If caffeine isn't present, the "energy" stimulation may derive from natural substances like guarana or ginseng. (1 gram of guarana is the equivalent of 40 milligrams of caffeine.) Neither of these substances is dangerous per se, but their overall effects haven't been fully determined. The site www.fact-pro-energydrinks.pdf from the University of California at Davis lists the individual ingredients of the more popular energy drinks.

DANGEROUS DOSES

In addition to caffeine's tendency to raise the heart rate and blood pressure, using an energy drink while exercising may also result in excessive dehydration due to fluid loss and the diuretic propensities of caffeine.

Like sports drinks, energy products contain a high caloric component, distorting a balance of nutritional sources. A reinforcing cycle of symptoms can occur when a rapid pulse rate leads to a sense of anxiety, which can result in sleep deprivation if it isn't alleviated. Prolonged use may elevate stomach acid levels, resulting in digestion problems, which may adversely affect metabolic systems. These concerns do not mean that energy products should be unnecessarily restricted. Still, full awareness of dosage, frequency, and other variables should be a part of someone's decision to use sports drinks. The proprietary claims by various manufacturers have made it difficult to determine what the drink contains, and alcoholic energy drinks are not required to disclose nutrition facts on the container. The US Food and Drug Administration (FDA) has required removing stimulants from drinks containing alcohol and caffeine. Still, combining alcoholic beverages with energy drinks includes young adults, for whom it can be particularly dangerous.

—*Leon Lewis*

Further Reading

Maugham, R. J., and R. Murray. *Sports Drinks: Basic Science and Practical Aspects*. CRC Press, 2001.

Migala, J. "The Strange Effect of Your Sports Drink." *Men's Health*, 19 May 2014, www.menshealth.com.

Neiman, D. *Exercise Testing and Prescription: A Health-Related Approach*. 7th ed., McGraw-Hill, 2011.

Schneider, M. B., and H. J. Benjamin. "Sports Drinks and Energy Drinks for Children and Adolescents: Are They Appropriate?" *American Academy of Pediatrics*, vol. 127, no. 6, 2011, pp. 1182-1189.

Sports and Fitness Performance

Category: Condition

Specialties and related fields: Alternative and complementary medicine, athletic training, chiropractic, dietetics, nutrition, personal training, strength and conditioning

Related term: Ergogenic aids

Definition: treatment to enhance athletic performance and fitness

KEY TERMS

coenzymes: organic compounds required by many enzymes for catalytic activity

creatine: an amino acid located mostly in the muscles and brain that regenerates adenosine triphosphate (ATP)

ginseng: an herbal remedy used in Asian countries to help develop strength, also helps reduce fatigue

hydroxymethyl butyrate (HMB): a dietary supplement and ingredient in certain medical foods that promote wound healing and provide nutritional support for people with muscle wasting due to cancer or human immunodeficiency virus (HIV) infections

minerals: nutrients needed in small amounts to keep the body healthy

stimulants: substances that speed up messages traveling between the brain and body and make a person feel more awake, alert, confident, or energetic

supplements: a substance or product that is added to a person's diet to make sure they get all the nutrients they need

vitamins: nutrients that are precursors of coenzymes that the body needs in small amounts to function and stay healthy

INTRODUCTION

In the competitive world of sports, the smallest advantage can make an enormous difference in the outcome of a contest. A substance that improves an athlete's strength, speed, or endurance is sometimes called an "ergogenic aid."

The most effective ergogenic aids (stimulants, anabolic steroids, and human growth hormone) are dangerous and illegal. Numerous natural options are marketed as alternatives. Some of the many supplements used to improve sports performance are discussed here.

PRINCIPAL PROPOSED NATURAL TREATMENTS

Two natural supplements have shown promise as ergogenic aids: creatine and hydroxymethyl butyrate.

Creatine. One of the best-selling and best-documented supplements for enhancing athletic performance, creatine is a naturally occurring substance that plays an important role in the production of energy in the body. The body converts creatine to phosphocreatine, a form of stored energy used by muscles. In theory, taking supplemental creatine will build up a reserve of phosphocreatine in the muscles to help them perform on demand. Supplemental creatine may also help the body make new phosphocreatine faster when it has been used up by intense activity. However, the balance of evidence suggests that if creatine supplements have any benefit for sports performance, it is slight and limited to highly specific forms of exercise.

Several small double-blind studies have found that creatine can improve performance in exercises that involve repeated short bursts of high-intensity activity with intervening rest periods of adequate length. A double-blind, placebo-controlled study investigated creatine and swimming performance in eighteen men and fourteen women. Men taking the supplement had significant speed increases when doing six bouts of 50-meter swims started at three-minute intervals, compared to men taking a placebo. However, their speed did not improve when swimming ten sets of 25-yard lengths started at one-minute intervals. Researchers theorize that the shorter rest time between laps was insufficient for the swimmers' bodies to resynthesize phosphocreatine.

None of the women in the study showed any improvement with the creatine supplement. The authors of this study noted that women normally have more creatine in their muscle tissue than men, so perhaps creatine supplementation (at least at this level) is not as beneficial to women as it appears to be for men. Further research is needed to fully understand the difference between the genders in response to creatine.

In an earlier double-blind study, sixteen physical education students carried out ten six-second bursts of extremely intense exercise on a stationary bicycle, separated by thirty seconds of rest. The results showed that the students who took 20 grams (g) of creatine for six days could maintain cycle speed throughout the repetitions. Many other studies have shown similar improvements in performance capacity involving repeated bursts of action. However, there have been negative results, too; in general, minimal to no benefits have been seen in studies involving athletes engaged in normal sports rather than contrived laboratory tests.

In contrast, endurance or nonrepetitive aerobic-burst exercise studies generally have not shown creatine supplementation benefits. Therefore, creatine probably will not help with marathon running or single sprints.

In addition to repetitive burst exercise, creatine has also shown promise for increasing isometric exercise capacity (pushing against a fixed resistance). Also, two double-blind, placebo-controlled studies, each lasting twenty-eight days, provide evidence that creatine and creatine plus hydroxymethyl butyrate can increase lean muscle and bone mass. However, one double-blind trial failed to find creatine helpful for enhancing general fitness, including resistance exercise performance, in older adults. The contradictory results seen in these small trials suggest that

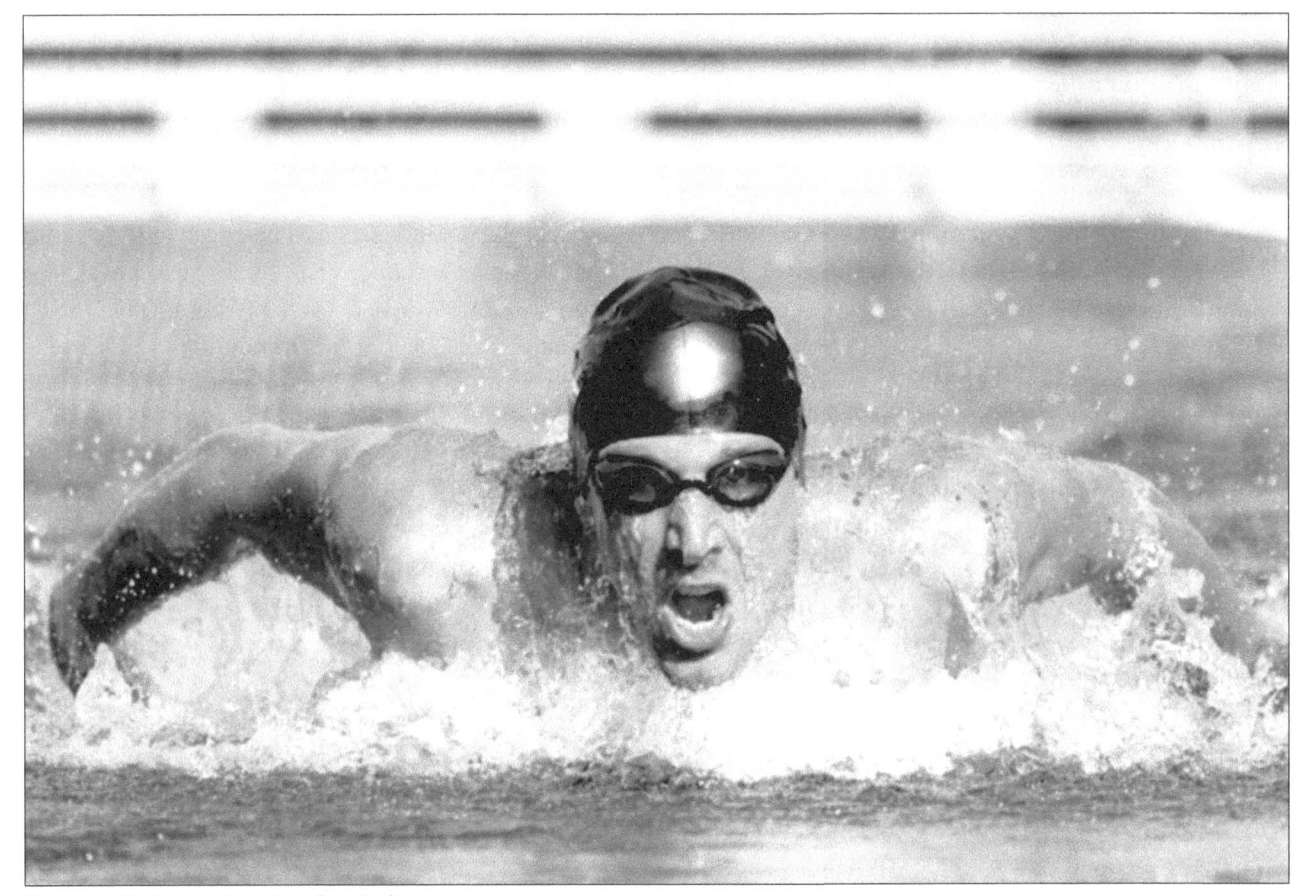

Photo via iStock/amriphoto. [Used under license.]

creatine offers at most a very modest sports performance benefit.

Hydroxymethyl butyrate. Beta-hydroxy beta-methylbutyric acid, or hydroxymethyl butyrate (HMB), is a chemical that occurs naturally in the body when the amino acid leucine breaks down. Leucine is found in particularly high concentrations in muscles. During athletic training, damage to the muscles leads to the breakdown of leucine and increased HMB levels. Some evidence suggests that taking HMB supplements might signal the body to slow down the destruction of muscle tissue. On this basis, HMB has been studied as a sports performance supplement for enhancing strength and muscle mass.

According to many of the small double-blind trials that have been reported, HMB appears to improve muscle-growth response to weight training. For example, in a controlled study, forty-one male volunteers aged nineteen to twenty-nine were given either 0, 1.5, or 3 g of HMB daily for three weeks. The participants also lifted weights three days per week according to a defined (and rather severe) schedule. The results suggested that HMB can enhance strength and muscle mass in direct proportion to intake.

In another controlled study reported in the same article, thirty-two male volunteers took either 3 g of HMB or a placebo daily. They then lifted weights for two or three hours daily, six days per week, for seven weeks. The HMB group saw a significantly greater increase in bench-press strength than the placebo group. However, there was no significant difference in body weight or fat mass by the end of the study.

Similarly, a double-blind, placebo-controlled trial of thirty-nine men and thirty-six women found that HMB supplementation improved response to weight training in four weeks. Two placebo-controlled studies of women found that 3 g of HMB had no effect on lean body mass and strength in sedentary women. Still, it did provide an additional benefit when combined with weight training. Also, a double-blind study of thirty-one men and women, all seventy years old and undergoing resistance training, found significant improvements in fat-free mass attributable to the use of HMB (3 g daily).

However, there have been negative studies too, but all were small, so their results are ultimately unreliable. Larger studies will be necessary to truly establish whether HMB is helpful for power athletes working to enhance strength and muscle mass.

OTHER PROPOSED NATURAL TREATMENTS

Numerous other supplements are marketed as ergogenic aids to improve speed, strength, or endurance. However, the evidence that they work is marginal at best. In many cases, the best available evidence indicates that these substances are ineffective.

Ginseng. There are three different herbs commonly called "ginseng": Asian or Korean ginseng (Panax ginseng), American ginseng (Panax quinquefolius), and Siberian ginseng (Eleutherococcus senticosus). The latter is not truly ginseng, but the Russian scientists responsible for promoting it believed it functioned identically and named it ginseng. According to some experts, a fourth herb, ciwujia, is actually Eleutherococcus. In contrast, others claim it is a related but different species.

Ginseng has shown some promise as a mild ergogenic aid, but published evidence remains at best incomplete and contradictory. Other forms of ginseng generally lack any meaningful supporting evidence.

For example, an eight-week, double-blind, placebo-controlled trial evaluated the effects of *P. ginseng* with and without exercise in forty-one people. The participants were given either *P. ginseng* or a placebo and then underwent exercise training or remained untrained throughout the study. The results showed that ginseng improved aerobic capacity in people who did not exercise but did not benefit those who did exercise.

In a nine-week, double-blind, placebo-controlled trial of thirty highly trained athletes, treatment with *P. ginseng* or *P. ginseng* plus vitamin E significantly improved aerobic capacity. Another double-blind, placebo-controlled trial of thirty-seven participants also found some benefits. Also, a double-blind, placebo-controlled study of 120 people found that P. ginseng gradually improved reaction time and lung function in a twelve-week treatment period among participants from forty to sixty years of age. (No benefits were seen in younger people.)

However, in an eight-week double-blind trial that followed sixty healthy men in their twenties, no benefit with *P. ginseng* could be demonstrated. Many other small trials of *P. ginseng* have failed to find evidence of benefit. These mixed outcomes suggest that ginseng is only slightly effective at best.

A double-blind study of twenty endurance athletes in eight weeks failed to find evidence of benefit with a standard *Eleutherococcus* formulation. Furthermore, in a small, double-blind, placebo-controlled trial of endurance athletes, *Eleutherococcus* increased physiologic signs of stress during intensive training. Ciwujia has not yet been studied in meaningful double-blind trials.

Medium-chain triglycerides. Medium-chain triglycerides (MCTs) are fats with an unusual chemical structure that allows the body to digest them easily. Most fats are broken down in the intestine and reassembled into a special form that can be transported in the blood. However, MCTs are absorbed intact and taken to the liver, where they are used directly for energy. In this sense, they are processed like carbohydrates. For that reason, MCTs have been proposed as an alternative to carbo-loading (consuming a large quantity of carbohydrates before intense physical exercise) for providing a concentrated source of easily utilized energy.

Several double-blind studies have evaluated MCTs' effects on high-intensity or endurance exercise performance, but the results have been thoroughly inconsistent. These results are not surprising because all of the studies were too small to eliminate the effects of chance properly.

Iron. Most athletes are probably not iron-deficient, and people should not take iron supplements if they already have enough iron in their bodies. However, iron supplements may enhance athletic training if a person is deficient in this essential mineral.

A double-blind, placebo-controlled trial of forty-two nonanemic women with evidence of slightly low iron reserves found that iron supplements significantly increased the benefits gained from exercise. Participants were put on a daily aerobic training program for the last four weeks of this six-week trial. At the end of the trial, those receiving iron showed significantly greater gains in speed and endurance than those given placebo. In addition, a double-blind, placebo-controlled study of forty nonanemic elite athletes with mildly low iron stores found that twelve weeks of iron supplementation enhanced aerobic performance.

Other double-blind trials also observed benefits with iron supplementation for marginally iron-depleted athletes. However, several other studies failed to find significant improvements. These contradictory results suggest that the benefits of iron supplements for nonanemic, iron-deficient athletes are small at most.

Colostrum. Colostrum is the fluid new mothers' breasts produce during the first day or two after birth. Colostrum contains growth factors, such as insulin-like growth factor 1 (IGF-1) that could enhance muscle development. On this basis, it has been tried as a sports supplement.

An eight-week double-blind study found that the use of colostrum enhanced sprinting performance. Other double-blind studies found improvements in rowing performance and vertical jump. In addition, one small double-blind study found that colostrum, compared to whey protein, increased lean mass in healthy men and women undergoing aerobic and resistance training. However, no improvements in performance were seen in this trial. In a double-blind, placebo-controlled study, the use of colostrum in an eight-week training period did not improve performance on an exercise-to-exhaustion test; however, it did improve performance on a repeat bout twenty minutes later.

Research suggests that the growth factor IGF-1 in colostrum is not directly absorbed into the body. Yet, consumption of colostrum nonetheless increases IGF-1 levels in the blood, perhaps by stimulating its natural release.

Pyruvate. Pyruvate, also called "dihydroxyacetone pyruvate," supplies the body with pyruvic acid. This natural compound plays important roles in the manufacture and use of energy. Pyruvate supplements have become popular with bodybuilders and other athletes based on slim evidence that pyruvate can improve body composition. However, the evidence regarding pyruvate as an ergogenic aid is weak and contradictory at best. One study failed to find that pyruvate supplements improved body composition or exercise performance; furthermore, pyruvate appeared to negate the beneficial effect of exercise on cholesterol profile.

Policosanol. Policosanol is a mixture of waxy substances manufactured from sugarcane. It contains octacosanol, which is also made from wheat germ oil. Both are marketed as performance-enhancing dietary supplements said to increase muscle strength and endurance and improve reaction time and stamina. However, the only evidence for policosanol as a performance enhancer comes from one small double-blind trial with marginal results.

Phosphatidylserine. Phosphatidylserine (PS) is a phospholipid and a major component of cell membranes. Good evidence suggests that PS can improve mental function, especially in the elderly. However, PS has also been marketed as a sports supplement to help bodybuilders and power athletes develop larger and stronger muscles. This claim is based on modest evidence indicating that PS slows the release of cortisol following heavy exercise.

Cortisol is a hormone that causes muscle tissue to break down. For unclear reasons, the body produces cortisol levels after heavy exercise. Strength athletes who believe natural cortisol release works against their efforts to rapidly build muscle mass hope that PS will help them advance more quickly. However, only two double-blind, placebo-controlled studies of PS as a sports supplement have been reported, and neither found effects on cortisol levels. Of these small trials, one found a possible ergogenic benefit, and the other did not.

Another study evaluated the use of phosphatidylserine for improving the performance of golfers. While improvement in perceived stress levels failed to reach statistical significance, participants who were given phosphatidylserine did tee-off successfully at a greater rate than those given placeboes.

Branched-chain amino acids. Amino acids are molecules that form proteins when joined together. Three (leucine, isoleucine, and valine) are called branched-chain amino acids (BCAAs). This term describes the shape of the molecules. Muscles have a particularly high BCAA content.

Both strength training and endurance exercise use greater amounts of BCAAs than normal daily activities, perhaps increasing an athlete's need for dietary intake of these amino acids. Sports such as mountaineering and skiing may cause even greater depletion of BCAAs because of metabolic changes at higher altitudes. Athletes have tried BCAA supplements to build muscle, improve performance, postpone fatigue, and cure overtraining syndrome (prolonged fatigue and other symptoms caused by excessive exercise). However, most evidence suggests that BCAAs are not helpful for these purposes.

Whey protein is rich in BCAAs, and on this basis, it has also been proposed as a bodybuilding aid. However, there is little evidence that whey protein is more effective than any other protein. One small double-blind study found evidence that casein and whey protein were more effective than placebo at promoting muscle growth after exercise. Still, whey was no more effective than the far less expensive casein. Another study failed to find benefits with combined whey and soy protein supplementation. However, a small study found more ergogenic benefits with whey than casein.

Other amino acids. Besides BCAAs, athletes use several other amino acids, sometimes individually and sometimes in combination. Amino acids believed by some to have ergogenic effects include arginine, glutamine, and ornithine (ornithine and glutamine combined form ornithine alpha-ketoglutarate), and the branched-chain amino acids leucine, isoleucine, and valine. However, evidence supporting the use of amino acids as ergogenic aids is sparse to nonexistent. The few clinical trials performed generally do not show positive results.

Carnitine. Carnitine, a substance closely related to amino acids, is used by the body to convert fat into energy. Even though the body can manufacture all it needs, supplemental carnitine could, in theory, improve the ability of certain tissues to produce energy, leading to its promotion as a sports performance enhancer. However, there is no meaningful evidence that this is the case.

Chromium. The mineral chromium has been sold as a "fat burner" and is also said to help build muscle tissue. However, studies evaluating its benefits as a performance enhancer and assessing its effectiveness as an aid to bodybuilding have yielded almost entirely negative results.

Coenzyme Q10. Coenzyme Q10 (CoQ10) is a natural substance that plays a fundamental role in the mitochondria, the parts of the cell that produce energy from food. On this basis, CoQ10 has been proposed as a performance enhancer for athletes. However, most clinical trials have found no significant improvement with using CoQ10.

Inosine. Inosine is an important chemical found throughout the body. It plays many roles, one of which is helping to make adenosine triphosphate (ATP), the body's main form of usable energy. Inosine supplements have been proposed as an energy booster for athletes based on this fact. However, most of the available evidence suggests that it does not work.

Ribose. Ribose is a carbohydrate that is also vital for the manufacture of ATP. Ribose has shown some promise for improving exercise capacity in people with certain enzyme deficiencies and other rare conditions that cause muscle pain during exertion. On this basis, it has been touted as an athletic performance enhancer; however, six small, double-blind, placebo-controlled human trials failed to find any benefit. In one of these studies, dextrose (a form of ordinary sugar) proved effective, while ribose did not.

Gamma oryzanol. Preliminary evidence suggests that gamma oryzanol, derived from rice bran oil, may increase endorphin release and aid muscle development. These findings have created interest in using gamma oryzanol as a sports supplement. However, a nine-week, double-blind, placebo-controlled trial of twenty-two weight-trained males found no difference between placebo and 500 mg daily of gamma oryzanol in terms of performance, body composition, or hormone levels.

Trimethylglycine. Trimethylglycine (TMG) is a naturally occurring compound that may help prevent atherosclerosis. It is, therefore, sometimes taken as a supplement. During its metabolism in the body, TMG is turned into another substance, dimethylglycine (DMG).

In Russia, DMG has been used extensively as an athletic performance enhancer and has become popular among American athletes. Trimethylglycine is less expensive and may have the same effects as DMG since it changes into DMG in the body. However, there is no evidence that DMG is effective and even some evidence that it is not.

Dehydroepiandrosterone. Athletes have used dehydroepiandrosterone (DHEA) on the belief that (like phosphatidylserine) it might limit the body's response to cortisol and thereby cause an increase in muscle tissue growth. However, study results have not established whether or not DHEA interferes with cortisol. Furthermore, studies of DHEA as an aid to increasing muscle mass or enhancing sports performance have produced mixed results at best.

Tribulus terrestris. Tribulus terrestris is a tropical plant with a long history of medicinal use. It has been tried for low libido in men and women, impotence, and female infertility.

One theory regarding how *T. terrestris* might help with sexual disorders is that a component from the plant called "protodioscin" is converted into the hormone DHEA in the body. The body uses DHEA as a building block for testosterone, estrogen (and other hormones). This finding has led bodybuilders and strength athletes to try *T. terrestris* for increasing muscular development. However, the scientific evidence seems to be against it. These results are not surprising because DHEA itself has not been found effective as a sports supplement.

One study involving fifteen men compared the effects of *T. terrestris* (3.21 mg per kilogram of body weight; for example, 292 mg daily for a two-hundred-pound man) with a placebo on body composition and endurance among men engaged in resistance training. At the end of the eight-week study, the only significant difference between the treatment and placebo groups was that the placebo group showed greater gains in endurance.

Another double-blind, placebo-controlled study, which enrolled twenty-two athletes and followed them for five weeks, failed to find benefit. The dose used in this trial was fixed at 450 mg daily for all participants.

Phosphate. Because phosphate plays a fundamental role in the body's energy-producing pathways, it has been suggested that taking high doses of phosphate (phosphate loading) before athletic activities might enhance performance. Phosphate-containing chemicals are also part of the process that allows oxygen release from hemoglobin. This fact has also intrigued researchers looking for ergogenic aids. However, while some studies have found that phosphate loading improves maximum oxygen utilization, others have not. Flaws in study design cast doubt on the positive results.

Commercial preparations. A small double-blind study of a mixture of various herbs and supplements marketed as SPORT found no evidence that it can improve sports performance in trained athletes.

Stimulants. Some athletes have used several plant-derived stimulants to improve their performance. These stimulants include ephedrine from the Chinese herb ma huang (also called "ephedra") and caffeine from coffee, tea, maté, cola, or guarana (a plant native to South America). Both ephedrine and caffeine are central nervous system stimulants. Caffeine also appears to change the way the body burns calories, possibly allowing it to burn fats first and preserve muscle glycogen for later in athletic performances (in a way, "saving the best for last").

Caffeine does appear to improve performance during endurance-type exercises. The International Olympic Committee has set a tolerance limit for caffeine in the urine at 12 micrograms per milliliter.

Ephedrine's value in enhancing sports performance has not been established; at the same time, serious safety issues are associated with its use. Some sports federations have determined that specific amounts of ephedrine in an athlete's system are grounds for disqualification.

Other. One small double-blind trial found that using the herb Rhodiola rosea improved endurance exercise performance. However, another study failed to find benefits from combining Cordyceps and Rhodiola.

A variety of antioxidants have been proposed for enhancing recovery after heavy exercise. One study found weak evidence that a combination of vitamin E (400 mg daily) and vitamin C (1,000 mg daily) taken for three weeks can improve aerobic performance.

Heavy exercise causes increased calcium loss through sweat; the body does not compensate for this by reducing calcium loss in the urine. The result can be a net calcium loss great enough that it presents health concerns for menopausal women, who are already at risk for osteoporosis. One study found that using an inexpensive calcium supplement (calcium carbonate), taken at a dose of 400 mg twice daily, is sufficient to offset this loss.

A small study found endurance exercise benefits with the herb *Panax notoginseng*. Another small trial suggests that acupuncture may enhance peak performance capacity. Weak evidence hints that arachidonic acid supplements might enhance response to resistance training.

Using a low-glycemic-index snack three hours before endurance running may be more helpful than a high-glycemic-index (carbohydrate) snack. However, another study failed to find benefits.

Galactose is a sugar that the body combines with glucose to create lactose ("milk sugar"). For various theoretical reasons, it has been hypothesized that using galactose might enhance endurance exercise performance. However, the one small study designed to test this hypothesis found that the consumption of galactose before endurance exercise proved detrimental.

A small double-blind study failed to find any performance or training-enhancing benefits with a newly marketed silicate product. Clinical trials also failed to show benefits with astaxanthin, fish oil, N-acetylcysteine, soy isoflavones, and tyrosine supplements.

Numerous other natural substances have been marketed as ergogenic aids, despite an essentially absolute absence of evidence that they help. These substances include *Cordyceps*, *Cystoseira canariensis*, deer antler velvet, ipriflavone, lipoic acid, methoxyisoflavone, nicotinamide adenine dinucleotide, and suma. One study found that L-citrulline, another purported ergogenic aid, actually decreases exercise capacity.

Many marketers sell products that they claim will act like human growth hormone, often called "HGH enhancers." However, these products are entirely speculative because there are no natural treatments proven to raise human growth hormone levels. Similarly, no herbs or supplements are known to act as "natural anabolic steroids."

One small study failed to find benefits with a liquid multivitamin-multimineral supplement. Also, the amino acid beta-alanine is said to raise levels of carnosine, which is hypothesized to enhance performance in athletes undergoing resistance training. However, a double-blind study of twenty-six athletes failed to find benefit with 6 g of alanine daily.

TREATMENTS NOT RECOMMENDED

Three commonly recommended supplements are not recommended for athletes: vanadium, boron, and androstenedione. The mineral vanadium has been suggested for use by bodybuilders based on its effects on insulin. Still, there is no evidence that it helps. A double-blind, placebo-controlled study involving thirty-one weight-trained athletes found no benefit of supplementation at more than one thousand times the recommended dose. Furthermore, there are serious safety concerns about taking vanadium at such high doses.

The mineral boron has been proposed as a sports supplement because it is thought to increase testosterone levels. However, studies have failed to provide meaningful evidence that it helps increase muscle mass or enhance performance. Furthermore, clinical studies suggest that boron supplementation is more likely to increase estrogen than testosterone. Increased estrogen is not likely to have a sports performance benefit in men. In women, it might increase the risk of breast cancer. Therefore, supplemental boron is not recommended as a sports supplement.

The hormone androstenedione enhances athletic performance and strength by increasing testosterone production, thereby building muscle. However, in double-blind studies, when androstenedione was given to men, it neither altered total testosterone levels nor improved sports performance, strength, or lean body mass. However, it increased estrogen levels, an effect that would not be considered favorable. Androstenedione does appear to raise testosterone levels in women, but it is unclear whether this would produce favorable results.

—*EBSCO CAM Review Board*

Further Reading

Candow, D. G., et al. "Effect of Whey and Soy Protein Supplementation Combined with Resistance Training in Young Adults." *International Journal of Sport Nutrition and Exercise Metabolism*, vol. 16, no. 3, 2006, pp. 233-44.

Carpenter, K. C., et al. "Baker's Yeast Beta-Glucan Supplementation Increases Monocytes and Cytokines Post-Exercise: Implications for Infection Risk?" *The British Journal of Nutrition*, vol. 109, no. 3, 2013, pp. 478-86.

Chilibeck, P. D., et al. "Effect of Creatine Ingestion After Exercise on Muscle Thickness in Males and Females." *Medicine and Science in Sports and Exercise*, vol. 36, no. 10, 2004, pp. 1781-88.

"Creatine." *MedlinePlus*, 4 Jan. 2020, medlineplus.gov/druginfo/natural/873.html. Accessed 30 June 2020.

De Bock, K., et al. "Acute Rhodiola rosea Intake Can Improve Endurance Exercise Performance." *International Journal of Sport Nutrition and Exercise Metabolism*, vol. 14, no. 3, 2004, 298-307.

"Dietary Supplements for Exercise and Athletic Performance." *National Institutes of Health, Office of Dietary Supplements*, US Department of Health and Human Services, 4 Oct. 2017, ods.od.nih.gov/factsheets/ExerciseAndAthleticPerformance-Consumer/. Accessed 30 June 2020.

Earnest, C. P., et al. "Low vs. High Glycemic Index Carbohydrate Gel Ingestion during Simulated 64-km Cycling Time Trial Performance." *The Journal of Strength and Conditioning Research*, vol. 18, no. 3, 2004, pp. 466-72.

Fry, A. C., et al. "Effect of a Liquid Multivitamin/Mineral Supplement on Anaerobic Exercise Performance." *Research in Sports Medicine*, vol. 14, no. 1, 2006, pp. 53-64.

Igwebuike, A., et al. "Lack of DHEA Effect on a Combined Endurance and Resistance Exercise Program in Postmenopausal Women." *The Journal of Clinical Endocrinology and Metabolism*, vol. 93, 2008, pp. 534-38.

Kendrick, I. P., et al. "The Effects of Ten Weeks of Resistance Training Combined with Beta-Alanine Supplementation on Whole Body Strength, Force Production, Muscular Endurance, and Body Composition." *Amino Acids*, vol. 34, no. 4, 2008, pp. 547-54.

Martin, B. R., et al. "Exercise and Calcium Supplementation: Effects on Calcium Homeostasis in Sportswomen." *Medicine and Science in Sports and Exercise*, vol. 39, no. 9, 2007, pp. 1481-86.

Murphy, M., et al. "Whole Beetroot Consumption Acutely Improves Running Performance." *Journal of the Academy of Nutrition and Dietetics*, vol. 112, no. 4, 2012, 548-52.

Rogerson, S., et al. "The Effect of Five Weeks of *Tribulus terrestris* Supplementation on Muscle Strength and Body Composition During Preseason Training in Elite Rugby League Players." *The Journal of Strength and Conditioning Research*, vol. 21, no. 2, 2007, pp. 348-53.

Sellami, Maha, et al. "Herbal Medicine for Sports: A Review." *Journal of the International Society of Sports Nutrition*, vol. 15, no. 14, 2018, doi:10.1186/s12970-018-0218-y.

Senchina, David. "Athletics and Herbal Supplements." *American Scientist*, vol. 101, no. 2, Mar.-Apr. 2013, doi:10.1511/2013.101.134.

Smith, W. A., et al. "Effect of Glycine Propionyl-L-Carnitine on Aerobic and Anaerobic Exercise Performance." *International Journal of Sport Nutrition and Exercise Metabolism*, vol. 18, no. 1, 2008, pp. 19-36.

Wu, C. L., and C. Williams. "A Low Glycemic Index Meal Before Exercise Improves Endurance Running Capacity in Men." *International Journal of Sport Nutrition and Exercise Metabolism*, vol. 16, no. 5, 2006, pp. 510-27.

SUPPLEMENTS

Category: Treatment
Specialties and related fields: Alternative medicine, family medicine, internal medicine, nutrition
Definition: chemical compounds, concentrated into pills, powders, and capsules, are used to prevent or treat diseases

KEY TERMS

coenzymes: a nonprotein compound that is necessary for the functioning of an enzyme

photonutrients: any chemical or nutrient derived from a plant source that absorbs light

phytonutrients: a substance found in certain plants which is believed to be beneficial to human health and help prevent various diseases

vitamins: an organic molecule that is an essential micronutrient that an organism needs in small quantities for the proper functioning of its metabolism

THE ROLE OF SUPPLEMENTS

Adequate nutrition is the foundation of good health. Everyone needs the four basic nutrients: water, carbohydrates, proteins, and fats. It is important to choose the proper foods to deliver these nutrients and, as necessary, to complement the diet with supplements.

Health-conscious adults have heard the message repeatedly that they can get the vitamins they need from the foods they eat. Still, surveys have shown that people in many countries fail to eat adequate amounts of fruit, vegetables, whole grains, and low-fat dairy foods. Should public health officials or registered dieticians recommend that people take supplements to compensate for poor eating habits? The answer to this question can be found in a discussion of vitamin supplements.

The 1990s brought to light much new information about human nutrition, its effects on the body, and its role in disease. The fuel for the body's engine comes directly from the food one eats, which contains many vital nutrients. Nutrients come in the form of vitamins, minerals, enzymes, water, amino acids, carbohydrates, and lipids (fats). These nutrients provide people with the basic materials that human bodies need to sustain life.

One of the latest types of dietary supplements is nutraceuticals. These supplements are obtained from naturally derived chemicals in plants, called "photonutrients," that make the plants biologically active. They are not nutrients in the classic sense. They determine a plant's color, ability to resist disease and flavor.

Nutritionists have discovered that fruits and vegetables, grains, and legumes contain other healthful nutrients called "phytochemicals." Researchers have identified thousands of phytochemicals that can remove these chemical compounds and concentrate them into pills, powders, and capsules. Phytochemicals are believed to be powerful ammunition in the war against cancer and other cellular mutations. In simple terms, cancer is a mutation of body cells through a multistep process. Phytochemicals are hypothesized to fight that disease by stopping one or more steps leading to cancer. For example, a cancer process can be kindled when a carcinogenic molecule invades a cell, possibly from foods eaten or air breathed. Sulforaphane, a phytochemical commonly found in broccoli, is then hypothesized to activate an enzyme process that removes the carcinogen from the cell before harm is done.

Researchers and pharmaceutical companies sell concentrated forms of various phytochemicals in vegetables such as broccoli, brussels sprouts, cauliflower, and cabbage. Tomatoes, for example, are believed to contain an estimated ten thousand different phytochemicals. Because no single supplement can compete with nature, some nutritionists recommend a shopping basket full of fruits and vegetables instead of expensive bottled supplements.

In general, natural food supplements are composed of byproducts of foods that can provide a multitude of health benefits. Natural food supplements can be high in certain nutrients. Examples are aloe vera, bee pollen, fish oils, flaxseed, primrose oil, ginseng, ginkgo Biloba, garlic, and oat bran. However, one caution is that supplements of this type may not have the same quality control or oversight as medications prescribed by a doctor and bought from a pharmacy. As such, the effects of supplements may vary from pill to pill and bottle to bottle.

THE PROMISE OF ANTIOXIDANTS

No discussion of supplements would be complete without the mention of antioxidants. They are a group of vitamins, minerals, and enzymes that help to protect the body from forming free radicals. Free radicals are groups of atoms that can cause damage to cells and thus impair the immune system. This damage is also thought to be the basis for the aging process. Free radicals are believed to be formed through exposure to radiation and toxic chemicals such as cigarette smoke and overexposure to the sun's rays.

Some common antioxidants are vitamin A, and its precursor, beta carotene; vitamin C; and vitamin E. Zinc and the trace mineral selenium are thought to play an important role

IN THE NEWS: DIETARY SUPPLEMENT CRACKDOWNS BY THE FDA

In the past, the dietary supplement industry has been loosely regulated. Even though the Food and Drug Administration (FDA) required all the ingredients to be label-listed, there were no rules that limited the manufacturers' recommendations regarding serving sizes or the actual content amount of the nutrients. Moreover, no proof was required to guarantee product safety. However, as a result of the increasing problem of cross-contamination and misleading labeling of dietary supplements, coupled with adverse health outcomes, in March 2003, the FDA proposed new labeling and manufacturing standards. A final rule was announced in June 2007, indicating that the current Good Manufacturing Practices (cGMPs) would apply to the dietary supplement business. These standards were already in effect for the pharmaceutical and veterinary industries. The new rulings will establish industry-wide standards to guarantee consistent manufacturing standards, assure the public that the dietary supplement industry is safe, and provide pure products with known strengths and compositions.

The FDA had been averaging about 550 supplement-related adverse event reports yearly since 1993; however, that figure doubled in 2002. For instance, dietary supplements had to be recalled by one manufacturer because of excessive lead contamination. Another manufacturer of niacin supplements mistakenly marketed a product that contained ten times the safe limit of niacin, which was not reflected on the label. The product was recalled after postmarketing research reported nausea, vomiting, and liver damage episodes. Dietary supplements containing ephedra, used for weight loss, increased energy, and athletic performance enhancement, have been linked to several deaths, resulting in the banning ephedra-enhanced products. A sports supplement abuse case involved the use of vitamins by a world-class athlete who failed a drug doping test; the results were later reversed when the product was tested and found to be cross-contaminated by an anabolic steroid compound also manufactured at the same laboratory where the vitamins were packaged.

Under the cGMPs ruling, manufacturers must document the identity, composition, purity, quality, and strength of the ingredients in dietary supplements. If the product deviates from what the manufacturer has claimed to be the ingredients, the FDA considers the product adulterated. The minimum standards require physical plants to be constructed to ensure proper manufacturing operations, facility maintenance and cleaning, quality control procedures, final product testing before going to market, and better methods for handling and resolving consumer complaints. These rulings do not limit consumers' access to dietary supplements but ensure a safer product.

—*Bonita L. Marks*

in neutralizing free radicals. Each vitamin or mineral has a recommended daily allowance (RDA).

Some in the field of nutrition have recommended higher supplementation doses of antioxidants, and specific use of four antioxidant supplements—vitamins C and E, selenium, and mixed carotenes—to protect the immune system even further. Recommendations such as this are numerous and related to different kinds of supplement use. People must weigh them carefully against data obtained from controlled clinical trials. While many of the substances touted as beneficial to health may have some benefits, supplements can be harmful in the wrong person, at the wrong dose, if taken in combination with the wrong medications or diet, or if taken in the presence of certain health conditions. For example, it is possible to overdose on vitamins such as A, B, and E or iron supplements. Some supplements, like St. John's wort, may create a side effect of light sensitivity, and discontinuing drugs such as valerian root can lead to heart problems. Also, it is easy to succumb to the temptation to seek "health in a bottle" instead of engaging in proven preventive practices. For these reasons, careful consideration and consultation with one's doctor should occur before embarking on any regimen of supplements.

PERSPECTIVE AND PROSPECTS

Natural supplements have been used for centuries in many parts of the world as alternative medicines. The use of supplements is based on modern research and development and discoveries by mainstream scientists about the benefits of various substances. Substances such as garlic and aloe vera are examples of home remedies that have shown some promise for different kinds of ailments.

Considered and careful examination of supplement regimens in controlled clinical trials will serve as the ultimate test of the utility of these substances for health purposes. Simultaneously, consumers must remain aware that personal use of these supplements may sometimes be somewhat experimental. Quality control concerns and interactions between supplements and prescribed medications are important considerations. Additionally, knowledge of the supplements found in pills or popular beverages and how they may interact with street drugs of different types is also important to avoid unnecessary harm. Such considerations are especially true for children and elders.

—*Lisa Levin Sobczak, Nancy A. Piotrowski*

Further Reading

Balch, James F., and Phyllis A. Balch. *Prescription for Nutritional Healing: A Practical A to Z Reference to Drug-Free Remedies Using Vitamins, Minerals, Herbs, and Food Supplements*. 4th rev. ed., Avery, 2008.

Hendler, Sheldon Saul. *The Doctors' Vitamin and Mineral Encyclopedia*. Simon & Schuster, 1990.

Murray, Michael. *The Pill Book Guide to Natural Medicines: Vitamins, Minerals, Nutritional Supplements, Herbs, and Other Natural Products*. Bantam, 2002.

The PDR Family Guide to Nutritional Supplements: An Authoritative A-to-Z Resource on the One Hundred Most Popular Nutritional Therapies and Nutraceuticals. Ballantine Books, 2001.

Weil, Andrew. *Eight Weeks to Optimum Health: A Proven Program for Taking Full Advantage of Your Body's Natural Healing Power*. Rev. ed., Ballantine Books, 2007.

VITAMINS AND MINERALS

Category: Biology
Specialties and related fields: Endocrinology, family medicine, internal medicine, nutrition
Definition: chemicals that supply the body with the means of metabolizing (extracting and using the energy from) the macronutrients (fats, carbohydrates, and proteins) it ingests; essential diet ingredients

KEY TERMS

fat-soluble vitamins: vitamins that, because of their structure and solubility, migrate to fatty tissues in the body, where they are stored

macronutrients: materials ingested in large amounts to supply the energy and materials for physical bodies

megadose: ten or more times the recommended daily allowance of a nutrient

micronutrients: substances of which only milligrams are needed in the daily diet, such as vitamins and minerals

mineral: an inorganic salt of particular metals or elements needed for good health

recommended daily (or dietary) allowance (RDA): the intake levels of the essential nutrients that are considered adequate to meet the known nutritional needs of most healthy persons

trace elements: elements needed in the diet at levels of less than 100 milligrams per day

vitamin: an organic compound constituent of food that is consumed in relatively small amounts (less than 0.1 gram per kilogram of body weight per day) and that is essential to the maintenance of life

water-soluble vitamins: vitamins that, because of their structure, show strong solubility in water; they normally pass through the body in a relatively short time

STRUCTURE AND FUNCTIONS

Vitamins are organic compounds (compounds made up of carbon, oxygen, nitrogen, sulfur, or hydrogen) that are constituents of food and crucial to the maintenance of life and good health. They make possible the production of energy and the formation of coherent body tissues from the macronutrients normally consumed in a regular diet. They are, among other things, coenzymes that serve as oxidizing, reducing, and transferring chemicals at the active sites of enzymes. Vitamins are part of the one hundred or so organic compounds that are of the proper size and stability to be absorbed from the digestive tract into the bloodstream without digestion or breakdown. Nevertheless, they are not produced in the body in large amounts to keep a person healthy since they have always been available in food; there was probably no need for the human metabolism to produce them. Plants synthesize vitamins; therefore, plants constitute the principal natural source of these compounds.

Vitamins are divided into two main groups: water-soluble and fat-soluble vitamins. Structural differences account for the two types of solubility. Fat-soluble vitamins (such as vitamins A, D, E, and K) consist mainly of hydrocarbon groupings (nonpolar hydrocarbon chains and rings compatible with nonpolar oil and fat). They are structurally similar to fats, whereas water-soluble vitamins have polar hydroxyl (-OH) and carboxyl (-COOH) groups that are attracted to and form hydrogen bonds with water. One of the most important differences between vitamins is the result of their solubility: Fat-soluble vitamins are stored in the body tissues and organs for relatively long periods, while water-soluble vitamins are eliminated from the body in a relatively fast manner, sometimes in a matter of hours.

Vitamin A (retinol) maintains the health of the eyes, skin, and mucous membranes and is particularly important for good vision in dim light. There are various physiological equivalents to vitamin A, compounds with closely related structures that can be used as the vitamin itself. Beta carotene is a provitamin (a substance that can be easily converted to a vitamin) of vitamin A found in carrots. The vitamin can also be found in liver and liver oils. Lack of vitamin A can cause night or total blindness.

The B vitamins are often considered a group called the "B complex" because they work together as coenzymes in biochemical reactions leading to growth and energy production. They are water-soluble and easily eliminated from food in the cooking process. They are present in various foods, especially meat and dairy products. Members of this group include pyridoxine (B_6), involved in at least sixty enzyme reactions (mostly in the metabolism and synthesis of proteins); thiamine (B_1), a coenzyme in carbohydrate metabolism and involved in energy production, digestion, and nerve activity; riboflavin (B_2), used in obtaining energy from foods; pantothenic acid (B_3), needed for proper growth; niacin (B4), needed for the production of healthy tissues; cobalamin (B_{12}), involved in the production and growth of red blood cells; and folic acid (B_9), also involved in the production of red blood cells and metabolism. Deficiency symptoms include anemia, skin disorders, and nervous system disorders.

Vitamin C, or ascorbic acid, is involved in the destruction of invading bacteria, in the synthesis and activity of interferon (which prevents entry of viruses into cells), in decreasing the effect of toxic substances (such as drugs and pollutants), and in the formation of connective tissue. Humans are one of the few species of animals for which ascorbic acid is a vitamin since other species produce it in their metabolic processes. Vitamin C is found mostly in citrus fruits. Deficiency symptoms include the degeneration of tissue and scurvy.

Vitamin D (calciferol) promotes the absorption of calcium and phosphorus through the intestinal wall and into the bloodstream. Its deficiency induces the disease rickets and, in adults, the malformation of bones. Unlike other vitamins, it forms in the body through the action of the sun's ultraviolet light. As with the vitamin B complex, vitamin D has a set of closely related molecular structures called D1, D2, D3, and so on. All these structures have the same physiological function. Because of limited sun exposure, copious clothing, and indoor living and working conditions, humans need to add vitamin D to their diet, as in fortified milk, cod liver oil, or vitamin supplements.

Vitamin E (alpha-tocopherol) is an antioxidant of polyunsaturated fatty acids (fatty acids with numerous double bonds). These fatty acids readily form particularly damaging peroxides that can lead to runaway oxidation in cells. Vitamin E protects the integrity of cell membranes, which contain considerable amounts of fat. It also helps maintain the integrity of the circulatory and central nervous systems; is involved in the functioning of the kidneys, lungs, liver, and genitalia; and detoxifies poisonous materials absorbed by the body. Aging, in some theories, is considered to be the cumulative effect of free radicals (reactive atoms) running wild in the body. The antioxidant properties of vitamin E may make it a good candidate for inhibiting aging or at least preventing premature aging. Its deficiency symptoms in humans are unknown. Vitamin E is present in various foods, especially in grain oils.

Biotin (also called "vitamin H") participates in metabolism by acting as a carboxyl carrier for several enzymes. Its sources are liver, cereals, and egg yolks. Deficiency symptoms include alopecia (the loss or absence of hair) and skin rashes.

Vitamin K completes the list of vitamins. This vitamin is commonly found in plants and vegetables. It participates in blood clotting, and its deficiency can cause bleeding and liver damage.

The term "minerals," when used in a nutritional context, includes all the nutritional, chemical elements of foods obtained from macronutrients, except for carbon, hydrogen, nitrogen, oxygen, and sulfur. This term also refers to metal elements combined with others in compounds such as soluble inorganic salts. In this combined form, they serve vital functions in the body.

Among their many functions, minerals are components of enzymes, are structural components of body parts such as bones, are involved in maintaining the electrolyte balance in body fluids, and transport materials, as hemoglobin does in blood. Minerals pass slowly through the body and are excreted in the feces, urine, and sweat. Therefore, people must continuously replace them to maintain an appropriate mineral balance in their bodies. Because living beings cannot generate minerals in their bodies, they must obtain them from foods or supplements. Plants pick up minerals directly from the soil, and animals get them from the plants they ingest. As opposed to vitamins, which plants synthesize, people cannot acquire minerals from their diets if they are not in the soil.

There are seventeen known minerals, although many others may exist. Since most of them are present in the body in relatively small amounts, their functions have been determined through the symptoms of various dietary deficiencies. Minerals can be grouped into two classes. The major elements-calcium, phosphorus, and magnesium, are required in amounts of 1 gram or more per day. The trace elements include chlorine, chromium, cobalt, copper, fluorine, iodine, iron, manganese, molybdenum, nickel, selenium, sulfur, vanadium, and zinc and are needed in milligram or microgram quantities each day.

Calcium, probably the best-known mineral, is the most abundant mineral in the body: up to 1.5 or 2.0 percent of total body weight, with 99 percent of it in bones and teeth. In the nervous system, it is used to slow down the heartbeat. It is metabolized by a hormone synthesized from calciferol (vitamin D). Excess calcium can give rise to kidney stones. Its deficiency is common in postmenopausal women, who produce less estrogen. This decrease encourages bone dissolution, and when bones are dissolved, calcium is lost. Calcium is found in milk, dairy products, fish, and green vegetables. Phosphorus, the second most common mineral, is a structural component of bones and soft tissue. It is found in nearly all foods.

Sodium and potassium cations (positively charged atoms) are components of many minerals. They work in the conservation of electrolytic balance in cell fluids. Potassium governs the activity of many cellular enzymes. At the same time, sodium keeps the water content of cellular fluids in a healthy balance. For the body to work properly, it needs the appropriate sodium to potassium ratio. Potassium ions concentrate inside the cell, while sodium ions concentrate outside the cell. Natural, unprocessed foods have high sodium-to-potassium ratios. Because sodium and potassium compounds are very soluble in water, they dissolve during processing and cooking and are discarded. Sodium is replenished by adding salt to food, but this is not the case with potassium, which is not added to food. Care must be taken in this matter, either by eating more fresh foods or using a specialized table salt containing a mixture of sodium chloride and potassium chloride. The retention of sodium leads to water retention, edema (swollen legs and ankles), and high blood pressure in some individuals. Sodium is mostly in table salt, and potassium is in meat, dairy products, and fruit.

Magnesium and chloride ions are the most common minerals in cell fluids, as they regulate fluid balances and electrical charges. Magnesium controls the formation of proteins inside the cell and the transmission of electrical signals from cell to cell. Chloride is present in the stomach as hydrochloric acid or stomach acid. Magnesium is found in whole-grain cereals, dried fruits, and leafy green vegetables, and chloride is found in table salt.

Trace elements work in various ways, with most of them incorporated into the structure of enzymes, hormones, and related molecules or acting in conjunction with vitamins. Among the trace elements, one of the more important ones is iron, a critical part of the hemoglobin molecule of red blood cells and involved in oxygen transport. Fluoride, another trace element, helps harden the enamel of teeth to make them resistant to decay; zinc plays an important role in growth, the healing of wounds, and the development of male sex glands, and manganese is needed for healthy bones and a well-functioning nervous system. Iodine is involved in the proper operation of the thyroid gland, chromium is important in glucose metabolism, and cobalt aids in cell function. Copper and selenium are other trace elements needed by the body. Most trace elements are found in fish, meat, fruits, and vegetables.

RELATED DISEASES
A well-balanced diet provides ample vitamins of all kinds. Vitamin deficiencies are not common in the United States and other Western countries. Megadoses of vitamins can create harmful effects; however, a toxic dose exists for many vitamins. For example, when taken in excess, vitamin A can cause headache, nausea, vomiting, fatigue, swelling, bleeding, pain in the arms and legs, and congenital disabilities. However, an acute deficiency of the vitamin can impair vision and eventually cause blindness. Consequently, there must be a balance in vitamin intake. People can achieve this balance by following the recommended daily (or dietary) allowances (RDAs).

In the United States, the Food and Nutrition Board of the National Academy of Sciences and the National Research Council determined the daily needs for some vitamins and minerals. The Food and Drug Administration (FDA) made these findings the basis for its list of RDAs. These allowances are presented in units of grams or milligrams, and these amounts are determined using international units of biological activity. (Some vitamins come in several forms, all of which are physiologically equivalent.) Recommended daily allowances do not cover every single vitamin and mineral needed for good health nor the more extreme nutritional requirements that result from illness or unusual genetic makeup. They serve as general guidelines for healthy individuals. For some substances lacking specific RDAs, such as chromium and a handful of other elements, the FDA lists the daily ranges of these micronutrients that it considers safe and effective. Recommended daily allowances depend on gender, age, weight, and other conditions. They are normally presented on food labels as percentages of the daily dietary requirement.

In 2005, the US Department of Agriculture (USDA) updated the Food Guide Pyramid. The new pyramid emphasizes the need for physical activity (thirty minutes of moderate or vigorous exercise per day) and the importance of variety in the diet. Unlike the older food pyramids, the 2005 version suggests food quantities in cups and ounces rather than as servings, which was ambiguous and confusing to consumers. For example, for a 2,000 calorie per day diet, the recommendations are six ounces of whole grains, two and a half cups of vegetables, two cups of fruit, three cups of dairy, and five and a half ounces from the meat and bean subgroup. Consumers can get personalized recommendations based on their age and gender at MyPyramid.gov.

The main criticisms of the 2005 food recommendations are that they do not mention any specific foods from which to abstain, that people who do not have web access cannot obtain personalized recommendations, and that the beef and dairy industry lobbies play a role in the USDA's decisions about these matters. Consumers should remember that the USDA's primary role is to promote agriculture in the United States. Politics are embedded in decisions about diets, and recommending that people eat less is not good for business. Some nutritionists and scientists believe that diet matters should be under the auspices of a more neutral party, such as the National Institutes of Health (NIH).

The activity of a vitamin or mineral depends only on its molecular structure, not on its source. Therefore, the synthetic vitamins found in food supplements provide the same nutrients as naturally occurring ones. However, it is crucial to remember that other substances or nutrients are present in food that help people obtain the necessary vitamin and mineral requirements. Authentic food often contains additional substances that enhance the absorption and utilization of its nutrients. For example, the calcium naturally present in food is more likely to carry with it any vitamin D or phosphorus that the body might need for its optimum use than is the calcium found in an antacid tablet or a food supplement. A balanced diet provides a diversity of nutrients that no pills can match.

Supplementation is commonly thought of as a means of maintaining nutritional equilibrium in the body. The major medical use of the vitamins is in curing the deficiency diseases caused by their absence from the diet. An FDA panel has judged nine vitamins as safe and effective over-the-counter drugs.

Many different analytical methods, such as ultraviolet-visible and infrared spectroscopy, paper, thin-layer, gas-liquid chromatography, mass spectroscopy, and biological assays, have been used to detect and identify vitamins. They have greatly helped to explain the complex structures of these compounds. These methods are also used to determine the vitamin content of a particular food item, providing the consumer with valuable nutritional information.

PERSPECTIVE AND PROSPECTS

Vitamin deficiency diseases such as scurvy, beriberi, and pellagra have plagued the world since the existence of written records. The concept of a vitamin or "accessory growth factor" was developed early in the twentieth century. In 1912, Casimir Funk, a Polish biochemist, isolated a dietary growth factor from the outer covering of rice grains and found that, when added to the food of those who had beriberi, it cured the disease. The factor was an organic compound called an "amine" (i.e., a compound containing nitrogen combined with carbon and hydrogen). Funk coined the term "vitamin" (meaning "life-giving amine") for the compound, which is now called "thiamin" or "vitamin B_1." In the next five decades, there was an exciting era of the isolation, identification, and synthesis of vitamins. Nutritional researchers discovered that not all vitamins are amines and changed the term to "vitamins." As biochemists obtained more information on the structure of vitamins, names changed from general ones (such as vitamin C) to more specific ones (such as ascorbic acid). These discoveries led to the availability of inexpensive synthetic vitamins and a dramatic reduction in overt vitamin deficiency diseases.

Small amounts of vitamins are essential for good health. However, the benefits of taking megadoses of certain vitamins to prevent or cure certain ailments are often debated. Even so, there is evidence that high levels of vitamins can prevent or alleviate several diseases. Improvements in the analytical methods used in detecting and identifying vitamins have led to better and more sensitive detection limits for these compounds. The result has been increased knowledge of vitamins and minerals and their function.

In 2002, the American Medical Association endorsed the notion that adults should take a multivitamin daily. This endorsement reversed the organization's long-standing antivitamin stance that vitamins were a waste of time and money for all except pregnant women and some people with chronic illnesses. The current recommendation, published in the Journal of the American Medical Association, acknowledges that vitamins may prevent chronic diseases, such as heart disease, cancer, and osteoporosis. Nevertheless, the efficacy and safety of regular intake of multivitamins remain a subject of debate in the medical community. In a 2013 book entitled *Do You Believe in Magic?: The Sense and Nonsense of Alternative Medicine*, Dr. Paul Offit of the University of Pennsylvania cites several studies suggesting that regular intake of vitamin supplements increases the risk of disease. However, critics like Dr. Dallas Clouatre of the American College of Nutrition argue that many vitamin studies rely on unscientific data, such as self-reporting through questionnaires.

—*Maria Pacheco, Lisa Levin Sobczak, LeAnna DeAngelo*

Further Reading

Balch, James F., and Phyllis A. Balch. *Prescription for Nutritional Healing: A Practical A to Z Reference to Drug-Free Remedies Using Vitamins, Minerals, Herbs, and Food Supplements.* 4th Rev. ed., Avery, 2008.

Duyff, Roberta Larson. *American Dietetic Association Complete Food and Nutrition Guide.* 3rd ed., John Wiley & Sons, 2007.

Lieberman, Shari, and Nancy Bruning. *Real Vitamin and Mineral Book.* 4th ed., Avery, 2007.

Murray, Michael. *The Pill Book Guide to Natural Medicines: Vitamins, Minerals, Nutritional Supplements, Herbs, and Other Natural Products.* Bantam, 2002.

Offit, Paul A. *Do You Believe in Magic?: The Sense and Nonsense of Alternative Medicine.* Harper, 2012.

Preidt, Robert. "Too Little Vitamin D May Hasten Disability as You Age." *HealthDay*, 17 July 2013, consumer.healthday.com/senior-citizen-information-31/misc-aging-news-10/too-little-vitamin-d-may-hasten-disability-as-you-age-678337.html.

Shelton, C. D. *Vitamins, Minerals & Supplements: Essential or Over-Hyped?* Amazon Digital Services Inc., 2013.

Weil, Andrew. *Eight Weeks to Optimum Health: A Proven Program for Taking Full Advantage of Your Body's Natural Healing Power.* Rev. ed., Ballantine Books, 2007.

Injuries

No one likes getting hurt, but you should seek help quickly when you do. Athletes are at high risk for injury. The hazards of contact sports are obvious, but factors such as inadequate nutrition, overtraining, and improper exercise technique carry less apparent but similar potential for harm. Healthcare professionals who specialize in rehabilitation can help the healing process. This section delves into some of the techniques they might use, as well as detailing common sports-related injuries. Topics discussed include: back pain, concussion, muscle sprains, repetitive strain injuries, tendon disorders, and traumatic brain injury.

Back Pain

Category: Disease/Disorder
Also known as: Backache
Specialties and related fields: Alternative medicine, anesthesiology, emergency medicine, exercise physiology, family medicine, general surgery, geriatrics and gerontology, neurology, nursing, obstetrics, occupational health, orthopedics, osteopathic medicine, physical therapy, preventive medicine, radiology, rheumatology, sports medicine
Definition: acute or chronic and usually severe pain centered along the spine, usually in the lower back and common in the neck and upper back

KEY TERMS

annular bulge: protrusion of a disk beyond its normal circumference, usually because of compression caused by gravity, the strain on the spine, or aging

cervical spine: the highest of three parts of the spine, consisting of seven vertebrae, named C1 (top of the neck) to C7, in a natural lordosis

herniated disk: prolapse of the nucleus through a rupture or weakness in the annulus

intervertebral disk: the flexible, cylindrical pad between every two vertebrae, consisting of the nucleus pulposis (gelatinous center) and the annulus fibrosis (concentric rings of cartilage); the flexibility, moistness, and thickness of the disk decreases naturally with age

kyphosis: backward curvature of the spine or a section of the spine

lordosis: forward curvature of the spine or a section of the spine

lumbar spine: the lowest of three parts of the spine, consisting of five vertebrae, named L1 to L5 (just above the sacrum), in a natural lordosis

radiculopathy: also called "nerve root entrapment" or "pinched nerve"; irritation or compression of the root of a spinal nerve between vertebrae, caused by an annular bulge, herniated disk, or spinal injury

referred pain: any pain whose origin is elsewhere in the body from where it is felt; with radiculopathy in the lumbar spine, the pain is typically in the leg

sciatica: intense pain in one buttock and down the back of that leg, caused by inflammation of the sciatic nerve, the largest nerve in the body; in some cases, this inflammation is referred pain from radiculopathy where the sciatic nerve originates between L4 and the sacrum

scoliosis: sideways curvature of the spine or a section of the spine

thoracic spine: the middle of three parts of the spine, consisting of twelve vertebrae, named T1 (top of the chest) to T12, in a natural kyphosis

CAUSES AND SYMPTOMS

Intervertebral disk problems cause most back pain. However, the disk problems themselves have various causes and manifestations. Annular bulges, disk herniation, muscular spasms, and strain from overexertion are just a few causes. Among these manifestations are sudden and persistent attacks of sharp, debilitating pain that exaggerate spinal kyphosis, may create scoliosis, and make standing up or bending over without assistance either impossible or very difficult.

Information on Back Pain

Causes: Usually disk disorders (herniation, muscular spasms, strain from overexertion, or poor posture)

Symptoms: Sudden and persistent attacks of sharp, debilitating pain

Duration: Acute or chronic

Treatments: Good posture and habits, painkillers, muscle relaxants, physical therapy; surgery in extreme cases

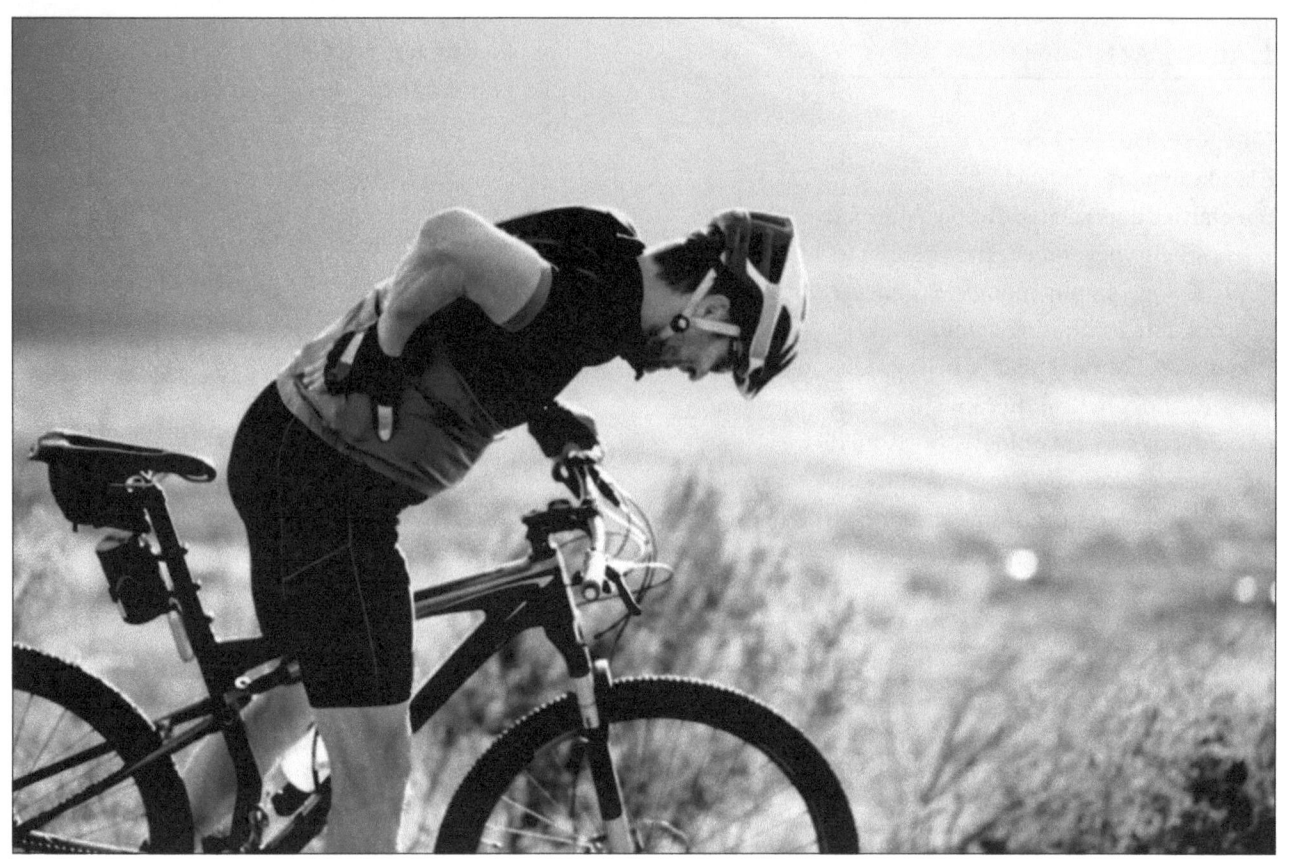

Back pain, common in athletes, can be caused by overworking muscles. Photo via iStock/:Mikolette. [Used under license.]

The more the lumbar spine approaches either kyphosis or scoliosis, the more out of alignment the natural curvature of the whole spine and the more pain results. Scoliosis or uncontrollable listing to one side is a frequent symptom of disk damage, usually either annular bulge or herniation.

Referred pain may appear from any lumbar radiculopathy. Still, the two most common presentations are in the thigh, from pinching the femoral nerve between L2 and L4 vertebrae, and sciatica, from pinching the sciatic nerve between L4 and the sacrum. Shooting pains elsewhere in the leg, genital dysfunction, incontinence, and other urinary or bowel complications may result from radiculopathy of several other lumbar, sacral, or lower thoracic nerves. In severe cases, partial paralysis or constant, intolerable pain may occur.

TREATMENT AND THERAPY

Many ways of treating back pain exist, and the program of treatment must be adapted to each patient's particular situation. Good posture is always essential. Learning to sit up straight, perhaps with a lumbar support roll, or a change of habits, such as learning to lift with the legs rather than the back, may be advised. Sometimes drug therapy with painkillers or muscle relaxants, or physical therapy with manipulation and exercises, is the only additional treatment required. As a last resort and in extreme cases, including emergency cases of incontinence or paralysis, surgery to repair a disk may be indicated.

Treatment options come not only from regular medicine but also from alternative, complementary, or allied health-care systems. Techniques drawn from chiropractic, osteopathy, yoga, acupuncture, and other therapy styles have sometimes provided either temporary or permanent relief. The McKenzie method of bending the spine backward, thus emphasizing lumbar lordosis, has proved successful.

PERSPECTIVE AND PROSPECTS

Low back pain seems to be equally prevalent in all eras and countries. Despite socioeconomic improvements in the lives of physical laborers, and even though a decreasing proportion of people worldwide make their living from physical labor, no concomitant decrease in new low back pain cases has been observed. If anything, there may be a slight increase in the percentage of low back pain cases in industrialized nations since the mid-twentieth century. People with desk-bound occupations and sedentary habits are at great risk for developing low back pain, especially if they slump in their chairs or fail to protect the natural lordosis of the lumbar spine.

Physicians no longer consider typical low back pain an injury or a disease. Since the late twentieth century, they have understood it as a natural degenerative condition that can usually be delayed by good posture and managed by physical therapy, painkilling drugs, and lifestyle changes.

—*Eric v.d. Luft*

Further Reading

Borenstein, David G., et al. *Low Back and Neck Pain: Comprehensive Diagnosis and Management*. 3rd ed., W. B. Saunders, 2004.

Brennan, Richard. *Back in Balance: Use the Alexander Technique to Combat Neck, Shoulder, and Back Pain*. Watkins, 2013.

Burn, Loic. *Back and Neck Pain: The Facts*. Oxford UP, 2006.

Cailliet, Rene. *Low Back Pain Syndrome: A Medical Enigma*. Lippincott Williams & Wilkins, 2003.

Chevan, Julia, and Phyllis A. Clapis. *Physical Therapy Management of Low Back Pain: A Case-Based Approach*. Jones Bartlett Learning, 2013.

Hodges, Paul W., et al. *Spinal Control: The Rehabilitation of Back Pain-State of the Art and Science*. Churchill Livingstone/Elsevier, 2013.

McGill, Stuart. *Low Back Disorders: Evidence-Based Prevention and Rehabilitation*. Human Kinetics, 2002.

McKenzie, Robin, and Craig Kubey. *Seven Steps to a Pain-Free Life: How to Rapidly Relieve Back and Neck Pain Using the McKenzie Method*. Dutton, 2000.

Owen, Liz, and Holly Lebowitz Rossi. *Yoga for a Healthy Lower Back: A Practical Guide to Developing Strength and Relieving Pain*. Shambhala, 2013.

Twomey, Lance T., and James R. Taylor, editors. *Physical Therapy of the Low Back*. Churchill Livingstone, 2000.

Waddell, Gordon. *The Back Pain Revolution*. 2nd ed., Churchill Livingstone/Elsevier, 2004.

BRUISES

Category: Disease/Disorder
Also known as: Ecchymoses, contusions, hematomas
Specialties and related fields: Emergency medicine, family medicine, hematology, pediatrics, vascular medicine, wound medicine
Definition: a bruise is an area of skin that has become discolored, usually due to trauma (a fall or hit to the affected area)

KEY TERMS

subcutaneous: beneath the skin
intramuscular: in underlying muscle
periosteal: in the bone

CAUSES AND SYMPTOMS

A bruise is a usually benign condition that happens when an individual has some injury. It may be a fall or a direct blow to any body part. As a result of the trauma, the affected body part undergoes various changes. A bruise can also occur spontaneously (a more serious illness or disease state) or from an allergic reaction. In most cases, bruises are not serious and resolve without medical treatment.

Bruises occur when small blood vessels just beneath the skin are broken. These broken blood vessels leak their contents (blood) into the surrounding soft tissue underneath the skin, which produces the characteristic black-and-blue discoloration. There are three types of bruises: subcutaneous (just beneath the skin), intramuscular (in the underlying muscle), and periosteal (in the bone). Bruises can last from several days to months. The typical black-and-blue mark begins to fade as the blood leaked into the surrounding tissue is reabsorbed. The discoloration turns to a light yellowish-green and then fades completely.

TREATMENT AND THERAPY
The initial treatment of bruises should include decreasing the bleeding, minimizing any swelling, and controlling the pain. Ice is very effective and should be applied to the affected area for thirty to sixty minutes at a time. The individual can ice their injury several times a day for two to three days. The ice should be in a container and covered by a towel to prevent damage to the skin. If possible, they should elevate the affected area above heart level. Wound elevation helps minimize swelling, which also helps decrease pain. If there is still discomfort after this period, then heat can be applied for twenty minutes at a time. The application of heat will help the blood be reabsorbed into the tissue. The last component of the treatment regimen should include pain control. Pain is easily controlled by using acetaminophen (Tylenol) or ibuprofen (Advil or Motrin).

Medical care should be sought if there is increased pain, decreased function (the affected part can no longer be used), headache, dizziness, fever (101° Fahrenheit or more), or a noticeable change in vision, or if the symptoms continue.

PERSPECTIVE AND PROSPECTS
Bruises are benign conditions that usually resolve without treatment. However, bruises are significant

> **INFORMATION ON BRUISES**
>
> **Causes**: Bleeding under the skin following injury; sometimes an allergic reaction or clotting disorder
>
> **Symptoms**: Black-and-blue skin discoloration, pain, swelling
>
> **Duration**: Acute
>
> **Treatments**: Ice, analgesics, sometimes heat

in an individual experiencing bruising without any clear reason for the occurrence. In this case, bruises can indicate something more serious, such as clotting disorders or other diseases. Simple self-care therapies will generally decrease discomfort and aid in a complete return to normal.

—*Rosslynn S. Byous*

Further Reading
"Bruise." *MedlinePlus*, 16 Nov. 2016, medlineplus.gov/bruises.html. Accessed 30 May 2022.
"Bruise: First Aid." *Mayo Clinic*, 12 Nov. 2020, www.mayoclinic.org/first-aid/first-aid-bruise/basics/art-20056663. Accessed 30 May 2022.
The Doctors Book of Home Remedies. Rev. ed., Bantam Books, 2009.
Gottlieb, William. *Alternative Cures: More than One Thousand of the Most Effective Natural Home Remedies*. Rodale, 2008.
Griffith, H. Winter. *Complete Guide to Sports Injuries: How to Treat Fractures, Bruises, Sprains, Strains, Dislocations, Head Injuries*. 3rd ed., Body Press/Perigee, 2004.
Moake, Joel L. "Bruising and Bleeding." *Merck Manual Consumer Version*, Nov. 2021, www.merckmanuals.com/home/blood-disorders/blood-clotting-process/bruising-and-bleeding. Accessed 30 May 2022.

Chronic Traumatic Encephalopathy (CTE)

Category: Condition
Specialties and related fields: Neurology, psychology, psychiatry, sports medicine, sports psychology

Definition: a progressive brain condition caused by repeated blows to the head and repeated concussions; it is commonly associated with contact sports, such as boxing or American football

KEY TERMS

dementia pugilistica ("punch drunk syndrome"): former name of CTE, first described in the 1920s as a condition that afflicted boxers

tau protein: a protein that helps stabilize the internal skeleton of neurons in the brain; a buildup of tau proteins is associated with neurodegenerative diseases

INTRODUCTION

Chronic traumatic encephalopathy (CTE) is a gradually progressing brain disease that occurs most frequently in athletes and other individuals who have experienced repeated blows, including concussions, to the head. The condition first became known in the 1920s as a disease affecting boxers. Additional cases mostly involving athletes were reported over the following decades. Still, broad recognition of CTE did not occur until the early 2000s. After being discovered in a deceased professional football player in the United States, it made headlines. In CTE, repetitive brain trauma sparks a progressive degeneration of brain tissue and an excessive buildup of a "tau protein" that can occur over months, years, or even decades. The progression continues even after the trauma incidents have stopped, leading to potential memory loss, confusion, depression, aggression, impaired judgment, problems with impulse control, and dementia.

BRIEF HISTORY

Chronic traumatic encephalopathy was initially dubbed *dementia pugilistica*, or "punch drunk syndrome," when first described in the 1920s as a condition that afflicted a group of boxers. A smattering of similar cases was reported in the subsequent years. In the 1960s, neurologists changed the condition's name to chronic traumatic encephalopathy. However, it was still largely considered a disease in the boxing community. That view changed in 2002 when a neuropathologist named Bennet Omalu documented and published the first evidence of CTE in a football player, American Hall of Famer Mike Webster of the Pittsburgh Steelers. Webster was only fifty years old at the time of his death. Still, his brain was ravaged by the toll CTE had taken over the years due to contact injuries suffered during his career on the field.

Since then, CTE has been diagnosed postmortem in several cases that garnered significant media attention, including the suicide deaths of National Football League (NFL) player Junior Seau and professional wrestler Chris Benoit, who hanged himself after killing his wife and son in a violent act of aggression. Debilitating depression and unchecked aggression are both common symptoms of late-stage CTE.

As a CTE-afflicted brain slowly degenerates, it will lose vital mass. As that happens, some brain areas are likely to atrophy while others are more apt to enlarge. Some areas of the brain will also undergo a buildup of tau protein, which is a molecule that traditionally steadies cellular structure in the neurons. However, suppose the tau protein becomes unbalanced or defective due to CTE. In that case, it can cause substantial interference with neuron function, inhibiting normal brain behavior and response.

OVERVIEW

The symptoms of CTE can be incapacitating for those affected. They may dramatically alter the lives of the person with CTE and that person's family and friends.

Some of the most frequently experienced symptoms of CTE are loss of memory, struggling to control impulsive and erratic behavior, impaired judgment, depression and aggression, problems with balance, and eventual signs of dementia. As the disease is still being studied and is often complicated to diagnose, some of the symptoms of CTE are often presumed to be part of the normal process of aging, or sometimes CTE is incorrectly diagnosed as other neurological disorders, such as Alzheimer or Parkinson's disease.

As of 2022, CTE can only be diagnosed after death during an autopsy examination of the brain. Funded by a grant from the Brain Injury Research Institute, the University of California in Los Angeles has embarked on research that may discover a means for diagnosing CTE in living patients. The idea is to use a biomarker to detect tau protein concentrations to identify CTE among the living. Other institutions have also set up centers, such as the prominent site at Boston University (BU), dedicated, in part, to study a method for determining evidence of CTE in living people, particularly through the use of magnetic resonance imaging (MRI). Diagnostic testing that can help identify potential CTE at its early stages would mean that it could be possible to screen professional athletes, military personnel, and other susceptible individuals who are at risk for developing CTE to safeguard them against further injury and help them to be proactive in identifying symptoms and dealing with the progressive disease. Eventually, the research aims to find ways to cure CTE, but the focus is on early detection for now.

Widespread concerns about head injuries and their association with the progressive degenerative disease of CTE have placed greater scrutiny and onus on contact sports. Under pressure, the NFL finally issued an official acknowledgment in March 2016, recognizing an indisputable link between CTE and head trauma sustained in football. The NFL had denied the connection for years despite the numerous players in whom CTE was discovered during an autopsy. According to some estimates, the incidence of CTE in professional football players may be as high as 90 percent. A study published in the *Journal of the American Medical Association (JAMA)* in 2017 examined the brains of 111 deceased NFL players and found that 110 had CTE. The *JAMA* study was the largest of its kind conducted at that time. In January 2018, Washington State University quarterback Tyler Hilinski committed suicide at twenty-one. After his death, Hilinski's family agreed to give his brain to Minnesota's Mayo Clinic for an autopsy. The autopsy revealed that Hilinski had CTE at the time of his death. According to the medical examiner, Hilinski's brain looked like a sixty-five-year-old due to the condition.

Cases of the potentially tragic effects of CTE continued into the 2020s. After performing an autopsy on former NFL player Phillip Adams, who had killed himself following a period on a day in April 2021 during which he shot and killed six people, experts reported finding a level of CTE that had been atypical in its severity. In December of that year, an autopsy report of former NFL wide receiver Vincent Jackson, who had been discovered dead in a hotel room in February, indicated that the direct cause of his death had been chronic alcohol use. At the same time, his brain showed signs of Stage 2 CTE, which physicians and his family speculated had likely contributed in a major way to his abuse of alcohol. Additionally, BU's CTE Center released findings that same December from a large study conducted to determine the risk of football players developing amyotrophic lateral sclerosis disease (ALS), tentatively connected with CTE. According to their results, NFL players have a four-times higher chance of developing and dying from ALS than the overall adult male population.

At the same time, CTE is not confined to football or boxing. Anyone who plays a rigorous sport that involves repeated or significant contact to the head is at risk, as are individuals who engage in activities or professions with a high likelihood of head trauma. Several professional ice hockey players have been diagnosed with CTE postmortem or have exhibited symptoms of the disease; this is particularly common in players who have a record of fighting on the ice. Some professional athletes from the ranks of racing, soccer, baseball, football, and wrestling have announced to the press that they intend to donate their brains after death to aid in the research toward diagnosing and eventually treating CTE.

—*Shari Parsons Miller*

Further Reading

Abrams, Jonathan. "Phillip Adams Had Severe C.T.E. at the Time of Shootings." *New York Times*, 14 Dec. 2021, www.nytimes.com/2021/12/14/sports/football/phillip-adams-cte-shootings.html. Accessed 25 Jan. 2022.

Belson, Ken. "'It's Not the Ending He Wanted.'" *New York Times*, 16 Dec. 2021, www.nytimes.com/2021/12/16/sports/football/vincent-jackson-death-cte.html. Accessed 25 Jan. 2022.

Grafman, Jordan, and Andres M. Salazar. *Handbook of Clinical Neurology: Traumatic Brain Injury, Part 1*. Elsevier, 2015.

Hernandez, Joe. "NFL Players Are 4 Times More Likely to Develop ALS, a New Study Shows." *NPR*, 16 Dec. 2021, www.npr.org/2021/12/16/1064850108/nfl-players-als-study. Accessed 25 Jan. 2022.

McKee, Ann C., et al. "Chronic Traumatic Encephalopathy in Athletes: Progressive Tauopathy after Repetitive Head Injury." *Journal of Neuropathology and Experimental Neurology*, vol. 68, no. 7 (2009): 709-35.

Mez, Jesse, et al. "Clinicopathological Evaluation of Chronic Traumatic Encephalopathy in Players of American Football." *Journal of the American Medical Association*, vol. 319, no. 4, 2017, pp. 360-70.

Petraglia, Anthony L., Julian E. Bailes, and Arthur L. Day. *Handbook of Neurological Sports Medicine: Concussion and Other Nervous System Injuries in the Athlete*. Human Kinetics, 2015.

Reddy, Luke. "Larry Johnson: Ex-NFL Player on Battle with What He Thinks Is Chronic Traumatic Encephalopathy." *BBC Sport*, 15 Dec. 2017, www.bbc.com/sport/american-football/42364622. Accessed 3 Jan. 2018.

COMMON SHOULDER INJURIES

Category: Injury
Specialties and related fields: Occupational therapy, orthopedics, physical therapy, sports medicine
Definition: damage to the shoulder that causes pain during movement

KEY TERMS

bursitis: inflammation of the fluid-filled pads (bursae) that act as cushions at the joints

osteoarthritis: degeneration of joint cartilage and the underlying bone, most common from middle age onward. It causes pain and stiffness, especially in the hip, knee, and thumb joints

psoriatic arthritis: a chronic, inflammatory disease of the joints and the places where tendons and ligaments connect to bone, usually associated with plaque psoriasis that affects the skin

rheumatoid arthritis: a chronic progressive disease, causing inflammation in the joints and resulting in painful deformity and immobility, especially in the fingers, wrists, feet, and ankles

rotator cuff: a capsule with fused tendons that supports the arm at the shoulder joint and is often subject to athletic injury

tendinitis: inflammation of a tendon, most commonly from overuse but also from infection or rheumatic disease

INTRODUCTION

Common shoulder injuries are frequently occurring problems relating to the human shoulder. The shoulder is composed of bones, muscles, and connective tissues. Millions of people suffer injuries to their shoulders every year. Many of these injuries—such as separations, dislocations, and fractures—result from sudden trauma. Many other problems—including frozen shoulder, arthritis, and rotator cuff damage—are more often the result of old age, disease, or general wear and tear on the shoulder. Physicians may prescribe a wide range of treatments for these ailments, including rest, ice, stretching, medication, and surgery.

SHOULDER PARTS AND INJURIES
The shoulder comprises several parts that work together to allow movement while maintaining stability. The bone structure of the shoulder consists of three parts, the humerus (upper arm bone), the clavicle (collarbone), and the scapula (shoulder blade). These bones form a ball-and-socket joint with a wide range of motion. Around these bones are muscles, tendons, and ligaments. Tendons and ligaments are both forms of strong connective tissue, but their functions in the body differ. Tendons connect muscles with bones and help to facilitate movement. Ligaments connect bones with other bones and help the body stay strong and stable.

Shoulders can move more freely than any other joints in the body. An intricate system of parts safeguards their function. These factors make shoulders immensely useful, but they also present many opportunities for injuries and other disorders. People of all ages, genders, sizes and backgrounds may develop shoulder problems. According to the American Academy of Orthopaedic Surgeons, about 7.5 million people in the United States sought medical attention for shoulder-related problems in 2006.

Many shoulder-related problems are caused by sudden injuries, while many others result from con-

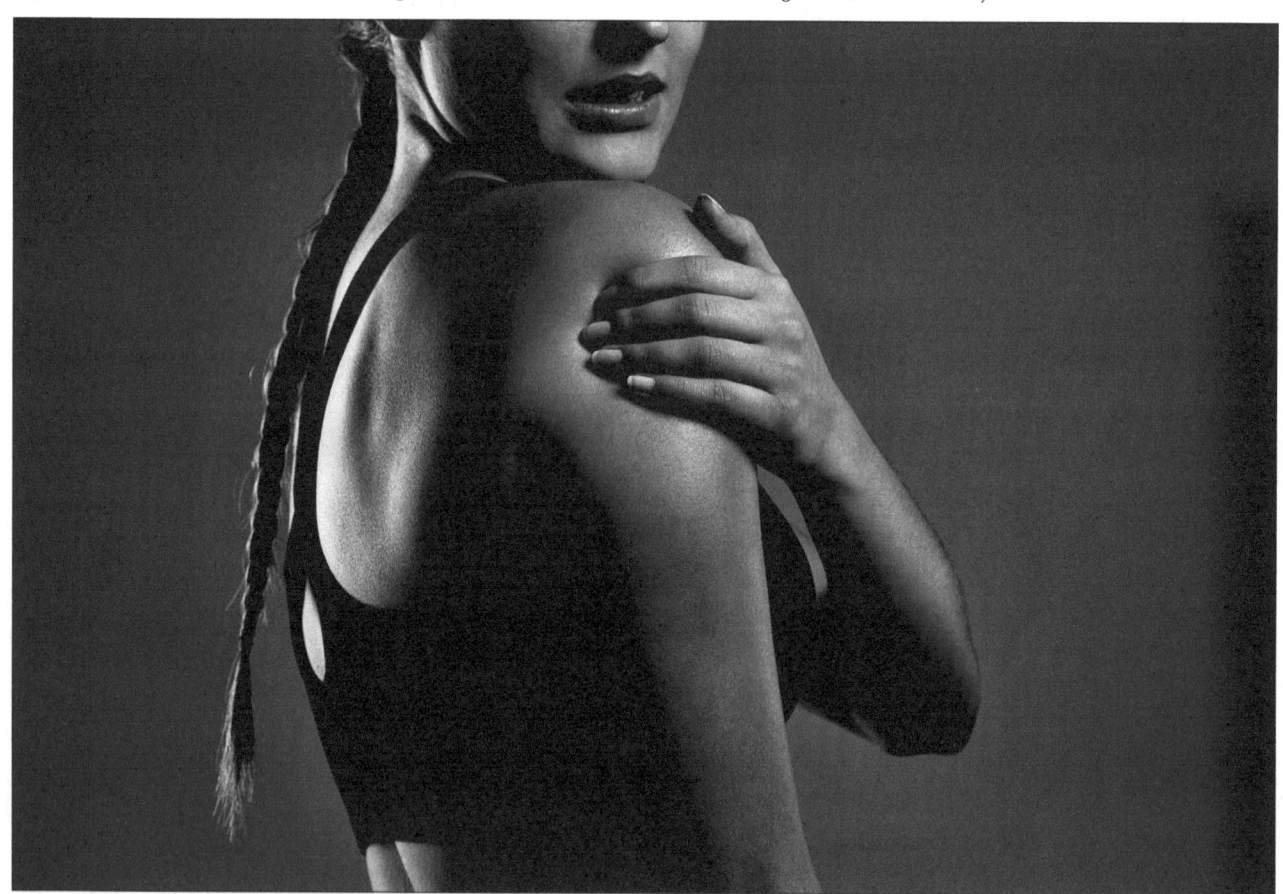

Photo via iStock/PeopleImages. [Used under license.]

sistent overuse of the shoulders. In both cases, athletes are particularly at risk for shoulder problems. According to a study published in 2009 in the *Journal of Athletic Training*, a group of high school athletes experienced shoulder injuries most often during football, wrestling, and baseball activities. Of these injuries, most were not serious, with athletes able to return to their sports in less than a week. However, a small percentage (6.2 percent) of the cases required surgery.

The pain from shoulder injuries varies greatly. In some cases, patients feel one concentrated area of pain. The pain extends over a large region or even the entire arm in other cases. Various diseases and nerve reactions can greatly alter and generally worsen the effects of shoulder injuries.

INJURIES FROM SUDDEN TRAUMA

Many kinds of common shoulder injuries exist. Some types are generally caused by sudden trauma such as falls, automobile accidents, and mishaps during sporting events. This group of injuries includes separation, dislocation, and fracture.

Separation involves serious injury to the ligaments that connect the scapula and clavicle bones. People most often suffer this injury due to falls, blows, or other forms of sudden trauma. In most cases, with rest, simple treatments such as applying ice, and possibly a medical sling, the injury will heal itself. However, surgery may be necessary to repair torn ligaments in serious cases.

A dislocation occurs when the ball-shaped end of the humerus comes out of the socket at the shoulder joint. This injury most frequently occurs if the arm is pulled or twisted in a manner that puts too much pressure on the shoulder. Although dislocation may be very painful and upsetting, the treatment is relatively simple. A physician can usually push the humerus back into place and repair the joint, leaving the patient with no lasting ill effects except temporary soreness. In some instances, however, severe dislocations may cause lasting damage to tendons, ligaments, or nerves or ongoing weakness of the joint that may contribute to future injuries.

A shoulder fracture is an injury in which one or more of the shoulder bones are cracked, usually by falls or other trauma. Fractures may vary in severity. The most commonly fractured bones in the shoulder are the humerus and clavicle. Usually, a doctor can set the bones back together and allow them to heal; if this treatment is not successful, surgery may be necessary. After the initial treatments, patients usually wear a sling to keep the damaged bones in place while they heal.

OTHER INJURIES AND PROBLEMS

Some kinds of common shoulder ailments are not typically associated with sudden trauma. These shoulder maladies include frozen shoulder, arthritis, and rotator cuff problems. These shoulder problems may be caused by old age, disease, or repeated wear and tear over a long period.

Frozen shoulder is a medical problem that occurs when the shoulder no longer moves easily, or the range of movement is restricted. People may experience frozen shoulder due to abnormal growths in the shoulder, diseases, or too much friction in the joint. This condition may also develop if a person does not move their shoulder for a long time. As with other ailments, surgery may be necessary, but often frozen shoulder will clear up with medicine, injections, and careful exercises.

Arthritis is a disease that harms the joints, sometimes including the shoulder. Different forms of arthritis may be caused by autoimmune disorders or by ongoing wear and damage to the cartilage of a joint. Medication, exercise, and physical therapy are among the most commonly prescribed treatments for arthritis. However, in serious or advanced cases, they may need surgery.

Some of the most common injuries and problems relating to the shoulder occur in the rotator cuff, an assortment of tendons and muscles that help the shoulder function. The rotator cuff tendons may suffer a tear due to repeated use, injury, or the degenerative effects of aging. They may also be affected by diseases such as bursitis and tendinitis, which irritate parts of the shoulder. Medication, electrical and ultrasound treatments, and rest are often prescribed for rotator cuff ailments.

—*Mark Dziak*

Further Reading

Bonza, John E., et al. "Shoulder Injuries Among United States High School Athletes During the 2005-2006 and 2006-2007 School Years." *Journal of Athletic Training*, vol. 44, no. 1, 2009, pp. 76-83, www.ncbi.nlm.nih.gov/pmc/articles/PMC2629044/.

"Common Shoulder Injuries." *OrthoInfo*, July 2009, orthoinfo.aaos.org/topic.cfm?topic=a00327.

"Shoulder Problems and Injuries." *WebMD*, 16 Jan. 2015, www.webmd.com/a-to-z-guides/shoulder-problems-and-injuries-topic-overview.

"What Are Shoulder Problems?" *National Institute of Arthritis and Musculoskeletal and Skin Diseases*. National Institutes of Health, June 2010, www.niams.nih.gov/Health_Info/Shoulder_Problems/shoulder_problems_ff.asp.

Concussion

Category: Disease/Disorder
Specialties and related fields: Critical care, emergency medicine, neurology, sports medicine
Definition: mild brain injury that briefly impairs neurological functions

KEY TERMS

amnesia: memory loss
disorientation: lack of comprehension of reality
unconsciousness: lack of awareness of one's surroundings

CAUSES AND SYMPTOMS

Various traumatic events can cause concussions: motor vehicle accidents, penetrating injuries, sports injuries, and falls. Recent studies indicate that the number of concussions from motor vehicle accidents and falls has decreased while penetrating injuries (gunshot wounds) and sports-related injuries are increasing. A concussion is a common athletic injury experienced by approximately 300,000 youths annually. Recent information suggests that children heal more slowly than adults following head trauma. Although concussions are the mildest traumatic brain injuries, they can result in irreversible damage or death if a person suffers another head trauma before recovering fully from the initial injury.

People who have experienced head trauma that disrupts brain activity and sometimes causes brief unconsciousness, ranging from several seconds to minutes immediately after an impact, are considered to have sustained a concussion. Direct, sudden, powerful blows to the head or an impact to the body that jars the head cause the brain to bounce inside the skull and suffer tissue bruising. Nerve fibers tear, and chemical reactions are altered.

Concussions are described as mild, moderate, or severe. However, there is a lack of standardized definitions for each type of concussion. A mild concussion may or may not involve a brief period of unconsciousness; the brain generally recovers quickly and without long-term damage. However, approximately 15 percent of those injured will continue to experience symptoms one year after the initial injury. These symptoms may range from headaches to emotional or behavioral problems. The US Centers for Disease Control and Prevention (CDC) and the National Center for Injury Prevention and Control have developed recommendations for standardized terminology, treatment, and prevention of mild traumatic brain injuries. A severe concussion is considered an emergency and requires an extended time for recovery.

Headache, dizziness, nausea, and disorientation immediately following the injury are considered risk factors for long-term complications from the head injury. Each person's brain and injury are unique. Therefore, a wide variety of symptoms may occur. Patients may experience double vision and suffer hearing problems. People with concussions also report becoming uncoordinated and sensitive to light and noises. They may experience sensory changes in smell and taste. Patients may become moody, cognitively impaired, unable to concentrate, or exhausted.

Researchers have determined that the major neuropsychological complications of concussion may occur in the brain's memory, learning, and planning functions. Some concussion patients taking tests, such as the Wechsler Abbreviated Scale of Intelligence, have revealed decreased concentration, reaction, and processing skills in performing intellectual tasks. Their strategies to solve problems are impaired compared to people who have not suffered concussions.

Medical professionals assess patients with a head injury by physical examination, radiological tests, and a standardized scale that measures the level of consciousness called the "Glasgow Coma Scale." Computed tomography (CT) and magnetic reso-

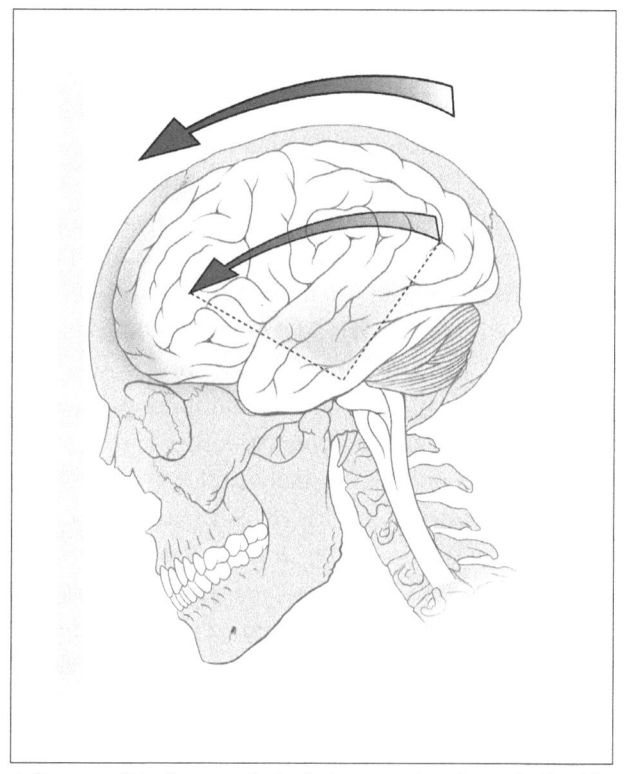

A diagram of the forces on the brain in concussion. Image by Patrick J. Lynch, medical illustrator, via Wikimedia Commons.

nance imaging (MRI) scans may also be used. The American Academy of Neurology emphasizes the duration of loss of consciousness to determine the severity of concussions. Evaluations also consider orientation and posttraumatic amnesia. Medical professionals assess patients' responses to stimuli and memory of incidents before their injury, defining the concussion according to the level of confusion, amnesia, and duration of loss of consciousness. Physicians ask patients questions about who and where they are and the time and date. The duration of amnesia after the brain trauma helps medical professionals to determine the extent of the injury and treatments that would be most effective to heal the brain. The Colorado Medical Society developed a popular system, assigning Grades 1 (mild), 2 (moderate), and 3 (severe) to concussions, to guide athletic personnel in examining players who suffer

---

Information on Concussion

Causes: Brain trauma from car accidents, falls, sports injuries, etc.

Symptoms: Unconsciousness, memory loss, headache, dizziness, nausea, disorientation, double vision, hearing problems, lack of coordination, sensitivity to light and noises, sensory changes in smell and taste

Duration: Ranges from several seconds to minutes immediately after impact

Treatments: Dependent on severity; none (mild), rest and alleviation of symptoms (moderate), neck immobilization and hospitalization (severe)

concussions during games and deciding how long they must refrain from participation to prevent additional damage.

Brain damage and death can result from serial concussions. Postconcussion complications may include second impact syndrome: If a patient suffers another concussion before healing is complete following the first injury, then the second concussion can be the catalyst for rapid cerebral swelling that causes increased pressure within the brain's structure. This pressure can cause the brain to press on the brain stem and result in respiratory failure and death. This condition is usually fatal.

Postconcussive syndrome (PCS) is more common. It consists of such cognitive and physical symptoms as headache, anxiety, vertigo, nausea, and hallucinations. An estimated 30 percent of professional football players suffer from PCS. Researchers have determined that people who experience several concussions, such as athletes and soldiers, are more vulnerable to becoming clinically depressed.

TREATMENT AND THERAPY
Research has found that patients who rest for one week following a concussion, with a slow return to previous activities to allow the brain to heal, have fewer long-term complications than do patients who resume activities more quickly. However, most patients recover, but some experience long-term concussion-related conditions, such as memory loss and neurological impairment.

Severe concussions with increased brain pressure require hospitalization, often in a neurological intensive care unit. The patient's head is maintained in a neutral position. The patient is at risk for stopped breathing due to increased brain pressure. This risk is decreased by placing the patient on a mechanical ventilator. The patient may have suffered internal bleeding in the brain because of the injury, and blood clots can form there. The patient may require surgery to remove these clots. Patients with preexisting conditions such as epilepsy and diabetes may develop complications related to those diseases and require longer recovery times.

Physicians recommend wearing helmets to absorb shocks sustained during athletic activities involving the risk of head injury to prevent or minimize concussions. The American Academy of Neurology has demanded a ban on boxing because the sport involves knocking out opponents by inflicting concussions. Boxers often suffer permanent brain damage and are at a heightened risk for neurological diseases.

PERSPECTIVE AND PROSPECTS
Concussions were first described in medical literature by Muslim physician Rhazes (850-923). He differentiated between a head injury that caused neurological symptoms and those that resulted in lesions and structural damage. In the nineteenth century, medical researchers developed hypotheses, often controversial, regarding concussion symptoms' physical and emotional influences. Second impact syndrome was first defined in 1984.

The development of sports medicine increased the interest in studying concussions. However, the understanding of the internal brain damage involved in concussions did not significantly advance until neuroimaging technologies such as CT scanning and MRI were developed in the late twentieth century. In the twenty-first century, medical professionals utilize those techniques to view brain tissues and observe the physiological reactions to concussion-causing trauma. Positive emission tomography (PET) has been developed to measure chemical changes in the brain. In the case of concussion, the PET scan can evaluate changes that signal areas of injury in the brain. These technologies will likely yield more accurate diagnostic exams for concussions.

—*Elizabeth D. Schafer, Amy Webb Bull*

Further Reading

Arbogast, Kristy B., et al. "Cognitive Rest and School-Based Recommendations Following Pediatric Concussion: The Need for Primary Care Support Tools." *Clinical Pediatrics*, vol. 52, no. 5, 2013, pp. 397-402.

Evans, Randolph W., editor. *Neurology and Trauma*. 2nd ed., Oxford UP, 2006.

Kennedy, Jan, et al. "A Survey of Mild Traumatic Brain Injury Treatment in the Emergency Room and Primary Care Medical Clinics." *Military Medicine*, vol. 171, no. 6, 2006, pp. 516-21.

Kerr, Mary, and Elizabeth Crago. "Acute Intracranial Problems." In *Medical-Surgical Nursing*, edited by Sharon Lewis, Margaret Heitkemper, and Shannon Dirksen, 6th ed., Mosby, 2004.

Metzl, Jordan. "Concussion in the Young Athlete." *Pediatrics*, vol. 117, no. 5., 2006, p. 1813.

National Center for Injury Prevention and Control. *Report to Congress on Mild Traumatic Brain Injury in the United States: Steps to Prevent a Serious Public Health Problem.* Centers for Disease Control and Prevention, 2003.

Shannon, Joyce Brennfleck, editor. *Sports Injuries Sourcebook*. 4th ed., Omnigraphics, 2012.

Wrightson, Philip, and Dorothy Gronwall. *Mild Head Injury: A Guide to Management*. Oxford UP, 1999.

Zimlich, Rachael, and Donald Collins. "Concussion: Symptoms, Causes, Diagnosis, & Treatment." Healthline, 1 Mar. 2022, www.healthline.com/health/concussion.

Fracture and Dislocation

Category: Disease/Disorder
Specialties and related fields: Emergency medicine, orthopedics, sports medicine
Definition: a fracture is a break in a bone, which may be partial or complete; a dislocation is the forceful separation of bones in a joint

KEY TERMS

anesthesia: a state characterized by loss of sensation, caused by or resulting from the pharmacological depression of normal nerve function

callus: a hard, bone-like substance made by osteocytes found in and around the ends of a fractured bone; it temporarily maintains bony alignment and is resorbed after complete healing or union of a fracture occurs

ecchymosis: a purplish patch on the skin caused by bleeding; the spots are easily visible to the naked eye

embolus: an obstruction or occlusion of a vessel (most commonly, an artery or vein) caused by a transported blood clot, vegetation, mass of bacteria, or other foreign material

epiphysis: the part of a long bone from which growth or elongation occurs

instability: excessive mobility of two or more bones caused by damage to ligaments, the joint capsule, or fracture of one or more bones

ischemia: local anemia or area of diminished or insufficient blood supply due to a mechanical obstruction, commonly narrowing of an artery

kyphoplasty: similar to vertebroplasty but uses a special balloon to restore vertebral height and lessen spinal deformity

osteoblast: a bone-forming cell

osteocyte: a bone cell

paralysis: the loss of power of voluntary movement or other function of a muscle as a result of disease or injury to its nerve supply

petechiae: minute spots caused by hemorrhage or bleeding into the skin; the spots are the size of pinheads

prone: the position of the body when face downward, on one's stomach and abdomen

pulse: the rhythmical dilation of an artery, produced by the increased volume of blood forced into the vessel by the contraction of the heart

transection: a partial or complete severance of the spinal cord

vertebroplasty: a medical procedure where acrylic cement is injected into the body of the vertebra for stabilization

CAUSES AND SYMPTOMS

A fracture is a linear deformation or discontinuity of a bone produced by applying a force that exceeds the modulus of elasticity (ability to bend) of a bone. Normal bones require excessive force to fracture. Disease, tumor-related diseases, or tumors themselves weaken the physical structure of bones, which reduces their ability to withstand an impact. Bones respond to stresses placed upon them and can thus be strengthened through physical conditioning and made more resistant to fracture. This is a normal part of training in many athletic activities.

Fractures are classified according to the type of break or, more correctly, by the plane or surface that is fractured. A break at a right angle to the axis of the bone is called "transverse." An oblique fracture is similar but is found at any angle other than perpendicular to the main axis of the bone. If a twisting force is applied, the break may be spiral or twisted. A comminuted fracture is a break that results in two or more fragments of bone. If the pieces of bone remain in their original positions, the fracture is undisplaced. In a displaced fracture, the portions of bone are not properly aligned.

When bones protrude through the skin, the fracture is an open, or compound, fracture. The fracture is closed or simple if bones do not penetrate the skin. Other types of fractures are associated with pathologic or disease processes. Stress fractures result from repeated stress or trauma to the same site of a bone. None of the individual stresses is sufficient to cause a break. If these stresses cause

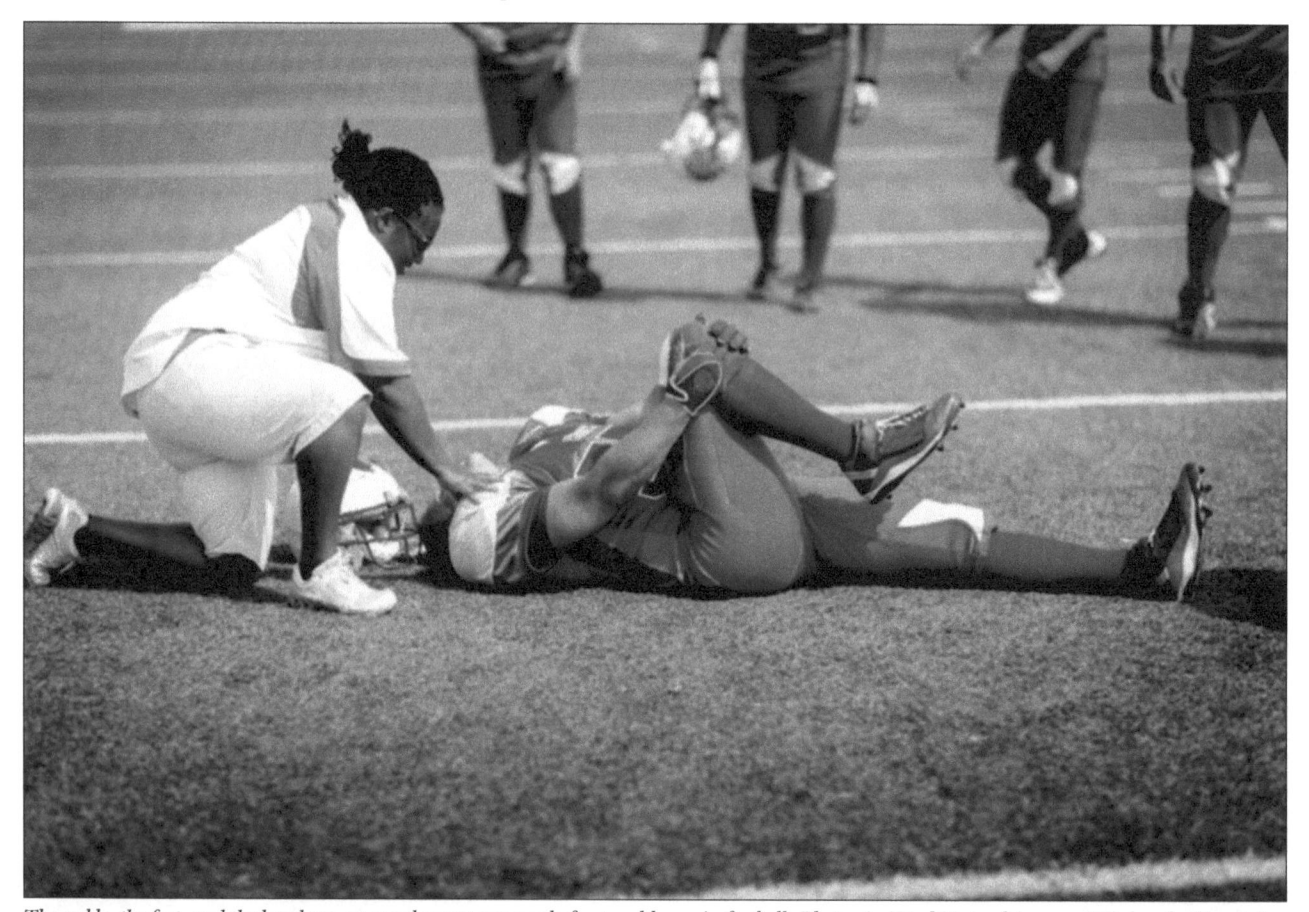

The ankle, the foot, and the hand are among the most commonly fractured bones in football. Photo via iStock/stevecoleimages. [Used under license.]

a callus to form, the bone will be strengthened, and the actual separation of fragments will not occur. A pathologic fracture occurs at the site of a tumor, infection, or other bone diseases. A compression fracture results when a bone is crushed; the force applied is greater than the ability of the bone to withstand it. A greenstick fracture is incomplete separation of bone.

The diagnosis of a fracture is based on several criteria: instability, pain, swelling, deformity, and ecchymosis. The most reliable diagnostic criterion is instability. The deformity is obvious with open fractures but may not be apparent with other, undisplaced breaks. Pain is not universally present at a fracture site. Swelling may be delayed and occur at some time after a fracture is sustained.

Ecchymosis is a purplish patch caused by bleeding into the skin; it will not be present if blood vessels are not broken. A definitive diagnosis is made with two-plane film X-rays taken at the fracture site at right angles to one another. If the fracture site is visually examined and palpated shortly after the injury occurs, an accurate tentative diagnosis may be made; this should be confirmed with X-rays as soon as it is convenient. Occasionally, an X-ray will not show undisplaced or chip fracture. Suppose a patient experiences symptoms of pain, swelling, or ecchymosis but has a negative X-ray for a fracture. In that case, the site should be immobilized and X-rayed again in two to three weeks.

Fractures occur most commonly in the extremities: arms or legs. Such fractures must be evaluated to determine if injuries have occurred to other tissues such as nerves or blood vessels. The presence of bruising or ecchymosis indicates blood vessel damage. The absence of peripheral pulses with severe bruising indicates that the major arteries are injured. Venous flow is more difficult to evaluate. Venous circulation is a lower pressure system than arterial, so venous bleeding can be considered less important and, therefore, temporarily tolerated.

> **INFORMATION ON FRACTURE AND DISLOCATION**
>
> **Causes**: Usually injury, sometimes disease or infection
>
> **Symptoms**: Varies widely; typically inflammation, pain, swelling, deformity, bruising
>
> **Duration**: Acute or chronic depending on severity
>
> **Treatments**: Reduction (return of fractured bone to normal position), immobilization, surgery, orthopedic appliances

Neurologic functioning may be assessed by the ability of the patient to contract muscles or sense skin touches or pinpricks. Temporary immobilization may be necessary before nerve status can be evaluated accurately.

An open fracture creates a direct pathway between the skin surface and underlying tissues. If bacteria contaminate the site, an opportunity for osteomyelitis (infection of the bone) to form is created. Inadequate treatment by the initial surgeon may result in skin loss, delayed union, loss of joint mobility, osteomyelitis, and even amputation.

Skin damage may or may not be related to a fracture. Bone involvement must be assumed when skin integrity is broken over or near a fracture site. If there is an infection of the fracture site, appropriate antibiotics are normally administered. If skin damage is extensive, the final surgical reduction of the underlying fracture may have to be delayed until the skin is healed.

Delayed union refers to the inability of a fractured bone to heal. This is a potentially serious problem, as normal stability is impossible as long as a fracture exists. Joints may not function normally in the presence of a fracture. If a fracture heals improperly, bones may be misaligned and cause pain with movement, leading to limitations of motion. If the bones are affected by osteomyelitis, the infection may spread to the joint capsule and reduce the normal range of motion for the bones or the joint. Amputation may become necessary if the infection becomes extensive in the area of a fracture. An infection, which becomes firmly established in bones or spreads widely into adjacent muscle tissue, may lead to cellulitis or gangrene and compromise a portion of an extremity. Amputation may be performed if the pathologic process cannot be treated with antibiotics and surgery.

Adequate blood supply to tissues is critical for survival. In an extremity, the maximum time limit for complete ischemia (lack of blood flow) is six to eight hours; after that time, the likelihood of later amputation increases. Pain, pallor, pulselessness, and paralysis are indicators of impaired circulation. When two of these signs are present, the possibility of vascular damage must be thoroughly explored.

Dislocations occur at joints and are caused by an applied force greater than the ligaments and muscles' strength that keeps a joint intact. The result is a stretching deformity or injury to a joint and an abnormal movement of a bone out of the joint. Accidental trauma, commonly the result of an athletic injury or automobile accident, is the most common cause of dislocation. The frequently dislocated joints include the shoulder and digits (fingers and toes). Dislocations of the ankle and hip are infrequent but serious; they require immediate management. Dislocations may accompany fractures, but the two injuries need not occur together.

When dislocations are reduced, the joint bones are returned to normal position. Reduction of a dislocation is accomplished by relaxing adjacent muscles and applying traction (pulling force) to the bone until it returns to its normal position within the joint. For most shoulder dislocations, the victim lies prone, and the dislocated arm hangs down freely. Gradual traction is applied until reduction occurs. This can be accomplished by bandaging a pail to the arm and slowly filling it with water. Alternatively, the victim can hold a heavy book while the muscles of the arm are allowed to relax until the dislocation is reduced. Such treatments are usually reserved for situations in which medical assistance is unavailable. Digits are reduced similarly by gently pulling the end of the finger or toe. Ankle and hip dislocations are potentially more serious because these joints are more complex and have extensive blood supplies. Reduction of dislocated ankles and hips should be undertaken by qualified medical personnel in an expedited manner.

After reduction, competent medical personnel should evaluate all dislocations. With dislocated digits, long-term damage is relatively unlikely. Still, it can occur because of ligament damage sustained in the initial injury. Dislocations of the shoulder may be accompanied by a fracture of the clavicle or collarbone. They may involve nerve damage in the shoulder joint. Dislocations of the ankle and hip may lead to avascular necrosis (damage to the bone due to inadequate blood supply) if not evaluated and reduced promptly.

TREATMENT AND THERAPY

Fractures are usually treated by reduction and immobilization. Reduction, which refers to returning the fractured bones to the normal position, may be either closed or open. Closed reduction is accomplished without surgery by manipulating the broken bone through overlying skin and muscles. Open reduction requires surgical intervention in which the broken pieces are exposed and returned to the normal position. Orthopedic appliances may be used to hold the bones in the correct position. The most common of these appliances are pins and screws, but metal plates and wires may also be employed. Orthopedic appliances are usually made of stainless steel. These may be left in the body indefinitely or may be surgically removed after healing is complete. Local anesthesia is usually used with closed reductions; open reductions are performed in an operating room under sterile conditions using general anesthesia.

Immobilization is generally accomplished using a cast. Casts are often made of plaster, but they may be inflatable plastic. It is important to hold bones in a rigid, fixed position for sufficient time for the broken ends to unite and heal. However, the cast must be loose enough to allow blood to circulate. Padding is usually placed before plaster is applied to form a cast. Whenever possible, the newly immobilized body part is elevated to reduce swelling in the cast, which would compromise the blood supply to the fracture site and the portion of the body beyond the cast. The doctor, nurse, or medical assistant should check the cast periodically to ensure that they do not impair circulation.

The broken bone and accompanying body part must be placed in an anatomically neutral position to minimize postfracture disability and improve the prospect of rehabilitation. The length of time a fractured bone is immobilized is highly variable and depends on several factors.

Traction may also be used to immobilize a fracture. Traction is the external application of force to overcome muscular resistance and hold bones in the desired position. Commonly, holes are drilled through bones, and pins are inserted; the ends of these pins extend through the skin's surface. Part of the body is fixed in position with a strap or weights, and wires are attached to the pins in the body part to be stretched. Weights or tension are applied to the wires until the broken bone parts move into the desired position. Traction is maintained until healing has occurred.

Individual ends of a single fractured bone are sometimes held in position by external pins and screws. Holes are drilled through the bone, and pins are inserted. The pins on opposite sides of the fracture site are then attached with threaded rods and locked by nuts. This process allows a fractured bone to be immobilized without using a cast.

Different bones require different amounts of time to heal. Furthermore, age is a factor in fracture healing. Fractures in young children heal more quickly than do broken bones in adults. The elderly typically requires even more time for healing. The availability of nutrients like calcium and vitamin D also affects how a fracture heals.

Delayed union of fractures is a term applied to fractures that either do not heal or take longer than normal to heal; there is no precise time frame associated with delayed union. Nonunion refers to fractures where healing is not observed and cannot be expected even with prolonged immobilization. X-ray analysis of a nonunion will show that the bone ends have sclerosed (hardened), that the ends of the marrow canal have become plugged, and that a gap persists between the ends of a fractured bone. The inadequate blood supply may cause nonunion to the fracture site, leading to cartilage formation instead of new bone between the broken pieces of bone. Nonunion may also be caused by injury to the soft tissues surrounding a fracture site. This damage impairs the formation of a callus and the reestablishment of an adequate blood supply to the fracture site; it is frequently seen in young children. Inadequate immobilization may also allow soft tissue to enter the fracture site by slipping between the bone fragments, leading to nonunion. Respect for tissue and minimizing damage in the vicinity of a fracture, especially with open reduction, will minimize problems of nonunion. Subjecting the nonuniting fracture site to a low-level electromagnetic field will stimulate osteoblastic (bone-forming cell) activity and healing.

The epiphyseal plate is the portion of bone where growth occurs. Bony epiphyses are active in children until they attain their adult height. At this time, the epiphyses become inactive and close. Once an epiphysis ceases to function, further growth does not occur. A fracture involving the epiphyseal plate is potentially dangerous in children because bone growth may be interrupted or halted. This situation can lead to inequalities in the length of extremities or impaired range of movement in joints. Accurate reduction of injuries involving an epiphyseal plate is necessary to minimize subsequent deformity. A key factor is the blood supply to the injured area: If adequate blood supply is maintained, epiphyseal plate damage is minimized.

Fractures of the spinal vertebrae are potentially very dangerous because they can cause injury to the nerves and tracts of the spinal cord. Fractures of the vertebrae are commonly sustained in automobile accidents, athletic injuries, falls from heights, and other situations involving rapid deceleration. When vertebrae are fractured, the spinal cord can be compromised. Spinal cord injury can be direct and cut all or a portion of the spinal nerves at the fracture site. The extent of the damage is dependent on the level of the injury. An accident that completely severs the spinal cord will lead to a complete loss of function for all structures below the level of injury. Since spinal nerves are arranged segmentally, cord damage at a lower level involves compromising fewer structures. As the level of injury becomes higher in the spinal cord, more vital structures are involved. Transection of the spinal cord in the neck usually leads to complete paralysis of the entire body; it can cause death if high enough to cut the lungs' nerves. Individuals in whom vertebral fractures and thus spinal cord injuries are suspected must have the spinal column immobilized before they are moved. Only a highly skilled professional should undertake the reduction of spinal cord fractures.

When bones having large marrow cavities such as the femur (thighbone) are fractured, fat globules may escape from the marrow and enter the bloodstream. A fat globule is then called an "embolus" (plural is emboli). Fat emboli are potentially dangerous in that they can become lodged in the lungs' capillaries. This causes pain and can lead to impaired blood oxygenation; a condition called "hypoxemia." About 10 to 20 percent of individuals sustaining a fractured femur also have central nervous system depression, skin petechiae (minute spots caused by hemorrhage or bleeding into the skin), and hypoxemia two to three days after the injury. This triad of signs is called "fat embolism syndrome." It is treated medically with oxygen, steroids, and anticoagulant drugs.

PERSPECTIVE AND PROSPECTS

Fractures rarely threaten a patient's life directly, and injuries to the brain, heart, circulatory system, and abdominal cavity must receive priority in treatment. However, it is imperative not to move a patient in whom a fracture is suspected without first immobilizing the potential fracture site. This is especially true with suspected fractures of the spine. Instability may not be apparent when a patient is lying down but can become catastrophic if the person is moved without proper preparation and immobilization.

Crush injuries of the spinal cord are relatively common among people living with osteoporosis. Osteoporosis is a pathological syndrome defined by a decrease in the density of a bone below the level required for mechanical support. It is frequently associated with a deficiency of calcium, problems related to calcium in the body, or a rate of bone cell breakdown greater than the rate of bone cell remodeling. Crush fractures occur when the bones become so weak that the weight of the upper portion of the body is greater than the ability of the vertebrae to support it. These crush injuries may occur slowly over time and cause no serious injury to the underlying spinal cord. The resulting deformity of the spine, however, impairs movement. There are limited treatments for osteoporotic crush fractures of the vertebrae. Most treatments aim to strengthen nearby muscles and aid in nutritional deficiencies causing osteoporosis. However, surgeries such as vertebroplasty, balloon kyphoplasty, and spinal fusion are available as last-line treatments for reoccurring or nonhealing (painful) vertebral fractures.

Occupational exposures may lead to fractures and dislocations. Professional athletes are clearly at increased risk for skeletal injuries. However, these individuals are also usually well-conditioned and so can withstand increased impacts and blows to the body. Many are also trained in methods that minimize the force of impact; they know how to fall properly.

The vast proportions of workers are not conditioned and are given minimal training to avoid situations that lead to fractures. Accident analysis reveals that carelessness is the most common predisposing factor. Workers operating without safety equipment such as belaying lines or belts may become overconfident. Slips or falls can occur in such a situation, and fractures result. Unsafe equipment can lead to hazardous situations and cause fractures or dislocations. Machinery that is not properly maintained can fail; parts may become detached, hit nearby workers, and cause fractures.

Recreational activities also result in fractures. Individuals who once were well-conditioned may engage in sports without proper equipment and sustain fractures or dislocations. Contact sports such as hockey, football, and basketball are primary examples of such activities. Riding bicycles and motorized recreational vehicles without proper safety equipment can lead to serious skeletal injuries. Activities such as rock climbing are inherently dangerous. Proper training and the use of safety equipment can reduce or minimize accidents. The keys to avoiding fractures and dislocations when participating in recreational activities are receiving proper instruction and training, employing adequate safety equipment, and using common sense by avoiding difficult or hazardous situations beyond one's physical abilities or skill level.

—*L. Fleming Fallon Jr., Mikhail Varshavski*

Further Reading

Brunicardi, F. Charles, et al., editors. *Schwartz's Principles of Surgery*. 9th ed., McGraw-Hill, 2010.

Currey, John D. *Bones: Structures and Mechanics*. Princeton UP, 2006.

Doherty, Gerard M., and Lawrence W. Way, editors. *Current Surgical Diagnosis and Treatment*. 13th ed., Lange Medical Books/McGraw-Hill, 2009.

Egol, Kenneth, Kenneth J., et al., editors. *Handbook of Fractures*. 4th ed., Lippincott Williams and Wilkins, 2010.

Marieb, Elaine N., and Katja Hoehn. *Human Anatomy and Physiology*. 9th ed., Pearson/Benjamin Cummings, 2012.

Townsend, Courtney M., Jr., et al., editors. *Sabiston Textbook of Surgery*. 19th ed., Saunders/Elsevier, 2012.

INJURIES, MINOR

Category: Condition
Specialties and related fields: Alternative and complementary medicine
Related terms: Bruises, contusions, joint injuries, ligament injuries, minor sports injuries, muscle injuries, sports injuries, sprains, strains
Definition: treatment of minor injuries, specifically bruises, minor fractures, and sprains

KEY TERMS

bioflavonoids: a group of compounds occurring mainly in citrus fruits and black currants, formerly regarded as vitamins

herb: any plant with leaves, seeds, or flowers used for flavoring, food, medicine, or perfume

injury: damage to the body

proteolytic enzymes: enzymes that catalyze proteolysis by breaking down proteins into smaller polypeptides or single amino acids and spurring the formation of new protein products

INTRODUCTION

All people are likely to injure themselves sometime during their lives. Although minor injuries such as bruises and sprains will heal without treatment, they can be quite unpleasant. Discussed here are injuries such as bruises, minor fractures, and sprains. However, there are other forms of minor injury, including minor burns, minor wounds, back pain, and more chronic soft tissue injuries.

Conventional treatment for minor sprains and strains involves anti-inflammatory drugs, icing, and, in some cases, physical therapy. Bruises are sometimes treated with ultrasound, although there is no meaningful evidence that it helps.

PRINCIPAL PROPOSED NATURAL TREATMENTS

Proteolytic enzymes help digest the proteins in food. The pancreas produces the proteolytic enzymes trypsin and chymotrypsin, and others, such as papain and bromelain, are found in foods. Proteolytic enzymes are primarily used as digestive aids for people who have trouble digesting proteins. When taken by mouth, proteolytic enzymes appear to be absorbed internally to a certain extent, and they might reduce inflammation and swelling. Several small studies have found proteolytic enzyme combinations helpful for treating minor injuries. However, the best and largest trial failed to find benefits. Most studies have involved proteolytic enzymes combined with citrus bioflavonoids, which are also thought to decrease swelling.

A double-blind, placebo-controlled study of forty-four persons with sports-related ankle injuries found that treatment with a proteolytic enzyme and bioflavonoid combination resulted in faster healing and reduced the time away from training by about 50 percent. Based on these and other results, a large (721-participant) double-blind, placebo-controlled trial of people with ankle sprains was undertaken to compare placebo with bromelain, trypsin, or rutin (a bioflavonoid), separately or in combination. None of the treatments, alone or together, proved more effective than the placebo.

Researchers found that treatment with a proteolytic enzyme combination significantly speeded recovery. Three other small double-blind studies involving about eighty athletes found that treatment with proteolytic enzymes significantly speeded the healing of bruises and other mild athletic injuries compared with placebo. In another double-blind trial, one hundred people were given an injection of their blood under the skin to simulate bruising following an injury. However, most of these older studies fall beneath modern standards in design and reporting.

OTHER PROPOSED NATURAL TREATMENTS

Oligomeric proanthocyanidins (OPCs), substances found in grape seed and pine bark, have shown promise for treating minor injuries. A ten-day, double-blind, placebo-controlled study of fifty people found that OPCs improved the rate at which edema disappeared following sports injuries. Also, a double-blind, placebo-controlled study of sixty-three women with breast cancer found that 600 milligrams of OPCs daily for six months reduced postoperative edema and pain. Similarly, in a double-blind, placebo-controlled study of thirty-two people who had cosmetic surgery on the face, swelling disappeared much faster in the treated group.

Preliminary evidence from a poorly reported double-blind trial of forty college football players suggests that a combination of vitamin C and citrus bioflavonoids taken before practice can reduce the severity of athletic injuries. A double-blind study of people recovering from minor injuries, including minor surgery, found that the bioflavonoid-like substances called "oxerutins" have similar effects. Another small placebo-controlled study suggests that an oral combination product containing vitamin C, calcium, potassium, proteolytic enzymes, rutin, and OPCs can slightly accelerate the healing of skin wounds.

The herb horse chestnut is thought to have properties similar to citrus bioflavonoids. The active ingredient in horse chestnut is a substance called "aescin." One double-blind study of seventy people found that about 10 grams of 2 percent aescin gel, applied externally to bruises in a single dose five minutes after the bruises were induced, reduced the tenderness of those bruises.

The herb comfrey is unsafe for internal use because of the presence of liver-toxic pyrrolizidine alkaloids. However, topical use is believed to be safe. In a double-blind, placebo-controlled study of 142 people with an ankle sprain, the use of comfrey gel resulted in more rapid recovery than placebo gel, according to pain, swelling, and mobility measurements.

The supplement creatine has shown some promise in preventing muscle weakness, commonly occurring when a limb is immobilized following injury or surgery. However, one study failed to find creatine helpful for restoring strength following arthroscopic knee surgery.

The supplement glucosamine might be helpful for people who experience knee pain from cartilage injury. In addition, one study found somewhat inconsistent evidence hinting that glucosamine might aid recovery from acute knee injuries experienced by competitive athletes. A small, double-blind, placebo-controlled study suggests that using calcium (1 gram daily) plus vitamin D (800 international units daily) may speed bone healing after fracture in people with osteoporosis. Another study found that using relaxation therapies to manage stress reduced the number of injury and illness days among competitive athletes.

One study failed to find that onion extract can help reduce scarring in the skin. Also, homeopathic forms of the herb Arnica are popular as a treatment for injuries. Still, studies suggest they are no more effective than a placebo.

—*EBSCO CAM Review Board*

Further Reading

Braham, R., et al. "The Effect of Glucosamine Supplementation on People Experiencing Regular Knee Pain." *British Journal of Sports Medicine*, vol. 37, 2003, pp. 45-49.

Brown, S. A., et al. "Oral Nutritional Supplementation Accelerates Skin Wound Healing." *Plastic and Reconstructive Surgery*, vol. 114, 2004, pp. 237-44.

Hespel, P., et al. "Oral Creatine Supplementation Facilitates the Rehabilitation of Disuse Atrophy and Alters the Expression of Muscle Myogenic Factors in Humans." *Journal of Physiology*, vol. 536, 2001, pp. 625-33.

Kerkhoffs, G. M., et al. "A Double-Blind, Randomised, Parallel-Group Study on the Efficacy and Safety of Treating Acute Lateral Ankle Sprain with Oral Hydrolytic Enzymes." *British Journal of Sports Medicine*, vol. 38, 2004, pp. 431-35.

Ostojic, S. M., et al. "Glucosamine Administration in Athletes: Effects on Recovery of Acute Knee Injury." *Research in Sports Medicine*, vol. 15, 2007, pp. 113-24.

Perna, F. M., et al. "Cognitive-Behavioral Stress Management Effects on Injury and Illness Among Competitive Athletes." *Annals of Behavioral Medicine*, vol. 25, 2003, pp. 66-73.

Stevinson, C., et al. "Homeopathic Arnica for Prevention of Pain and Bruising." *Journal of the Royal Society of Medicine*, vol. 96, 2003, pp. 60-65.

Tyler, T. F., et al. "The Effect of Creatine Supplementation on Strength Recovery After Anterior Cruciate Ligament (ACL) Reconstruction." *American Journal of Sports Medicine*, vol. 32, 2004, pp. 383-88.

Muscle Sprains, Spasms, and Disorders

Category: Disease/Disorder
Also known as: Myopathies
Specialties and related fields: Exercise physiology, family medicine, osteopathic medicine, physical therapy, sports medicine
Definition: injuries, defects, or disorders of the muscles of the body

KEY TERMS

myopathies: neuromuscular disorders in which the primary symptom is muscle weakness due to dysfunction of muscle fiber

spasm: a sudden contraction of a muscle or group of muscles, such as a cramp

sprain: a stretched or torn ligament

strain: an injury to a muscle or tendon from overuse

CAUSES AND SYMPTOMS

The human body has three kinds of muscle tissue: smooth muscle, cardiac muscle, and striated muscle. Smooth muscle tissue is found around the intestines, blood vessels, and bronchioles in the lung, among other areas. These muscles are controlled by the autonomic nervous system, meaning their movement is not subject to voluntary action. They have many functions: They maintain the airway in the lungs, regulate the tone of blood vessels, and move foods and other substances through the digestive tract. Cardiac muscle is found only in the heart. Striated muscles are those that move body parts. They are also called "voluntary muscles" because they must receive a conscious command from the brain to work. They supply the force for physical activity, prevent movement and stabilize body parts.

Muscles are subject to many disorders: Muscle sprains, strains, and spasms are common events in everyone's life, and, for the most part, they are harmless, if painful, results of overexercising, accidents, falls, bumps, or countless other events. Yet these symptoms can signal serious myopathies or disorders within muscle tissue.

Myopathies constitute a wide range of diseases. They are classified as inflammatory myopathies or metabolic myopathies. Inflammatory myopathies include infections by bacteria, viruses, or other microorganisms, as well as other diseases that are possibly autoimmune in origin (resulting from and directed against the body's own tissues). In metabolic myopathies, there is some failure or disturbance in the body's ability to maintain a proper metabolic balance or electrolyte distribution. These conditions include glycogen storage diseases, in which there are errors in glucose processing; disorders of fatty acid metabolism, in which there are derangements in fatty acid oxidation; mitochondrial myopathies, in which there are biochemical and other abnormalities in the mitochondria of muscle cells; endocrine myopathies, in which an endocrine disorder underlies muscular symptoms; and the periodic paralyses, which can be the result of inherited or acquired illnesses. This is only a partial list of myopathies, the symptoms of which include weakness and pain.

Muscular dystrophies are a group of inherited disorders in which muscle tissue fails to receive nourishment. The results are progressive muscular weakness and the degeneration and destruction of muscle fibers. The symptoms include weakness, loss of coordination, impaired gait, and impaired muscle extensibility. Over the years, muscle mass decreases, and the arms, legs, and spine become deformed.

Neuromuscular disorders include various conditions in which muscle function is impaired by the faulty transmission of nerve impulses to muscle tissue. These conditions may be inherited; they may be attributable to toxins, such as food poisoning (botulism) or pesticide poisoning; or they may be side effects of certain drugs. The most commonly seen neuromuscular disorder is myasthenia gravis.

Injuries sustained during sports and games have become so significant that sports medicine has become a recognized medical subspecialty. The most common muscular disorders are those that result from overexertion, exercise, athletics, accidents, and trauma. Besides the muscles, the parts of the body involved in these disorders include tendons (tough, stringy tissue that attaches muscles to bones), ligaments (tissue that attaches bone to bone), synovia (membranes enclosing a joint or other bony structure), and cartilage (soft, resilient tissue between bones). A sprain is an injury in which ligaments are stretched or torn. In a strain, muscles or tendons are stretched or torn. A contusion is a bruise that occurs when the body is subjected to trauma; the skin is not broken, but the capillaries underneath are, causing discoloration. A spasm is a short, abnormal contraction in a muscle or group of muscles. A cramp is a prolonged, painful contraction of one or more muscles.

Sprains can be caused by twisting the joint violently or forcing it beyond its range of movement, and the ligaments that connect the bones of the joint stretch or tear. Sprains occur most often in the knees, ankles, and arches of the feet. There is pain and swelling and at least some immobilization of the joint.

A strain is also called a "pulled muscle." When too great a demand is placed on a muscle, it and the surrounding tendons can stretch or tear. The main symptom is pain; swelling and muscle spasms may also occur.

Muscle spasms and cramps are common. Sometimes they occur spontaneously, such as the calf muscle cramps at night. Sometimes they are attributable to muscle strain (the charley horse that tightens thigh muscles in runners and other athletes). Muscles used often will go into spasm, such as those in the thumb and fingers of writers (writer's cramp), as can muscles that have remained in one position for too long. Muscle spasms and cramps can also occur as direct consequences of dehydration; they are common in athletes who sweat excessively during hot weather.

Some injuries to muscles and joints occur so regularly that they are named for their associated activities.

A good example is tennis elbow, a condition resulting from repeated, vigorous arm movement, such as swinging a tennis racket, using a paintbrush, or pitching a baseball. Runners' knee can afflict joggers and other athletes. Sprains usually cause it in the knee ligaments; there is pain, and there may be partial or total immobilization of the knee. As the name suggests, Achilles tendinitis is inflammation of the Achilles tendon in the heel. It is usually the result of excessive physical activity that causes small tears in the tendon. Pain and immobility are symptoms. Tendinitis can also occur in other joints; elbows and shoulders are common sites. Tenosynovitis is inflammation of the synovial membrane that sheathes the tendons in the hand. It may be caused by a bacterial infection or may be attributable to overexertion.

Tumors and cancerous growths in muscle tissue are rare. If a lump appears in muscle, it is usually a lipoma, a benign fatty deposit. However, one tumor, called "rhabdomyosarcoma," is malignant and can be fatal.

> **INFORMATION ON MUSCLE SPRAINS, SPASMS, AND DISORDERS**
>
> **Causes**: Injury, overexercise, disease, toxin or pesticide exposure, neurological or endocrine disorders, hereditary factors
>
> **Symptoms**: Vary; can include bruising, pain, inflammation, muscle spasms or cramps, progressive muscle weakness, loss of coordination, impaired gait
>
> **Duration**: Acute to chronic
>
> **Treatments**: Depends on the condition; may include physical therapy, surgery, medications (analgesics, steroids, corticosteroids, anti-inflammatory drugs), rest-ice-compression-elevation (R-I-C-E) formula

TREATMENT AND THERAPY

Myopathies are a wide group of diseases, and treatment varies considerably among them. The muscular dystrophies also vary in their treatment methods. Physical therapy is recommended to prevent contractures, the permanent, disfiguring muscular contractions that are a disease feature. Orthopedic appliances and surgery are also used. Because these diseases are genetic, it is sometimes recommended that people with a familial history of muscular dystrophy be tested for certain genetic markers that would suggest the possibility of disease in their children.

Myasthenia gravis is treated with drugs that increase the number of neurotransmitters available where nerves and muscles come together. The drugs help improve the transmission of information from the brain to the muscle tissue. In some cases, plasmapheresis is used to eliminate blood-borne substances that may contribute to the disease. Surgical removal of the thymus gland helps alleviate symptoms in some patients.

The R-I-C-E formula is recommended to treat the many muscle disorders caused by athletic activity and excessive wear and tear on the muscle. The acronym stands for rest-ice-compression-elevation: The patient must rest and not use or exercise the limb or muscle involved; an ice pack is applied to the injury; compression is supplied by wrapping a moist bandage snugly over the ice, reducing the flow of fluids to the injured area; and the injured limb is elevated. If a fracture is involved, the limb must be properly splinted or otherwise immobilized before elevation. The ice pack is held in place for twenty minutes and removed, but the bandage is held in place. Ice therapy can be resumed every twenty minutes.

Heat is also part of the therapy for strains and sprains. Still, it is not applied until after the initial swelling has gone down, usually after forty-eight to seventy-two hours. Heat raises the metabolic rate in the affected tissue. Increases local metabolism brings more blood to the area, carrying nutrients needed for tissue repair. Moist heat is preferred, and it can be supplied by an electrical heating pad, a chemical gel in a plastic bag, or hot baths and whirlpools. In using pads and chemical gels, there should be a layer of toweling or other material between the heat source and the body. A whirlpool or hot bath temperature should be about 106 degrees Fahrenheit. Only the injured part should be immersed, if possible. As in the ice treatments, heat should be applied for twenty minutes and can be repeated after twenty minutes of rest.

Analgesics are given for pain. Over-the-counter preparations such as aspirin, acetaminophen, or ibuprofen are often used. Sometimes, when pain is severe, more potent medications are required. Steroids are sometimes prescribed to reduce inflammation, and nonsteroidal anti-inflammatory drugs (NSAIDs) can alleviate pain and inflammation. Surgery may be required if a strained muscle or tendon is seriously torn or otherwise damaged. Similarly, if a sprain involves torn or detached ligaments, they may have to be surgically repaired.

Muscle spasms and cramps may require manipulation and applying heat or cold. Massage and immersion in a hot bath are useful, as are cold packs. The affected limb is gently extended to stretch the contracted muscle.

Tennis elbow, runner's knee, and tendinitis respond to RI-C-E therapy. Ice is applied to the injured site, and the limb is elevated and allowed to rest. When tenosynovitis is caused by bacterial infection, prompt antibiotic therapy may be necessary to avoid permanent damage. When it is attributable to overexertion, analgesics may help relieve pain and inflammation. Rarely a corticosteroid is used when other drugs fail.

Often, the injured site requires physical therapy for the full range of motion to be restored. The physical therapist analyzes the patient's capability and develops a regimen to restore strength and mobility to the affected muscles and joints. Physical therapy may involve massage, hot baths, whirlpools, weight training, or isometric exercise. Orthotic devices may be required to help the injured area heal.

An important aspect of sports medicine and the treatment of sports-related muscle disorders is prevention. Many painful, debilitating, and immobilizing episodes can be avoided by proper training and conditioning, intelligent exercise practice, and restriction of exertion. Before undertaking any sport or strenuous physical activity, the individual is advised to warm up by gentle stretching, jogging, jumping, and other mild muscular activities. Arms can be rotated in front of the body, over the head, and in circles perpendicular to the ground. Knees can be lifted and pulled up to the chest. Shoulders should be gently rotated to relax upper-back muscles. Neck muscles are toned by gently and slowly moving the head from side to side and in circles. Back muscles are loosened by bending forward and continuing around in slow circles.

If a joint has been injured, it is important to protect it from further damage. Physicians and physical therapists often recommend that athlete's tape, brace, or wrap susceptible joints, such as knees, ankles, elbows, or wrists. Sometimes a simple commercial elastic bandage, available in various configurations specific to parts of the body, is all that is required. Neck braces and back braces are used to support these structures.

Benign muscle tumors require no treatment or may be surgically removed. Malignant tumors may require surgery, radiation, and chemotherapy.

PERSPECTIVE AND PROSPECTS
With the increased interest in physical exercise in the United States has come increasing awareness of the dangers of muscular damage that can arise from improper exercise, as well as of the cardiovascular risks that lie in wait for weekend athletes. Warm-up procedures are universally recommended. Individual exercisers, those in gym classes, professional athletes, and schoolchildren are routinely taken through procedures to stretch and loosen muscles before they start a strenuous activity.

Greater attention is being paid to the special needs of young athletes, such as gymnasts. Over the years, new athletic toys and devices have constantly been developed for the young: Skateboards, skates, scooters, and bicycles expose children to a wide range of bumps, falls, bruises, strains, and sprains. Protective equipment and devices have been designed especially for them: Helmets, padding, and special uniforms give children more security in accidents. Similarly, adults should take the time and trouble to outfit themselves correctly for the sports and athletics they engage in: Joggers should tape, wrap, and brace their joints, and cyclists should wear helmets.

Nevertheless, the incidence of sports- and athletics-related muscular damage is relatively high, indicating the necessity for increased attention to prevention. The growth of sports medicine as a medical specialty helps considerably in this endeavor. Physicians and nurses in this area are trained to deal with the various problems that arise and are often expert commentators on the best means to prevent them.

—*C. Richard Falcon*

Further Reading
Brukner, Peter, and Karim Khan. *Brukner & Khan's Clinical Sports Medicine*. 4th ed., McGraw-Hill, 2010. Print.
Kirkaldy-Willis, et al., editors. *Managing Low Back Pain*. 4th ed., Churchill Livingstone, 1999.
Litin, Scott C., editor. *Mayo Clinic Family Health Book*. 4th ed., Harper Resource, 2009.
MacAuley, Domhnall. *Oxford Handbook of Sport and Exercise Medicine*. 2nd ed., Oxford UP, 2012.
Marieb, Elaine N., and Katja Hoehn. *Human Anatomy and Physiology*. 9th ed., Pearson/Benjamin Cummings, 2010.
McArdle, William, et al. *Exercise Physiology: Energy, Nutrition, and Human Performance*. 7th ed., Lippincott Williams & Wilkins, 2010.
Rouzier, Pierre A. *The Sports Medicine Patient Advisor*. 3rd ed., Sports Med Press, 2010.
Salter, Robert Bruce. *Textbook of Disorders and Injuries of the Musculoskeletal System*. 3rd ed., Williams & Wilkins, 1999.

Post-Concussion Syndrome

Category: Injury
Specialties and related fields: Neurology, psychiatry, psychology
Definition: a sequel to concussions when concussion symptoms last beyond the expected recovery period after the initial injury

KEY TERMS

amnesia: partial or total memory loss
concussion: temporary unconsciousness or confusion caused by a blow on the head
dizziness: a sensation of spinning around and losing one's balance
headaches: a continuous pain in the head

INTRODUCTION

Post-concussion syndrome (PCS) is a condition that occurs following a head injury, usually a concussion. The condition presents varying symptoms ranging from minor headaches to memory loss. These symptoms can last for days, weeks, or months. In some cases, PCS can persist for years. However, a head injury is the primary cause of PCS, and not all patients who experience head trauma develop PCS. Treatment for the condition depends on the severity and persistence of symptoms. Many experts believe PCS is caused by structural damage to the brain and a disruption of the brain's neural networks. Health-care professionals also note a connection between underlying psychological conditions and PCS development following head trauma.

BACKGROUND

Post-concussion syndrome usually develops following a concussion, the least serious and most common type of traumatic brain injury caused by a sudden impact on the head. This impact shakes the brain; sometimes, the brain moves around inside the skull. This movement can cause bruising, blood vessel damage, and nerve injuries, leading to several symptoms.

Individuals who have suffered previous concussions or head trauma are more likely to experience PCS than those who have not. Patients with a history of headaches are more prone to developing the condition. Age is also a risk factor in developing PCS. Women, the elderly, and younger patients have a higher risk of developing PCS following head trauma.

Most experts agree that both physiological and emotional factors play an important role in PCS occurrence. Many medical experts believe PCS is primarily caused by the impact itself, which causes structural or nerve damage to the brain. These physical problems are thought to lead to the common symptoms associated with PCS. Other health-care professionals believe PCS symptoms are psychological. Many common symptoms resemble those experienced by individuals with depression, anxiety, and post-traumatic stress disorder (PTSD).

Researchers have not determined why some patients with previous instances of head trauma develop persistent PCS while others do not, however. Studies have not shown a connection between the head injury's seriousness and persistent PCS's emergence. However, some studies have found that certain medical diagnoses are more common in head trauma patients who develop PCS than in patients who do not. For instance, patients with a history of depression, anxiety, and PTSD more commonly develop PCS. The condition is also more likely to develop in individuals experiencing major life stressors and those who lack a good social support system and coping skills.

OVERVIEW

Patients experiencing PCS usually begin showing symptoms within the first seven to ten days after experiencing head trauma. PCS symptoms can last from a few days to a few months; in some cases, patients experience symptoms for years. Patients with PCS commonly report experiencing headaches, dizziness, sleep disorders, mental symptoms such as depression and anxiety, and memory and concentration problems. Other symptoms include fatigue, ringing in the ears, blurred vision, noise and light sensitivity, and in rare instances, a loss of smell and taste. Patients who report headaches often describe them as being tension or migraine-like. Some experts believe such headaches are a symptom of a neck injury sustained with a concussion or head injury.

Although no definitive test exists to show a patient has developed PCS, doctors often suggest brain scans such as computerized tomography (CT) scan or magnetic resonance imaging (MRI) to look for brain abnormalities. Patients experiencing dizziness may also be referred to an ear, nose, and throat (ENT) doctor. Doctors recommend that patients exhibiting depression, anxiety, or memory loss visit a psychologist or licensed counselor for proper diagnosis.

No single treatment effectively resolves all cases of PCS. Treatment for PCS is specific to the symptoms each patient presents. Many patients simply need rest and a reduction in stress to recover fully. Health professionals also treat PCS by the symptom. For headaches, doctors often prescribe medications used for tension or migraine headaches. Other medicines that appear to be effective at treating PCS headaches include antidepressants, antihypertensive agents, and antiepileptic agents. However, patients are warned not to overuse these medications, as it can lead to persistent PCS headaches.

Patients who experience problems such as memory loss and lack of concentration following head trauma are advised to keep rested and wait to see if the symptoms dissipate or worsen. Since stress can aggravate the cognitive symptoms of PCS, patients are sometimes advised to learn stress-management techniques. These symptoms often dissolve on their own within a few weeks or months. Some doctors recommend cognitive therapy to help strengthen cognitive areas affected during the head trauma. Some patients will require occupational or speech therapy to restore various physiological functions.

Individuals who develop psychological symptoms such as anxiety or depression are encouraged to visit a psychologist or psychiatrist. These professionals help people with PCS cope with the effects and provide medications such as antidepressants or antianxiety pills to help ease symptoms.

Health-care professionals recommend avoiding head injuries at all costs to curtail PCS. Although it is not always possible to prevent head trauma, individuals can avoid certain activities to decrease their chances of getting a head injury. Common activities that can lead to head trauma include football, baseball, skiing, and snowboarding. Riding a bicycle or motorcycle can also lead to a head injury. People engaging in certain sports and high-speed activities are advised to wear a helmet to protect the head in an accident.

—*Cait Caffrey*

Further Reading

Bowman, Joe. "Post-Concussion Syndrome." *Healthline*, 28 Aug. 2019, www.healthline.com/health/post-concussion-syndrome#causes3. Accessed 30 Oct. 2017.

"Concussion (Traumatic Brain Injury)." *WebMD*, 25 Aug. 2020, www.webmd.com/brain/concussion-traumatic-brain-injury-symptoms-causes-treatments#1. Accessed 30 Oct. 2017.

Leddy, John J., et al. "Rehabilitation of Concussion and Post-concussion Syndrome." *Sports Health*, vol. 4, no. 2, 2012, pp. 147-54, www.ncbi.nlm.nih.gov/pmc/articles/PMC3435903/.

"Mind, Body and Sport: Post-Concussion Syndrome." *National Collegiate Athletic Association*, n.d., www.ncaa.org/sport-science-institute/mind-body-and-sport-post-concussion-syndrome.

"Post-Concussion Syndrome." *Mayo Clinic*, 6 Oct. 2020, www.mayoclinic.org/diseases-conditions/post-concussion-syndrome/symptoms-causes/syc-20353352. Accessed 30 Oct. 2017.

"Post-Concussion Syndrome." *WebMD*, 19 Apr. 2021, www.webmd.com/brain/post-concussion-syndrome. Accessed 30 Oct. 2017.

"Postconcussive Syndrome in the ED." *MedScape*, 24 Sept. 2018, emedicine.medscape.com/article/828904-overview?pa=KwZqvW%2FA7DuAHx67PMGl7hi9c58jxFhRd2Zx%2BUzZm%2FaYsSfkvLYCg1JVxbMrw1SmBxE%2FchwRMJ0Z5P4D5Tj5%2FQ8oyMK1o%2FrQdMeQkhfWxCQ%3D. Accessed 30 Oct. 2017.

"What Is PCS?" *Concussion Legacy Foundation*, n.d., concussionfoundation.org/PCS-resources/what-is-PCS. Accessed 30 Oct. 2017.

REPETITIVE STRAIN INJURY (RSI)

Category: Injury

Definition: impairment of loss of function in tendons and muscles, typically in the hands, caused by the repetitive performance of certain actions

KEY TERMS

bursitis: inflammation of the fluid-filled pads (bursae) that act as cushions at the joints, typically in the knee, elbow, or shoulder

epicondylitis: inflammation of the tendons surrounding the elbow, typically due to overuse and repetitive motions of the forearm

sprain: wrench or twist the ligaments of (an ankle, wrist, or other joint) violently to cause pain and swelling but not dislocation

strain: a stretching or tearing of a muscle or a tissue connecting muscle to bone

tendonitis: inflammation of a tendon, most commonly from overuse but also from infection or rheumatic disease

INTRODUCTION

A repetitive strain injury (RSI) is a condition that occurs due to repetitive motions, such as assembly-line work, computer work, or activities like playing musical instruments, sewing, or playing tennis. Such injuries affect muscles, nerves, tendons, and other soft tissues and may be very painful. Repetitive strain injury is also known as: cumulative trauma disorder, occupational overuse syndrome, regional musculoskeletal disorder, repetitive motion injury, repetitive motion disorder, and stress injury.

Repetitive strain injury may be caused by many actions, such as awkward or sustained positions, mechanical compression (pressing against hard surfaces), and repetitive tasks. Types of RSI include bursitis, carpal tunnel syndrome, epicondylitis, ganglion cyst, tendinitis, tenosynovitis, tennis elbow, and trigger finger.

OVERVIEW

Experts have identified two types of RSI. Type 1 includes carpal tunnel syndrome and tendinitis and is usually caused by repetitive tasks. Type 2 is often called "nonspecific pain syndrome." Patients feel pain, but a medical exam does not find evidence of inflammation or swelling.

Some examples of RSI include the following:

- Bursitis is inflammation of the bursa, a sac filled with fluid. Bursae cushion bones, joints, tendons, and muscles.
- Carpal tunnel syndrome (CTS) occurs when the median nerve is compressed in the carpal tunnel, which is in the wrist area. Individuals with CTS may experience numbness and pain in the hand.
- Epicondylitis, which includes tennis elbow and golfer's elbow, results from overusing the muscles and tendons in a joint. Rotator cuff syndrome is a similar condition that occurs in the shoulder.

- Tendinitis is inflammation of a tendon.
- A condition commonly called "writer's cramp" is a type of RSI caused by computer use. Experts say this condition has been rising for some time as computer work has become more common.

Repetitive strain injury often affects parts of the arm—including the elbow, forearm, hand, and wrist—and is frequently related to workplace activities. Some causes of RSI include overuse of muscles in the arms, back, hands, neck, shoulders, and wrists; repetitious actions, often performed daily for a long time; a cold work environment; vibrating equipment; poorly designed equipment or poorly organized work areas; forceful movement; infrequent rest breaks; and awkward posture.

Experts are not sure why RSI affects some people but not others. Not everyone who performs the same job or does the same activities gets RSI. Researchers are examining psychosocial factors in the workplace, such as stress, to see if they factor into RSI development. One theory is that stress causes muscle tension, which might cause pain sensitivity.

SIGNS, SYMPTOMS, AND TREATMENT

An individual may report symptoms, such as pain. Other people, including medical professionals, may observe symptoms, such as a rash or swelling. Symp-

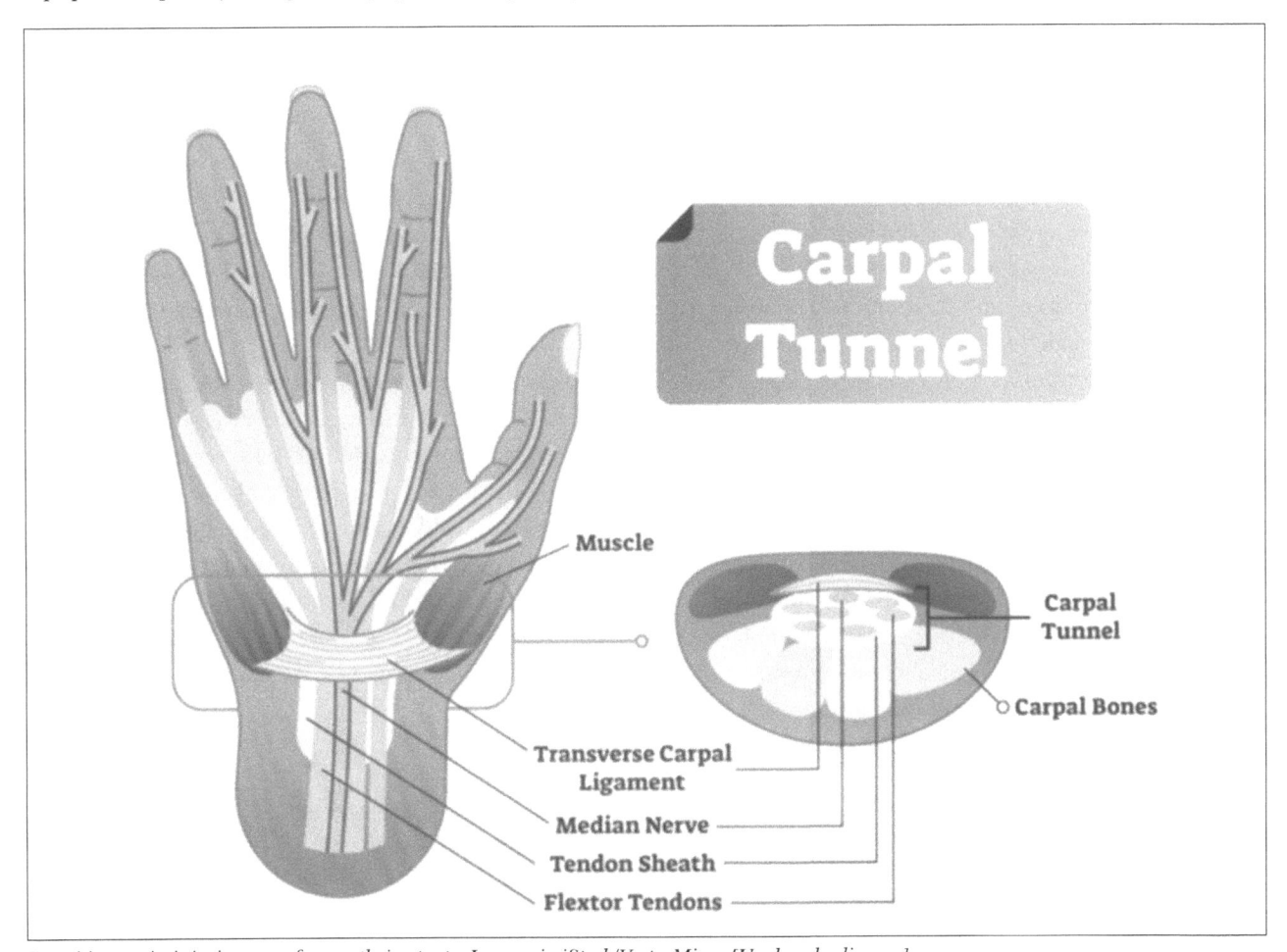

Repetitive strain injuries occur frequently in sports. Image via iStock/VectorMine. [Used under license.]

toms may be transitory. For example, they may only be experienced at certain times, such as when the patient moves a body part in a certain way. Sometimes they become worse over time and become constant. Common RSI signs and symptoms include pain and tenderness, throbbing, tingling (also called "pins and needles"), and loss of sensation and strength.

Early treatment may prevent further damage, but serious injury may be permanent. The goal of treatment is usually pain relief and improved mobility and strength. Pain may be treated with anti-inflammatory painkillers, such as ibuprofen and heat or cold packs. Elastic wraps may be used to support the affected area, and splints may be needed to immobilize the area. In some cases, steroid injections may also be used to treat inflammation.

Some patients may benefit from physical therapy, which often includes exercises such as walking and swimming. Physical therapists sometimes offer patients tips regarding posture to help them prevent further injury. Patients may also benefit from yoga, tai chi, other activities, and meditation. For some, electrotherapy, which targets painful areas with small electrical impulses, may offer pain relief. However, some patients with severe injuries may need surgery.

Occupational therapy (OT) involves assessing the workplace or activity that led to the RSI. Occupational therapists may discuss work environment issues, such as chair height, keyboard position, and equipment such as mouse devices and pen tablets. Occupational therapy may also include identifying stressors in the workplace and examining work habits, such as scheduling regular breaks from the activity.

PREVENTION

Experts have identified several ways to avoid RSI. Computer station RSI may be the result of poor posture. Chairs should be adjusted so users' forearms are horizontal to their desks. Thighs should be level, and feet should be flat on the floor or a footrest. The top of the computer screen should be level with an individual's eyes. Equipment such as standing or adjustable desks have also been proposed to help avoid the postures and repetition that can lead to RSI.

Computer keyboards may cause strain on the user. New keyboards have been developed to allow users to position their hands more naturally. Software features such as autocorrect may eliminate frequent keystrokes to correct mistakes. Combination keystrokes should be made using both hands rather than by contorting the fingers of one hand to hit both keys. A keyboard should be adjusted, so it tilts away from the user, and the wrists should not rest on a wrist pad. Workers should occasionally stretch their fingers and wrists.

A standard mouse also may cause or aggravate RSI, so some users may benefit from trying out other types of equipment or using keyboard shortcuts instead of the mouse. Mouse tool software or voice recognition software may eliminate the need for a mouse.

Experts believe people should take ten-minute breaks every hour when performing repetitive activities. Workers might schedule tasks such as photocopying throughout the day to take breaks from repetitive actions like typing. They might also take time to stretch their fingers and hands or get up and walk around to help loosen the muscles in the shoulders and neck.

—*Josephine Campbell*

Further Reading

Hendrickson, Mark. "Repetitive Stress Injury." *Cleveland Clinic*, 2018, my.clevelandclinic.org/health/diseases/17424-repetitive-stress-injury. Accessed 23 Feb. 2018.

"NINDS Repetitive Motion Disorders Information Page." *National Institute of Neurological Disorders and Stroke*, 11 July 2013, www.ninds.nih.gov/disorders/repetitive_motion/repetitive_motion.htm. Accessed 30 Jan. 2015.

Nordqvist, Christian. "What Is Repetitive Strain Injury (RSI)? What Causes Repetitive Strain Injury?" *Medical News Today*. MediLexicon International Limited, 19 Jan. 2010, www.medicalnewstoday.com/articles/176443.php. Accessed 19 Jan. 2010.

"Prevent RSI." *National Health Service*. Gov.UK, 10 Oct. 2013, www.nhs.uk/Livewell/workplacehealth/Pages/rsi.aspx.

"Preventing RSI." *Harvard RSI Action*. Harvard University, www.rsi.deas.harvard.edu/preventing.html. Accessed 2 Feb. 2015.

"Repetitive Strain Injury (RSI)." *NHS Choices*. Gov.UK, 27 Jan. 2016, www.nhs.uk/conditions/repetitive-strain-injury-rsi/. Accessed 23 Feb. 2018.

Soft Tissue Pain

Category: Condition
Specialties and related fields: Athletic training, chiropractic, occupational therapy, orthopedics, physical therapy
Definition: the result of trauma or overuse occurs of muscles, tendons, or ligaments

KEY TERMS

pain relief: techniques or medications that prevent or reduce pain

therapeutic massage: manipulation of the body's soft tissues to treat body stress or pain

transcutaneous electrical nerve stimulation (TENS): the use of electric current produced by a device to stimulate the nerves for therapeutic purpose

INTRODUCTION

When specific causes of symptoms are unknown, doctors sometimes refer to conditions simply by naming the symptoms. Such is the case for soft tissue pain. The term "soft tissue pain" refers to discomfort in the interconnected system of muscles, tendons, and ligaments, as opposed to the bones, and says nothing about the particular cause.

The most commonly used conventional treatments for soft tissue pain consist primarily of drugs that relieve pain and inflammation, such as ibuprofen, acetaminophen, and muscle relaxants. Physical therapy methods are commonly recommended for selected forms of soft tissue pain. Still, there is little to no reliable scientific evidence that they help. Other methods, such as therapeutic exercises, may help. Still, most reported studies are significantly flawed by the lack of a credible placebo treatment.

A similar lack of reliable evidence exists regarding other nonsurgical, nondrug methods used to control soft tissue pain, such as injection therapy, radiofrequency denervation, and transcutaneous electrical nerve stimulation (TENS). Surgery may be useful for certain selected forms of soft tissue pain, although the supporting research evidence is generally incomplete.

PROPOSED NATURAL TREATMENTS

Natural soft tissue pain treatments include back pain, bursitis, fibromyalgia, neck pain, rotator cuff injury, sciatic pain, sports injuries, sprains, tendonitis, and tension headache. Alternative therapies that may be useful for soft tissue pain, in general, include acupuncture, biofeedback, chiropractic, hypnosis, magnet therapy, massage, prolotherapy, and relaxation therapy. Herbs and supplements that may have a general pain-relieving effect include Boswellia, butterbur, devil's claw, D-phenylalanine, proteolytic enzymes, and white willow.

—*EBSCO CAM Review Board*

Further Reading

Bisset, L., et al. "A Systematic Review and Meta-analysis of Clinical Trials on Physical Interventions for Lateral Epicondylalgia." *British Journal of Sports Medicine*, vol. 39, 2005, pp. 411-22.

Frost, H., et al. "Randomised Controlled Trial of Physiotherapy Compared with Advice for Low Back Pain." *British Medical Journal*, vol. 329, 2004, p. 708.

Hayden, J. A., et al. "Meta-analysis: Exercise Therapy for Nonspecific Low Back Pain." *Annals of Internal Medicine*, vol. 142, 2005, pp. 765-75.

Khadilkar, A., et al. "Transcutaneous Electrical Nerve Stimulation (TENS) for Chronic Low Back Pain." *The Cochrane Database of Systematic Reviews*, vol. 3, no. CD003008, 2005, doi:10.1002/14651858.CD003008.pub2.

Niemisto, L., et al. "Radiofrequency Denervation for Neck and Back Pain." *The Cochrane Database of Systematic Reviews*, vol. 1, no. CD004058, 2003, doi:10.1002/14651858.CD004058.

Robertson, V. J., and K. G. Baker. "A Review of Therapeutic Ultrasound: Effectiveness Studies." *Physical Therapy*, vol. 81, 2001, pp. 1339-50.

Sports-Related Wrist and Hand Injuries

Category: Injury
Specialties and related fields: Orthopedics, orthopedic surgery, physical therapy, sports medicine
Definition: strains, sprains, fractures, or tears of the tendons, ligaments, muscles, or bones of the hand or wrist due to overuse, trauma, or aging

KEY TERMS

ligaments: a short band of tough, flexible fibrous connective tissue which connects two bones or cartilages or holds together a joint

sprain: a stretching or tearing of ligaments, the fibrous tissue that connects bones and joints

strain: a stretching or tearing of a muscle or a tissue connecting muscle to bone (tendon)

tendons: a flexible but inelastic cord of strong fibrous collagen tissue attaching a muscle to a bone

tendinitis: inflammation of a tendon, most commonly from overuse but also from infection or rheumatic disease

tendinosis: degeneration of the tendon's collagen in response to chronic overuse

INTRODUCTION

Sprains are damage to ligaments. A ligament is a type of tissue that connects bone to bone. There are different grades of sprain, from minor tear to complete rupture. Treatment and recovery time will depend on the grade of the sprain.

While hand and wrist injuries are very common among all types of athletes, some never seek treatment. However, delaying the diagnosis and treatment may result in long-term problems or permanent disability. Here is a list of some of the most common hand and wrist injuries that athletes experience.

SPRAINS

Sprains are damage to ligaments. A ligament is a type of tissue that connects bone to bone. There are different grades of sprain, from minor tear to complete rupture. Treatment and recovery time will depend on the grade of the sprain.

THUMB SPRAINS

Breaking a fall with the palm of your hand or taking a spill on the slopes with your hand strapped to a ski pole could leave you with a painful thumb injury. The ulnar collateral ligament acts like a hinge and helps your thumb function properly. If you sprain your thumb, you could lose some or all of your ability to grasp items between your thumb and index finger or to grasp well with the entire hand.

WRIST SPRAINS

A wrist sprain occurs when you stretch or tear the ligaments that connect the bones in your wrist. This can happen when you break a fall by landing on the palm of your hand. This may result in an overextension of your wrist, causing a sprain.

INJURIES TO THE BONE

Bones can be fractured and dislocated. A fracture is a crack or break in a bone. A dislocation occurs when a bone is pushed out of place and no longer lines up correctly at the joint. Both injuries decrease the ability to move and cause pain.

HAND FRACTURES

Fractures of the hand include breaking the bones of the hand between your wrist and knuckles, as well as your fingers. The most hand fracture is called a "boxer's fracture." A boxer's fracture usually occurs when you strike an object with your closed fist, injuring the long bone that connects the little finger to the wrist. This fracture also results in damage to the surrounding soft tissues.

WRIST FRACTURES

Scaphoid fractures account for many wrist fractures. The scaphoid bone is one of eight small bones that make up the wrist. The scaphoid bone lies at the base of the thumb adjacent to the radius, one of two large bones that make up the forearm.

Wrist fractures are common both in sports and motor vehicle accidents. The break usually occurs during a fall on the outstretched hand. The angle at which the palm hits the ground may determine the type of injury. The more the wrist is bent back (extension), the more likely the scaphoid bone will break. With less wrist extension, it is more likely the radius will break.

Scaphoid fractures are not always immediately obvious. Many people with a fractured scaphoid think they have a sprained wrist instead of a broken bone because there is no obvious deformity and very little swelling.

DISLOCATIONS OF THE PIP JOINT

One of the most common injuries to an athlete's hand is an injury to the joint above the knuckle, the proximal interphalangeal (PIP) joint. Injuries to the PIP joint occur when the finger is forced backward or downward into a bent position. Injuries to the PIP joint may include fractures, dislocations, and fracture-dislocations.

SOFT TISSUE AND CLOSED TENDON INJURIES

Tendons are a type of connective tissue that attaches muscle to bone. Tendon injuries may result from:
- **Tendinitis**—inflammation of the tendon associated with acute injury
- **Tendinosis**—microtears in the tendon tissue with no significant inflammation, associated with chronic injury

DEQUERVAIN'S SYNDROME

DeQuervain's syndrome is a common injury in racquet sports and athletes who use a lot of wrist motion, especially repetitive rotating and gripping.

The overuse of the hand may eventually irritate the tendons found along the thumb side of the wrist. This irritation causes the lining around the tendon to swell, making it difficult for the tendons to move properly.

ECU TENDINITIS

Extensor carpi ulnaris (ECU) tendinitis is another common sports-related closed tendon injury. ECU tendinitis is an inflammation of the tendon that runs along the back of the wrist and is caused by repetitive twisting and backward flexion. It is most commonly seen in basketball players and those playing racquet sports.

BASEBALL FINGER

A baseball finger (or mallet finger) is an injury commonly occurring at the baseball season's beginning. It occurs when a ball hits the tip of your finger, bending it down. Normally, the tip of your finger can bend toward the palm of your hand about 60-70 degrees. However, add the force of a ball that has been batted through the air, and it can push your finger beyond that limit, tearing the extensor tendon that controls muscle movement in the affected finger. If the force is great enough, it may even pull tiny pieces of bone away.

JERSEY FINGER

A Jersey finger is the opposite of a mallet finger. It occurs when the fingertip, usually the ring finger, is forcibly extended, such as if your finger gets caught in an opponent's jersey. This causes the flexor tendon, which bends the fingertip, to be pulled away from the bone and will leave you unable to bend your finger without assistance.

BOUTONNIERE DEFORMITY

Boutonniere deformity is an injury to the tendons that straighten your fingers. It occurs when your finger receives a forceful blow when it is bent. Several tendons running along the side and top of your finger work together to straighten the finger. Suppose the tendon on the top that attaches to the middle bone of the finger (the central slip of the tendon) is injured by a forceful blow. In that case, it can sever the central slip from its attachment to the bone, in some cases, even popping the bone through the opening. The tear looks like a buttonhole. If you have a boutonniere deformity, the middle joint of your finger will bend downward, and the fingertip end joint bends back. People with a boutonniere deformity cannot fully straighten their finger.

PREVENTING SPORTS-RELATED HAND AND WRIST INJURIES

The best ways to prevent sports-related hand, wrist, and upper extremity injuries include:

- **Take your time**: Gradually work yourself into shape for any new activities. Slowly increase the length of time and intensity of all activities.
- **Wrist guards**: If your sport is rollerblading, street hockey, or skateboarding, wrist guards may help protect you from bone fractures and hand scrapes if you fall or slide.
- **Gloves**: Use gloves to protect your hands, particularly if you are a bicyclist or skateboarder. In addition to protecting your nerves, gloves can protect your skin from direct wounds and cuts. The gloves will help protect your hands if the palm suffers a direct blow.
- **Warm-up**: Before playing sports, include a warm-up routine to focus on light stretching and improving your flexibility. Warm-ups should also include light running, walking, or biking to elevate your heart rate and loosen your muscles.

—Elizabeth Peterson

Further Reading

"8 Minute Stretching Routine for Women!" *YouTube*, uploaded by fabulous50s, 6 Sept. 2019, www.youtube.com/watch?v=6CfUWws9IYs.

Aronowitz, E. R., and J. P. Leddy. "Closed Tendon Injuries of the Hand and Wrist in Athletes." *Clinics in Sports Medicine*, vol. 17, no. 3, 1998, pp. 449-67.

Brown, H. C. "Common Injuries of the Athlete's Hand." *Canadian Medical Association Journal*, vol. 117, no. 6, 1977, pp. 621-25.

Chen, N. C., J. B. Jupiter, et al. "Sports-Related Wrist Injuries in Adults." *Sports Health*, vol. 1, no. 6, 2009, pp. 469-77.

"Flexor Tendon Injuries." *OrthoInfo*, Jan. 2022, orthoinfo.aaos.org/en/diseases—conditions/flexor-tendon-injuries/.

"Hand Fractures." *OrthoInfo*, May 2022, orthoinfo.aaos.org/en/diseases—conditions/hand-fractures.

Morgan, W. J., and L. S. Slowman. "Acute Hand and Wrist Injuries in Athletes: Evaluation and Management." *Journal of the American Academy of Orthopaedic Surgeons*, vol. 9, no. 6, 2001, pp. 389-400.

Shehab, Ramsey, and Mark H. Mirabelli. "Evaluation and Diagnosis of Wrist Pain: A Case-Based Approach." *American Family Physician*, vol. 87, no. 8, 2013, pp. 568-73.

"Sprained Thumb." *American Society for the Surgery of the Hand*, 2015, www.assh.org/handcare/condition/sprained-thumb.

"Wrist Sprains." *OrthoInfo*, Apr. 2018, orthoinfo.aaos.org/en/diseases—conditions/wrist-sprains.

STRENGTH TRAINING

Category: Procedure
Anatomy or system affected: Musculoskeletal
Specialties and related fields: Physiology, fitness, gerontology
Definition: strength training is a type of physical exercise specializing in the use of resistance to induce muscular contraction, which builds the strength, anaerobic endurance, and size of skeletal muscles

KEY TERMS

anabolism: the repair/growth stage of muscle development
body weight: the use of the person's natural weight as the form of resistance while exercising
catabolism: damage to muscles
free weight: a freestanding object whose weight is used as resistance while exercising
spotter: a person who assists with a person exercising to ensure proper technique and injury prevention; this can be hands-on, by being in a physical position to prevent accidents, or hands-off by watching the exercising person and being ready to assist as needed
stretchable tubing: elastic workout object with little to no weight that uses tension to create resistance for exercise
weight machine: a stationary machine used for exercise that uses attached weights and gravity to offer resistance

INTRODUCTION

Strength training, also called "resistance training" or weight lifting, is a type of exercise that uses resistance to build strength, muscle mass, and endurance. Resistance may be in the form of weights, weight machines, stretchable tubing, or body weight. Using resistance causes muscles to contract or shorten, strengthening them.

When a person creates resistance on a muscle, tiny tears damage the muscle cells. After strength training, hormones, nutrients, and proteins in the body repair and replenish muscles, helping them grow. The damage to the muscles is called "catabolism," and the repair/growth stage is called "anabolism." Building muscle has many positive health effects. It has been shown to help people manage their weight, strengthen their bones, and build their stamina.

TYPES OF STRENGTH-TRAINING EXERCISES

Fitness experts classify strength-training exercises by the type of resistance used. Athletes can perform these exercises using free weights or items found in the home, specialized machines found at gyms, resistance tubing, or even one's body weight. People can use a combination of different strength-training exercises and cardiovascular exercise to achieve maximum health and performance.

FREE WEIGHTS

Free weights, such as barbells and dumbbells, can be used to provide resistance. Lifting free weights has many advantages. People do not need expensive equipment or even a gym membership to lift free weights. At home, they can use heavy objects such as canned goods, bricks, or water bottles to exercise their muscles.

Moving and controlling free weights takes great focus and helps people improve their coordination skills. People with injuries or limited movement can adjust how they lift free weights to accommodate their needs. In addition, lifting free weights exercises many muscles at once, even ones that are not specifically targeted. For example, if people stand and raise weights in front of them, the muscles in the abdomen and back will help keep the body steady.

Nevertheless, there are some disadvantages to lifting free weights. People who do not use proper form while lifting weights may risk serious injury. To prevent injury, people should not lift weights that are too heavy. Furthermore, they should always lift weights—especially heavy weights—with another person, known as a "spotter," to ensure they are using the correct form. Other disadvantages involve the storage and cost of free weights. Storing free weights and designating an area to lift can be an issue in homes with little free space. Free weights can also be costly if people purchase multiple pieces of equipment, such as weight benches, bars, and weight plates.

WEIGHT MACHINES

Weight machines are relatively easy to use. They are safer than free weights and do not require as much coordination. People position themselves on the machines, move a pin in the weight stack to the desired weight, and then move the machine by either pushing or pulling on handles or bars. Still, people must use good form on the machines, so they do not injure themselves, and they should avoid lifting weights that are too heavy.

Using weight machines has several disadvantages. They are large and expensive, so most people must join a gym to use them. Machines usually target only one set of muscles, which means a person must use multiple machines to work different muscle groups. People not of average size may have difficulty using the machines correctly. Additionally, since most machines cannot be adjusted, they might not properly accommodate people with limited movement or injuries.

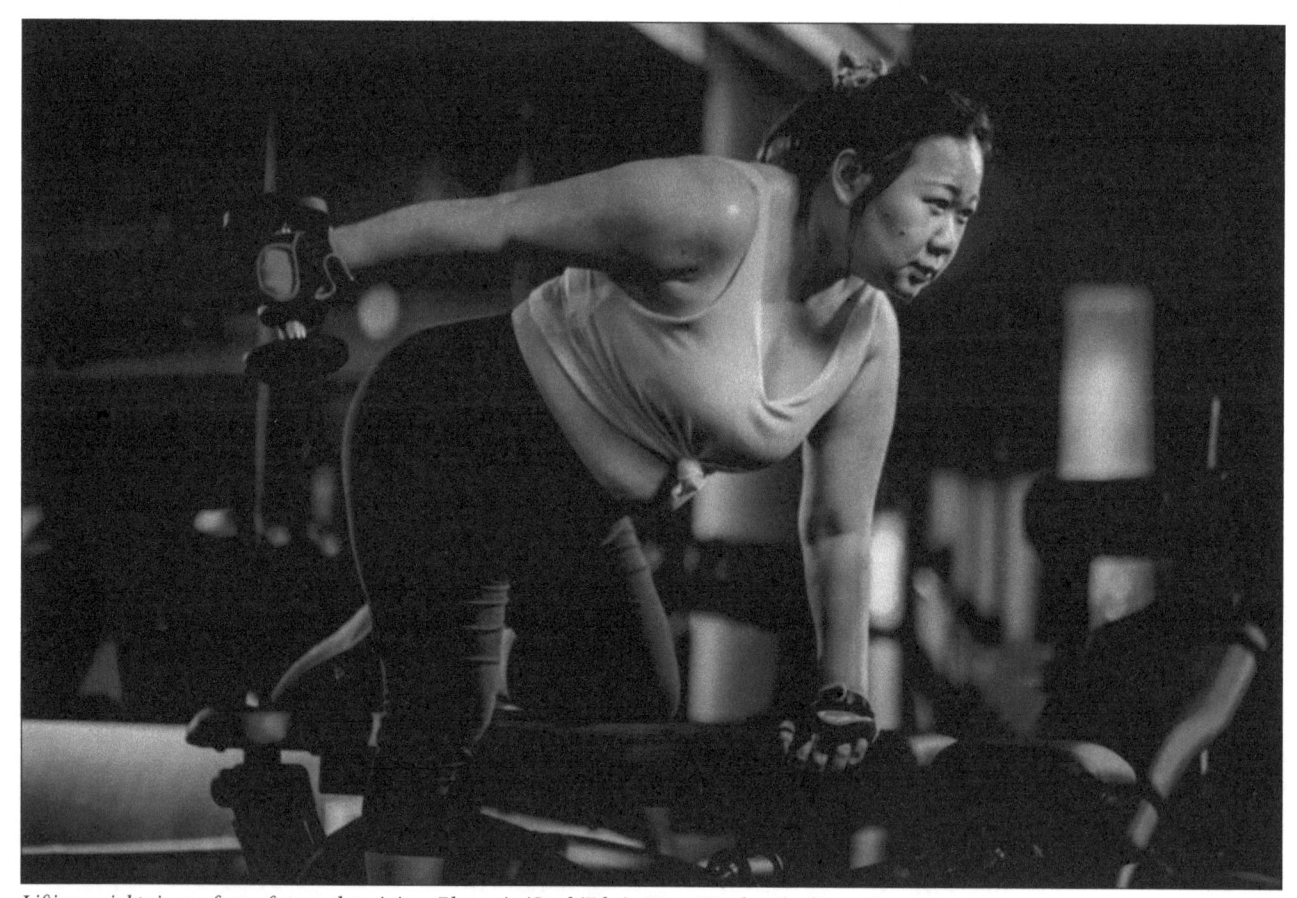

Lifting weights is one form of strength training. Photo via iStock/Edwin Tan. [Used under license.]

STRETCHABLE TUBING

Stretchable or resistance tubing is made of elastic tubes that stretch to provide resistance. They come in different sizes and thicknesses, creating more or less tension. To use them, people put them around a body part and pull on them to create tension. This causes the muscle to contract. Stretchable tubes are inexpensive, portable, easy to use, and take up little space. They can also target a variety of muscle groups. However, these tubes lose elasticity over time and may need replacement. Additionally, they can snap and cause injury.

BODY WEIGHT

People do not need free weights, machines, or stretchable tubing to strength train. They can use their own body weight as resistance to perform exercises such as abdominal crunches, leg squats, lunges, pull-ups, push-ups, and more. These types of exercises use the weight of a person's body as resistance. The major advantage to using one's body weight is that it is free. No special equipment is needed. Also, exercises that rely on body weight can be performed anywhere. A disadvantage to this form of strength training is that the resistance cannot be decreased. Yet, resistance may be increased by altering how some exercises are performed.

BENEFITS OF STRENGTH TRAINING

Strength training has many benefits. These benefits include improved athletic performance, injury rehabilitation, weight loss and stress, and combat effects of aging. According to the American College of Sports Medicine, a person should work out all the muscle groups to fatigue at least two to three days a week with rest days between active workout days to achieve maximum results. The major muscle groups include the abdominals, arms, back, chest, legs, and shoulders. Working out a muscle to fatigue means people should perform an exercise with weights that are heavy enough so that they can only perform eight to twelve repetitions. This is just an average number and can change depending on several factors, such as a person's age, health, goals, and strength.

Strength training is one of the primary methods people use to improve athletic performance. Strength training programs can improve an athlete's muscle power and economy. An improvement in the economy allows an athlete's body to burn through less energy at lower levels of intensity, as well as slowing down the draining of carbohydrate stores. An improvement in muscle power allows an athlete to increase the amount of force produced, improving performance.

Injury rehabilitation, facilitated by a physical therapist, often utilizes body weight, resistance bands, and weight machines to regain muscle strength and function in later stages. Regaining muscle strength is accomplished through a focus on stabilizing muscles. An increased function is accomplished through a program designed to increase the muscle's range of motion.

Research has indicated that the average American does not move enough and leads a sedentary lifestyle. Many people have jobs that keep them inactive during the day. In addition, many people spend much of their free time doing sedentary activities, such as watching television or playing on computers, instead of physically exercising. These conditions can lead to weight gain and stress. Strength training releases the brain neurotransmitters dopamine and serotonin, which, when released, help combat depression. Muscles during strength training also burn through carbohydrates, which when combined with a healthy diet, results in weight loss.

Research has shown that specific effects of aging on the brain, muscle strength, and muscle density can be slowed down by incorporating strength training. Strength training increases neurogenesis, neuroplasticity, and cognition performance, slowing down the deterioration of brain function. After the age of thirty, people lose five pounds of muscle every decade. In addition, people lose bone density as they age. Research has proven that resistance exercises can help slow or even reverse age-related muscle and bone loss. Strength training also helps to reduce the loss of motor.

RISKS OF STRENGTH TRAINING

Strength training can also have harmful effects on the body. These effects usually occur due to overtraining or improper technique. Proper research and consulting with strength and conditioning professionals can greatly reduce the risks of strength training.

Overtraining occurs when the intensity and frequency of strength training routines over an extended period doesn't allow the body significant time to recover. Overtraining has a variety of negative consequences, including muscle weakness, decreased athletic performance, reduction in quality of sleep, and increased resting heart rate. Overtraining is easily preventable by recognizing body fatigue and allowing ample time for the body to recover following strength training.

Improper technique occurs when a strength training exercise is done incorrectly. Poor exercise form can have immediate and long-term effects on the body. Improper technique adds additional pressure on joints and muscles, stretching of soft-tissue muscle, and can make preexisting injuries worse. Ways to avoid improper technique involve the use of a spotter to monitor exercise, proper research on exercises, and avoiding continuing exercise when muscle fatigue occurs.

—*Bradley R. A. Wilson*

Further Reading

Collins, A. *Strength Training Over 40: A 6-Week Program to Build Muscle and Agility*. Rockridge Press, 2020.

Haff, G. Gregory, and N. Travis Triplett. *Essentials of Strength Training and Conditioning*. 4th ed., Human Kinetics, 2016.

Hunt, K. *Beginner's Guide to Weight Lifting: Simple Exercises and Workouts to Get Strong*. Rockridge Press, 2020.

———. *Bodybuilding for Beginners: A 12-Week Program to Build Muscle and Burn Fat*. Rockridge Press, 2019.

———. *Strength Training for Beginners: A 12-Week Program to Get Lean and Healthy at Home*. Rockridge Press, 2020.

Noelle, B. *Weight Training for Women: Exercises and Workout Programs for Building Strength with Free Weights*. Rockridge Press, 2020.

"Strength Training." *Salem Press Encyclopedia of Health*. Salem Press. Accessed 15 May 2021.

"Strength Training: Get Stronger, Leaner, Healthier." *Mayo Clinic*. Mayo Foundation for Medical Education and Research, www.mayoclinic.org/healthy-living/fitness/in-depth/strength-training/art-20046670.

TENDINITIS

Category: Disease/Disorder

Also known as: Epicondylitis, tendinosis, tendon overuse syndrome, tendonitis

Specialties and related fields: Exercise physiology, family medicine, occupational health, orthopedics, physical therapy, preventive medicine, sports medicine

Definition: an inflammation of a tendon or tendon sheath

KEY TERMS

collagen: strengthening protein in tendon tissue

ergonomics: the science of the relationship between the human form and its biomechanical environment

extracorporeal: pertaining to something occurring outside the body, such as therapy

inflammation: a condition of tenderness and disturbed function of an area of the body, caused by a reaction of tissue to injury or infection

tendinopathy: a general term referring to any tendon disorder

CAUSES AND SYMPTOMS

Tendons are fibrous cords that attach muscles to bones. Their function is to transmit force and coordinate the activity between muscles and bones. When too much stress is placed upon the tendons, they may become inflamed (tendinitis), damaged, or both from the chronic degeneration of tendon collagen (tendinosis). The cause of such stress is usually poor technique, overuse, or repetitive movements in sports, recreational, and occupational activities. The injury usually follows the progression of multiple microscopic tears in the tendon tissue, eventually leading to acute inflammation and pain. The areas most commonly affected are the rotator cuff of the shoulder, the elbow ("tennis elbow" or "golfer's elbow"), the wrist/thumb (de Quervain's disease), the knee ("jumper's knee"), and the ankle (Achilles tendinitis).

Many athletic activities, such as racquet sports, baseball, running, and weight training, involve repetitive movements that may stress the tendons. Many occupations also pose a risk; examples include performing assembly-line work, playing a musical instrument, and using a keyboard. Tendinitis may also be caused by infection or by a buildup of calcium deposits (calcific tendinitis) or other joint materials resulting from a chronic illness such as diabetes or arthritis.

Pain is the usual complaint. It occurs when the patient moves the affected joint but may sometimes persist when the joint is at rest. The affected area may also have swelling, warmth, and redness. In severe cases, simple activities such as raising a coffee cup or brushing teeth may cause pain.

TREATMENT AND THERAPY

The term "tendinitis" has traditionally been used as a blanket term for all tendinopathies. However, medical professionals emphasize that tendinitis and tendinosis, often occurring hand-in-hand, are different conditions and must be treated accordingly. Tendon overuse conditions have been generally considered inflammatory processes (tendinitis), and therapy has been administered based on that conception. However, it is important to recognize that overuse tendon conditions are frequently caused by collagen damage and degeneration of tendon tissue (tendinosis), eventually leading to an acute inflammatory condition. Tendinosis requires a different approach to therapy once the initial inflammation is treated.

True tendinitis conditions are treated with therapy aimed at reducing inflammation. Rest and avoidance of the causative activity, alternative application of ice and heat, compression and elevation of the affected extremity, and immobilization with slings and splints are all practical measures. Health-care providers may suggest over-the-counter anti-inflammatory medications such as ibuprofen. A method exists for delivering medication to inflamed tissue: iontophoresis, whereby a small electrical current delivers anti-inflammatory medication, such as dexamethasone, through the skin to the inflamed tissue. More severe cases may require corticosteroid injections. Tendinitis caused by infection is treated with antibiotics and sometimes surgery if first-course therapy is not effective. Recovery from tendinitis varies from a few to several weeks.

Tendinosis therapy is aimed at allowing the injured tendon tissue to heal. Rest and avoidance of the offending activity are most important. Icing, ultrasound, and electrical stimulation may enhance collagen production. Once the initial inflammation has been treated, anti-inflammatory medications and corticosteroid injections are not indicated and may impede healing. Ergonomic changes in the workplace and the correction of improper techniques in sports activities are important. Physical therapy and strengthening exercises play key rehabilitative roles by helping prevent future injury.

> **INFORMATION ON TENDINITIS**
>
> **Causes**: Stress on tendons resulting from poor technique, overuse, or repetitive movements in sports, recreational, or occupational activities; buildup of calcium deposits from chronic illness such as diabetes or arthritis
>
> **Symptoms**: Pain, swelling, warmth, and redness in the affected area
>
> **Duration**: A few to several weeks; sometimes recurrent
>
> **Treatments**: Rest, avoidance of causative activity, alternative application of ice and heat, compression and elevation of the affected extremity, immobilization with slings and splints, anti-inflammatory drugs (ibuprofen, corticosteroid injections), antibiotics, sometimes surgery

They may also improve collagen formation and thus speed healing. Surgery to remove damaged tissue is used only as a last resort when conservative management has failed. Recovery from tendinosis may take up to several months.

PERSPECTIVE AND PROSPECTS

Tendinopathies have been regarded as conditions often recalcitrant to therapy, becoming chronic or frequently reoccurring. This difficulty may be partly attributable to the lack of distinction between tendinitis and tendinosis. It has been postulated that some of the therapies for tendinitis, when used on tendinosis, may cause further tissue deterioration and thus contribute to the chronic nature of the disorder. Additionally, once the initial inflammation is treated and pain is no longer felt, the injured individual will often begin the offending activity before healing is complete. This leads to further damage and weakened tissue, creating a frustrating cycle. Therefore, it is crucial that a proper diagnosis is made before treatment begins and that the injured individual follow the full course of therapy and rest to ensure optimal healing.

The investigation of new treatment modalities is ongoing. Extracorporeal shock wave therapy has been shown to have some positive benefits for both tendinosis and calcific tendinitis. The use of ultrasound and electrical stimulation has gained acceptance by some professionals.

Preventive measures can greatly reduce the risk of developing overuse tendinopathies. This approach is becoming more evident in the workplace, where proper ergonomic environments help decrease employee injury, increase productivity, and reduce injury and absences. Conditioning and emphasis on correct technique in sports and recreational activities will greatly reduce the incidence of tendon overuse disorders.

—*Barbara C. Beattie*

Further Reading

El-Bogdadi, Daniel. "Tendinitis and Bursitis." *Arthritis and Rheumatism Associates, P.C.*, n.d., arapc.com/tendonitis-and-bursitis/.

Hecht, Marjorie. "Understanding Tendinopathy." *Healthline*, 8 Nov. 2018, www.healthline.com/health/tendinopathy.

Khan, Karim M., et al. "Overuse Tendinosis, Not Tendinitis: A New Paradigm for a Difficult Clinical Problem." *Physician and Sports Medicine*, vol. 28, no. 5, 2000, pp. 38-45.

———. "Time to Abandon the 'Tendinitis' Myth: Painful, Overuse Tendon Conditions Have a Non-inflammatory Pathology." *British Medical Journal*, vol. 324, no. 7338, 2002, pp. 626-27.

Porter, Robert S., et al., editors. *The Merck Manual Home Health Handbook*. Merck Research Laboratories, 2009.

Standish, William D., et al. *Tendinitis: Its Etiology and Treatment*. Oxford UP, 2000.

"Tendinitis." *MedlinePlus*, 16 Mar. 2017, medlineplus.gov/tendinitis.html.

"Tendinitis and Bursitis." *American College of Rheumatology*, Dec. 2021, www.rheumatology.org/I-Am-A/Patient-Caregiver/Diseases-Conditions/Tendinitis-Bursitis.

Tendon Disorders

Category: Disease/Disorder
Specialties and related fields: Occupational health, orthopedics, physical therapy, podiatry, sports medicine
Definition: inflammation or tearing of the tendons

KEY TERMS

collagen: the main structural protein found in skin and other connective tissues, widely used in purified form for cosmetic surgical treatments

epicondylitis: irritation of the tissue connecting the forearm muscle to the elbow

shin splints: pain caused by overuse along the shinbone, the large front bone in the lower leg

tendinitis: a condition in which the tissue connecting muscle to bone becomes inflamed

INTRODUCTION

Tendons are the tough, white, fibrous cords that connect muscles to movable structures such as bone or cartilage. The presence of tendons allows muscles to act at a distance and concentrates the force of the muscle into a small area. Sometimes tendons can change the direction of a muscle's pull, thus allowing the muscle to act around a joint. The structure of a tendon consists of parallel bundles of collagen fibrils, making it extraordinarily strong. A sheath, or vagina fibrosa, surrounds the tendon and is responsible for holding it in place. Between the fibrils and the sheath lie a lymphatic network and a fluid that allows tendon movement without excessive friction. Because of the vital functions of tendons, diseases and injuries can be debilitating and painful. Damaged tendons heal slower than epithelial tissue, for example, because tendons have a lower blood supply than other soft tissues.

Trauma to tendons usually occurs in conjunction with impact, twisting, overstretching, or the simple overuse of a joint. These actions commonly result in partial or complete tears of the fibrous cord. Only if a tendon has not been stretched more than 4 percent of its original length will it return to its normal state once the force is released. When it is stretched from 4 to 8 percent of its normal length, the molecular bonds between individual collagen fibers begin to fail, and the fibers slide past one another. At 8 to 10 percent strain, the tendon is in danger of tearing because individual fibers rupture, placing even more force on the remaining intact fibers. Although Golgi tendon organs send signals to the brain regarding excessive strain on tendons, such tearing usually occurs quickly during physical activities. Pain, swelling, and abnormal motion at the joint follow the damage. Tendinitis is the name given to the inflammation of a tendon.

TENDON DISORDERS OF THE UPPER BODY

Tennis elbow, or lateral epicondylitis, involves the elbow joint and can be attributed to excessive extensor movements in the wrist joint and a sustained gripping of objects such as a tennis racket. There is great diversity in opinion regarding the development of this disorder and its treatment. The latter includes rest, stretching, icing, heat, ultrasound, bracing, and surgery. Golfer's elbow is less often seen but is similar to tendinitis of the common flexor tendon.

Supraspinatus tendinitis, or swimmer's shoulder, is seen in athletes participating in swimming, tennis, and other activities involving overhead arm movement. Repeated overhead arm swings impinge and sometimes tear the supraspinatus tendon between the acromion and the proximal end of the humerus. The disorder has also been termed impingement syndrome. Treatments include icing, stretching, modifying stroke technique in swimmers, anti-inflammatory drugs, and surgery.

Bicipital tendinitis usually stems from sports that require throwing or paddling. This type of tendon

> **INFORMATION ON TENDON DISORDERS**
>
> **Causes:** Disease, trauma, injury, overuse
>
> **Symptoms:** Inflammation, pain, abnormal motion
>
> **Duration:** Acute or recurrent episodes
>
> **Treatments:** Rest, appropriate stretching, icing, heat, ultrasound, braces, surgery, anti-inflammatory drugs

disorder is similar to the supraspinatus type in that pinching of a tendon is involved. The narrow tendon connecting the long head of the bicep muscle to the scapula lies in a groove and is restrained by a ligament therein. Pain occurring while a physician applies pressure to this groove and moves the patient's arm is diagnostic for this tendinitis. Treatments are the same as for supraspinatus tendinitis and are almost always successful.

Vigorous throwing can cause triceps tendinitis. Other tendons prone to injury are those attaching the infraspinatus, teres minor, and teres major muscles. Indeed, any tendon may incur damage depending on an individual's specific activities.

Synovitis of the wrist extensor tendons results from friction between the tendon, its surrounding sheath, and bone processes. Tenosynovitis brings about a thickening of the tendon sheath, and at times a rubbing sound can even be heard during movement. An aching pain develops and may be relieved by methods applied in tendinitis cases. In addition, ultrasound therapy in water is highly successful. The abductor pollicis longus and the extensor pollicis brevis muscles are most often affected.

TENDON DISORDERS OF THE LOWER BODY

Tendons of the lower body undergo greater stress than tendons of the torso because a greater weight is moved, and a more continuous motion is involved. Achilles tendinitis often occurs in people participating in sports involving running and jumping. This type of inflammation has become the most common athletic injury. When great tensile strength is needed, the tendon tends to be long compared with the muscle to which it attaches. The Achilles tendon is long and durable but twists as it descends the lower leg, making certain areas of the tendon vulnerable to the concentration of stress. Quality footwear with slight heel elevation and padding can reduce the tearing effect on this tendon. Stretching the gastrocnemius and soleus muscles before athletic exertion ensures that these muscles absorb a greater portion of the force that would otherwise be transferred to the tendon.

Jumper's knee, or patellar tendinitis, is fairly common in basketball and volleyball players; it is often mistaken for arthritis of the knee. Repetitive extending of the leg at the knee causes microtearing in the kneecap tendon; thus, the torn fibers fray and eventually degenerate. More stress is then placed on the remaining intact fibers, resulting in the likelihood of their failure.

Many other lower-body injuries may involve tendons. A groin pull is most frequent in soccer players because of the sudden stresses involved in kicking and changing direction by planting cleats firmly into the ground and jolting the body into a new configuration. Hamstring pull occurs during bursts of sprinting because the hamstring functions in the forward movement of a leg after a stride are completed. During extremely fast running, the hamstring requires great force to keep pace; thus, damage to the connecting tendon and the muscle itself is likely to occur if attention is not given to proper stretching techniques before the exertion.

The term "shin splints" refers to several painful injuries to the lower leg. Indicative of shin splints is pain and tenderness along the tibia (shinbone) and the middle one-third of the leg. The condition develops in athletes who do not use sufficient padding in their shoes or who run and play on hard surfaces. Genuine shin splints do not involve tendons directly;

fortunately, tendinitis of the tibial muscles can be differentiated from true shin splints because tendinitis pain is located higher up on the leg.

COMPARTMENT SYNDROME

Compartment syndrome is most frequently seen in runners. The leg is divided into three compartments, each encompassed by a tight fascial sheath. When an injury occurs to muscles or tendons of a certain compartment, swelling accompanied by a cutting off the blood supply can cause further problems. Even the sudden growth of muscles as a result of physical activity can impair the function of muscles and nerves deeper in the leg.

—*Ryan C. Horst, Roman J. Miller*

Further Reading

Delforge, Gary. *Musculoskeletal Trauma: Implications for Sport Injury Management*. Human Kinetics, 2002.

El-Bogdadi, Daniel. "Tendinitis and Bursitis." *Arthritis and Rheumatism Associates, P.C.*, n.d., arapc.com/tendonitis-and-bursitis/.

Józsa, László, and Pekka Kannus. *Human Tendons: Anatomy, Physiology, and Pathology*. Human Kinetics, 1997.

Stanish, William D., et al. *Tendinitis: Its Etiology and Treatment*. Oxford UP, 2000.

"Tendinitis." *MedlinePlus*, 16 Mar. 2017, medlineplus.gov/tendinitis.html.

"Tendinitis and Bursitis." *American College of Rheumatology*, Dec. 2021, www.rheumatology.org/I-Am-A/Patient-Caregiver/Diseases-Conditions/Tendinitis-Bursitis.

Weintraub, William. *Tendon and Ligament Healing: A New Approach to Sports and Overuse Injury*. 2nd Rev. ed., Paradigm, 2003.

TENNIS ELBOW (LATERAL EPICONDYLITIS)

Category: Disease/Disorder
Specialties and related fields: Athletic training, orthopedics, personal training, physical therapy, sports medicine, strength and conditioning

Definition: inflammation or, in some cases, microtearing of the tendons that join the forearm muscles on the outside of the elbow

KEY TERMS

extensor: any of the muscles that increase the angle between members of a limb, as by straightening the elbow or knee or bending the wrist or spine backward

flexor: any of the muscles that decrease the angle between bones on two sides of a joint, as in bending the elbow or knee

humerus: long bone of the upper limb or forelimb of land vertebrates that forms the shoulder joint

lateral epicondyle: a large eminence on the lateral side of the proximal end of the humerus that is an attachment site for the radial collateral ligament at the elbow joint and the common tendon of the supinator and extensor muscles

CAUSES AND SYMPTOMS

Lateral epicondylitis results from chronic inflammation of the muscles that extend the wrist. This condition is most commonly due to excessive wrist pronation/supination and extension motions. For example, performing a backhand swinging motion, such as while playing tennis, involves the use of the extensor muscles of the wrist. Chronic overuse of these wrist extensor muscles can cause inflammation and pain. However, although lateral epicondylitis may be observed in individuals who play tennis for more than two hours daily, this condition does not exclusively affect tennis players. Any motion that involves repetitive wrist extension can elicit symptoms of lateral epicondylitis. The risk of developing lateral epicondylitis increases with age. This condition may also be idiopathic or occur without any identifiable cause.

The pathophysiology of this condition results from overuse and repetitive motions. Three primary muscles are involved in wrist extension and originate at the lateral epicondyle of the humerus: the extensor carpi radialis brevis, the extensor digitorum with extensor digiti minimi, and the extensor carpi ulnaris. Lateral epicondylitis has been observed in tennis players due to the repetitive rapid and forceful movements as the muscle-tendon unit is lengthened or in eccentric motion. As these muscles are overexerted, microscopic tears form. The healing process of microscopic muscle tears will lead to stronger and larger muscles. However, excessive muscular use results in microtears that do not have time to repair themselves, thus resulting in improper healing. This increased breakdown of the muscle and tendons results in chronic inflammation of these structures. Chronic inflammation results from neovascularization of the affected area to bring nutrients to the damaged tissues. This process of neovascularization in these extensor muscles causes the pain associated with lateral epicondylitis.

Some common symptoms exist when patients present with lateral epicondylitis. The pain in this condition is typically located on the lateral aspect of the elbow about 1.5 centimeter distal to the lateral epicondyle, and may or may not radiate to the hand. Patients often report an insidious onset of elbow pain. Still, they can relate it to a particular activity twenty-four to seventy-two hours earlier with no associated trauma to the joint. The level of pain reported by patients with lateral epicondylitis is variable depending on how far the condition has progressed. Some patients present with mild pain with occasional aggravation on certain movements. In contrast, others report severe pain limiting daily activities like holding objects.

The diagnosis of lateral epicondylitis is typically clinical; the physician relies on history and physical exam findings to make the diagnosis. History of overuse and repetitive wrist movements due to sports or work is common. Pain on palpation of the lateral epicondyle or proximal wrist extensor muscles or pain with resisted wrist extension or flexion while the elbow is in full extension suggests lateral epicondylitis. However, if the clinician is unsure if a patient has elbow pain related to lateral epicondylitis, an MRI (magnetic resonance imaging) or ultrasound scan can be performed to see if there is any muscle damage to the area distal to the lateral epicondyle. The clinician can also order a three-view X-ray to rule out osteophytes or an alternative diagnosis.

TREATMENT AND THERAPY

The treatment goals of lateral epicondylitis include pain control, preservation of a range of motion and grip strength, prevention of further disease progression, and return to baseline function. Initial treatment for patients with lateral epicondylitis is with conservative measures. These treatments include rest, nonsteroidal anti-inflammatory drugs, ice, and activity modification. A counterforce brace placed distal to the lateral epicondyle may also be used during the first six weeks of injury. The brace can help relieve pain by reducing muscle and tendon strain of the forearm extensor muscles. Suppose the pain does not improve at six weeks of conservative treatment. In that case, the patient is sent to physical

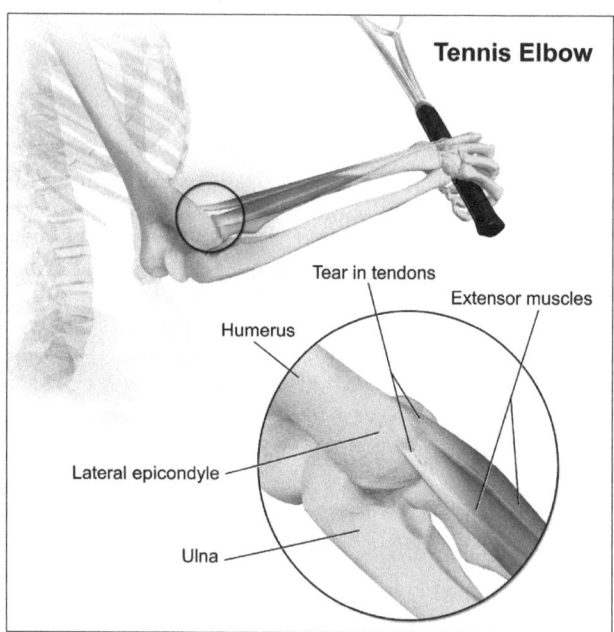

Image by BruceBlaus, via Wikimedia Commons.

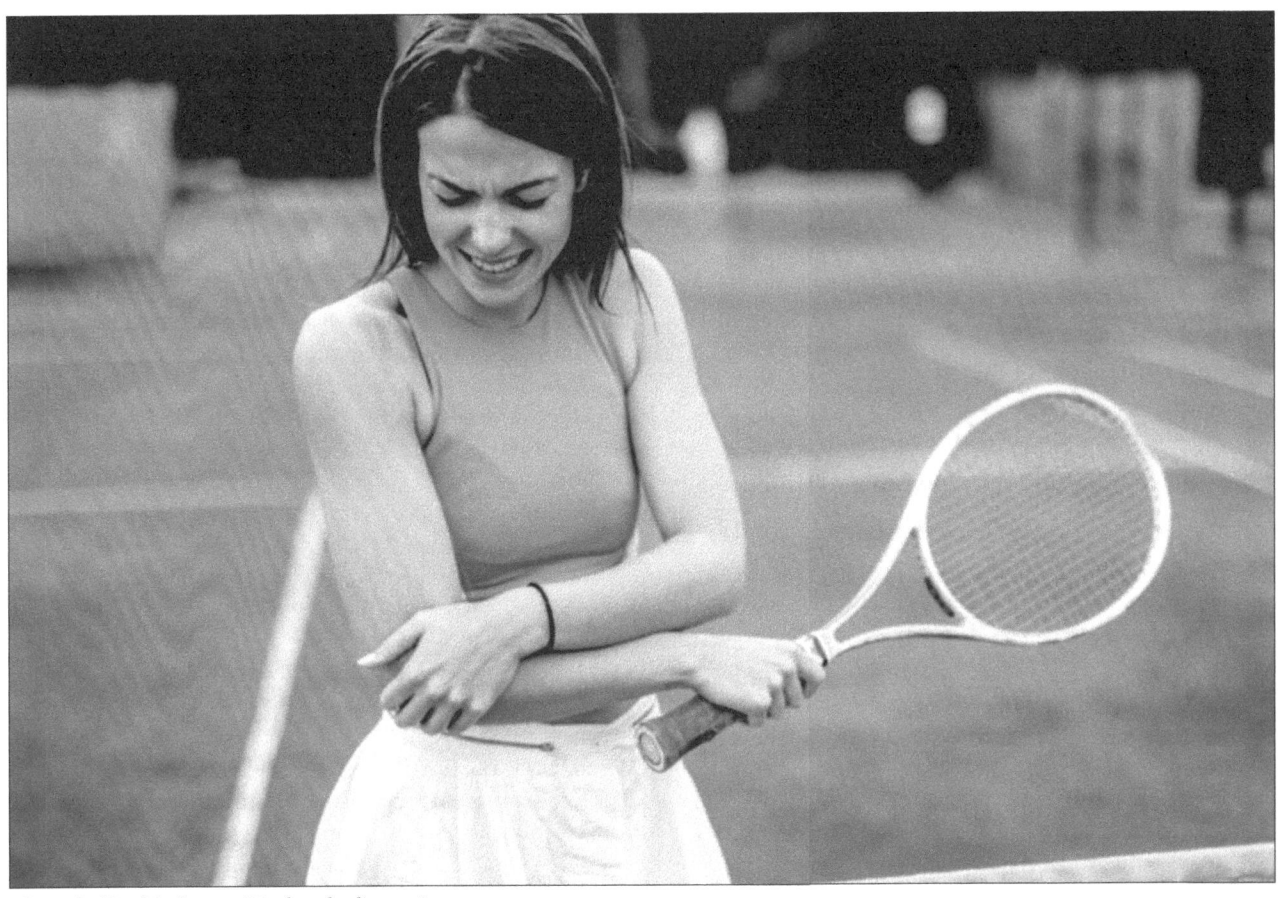

Photo via iStock/urbazon. [Used under license.]

therapy as a second-line treatment. Physical therapy focusing on gradual eccentric and isometric muscle strength training helps improve the symptoms associated with this condition.

If symptoms are not improved after six to twelve months, then other more complex treatments are considered. A corticosteroid injection to the elbow can dampen the inflammatory process and provide short-term relief. Since corticosteroid injections do not prevent the recurrence of pain from lateral epicondylitis and may cause skin changes at the injection site, this treatment is frequently used as a part of comprehensive therapy rather than as a primary treatment. Health-care providers can also inject autologous blood or separate the blood into platelet-rich plasma (PRP) for injection to the affected area. Studies have shown that PRP and autologous blood leads to improved healing of the damaged tissue. Other options include acupuncture, injection of botulinum toxin, or prolotherapy, but these treatments are not as well studied as other therapies. Extracorporeal shockwave therapy, which is a treatment that uses acoustic waves, may also be considered. However, this type of therapy may cause discomfort to the patient. More studies must be conducted to investigate its clinical efficacy and benefits further. Patients are still encouraged to keep up with physical therapy and other conservative treatment while undergoing second-line interventions.

Most lateral epicondylitis cases resolve with either first-line or second-line treatment. However, suppose the patient continues to have refractory lateral elbow pain after exhausting all other options. In that case, surgical referral to orthopedics may be considered. Patients are referred for surgery consultation if they have unimproved symptoms or function despite a trial of nonoperative treatments for six to twelve months. Surgical referral should be considered for patients with chronic elbow tendinopathy who do not wish to attempt nonsurgical treatments. The role of surgery in these cases is to perform a debridement of the affected arm to remove any offending particles or substances that could be the source of the patient's pain. Patients should know that surgical intervention is not a definitive treatment, and they could still have pain after surgery.

—*Jason Pyon, Marichelle Pita*

Further Reading

Ahmad, Z., et al. "Lateral Epicondylitis: A Review of Pathology and Management." *Bone Joint Journal*, vol. 95B, no. 9, 2013, pp. 1158-64, doi:10.1302/0301-620X.95B9.29285. PMID:23997125.

Bisset L. M., and B. Vicenzino. "Physiotherapy Management of Lateral Epicondylalgia." *Journal of Physiotherapy*, vol. 61, no. 4, 2015, pp. 174-81, doi:10.1016/j.jphys.2015.07.015.

Coombes, B. K., et al. "Management of Lateral Elbow Tendinopathy: One Size Does Not Fit All." *Journal of Orthopaedic & Sports Physical Therapy*, vol. 45, no. 11, 2015, pp. 938-49, doi:10.2519/jospt.2015.5841.

Dingemanse, R., et al. "Evidence for the Effectiveness of Electrophysical Modalities for Treatment of Medial and Lateral Epicondylitis: A Systematic Review." *British Journal of Sports Medicine*, vol. 48, no. 12, 2014, pp. 957-65, doi:10.1136/bjsports-2012-091513.

Johnson, Greg W. "Treatment of Lateral Epicondylitis." *American Family Physician*, vol. 76, no. 6, 15 Sept. 2007, pp. 843-48.

Landesa-Martínez, L., and R. Leirós-Rodríguez. "Physiotherapy Treatment of Lateral Epicondylitis: A Systematic Review." *Journal of Back and Musculoskeletal Rehabilitation*, 4 Aug. 2021, doi:10.3233/BMR-210053. PMID:34397403.

Sims, S. E., et al. "Non-surgical Treatment of Lateral Epicondylitis: A Systematic Review of Randomized Controlled Trials." *HAND*, vol. 9, no. 4, 2014, pp. 419-46.

Testa, G., et al. "Extracorporeal Shockwave Therapy Treatment in Upper Limb Diseases: A Systematic Review." *Journal of Clinical Medicine*, vol. 9, no. 2, 6 Feb. 2020, doi:10.3390/jcm9020453. PMID: 32041301; PMCID: PMC7074316.

Thanasas, Christos, et al. "Platelet-Rich Plasma Versus Autologous Whole Blood for the Treatment of Chronic Lateral Elbow Epicondylitis: A Randomized Controlled Clinical Trial." *American Journal of Sports Medicine*, vol. 39, no. 10, 2011, pp. 2130-34.

Thompson, Jon C. *Netter's Concise Orthopaedic Anatomy*. 2nd ed., Elsevier, 2015.

Walrod, Bryant James. "Lateral Epicondylitis." *Medscape*, 8 Mar. 2021, emedicine.medscape.com/article/96969-overview. Accessed 19 Aug. 2017.

Weber C., et al. "Efficacy of Physical Therapy for the Treatment of Lateral Epicondylitis: A Meta-analysis." *BMC Musculoskeletal Disorders*, vol. 16, no. 1, 2015, p. 223, doi:10.1186/s12891-015-0665-4.

Yao, G., J. Chen, Y. Duan, and X. Chen. "Efficacy of Extracorporeal Shock Wave Therapy for Lateral Epicondylitis: A Systematic Review and Meta-Analysis." *BioMed Research International*, 18 Mar. 2020, p. 2064781, doi:10.1155/2020/2064781. PMID: 32309425; PMCID: PMC7106907.

Traumatic Brain Injury

Category: Disease/Disorder

Specialties and related fields: Emergency medicine, neurology, neurosurgery, occupational therapy, physical therapy, psychiatry, psychology, sports medicine

Definition: brain dysfunction, or other pathologies, caused by an external force to the head

KEY TERMS

arachnoid mater: the fine, delicate membrane, the middle one of the three membranes or meninges that surround the brain and spinal cord, situated between the dura mater and the pia mater

aspiration: breathing in foreign objects, such as sucking food particles or saliva into the airway

brain herniation: a phenomenon that occurs when increased pressure inside the skull due to bleeding, a stroke, head injury, or tumor moves brain tissues, causing neurological dysfunction or neuronal death

brain parenchyma: the functional tissue of the brain consisting of cells for cognition and controlling the rest of the body and stroma, or supportive tissue

closed head injury: an injury to the brain that arises from a problem within the cranium

cognitive functions: mental functions such as reasoning, language, memory, and problem-solving

computerized tomography (CT) scan: a visual diagnostic technology using X-rays that can detect brain abnormalities

dura mater: the tough outermost membrane enveloping the brain and spinal cord

hematoma: A pool of mostly clotted blood that forms in an organ, tissue, or body space

magnetic resonance imaging (MRI): a visual diagnostic technology that can create high-resolution pictures of brain structures

pai mater: the delicate innermost membrane enveloping the brain and spinal cord

traumatic brain injury: an injury to the brain caused by blunt force

EPIDEMIOLOGY

Few injuries instill more fear in parents, coaches, athletes, and colleagues than traumatic brain injuries. Except for paralyzing spinal injuries, traumatic brain injuries constitute a major source of health loss and disability worldwide. The economic impact of traumatic brain injuries in the United States in 2010 was estimated to be $76.5 billion in direct and indirect costs.

It is difficult to estimate the global burden of traumatic brain injury because of the varied quality of the available data. High-income countries tend to have high-quality epidemiological data. Low-income countries, however, do not, on average, have high-quality epidemiological data, and most of the world's population resides in low- and middle-income countries. The estimated global prevalence (or likeliness of having the condition) of traumatic brain injury in 2016 was 759 cases per one hundred thousand people. The estimated annual global incidence (or frequency of occurrence) of traumatic brain injury in 2016 was 27.08 million, with an incidence rate of 369 cases per 100,000 people. Falls are the single most common cause of traumatic brain injury, and traffic accidents are the second most common cause. The incidence of traumatic brain injury in the United States in 2016 was 1.11 million, and the prevalence was 2.35 million. The highest rates of emergency room visits for traumatic brain injury occur in older adults (≥75 years; 1682 per 100,000), the very young (0 to 4 years; 1619 per 100,000), and young adults (15 to 24 years; 1,010 per 100,000). Alcohol and illicit drug abuse increase the risk of traumatic brain injuries.

CAUSES AND SYMPTOMS

Six different types of external force may result in traumatic brain injury. They include: (1) the head being struck by an object; (2) the head striking an object; (3) acceleration/deceleration of the brain without direct external impact; (4) a foreign object penetrating the brain; (5) the force from a blast or explosion; and (6) other forces yet to be defined.

The head trauma that causes a traumatic brain injury may cause primary injuries. Such primary injuries include skull fractures, blood vessel injuries, such as an epidural or subdural hematoma, a subarachnoid or intracerebral hemorrhage, and brain parenchymal injuries like brain contusions and diffuse axonal injury. Head trauma-induced primary injuries may cause secondary injuries like cerebral herniation, seizures, and increased intracranial pressure.

Skull fractures are easily seen during imaging. Skull fractures consist of linear fractures, depressed fractures, and basilar skull fractures. A linear skull fracture is a single fracture that runs through the entire skull thickness. Depressed skull fractures occur when fragmented pieces of the skull bend directly into the brain and damage the underlying brain tissue. Basilar skull fractures usually require significant force and carry a high risk of cervical spine injury and bleeding within the skull (hematoma). Basilar skull fractures consist of damage to one or more bones at the skull base. These bones include the orbital plate of the frontal bone, the petrous or squamous portion of the temporal bone, the occipital and sphenoid bones, and the cribriform plate of the ethmoid bone. Fractures of these bones at the base of the skull may cause cerebrospinal fluid to escape through the ear and nose. Cerebrospinal leaks mixed with blood tend to form a "halo" on a Kleenex because the three most spinal fluid, which does not clot and is thinner than blood, runs faster than blood. One to three days after the injury, the patient may also experience two black eyes (i.e., "raccoon eyes" or periorbital ecchymosis) and a "Battle sign" or bruise just behind the ear.

If someone has had head trauma, they must undergo an initial evaluation known as the "ABCDE" assessment:

"A" stands for airway. People unfortunate enough to have experienced a traumatic brain injury may not be able to control their breathing appropriately. They are at risk for aspiration and suboptimal respiration. Poor respiration deprives the tissues of oxygen, a condition known as "hypoxia," which worsens brain injury. Suppose the brain is deprived of oxygen and glucose for more than six or seven seconds. In that case, a person usually becomes unconscious, and brain cells begin to die. Under such circumstances, an individual may require mechanical ventilation or endotracheal intubation.

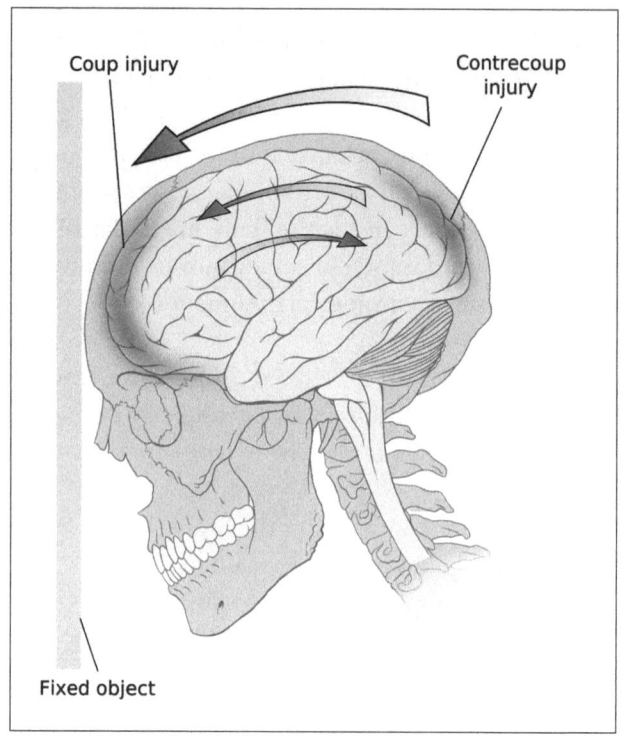

Figure 1. The coup-contrecoup phenomenon may be caused by ricochet of the brain. Photo by Patrick J. Lynch, via Wikimedia Commons.

"B" stands for breathing. If the individual has increased intracranial pressure, they may have an irregular breathing pattern. Abnormal breathing patterns are part of the so-called Cushing triad.

"C" is for circulation. Abnormally low blood pressure (hypotension) may significantly reduce blood circulation through the brain. Hypertension (high blood pressure) and bradycardia (an abnormally slow heart rate; <60 bpm) are the two remaining features of Cushing's triad.

"D" is for disability. Anyone who has experienced head trauma is assessed with a fifteen-point Glasgow Coma Scale (GCS). The maximum score for the GCS is fifteen, and the minimum is three. The GCS score is three parts: motor response, verbal response, and eye movement. If the person spontaneously opens their eyes, they receive four points. If they open their eyes only when asked to do so, they receive three points, and if they open their eyes in response to mild pain, they receive two points. If they do not open their eyes, they receive one point. To assess the verbal response, the health-care worker asks the patient what year it is. Should they respond appropriately, five points and four points if they respond but get the year wrong. Suppose they respond with words that make no sense (the patient says something like "window" or "hot dog"), three points. If they respond with a more like a moan, they are given two points, and if the patient does not respond at all, one point. The health-care provider gives the patient a command to assess the motor response. She may ask the patient something like, "show me four fingers." If they execute the command successfully, they are awarded six points. If the individual's consciousness prevents such a test, then rubbing the orbit of the eye may cause them to smack the hand out of the way. That will give the patient five points. If they fail that test, then pricking the tip of the finger with a toothpick should cause them to withdraw their hand. If the patient withdraws her hand, they receive four points. If that does not work, determine if the upper limbs are flexed, and the lower limbs are extended. If that is the case, then the patient gets three points. The patient receives two points if the upper and lower limbs are extended. If there is no muscle tone, the individual receives one point.

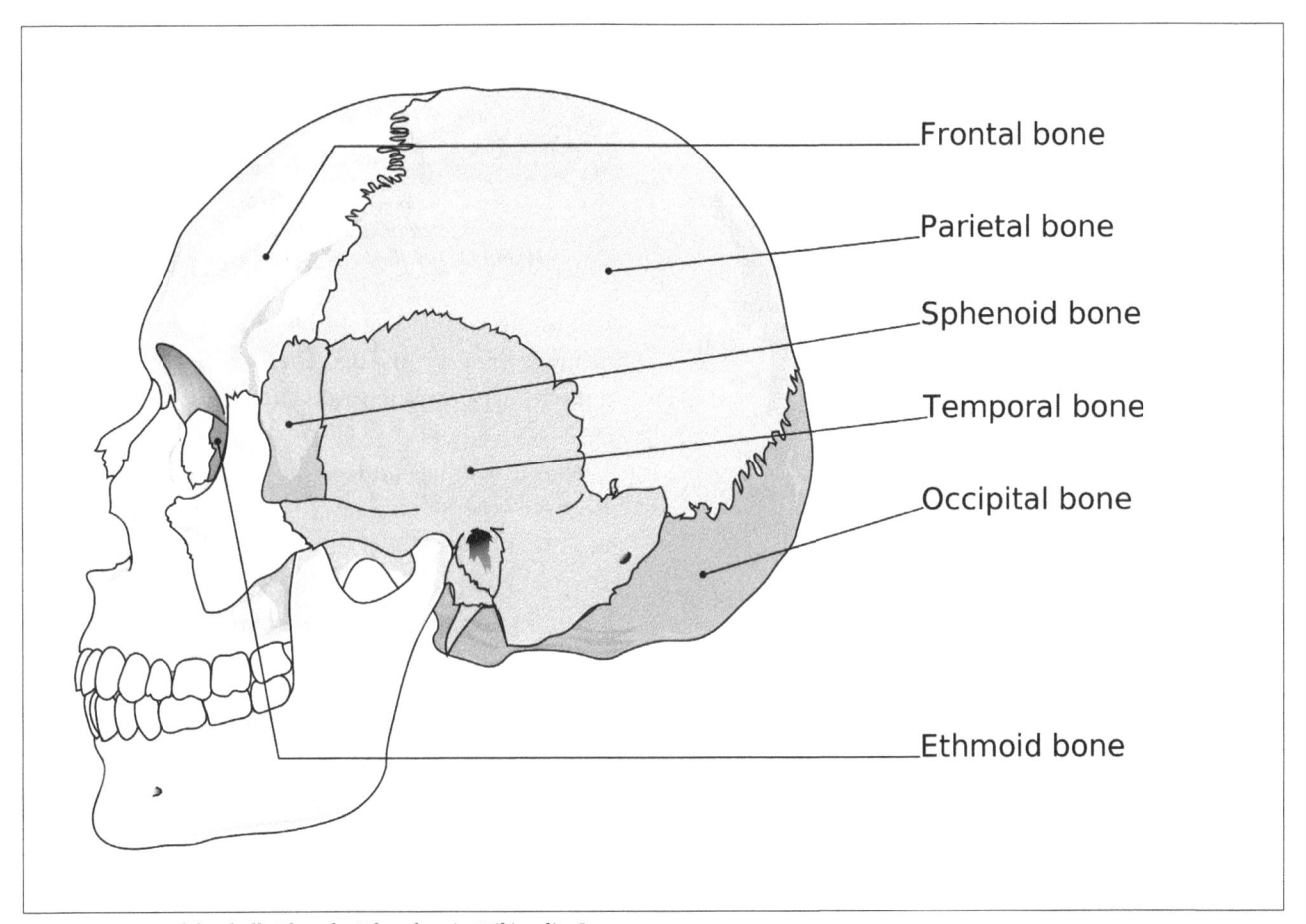

Figure 2. Bones of the skull. Photo by Edorado, via Wikimedia Commons.

"E" stands for exposure. Rolling the individual onto their stomach exposes the back and helps identify other injuries like spinal cord fractures.

After the ABCDEs assessments, the patient's medical history and physical status are examined with the AMPLE assessment:

"A" stands for allergies to medications, latex, foods, or other chemicals.

"M" stands for medications like antiplatelet and anticoagulant medications that increase the risk of intracranial bleeding.

"P" stands for pregnancy and past medical history.

"L" stands for last meal.

"E" stands for the events that cause the head trauma.

Traumatic brain injury classification depends on the GCS score. A mild traumatic brain injury is also known as a "concussion." Individuals with concussions usually have a GCS of 13 to 15 and a complete loss of consciousness for less than thirty minutes. Any posttraumatic memory loss (amnesia) or any changes in the level of consciousness (confusion or lethargy) last for less than one day. Concussions are graded regarding their symptoms. A grade one concussion occurs if there is no loss of consciousness and no amnesia. Someone suffers from a grade 2 concussion if they have experienced a loss of consciousness but no amnesia. A grade 3 concussion occurs if the person experiences loss of consciousness and amnesia.

A moderate traumatic brain injury has a GCS of 9 to 12. These individuals experienced a loss of consciousness for thirty minutes to twenty-four hours. They also may have posttraumatic amnesia for one to seven days and some change in the level of consciousness for more than twenty-four hours. A severe traumatic brain injury has a GCS less than or equal to eight. Such people typically cannot maintain their airways and require intubation. Severe traumatic brain injuries have a loss of consciousness for more than twenty-four hours and posttraumatic amnesia for more than seven days. They also have a change in the level of consciousness of more than twenty-four hours.

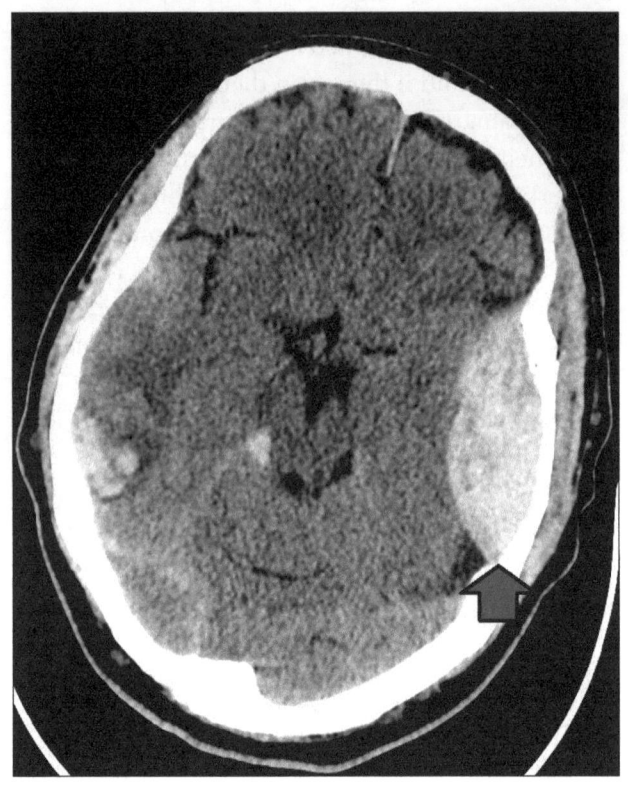

Figure 3. Epidural hematoma on the persons left (images right) with an associated skull fracture. Also has some bleeding on the person's right. Photo by James Heilmann, M.D., via Wikimedia Commons.

Anyone who has undergone head trauma should also have several laboratory tests. A complete blood count (CBC) should ensure that the individual has at least 100,000 platelets per microliter (the minimum threshold for neurosurgery) and normal red blood cell counts to ensure adequate oxygen delivery to the brain. Blood clotting tests, the prothrombin (PT), international standardized ratio (INR), and partial thromboplastin time (PTT) tests to check that the patient's bleeds will not worsen. Blood alcohol, blood glucose level measurements, and urine toxicology assays are important to identify or rule out other potential causes of an altered mental status.

Brain imaging is the most direct way to observe brain injury. A non-contrast brain computerized tomography (CT) scan can detect any shift in the brain's midline due to mass effect. Blood collecting inside the skull that compresses the brain causes this mass effect. Brain compression can cause cerebral herniation, which is life-threatening. The CT scan must be done without contrast because both blood and contrast dye or white, making it difficult to detect a bleed within the skull. The CT scan is usually normal but moderate, and abnormal brain CT scans usually accompany severe traumatic brain injuries in a mild traumatic brain injury.

Because increased intracranial pressure can damage the brain, health-care providers must immediately act to lower the intracranial pressure in patients with a head injury. The cerebral perfusion pressure (CPP) is an indirect measure of blood flow through the brain. Cerebral perfusion pressure equals the mean arterial pressure (MHP) minus the intracranial pressure (ICP). It is impossible to measure cerebral blood flow directly. Therefore, hospitals use the CPP to represent cerebral blood flow. The CPP must be above 60 mmHg to ensure that the brain gets enough blood. Therefore, the systolic blood pressure must remain above 100 mmHg. Blood transfusions and getting intravenous fluids can help maintain the systolic blood pressure.

Hospitals use an intracranial ICP monitor to measure ICP. Intracranial ICP monitors are placed in the lateral or third ventricle of the brain, the epidural or subdural space, or the brain parenchyma. Intracranial ICP monitors are typically used in people with a GCS ≤ 8 and an abnormal CT scan. A normal ICP is approximately ten mmHg and must be kept <20 mmHg. Elevating the head of the bed to thirty degrees lowers the ICP by increasing venous outflow from the brain. Raising the head of the bed cannot be done in an individual with a cervical spine injury.

The signs and symptoms of increased intracranial pressure include a diminishing level of consciousness (early sign), headache, nausea, vomiting, ocular palsies, dilated pupils (mydriasis), swelling of the optic disc (papilledema), difficult or labored breathing (dyspnea), back pain, and decorticate/decerebrate posturing.

Linear skull fractures usually do not require treatment unless they break an underlying blood vessel. The middle meningeal artery lies underneath a skull region where four bones converge: the frontal, parietal, sphenoid, and temporal bones. A fracture that breaks the middle meningeal artery causes an epidural hematoma. Depressed skull fractures directly damage the underlying brain and usually require surgery. Basilar skull fractures may cause damage to cranial nerves III (oculomotor), IV (trochlear), and VI (abducens). Damage to cranial nerve III causes double vision (diplopia), dilation of the pupil that does not respond to light (pupil mydriasis), and drooping of the upper eyelid (upper eyelid ptosis). Cranial nerve IV damage prevents the eyes from moving toward the nose (adduction). When the person tries to move the affected eye toward their nose, it turns upward. Damage to cranial nerve VI prevents the eyes from moving away from the midline (abduction).

Brain injuries may accompany skull fractures. Extra-axial injuries occur within the skull but do not include the brain. Intra-axial injuries involve the brain parenchyma, including intracerebral hemorrhage, cerebral contusions, and diffuse axonal injury. Examples of extra-axial injuries include epidural and subdural hematomas and subarachnoid hemorrhages.

An epidural hematoma results when blood collects between the dura mater and the skull bones. Epidural hematomas result from skull fractures that tear open the middle meningeal artery and cause profuse bleeding. Epidural hematomas tend to require blows to the head with substantial force.

Therefore, they are more common in head trauma from sports injuries (e.g., a golf ball or baseball striking the skull) or fights. People unfortunate enough to experience an epidural hematoma may lose consciousness and then recover and seem normal. Rapid growing epidural hematomas can put substantial pressure on the brain and lead to brain herniation. A head CT scan usually shows an overly dense collection of blood shaped like a lens.

Subdural hematomas result when blood collects between the dura and arachnoid mater. Tearing the bridging veins that connect the venous sinuses with the skull's superficial veins causes subdural hematomas. The bleeding is slower in a subdural hematoma since the source of the bleeding is veins rather than arteries. Symptoms depend on how fast blood accumulates. An acute subdural hematoma occurs within two days after head trauma. A subacute subdural hematoma occurs between two days to two weeks after experiencing head trauma, and a chronic subdural hematoma occurs over two weeks after head trauma. Whereas epidural hematomas require a high-force blow to the head, even minor head trauma, like walking into a wall or door, can cause a subdural hematoma. Subdural hematomas are more common in those with brain atrophy since brain shrinkage stretches the bridging veins, increasing their tendency to tear. The elderly and alcoholics are at the highest risk for subdural hematomas. Subdural hematomas in children often result from child abuse. Children have large heads and small brains, and shaking them causes subdural hematomas and rental hemorrhages. Subacute subdural hematomas on a head CT scan show a crescent-shaped area of high density that crosses suture lines. This distinguishes it from epidural hematomas, which do not cross suture lines. Subacute subdural hematomas have bleeding that blends in with the scan's background, making them easy to miss.

Bleeding between the arachnoid and pia mater causes a subarachnoid hemorrhage. The most common cause of subarachnoid hemorrhages is head trauma. However, nontraumatic subarachnoid hemorrhage can result from the spontaneous rupture of an intracranial berry aneurysm. Head CT scans in cases of a subarachnoid hemorrhage show blood in the sulci, the fissures between the cerebral hemispheres, and the ventricular cisterns. The more blood detected in a head CT scan, the worse prognosis for the patient. A lumbar puncture and subsequent cerebrospinal fluid analysis reveal red blood cells (xanthochromia) in the CSF if the head CT scan fails to show blood in the brain. In cases of traumatic subarachnoid hemorrhage, a lumbar puncture is contraindicated since the high intracranial pressure increases the risk of cerebral herniation.

Intra-axial injuries are injuries to the brain parenchyma. Intracerebral hematomas result when external shear forces tear the arterioles underneath the pia mater and cause a small bleed to form. Intracerebral hematomas tend to occur with extra-axial injuries. On a brain CT scan, intracerebral hematomas have a regular shape and a well-defined border. These bleeds occur deep within the brain and have a high mortality rate.

A cerebral contusion, or "brain bruise," tends to occur near the brain's surface, does not have a regular shape on a head CT, and has a poorly defined border. If a cerebral contusion occurs on the same side as the head trauma, it is called a "coup" injury. If it occurs on the side opposite the impact, it is called a "contrecoup" injury. Cerebral contusions may have swelling (edema) surrounding them. If this brain swelling increases, surgical relief of the increased pressure might be necessary.

The most common intra-axial injury is diffuse axonal injury (DAI). Diffuse axonal injuries result from shear forces on the axons in the brain, causing them to stretch and potentially tear. A DAI may cause posttraumatic coma (>6 hours) that is not caused by a cerebral contusion or large hematoma. Those who recover from posttraumatic comas may have lasting cognitive challenges such as language problems (aphasias) on memory loss (amnesia). A brain CT scan usually shows many small, dense, hole-like lesions near the gray-white matter junction. Diffuse axonal injuries are better seen with a brain magnetic resonance imaging scan (MRI). Magnetic resonance imaging scans provide better resolution and detect DIAs more accurately.

Traumatic brain injuries may cause chronic complications. Posttraumatic seizures may occur up to a week after a moderate or severe traumatic brain injury. Posttraumatic epilepsy may develop months to years after the head injury. Prolonged increased intracranial pressure can cause a Cushing ulcer. Cushing ulcers are stress gastric ulcers that may also include proximal duodenum or distal esophagus ulcers.

A complication of multiple concussions is chronic traumatic encephalopathy (CTE). Athletes who experience repetitive head trauma in contact sports are at the highest risk for CTE, including those who play American football, boxers, and soccer players. Chronic traumatic encephalopathy develops eight to ten years after initial head trauma, but the amount of head trauma required to cause CTE remains unknown. In its early stages, CTE causes mood and behavioral changes. In its later stages, it affects cognition, causing memory and processing deficits.

TREATMENT AND THERAPY

Traumatic brain injury treatment begins with assessing the cause and severity of the injury. Medical imaging technologies, such as CT and MRI scans, can visualize the brain structures and potential pathologies.

Visual diagnostics alone usually cannot determine the specific impact on mental processes and functions. Neuropsychological procedures, often admin-

> **INFORMATION ON BRAIN DAMAGE**
>
> **Causes**: Accidents (automobile collisions, falls, sports injuries); strokes
>
> **Symptoms**: Motor control problems, paralysis, balance, and sensory problems; often speech and language difficulties, memory loss, concentration, and attention problems; if extensive, loss of consciousness, coma, and death
>
> **Duration**: Acute
>
> **Treatments**: Depends on the cause; may include surgery (hemorrhage, tumor) or drug therapy (swelling, blockage, infection)

istered in a particular array or test battery, along with visual imaging, provide the best assessment of how the damage affects brain function. Specialized neuropsychological tests are used to determine the extent of deficits in thinking, such as language processing, memory, decision-making, sensory perception, and motor functioning.

Increased ICP increases the risk of mortality and poor outcomes. Therefore, maintaining normal ICP and lowering an elevated ICP is a high priority in managing a patient with traumatic brain injury. If the patient has a ventricular catheter, cerebrospinal fluid drainage is a first-line intervention for lowering the ICP. Continuous cerebrospinal fluid drainage is recommended for patients with low GCS scores (<6).

Drugs called "osmotic diuretics" (e.g., mannitol, hypertonic saline) extract water from neurons and lower the ICP. Sedatives like propofol also lower the ICP by decreasing cerebral activity and metabolic demand and reducing cerebral blood flow. Propofol, however, can cause hypotension, and, therefore, the nurse should closely monitor the patient's blood pressure.

Blood levels of carbon dioxide also influence cerebral blood flow. When blood levels of carbon dioxide ($PaCO_2$) increase, the blood vessels surrounding the brain dilate, increasing cerebral blood flow and ICP. When the carbon dioxide levels in the blood are low, the blood vessels in the brain constrict, and cerebral blood flow decreases, decreasing the ICP. The goal is for patients to have a normal blood level of carbon dioxide between thirty-five and 45 mmHg. This $PaCO_2$ range lowers the ICP and maintains adequate blood flow to the brain.

More extreme methods of lowering the ICP include therapeutic hypothermia or pentobarbital administration to induce a coma (barbiturate coma). A barbiturate coma pharmacologically lulls the brain to sleep and lowers its metabolic rate. Therapeutic hypothermia cools the body, lowers the ICP, and protects the brain against any secondary injuries. If elevated ICP does not respond to these therapies, neurosurgery is necessary.

Linear skull fractures require no treatment unless they tear an underlying blood vessel. Disruption of the middle meningeal artery causes an epidural hematoma. Depressed skull fractures and penetrating injuries require removing dead or irreparably damaged tissue (debridement) and repairing injured tissues. Foreign body removal is an important treatment for penetrating injuries. Prophylactic antibiotic treatments significantly reduce postsurgical and posttrauma infections. Basilar skull fractures that cause cerebrospinal fluid to leak through the nose and ears increase the risk of meningitis, and require prophylactic antibiotic treatments

Epidural and subdural hematomas and intracerebral hematomas are medical emergencies. The main treatment is "decompressive craniectomy." The neurosurgeon removes a portion of the skull to drain the hematoma and relieve pressure on the brain. In emergency circumstances, surgeons can drill a hole in the skull (Burr hole trephination) to relieve intracranial pressure. Nonsurgical treatments for smaller hematomas that meet specific criteria are also available.

A complication of subarachnoid hemorrhages is posttraumatic vasospasm of the subarachnoid vessels. This complication occurs two days to two weeks after the initial hemorrhage. Vasospasm of the subarachnoid vessels causes cerebral ischemia. Those with subarachnoid hemorrhages are given a calcium channel blocker called "nimodipine" to prevent this complication. Nimodipine relaxes the smooth muscles that surround the subarachnoid blood vessels. A three-week course of nimodipine is given within four days of the subarachnoid hemorrhage.

Prophylactic use of antiepileptic medications can also prevent posttraumatic epilepsy. Traumatic brain injury patients are given the antiepileptic drug phenytoin for one week to prevent posttraumatic seizures. Cushing ulcers are treated with proton pump inhibitors.

Concussions are usually treated with rest, pain relief medications, and observation. A brain CT scan is only recommended if the person has a worsening headache, persistent confusion, or other neurological deficit. Complete recovery from a concussion may take a few weeks. If the individual experiences headaches, confusion, dizziness, depression, or any decline in cognitive function that persists beyond two weeks, they suffer from so-called post-concussive syndrome. Post-concussive syndrome is treated symptomatically. Analgesics are usually given for headaches, and any depression is treated with selective serotonin reuptake inhibitors.

Athletes who have experienced a grade one concussion should sit out the rest of the game. Any athlete who has suffered from a grade 2 concussion should set out for at least the remainder of the week. Athletes who have experienced a grade 3 concussion should sit out the rest of their athletic season. Convincing athletes to sit out the rest of their athletic season may be difficult. Nevertheless, the athlete must comply with this requirement. A second blow to the head after a concussion may be fatal. This phenomenon, known as "second-impact syndrome," occurs because a concussion weakens cerebral blood vessels and makes them leaky. A second blow to the head may cause massive and potentially fatal brain swelling.

PERSPECTIVE AND PROSPECTS

Although brain injuries have occurred since the beginning of humankind, the question of what the brain does and how it contributes to behavior has only been partially answered. There is evidence from human skull remains that small holes were drilled as a form of crude brain surgery in 2000 BCE. The purpose of the procedure is unknown; however, it could have helped an injured person by relieving brain swelling. Before the first century CE, intellectuals did not widely accept that the brain was the center for reasoning, emotions, and movement. During early human history, scientists believed the heart ruled thoughts and emotions. Galen of Pergamum (130-01 CE), a Roman physician, was influential in bringing forth the notion that the brain, and not the heart, gave rise to behavior. He learned much about the brain and its impact on behavior by observing injured gladiators who survived fierce battles in the Roman coliseum. Prospects for future therapies to compensate for brain damage include stem cell tissue transplantation to stimulate new brain cell development. Also, refined brain imaging technologies produce clearer pictures that allow practitioners to make more accurate diagnoses.

—*Michael A. Buratovich*

Further Reading

"Brain Injury Diagnosis." *Brain Injury Association of America*, 2022, www.biausa.org/brain-injury/about-brain-injury/diagnosis. Accessed 30 May 2022.

"Concussion." *MedlinePlus*, n.d., medlineplus.gov/ency/article/000799.htm. Accessed 30 May 2022.

Daugherty, J., et al. "Traumatic Brain Injury-Related Deaths by Rae/Ethnicity, Sex, Intent, and Mechanism of Injury—United States, 2000-2017." *MMWR Morbidity and Mortality Weekly Report*, vol. 68, 2019, pp. 1050-56, doi.http://dx.doi.org/10.15585/mmwr.mm6846a2.

Landau, Elaine. *Head and Brain Injuries*. Enslow, 2002.

"Traumatic Brain Injury." *MedlinePlus*, 21 Feb. 2020, medlineplus.gov/traumaticbraininjury.html. Accessed 30 May 2022.

Zasler, Nathan D., et al. *Brain Injury Medicine*. 2nd ed., Demos Medical Publishing, 2013.

Zollman, Felise S. *Manual of Traumatic Brain Injury: Assessment and Management*. 2nd ed., Springer Publishing, 2016.

WOUNDS

Category: Injury

Specialties and related fields: Critical care, emergency medicine, family medicine, internal medicine

Definition: a breakdown in the skin's protective function, resulting in disruptions or breaks in the continuity of any body tissue

KEY TERMS

abrasion: an injury that results from scraping that removes or damages the skin layer

avulsion: a wound caused by tearing of the skin and underlying tissue

contusion: a wound that typically does not break the skin but causes bruising

incision: a wound or injury that results from the slicing motion of a sharp edge

THE NATURE OF WOUNDS

Wounds might arise because of violence, accident, or intentional procedure, such as surgery. They may be classified according to the instrument responsible, such as a knife, bullet, or shrapnel, or how they occurred, such as a burn or a crushing wound.

Surgeons describe wounds according to their general appearance. A wound may be described as incised when a sharp cutting instrument is involved;

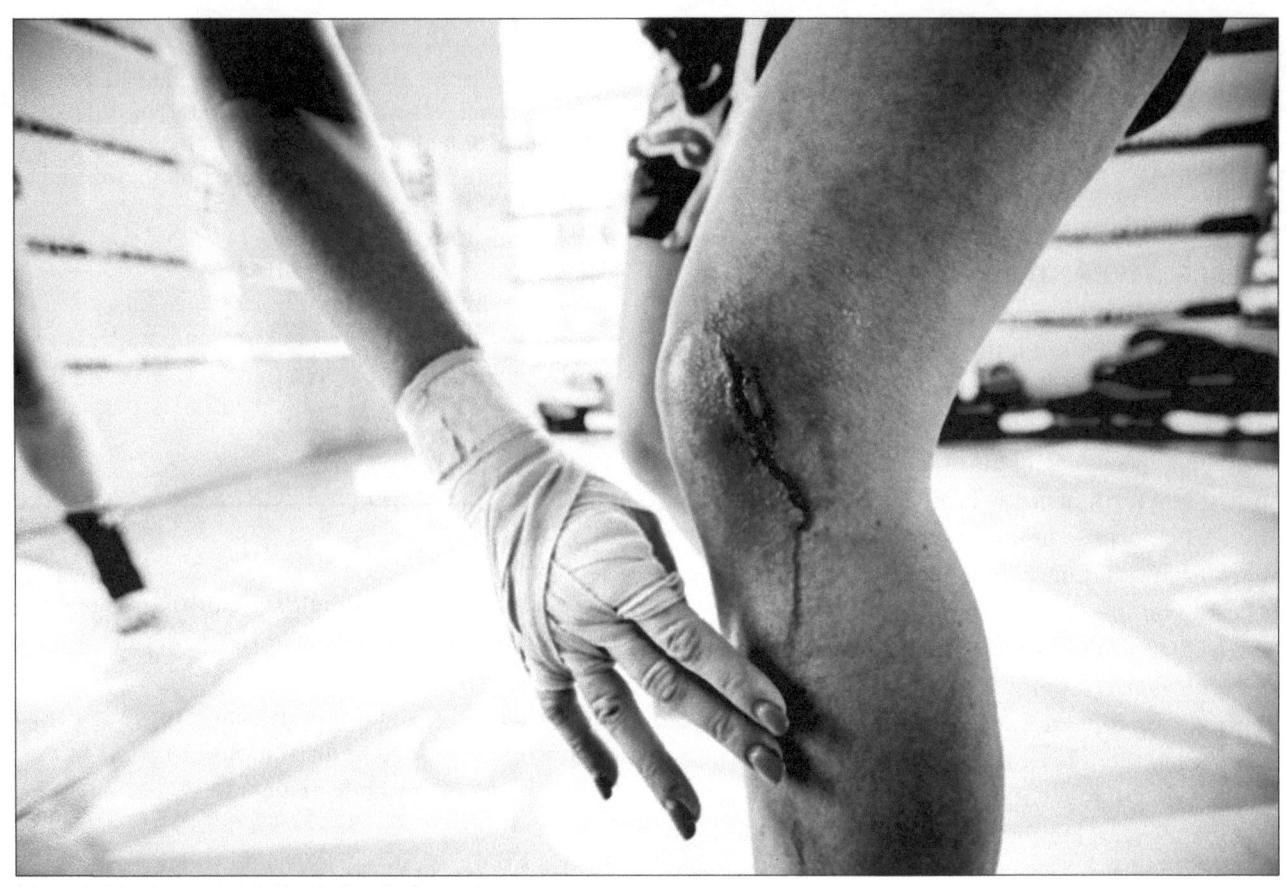

Photo via iStock/Dean Mitchell. [Used under license.]

lacerated, when the tissue is damaged, cut, or torn; abrasion, when a superficial layer of skin is removed; contused, when a forceful blow to the tissue leaves the skin intact, causing bluish/blackish discoloration; avulsed, when part of the tissue is torn apart; punctured, when the outer opening is rather small; penetrating; and nonpenetrating when the external tissue remains intact. Fractures are also classified in several terms, such as incomplete, complete, closed, or open. The depth of the tissue injury classifies burns as a first, second, or third degree.

Generally, wounds may be classified as open or closed. Closed wounds involve no external hemorrhage. Their degree of seriousness is related to the force of the blow and its direction, the victim's age, and other physiological and anatomical factors. Normally, internal hemorrhage stops abruptly or by applying direct pressure, with the blood and fluid absorbed within a few days. More bleeding occurs when larger internal vessels are damaged, with subsequent blood collection in tissues, forming a hematoma that may take several weeks to be absorbed. The impact on a body part may damage a part that is not directly involved at the time of impact. Thus, a fall on an outstretched hand may injure the flesh and bones of the hand itself and the scaphoid part of the wrist or even the elbow or shoulder. During a car accident, a stationary body part may be heavily affected by the transmission of impact from a relatively mobile part; when occurring in the neck, this type of injury is commonly known as "whiplash." First aid procedures for fractures, sprains, and strains include ice packs, crutches, elevation, and splinting.

INFECTIONS RESULTING FROM WOUNDS

Open wounds occur when the skin or mucous membranes are broken, thus allowing the invasion of hazardous foreign material, such as bacteria or dirt, into the tissues. This invasion may lead to infection, which is particularly serious when the disruption of the skin is considerable. Generally, injuries from sharp instruments (such as a needle, knife, or bullet) cause little tissue damage, except to the part they penetrate. The great danger lies in the injury of a vital organ and from the foreign objects on the instrument's surface. Injuries from irregular objects (such as bomb fragments or a jagged knife) create much more damage, which leads to longer recuperation periods. Skin is elastic and well supplied with blood, which means that superficial cuts heal easily. The subcutaneous fatty tissues and muscles are not as rich in blood supply. Their damage is more serious and long-lasting, especially because it is easier for infection to occur.

Injuries to joints, nerves or major capillaries (such as arteries) will complicate the state of the open wound. Fragmentation of bone in an open wound is particularly troublesome. The fragments cannot survive without blood and will act as foreign substances, thus creating a serious infection.

The contamination of the wound may start immediately after the causative incident. Nonbacterial contamination is more serious when organic substances are involved. In bacterial contamination, the most serious results are seen with virulent bacteria that are nourished by dead tissue and foreign organic material, sometimes leading to gas gangrene. Such infection spreads unchecked and can be stopped only by surgical removal or amputation to avoid death. Streptococcal and staphylococcal bacteria cause other infections. They are characterized by the local production of swelling, redness, and pus.

Finally, tetanus is another type of wound infection. It starts with serious muscle spasms a few days after the injury and, left untreated, often leads to death.

THE HEALING PROCESS

When an open wound occurs, the tissues are cut and the edges of the wound separate, pulled apart by the skin's elasticity. Blood flowing from the wound fills the resulting cavity, fibrinogen, and fibrin are produced, and the blood clots, creating a scab. During the first twenty-four hours after the injury, the scab shrinks, drawing the edges of the skin together. Special cells called "histiocytes" and "macrophages" digest the debris in the wound, such as blood seepage, dead cells, and other foreign bodies, two to three days after the injury. Connective tissue cells called "fibroblasts" grow inward from the margins of the wound to close the cavity 3 to 5 days after injury. The fibroblasts produce a collagen protein that provides strength to the new skin.

The red-colored capillaries slowly disappear and are replaced by white collagen. Thus, upon removing the scab, a layer of reddish granulation tissue appears, covering the subcutaneous tissue. A thin, gray membrane extends outward from the skin edges and covers the whole surface. Contraction brings the epithelial sheets from the two sides together, and eventually, the skin around the wound is reproduced. Wounds that cross normal skin creases become depressed below the level of the surrounding skin. The resulting scars, which are very low in capillaries, do not become tanned with sunlight exposure. They produce neither hair nor sweat, which indicates less than fully functional skin. They are much whiter than the surrounding skin.

TREATMENT

Medical treatment of wounds requires first the control of bleeding by direct pressure or bandaging. In the case of small cuts, local irrigation and disinfection include the external use of oxidizing agents (such as hydrogen peroxide) and nonpolar ointments (such as petroleum jelly) to combat invading polar bacteria. A large area of injury or dead tissue is managed surgically, either by debridement or amputation. The skin around any surgery is treated with antiseptics and is carefully protected with a sterilized cloth. Sutured wounds heal faster because stitches bring the skin edges together. Foreign surgical material introduced in a wound may be absorbed by the tissues, which happens when catgut is used to close the wounded tissue. Body factors are also crucial in the overall healing; these include age, the simultaneous presence of diseases such as uncontrolled hypertension and diabetes, and nutrition that includes adequate quantities of protein and antioxidants, such as vitamin C. Hospitals take elaborate precautions to prevent infections through sterilization, hand sanitation, good air filtration, the use of ultraviolet light to kill bacteria in the operating room, and the administration of antibiotics.

—*Soraya Ghayourmanesh*

Further Reading

Collier, Mark. "Understanding Wound Inflammation." *Nursing Times*, vol. 99, no. 25, 2003, pp. 63-64.

Cutting, K. F., and K. G. Harding. "Criteria for Identifying Wound Infection." *Journal of Wound Care*, vol. 3, no. 4, 1994, pp. 198-201.

Gulli, Benjamin, Les Chatelain, and Chris Stratford, editors. *American Academy of Orthopaedic Surgeons. Emergency Care and Transportation of the Sick and Injured.* 9th ed., Jones and Bartlett, 2005.

Handal, Kathleen A. *The American Red Cross First Aid and Safety Handbook*. Little, Brown, 1992.

Krohmer, Jon R., editor. *American College of Emergency Physicians First Aid Manual*. 2nd ed., DK, 2004.

Marsh, J. L., et al. "Fracture and Dislocation Classification Compendium-2007: Orthopaedic Trauma Association Classification, Database and Outcomes Committee." *Journal of Orthopedic Trauma*, vol. 21, Nov./Dec. 2007, pp. 1-133.

Subbarao, Italo, et al., editors. *American Medical Association Handbook of First Aid and Emergency Care*. Rev. ed., Random House Reference, 2009.

Thygerson, Alton L. *First Aid and Emergency Care Workbook*. Jones and Bartlett, 1987.

Youngson, R. M. *First Aid*. HarperCollins, 2003.

Diagnostic Techniques

If you break your wrist, how does the doctor know how to set your arm? If you sustain a head injury, how do they know if you will be alright? The diagnostic technologies discussed here tell you how. Genetic testing can assess risk of injury, while MRI is an indispensable noninvasive tool for evaluating sports injuries. Other techniques discussed in this segment are ultrasonography and genomics.

Genetic Testing

Category: Human genetics and social issues
Specialties and related fields: Cardiology, genetic counseling, obstetrics and gynecology, oncology, pediatrics, perinatology, reproductive specialist
Definition: any procedure used to detect the presence of a genetic disorder or a defective gene in a fetus, newborn, or adult

KEY TERMS

genetic disorder: a disorder caused by a mutation in a gene or chromosome

genetic marker: a distinctive deoxyribonucleic acid (DNA) sequence that shows variation in the population and can therefore potentially be used for identification of individuals and discovery of disease genes

PRENATAL DIAGNOSIS

Prenatal diagnosis is the testing of a developing fetus in the womb or uterus for the presence of a genetic disorder. This type of genetic screening aims to inform a pregnant woman of the chances of having a baby with a genetic disorder. Prenatal diagnosis is limited to high-risk individuals and is usually only recommended if a woman is thirty-five years of age or older, if she has had two or more spontaneous abortions, or if she or her partner has a family history of a genetic disorder. Hundreds of genetic disorders can be tested in a fetus. One of the most common genetic disorders screened for is Down syndrome, or trisomy 21, caused by having an extra copy of chromosome 21. The incidence of Down syndrome increases sharply in children born to women over the age of forty.

One technique used for prenatal diagnosis is amniocentesis. It is typically performed between the sixteenth and eighteenth weeks of pregnancy. Amniocentesis involves the insertion of a hypodermic needle through the abdomen into a pregnant woman's uterus. The insertion of the needle is guided by ultrasound. Ultrasound machines use high-frequency sound waves to locate a developing fetus or internal organs and present a visual image on a video monitor. A small amount of amniotic fluid is withdrawn. The amniotic fluid surrounds and protects the fetus and contains fetal secretions and cells sloughed from the fetus. These cells are analyzed for genetic abnormalities. Amniocentesis detects gross chromosomal disorders such as Down syndrome, Edwards syndrome (trisomy 18), and Patau syndrome (trisomy 13) by examining the chromosome number of the fetal cells. Certain biochemical disorders such as Tay-Sachs disease, a progressive disorder characterized by a startle response to sound, blindness, paralysis, and death in infancy, can be determined by testing for the presence or absence of specific enzyme activity in the amniotic fluid. Amniocentesis can also determine the sex of a fetus and detect common congenital disabilities such as spina bifida (an open or exposed spinal cord) and anencephaly (partial or complete absence of the brain) by measuring levels of alpha-fetoprotein in the amniotic fluid. The limitations of amniocentesis include the inability to detect most genetic disorders, possible fetal injury or miscarriage, infection, and bleeding.

Chorionic villus sampling (CVS) is another technique used for prenatal diagnosis. It is performed earlier than amniocentesis (between the eighth and twelfth weeks of pregnancy). Under ultrasound guidance, a catheter is inserted into the uterus via the cervix to obtain a sample of the chorionic villi. The chorionic villi are part of the fetal portion of the placenta, the organ that nourishes the fetus. The chorionic villi can be analyzed for chromosomal and biochemical disorders but not for congenital disabilities like spina bifida and anencephaly. The limitations of this technique are inaccurate diagnosis and a slightly higher chance of fetal loss than in amniocentesis.

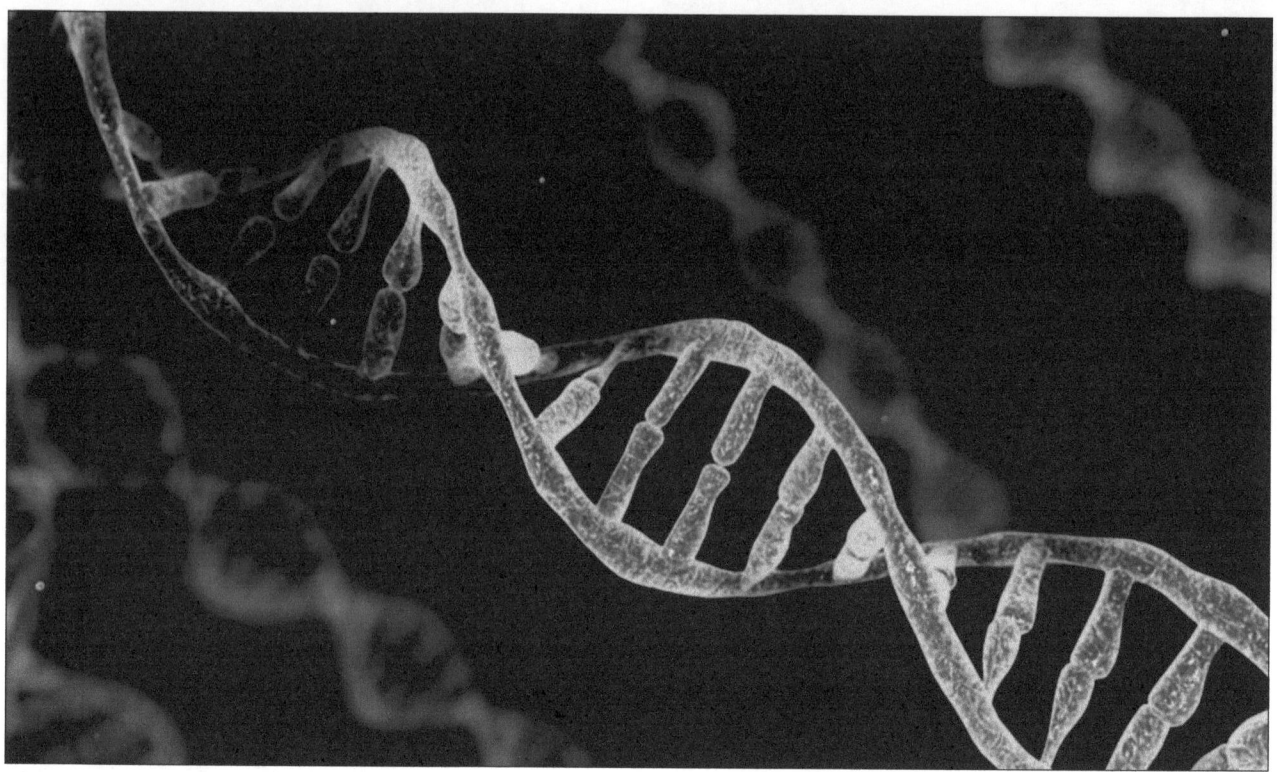

Photo via iStock/Shutter2U. [Used under license.]

Cell-free fetal deoxyribonucleic acid (DNA) testing became available in 2011 in the United States. Cell-free fetal DNA testing involves a simple blood draw from a pregnant woman; the blood is then analyzed for fragments of fetal DNA that have passed into the pregnant mother's bloodstream. Cell-free fetal DNA testing carries fewer risks than amniocentesis or CVS but does not offer a complete diagnosis. A growing number of pregnant women are opting for cell-free fetal DNA testing first and then undergoing amniocentesis if the results of the cell-free test indicate there is a risk for a genetic disorder to get an accurate diagnosis.

NEONATAL TESTING

The most widespread genetic testing is the mandatory testing of every newborn infant for the inborn error of metabolism (a biochemical disorder caused by mutations in the genes that code for the synthesis of enzymes) phenylketonuria (PKU), a disorder in which the enzyme for converting phenylalanine to tyrosine is nonfunctional. This type of testing aims to initiate early treatment of infants to prevent brain damage and permanent intellectual disabilities. A blood sample is taken by heel prick from a newborn in the hospital nursery, placed on filter papers as dried spots, and subsequently tested, using the Guthrie test, for abnormally high phenylalanine levels. In infants who test positive for PKU, a diet low in phenylalanine is initiated within the first two months of life. Newborns can be tested for many other disorders, such as sickle-cell disease and galactosemia (accumulation of galactose in the blood). By the mid-2010s, all US states screened newborns for at least twenty-nine disorders. The most thorough state newborn screening programs checked for nearly sixty disorders.

CARRIER TESTING

A healthy couple contemplating having children can be tested voluntarily to determine if they carry a gene for a disorder that runs in the family. This type of testing is known as "carrier testing." It is designed for carriers (individuals who have a normal gene paired with a defective allele of the same gene but have no symptoms of a genetic disorder). Carriers of the genes responsible for Tay-Sachs disease, cystic fibrosis (accumulation of mucus in the lungs and pancreas), Duchenne muscular dystrophy (wasting away of muscles), and hemophilia (uncontrolled bleeding caused by lack of blood clotting factor) can be detected by DNA analysis.

DNA samples from patients are removed by an eight-needle apparatus and deposited into a tray for genetic testing at Myriad Genetics in Salt Lake City. When the gene responsible for a specific genetic disorder is unknown, linkage analysis can identify the location of the gene on a chromosome. Linkage analysis is a technique in which geneticists look for consistent patterns in large families where the mutated gene and a genetic marker always appear together in affected individuals and those known to be carriers. Suppose a genetic marker lies close to the defective gene. In that case, it is possible to locate the defective gene by looking for the genetic marker. The genetic markers used for linkage analysis are restriction fragment length polymorphisms (RFLPs). When human DNA is isolated from a blood sample and digested at specific sites with special enzymes called "restriction endonucleases," RFLPs are produced. Restriction fragment length polymorphisms are found scattered randomly in human DNA and are of different lengths in different people, except in identical twins. They are caused by mutations or the presence of varying numbers of repeated copies of a DNA sequence and are inherited. RFLPs are separated by gel electrophoresis, a technique in which DNA fragments of varying lengths are separated in an electric field according to their sizes. The separated DNA fragments are blotted onto a nylon membrane, a process known as "Southern blotting." The membrane is probed and then visualized on X-ray film. The characteristic pattern of DNA bands visible on the film is similar to the bar codes on grocery items.

An early successful example of linkage analysis involved searching for the gene that causes Huntington's disease. This always-fatal neurological disease typically onset after thirty-five or forty years of age. In 1983, James Gusella, Nancy Wexler, and Michael Conneally reported a correlation between one specific RFLP they named G8 and Huntington's disease (Huntington's chorea). After studying numerous RFLPs of generations of an extended Venezuelan family with a history of Huntington's disease, they discovered that G8 was present in members afflicted with the genetic disorder and was absent in unaffected members.

High-risk individuals or families can be tested voluntarily for a mutated gene that may indicate a predisposition to a late-onset genetic disorder such as Alzheimer's disease or other conditions like hereditary breast, ovarian, and colon cancers. This type of testing is called "predictive testing." Unlike tests for many of the inborn errors of metabolism, predictive testing can give only a rough idea of how likely an individual may be to develop a particular disease. It is not always clear what people should do with such information, but at least in some cases, lifestyle or therapeutic changes can be instituted to lessen the likelihood of developing the disease.

IMPACT AND APPLICATIONS

Genetic testing has had a significant impact on families and society at large. It provides objective information to families about genetic disorders or congenital disabilities. It provides an analysis of the risks for genetic disorders through genetic counseling. Consequently, many prospective parents can make informed and responsible decisions about conception and birth. Some choose not to bear children, some terminate the pregnancy after prenatal diagnosis, and some may opt to use in vitro fertilization with preimplantation genetic screening. Genetic testing can have a profound psychological impact on an individual or family. A positive genetic test could cause a person to experience depression. In contrast, a negative test result may eliminate anxiety and distress. Questions have been raised in the scientific and medical community about tests' reliability and high costs. There is concern about whether genetic tests are stringent enough to ensure errors are not made. DNA-based diagnosis can lead to errors if DNA samples are contaminated. Such errors can be devastating to families. People at risk for late-onset disorders such as Huntington's disease can be tested to determine if they are predisposed to developing it. There is, however, controversy over whether it is ethical to test for diseases for which there are no known cures or preventive therapies. The question of testing also creates a dilemma in many families. Unlike other medical tests, predictive testing involves the participation of many family members. Some family members may wish to know their genetic status, while others may not.

While there has been great enthusiasm over genetic testing, social, legal, and ethical issues include discrimination, confidentiality, reproductive choice, and abuse of genetic information. Insurance companies and employers may require prospective customers and employees to submit to genetic testing or may inquire about a person's genetic status. Individuals may be denied life insurance coverage because of their genetic status, or a prospective customer may be forced to pay exorbitant insurance premiums. The potential for discrimination concerning employment and promotions also exists. For example, due to the sickle-cell screening programs of the early 1970s, many African Americans with sickle-cell disease were denied employment and insurance coverage, and some were denied entry into the US Air Force. The Americans with Disabilities Act, signed into federal law in 1990, contained provisions safeguarding employees from genetic discrimination by employers. By 1994, companies with fifteen or more employees had to comply with the law, which prohibits employment discrimination because of genetic status and prohibits genetic testing by employers. The Patient Protection and Affordable Care Act, commonly known as "Obamacare," was signed into law in 2010 and prevented health insurance companies from denying coverage to or raising rates on individuals with preexisting conditions, offering protection to individuals with a genetic predisposition for developing certain diseases.

As genetic testing becomes standard practice, the potential for misuse of genetic tests and genetic information will increase. Prospective parents may potentially use the prenatal diagnosis to ensure the birth of a "perfect" child. Restriction fragment length polymorphism analysis, used in genetic testing, has applications in DNA fingerprinting or DNA typing. DNA fingerprinting is a powerful tool for identifying individuals used to generate patterns of DNA fragments unique to each individual based on differences in the sizes of repeated DNA regions in humans. It is used to establish identity or nonidentity in immigration cases and paternity and maternity disputes; it is also used to exonerate the innocent accused of violent crimes and link a suspect's DNA to body fluids or hair left at a crime scene. Several states in the United States have been collecting blood samples from various sources, including newborn infants during neonatal testing and individuals convicted of violent crimes. They have been storing genetic information derived from them in DNA databases for future reference. Unauthorized people could misuse such information.

—*Oluwatoyin O. Akinwunmi, Bryan Ness*

Further Reading

Arribas Ayllon, M., et al. *Genetic Testing: Accounts of Autonomy, Responsibility, and Blame*. Routledge, 2011.

Boslaugh, Sarah. *Genetic Testing*. Greenwood, 2020.

Bourn, David. *Diagnostic Genetic Testing: Core Concepts and the Wider Context for Human DNA Analysis*. Springer, 2021.

Cowan, Ruth Schwartz. *Heredity and Hope: The Case for Genetic Screening*. Harvard UP, 2008.

Greenfield Boyce, Nell. "DNA Blood Test Gives Women a New Option for Prenatal Screening." *NPR*. Shots, 24 Feb. 2015. Accessed 2 Feb. 2016.

Griffin, Darren K., and Gary L. Harton, editors. *Preimplantation Genetic Testing: Recent Advances in Reproductive Medicine*. CRC Press, 2020.

Juth, Niklas, and Christian Munthe. *The Ethics of Screen in Healthcare and Medicine: Serving Society or Serving the Patient?* Springer, 2012.

Milligan, Eleanor. *The Ethics and Choice in Prenatal Screening*. Cambridge Scholars Publishing, 2011.

Milunsky, Aubrey, and Jeff M. Milunsky. *Genetic Disorders and the Fetus: Diagnosis, Prevention, and Treatment*. 7th ed., Wiley, 2015.

Sharpe, Neil F., and Ronald F. Carter. *Genetic Testing: Care, Consent, and Liability*. Wiley-Liss, 2006.

Teichler-Zallen, Doris. *To Test or Not to Test: A Guide to Genetic Screening and Risk*. Rutgers UP, 2008.

Wade, Christopher H., et al. "Effects of Genetic Risk Information on Children's Psychosocial Wellbeing: A Systematic Review of the Literature." *Genetics in Medicine*, vol. 12, no. 6, 2010, pp. 317-26.

Genomics

Category: Specialty

Specialties and related fields: Bacteriology, biochemistry, biotechnology, cytology, embryology, ethics, genetics, microbiology, pharmacology

Definition: the study of whole genomes; a genome is the complete set of genetic information found in a particular organism

KEY TERMS

bioinformatics: a computational discipline that provides the tools needed to study whole genomes and proteomes

DNA microarrays: solid supports which contain many or all genes from a given genome, enabling the expression of these genes to be monitored simultaneously

DNA sequencing: determining the order of deoxyribonucleic acid (DNA) bases in a particular unit of genetic information

orthologues: similar genes from different species that are thought to be related by evolution

proteomics: the study of proteomes; a proteome is the complete set of proteins in a particular cell type

synteny: when whole regions of chromosomes from different species are similar in structure

A NEW SCIENTIFIC DISCIPLINE

Genomics grew out of the field of genetics, the study of heredity. Until the late twentieth century, it was impossible to study the complete set of genetic information in a living organism. Genetics traces its roots to the 1860s when the Austrian monk Gregor Mendel performed experiments on the mechanism of heredity in pea plants. However, the field of genomics is much younger, dating from the 1980s. In this decade, American geneticist Thomas Roderick used the term genomics to name a new scientific journal that dealt with the analysis of genomic information. In Mendel's time, while organisms were seen to exhibit certain traits, it was not known how these traits were determined. By the early twentieth century, it was recognized that traits are inherited in units of information called "genes." However, the chemical nature of the gene was still unknown. It took until the middle of that century to recognize that genes were made up of deoxyribonucleic acid (DNA), the structure of which was first identified by American biologist James Watson and British biophysicist Francis Crick in 1953.

Deoxyribonucleic acid is made up of four different deoxyribonucleotides, commonly referred to as bases: adenine (A), cytosine (C), guanine (G), and thymine (T). Together, they spell out a chemical code used by the cell to make proteins. Since the set of proteins contained within a cell gives that cell its unique properties, determining the order of DNA bases in a given genetic unit will reveal what types of proteins are encoded by this information, a procedure known as "DNA sequencing." While a gene has been defined as the amount of DNA needed to encode one protein, a genome is the entire set of genes found in an organism, including any noncoding DNA found between genes. The number of genes present in an organism varies from fewer than two hundred in some obligately parasitic bacteria to about twenty-three thousand (in the simple flowering plant Arabidopsis); humans were found to have slightly fewer than this number.

During the 1980s, a public consortium, the International Human Genome Sequencing Consortium, was formed to sequence the human genome by 2005. As this effort was called, the Human Genome Project also aimed to sequence the genomes of several model organisms that scientists have used to help understand biological complexity. These model organisms, including the *Escherichia coli* bacterium, yeast, *Caenorhabditis elegans* (a roundworm), Drosophila (the fruit fly), and the mouse, also served as trial runs to improve the efficiency of DNA sequencing over time gradually. *E. coli*, like most bacteria, has a genome that numbers in the millions of bases—usually abbreviated bp (for base pair) since each base in DNA is paired with its complementary base, A to T and G to C—while yeast has a genome of approximately 10 million bp and the next three organisms have genomes that number in the hundreds of millions of bp. Mice, like humans, have genomes that are three3 billion bp in size. Steady progress was made around the turn of the twentieth century on the genome efforts described above. The sequence of each respective genome was determined and made publicly available via computer databases. The completion of the human genome was announced in April 2003, the month of the fiftieth anniversary of Watson and Crick's first description of the structure of DNA.

Does the field of genomics represent a new scientific discipline in and of itself, or is it just another extension of genetics? Other than the sheer size of genetic information being analyzed in genomics, another major difference would support the former possibility. Ever since Mendel's time, genetics has taken a reductionist approach. Since Mendel could not have dreamed of understanding the pea plant as a whole, he limited his investigation to several easily characterized traits, such as plant height and seed color. Since that time, many scientists have sought to understand complex biological processes by breaking them into manageable pieces. Genomics attempts a different, expansionist approach. In the postgenomics era (as some scientists have called the twenty-first century), the questions being posed are holistic: they attempt for the first time to understand an organism as a whole using its complete set of genetic information as a guide. Genomics has spawned a new set of fields that end in "-omics," denoting that they attempt to study the complete set of particular molecules in an organism or cell type. Proteomics is the study of the complete set of proteins in a cell type. At the same time, metabolomics studies the complete set of metabolic reactions in a cell.

New approaches to science also require new tools. The tools on which geneticists have relied over the years have largely proved insufficient for studying entire genomes. Bioinformatics is a subdiscipline of computational biology that has arisen to provide such tools. Bioinformatics includes the computational methods required to find patterns in the huge genomic databases that have been produced, track the expression of genes using DNA microarrays, identify all the proteins in a cell, and model the protein interactions involved in cell metabolism, among other things.

DIVISIONS WITHIN THE FIELD

In addition to producing the "-omics" disciplines, the field of genomics can itself be subdivided. The main divisions of genomics are structural, functional, and comparative genomics. Although these divisions are somewhat artificial, they help illustrate the different goals of genomics research.

Structural genomics is concerned with the structure of genetic information. Determining the number, location, and order of genes on a particular chromosome is one pursuit of this field. While bacterial genomes are typically contained within a single circular chromosome, humans have twenty-three pairs of chromosomes, and some organisms have even more. Studying regions of DNA between genes, or intergenic regions, is also the realm of structural genomics. Intergenic regions are often composed of a highly repetitive DNA sequence that does not code for any protein. In the early twenty-first century, the precise function of these regions still eluded scientists. Although noncoding sequences are relatively rare in bacteria, it makes up a major portion of many multicellular organisms, including about 98 percent of the human genome. A separate goal of structural biology is to determine the three-dimensional (3D) structure of all the proteins encoded by a genome; an endeavor called "structural proteomics."

Functional genomics is less concerned with the structure of a genome and more concerned with its function. This division of genomics tends to be of more interest to pharmaceutical companies and the medical community. Functional genomics asks questions such as, "What do the products of individual genes do?" and "How does the perturbation of gene function lead to disease states?" However, determining the function of a gene is not as straightforward as it might appear. By the early twenty-first century, determining the structure of a given genome was relatively easy. Still, the function of up to half the genes in a typical sequenced genome remained undetermined. Even determining the 3D structure of a protein produced by a specific gene does not guarantee that its function can be discerned. Still, scientists are hopeful that this will lead to conjecture concerning its function.

Another clue concerning gene function can be derived by determining where and when a particular gene is expressed (activated to produce its corresponding protein). While gene expression has traditionally been monitored one gene at a time using molecular genetic techniques, around the turn of the twenty-first century, researchers began experimenting with DNA microarrays., or "gene chips," which include copies of many, if not all, genes from a given genome attached to a solid support such as a glass slide. The expression of these genes can be monitored at any given time by binding fluorescently tagged sequences of DNA that are complementary to the genes in question. An automated scanner then measures the fluorescence of each spot and records the data into a computer.

The final division of genomics, comparative genomics, encompasses the goals of the other two divisions but achieves these goals by making comparisons between two or more different genomes. For example, the structure of a given genome may not appear significant until the same basic structure is detected in another species. Regions of chromosomes from two different species that are similar in structure are said to display synteny. Comparative genomics as a discipline was not possible until the mid-1990s when computing technology had developed to the point where huge databases of genomic information could be stored and compared quickly and accurately. Comparative genomics has also aided in the quest to determine gene function. One of the most common techniques of determining gene function is searching for orthologues in related species. Orthologues are genes from different species that are thought to be related by evolution; they often encode similar, but not identical, proteins with related functions.

PERSPECTIVE AND PROSPECTS

Genomics can trace its origins to the development of techniques used to determine the sequence of DNA. In 1977, British biochemist Frederick Sanger and colleagues published a sequencing method based on the principle of chain termination. In this method, the target DNA sequence is determined by enzymatically producing a complementary strand of DNA. In "Sanger sequencing," as it is now called, a molecular "poison" is included in a given reaction mixture so that the newly synthesized complementary chain is terminated at specific bases. Sanger's method was then modified in the 1990s to include fluorescent dyes on the chain-terminating bases so that the DNA sequence could be read using a scanner and recorded directly into a computer. Some have claimed that Sanger and colleagues were the first group to sequence a genome since they published a viral genome sequence in the same year that they described their revolutionary technique. Viruses, however, are not free-living organisms, and their genomes are thousands of times smaller than the typical bacterial genome.

The Human Genome Project was first proposed in 1986. It was funded two years later at an expected cost of $3 billion. The project officially got underway in 1990 as sequencing began in earnest on some of the smaller model genomes. In 1995, as some of these sequencing efforts were nearing completion, American pharmacologist Craig Venter and his colleagues at a private, not-for-profit institute, the Institute for Genome Research, published the genome sequence of the bacterium *Haemophilus influenzae*, the first free-living organism to have its genome sequenced.

While the public consortium had been working on sequences using established techniques, Venter and colleagues had developed a faster technique for determining the sequence of whole genomes. While this technique still used the basic Sanger-style chain termination procedure, it simplified an earlier step

---

In the News: Last Human Chromosome Sequenced

In May 2006, British molecular biologist Simon G. Gregory, along with more than 160 of his colleagues, published in the journal nature the sequence of human chromosome 1, the last human chromosome to have its deoxyribonucleic acid (DNA) sequenced. Although largely ignored in the popular press, this event officially brought the Human Genome Project to an end. Perhaps the lack of fanfare can be linked to the fact that the project had already celebrated a few widely publicized conclusions. In June 2000, US President Bill Clinton and British prime minister Tony Blair announced the completion of a "rough draft" of the human genome sequence. This meant that 90 percent of the genome had been completed, with an error rate of 1 in 1,000 base pairs, even though more than 150,000 gaps in the sequence were still present. This rough draft was published in Nature and the journal Science about six months after this announcement. The "final" sequence was published in these same journals in April 2003. In this case, "final" meant that 99 percent of the genome had been completed, with an error rate of 1 in 10,000 base pairs, and fewer than 400 gaps were left.

Raw DNA sequence, however, is not as useful to scientists as a fully annotated sequence. Annotation involves the identification of potential genes as well as making an educated guess at their function. The first annotated sequence of a human chromosome (number 22) was published in *Nature* in December 1999. The number of human chromosomes had originally been established using cytology. At that time, the twenty-two pairs of autosomal (nonsex) chromosomes had been numbered from 1 to 22, based on their apparent size from largest to smallest. Modern techniques have shown that the two penultimately numbered chromosomes are the largest and smallest chromosomes, namely chromosomes 2 and 21, respectively. Although chromosome 1 was ultimately not the largest human chromosome, it does contain the greatest number of genes (3,141). It has the most known genetic diseases associated with it, including Alzheimer's and Parkinson's diseases, certain forms of autism and mental retardation, and several cancers. Gregory and colleagues published "The DNA Sequence and Biological Annotation of Human Chromosome 1," and the Human Genome Project was (once again) brought to completion.

—*James S. Godde*

in the process in which large numbers of clones of genomic fragments were made before sequencing could begin. Venter had circumvented this cloning step; he called his approach "whole-genome shotgun sequencing." During the next two years, the public consortium published the sequences of yeast and *E. coli*, respectively, and in 1998 announced that the sequence of *C. elegans* was complete. That same year, Venter announced that he was starting a for-profit company, Celera Genomics, which would complete the human genome within three years using shotgun sequencing. However, Venter had only demonstrated this approach using bacterial genomes until this time. To demonstrate the validity of the shotgun approach on large genomes and gear up for sequencing the human genome, Celera sequenced the 170 million bp genome of the fruit fly in 2000; at that time, the largest genome ever sequenced.

During the final years of the twentieth century, spurred on by the competition from the private sector, the public consortium had redoubled its efforts on the human genome. In February 2001, the race to sequence the human genome ended in a tie. Both sequencing efforts, public and private, published their draft sequence of the human genome at this time. In April 2003, the two efforts together announced the final completed sequence. The mouse genome sequence was also published in 2003. In fact, by mid-2003, about 150 genomic sequences had been determined (the vast majority of which were bacterial genomes), and almost 600 more were underway, including many more multicellular organisms.

Are the time, effort, and money that have been spent on various genome-sequencing projects worth it? One promise that genomics may hold for the future is the identification of all human disease genes. While this has been one of the main justifications for the Human Genome Project, one should keep in mind that identifying the gene that causes a particular disease is not always equivalent to finding a cure. Another potential benefit of genomic research is the development of better treatments for bacterial and parasitic infections. Many disease-causing bacteria have already been the subject of genome sequencing efforts, including the causative agents of bubonic plague, anthrax, and tuberculosis, to name a few. Some indirect benefits of genomics (which may, in time, prove just as valuable) include a better understanding of evolutionary relationships between species and a firmer grasp of basic cellular function. In all, the field of genomics promises to be a powerful means of scientific inquiry well into the future.

—*James S. Godde, Jeffrey A. Knight*

Further Reading

Archibald, John M. *Genomics: A Very Short Introduction*. Illustrated ed., Oxford UP, 2018.

Beery, Theresa, et al. *Genetics and Genomics in Nursing and Health Care*. 2nd ed., F. A. Davis Company, 2018.

Campbell, A. Malcolm, and Laurie J. Heyer. *Discovering Genomics, Proteomics, and Bioinformatics*. 2nd ed., CSHL Press, 2009.

Centers for Disease Control. "Genomics & Health Impact Update: August 6, 2013." *CDC Public Health Genomics*, Aug. 1-8, 2013.

Lesk, Arthur. *Introduction to Genomics*. 3rd ed., Oxford UP, 2017.

McCarthy, Jeanette, and Bryce Mendelsohn. *Precision Medicine: A Guide to Genomics in Clinical Practice*. McGraw Hill/Medical, 2016.

Olson, Steve, and Institute of Medicine (US). *Integrating Large-Scale Genomic Information into Clinical Practice: Workshop Summary*. National Academies Press, 2012.

Pevsner, Jonathan. *Bioinformatics and Functional Genomics*. 3rd ed., Wiley-Blackwell, 2015.

Snyder, Michael. *Genomics and Personalized Medicine: What Everyone Needs to Know*. Illustrated ed., Oxford UP, 2016.

Wei, Liping, et al. "Comparative Genomics Approaches to Study Organism Similarities and Differences." *Journal of Biomedical Informatics*, vol. 35, 2002, pp. 142-50.

Magnetic Resonance Imaging (MRI)

Category: Procedure
Specialties and related fields: Biotechnology, nuclear medicine, radiology
Definition: a noninvasive, nonradiological method of obtaining detailed information concerning normal and diseased tissue

KEY TERMS

electromagnetic waves: a convenient way of understanding energy as a wave; visible light, X-rays, and radio waves, which have the longest wavelength and lowest energy, are the most familiar examples

Fourier transform: a mathematical method that allows magnetic resonance imaging (MRI) to utilize one radio frequency pulse and thereby examine all wavelengths, as opposed to examining each wavelength individually with a continuous wave

nucleus: the dense, positively charged, central core of an atom, containing its massive protons and neutrons

zeugmatography: a name applied to MRI characterizing the close relationship of nuclear magnetic forces and electromagnetic waves (from the Greek *zeugma*, meaning "to yoke together")

INDICATIONS AND PROCEDURES

In 1901, Wilhelm Conrad Röntgen won the first Nobel Prize in Physics for his discovery of X-rays. Twenty-first-century applications of this radiation have produced medical miracles. Magnetic resonance imaging (MRI), often called nuclear magnetic resonance (NMR) imaging, differs fundamentally from X-rays and other imaging methods. It can produce a far richer array of three-dimensional images without the dangers attendant on ionizing radiation or the introduction of radioactive chemicals. Magnetic resonance imaging allows both safe diagnosis and study in healthy subjects. Furthermore, radiologists can use the method to examine flowing matter, such as in the circulatory system.

MRI SCANNING

This diagnostic imaging technique employs a powerful magnet to generate a magnetic field that is capable of aligning the protons in the body's hydrogen atoms, which are then knocked out of alignment by radio-wave pulses; as the protons realign, they emit radio signals that can be detected and used to create a cross-sectional image of the body.

The nuclei of hydrogen atoms behave like tiny magnets when placed in a magnetic field. When radio waves are superimposed on the magnetic waves, hydrogen atoms can be made to change their alignment with the magnetic field. The time required for the atoms to return to their original orientation after the radio waves cease varies with the nature of the tissue in which the hydrogen atoms reside. This combination of natural circumstances and the marvels of modern electronics has made it possible to obtain detailed images of brain tumors, spinal fluid, and blood vessels.

The discovery, in the mid-1940s, by Edward M. Purcell and Felix Bloch of the basic nuclear magnetic resonance techniques won them the 1952 Nobel Prize in Physics. Their innovation changed the practice of chemistry, biochemistry, and biology dramatically. Following new theoretical and practical contributions, diagnostic medicine participates fully in this revolution.

Both permanent magnets and electromagnets are used, and each has advantages, but the superconducting magnet is rapidly becoming the standard. The essential factors in producing detailed images are constant field strength and a highly uniform field. A transmitter connected to a radio frequency transmitter-receiver broadcasts and receives the signal returned from the patient. A short but intense pulse of radio frequency power is required, and its duration is critical to control electronic noise, which obscures the signal required to form the final image. These signals must be processed by complex computer methods to allow the final image to be displayed.

During the 1970s, several innovations were introduced that allowed broad application of the MRI technique. Paul Lauterbur demonstrated the generation of spatial maps by rotating the object to obtain a series of projections from which an image can be reconstructed. His method, called "NMR zeugmatography," introduced a radically new approach to MRI. By superimposing a magnetic field gradient on the main magnetic field, it is possible to make the resonance frequency a function of the spatial origin of the signal. Later, Richard R. Ernst built on his earlier introduction of Fourier-transform NMR to develop methods of two-dimensional NMR. Such techniques provide detailed information concerning the local structure of large molecules of biological importance. He was awarded the 1991 Nobel Prize in Chemistry because this same method laid the groundwork for the clinical use of MRI. Methods are now available for creating three- and four-dimensional MRIs, which are important in protein studies and will pave the way for future applications in nonchemical research.

USES AND COMPLICATIONS

Magnetic resonance imaging has been used to evaluate a wide variety of medical situations. The earliest uses involved the brain and the spinal cord, where it is necessary to avoid high-energy radiation or radioactivity. Since an MRI can provide excellent soft-tissue images and penetrating bony and air-filled structures, it is also well suited to the examination of the chest and abdomen. In these applications, it was first necessary to overcome motion-related problems. A further important modification, the flow imaging technique, allows the use of MRI in studies of the vascular system and has led to magnetic reso-

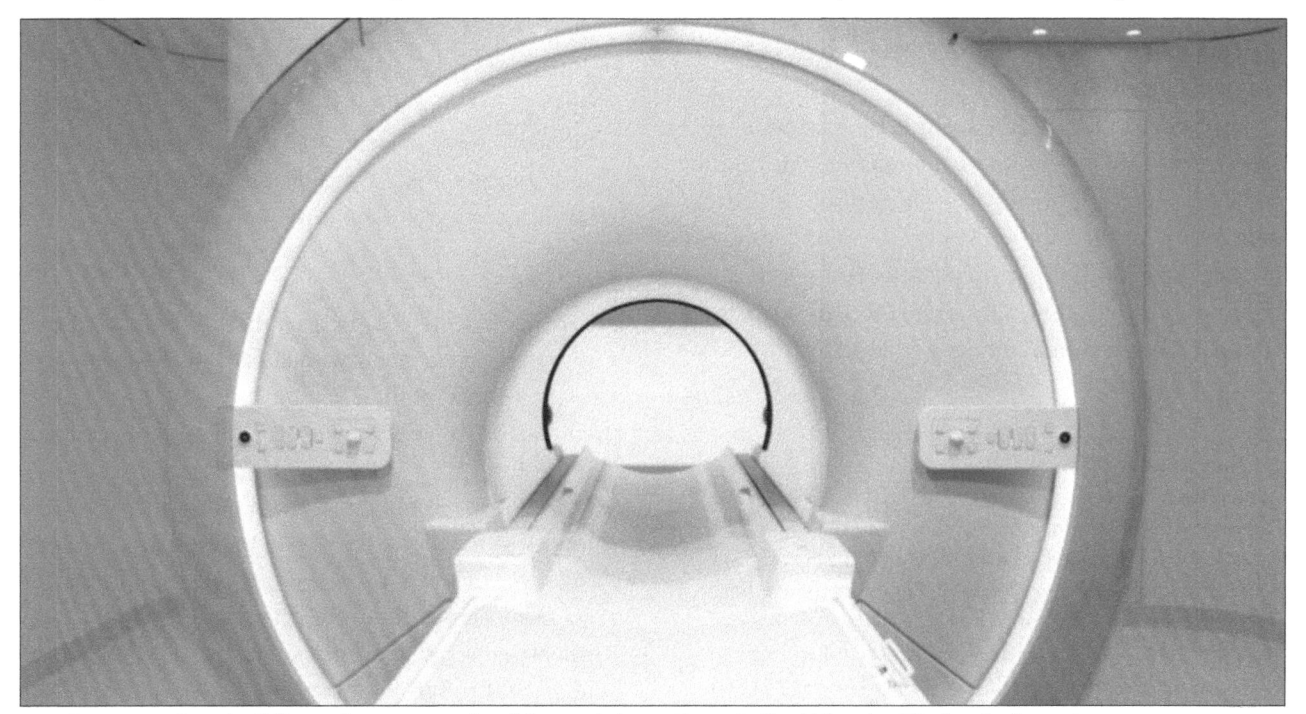

MRI images can show the difference between normal and damaged tissue. Photo via iStock/simonkr. [Used under license.]

nance angiography. This latter approach has clear advantages over the invasive X-ray procedure. Additional modifications allow the direct study of tissues of various living organisms under physiological conditions.

Functional MRI is a developing technology that allows neuroradiologists and neurosurgeons to evaluate the activity of the brain and cerebral blood vessels in real-time, observing brain activity. At the same time, the patient is asked questions or asked to perform various functions. This technique is especially helpful in coma patients or patients in a persistent vegetative state. There are even rare instances of functional MRI demonstrating active brain function in paralyzed patients thought to be brain dead or unconscious.

Despite the broad applicability of MRI, there are limitations. Other imaging techniques must evaluate patients on life-support systems or with unstable physiological conditions. The presence of a magnetic metal apparatus in the body is another limitation. There have also been discussions concerning effects related to the electrical currents induced by magnetic gradient fields.

This diagnostic imaging technique employs a powerful magnet to generate a magnetic field that is capable of aligning the protons in the body's hydrogen atoms, which are then knocked out of alignment by radio-wave pulses; as the protons realign, they emit radio signals that can be detected and used to create a cross-sectional image of the body.

—*K. Thomas Finley*

Further Reading

"Body MRI." *RadiologyInfor.org: For patients*, 15 June 2020, www.radiologyinfo.org/en/info/bodymr.

Bongard, Frederick, et al., editors. *Current Diagnosis and Treatment: Critical Care*. 3rd ed., McGraw-Hill Medical, 2008.

Bushong, Stewart C., and Geoffrey Clarke. *Magnetic Resonance Imaging: Physical and Biological Principles*. 4th ed., Mosby, 2014.

Buxton, Richard B. *An Introduction to Functional Magnetic Resonance Imaging: Principles and Techniques*. 2nd ed., Cambridge UP, 2009.

Griffith, H. Winter. *Complete Guide to Symptoms, Illness, and Surgery*. 5th ed., Perigee, 2006.

Kelley, Lorrie L., and Connie Petersen. *Sectional Anatomy for Imaging Professionals*. 4th ed., Mosby, 2018.

"MRI (Magnetic Resonance Imaging)." US Food and Drug Administration, 29 Aug. 2018, www.fda.gov/radiation-emitting-products/medical-imaging/mri-magnetic-resonance-imaging. Accessed 12 June 2022.

"MRI Scans." *MedlinePlus*, 22 Dec. 2016, medlineplus.gov/mriscans.html. Accessed 12 June 2022.

Pagana, Kathleen Deska, and Timothy J. Pagana. *Mosby's Diagnostic and Laboratory Test Reference*. 15th ed., Mosby, 2020.

SINGLE-PHOTON EMISSION COMPUTED TOMOGRAPHY (SPECT)

Category: Procedure

Specialties and related fields: Cardiology, nuclear medicine, psychiatry, pulmonary medicine, radiology

Definition: a nuclear imaging test used to provide three-dimensional information about the flow of blood through arteries and veins to diagnose a wide range of health conditions, including strokes, epilepsy, dementia, and tumors

KEY TERMS

gamma rays: electromagnetic radiation emitted during radioactive decay with short wavelengths

ischemia: reduced blood flow

myocardial perfusion imaging (MPI): a type of cardiac stress test

neurotransmitter: a chemical that communicates nerve impulses from one nerve cell to another

photons: particles that travel at the speed of light

tracer: a substance that is injected into the body and releases energy that allows it to be followed along its path through the circulatory system and metabolism pathways

INDICATIONS AND PROCEDURES

Single-photon emission computed tomography (SPECT) uses the radioisotopes xenon 133, technetium 99, and iodine 123 to acquire information about blood flow. A small amount of radioisotope is injected into a patient's vein to observe blood flow and metabolic pathways during the digestion of food. These radioisotopes are the radioactive forms of the naturally occurring elements of xenon, technetium, and iodine. These forms are referred to as radioactive because they emit gamma rays. A gamma-ray detector containing a series of crystals that convert the gamma rays to photons of light directly measures these gamma rays. Photomultiplier tubes amplify the photons into electrical signals, which are then converted by a computer into detailed three-dimensional visual images on a screen.

Single-photon emission computed tomography is one of several nuclear imaging techniques used in medicine for diagnosis. Imaging is important as a noninvasive method of seeing inside the body without requiring surgery. Other common techniques include X-rays, magnetic resonance imaging (MRI) scans, computed tomography (CT) scans, and ultrasound. The other nuclear imaging techniques include cardiovascular imaging, bone scanning, and positron emission tomography (PET). All these techniques assist in the detection of inadequate blood flow to tissues, aneurysms (weak locations in the walls of blood vessels), various blood cell disorders, and tumors.

Of these techniques, SPECT is the most similar to PET, but SPECT is less expensive and more readily available. Single-photon emission computed tomography radioisotopes emit single gamma rays with longer decay times than in PET and thus have the disadvantage of producing less detailed images than PET.

Tomography refers to the technique of using rotating X-rays to record an image within the body. With today's computers, the terminology of CT is used. The imaging process of SPECT combines CT with the use of radioisotopes. These radioisotopes are often referred to as tracers because they allow physicians to follow the pathway traveled by the blood through the body. Tracers emit gamma rays collected by a computer, which then translates the data into two-dimensional cross-sections that are added together to form a three-dimensional image. These radioactive tracers decay within minutes to hours and are eliminated in the urine, thus posing little harm to the body.

USES AND COMPLICATIONS

The sharp images that can be obtained using SPECT enable it to be a useful diagnostic tool for various cardiovascular, cerebrovascular, and neurological disorders. Single-photon emission computed tomography is more sensitive than an electrocardiogram (ECG) for detecting ischemia. Single-photon emission computed tomography scanning enhances myocardial perfusion imaging (MPI) after a patient exerts stress to compare images from before and after stress to assess blood flow and diagnose ischemic heart disease. Single-photon emission computed tomography has become an extensively used tool to diagnose coronary artery disease (CAD). Single-photon emission computed tomography has been widely used to detect tumors because it is such a useful tool for detecting reduced blood flow. For example, as part of diagnosing patients suspected of having aneurysms or tumors at the base of the skull, the internal carotid artery temporary balloon occlusion (TBO) test is enhanced by using SPECT to evaluate the cerebral blood flow. Single-photon emission computed tomography is also used to detect lymphoma tumors in the chest and abdomen, neuroendocrine tumors, stress fractures and stress reactions in the spine (known as "spondylolysis"), and liver lesions.

The high resolution of SPECT allows it to be a very useful tool for obtaining images of the striatum, a specific area of the brain containing the neurotransmitter dopamine. This dopamine activity can be monitored to help diagnose schizophrenia and various mood and movement disorders, including epilepsy, Alzheimer's disease, dementia, and obsessive-compulsive disorder.

PERSPECTIVE AND PROSPECTS

Although a SPECT scan exposes the body to less radiation than a CT or chest X-ray, pregnant or nursing women should not receive a SPECT scan. A nuclear medicine technologist will inject a patient with a small amount of radioactive tracer. After enough time is allowed for the tracer to travel to the brain (usually ten to twenty minutes), a special camera called a "gamma camera" is used to acquire multiple images from multiple angles by rotating around the head. This gamma camera detects the gamma radiation emitted by the radioactive tracers. Thus, the patient needs to remain motionless during the scanning process to obtain clear images. After the scanning process, the patient needs to drink fluids to remove the radioactive tracers from the body.

IN THE NEWS: USE OF SPECT TO DETECT PULMONARY EMBOLISM

Single-photon emission computed tomography has been shown by researchers to be useful in the diagnosis of pulmonary embolism. According to the study titled "Detection of Pulmonary Embolism with Combined Ventilation-Perfusion SPECT and Low-Dose CT: Head-to-Head Comparison with Multidetector CT Angiography," SPECT plus low-dose CT had a sensitivity of 97 percent and specificity of 100 percent. This diagnostic effectiveness was much greater than that of the multidetector CT angiography alone, which had a sensitivity of 68 percent and specificity of 100 percent.

Pulmonary embolism is a blockage in an artery in the lung caused by a blood clot. Diagnosis can be problematic because a seemingly healthy individual can develop this condition quickly, often with no symptoms. Furthermore, the mortality rate is estimated at a relatively high 30 percent.

The article published by researchers in Denmark in the December 2009 issue of the *Journal of Nuclear Medicine* is one of several recent articles describing additional applications of SPECT to diagnose these types of blood flow abnormalities as well as coronary heart disease and even to diagnose brain damage and cancer. Researchers in Houston, Texas, have found that using SPECT along with the coronary artery calcium score (CACS) is more effective in diagnosing coronary heart disease than either method alone. These results were published in November 10, 2009, *Journal of the American College of Cardiology* issue. ReGen Therapeutics has also reported that SPECT has shown the effectiveness of its drug zolpidem for treating brain damage.

—*Jeanne L. Kuhler*

Further Reading

"Assessment of Brain SPECT: Report of the Therapeutics and Technology Assessment Subcommittee of the American Academy of Neurology." *Neurology*, vol. 46, no. 1, 1996, pp. 278-85, doi:10.1212/wnl.46.1.278.

Frankle, W. G., et al. "Neuroreceptor Imaging in Psychiatry: Theory and Applications." *International Review of Neurobiology*, vol. 67, 2005, pp. 385-440.

Masdeu, J. C., et al. "Special Review: Brain Single Photon Emission Tomography." *Neurology*, vol. 44, 1994, pp. 1970-77.

Van Heertum, R. L., et al. "Single Photon Emission CT and Positron Emission Tomography in the Evaluation of Neurologic Disease." *Radiologic Clinics of North America* vol. 39, no. 5, 2001, pp. 1007-33, doi:10.1016/s0033-8389(05)70326-2.

Ultrasonography

Category: Procedure
Specialties and related fields: Cardiology, embryology, gynecology, internal medicine, obstetrics, radiology, urology, vascular medicine
Definition: a technique that directs ultrasonic waves into body tissues and uses the reflections to create visual images, making it possible to view the anatomy of organs and blood vessels and evaluate the dynamics of blood flow

KEY TERMS

Doppler effect: the relationship of the apparent frequency of waves, such as sound waves, to the relative motion of the source of the waves and the observer or instrument; the frequency increases as the two approach each other and decreases as they move apart; an effect also known as the "Doppler shift"

duplex scan: an ultrasound representation of echo images of tissues and blood vessels combined with a Doppler representation of blood flow patterns

frequency: the number of complete cycles, such as sound cycles, produced by an alternating energy source; sound is measured in cycles per second, and one cycle per second is equal to 1 hertz

oscilloscope: an instrument that displays a visual representation of electrical variations on the fluorescent screen of a cathode-ray tube

transducer (probe): a device designed to transfer ultrasound waves into the body noninvasively, receive the returning echoes, and transform those echoes into electrical voltages

ultrasonic: referring to any frequency of sound that is higher than the audible range—that is, higher than 20,000 cycles per second (20 kilohertz)

INDICATIONS AND PROCEDURES

Sound waves are mechanical pressure waves that can propagate through liquids, solids, and, to some extent, gases. A sound wave is composed of cyclic variations that occur over time; 1 cycle per second is called 1 hertz (Hz). Ultrasound waves have a frequency of oscillation higher than 20,000 hertz, placing ultrasound above the audible range for humans. The useful frequency range for medical diagnostic ultrasound is between 1 and 10 megahertz (10 million hertz). However, surgical instruments often use carrier frequencies greater than 20 megahertz.

The basic ultrasound system has two principal components. The first, and perhaps more important, component is the transducer or probe. The transducer converts electrical pulses into mechanical pressure (sound) waves that are transmitted into the tissues. It then detects the echoes that are reflected from the tissues and transforms those echoes into electrical voltages. The second component is the audiovisual electronic component, which processes and displays the reflected echoes in the form of an image of internal organs and structures or an image of the movement of red blood cells.

Ultrasound waves are created when the crystalline material within the transducer is excited by an electrical voltage produced by the instrument's oscillator. Applying an electrical charge causes the crystalline particles to expand and contract, producing mechanical waves and pulses. These sound pulses pass from the face of the transducer into the body, where they strike the organs, bones, and blood vessels. The reflected echoes, in turn, strike the face of the transducer, again causing the crystalline particles to vibrate and produce an electrical charge. Such crystalline material is said to have piezoelectric (a combination of the Greek word *piesis*, meaning "pressure," and the word "electric") properties.

Ultrasound systems commonly employ sound in two modalities. The transducer uses sound waves to create an echo image of body structures. The audiovisual component uses the Doppler shift theory to analyze the range of velocities over which red blood cells are moving.

Millions of sound pulses must be transmitted into the body each second to create an echo image. For each transmitted pulse, the transducer crystal receives one line of echo information. The pulses are sent into the body from many angles as the sound beam is moved over the body surface to build up an image rapidly and depict the real-time motion of body structures. The depth of the echoes is displayed as a function of time, and a two-dimensional (2D) image is created by relating the sound's direction of propagation to the direction of the echo-image trace that appears on the instrument's oscilloscope.

The time required for a sound pulse to travel from the transducer to its target within the body, reflect, and return to the transducer measures the distance to the target, as radar does. In body tissues, sound travels at a speed of 1,540 meters per second. It takes approximately 13 microseconds for a sound pulse to travel 1 centimeter into the body and return to the transducer. With this information, the machine can determine the depth and orientation of the echoes.

As a sound beam travels through tissues, it is attenuated or reduced in amplitude and intensity. Attenuation occurs as the energy from the beam is absorbed by the tissues and transformed into heat. Additionally, a part of the beam may be reflected into the surrounding tissues at an angle away from the incident angle or backscattered as the long wavelength of the sound beam strikes the smaller red blood cells. Only a small fraction of the returning echoes reach the face of the transducer.

The echo intensity is dependent on the degree of change and impedance of each tissue through which the echo passes, the strength of the incident sound beam, and the degree of attenuation of the beam. Because the sound beam attenuates as the depth of penetration increases, the echoes that return from the deepest part of the image field are reduced in intensity compared to the echoes that return from the structures nearer the skin surface. To equalize the intensity of the echoes from all depths of the image field, the echoes that travel farthest and therefore take the longest time to reach the transducer are amplified over time using time-gain compensation methods.

For medical imaging applications, the returning echoes may be displayed in several ways. The amplitude mode (A-mode) depicts the returning echoes as deflections on the instrument's oscilloscope; the deflection height depends on the returned signal's strength, and the distance between the deflections depends on the depth of the signal. The brightness mode (B-mode) depicts the strength of the echoes as shades of gray, with the strongest echoes appearing the brightest. The B-mode display makes it possible to differentiate tissue texture characteristics. The time-motion mode depicts movement over time by moving the B-mode trace across the face of a high-persistence oscilloscope, showing the depth, orientation, and strength of echoes with respect to time.

The transducer crystal determines the sound beam's shape and focus and the sound waves' frequency. These features are important in resolving echo information into complex images. The beam may be divided into three parts: the near field, the focal zone, and the far field. The beam width, close to the face of the transducer, is equal to the width of the transducer. The beam converges as it travels away from the transducer and then diverges at its narrow focal zone. For tissue targets to be resolved into discrete image points, both the beam's lateral and axial planes must be narrow. The focusing of the beam is facilitated by placing convex acoustic lenses in front of the transducer crystal to shorten the near field to a narrow focal point, thereby increasing the lateral resolution.

Axial resolution is the ability to distinguish targets along the sound beam. Suppose a single pulse is emitted from the transducer. In that case, echo sources lying close together in the axial path of the beam may not be separated. Multiple short bursts of sound are used to separate the echo sources; each echo is captured as a discrete burst. Because the axial resolution is inversely proportional to the ultrasound pulse's duration (and the crystal's resonant frequency is inversely proportional to its diameter), small-diameter, high-frequency crystals are used to obtain maximum axial resolution.

Ultrasound may be used to determine the velocity of blood flow. According to the Doppler theory, this velocity is determined in relation to the frequency of the incident sound beam. Ultrasound technicians may use several different techniques to process and display the echoes from moving red blood cells. They may program the ultrasound system's computers to perform fast Fourier transform analysis, a complex mathematical method for ranking the speed of the echoes returning over time. The computer displays the signals either as spectral tracings of the range of Doppler frequency shifts, represented in the returned echoes recorded throughout the cardiac cycle or as color-coded Doppler-shifted signals from within the blood vessels, superimposed on a gray-scale image of the surrounding tissues.

USES AND COMPLICATIONS

High-resolution abdominal ultrasonography is a valuable technique for visualizing intra-abdominal organs and disease processes. For example, high-resolution abdominal ultrasonography can identify liver conditions such as parenchymal abnormalities, abscesses, hematomas, cysts, and cancerous lesions easily using this technique. B-mode and Doppler color-flow imaging are valuable technologies to evaluate the tissue characteristics and blood flow patterns of transplanted organs. An ultrasound examination of the gallbladder may reveal gallstones, obstruction of the common bile duct, or inflammatory disease. Ultrasound imaging of the pancreas can identify this organ's pancreatitis, pancreatic pseudocysts, and carcinoma. An ultrasound examination of the spleen may reveal splenomegaly or enlargement of the spleen in response to disease or trauma. Additionally, ultrasonography can evaluate the splenic volume and identify hematomas, congenital cysts, infarctions, and tumors within the organ. The technology is particularly well suited for studying tumors and abscesses within the abdomen. Ascites and other fluid collections may be recognized, and primary tumors and lymph node metastases within the abdominal cavity may be identified utilizing pulse-echo imaging.

Ultrasound has certain characteristics that make it particularly valuable for examining the kidneys and the genitourinary tract. The ability to image both native and transplanted kidneys noninvasively from the longitudinal and transverse planes provides additional diagnostic information in uremic patients for whom the injection of contrast agents is undesirable or may fail to provide sufficient information. Urologic ultrasonography may determine renal size and position or identify cysts and masses, kidney or bladder stones, obstruction of the ureters, and bladder contour.

Transabdominal scanning of the pelvic organs, which is used to determine the presence or absence of suspected lesions, makes possible the precise localization and quantitative mapping of pelvic abdominal masses, facilitating the determination of disease stages and the positioning of radiation ports. The technology is used to differentiate cysts from solid tumors and determine if pelvic tumors are of uterine, ovarian, or tubal origin.

The sonographic resolution of deep abdominal structures is achieved by internal scanning; endorectal or endovaginal approaches are used to reduce the distance between the transducer and the target organ. During these procedures, the transducer probe either is in direct contact with the genital organs or prostate gland or is separated from them by the thin walls of the bladder or rectum. The information obtained with these techniques is considered submacroscopic, observed at approximately twenty to thirty times light magnification.

Ultrasonography plays a major role in the evaluation of obstetrical cases. Ultrasonic imaging is used to study early pregnancy and high-risk cases and to confirm ectopic pregnancy (development of the fetus outside the uterus). In cases of spontaneous abortion, ultrasound procedures are used to indicate whether the fetus and placenta have been retained. Ultrasonography is often used to determine fetal growth rate and placental development and confirm intrauterine fetal death, threatened abortion, and fetal abnormalities. It is the best method for guiding amniocentesis (the sampling of placental fluids). A study published in the *Journal of the American Medical Association* in 2013 confirmed that ultrasound is the best detector of ectopic pregnancies.

Echocardiography, the ultrasound evaluation of the heart, is a reliable and useful tool for studying patients with congenital and acquired heart disease. The role of cardiac ultrasound in investigating cardiac dysfunction, tetralogy of Fallot, transposition of the great vessels, and atrial septal defect has been well-defined. Echocardiology is used to detect pericardial effusion; it is coupled with Doppler ultrasound to evaluate the pulmonic, mitral, tricuspid, and aortic valves; and is used to investigate primary myocardial disease and atrial tumors. Endoesophageal (transesophageal) imaging and Doppler color-flow technology improve the resolution of cardiac structures and blood flow patterns.

Combining pulse-echo imaging of the blood vessels and Doppler ultrasound detection of red blood cell movement effectively visualizes the body's vascular systems. This combined technology, known as "duplex scanning," not only offers information that is relevant to the anatomy and morphology of blood vessels but also—and this is, most important—provides, the opportunity to evaluate the dynamics of blood flow and the pathophysiology of vascular disease. Duplex technology is used to demonstrate the presence and characteristics of atherosclerotic disease and to define the severity of vascular compromise resulting from the progression of a disease or the presence of blood clots in vessels (thrombosis).

Applications of the technology have been extended to the evaluation of arteries and veins of the extremities, the abdomen, and the brain. Advances in computer technology have made it possible to color-code the Doppler-shifted signals returning from moving red blood cells within the vessels. Doppler color-flow imaging has facilitated the investigation of vascular disorders that result in slow or reduced blood flow (venous thrombosis or preocclusive narrowing of vessels) or that affect the vascularity of organs and tissues (tumors or transplanted organs). Therefore, vascular ultrasonography plays a major role in evaluating patients with arterial occlusive disease and those suspected of having thrombosis of the deep or superficial venous systems.

PERSPECTIVE AND PROSPECTS

Ultrasonic techniques have assumed a preferred role in diagnosing many diseases and have become an essential component of quality medical care. In contrast to the rapid development and use of X-ray technology in medical diagnosis, the application of diagnostic ultrasound has been relatively slow. Progress depended in large part on the development of high-resolution electronic devices and transducers. Early research into medical applications involved the adaptation of instruments that had been designed for industrial or military purposes.

The first attempts to locate objects with ultrasound probably occurred following the sinking of the *Titanic* in 1912. Improvements in the technology led to the widespread industrial and military use of ultrasound for detecting flaws in metals, determining the range and depth information, and navigation. The first application of ultrasound to medical diagnosis occurred in 1937 when K. T. Dussik attempted to image the cerebral ventricles by measuring the attenuation of a sound beam transmitted through the head. In 1947, Douglas H. Howry pioneered the ultrasonic imaging of soft tissues and constructed a pulse-echo system that utilized a transducer submerged in water. The system utilized surplus Navy sonar equipment, a high-fidelity recorder power supply, and a metal cattle-watering trough in which the patient and the transducer were immersed.

In the 1960s, Howard Thompson and Kenneth Gottesfeld performed obstetric and gynecologic examinations using the first contact scanner, produced in 1958 by Tom Brown, an engineer, and Ian Donald, a professor of midwifery, at Glasgow University in Scotland. The first commercial scanner marketed in the United States was designed by William L. Wright, an engineer at the University of Colorado.

The 2D scanning system was developed in 1953 by John Reid, an engineer, in cooperation with John Wild, a physician. He demonstrated that ultrasound could detect differences between normal tissues, benign tumors, and cancers. The collaboration between medicine and engineering has propelled diagnostic ultrasonography forward at a phenomenal rate of development since that time.

Inge Edler pioneered the field of echocardiography. She discovered in the 1950s that echoes from the moving heart could be received and displayed by using a time-motion ultrasonic flow detector. Edler used this technology to diagnose mitral stenosis, pericardial effusion, and thrombus in the left atrium.

S. Satomura first employed ultrasound to evaluate blood flow in 1959. This investigator observed that ultrasound could be transmitted through the skin to derive information about the blood flow velocity by using the Doppler effect to analyze the reflected signals from the moving blood cells. Researchers at the University of Washington in the 1960s developed the first transcutaneous continuous-wave Doppler system. The instrument was first used to detect fetal life by demonstrating the fetal heartbeat. This application of Doppler ultrasound spurred research under the guidance of Eugene Strandness Jr., which ultimately led to the development of duplex scanners. These instruments combine pulse-echo imaging with analysis of blood flow patterns derived from the Doppler effect. As a result of the efforts of these early investigators and others, diagnostic medical ultrasonography has evolved into a highly useful tool with diverse clinical applications.

—*Marsha M. Neumyer*

Further Reading

Bates, Jane A. *Abdominal Ultrasound: How, Why, and When.* 3rd ed., Churchill Livingstone/Elsevier, 2011.

Bernstein, Eugene F., editor. *Vascular Diagnosis.* 4th ed., Mosby, 1993.

Fletcher, Jenna. "What is a Doppler Ultrasound?" *MedicalNewsToday*, 28 Oct. 2019, www.medicalnewstoday.com/articles/326824.

Griffith, H. Winter, et al. *Complete Guide to Symptoms, Illness, and Surgery.* 6th Rev. ed., TarcherPerigee, 2012.

Hagan, Arthur D., and Anthony N. DeMaria. *Clinical Applications of Two-Dimensional Echocardiography and Cardiac Doppler.* 2nd ed., Little, Brown, 1989.

Kremkau, Frederick W. *Diagnostic Ultrasound: Principles and Instruments.* 7th ed., Saunders/Elsevier, 2006.

Pagana, Kathleen Deska, and Timothy J. Pagana. *Mosby's Diagnostic and Laboratory Test Reference.* 11th ed., Mosby/Elsevier, 2013.

"Ultrasound." *MedlinePlus*, 15 Dec. 2020, medlineplus.gov/lab-tests/sonogram/.

INJURY TREATMENTS—STANDARD

"A doctor should be a clown at heart, a scientist at brain and a mother at conscience."

—Abhijit Naskar, *Time to Save Medicine*

Can you explain what it takes to replace a knee or hip joint? If you can't, then you need to read the articles in this section, which will give you the how, why, and what-for in a clear and understandable manner. Sports injuries are generally treated using immobilization, injections to reduce swelling and pain, prescription anti-inflammatory drugs, or, as a last resort, surgery. Topics such as casts and splints, physical rehabilitation, braces, spinal cord injury, tendon repair, and hyaluronic acid injections highlight some of the usual approaches to addressing debilitating injuries.

Advances in Spinal Cord Injury Research

Category: Therapy
Specialties and related fields: Neurology, neurosurgery, orthopedics, regenerative medicine
Definition: a new treatment for severe spinal cord injuries that puts electrical impulses into the spine to restore blocked nerve impulses

KEY TERMS

physical rehabilitation: a set of interventions designed to optimize functioning and reduce disability in individuals with health conditions in interaction with their environment

spinal cord injury: damage to the tight bundle of cells and nerves that sends and receives signals from the brain to and from the rest of the body

INTRODUCTION

Spinal cord injury (SCI) is a complex condition that affects the entire body. The spinal cord and the brain make up what is known as the central nervous system (CNS). The spinal cord consists of a tight bundle of blood vessels, neural cells (neurons), and the specialized glial cells surrounding neurons, providing support and insulation. The neurons extend their nerve pathways (axons) from the base of the brain to the lower back. The spinal cord network receives information from the rest of the body and relays that information to the brain. The brain also sends messages through the network to all body parts. The network of nerves outside the brain and the spinal cord is known as the "peripheral nervous system." Damage to the spinal cord disrupts the delicate system of whole-body communication that assures well-being and overall functionality.

The injury occurs when the vertebrae that normally protect the cord's soft tissue (nerves) break or dislocate in ways that put pressure on the cord. Injury type and location determine likely outcomes. The more axons that remain intact, the greater the chance of function recovery. Loss of function occurs below the point of injury. Therefore, the higher the injury is on the cord, the greater the loss of function.

In a 2019 update, the National Institute of Neurological Disorders and Stroke (NINDS) estimated that 12,000 SCIs occur in the United States annually. More than a quarter of a million people live with an SCI. At least 36.5 percent of SCIs result from motor vehicle accidents (MVAs), and over one quarter are due to falls. Acts of violence, sporting accidents, and other factors make up the remainder of SCIs. Approximately 80 percent of SCI patients are male.

ELECTRICAL STIMULATION OFFERS HOPE AND NEW UNDERSTANDING

For generations, the prevailing attitude toward SCI was that injury to the spine was permanent. The belief has been that once the spine is broken, it cannot be repaired. People who suffered an SCI had little hope of partial recovery, let alone full functional recovery. Research and experimentation are revolutionizing the treatment for SCI.

In a 2018 article for *leapsmag*, author Karen Weintraub reported that recovery is possible, even years after the injury. According to Weintraub, researchers at the Kentucky Spinal Cord Injury Research Center have discovered that neurons that survive an injury can generate signals and initiate movement. Results at the center also indicate that the traditional practice of waiting to attempt treatment, consigning patients to wheelchairs or beds, is not the best practice. The team in Kentucky combined epidural electrical stimulation with physical rehabilitation. Patients receiving the treatment are standing independently, and many are walking. Others are using limbs they never expected to use again.

Researchers at the center believe that some form of physical therapy and treatment should begin as soon as possible for most SCI patients. The team believes that the electrical stimulation paired with physical therapy effectively kick-starts spinal cord nerve circuits into a functioning state. While the volume of nerve message output is lower after injury, there is reason to believe that stimulation trains neurons to respond to the lower volume. The success of this approach calls for a complete change in thinking about SCI.

DOES THE SPINAL CORD HAVE A BLOOD PRESSURE?

Researchers in Kentucky are not the only SCI specialists to realize prevailing beliefs about SCI are not entirely true. Encouraging research is coming out of Zuckerberg San Francisco General Hospital and Trauma Center, as doctors, there are proving spinal cord function can be recovered. According to a 2018 article for *MedicalXpress*, author Kathleen Masterson reports that Dr. Sanjay Dhall and colleagues have discovered important new factors in injury and recovery that have prompted a new treatment protocol. Their treatment protocol combines revised ways of evaluating injury with new treatments. Traditionally, evaluating injury included imaging and measuring feeling and movement in a patient's arms and legs. Dhall based the treatment on indications that the most important factor in SCI is spinal cord blood pressure (BP). Spinal BP is called "spinal cord perfusion." Because the spinal cord regulates BP throughout the body, injury to the cord affects the body's ability to maintain adequate BP. The new treatment involves measuring each patient's blood flow to the spine. Previously, doctors would artificially raise everyone's BP in the same way across different injuries, ages, and general health. Another aspect of the protocol is moving patients who need surgery into an operating room as soon as possible.

At the time of Masterson's article, Dr. Dhall's team had treated ten SCI patients with the new protocol. The results have been so encouraging that the new method has become the standard of care.

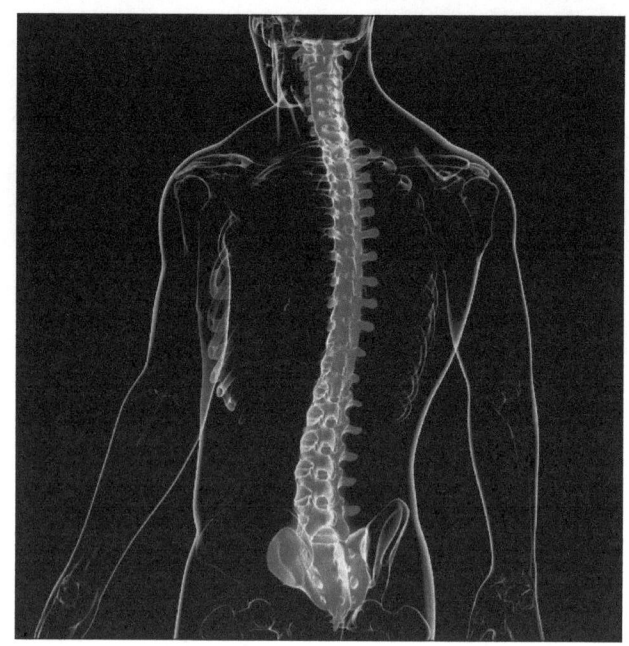

Image via iStock/magicmine. [Used under license.]

USING STEM CELLS TO TREAT SCI

The hope of using stem cells to treat SCI was born when stem cell research began. Stem cells can develop into specific cells the body needs. Thus, they are the hope of reparative and regenerative treatments. A 2019 article for the *Mayo Clinic News Network* suggests the hoped-for day of treating SCI with stem cell therapies has arrived. The article by Susan Lindquist reported the early results of a trial with ten SCI patients in Rochester, Minnesota. The Mayo Clinic team used stem cells from the patient's fat cells to regenerate spinal nerve cells.

The first patient treated has shown improvement in both sensation and motor function. However, not all the patients in the trial had the same response. Researchers hope the trial will answer important questions about ideal dosage, why patients respond differently to stem cell injections, and whether there are side effects to the treatment. This study is important to ongoing research into the effectiveness of stem cell therapies. In addition, it is especially important to regenerative medicine research. Scientists are learning. And what they are learning has life-changing potential for SCI patients now and in the future.

—Liam Hooper

Further Reading

Lindquist, Susan B. "Case Report: Stem Cells a Step Toward Improving Motor, Sensory Function after Spinal Cord Injury." *Mayo Clinic News Network*, 27 Nov. 2019, newsnetwork.mayoclinic.org/discussion/case-report-stem-cells-a-step-toward-improving-motor-sensory-function-after-spinal-cord-injury/. Accessed 31 Dec. 2019.

Masterson, Kathleen. "A New Spinal Cord Injury Treatment is Getting Patients Back on Their Feet." *MedicalXpress*, 10 Sept. 2018, medicalxpress.com/news/2018-09-spinal-cord-injury-treatment-patients.html. Accessed 31 Dec. 2019.

"Spinal Cord Injury: Hope Through Research." *National Institute of Neurological Disorders and Stroke*, 13 Aug. 2019, www.ninds.nih.gov/disorders/patient-caregiver-education/hope-through-research/spinal-cord-injury-hope-through-research. Accessed 31 Dec. 2019.

"Spinal Cord Research." *Christopher & Dana Reeve Foundation*, 2019, www.christopherreeve.org/research/spinal-cord-research. Accessed 31 Dec. 2019.

Weintraub, Karen. "Advances Bring First True Hope to Spinal Cord Injury Patients." *leapsmag*. Future Frontiers, 12 Nov. 2018, leapsmag.com/advances-bring-first-true-hope-to-spinal-cord-injury-patients. Accessed 31 Dec. 2019.

ARTHROPLASTY

Category: Procedure
Specialties and related fields: Anesthesiology, general surgery, geriatrics and gerontology, orthopedics, rheumatology, sports medicine, occupational and physical therapy

Definition: surgical reconstruction or replacement of a joint

KEY TERMS

acetabulum: the portion of the pelvic bone joining the femoral head to create the hip joint
cartilage: flexible connective tissue between bones
epidural: the injection of an anesthetic into the fluid around the spine or into the epidural space in the back
femur: the leg bone extending from the knee to the hip
orthopedics: a medical specialty emphasizing the prevention and correction of skeletal deformities
patella: the flat, triangular bone in the front of the knee; also called the "kneecap"
rheumatoid arthritis: a long-term autoimmune disorder that primarily affects joints resulting in warm, swollen, and painful joints
tibia: the shin bone
viscosupplementation injections: injections to add lubrication into the joint to make joint movement less painful

INDICATIONS AND PROCEDURES

Cartilage within a joint covers the ends of the bones, preventing bone from pressing on bone and allowing smooth, pain-free movement. Joints can become painful when cartilage on the end of each adjoining bone deteriorates, a process called "osteoarthritis." A fracture, trauma, or another medical condition such as rheumatoid arthritis can also cause joint pain and disability, any of which may lead an individual to consider arthroplasty. Should initial nonsurgical treatments such as medications, physical therapy, and joint injections prove to be unsuccessful, arthroplasty, a surgery undertaken to replace deteriorating joints, becomes an option, particularly among the elderly.

Arthroplasty may be performed on the fingers, wrists, shoulders, elbows, and ankles but the most common sites of the surgery are the hips and knees. Most patients requiring hip or knee replacements are over the age of fifty, but arthroplasty may be indicated for younger people who have suffered advanced joint deterioration or trauma. Specialists in sports medicine who are typically orthopedic surgeons also frequently prescribe arthroplasty.

The hip is a ball-and-socket joint comprising the top of the femur (ball) inserted into the acetabulum (socket). During walking, the top of the femur slides within the acetabulum. Cartilage of the hip joint normally covers both bones where they join permitting smooth, painless contact between the surfaces. When the cartilage deteriorates, bones rub against each other, causing pain and restriction in movement that is eventually best relieved by hip replacement surgery.

In hip surgery, an incision, varying in length from 2 to 12 inches, is made over the back of the hip (and more recently, the front of the hip, referred to as an anterior approach). Tissue and muscles are cut or pushed aside to expose the hip joint. The femur and acetabulum are separated. A cavity made in the acetabulum accommodates the replacement cup and allows for the insertion of a plastic-lined metal shell. The ball on the femur end of the joint is removed and replaced with a metal ball attached to a metal stem, usually made of titanium that is inserted into the femoral canal. The two parts are then cemented into place, making them adhere to the bone. Damaged muscles and tendons are repaired before the incision is closed with staples or sutures.

A similar situation can afflict the knee. In some instances, an orthopedist makes a small incision in the knee using a surgical instrument called an "arthroscope" or "endoscope." The device inserts a narrow, illuminated tube with a camera attached into the affected site for a visual examination viewed on a monitor. If this examination, as well as previous X-rays, reveal worn bone and cartilage, a knee replacement is potentially indicated.

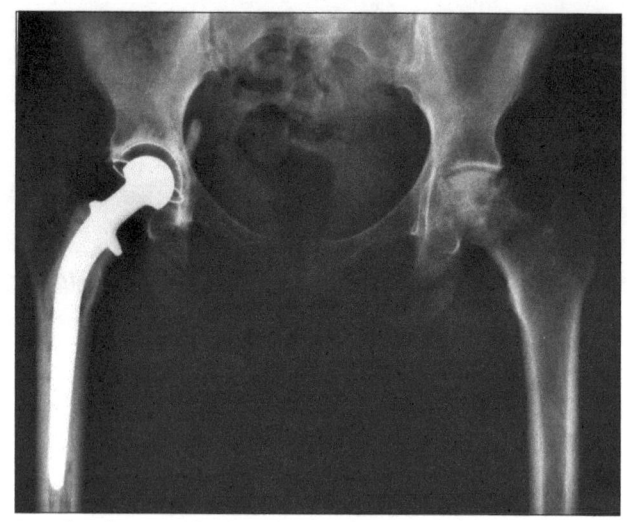

In arthroplasty, artificial implants replace part of the hip joint. Photo via Wikimedia Commons. [Public domain.]

Knee arthroplasty consists of the worn knee joint being replaced with metal and plastic components. In knee arthroplasty, a long incision is made in the front of the knee and the patella is removed to make the joint accessible. Holes are drilled into the lower femur to affix the metal replacement. Holes are also drilled in the upper tibia to anchor a plastic plate. The back part of the patella is excised to create a flat surface into which holes are drilled to receive a plastic button. In most cases, the prosthesis is secured with cement, and the incision closed, usually with sutures or staples. Because polymethylmethacrylate cement is usually used in both the hip and knee procedures, the individual, under the guidance of a physical therapist, can gradually place weight on the surgical limb and progress as tolerated. Knee and hip arthroplasties are performed without cement and use implants with a textured or coated surface that the new bone actually grows into. Such implants may also use screws or pegs to stabilize the implant until the completion of bone ingrowth. Since cementless implants depend on new bone growth for stability, they require a longer healing time than cemented replacements. Typically, hip and knee replacements are performed on patients under general anesthesia, although a local anesthetic, either spinal or epidural, is sometimes used. In most cases, general anesthesia is preferred because patients must remain completely still during this surgery and general anesthesia causes temporary paralysis.

USES AND COMPLICATIONS

Arthroplasty is used to relieve pain and restore mobility in patients who have been disabled by their conditions and are reasonable surgical risks. Because many such patients are elderly, extensive preoperative evaluation is necessary. Arthroplasty may be used when medical treatments no longer effectively relieve joint pain and disability. Some medical treatments for osteoarthritis tried before arthroplasty include physical therapy, cortisone joint injections, anti-inflammatory medicines, viscosupplementation injections, and pain medicines.

Conditions such as diabetes mellitus, hypertension, heart or lung disease, and anemia increase the surgical risk. Open lesions increase the risk of infection. Nerve damage can result from cutting muscles and tendons during surgery. Blood clots can form in the lungs or legs of patients undergoing arthroplasty, and this risk may continue for two months following surgery. Blood thinners are usually administered postoperatively. Infection and loosening of prosthetic parts are additional surgical risks and complications.

Physical therapy, essential following arthroplasty of any joint, usually begins two or three days after the surgery and continues for eight weeks. Most patients are completely ambulatory within six weeks postoperatively of hip or knee arthroplasty.

PERSPECTIVE AND PROSPECTS

Joint replacement is becoming more common, and more than 1 million Americans have a hip or knee replaced each year. Research has shown that despite increases in age, joint replacement can help overall mobility and general well-being. As life expectancy increases, incidence of joint problems is increasing exponentially. In the early twentieth century, many people who lived beyond their sixties were immobilized by chronic arthritis, osteoporosis, and painful joints. When an elderly person suffered a broken hip, it often marked the beginning of a physical decline with a fatal outcome. Medical advances made during World War II had a profound effect on treating many physical problems that, although experienced in combat by relatively young people, required treatment that was soon used in dealing with the joint problems of the elderly. Hip and knee surgery were once more disabling than they currently are. Hip surgery now requires incisions as small as 1-inch long, although 4-inch incisions are more common and 10-inch incisions are used by some surgeons.

Although arthroplasty usually involves a hospital stay of two days depending on the complexity of each individual case, some low-risk individuals without postoperative complications become outpatient procedures. The use of titanium in prostheses has extended the effectiveness of such surgery, with these devices currently expected to last for over two decades. People who have arthroplasty generally have substantial improvement in their joint pain, ability to perform activities, and quality of life.

— *R. Baird Shuman*

Further Reading

"Arthroplasty." *Johns Hopkins Medicine*, 2019, www.hopkinsmedicine.org/health/treatment-tests-and-therapies/arthroplasty.

Feng, James, et al. "Total Knee Arthroplasty: Improving Outcomes with a Multidisciplinary Approach." *Journal of Multidisciplinary Healthcare*, vol. 11, 2018, pp. 63-73, doi:10.2147/jmdh.s140550.

Gogineni, Hrishikesh C., et al. "Transition to Outpatient Total Hip and Knee Arthroplasty: Experience at an Academic Tertiary Care Center." *Arthroplasty Today*, vol. 5, no. 1, 2019, pp. 100-105, doi:10.1016/j.artd.2018.10.008.

Karachalios, Theofilos, et al. "Total Hip Arthroplasty." *EFORT Open Reviews*, vol. 3, no. 5, 2018, pp. 232-39, doi:10.1302/2058-5241.3.170068.

Lee, Yong Seuk. "Comprehensive Analysis of Pain Management after Total Knee Arthroplasty." *Knee Surgery & Related Research*, vol. 29, no. 2, 2017, pp. 80-86, doi:10.5792/ksrr.16.024.

Warwick, Hunter, et al. "Immediate Physical Therapy Following Total Joint Arthroplasty: Barriers and Impact on Short-Term Outcomes." *Advances in Orthopedics*, vol. 2019, 8 Apr. 2019, pp. 1-7, doi:10.1155/2019/6051476.

Weber, Markus, et al. "Predicting Outcome after Total Hip Arthroplasty: The Role of Preoperative Patient-Reported Measures." *BioMed Research International*, vol. 2019, 2019, pp. 1-9, doi:10.1155/2019/4909561.

Astym® Therapy

Category: Procedure
Specialties and related fields: Athletic enhancement, athletic training, occupational therapy, physical therapy, rehabilitation
Definition: a regenerative soft tissue therapy that rebuilds and heals the soft tissues of the body, noninvasively and without pharmaceuticals

KEY TERMS

soft tissue massage: a form of manual physical therapy involving hands-on techniques on muscles, ligaments, and fascia to break adhesions and optimize muscle function

tendonitis: inflammation or irritation of a tendon, the thick fibrous cords that attach muscle to bone

tendinopathy: degeneration of the collagen protein that forms the tendon

INDICATIONS AND PROCEDURES

Astym® treatment is regenerative soft tissue therapy that rebuilds and heals the soft tissues of the body, noninvasively and without pharmaceuticals. Astym® treatment safely and effectively stimulates internal scar tissue to be resorbed by the body and regenerates damaged soft tissues. This noninvasive therapeutic approach utilizes handheld instrumentation, applied topically to locate underlying dysfunctional soft tissue. Astym® then transfers specific pressures and shear forces via that instrumentation to the dysfunctional tissue through specific protocols and application patterns developed from scientific and clinical studies. These particular pressures and shear forces induce a cellular response that activates the synthesis of cellular mediators and growth factors. These signaling molecules activate scar tissue resorption, stimulate tissue turnover, and regenerate soft tissues.

Astym® therapy is typically provided in a physical or occupational therapy setting. However, elite athletes are frequently treated as part of their team care to optimize performance, and treatment may occur at the site of competitions. In addition, large employers and the military routinely have Astym® therapy provided in their facilities or in the field to minimize interruption by resolving injuries effectively and efficiently.

Astym® therapy engages the regenerative mechanisms of the body. It is consistently safe and effective in treating internal scar tissue that is causing pain or movement restriction, chronic tendonitis, traumatic soft tissue injury, postsurgical pain/restrictions, and other soft tissue dysfunctions. Astym® therapy was methodically developed from theories tested in basic scientific experiments and extended to clinical study and practice.

Tendinopathies and tendonitis are widespread problems and often challenge health-care professionals, in many cases remaining unresolved. Astym® treatment is highly effective in the treatment of tendinopathy, and clinical trials have demonstrated Astym® therapy to reduce pain and increase motion and functional ability in this population. Effective both as a first-line treatment and as a last resort when other treatments have failed, Astym® therapy is an attractive treatment option. It has a relatively short treatment course of four to six weeks (eight to ten visits). There are usually no restrictions on activity during treatment, which is a welcome change from other more restrictive treatment options. Randomized clinical trials have shown Astym® therapy to be more effective than the standard-of-care treatments for lateral elbow tendinopathy (tennis elbow), patellar (knee) tendinopathy, and Achilles tendinopathy.

Internal scar tissue may result from several factors, including overuse, problematic biomechanics, trauma, or surgery. Although Astym® therapy routinely demonstrates considerable success in treating conditions where scar tissue is present, extraordinary improvement has been shown when Astym® therapy is used postsurgically. Astym® therapy has also been found to reduce pain and increase function in cases where internal scar tissue is interfering with movement or causing pain.

There is also evidence that Astym® therapy can improve the brain-to-body connection by stimulating neuroplastic changes in damaged nervous systems. Such healing is critically important since Astym® therapy may alter the natural progression or prognosis for such disorders as cerebral palsy and brain injury, which has not yet been possible. A large, three-arm randomized controlled trial demonstrated the positive neural effects of Astym® therapy. This trial revealed that Astym® therapy immediately and significantly improves muscle performance after injury. These results are supported by other clinical studies indicating improvement in neural conditions such as carpal tunnel syndrome, restricted movement due to cerebral palsy, and brain injury.

USES AND COMPLICATIONS

Astym® therapy is generally well tolerated by patients. General contraindications include: compromised skin integrity; open wound(s); active infection; skin ulcerations; acute deep venous thrombosis (DVT); treatment involving the area of a pacemaker or internal defibrillator; active primary or metastatic tumor site; clotting disorders; and any medical condition or disorder that may be exacerbated by the application of topical pressures on the skin or underlying structures. The treating therapist/clinician should adjust the topical pressures and forces to be within each patient's tolerance.

It is important to confirm that the clinician is officially certified in Astym® therapy to receive proper treatment. Certification training educates clinicians on the scientifically developed protocols and specific treatment parameters studied in randomized controlled trials. Astym® therapy has consistently demonstrated safety and effectiveness in clinical study and is well tolerated by patients. Astym® therapy is distinctly different from instrument-assisted soft tissue mobilization (IASTM) interventions. It is important to recognize that IASTM interventions show neither the effectiveness nor the safety of Astym® therapy. Although the IASTM methods use tools to treat tissue, the methods and results are quite different from those of Astym® therapy. Instrument-assisted soft tissue mobilization methods use tooled cross-friction massage to, it is argued, break apart the tissue, whereas Astym® therapy engages the regenerative mechanisms of the body, aiming to repair damaged tissue and stimulate the resorption of scar tissue. However, IASTM methods are often not well tolerated by patients. A recent systematic review evaluated the research on IASTM. It concluded the research does not support the efficacy of IASTM for treating musculoskeletal pathologies.

PERSPECTIVE AND PROSPECTS

Historically, treatment for soft tissue disorders centered upon treating inflammation. However, with the discovery that tendinopathies and some other soft tissue conditions are primarily degenerative, scholars emphasize that treatment should now be focused on regeneration and restoration. Astym® therapy was the first conservative treatment scientifically developed to engage the body's regenerative mechanisms and has been proven to be effective in treating a variety of soft tissue disorders. Although many available treatments today still focus on reducing inflammation, they often have little to no scientific evidence supporting their effectiveness.

—*Thomas L. Sevier*

Further Reading

Cheatham, S. W., et al. "The Efficacy of Instrument Assisted Soft Tissue Mobilization: A Systematic Review." *Journal of the Canadian Chiropractic Association*, vol. 60, no. 3, 2016, pp. 200-211.

Chughtai, M., et al. "A Novel, Nonoperative Treatment Demonstrates Success for Stiff Total Knee Arthroplasty after Failure of Conventional Therapy." *Journal of Knee Surgery*, vol. 29, no. 3, 2016, pp. 188-93.

Davies, C. C., D. Brockopp, and K. Moe. "Astym® Therapy Improves Function and Range of Motion Following Mastectomy." *Breast Cancer: Targets and Therapy*, vol. 8, 2016, pp. 39-45.

Kivlan, B. R., et al. "The Effect of Astym® Therapy on Muscle Strength: A Blinded, Randomized, Clinically Controlled Trial." *BMC Musculoskeletal Disorders*, vol. 16, 2015, p. 325.

Ryan, S. L., and P. Wallace. "Use of Astym® Treatment to Improve Contractures and Dyskinesia in an Individual with Anoxic Encephalopathy." *Combined Sections Meeting, APTA*, Feb. 2009.

Scheer, N. A., et al. "Astym® Therapy Improves Bilateral Hamstring Flexibility and Achilles Tendinopathy in a Child with Cerebral Palsy: A Retrospective Case Report." *Clinical Medicine Insights: Case Reports*, vol. 9, 2016, pp. 95-98, doi:10.4137/CCRep.S40623.

Sevier, T. L., and C. W. Stegink-Jansen. "Astym® Treatment vs. Eccentric Exercise for Lateral Elbow Tendinopathy: A Randomized Controlled Clinical Trial." *PeerJ*, vol. 3, 2015, p. e967, doi.org/10.7717/peerj.967.

Wilson, J. K., et al. "Comparison of Rehabilitation Methods in the Treatment of Patellar Tendinitis." *Journal of Sport Rehabilitation*, vol. 9, no. 4, 2000, pp. 304-14.

Braces, Orthopedic

Category: Treatment
Specialties and related fields: Orthopedics, sports medicine
Definition: a device to aid a joint by immobilization, restriction of movement, movement assistance, weight-bearing support, or postural maintenance

KEY TERMS

abdominal binders: a compression belt that facilitates recovery after abdominal surgeries

back braces: an orthopedic device that limits spinal motion after a bone fracture or spinal fusion surgery.

cervical collars: also known as a "neck brace," this device supports a person's neck and protects the neck after a traumatic head or neck injury, and can be used to treat chronic medical conditions

orthopedic bracing: medical devices designed to properly align, correct the position, support, stabilize, and protect certain parts of the body

rib belt: a device applied to the thoracic and upper abdominal region to compress and bind the rib cage during rib fractures and postoperative care while allowing flexibility and comfortable breathing

INDICATIONS AND PROCEDURES

Orthopedic braces have been developed for virtually any joint of the human body. Braces are used to prevent injury, maintain function, or enhance rehabilitation. They are often used in sports-related activities. Individuals who are considered susceptible to a specific injury are given a brace to reduce the chances of injury. Some individuals may have had a previous injury that affects their performance or the ability to perform day-to-day activities. These people would be given braces to help them function normally or obtain closer-to-normal function. People recovering from an injury may also use braces to help speed up the recovery process and protect against further injury.

When professionals choose a specific brace, several factors must be considered, including the type of shoes worn, playing surface, type of activity, previous injuries, weather, and the individual's attitude about wearing braces. Selecting the appropriate brace is critical for protecting the body part or decreasing recovery time.

Orthopedic braces must be positioned properly, securely fastened, easy to put on, comfortable, and durable for orthopedic braces to perform well. Improper placement may increase the chances of injury. Adjustments to the brace during activity may also be necessary if the brace becomes loose and moves around. Many athletes do not like wearing braces because they find them uncomfortable, do not like to spend time putting them on, and believe they can negatively affect performance. Therefore, good braces generally are easy to apply and are made of comfortable, light materials. The durability of materials used in brace construction is also important because braces are often exposed to sweat, environmental elements, and impact with other objects during normal use.

USES AND COMPLICATIONS

Braces fall into one of two broad types: prophylactic and rehabilitative. Prophylactic braces protect joints from injuries during various activities, many of which fall in the category of competitive sports.

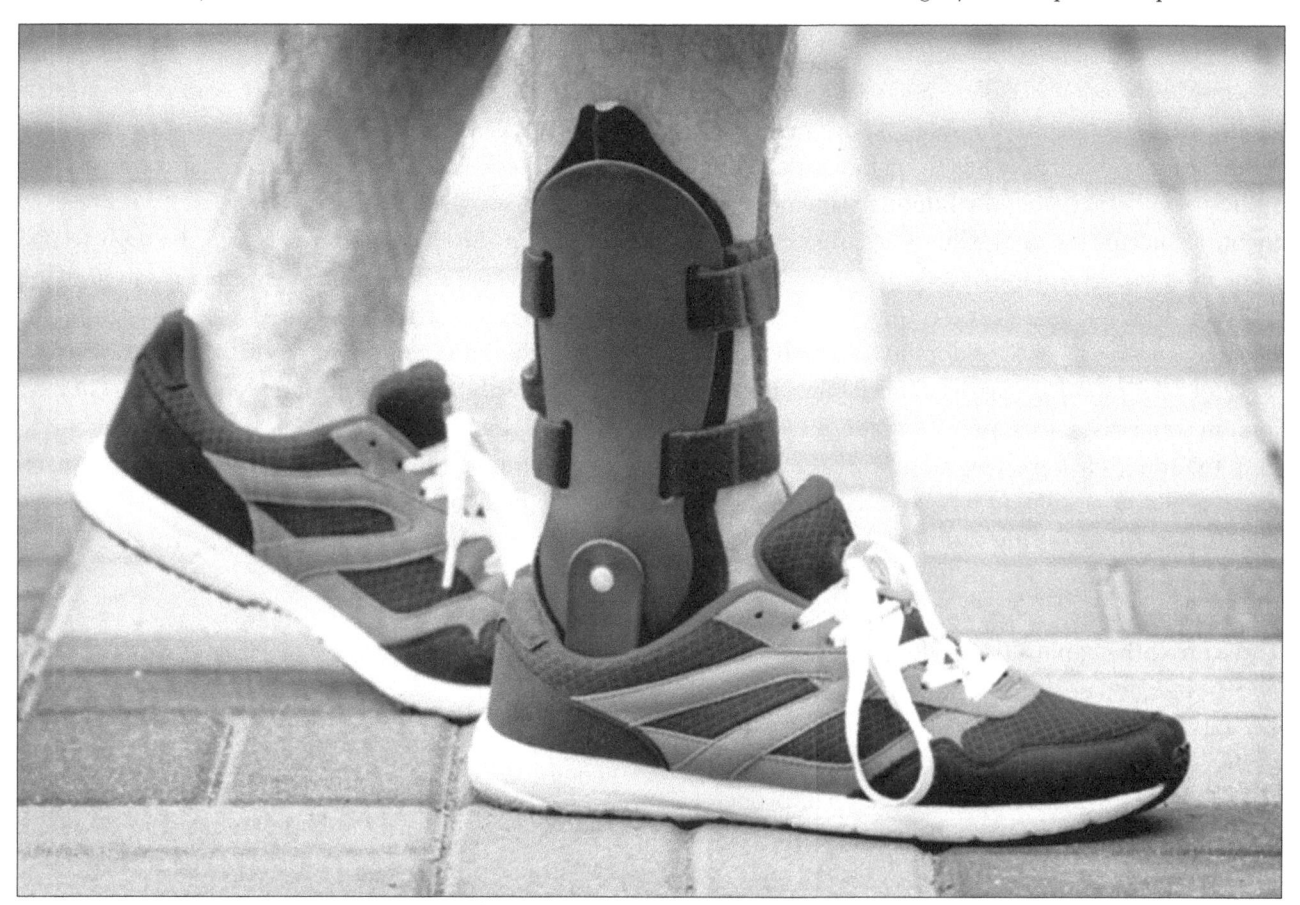

Photo via iStock/humonia. [Used under license.]

These braces stabilize the joint to protect it against contact forces, lateral movements, falls, or repetitive movements. Rehabilitative braces are used after an injury or surgery to support joints or limit movements and assist healing.

The most injured joint is the ankle. There are numerous ankle braces on the market, such as lace-up, elastic, and semirigid braces. Despite these numerous options, professionals do not agree on which method of ankle bracing is best. Still, it is common to see standard ankle taping as an injury prevention technique.

Another common joint injury is to the knee, especially the anterior cruciate ligament (ACL). Many knee braces have been designed, ranging from simple neoprene to more elaborate hinged braces. Although these braces cannot completely protect the knee, they help stabilize the joint.

Upper extremity braces are also used. Specialized braces are made for the shoulder, elbow, wrist, hand, and fingers. These braces include casts, cuffs, splints, and basic taping. By limiting some movements at specific joints, the joints are protected from some injuries or reinjuries.

Braces can be used to protect the core of the body, as with neck, back, abdominal, and rib braces. Neck or cervical collars are used to stabilize the neck and, in some cases, to limit movement. Back braces help to reduce back pain by supporting the back and abdominal muscles. Abdominal binders are generally used to compress the abdominal muscles, which incisions from surgery or childbirth may have weakened. Rib belts are used to compress the chest area and restrict the expansion of the rib cage. Rib belts benefit individuals with chest injuries such as broken ribs or chest infections.

Braces are noninvasive and present few complications to the individual if they are put on appropriately. They have been successfully used to prevent injuries and assist rehabilitation without major risks to the individuals using them.

PERSPECTIVE AND PROSPECTS

Advances in orthopedic braces are partly due to better materials and enhanced designs. A common brace many years ago was the plaster cast. These casts are very effective at immobilizing body parts. Still, athletes do not commonly use them because of their greater weight, limited durability, and hardness, which poses a danger to other athletes. Silicone rubber splints are used in competitive contact sports. They are rigid enough to stabilize the body part but soft enough that the injured athlete or opponents are not put at risk of injury from contact with the device.

Thermoplastics are materials that can be shaped when heated to fit a specific body part. Upon cooling, the material hardens to the limb's shape and helps protect it. However, the thickness is less than other braces, and thermoplastics cannot be used for recent fractures. One of the more common materials used in the construction of orthopedic braces is neoprene. Neoprene works well because it compresses the joint, which reduces pain, helps warm the joint (which aids healing), and helps train the body to react to external forces. Since neoprene is soft and light, it is comfortable to wear.

By combining new materials with better designs, orthopedic braces will continue to improve. They will be lighter, stronger, softer, easier to wear, and more durable. Most important, they will better protect the body parts from injury.

—*Bradley R. A. Wilson*

Further Reading

Beam, Joel W. *Orthopedic Taping, Wrapping, Bracing, and Padding*. 4th ed., F. A. Davis Company, 2021.

Perrin, David H. *Athletic Taping and Bracing*. 3rd ed., Human Kinetics, 2012.

Prentice, William E. *Arnheim's Principles of Athletic Training*. 14th ed., McGraw-Hill, 2011.

Street, Scott, Runkle, Deborah. *Athletic Protective Equipment: Care, Selection, and Fitting*. McGraw-Hill, 2000.

CASTS AND SPLINTS

Category: Treatment
Specialties and related fields: Emergency medicine, family medicine, general surgery, internal medicine, nursing, orthopedics, pediatrics, physical therapy, sports medicine
Definition: casts are solid, firm dressings formed with plaster of Paris or similar material around a limb or other body part to provide immobilization for healing; splints are orthopedic devices made from rigid metal or plaster or from flexible felt or leather that support, immobilize, or restrain any body part during the healing process

KEY TERMS

callus: a bony deposit formed between and around the broken ends of a fractured bone during healing

hematoma: a swelling that contains blood

ischemia: lack of blood supply resulting in tissue damage

INDICATIONS AND PROCEDURES

The general objectives of fracture management are to realign the bone fragments, maintain the alignment by immobilization, and restore function to the limb or part. Closed reduction is the manipulation of the bone fragments until the bone is realigned. Manual traction and rotation of the limb may be necessary. This type of reduction is done with a general anesthetic or sedation. The realigned bone is then immobilized by applying a cast or splint. Immobilization is essential after the fracture is realigned. If the bone fragments are not immobilized, the necessary hematoma and callus formation will be disrupted, and the bone will heal slowly, in poor alignment, or fail to heal. Restoration of function is accomplished by preventing complications during immobility and by rehabilitation methods that prepare the patient for mobility and maintain muscle strength, tone, and range of motion.

USES AND COMPLICATIONS

Complications of fractures include infection (osteomyelitis), problems of bone union, compartment syndrome, nerve damage, and cast syndrome. Delayed fracture union occurs when the bone does not unite in the usual amount of time. The delay may have various causes, including infection, poor circulation to the bone, and inadequate reduction. Nonunion is the failure of healing so that firm union does not occur. Malunion is a complication in which union occurs in a deformed or angulated position. Compartment syndrome occurs when swelling develops within a confined space. Tight splints and casts may cause pressure from outside the compartment, or inflammation and resulting edema or hemorrhage may cause pressure from within, compromising circulation in the extremity. Ischemia of the muscle occurs if enough pressure builds and leads to nerve damage. The first symptom of compartment syndrome is increased pain that is not unrelieved by narcotics. Other symptoms and signs include paralysis, paresthesias, and decreased or absent pulses. Irreversible damage begins in the muscles and nerves after six hours of ischemia. The extremity becomes useless after twenty-four to forty-eight hours with the loss of motor and sensory function. Nerve damage can result from the original injury itself or the casting. Cast syndrome, a complication of body casts, is caused by compression of part of the duodenum by the superior mesenteric artery, resulting in gastric or intestinal obstruction. The condition can become fatal if allowed to progress. Treatment includes gastrointestinal decompression, no intake of food or fluid by mouth, fluid, electrolyte intravenous replacement, and removal of the cast.

Nursing management of fracture patients involves efficient care of the cast. Analgesics are administered before cast application if needed. The

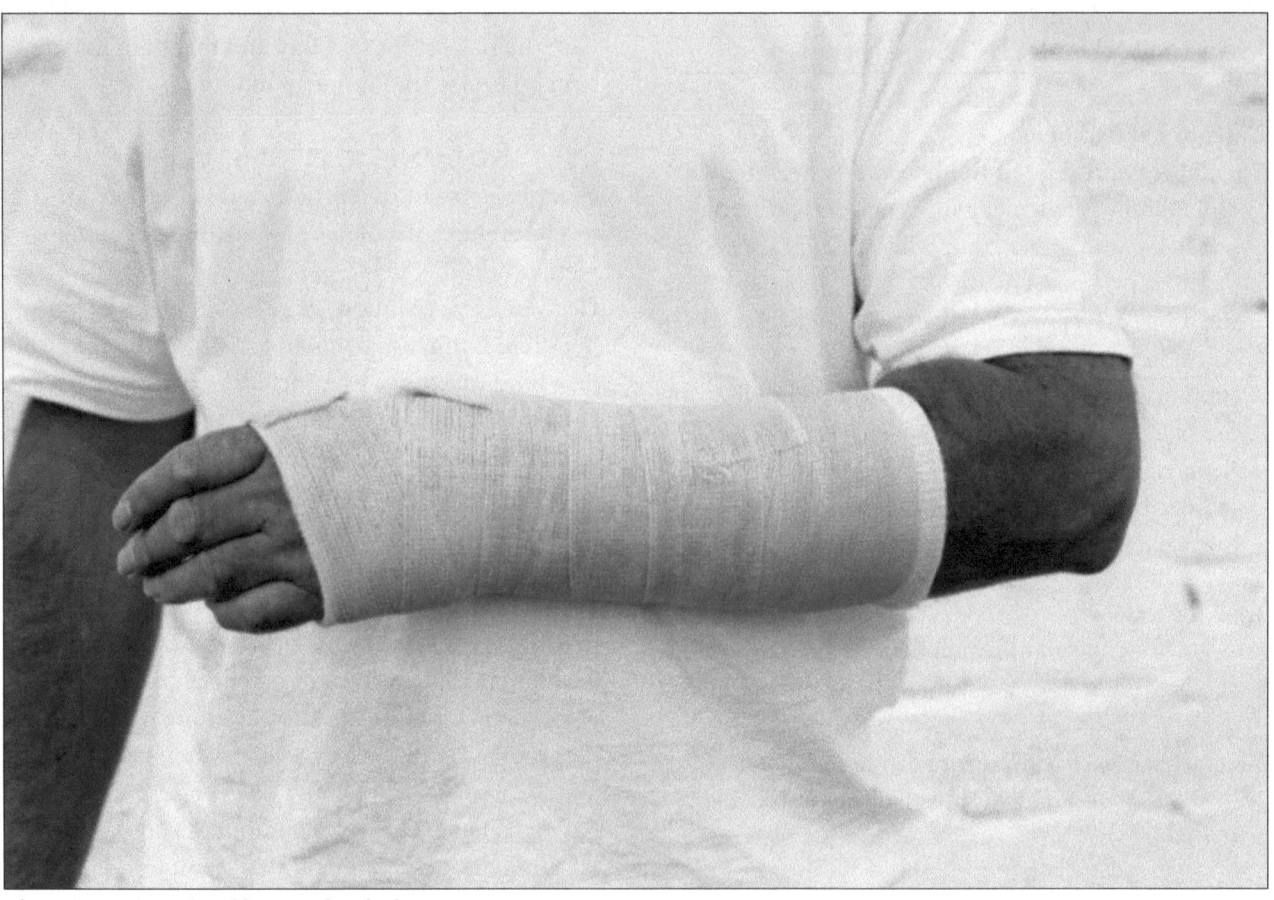

Photo via iStock/vandervelden. [Used under license.]

nurse will inspect the skin under the cast area for redness, abrasions, open lesions, or bruising. These areas will need careful evaluation through a cast window to determine that the skin is not breaking down. The skin will be cleaned and dried thoroughly. The nurse will apply a tubular stockinette long enough to extend beyond both cast edges to the limb. Rolls of a feltlike material are wrapped around the limb. Bony prominences are wrapped sufficiently to prevent friction and pressure from the cast when applied. The plaster cast is applied over the protective coverings. The orthopedist should order an X-ray to ensure proper bone alignment following cast application. The nurse will teach the patient to avoid allowing any objects or crumbs to fall under the cast, as such objects would become pressure points and could cause skin breakdown. The patient should be taught not to scratch under the cast with any object. If itching occurs, the patient may blow cool air from a hair dryer through the open end of the cast to alleviate the sensation. The nurse will monitor the casted limb for odors indicating infection. Hot spots along the cast may also indicate infection of the skin underneath. Drainage through the cast is a sign of infection or bleeding. A patient who believes that bleeding has occurred should circle the drainage area with ink and label the date and time on the cast. The nurse should remember to check the undersurface of the cast as drainage flows downward. Creating a cast window to expose the area of skin that requires care may be necessary.

Neurovascular assessment should be made frequently for the first twenty-four hours following application of a cast. If neurovascular impairment is not recognized early, then irreversible damage can result in loss of function or even loss of the extremity. These assessments include evaluating the circulatory status-color, temperature, capillary refill, edema, and pulses. Neurologic status includes sensation, mobility, presence of numbness and tingling, or pain. Patients should be taught to self-monitor and self-evaluate their casted extremity.

The cast is split with an electric cast remover that vibrates rather than cuts when the fracture is healed. The patient will feel only pressure, vibration, and heat. When the cast is removed, the extremity will appear thin and flabby, and the skin will be scaly and may be foul-smelling. The nurse should prepare the patient for the appearance of the limb, explaining that when the part begins to be used once again, the muscle will return to its former size. The weakened limb will need support when moved; it may be painful. The limb can swell if held in a dependent position. Patients will be instructed to continue to elevate the extremity. The nurse should reassure them that the tendency for swelling will subside with activity and exercise.

PERSPECTIVE AND PROSPECTS

Humans have had to contend with broken or malformed bones since prehistory. Ancient Egyptian hieroglyphics depict injured limbs wrapped and braced to heal normally. The earliest methods of holding a reduced fracture involved using splints. These are rigid strips laid parallel to each other alongside the bone. The Egyptians used wooden splints made of bark wrapped in linen. Plaster of Paris bandages were introduced in different forms by a surgeon in the Dutch army in 1851. The bandages hardened rapidly and provided an exact fit.

—*Jane C. Norman*

Further Reading
"Adult Forearm Fractures." *OrthoInfo*, Sept. 2021, orthoinfo.aaos.org/en/diseases—conditions/adult-forearm-fractures/.
"Care of Casts and Splints." *OrthoInfo*, Mar. 2020, orthoinfo.aaos.org/en/recovery/care-of-casts-and-splints/.
Clarke, Sonya, and Julie Santy-Tomlinson. *Orthopaedic and Trauma Nursing: An Evidence-Based Approach to Musculoskeletal Care*. Wiley-Blackwell, 2014.
"Elbow Fractures in Children." *OrthoInfo*, June 2019, orthoinfo.aaos.org/en/diseases—conditions/elbow-fractures-in-children/.
"Forearm Fractures in Children." *OrthoInfo*, June 2019, orthoinfo.aaos.org/en/diseases—conditions/forearm-fractures-in-children/.
Schoen, Delores Christina. *Adult Orthopaedic Nursing*. Lippincott Williams & Wilkins, 2000.
Tétreault, Patrice, and Hugue Ouellette. *Orthopedics Made Ridiculously Simple*. MedMaster, 2014.

Constraint-Induced Movement Therapy (CIMT)

Category: Therapy
Specialties and related fields: Neurology, occupational therapy, physical therapy, sports medicine, sports psychology
Definition: a form of rehabilitation therapy that improves upper extremity function in stroke and other central nervous system damage victims by increasing the use of their affected upper limb

KEY TERMS

adaptive task practice: a training method in which a motor or behavioral objective is approached in small steps by successive approximations or by making the task more difficult per the patient's motoric capabilities

learned nonuse: a motor learning phenomenon whereby limb movement is suppressed initially due to adverse reactions and failure of any activity attempted with the affected limb, resulting in the suppression of motor behavior

INTRODUCTION

Constraint-induced movement therapy (CIMT) is a series of rehabilitation techniques to help patients improve their ability to use limbs. Constraint-induced movement therapy has been used in patients with various medical issues, including those who have experienced strokes or traumatic brain injury, individuals with multiple sclerosis, and children with hemiplegia, or unilateral cerebral palsy, which means paralysis of one side of the body.

Constraint-induced movement therapy involves limiting the patient's use of the less affected limb—for example, by putting the less affected arm in a sling or mitt for most of the day—and having the patient use the other limb almost exclusively for two to three weeks. The patient also receives several hours of training daily using the more affected limb. Another treatment, modified CIMT (mCIMT), is similar but includes less daily training while the more affected limb is restricted.

Studies have found that CIMT can influence the brain. Imaging studies show that areas of the brain related to moving the more affected limb grow in patients engaged in CIMT. This phenomenon has been described as a rewiring of the brain.

BACKGROUND

Constraint-induced movement therapy is based on the research of behavioral neuroscientist Edward Taub and others at the University of Alabama at Birmingham. Taub first began the work earlier, however. He was a graduate student at Columbia University when he conducted laboratory work in a research institute at the Jewish Chronic Disease Hospital in New York. Researchers operated on monkeys to sever the spinal nerve connection allowing them to feel sensation in one or both front limbs. The monkeys used these limbs as supports to move around and grasp and manipulate items. Although the limbs were not affected in any other way—they still operated as before—the monkeys stopped using the limbs that lacked sensation.

Researchers persuaded the monkeys to use the affected limbs through several conditioning techniques. For example, the monkey could learn to move the limb when it hears a sound, such as a buzzer, because it receives a small electric shock if it fails to move the limb. Taub and the other researchers also tried a restraint method—the unaffected limb was restrained using a straitjacket, so the monkey could not use it, but the affected limb was left free. If the monkey did not use the affected limb, it was more or less helpless. Researchers placed food outside the monkeys' cages. Within a few hours, the monkeys began to use the unbound limbs. They reached out to pick up the food and managed to feed themselves. Some of the monkeys began using their unbound limbs to support their bodies as they moved around their cages. Their movements were clumsy because they did not have sensation in the limbs, but they could function well. After one week with the unaffected limbs bound, the monkeys continued to use the limbs that did not have sensation. This behavior continued and was found to be permanent. Taub and his colleagues began to publish papers on their monkey studies during the 1960s, although the work continued for decades.

The researchers worked to build on knowledge from earlier studies. Previous studies had concluded that a living creature could not move or use its limbs without sensory input. Taub's research proved this to be untrue. The work also disproved ideas about the adult brain. Previously, researchers believed only immature brains could adapt—they had plasticity—but the monkey experiments showed that adult primate brains were not rigid and set.

Researcher Larry Anderson, who had observed Taub's work, attempted to translate Taub's findings to human patients in 1967. Anderson immobilized the unaffected arms of three stroke patients. He sounded a tone. Patients who did not move their affected but unbound arms received mild electric shocks. After some success with his small study, Anderson applied his work to a larger group of twenty-four stroke patients. All the patients in this group saw improvement in their affected limbs. Taub began a series of experiments using human stroke patients in 1986.

OVERVIEW

CIMT is based on learned nonuse. This is the idea that when a person does not use a limb, their brain forgets how to use it.

Learned nonuse often arises when an individual does not try to use a weakened limb because it is just easier to use the other one. The less the affected limb is used, the greater the loss of mobility as the brain forgets how to use it; this leads the person to rely even more on the other limb, creating a cycle of nonuse. This prevents the individual from regaining strength and using an affected limb.

Physical therapists have found that the adage "use it or lose it" is true in recovery. Patients must regularly use the affected limbs to rewire the brain and regain control of the limbs. CIMT helps counteract learned nonuse by forcing the individual to use the affected limb. This use helps the brain relearn how to operate the limb.

Many stroke patients need to relearn using an affected arm and hand. A physical therapist often begins working with a stroke patient by restraining the functional arm for 90 percent of the patient's waking time. Next, the therapist puts a mitt on a stroke patient's functional hand for several hours a day. The patient performs repetitive tasks using the affected free hand. This exercise with the affected hand helps the brain repair the pathways required to use the limb. These repetitive tasks involve shaping or adaptive task practice (ATP). During ATP, the therapist breaks tasks down into manageable pieces, then changes one part of it at a time. For example, making a telephone call involves picking up the handset and dialing a number. Shaping might involve learning to grasp the handset first. After the patient repeatedly practices this action, the therapist might have the patient grasp the handset and bring it to their ear. After repeatedly practicing these steps, the patient would add another step, and so on.

When used soon after the event that caused paralysis, such as a stroke, CIMT can prevent patients from developing learned nonuse. Constraint-induced movement therapy is effective even long after patients have experienced a loss of limb control. Physical therapists advise patients to begin therapy no matter how much time has passed.

—*Josephine Campbell*

Further Reading

"CI Therapy Research Group." *University of Alabama at Birmingham Department of Psychology*, www.uab.edu/citherapy/. Accessed 29 Nov. 2017.

"Constraint Induced Movement Therapy." *Children's Hemiplegia and Stroke Association*, chasa.org/treatment/constraint-induced-movement-therapy/. Accessed 29 Nov. 2017.

"Constraint Induced Movement Therapy." *Physiopedia*, www.physio-pedia.com/Constraint_Induced_Movement_Therapy. Accessed 29 Nov. 2017.

"Edward Taub, PhD." *American Psychological Association*, www.apa.org/action/careers/health/edward-taub.aspx. Accessed 29 Nov. 2017.

McDermott, Annabel. "Constraint-Induced Movement Therapy—Upper Extremity." *Heart & Stroke Foundation Canadian Partnership for Stroke Recovery*, 22 Sept. 2016, www.strokengine.ca/intervention/constraint-induced-movement-therapy-upper-extremity/. Accessed 29 Nov. 2017.

"Neurological Rehabilitation." *Johns Hopkins Medicine*, www.hopkinsmedicine.org/healthlibrary/conditions/physical_medicine_and_rehabilitation/neurological_rehabilitation_85,P01163. Accessed 29 Nov. 2017.

Schwartz, Jeffrey M., and Sharon Begley. *The Mind and the Brain: Neuroplasticity and the Power of Mental Force*. HarperCollins, 2002, pp. 138-62.

Taub, Edward. "The Behavior-Analytic Origins of Constraint-Induced Movement Therapy: An Example of Behavioral Neurorehabilitation." *Behavioral Analysis*, vol. 35, no. 2, Fall 2012.

Wolf, Steven L., et al. "The EXCITE Stroke Trial: Comparing Early and Delayed Constraint-Induced Movement Therapy." *Stroke*, vol. 41, no. 10, Oct. 2010, pp. 2309-15.

EXERCISE-BASED THERAPIES

Category: Therapy or Technique
Specialties and related fields: Athletic training, occupational therapy, physical therapy
Definition: a regimen or plan of physical activities designed and prescribed to facilitate the patient's recovery from diseases and any conditions which disturb their movement and activity of daily life or maintain a state of well being

KEY TERMS

Alexander technique: a process that teaches how to properly coordinate body and mind to release harmful tension and to improve posture, coordination, and general health

Feldenkrais method: a system of gentle movements that promote flexibility, coordination, and self-awareness

Pilates: a system of physical conditioning involving low-impact exercises and stretches designed to strengthen muscles of the torso and often performed with specialized equipment

qigong: a Chinese system of breathing exercises, body postures, movements, and mental concentration intended to maintain good health and control the flow of vital energy

Tai Chi: Chinese martial art and form of stylized, meditative exercise characterized by methodically slow circular and stretching movements and positions of bodily balance

Trager approach: a combination of hands-on tissue mobilization, relaxation, and movement reeducation called "Mentastics"

yoga: comes from a Sanskrit word meaning "union;" yoga combines physical exercises, mental meditation, and breathing techniques to strengthen the muscles and relieve stress

OVERVIEW

According to a 2008 Centers for Disease Control and Prevention (CDC) health study, 7 percent of those surveyed engaged in what is considered exercise-based complementary and alternative medicine (CAM) activities. These activities are considered outside the scope of conventional exercise practices. Although pain relief was the most common reason for its use, exercise-based CAM is used throughout the spectrum of medical conditions. A survey of the medical literature revealed seven exercise-based CAM activities, namely yoga, Tai Chi, qigong, Pilates, the Alexander technique, the Feldenkrais method, and the Trager approach.

With an estimated 16 million participants in the United States, yoga is the most popular exercise-based CAM activity. A five-thousand-year-old practice that originated in India, yoga seeks to integrate the mind, body, and spirit through physical poses, breathing exercises, meditation, and spiritual philosophy. Pilates is another popular exercise system in the West. This one-hundred-year-old exercise is designed to strengthen core muscles while focusing on posture and proper breathing. Often, props and apparatus are used.

Originally conceived as a martial art in China five hundred years ago, Tai Chi is now practiced primarily for general physical fitness. Although many forms exist, Tai Chi uses a series of slow, graceful movements to enhance strength, stamina, and balance. Tai Chi is part of a larger, five-thousand-year-old system of traditional Chinese mental, spiritual, and physical training called "qigong." Other components of qigong include physical poses, meditation, and breathing exercises.

The Feldenkrais Method, the Alexander technique, and the Trager approach are lesser-known exercise-based CAM activities. These are movement therapies in which practitioners are guided in their posture and physical actions to improve balance, reduce pain, and increase emotional well-being.

MECHANISMS OF ACTION

Four of the seven forms of exercise-based CAM can be considered forms of general physical exercise. Yoga, Pilates, Tai Chi, and qigong involve various degrees of cardiovascular, strength, and flexibility training. Thus, they promote stamina, bone health, healthy weight, muscle tone, balance, and strength. Yoga, Tai Chi, and qigong also involve meditation. Although scientific research is ongoing, meditation decreases heart rate, increases blood flow to the organs, and improves mood regulation because of changes in the nervous system. No clinical data are available to determine the exact mechanism of action of the Alexander technique, the Feldenkrais method, or the Trager approach.

USES AND APPLICATIONS

Exercise-based CAM is most commonly used to improve and maintain overall fitness. Other common therapeutic uses are reducing stress, relieving pain, and improving flexibility. Exercise-based CAM experts claim, however, that these exercise systems help treat a variety of conditions, such as asthma, osteoporosis, menstrual pain, depression, cancer, high blood pressure, diabetes, arthritis, insomnia, neuromuscular disorders, fatigue, attention deficit disorder, gastrointestinal disorders, infertility, sinusitis, and heart disease.

SCIENTIFIC EVIDENCE

Determining whether exercise-based CAM is effective in managing and preventing illness is challenging. A limited number of well-designed clinical trials are available. The wide variety of practices within these different styles makes obtaining a consensus difficult.

In 2010, several large, well-designed studies showed that Tai Chi and qigong were beneficial in preventing osteoporosis in postmenopausal women and treating hypertension and heart disease. Additionally, these studies suggest that Tai Chi may be effective in enhancing the immune system of the elderly.

A review of the medical literature reveals promising evidence that yoga may help treat various medical conditions, including mood disorders, hypertension, insomnia, back pain, and osteoporosis, and may improve overall physical conditioning. In a 2008 randomized clinical trial in the journal Menopause, yoga reduced hot flashes in women by 30 percent. Furthermore, numerous studies have demonstrated that yoga diminishes sex performance anxiety and enhances female sexual desire. Many health practitioners use yoga in conjunction with conventional medicine to treat cancer to reduce anxiety, pain, and insomnia. However, scientists continue to debate the exact mechanisms of action involved.

A gap in the literature exists regarding the use of Pilates in treating medical conditions. Although experts in the Feldenkrais Method, the Alexander technique, and the Trager approach claim that their movement exercises reduce pain, prevent injury and improve balance, no well-designed clinical trials have been conducted to determine their efficacy. Experts agree that Pilates effectively improves strength, flexibility, and balance.

Regarding other medical claims about exercise-based CAM, no well-designed randomized controlled trials are available; a review of the medical literature did not support the claims.

CHOOSING A PRACTITIONER

Hundreds of exercise-based CAM instructor-training programs have been established in the United

States. None, however, include provider licensing requirements. Certification standards for yoga instruction are largely based on the style of yoga studied and practiced. One program, the Yoga Alliance, is a nonprofit organization in the United States that maintains standards for yoga teacher-training programs. Teacher certification with this program requires two hundred hours of training.

Several Tai Chi and qigong organizations provide teacher certification in the United States. Various levels of certification are offered based on hours of training and desired goals. Hundreds of Pilates training programs have been established in the United States, too. Although licensing is not required, the Pilates Method Alliance offers a national teacher's certification program through written examination. Instructors of the Feldenkrais Method, the Alexander technique, and the Trager approach must complete two-to-four-year training programs that encompass four hundred to sixteen hundred hours of class and fieldwork for certification.

SAFETY ISSUES

Exercise-based CAM is generally considered safe for those without serious health conditions or injuries. Persons with spine or joint disease, uncontrolled blood pressure, or severe balance abnormalities should avoid some exercise-based CAM activities. Although uncommon, spine and joint injuries have occurred during CAM exercise activities. To avoid such injuries, participants should adhere to the directions of a certified instructor. Pregnant women, who should exercise caution when considering CAM, typically require modification of certain practices. All potential participants, especially if pregnant, looking into exercise-based CAM as a form of therapy should consult with their health-care providers before joining any exercise-based program. It is advisable to choose a certified provider. Typically, a national association that confers the certification will have a list of qualified providers.

—Marie President

Further Reading

Abbott, Ryan, and Helen Lavretsky. "Tai Chi and Qigong for the Treatment and Prevention of Mental Disorders." *Psychiatric Clinics of North America*, vol. 36, no. 1, 2013, pp. 109-19, doi:10.1016/j.psc.2013.01.011.

Brämberg, Elisabeth Björk, et al. "Effects of Yoga, Strength Training and Advice on Back Pain: A Randomized Controlled Trial." *BMC Musculoskeletal Disorders*, vol. 18, no. 1, 29 Mar. 2017, doi:10.1186/s12891-017-1497-1.

Hillier, Susan, and Anthea Worley. "The Effectiveness of the Feldenkrais Method: A Systematic Review of the Evidence." *Evidence-Based Complementary and Alternative Medicine*, 8 Apr. 2015, pp. 1-12, doi:10.1155/2015/752160.

Klein, Penelope, et al. "Meditative Movement, Energetic, and Physical Analyses of Three Qigong Exercises: Unification of Eastern and Western Mechanistic Exercise Theory." *Medicines*, vol. 4, no. 4, 23 Sept. 2017, p. 69, doi:10.3390/medicines4040069.

Nichols, Hannah. "The Research-Backed Benefits of Yoga." *Medical News Today*, 23 Sept. 2019, www.medicalnewstoday.com/articles/326414.php.

Selhub, Eva. "The Alexander Technique Can Help You (Literally) Unwind." *Harvard Health*, 19 Nov. 2015, www.health.harvard.edu/blog/the-alexander-technique-can-help-you-literally-unwind-201511238652.

Solloway, Michele R., et al. "An Evidence Map of the Effect of Tai Chi on Health Outcomes." *Systematic Reviews*, vol. 5, no. 1, 27 July 2016, doi:10.1186/s13643-016-0300-y.

Teut, Michael, et al. "Qigong or Yoga Versus No Intervention in Older Adults with Chronic Low Back Pain—A Randomized Controlled Trial." *The Journal of Pain*, vol. 17, no. 7, 2016, pp. 796-805, doi:10.1016/j.jpain.2016.03.003.

Wells, Cherie, et al. "The Effectiveness of Pilates Exercise in People with Chronic Low Back Pain: A Systematic Review." *PLOS One*, vol. 9, no. 7, 1 July 2014, doi:10.1371/journal.pone.0100402.

Hyaluronic Acid Injections

Category: Procedure/Treatment
Specialties and related fields: Orthopedic surgery, family medicine/primary care, physician assistant/nurse practitioner under physician supervision, plastic surgery, dermatology
Definition: hyaluronic acid is a gel-like substance found in high amounts in joints to lubricate and help joints move smoothly; it is also found in the skin to help increase elasticity and other tissues in the body

KEY TERMS

arthralgia: joint pain

arthrofibrosis: scar tissue in a joint that develops after surgery, implant, or joint replacement

arthropathy: disease of a joint in the body

arthroscopy: a procedure where a surgeon uses an instrument called an "arthroscope" to look inside a joint

articulating: where a joint or juncture between bones or cartilages is present for motion

hyaluronan: a naturally occurring gel-like material that is found primarily in synovial fluid

hyaluronic acid: a substance present in body tissues, such as skin and cartilage. In joints, it serves to help lubricate the joints

intra-articular: occurring within a joint

joint effusion: a collection or buildup of fluid in a joint

knee cartilage defect: an area of damaged cartilage in the knee

osteoarthritis: a progressive disorder of the joints caused by gradual loss of cartilage which can result in the development of bone spurs and cysts at the margins of joints

synovial fluid: a clear fluid that serves as a lubricant in a joint, tendon sheath, or bursa

viscosupplementation: a treatment typically involving injection(s) of hyaluronic acid or related compounds; used in the treatment of osteoarthritis

INDICATIONS AND PROCEDURES

Hyaluronic acid injections (in a treatment group called "viscosupplementation") were approved by the United States Federal Drug Administration (FDA) in 1997 to treat osteoarthritis of the knee. It is a gel-like material made from hyaluronan, found in the combs on the tops of the heads of chickens or manufactured synthetically. Brand names include: Euflexxa, Gel-One, GelSyn-3, GenVisc 850, Hyalgan, Hyalgan L/L, Hymovis, Monovisc, Orthovisc, Supartz, Supartz FX, Synvisc, and Visco-3.

In March 2005, injectable hyaluronic acid injections were also approved to increase skin elasticity and decrease wrinkles in the face, enhance lips, and replace soft-tissue volume loss associated with aging facial wrinkles, etc. The hyaluronic acid gel works by temporarily adding volume and increasing elasticity to facial tissue to restore a smoother appearance to the face. It is injected into facial tissue to smooth wrinkles and folds, especially around the nose and mouth. The effect of the hyaluronic acid gel can last approximately six months. Most patients need one injection of hyaluronic acid to achieve the most favorable benefits of wrinkle-smoothing; about one-third of patients need more than one injection to get a satisfactory result.

Hyaluronic acid filler injections are usually given by a plastic surgeon, dermatologist, esthetician, or other trained health-care professional. Brand names include: Restylane, Juvederm, Belotero, Hylaform, and Captique, as well as others.

Although hyaluronic acid filler injections are now commonly used by health-care professionals today to smooth wrinkles at the request of the aging, young-appearance-oriented population, the primary use of hyaluronic acid injections is for the treatment of knee osteoarthritis.

Hyaluronic acid injections are used in individuals with knee pain caused by osteoarthritis of the knee that has not responded to physical therapy, anti-inflammatory drugs, or other treatment. They can also be used to control pain symptoms from damage to knee cartilage caused by repeated knee trauma or in individuals that have had prior arthroscopic surgery or cleaning the defective cartilage that has not been successful.

However, hyaluronic acid injections are not recommended in individuals with allergies to hyaluronan, chicken eggs, or feathers, sensitivity to bacterial proteins, or in patients with bleeding disorders, severe inflammation, infection, or joint effusion of the affected knee, or skin problems near the knee. However, once the inflammation or infection is treated and resolved, the injection may be possible based on an examination and evaluation by the physician.

Some brands of hyaluronic acid are not derived from animal proteins (e.g., Euflexxa), and patients may be eligible for injection with these brands.

Hyaluronic acid injections have not been studied in children or breastfeeding women. The relationship of age to the effects of hyaluronic acid injection in geriatric patients is not available.

Individuals should also check with their health insurance company to inquire about coverage for hyaluronic acid injections.

The largest study and review of the use of hyaluronic acid injections for knee pain from osteoarthritis was done by Nicholas Bellamy, and his team in 2006. They found that pain levels in the average patient who received these injections were reduced by 28 to 54 percent, which is about the percentage of relief from an individual taking nonsteroidal anti-inflammatory drugs (NSAIDs) for knee pain relief. However, the researchers also found that hyaluronic injections improved the ability of patients who received them to move about and perform daily activities by 9 to 32 percent. They also noted in their review that although cortisone injections for the knee may work more quickly for relief of knee pain and possibly improve function, hyaluronic acid injections tend to take longer to work (can be five to eight weeks for full effectiveness) but yield longer-lasting improvement.

Later analysis of treatments for knee osteoarthritis by Bannuru and others in 2015 reviewed research studies in which randomized trials of adults with knee osteoarthritis comparing two or more of the following—NSAIDs, cortisone injections, hyaluronic acid injections, and oral NSAIDs and hyaluronic acid injection placebos for treatment of osteoarthritis—were studied. Bannuru and his colleagues' analysis noted that articular treatments (cortisone and hyaluronic injections) improved the movement and functional ability of patients who received them and were superior to NSAIDs. All treatments except acetaminophen (Tylenol) improved pain control.

PROCEDURE

An orthopedic surgeon, primary care physician, or other health-care professional trained and supervised to provide the hyaluronic acid injection(s) will first clean the knee to be injected with an alcohol swab. Sometimes a local anesthetic spray or lidocaine injection is used to lessen patient discomfort before the physician inserts the needle with the hyaluronic acid. The needle is first placed in the intra-articular space of the affected knee, and a small amount of synovial fluid is withdrawn to assure correct placement.

Once the hyaluronic acid is injected into the knee, the health-care provider usually has the patient flex their knee three or four times to help circulate the hyaluronic acid in the knee. Depending on the hyaluronic acid brand used for the procedure, one injection or a series of three to five injections one week apart are given. The multi-injection and single-dose repeat injections can be given after six months if needed.

Strenuous exercise, for example, jogging, heavy lifting, racquetball, or prolonged standing, should be avoided for forty-eight hours or as advised by the health-care provider. Any moderate swelling or pain of the injected knee should have ice packs applied. However, any sharp or increased pain, locking, or swelling of the injected knee should be reported to the individual's health-care provider.

USES AND COMPLICATIONS

The most common side effects reported after hyaluronic acid knee injections are minor pain at the injection site, swelling, and a small buildup of fluid in the affected knee joint. These symptoms usually disappear within a few days.

Other issues that are less common but may occur include joint stiffness, warmth at the injection site, arthropathy, and gait disturbance.

As individuals grow older, joint issues—especially in the knees—can be challenging. In addition to the use of hyaluronic acid injections, other new procedures are being studied to restore or replace damaged knee cartilage and improve function and mobility while decreasing pain from osteoarthritis. Among treatments being researched are stem cells used to promote cartilage growth, novel anti-inflammatory drugs that inhibit inflammation in osteoarthritis, and growth factors for cartilage regrowth.

—*Joanne R. Gambosi*

Further Reading

Bannuru, R. R., et al. "Comparative Effectiveness of Pharmacologic Interventions for Knee Osteoarthritis: A Systematic Review and Network Meta-Analysis." *Annals of Internal Medicine*, vol. 162, no. 1, 2015, pp. 46-54, doi:10.7326/M14-1231.

"Hyaluronic Acid (Injection Route)." *Mayo Clinic*, 1 Feb. 2022, www.mayoclinic.org/drugs-supplements/hyaluronic-acid-injection-route/description/drg-20074557. Accessed 8 June 2022.

"Injections That May Ease Your Joint Pain." *Cleveland Clinic*, 2 Apr. 2021, health.clevelandclinic.org/injections-that-could-ease-your-joint-pain/. Accessed 8 June 2022.

Vad, Vijay. "Hyaluronic Acid Injections for Knee Osteoarthritis." *Arthritis-health*, 28 Mar. 2019, www.arthritis-health.com/treatment/injections/hyaluronic-acid-injections-knee-osteoarthritis. Accessed 8 June 2022.

"Viscosupplementation Treatment for Knee Arthritis." *OrthoInfo*, Feb. 2021, orthoinfo.aaos.org/en/treatment/viscosupplementation-treatment-for-knee-arthritis/. Accessed 8 June 2022.

KNEECAP REMOVAL

Category: Procedure
Specialties and related fields: Occupational therapy, orthopedics, physical therapy
Definition: the surgical removal of the kneecap

KEY TERMS

chondromalacia: degeneration of cartilage in the knee, usually caused by excessive wear between the patella and lower end of the femur

patella: the kneecap bone located anterior to the knee joint within the tendon of the quadriceps femoris muscle, providing an attachment point for both the quadriceps tendon and the patellar ligament

quadriceps muscle: a hip flexor and a knee extensor; it consists of four individual muscles; three vastus muscles and the rectus femoris; they form the main bulk of the thigh and collectively are one of the most powerful muscles in the body; it is located in the anterior compartment of the thigh

INDICATIONS AND PROCEDURES

The kneecap, or patella, is the triangular bone at the front of the knee. It is held in position by the lower end of the quadriceps muscle, which surrounds the patella and is attached to the upper part of the tibia by the patellar tendon. The role of the kneecap is to protect the knee.

Kneecap removal surgery, or patellectomy, is performed due to fracture, frequent dislocation, or painful arthritis in the kneecap. A fracture is usually caused by a direct or sharp blow to the knee. Dislocation of the patella is often linked to a congenital abnormality, such as the underdevelopment of the lower end of the femur or excessive laxity of the ligaments that support the knee. Painful degenerative arthritic conditions, such as retropatellar arthritis and chondromalacia patellae, inflame and roughen the undersurface of the kneecap. Arthritic pain often worsens with the climbing of stairs or bending of the knee.

Before surgery, a clinical examination is conducted, including blood and urine studies and X-rays of both knees. The knee is thoroughly cleansed with antiseptic soap. Anesthesia is administered either by local injection, spinal injection, or inhalation and injection (general anesthesia).

The surgery begins with an incision made around the kneecap. The skin is pulled back, exposing the muscle-covered kneecap. Surrounding muscle and connecting tendons attached to the kneecap are cut, and the kneecap is carefully removed. The remaining muscle is then sewn back together with strong suture material. Surgery is completed with the closing of the skin with sutures or clips. Full recovery takes about six weeks.

USES AND COMPLICATIONS

Following surgery, a scar will form along the incision. As the incision heals, the scar will recede gradually. Heating pads can alleviate pain from the incision. The surgical patient should elevate their affected leg with pillows. Frequent movement of the legs while resting in bed will decrease the likelihood of deep vein blood clots. General activity and returning to work are encouraged as soon as possible. Standing for prolonged periods, however, is not recommended during recovery. Following the approximate six-week recovery time, physical therapy is often used to restore strength to the knee.

Possible complications associated with kneecap removal include excessive bleeding and surgical wound infection. Additional complications can occur during recovery if general postoperative guidelines are not followed. Some loss of function can be expected.

—*Jason Georges*

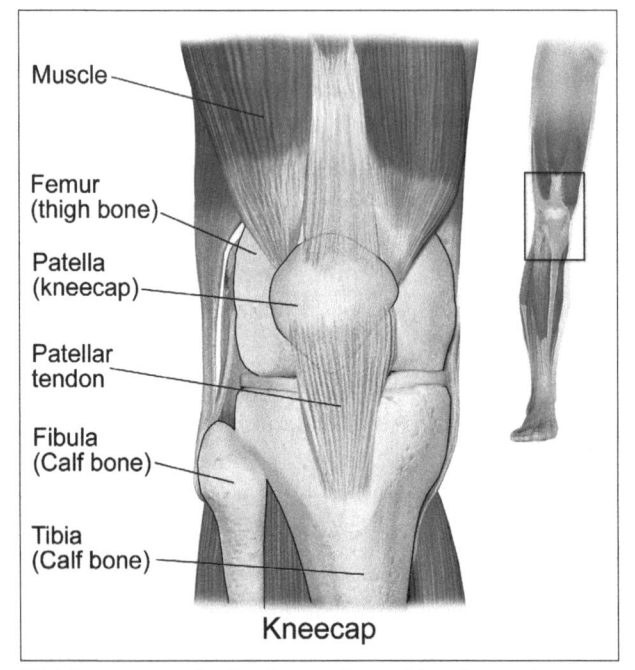

High-impact sports that involve running and jumping are prone to knee injuries. Image by BruceBlaus via Wikimedia Commons.

Further Reading
Doherty, Gerard M., and Lawrence W. Way, editors. *Current Surgical Diagnosis and Treatment.* 12th ed., Lange Medical Books/McGraw-Hill, 2006.
Halpern, Brian. *The Knee Crisis Handbook: Understanding Pain, Preventing Trauma, Recovering from Knee Injury, and Building Healthy Knees for Life.* Rodale Books, 2003.
Kwong, Yune, and Vikram V. Desai. "The Use of a Tantalum-Based Augmentation Patella in Patients with a

Previous Patellectomy." *Knee*, vol. 15, no. 2, 2008, pp. 91-94.

Mulholland, Michael W., et al., editors. *Greenfield's Surgery: Scientific Principles and Practice*. 4th ed., Lippincott Williams & Wilkins, 2006.

"Patella Fracture." *Cleveland Clinic*, 12 Nov. 2021, my.clevelandclinic.org/health/diseases/22081-patella-fracture. Accessed 9 June 2022.

Tapley, Donald F., et al., editors. *The Columbia University College of Physicians and Surgeons Complete Home Medical Guide*. Rev. 3rd ed., Crown, 1995.

Tierney, Lawrence M., et al., editors. *Current Medical Diagnosis and Treatment 2007*. McGraw-Hill Medical, 2006.

Yao, Reina, et al. "Does Patellectomy Jeopardize Function after TKA?" *Clinical Orthopaedics & Related Research*, vol. 471, no. 2, 2013, pp. 544-53.

PHYSICAL REHABILITATION

Category: Specialty

Specialties and related fields: Exercise physiology, orthopedics, osteopathic medicine, physical therapy, sports medicine

Definition: the discipline devoted to restoring normal bodily function, primarily of the muscles and skeleton

KEY TERMS

atrophy: a wasting away; a diminution in the size of a cell, tissue, organ, or part

cutaneous: pertaining to the skin

edema: the accumulation of an excessive amount of fluid in cells or tissues

electromyography: an electrodiagnostic technique for recording the extracellular activity (action and evoked potentials) of skeletal muscles at rest, during voluntary contractions, and during electrical stimulation

gangrene: necrosis (tissue death) caused by the obstruction of the blood supply; may be localized in a small area or may involve an entire extremity

goniometry: the measurement of angles, particularly those for the range of motion of a joint

ischemia: local anemia or area of diminished or insufficient blood supply caused by mechanical obstruction of the blood supply (commonly, narrowing of an artery)

musculoskeletal: pertaining to or comprising the skeleton and the muscles

physiatry: the branch of medicine dealing with the prevention, diagnosis, and treatment of disease or injury and the rehabilitation from resultant impairments and disabilities; uses physical agents such as light, heat, cold, water, electricity, therapeutic exercise, mechanical apparatus, and pharmaceutical agents

rehabilitation: the restoration of normal form and function after injury or illness; the restoration of the ill or injured patient to an optimal functional level in the home and community concerning physical, psychosocial, vocational, and recreational activity

vascular: relating to or containing blood vessels

SCIENCE AND PROFESSION

Physical rehabilitation has been defined as a scientific discipline that uses physical agents such as light, heat, water, electricity, and mechanical agents to manage and rehabilitate pathophysiological conditions resulting from disease or injury. Rehabilitation involves treating and training patients to maximize their potential for normal living physically, psychologically, socially, and vocationally.

Historical records indicate that the Chinese used rubbing as a therapeutic measure as early as 3000 BCE Hippocrates also advocated rubbing in writings dating from 460 BCE; subsequent Roman civilizations used it. The Roman poet Homer wrote about hydrotherapy as a cure for Hector. Immersion in the Nile and Ganges rivers as an aid to healing has been practiced for centuries. Peter Henry Ling developed and published a scientific basis for therapeutic massage in 1812. Modern physical therapy was established in 1917 with the creation of the Division of Special Hospitals and Physical Reconstruction. This effort was directed at persons injured in World War I and included educational and vocational training programs.

Physical rehabilitation is known for its work in restoring function to traumatized limbs. Practitioners in the field work with persons of all ages: with children to overcome congenital disabilities, with adults to restore muscular function lost from strokes, with the elderly to maintain as much normal functioning as possible in the face of advancing age, and with postoperative patients to accelerate healing and a return to normal activities. In addition, emphasis is placed on preventing and treating athletic injuries—prevention through the teaching of exercises to strengthen specific body parts and treatment through restoring normal bodily movements.

Prevention is defined as the avoidance of sickness, disability, or injury. There are three types or levels of prevention: primary, secondary, and tertiary. Primary prevention refers to complete avoidance before any problem has developed. A good example of primary prevention is being immunized for a specific disease. Secondary prevention refers to attempts to limit the extent of disease, disability, or pathological process. A convenient illustration of secondary prevention is an individual who quits smoking. Some damage may have been done to the lungs and other organs, but it is curtailed when an individual stops smoking. The extent of recovery for lost function depends on the degree of damage incurred before the cessation of the activity. Tertiary prevention refers to attempts to recover functions or abilities that have been lost or severely compromised. Physical rehabilitation is a form of tertiary prevention: Attempts are made to restore normality that has been lost as a result of an accident, disease process, or injury.

Physical rehabilitation employs individuals with a variety of training. Physiatrists are physicians who have specialized training in physical medicine and rehabilitation. They are usually the leaders of rehabilitation teams and direct many of the activities of other personnel.

Physiatrists supervise the assessment of injured patients and conduct invasive tests such as electromyography. Physical therapists are specialists with graduate-level training; in the United States, the scope of their activities is regulated by individual states and may vary from state to state. Typically, they operate alone but under the supervision or direction of a physiatrist. However, in some states, they can practice independently. Physical therapists carry out the treatment plan devised by a physiatrist and apply the therapeutic modalities. Speech and occupational therapists have specialized training to assist patients in these areas. Speech therapists concentrate on overcoming language and speech difficulties. In contrast, occupational therapists provide injured persons with skills and training for new jobs. Therapy aides assist these specialists in completing some of the more routine aspects of rehabilitation. Their education ranges from one to four years of training after high school.

DIAGNOSTIC AND TREATMENT TECHNIQUES
Individuals must be assessed before receiving physical rehabilitation. The assessment process begins with a complete history and physical examination. Subsequently, specific tests may be needed. Two common assessment tools are goniometry and electromyography. Goniometry refers to the measurement of joint motion. It is done by measuring angles of movement and is reported in degrees of arc. Electromyography is a technique that is used to evaluate the functioning of muscle units. Electrodes are placed in muscle groups. The nerve that controls the muscle is electrically stimulated, and the resultant muscle reaction is measured. Electromyography

yields information concerning the strength of muscle contractions and the speed of conduction along the nerve. These data help to pinpoint the basis of many muscular problems. As with all testing, patient-derived values are compared to standard norms to estimate pathology or lost function.

Other aspects of an injured patient are also assessed: speech and language, psychological makeup, and vocation. Speech and language are needed for communication. Strokes or other injuries can interfere with the ability to communicate. Depending on where they occur in the brain, strokes can have different effects; these must be identified. Language ability requires both neurological integrity and muscular control. Any deficit in either component can impair speech. A primary goal of rehabilitation is communication proficiency (both speech and language), which is a prerequisite for success in many jobs.

Psychological makeup is assessed to pinpoint personality problems that could impede normal interactions with the world or success in a job. Individuals requiring assistance in this area are referred to other professionals for specialized help. Vocational assessment is important because individuals sustaining strokes or serious injuries frequently cannot return to their previous jobs. When a vocational recommendation has been made for a patient, a specific rehabilitation course is created.

Four main therapeutic modalities are used in physical rehabilitation: heat, diathermy, cold, and hydrotherapy. Heat increases the rate of cellular metabolism, thus increasing blood flow. Heat also has a sedative effect, relaxing the body part. Tissue repair occurs more rapidly with increased metabolism and circulation. Stress on the injured area is reduced, allowing tissue repair to proceed unimpeded. The net effect is to speed healing.

Several methods supply heat. Compresses of cloth immersed in heated water have been used for centuries. Confining the heated water in a container provides heat in a dry form. Electric heating pads are more convenient because they can supply dry heat at a constant temperature for an unlimited time. Melted paraffin is occasionally used to concentrate heat in a specific location; a professional must apply this substance under controlled conditions. These modalities supply heat to the skin's surface; it penetrates passively, diminishing in intensity with increasing distance from the surface.

Infrared lamps provide heat that can penetrate greater depths than heat sources applied to the skin's surface. Additional advantages include dryness and being able to position the body to be heated. Because of its ability to penetrate, infrared light must be limited in exposure to avoid burns. It can also cause excessive drying of skin surfaces. Heat can also be supplied convectively, most often by immersion in warmed water. The stream of water can be directed at particular body parts, providing heat and stimulation.

Diathermy is defined as deep heating. Deep tissues are heated because superficial heating produces only a few mild physiologic reactions. The problem is to avoid burning superficial tissues while heating deep structures. Three main methods can achieve this effect: shortwave, ultrasound, and microwave energies. In all three methods, energy is transferred and finally converted into heat when it reaches deep tissues. With shortwave, energy is transferred into deeper tissues by a high-frequency current. Ultrasound uses high-frequency acoustic vibrations that penetrate deep tissues. Microwave uses electromagnetic radiation to heat deeper tissues. Diathermy exploits all the advantages of heat: locally elevated temperatures, increased circulation, and decreased sensitivity of nerve fibers, which increases the threshold of pain. Diathermy is most useful in treating relatively deep muscular injuries. It cannot be used safely with sensory impairment because burning can occur, nor can it be used in joints that have been replaced with prostheses.

Cold creates physiological effects that are opposite to those of heat. Cooling decreases tissue metabolism. The application of cold slows blood circulation, which, in turn, tends to reduce tissue swelling caused by edema. Cold is more penetrating than heat. Too much cold, however, can become a problem. Cooling a large surface area of skin or lowering the core temperature of a body induces shivering, which causes the production of heat.

Cooling affects the nervous system. With cooling, the first cutaneous sense to be lost is light touch. Motor power is lost next. Pain and gross pressure are eventually lost with a sufficiently long application of cold. When ice is applied, an individual subjectively experiences an appreciation of the cooling, followed by a sense of burning or aching and, eventually, by cutaneous anesthesia. The total time needed to induce cutaneous anesthesia is between five and seven minutes. Cooled underlying muscle fibers lose some of their power; thus, people are temporarily but noticeably weaker after cold is applied. The cooling of connective tissues around joints may diminish the ease and precision of movement.

Local cooling is used to reduce the unrestricted flow of fluid and blood into tissues after they have been traumatized. Cold reduces superficial and deep pain and reduces reflex spasticity of muscles. Cold tends to preserve and extend the viability of tissues with inadequate circulation, thus retarding the development of gangrene in an ischemic body part, which is most commonly seen in limbs.

There are reasons not to apply cold. Occasionally, individuals react to cold by abruptly increasing their arterial pressure. People who suffer from Raynaud's disease typically do not tolerate cold applied to their fingers or toes. The stiffness associated with rheumatoid arthritis is usually aggravated by cooling. Prolonged or excessive cooling can lead to frostbite. People who have experienced clinical hypothermia are must less tolerant of cold than those who have not had such an experience.

Several common methods exist for achieving therapeutic cooling: immersion, cold packs, cryokinetics, and a combination of local cooling and remote heating. Immersion is usually begun in cold water to which ice is steadily added. Total immersion is usually limited to ten or twenty minutes. The affected portion of the body is submerged in chilled water. Cooling to a temperature above that of ice water may reduce muscular spasticity. Cold packs are often made by wrapping ice in a wet towel or plastic bag and applying it to the skin. Frozen cold packs should not be applied directly to the skin because they can cause locally severe tissue damage.

Cryokinetics is a procedure that combines cooling and exercise. Cooling is first accomplished through immersion or rubbing the skin over the affected part of the body with ice for five to seven minutes, so-called ice massage. The cooling produces mild anesthesia that allows the individual actively exercise the cooled body portion without pain. This method is considered to be particularly effective in recent acute muscle strains. The simultaneous application of heat and cold is sometimes effective. Heating an uninvolved portion of the body maintains the core temperature, inhibiting shivering. At the same time, cold applied to the injured portion of the body reduces pain. In theory, this arrangement allows cold to be applied for longer periods than would otherwise be possible. Because it is difficult to control heating and to cool simultaneously, however, this technique is not frequently used.

Hydrotherapy is the external application of water for therapeutic purposes. The water temperature can range from cold to hot. With immersion, water provides buoyancy, relieving pressure on weight-bearing portions of the body. Water also provides resistance that is used in treating patients with motor weakness. Buoyancy alters the effect of exercises done in water by allowing a severely injured person to move; this provides psychological benefit and hope that they can perform the same motion out of the water. Brief application of cold has a tonic or stimulating effect, increasing blood pressure and the respiratory rate and stimulating shivering. Mild hot water provides sedation to irritated sensory and motor nerves, thus relieving pain caused by cramps and muscle spasms. It also reduces stress, calming agitated or excited persons. The most common method of hydrotherapy is a whirlpool bath, which combines buoyancy, heat, and mechanical stimulation to the affected body part.

Massage and movement are key components of applied physical rehabilitation. Massage is the systematic and scientific manipulation of body tissues; massage is best performed by the hands. Massage has a sedative effect when constantly and steadily applied, leading to decreased muscular tension. Combined with heat or cold, the resulting relaxation facilitates the movement of injured body parts. Mechanically, massage stimulates the circulatory system, enhancing blood flow. The applied force of massage is effective in stretching muscle groups and breaking the adhesions between individual muscle fibers that limit motion. This same action mobilizes fluid and promotes its elimination. Massage does not develop muscle strength and should not be used as a substitute for active exercise.

Therapeutic exercise is the performance of movement to correct an impairment, improve musculoskeletal function, or maintain a state of well-being. Movement is the key: The energy to accomplish the movement can be supplied passively by a therapist or actively by an individual. Muscles are stretched with passive movement or contracted during active flexion or contraction. Individuals with injuries that involve the nervous system may lose the function of any muscles supplied by the injured nerves. These muscles must be moved passively to avoid loss of muscle mass and function due to disuse atrophy. Muscles respond to stimulation. Thus, exercises are designed to strengthen injured muscles. Parts in adjacent body structures must be stabilized to maximize the benefit derived from exercise. Prolonged moderate stretching is more beneficial than momentary vigorous stretching. Movements and stretching should be within the patient's pain tolerance to avoid injury to blood vessels.

PERSPECTIVE AND PROSPECTS

Physical rehabilitation operates within a larger context of health-care provision. The need for primary prevention is addressed by teaching athletes and recreational fitness practitioners correct methods for strengthening muscle groups. Classes on first aid measures for treating common musculoskeletal injuries are taught by rehabilitation specialists such as physicians, therapists, and nurses. These classes are offered in schools and communities throughout the year. Physicians practicing occupational medicine also advocate primary prevention of musculoskeletal injuries associated with the work site. These professionals analyze working environments and recommend ways to restructure particular job tasks to reduce the chances of injury.

Professionals who treat injuries such as sprains, strains, and fractures provide secondary prevention in office and hospital settings. Care for acute injuries is usually accompanied by instruction in prevention in the hope that patients will avoid similar problems in the future. In the working environment, injured workers are provided with appropriate treatment and therapy and returned to work expeditiously, consistent with standards of proper care. This approach is usually best for all concerned, especially the injured worker. Such a case illustrates the many facets of rehabilitation. Normal physical functioning is returned with conventional therapy. Self-esteem is bolstered with a return to meaningful work and previous income-earning capacity. Economically, the employer also benefits by having a trained and experienced worker on the job rather than having a skilled individual on disability and a less capable replacement worker on the job, both receiving payment.

Tertiary prevention involves the traditional rehabilitation activities that begin after treatment for a massive injury or chronic disease process. Frequently, such rehabilitation returns only a portion of lost functions. Nevertheless, this treatment has value, improving an injured person's self-esteem and quality of life. It underscores, however, the greater importance of avoiding and preventing injuries.

Health can be viewed as being on a continuum. One end is defined by death, the final termination of health. All life constitutes the rest of the spectrum. Health is frequently defined as the absence of disease or infirmity. This definition is appealing in its simplicity but is difficult to use because it is based on the absence rather than the presence of something. The question of where good health ends and impaired health begins is probably highly individual and open for debate. However, the division point between good and bad or acceptable and unacceptable health status does provide a good beginning for the activities encompassed by physical rehabilitation. The recovery of lost or impaired function is the domain of this field. This goal is also consistent with the definition of tertiary prevention. Rehabilitation and prevention are complementary opposites. Together, they span the entire spectrum of health.

—*L. Fleming Fallon Jr.*

Further Reading

Cifu, David X. *Braddom's Physical Medicine and Rehabilitation*. 6th ed., Elsevier, 2020.

Frontera, Walter R., et al., editors. *DeLisa's Physical Medicine and Rehabilitation: Principles and Practice*. 6th ed., Lippincott Williams & Wilkins, 2019.

Garrison, Susan J., editor. *Handbook of Physical Medicine and Rehabilitation: The Basics*. 2nd ed., Lippincott Williams & Wilkins, 2003.

Gonzalez-Fernandez, Marlis, and Stephen Schaaf, editors. *Handbook of Physical Medicine and Rehabilitation*. Demos Medical, 2021.

Kisner, Carolyn, et al., editors. *Therapeutic Exercise: Foundations and Techniques*. 7th ed., F. A. Davis Company, 2017.

Neumann, Donald A. *Kinesiology of the Musculoskeletal System: Foundations for Rehabilitation*. 3rd ed., Mosby, 2016.

Oliver, Zayne. *Physical Medicine and Rehabilitation*. Larsen and Keller Education, 2017.

ROTATOR CUFF SURGERY

Category: Procedure
Specialties and related fields: Orthopedics, orthopedic surgery, physical therapy
Definition: a surgical procedure that repairs a torn tendon in the shoulder

KEY TERMS

acromion: the outward end of the spine of the scapula or shoulder blade

arthroscopy: minimally invasive surgical procedure on a joint in which an examination and sometimes treatment of damage is performed using an arthroscope, an endoscope that is inserted into the joint through a small incision

deltoid muscle: the muscle forming the rounded contour of the human shoulder

humeral: relating to the humerus bone, the bone of the upper arm or forelimb, forming joints at the shoulder and the elbow

rotator cuff: a capsule with fused tendons that supports the arm at the shoulder joint and is often subject to athletic injury

shoulder impingement: a common cause of shoulder pain, often caused by the repeated activity of the shoulder; also called "swimmer's shoulder"

tendonitis: inflammation of a tendon, often caused by overuse

INDICATIONS AND PROCEDURES

The shoulder, a ball and socket joint, is the most flexible joint in the human body. Because of its structure, a wide range of motion is permitted. The shoulder's structure predisposes it to a high risk of injury. The shoulder is stabilized by a group of four muscles, collectively known as the "rotator cuff": the subscapularis, the supraspinatus, the infraspinatus, and the teres minor.

The signs and symptoms of rotator cuff injuries are the same for men and women, including point tenderness around the region of the humeral head deep within the deltoid muscle, pain and stiffness within the shoulder region within a day of participating in activities that involve shoulder movements, and difficulty in producing overhead motions involving the upper arm. Pain often occurs at night due to sleeping positions that put excess pressure on the joint. Occasionally, a clicking noise can be heard from the joint upon movement, or the patient may experience a "sticking point" when shoulder movements are attempted. Injuries to the rotator cuff can mimic other common shoulder region problems, including bursitis (inflammation of a bursa, a soft, fluid-filled sac that helps cushion surfaces that glide over one another) and tendonitis (inflammation of a tendon). Injuries to the rotator cuff include impingement and tears.

Impingement occurs when the rotator cuff tendons are pinched because of narrowing the space between the acromion (shoulder blade) process and the rotator cuff. This narrowing commonly occurs with aging but can also be traumatically induced. Sports commonly stress the rotator cuff, including baseball, swimming, and tennis. Besides a traumatic injury, chronic impingement of the rotator cuff tendons can cause partial or complete tears. To evaluate the extent of shoulder dysfunction, the physician will conduct a physical examination to determine the range of motion and use

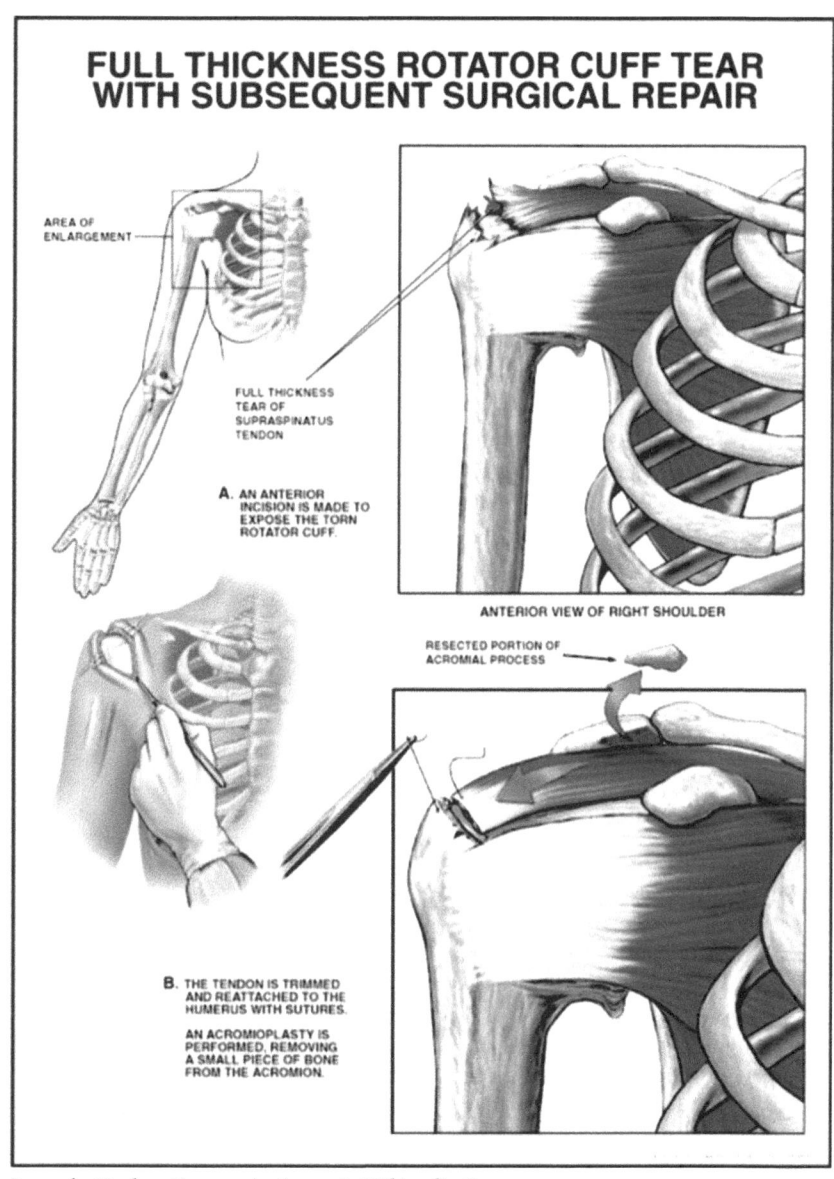

Image by Nucleus Communications, via Wikimedia Commons.

diagnostic procedures such as X-rays, an arthrogram (an X-ray after a tracer dye has been injected into the shoulder), magnetic resonance imaging (MRI), and ultrasound. Nonsurgical interventions include rest, ice immediately following an injury or heat twenty-four hours afterward, painkillers, anti-inflammatory medications, and physical therapy.

Rotator cuff surgery is usually recommended when there is little improvement in shoulder function or pain reduction after a course of noninvasive therapies. Surgery to correct rotator cuff tears is more successful if the procedure is performed within three months of injury. If the shoulder is surgically treated later, there is a complication of the torn tendons retracting from each other, increasing the difficulty of the surgery and decreasing the chances of a satisfactory outcome. Surgery can be a classic open procedure, requiring a 2- to 3-inch incision in the shoulder, or less traumatic arthroscopy, which requires only a small incision, half an inch or less, just large enough to accommodate the instruments and a video camera apparatus. Occasionally, the surgeon will use a combination of the open procedure and arthroscopy. Either general anesthesia, in which the patient is asleep, or local anesthesia, in which the region is "frozen" but the patient is awake, can be used for the procedure. Often a scalene block is also used, removing all extremity sensation that eventually returns shortly after surgery. A light sedative may also be used with local anesthesia to put the patient at ease but not asleep. Acromioplasty reduces the impingement of the rotator cuff tendons. In this procedure, a portion of the bone underneath the acromion is shaved to give the tendons more room to move and prevent them from becoming pinched. This process is often included in rotator cuff surgical repairs. The torn tendons are reattached to the humerus (upper arm bone) in rotator cuff repairs. The open surgical procedure requires a relatively large incision through the shoulder and cutting through the deltoid muscle. Any scar tissue that has formed is removed, and a small ridge is cut into the top of the humerus. Small holes are drilled into the bone, and the tendons are sutured to the bone using these holes as anchors. The surgeon will also correct any other problems, such as removing bone spurs, shaving down the acromion, or freeing up ligaments that may be pressing against the tendons.

The orthopedic surgeon can still perform most of these additional procedures during arthroscopic surgery. A thin tube is inserted after the small incision is made into the shoulder. This tube contains the surgical instruments and a video camera that is used to guide the repair procedure. Arthroscopic surgery is becoming more common and is preferred for small to larger tears, as it limits the amount of surgical intervention, reduces surgical risks, and quickens recovery time. If more extensive damage is discovered, the surgeon may choose to combine the arthroscopic procedure with open surgery. However, arthroscopic tear repair has advanced tremendously, to the point that tears previously thought to be irreparable or too extensive are now being completed with arthroscopy.

IMPACT ON WOMEN

Currently, literature provides limited consistent information on the impact of patients' gender on recovery after rotator cuff repair. One study investigated whether gender affects pain and functional recovery after rotator cuff repair in the early postoperative period. Eighty patients (forty men and forty women) were prospectively enrolled in the study. Pain intensity and functional recovery were evaluated using a visual analog scale (VAS) pain score and range of motion on the first five postoperative days, at two and six weeks, and at three, six, and twelve months after surgery. Perioperative medication-related adverse effects and postoperative complications were also assessed.

Results showed the mean VAS pain score was significantly higher for women than men two weeks after surgery ($p = 0.035$). There was no significant difference between men and women in VAS pain scores for all other periods. However, women had higher scores than men. Mean forward flexion in women was significantly lower than in men six weeks after surgery ($p = 0.033$). The mean degree of external rotation in women was significantly lower than in men at six weeks ($p = 0.007$) and three months ($p = 0.017$) after surgery. There was no significant difference in medication-related adverse effects or postoperative complications.

The authors of this study concluded women had more pain and slower recovery of shoulder motion than men during the first three months after rotator cuff repair. The findings can serve as guidelines for pain management and rehabilitation after surgery and help explain postoperative recovery patterns to patients with scheduled rotator cuff repair.

In another study, researchers wanted to determine the differences in disability between men and women and examine the relationship between factors that represent sex (biological factors) and gender (nonbiological factors) with disability and satisfaction with surgical outcomes six months after rotator cuff surgery.

Patients with impingement syndrome or rotator cuff tear who underwent rotator cuff surgery completed several standard assessment forms, such as the Quick Disabilities of the Arm, Shoulder and Hand (QuickDASH), which measures status before surgery and six months postoperatively. They also rated their satisfaction with surgery at their follow-up appointment. One hundred and seventy patients entered the study (85 men and 85 women). One hundred and sixty patients (94 percent) completed the six-month assessment. Women reported more disability both before and after surgery. Disability at six months was associated with a pain-limited range of motion, participation limitation, age, and strength. Satisfaction with surgery was associated with the level of reported disability, expectations for improved pain, pain-limited range of motion, and strength.

The researchers concluded that this study indicated women with rotator cuff pathology suffer from higher levels of pre-and postoperative disability, and sex and gender qualities contribute to these differences. Similar studies in the future regarding differences between men and women before and postoperative rotator cuff repair will help promote more effective and tailored care by health professionals.

USES AND COMPLICATIONS

The varying outcomes from rotator cuff surgery range from almost full recovery to no improvement. The degree of recovery depends upon the extent of damage to the rotator cuff and patient compliance with physical therapy after surgery. If the tendon has been torn for a long time, it may not be reparable.

As with all surgical procedures, the patient may have an adverse reaction to the anesthesia. This risk is greater if the person is obese or has a cardiovascular, pulmonary, or metabolic condition. Surgical incisions always have the risk of infection. Still, this risk is minimized with the arthroscopic procedure because of the small incision size and the relatively short operative time (one to two hours). In rare instances, there is also the risk of nerve damage resulting in partial paralysis or temporary numbness at the incision area.

After surgery, the recovering arm will be put in a sling with a small shock-absorbing pillow placed behind the elbow. In the first three months following surgery, the patient should take extreme care with shoulder movements. Reaching and lifting objects above the head should be avoided during this period. Passive range of motion exercises, in which the physical therapist moves the arm, should be started as soon as possible to prevent scar tissue formation and resultant stiffness. Exercises should be done several times a day so that within two to three weeks, the range of motion (flexibility) of the repaired shoulder should be equivalent to that of the uninjured shoulder. After six weeks, more advanced exercises are recommended to strengthen the rotator cuff and the surrounding shoulder muscles. Full recovery and rehabilitation from rotator cuff surgery can take up to a year.

—*Bonita L. Marks, Jeffrey P. Larson*

Further Reading

Codsi, Michael, and Chris R. Howe. "Shoulder Conditions: Diagnosis and Treatment Guideline." *Physical Medicine and Rehabilitation Clinics of North America*, vol. 26, no. 3, 2015, pp. 467-89, doi:10.1016/j.pmr.2015.04.007.

Pfeiffer, Ronald P., and Brent C. Mangus. *Concepts of Athletic Training*. 6th ed., Jones and Bartlett, 2012.

"Rotator Cuff Repair." *MedlinePlus*, n.d., www.nlm.nih.gov/medlineplus/ency/article/007207.htm.

"Rotator Cuff Tears." *American Academy of Orthopedic Surgeons*, June 2022, orthoinfo.aaos.org/topic.cfm?topic=A00064.

"Rotator Cuff Tears." *Cleveland Clinic*, 28 Jan. 2021, my.clevelandclinic.org/health/diseases/8291-rotator-cuff-tears-overview.

"Shoulder Joint Replacement." *OrthoInfo*, Sept. 2021, orthoinfo.aaos.org/en/treatment/shoulder-joint-replacement/.

Simons, Stephen M., and Michael Roberts. "Patient Education: Rotator Cuff Tendinitis and Tear (Beyond the Basics)." *UpToDate*, May 2022, www.uptodate.com/contents/rotator-cuff-tendinitis-and-tear-beyond-the-basics.

Tendon Repair

Category: Procedure
Specialties and related fields: General surgery, occupational health, orthopedics, podiatry, sports medicine
Definition: the surgical repair of tendons, the bands of tissue that attach muscle to bone

KEY TERMS

Achilles tendon: the tendon connecting calf muscles to the heel

collagen: the principal protein of the skin, tendons, ligaments, cartilage, bone, and connective tissue that is the major insoluble fibrous protein in the extracellular matrix and connective tissue

patellar tendon: a structure that attaches the bottom of the kneecap (patella) to the top of the shinbone (tibia)

suture: also known as a "stitch" or "stitches," is a medical device used to hold body tissues together and approximate wound edges after an injury or surgery

INDICATIONS AND PROCEDURES

Tendons are straps of collagenous tissue that attach muscles to bone. They are strong and flexible; a tendon approximately 0.5 inches- (1.3 centimeters-) thick can support a ton. Tendons are most prominently observed in the hands, where they are associated with the muscles that move the fingers and thumbs, and in the heel, where the Achilles tendon joins the muscles and bones of the foot. The Achilles tendon is the longest and thickest tendon in the body.

Tendon injuries can be of several types. If the hand or foot is badly cut, the slice may enter or sever the tendon, resulting in an inability to move the fingers or toes. Tendons have also ruptured during physical activity; the Achilles tendon is at particular risk during certain running or jumping exercises. Severance of the Achilles tendon is indicated by an inability to stand on tiptoe. The sensation that the patient experiences with the initial tear has been likened to a kick.

More often, the Achilles tendon may become inflamed by activity. Such inflammation is usually indicated by pain that develops at the beginning and end of a run but seems to improve during the exercise. Often, the pain becomes worse at night. Treat-

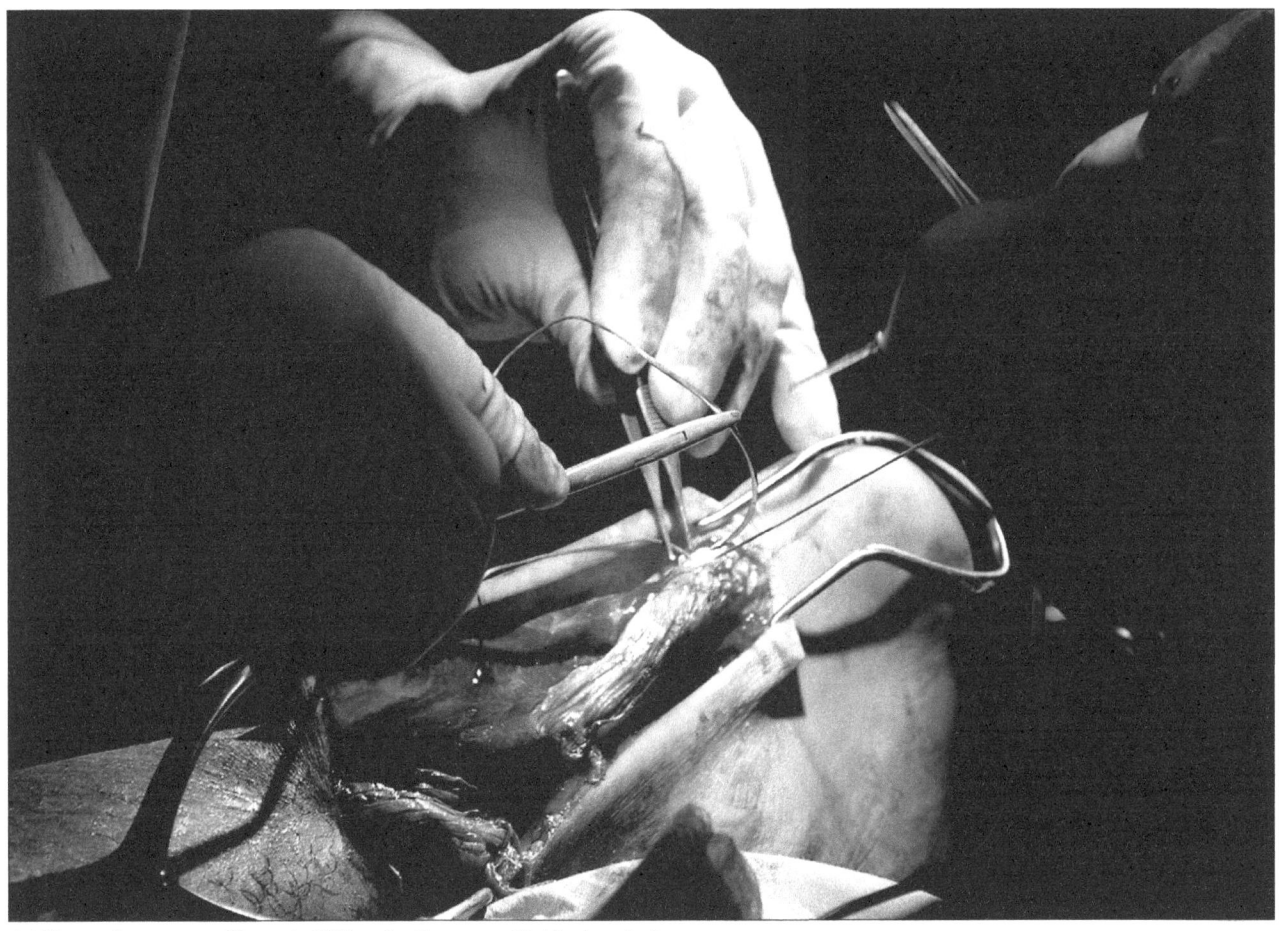

Achilles tendon surgery. Photo via Wikimedia Commons. [Public domain.]

ment of minor inflammation generally involves rest or cessation of the activity. A physician may administer corticosteroids to relieve the inflammation.

Surgery is often required for proper repair if a tendon has been cut or severed. The surgeon makes an incision through the affected area, whether hand or foot and sutures the ends of the tendon together. Since tendons are under great tension, they may snap or regress from the site of the injury.

USES AND COMPLICATIONS

If carried out properly and quickly, tendon repair is generally satisfactory. The patient may be immobilized for weeks, and some permanent stiffness is common. Because the blood supply to tendons is poor, healing may be a problem. One new method for repairing tendons is platelet-rich plasma therapy. Platelets produce growth factors, proteins that take part in the healing process. Blood is drawn from the patient being treated. The blood is spun down using a centrifuge to separate the plasma-containing platelets from the red and white blood cells. The resulting platelet-rich plasma is injected into the site of tendon damage, supplying the tendon with healing growth factors. These healing growth factors had been lacking because of the poor blood supply.

—*Richard Adler*

Further Reading

Garrick, James G., and David R. Webb. *Sports Injuries: Diagnosis and Management*. 2nd ed., W. B. Saunders, 1999.

Irvin, Richard, et al. *Sports Medicine: Prevention, Evaluation, Management, and Rehabilitation of Athletic Injuries*. 2nd ed., Allyn & Bacon, 1998.

"Patellar Tendon Tear." *OrthoInfo*, Sept. 2021, orthoinfo.aaos.org/en/diseases—conditions/patellar-tendon-tear/.

"Quadriceps Tendon Tear." *OrthoInfo*, Oct. 2021, /orthoinfo.aaos.org/en/diseases—conditions/quadriceps-tendon-tear/.

Scuderi, Giles R., and Peter D. McCann, editors. *Sports Medicine: A Comprehensive Approach*. 2nd ed., Mosby/Elsevier, 2005.

Small, Eric, et al. *Kids and Sports: Everything You and Your Child Need to Know About Sports, Physical Activity, and Good Health*. Newmarket Press, 2002.

"Tendon Repair." *MedlinePlus*, n.d., medlineplus.gov/ency/article/002970.htm.

Weintraub, William. *Tendon and Ligament Healing: A New Approach to Sports and Overuse Injury*. Rev. ed., Paradigm, 2003.

Tommy John Surgery

Category: Procedure

Specialties and related fields: Athletic training, orthopedics, physical therapy, strength and conditioning

Definition: a surgical procedure in which a healthy tendon extracted from an arm (or sometimes a leg) is used to replace an arm's torn ligament; the healthy tendon is threaded through holes drilled into the bone above and below the elbow

KEY TERMS

ulnar collateral ligament: a ligament that runs on the inner side of the elbow to help support it when performing certain motions, such as throwing

valgus: a deformity involving oblique displacement of part of a limb away from the midline

INDICATIONS AND PROCEDURES

Tommy John surgery is the operative repair of the elbow's ulnar collateral ligament (UCL). The UCL is located on the medial side of the elbow and connects the ulna to the humerus. The mechanism of a UCL tear is due to increased valgus stress on the arm. The predominant method of increasing stress on the UCL is through throwing motions. Repetitive throwing motions or throwing at high-velocity cause microtrauma to the UCL, increasing the odds of a full-thickness tear. However, the actual tearing of the ligament is called a "traumatic injury" and involves a specific event. In many cases, only rest and physical therapy are needed to correct a UCL tear. However, in athletes who rely on throwing motions, a surgical repair is indicated to return to play earlier and at a preinjury level of performance.

Surgical repair of the UCL is a relatively new operation. The first instance of UCL repair happened in 1974 to professional baseball player Tommy John, giving the procedure its name. The instance of athletes who elect to have Tommy John surgery has grown in the past several years to the point where high school and little league pitchers are having the procedure.

During a Tommy John surgery, tendons from the wrist are sacrificed and sutured onto the humerus and ulna to act as a collateral ligament and repair the UCL. Since 1974, the operative technique has evolved to make the procedure less invasive, resulting in better operative outcomes. The initial technique sacrificed the muscles of finger flexion and arm pronation by ligating them from the medial epicondyle of the humerus. Then, the ulnar nerve, which runs alongside the medial epicondyle in the elbow, was displaced posteriorly and submuscularly to avoid obstructing the surgical field and preventing unintentional injury. After nerve repositioning, two holes were drilled into the humerus and two into the ulna to prepare for the anchoring of the new ligament. The palmaris longus tendon in the wrist was harvested and used as the new UCL. The tendon was threaded into the predrilled holes in the humerus and ulna in a figure-of-eight fashion. This technique added extra strength to the ligament. The graft would then be sutured onto itself to complete the procedure. The initial procedure had a sixty percent success rate. As more orthopedic surgeons began performing the procedure, they made modifications to increase their success rate. Presently, the flexor and pronator muscles of the forearm are split and not dissected from the epicondyle, decreasing morbidity. Also, the palmaris longus tendon is attached in a triangular pattern instead of a figure-eight, increasing the stability of the graft and decreasing the number of bone anchor holes. Lastly, the ulnar nerve is repositioned subcutaneously instead of submuscularly, reducing the risk of nerve damage. As a result of these improvements, the success rate of Tommy John surgery is now approaching the high nineties.

USES AND COMPLICATIONS

Outcomes of Tommy John Surgery involve the athlete's ability to return to preinjury strength and activity levels within one year of surgery. Postprocedure, athletes will begin the rehabilitation process. On average, the initial phase of rehab takes twenty-four weeks to complete. However, achieving activity without restriction will take longer, usually about eleven months to a year postprocedure.

There are several risks to the repair of the UCL. Since the ulnar nerve has to be repositioned out of the surgical field, some component of nerve injury might occur, with patients complaining of numbness along the ulnar side of the hand. Some athletes complain of elbow joint stiffness secondary to the healing process. There is also a possibility of feeling instability of the joint relating to how the new medial ligament healed. Lastly, there are also risks of graft failure due to a fracture of the bone at the location of the anchor holes.

Since pitcher Tommy John had his UCL repaired in 1974, the surgery has been growing in popularity. Tommy John surgery is a safe procedure that takes the palmaris longus tendon to reattach to the medial elbow to stabilize the joint against valgus stress. This procedure has a high success rate, with many athletes returning to full participation within one year.

—*Nick Feo*

Further Reading

Andrews, James R., et al. "The Ulnar Collateral Ligament Procedure Revisited: The Procedure We Use." *Sports Health*, vol. 4, no. 5, 2012, pp. 438-41.

Hyman, John, et al. "Valgus Instability of the Elbow in Athletes. *Clinics in Sports Medicine*, vol. 20, no. 1, 2001, pp. 25-45.

Jobe, Frank, W., et al. "Reconstruction of the Ulnar Collateral Ligament in Athletes." *Journal of Bone & Joint Surgery*, vol. 68, no. 8, 1986, pp. 1158-63.

Liu, Joseph, N., et al. "Outcomes in Revision Tommy John Surgery in Major League Baseball Pitchers." *Journal of Shoulder and Elbow Surgery*, vol. 25, no. 1, 2016, pp. 90-97.

Makhni, Eric C., et al. "Performance, Return to Competition, and Reinjury After Tommy John Surgery in Major League Baseball Pitchers." *The American Journal of Sports Medicine*, vol. 42. no. 6, 2014, pp. 1323-32.

Injury Treatments—Alternative/Experimental

"You don't need treatment. The fever, inflammation, coughing, etc., constitute the healing process. Just get out of their way and permit them to complete their work. Don't try to 'aid' nature. She doesn't need your puny aid—she only asks that you cease interfering."

—Herbert M. Shelton, *Getting Well*

All standard medical treatments began as experimental treatments. Likewise, some modern treatments were, at one time, alternative treatments. For example, the modern sleep aid melatonin began as an alternative treatment. Nevertheless, many alternative treatments have little to no high-quality evidence for efficacy and are a waste of time and money. This section takes a hard look at alternative and experimental injury treatments. Subjects include: acupressure, applied kinesiology, cupping, diet-based therapy, prolotherapy, and tissue engineering.

Acupressure

Category: Therapy or technique
Specialties and related fields: Alternative health practitioner, traditional Chinese medicine

KEY TERMS

meridians: each of a set of pathways in the body along which vital energy is said to flow; there are twelve such pathways associated with specific organs

moxibustion: a type of heat therapy in which an herb is burned on or above the skin to warm and stimulate an acupuncture point or affected area

pressure points: a point on the surface of the body sensitive to pressure

qi: the circulating life energy that in Chinese philosophy is thought to be inherent in all things; in traditional Chinese medicine, the balance of negative and positive forms in the body is believed to be essential for good health

OVERVIEW

Acupressure is sometimes thought of as acupuncture without needles. Acupressure conveys the care and empathy necessary for healing, like other touch therapies. Because acupressure and acupuncture support the body's natural healing powers, many conditions can be improved, corrected, or eliminated. As such, holistic therapies like acupressure are appropriate for problems best suited to a biopsychosocial approach.

Acupressure is part of the healing system of traditional Chinese medicine (TCM), a unique and comprehensive system for diagnosing and treating disease, preventing illness, and promoting wellness. Originating in China thousands of years ago, TCM continues to be practiced worldwide. Traditional Chinese medicine encompasses many diverse health-enhancing and energy-balancing therapies, including acupuncture, herbal medicine, Tai Chi Chuan, qigong, Gua Sha, cupping, moxibustion, and Tui na acupressure. All these techniques, and many others, manipulate qi, the vital energy of life. Modern sciences such as biology, physiology, and biochemistry have not confirmed the existence of qi. Consequently, its existence is widely disbelieved in modern medicine.

To understand acupressure, one should study some basic principles of TCM. One theory, in particular, necessitates elaboration: the notion that human beings are governed by opposing but complementing forces, yin and yang, a notion at the heart of Daoism, which forms the basis of TCM. According to Daoism, this balance of forces infiltrates and influences the entire universe, including those within. One of the basic aims of TCM is to correct imbalances of yin and yang to prevent sickness and restore health. Fully comprehending the principles behind yin and yang (and many other concepts) permits Chinese medical practitioners to diagnose accurately and treat effectively.

In short, TCM offers alternative explanations for how health problems develop in the first place, and it provides many approaches for treating these problems. Depending on a person's clinical presentation, acupressure and other modalities used alone or with allopathic methods can benefit many health conditions.

MECHANISM OF ACTION

Acupressure relies on touch rather than needles to manipulate the flow of qi in the body. Specifically, qi is thought to move through the body through a complex system of meridians or energy channels. These meridians are known by the names of body organs (the bladder channel or liver channel) and refer to energetic patterns with specific characteristics based on TCM principles and practice.

Specific areas on the skin where the meridians pass and allow the manipulation of qi are referred to as acupoints or acupressure points. These points are pressed, rubbed, tapped, or otherwise touched during a typical acupressure session to influence qi to bring about desired results. The effects of acupressure are reinforced through a healthy diet, herbal formulas, exercise, fresh air, meditation, and spirituality. However, no imagining techniques or laboratory tests have established the existence of meridians or qi.

USES AND APPLICATIONS

According to the World Health Organization data, TCM is helpful for ophthalmological, respiratory, gastrointestinal, neurological, and musculoskeletal disorders and disorders of the ear, nose, and throat. In the United States, acupressure (and acupuncture) is used mostly to treat painful conditions such as headaches, arthritis, bursitis, injuries, and postsurgical pain.

Unfortunately, the evidence base for acupressure treatments remains scant. For example, a randomized controlled trial by Eric Noll and colleagues, published in the *European Journal of Anesthesia*, examined 163 postoperative patients, dividing them into three groups. The first group received acupressure for six minutes, three times a day for two days after their surgical procedure, the second group received sham acupressure treatments, and the third group received no such interventions. Pain levels in all three groups were not significantly different between the three groups. Well-controlled trials like this one usually fail to demonstrate any benefit to acupressure.

The effectiveness of TCM, in general, extends beyond controlling pain. More recently, acupressure is being used to treat chronic fatigue, anxiety, stress, insomnia, depression, addictions, smoking, eating disorders, irritable bowel syndrome, hypertension, sexual dysfunctions, premenstrual and menopausal symptoms, and many other conditions. Also, acupressure appears to improve circulation, boost immune functioning, help eliminate metabolic waste products, promote relaxation, enhance self-esteem, and create a general sense of well-being.

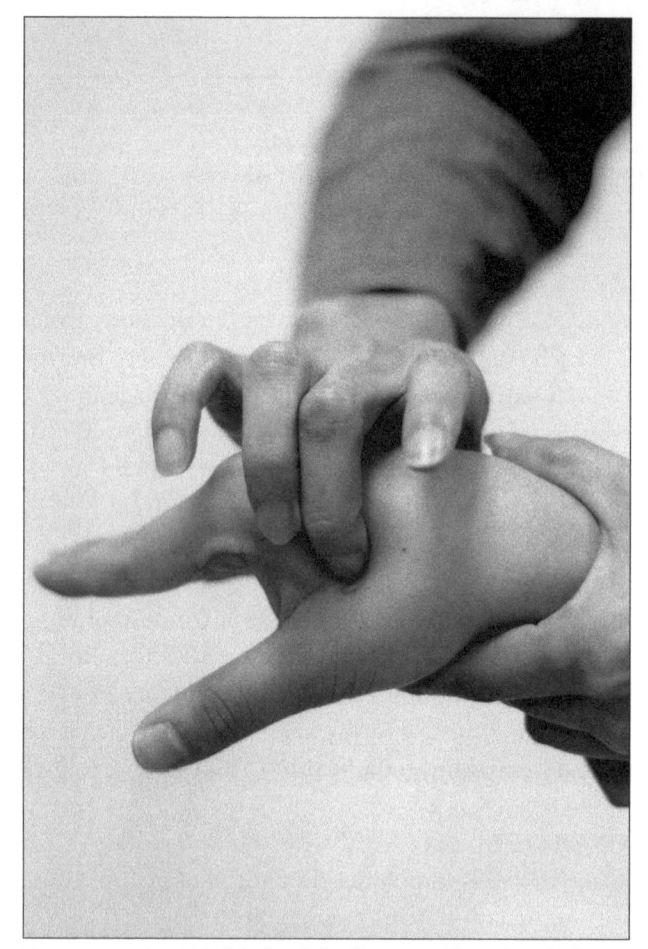

Pressure may be applied by hand, by elbow, or with various devices. Photo by Mk2010, via Wikimedia Commons.

However, in its most crucial role, TCM presents a theoretical and practical framework for engaging in a holistic understanding of health and illness.

SCIENTIFIC EVIDENCE

Controlled double-blind studies into the efficacy of acupressure have failed to provide solid evidence of efficacy. However, some smaller studies may affirm the positive role of acupressure in such conditions as pain, stroke, heart disease, cancer, smoking, obesity, insomnia, allergies, and menstrual disorders. The quality of these studies varies, however. For example, a study by Marayam Narimani and others in the journal *Anesthesiology and Pain Medicine* presented evidence that acupressure decreased pain levels in patients who had received coronary artery bypass graft (CABG) surgery. However, these authors called this study a "double-blinded" study, even though it was not since the patients whether pressure was being applied as did the acupressure therapist. Second, all the control group patients received more anesthetics than the acupressure group, confounding the overall results. A second systematic review in the *World Journal of Psychiatry* by Jingxia Lin and others found evidence that acupressure effectively treats depression. Regrettably, this review included several studies in its meta-analysis that did not control for the placebo effect of administering acupressure or check for blinding success. These shortcomings make it likely that many patients knew what treatment they received. Therefore, any results reported by these studies were probably mostly due to placebo effects. Unfortunately, clinical trials that evaluate acupressure tend to suffer from such methodological problems. The efficacy of acupressure remains unproven.

Additionally, proponents of acupressure also point to millennia of observational information gathered throughout China, Japan, Korea, and other Asian countries. Still, much of this evidence is admittedly anecdotal.

CHOOSING A PRACTITIONER

TCM is certainly more complex than the beginner or casual observer might think. This ancient discipline specifically emphasizes concepts of wellness, illness, and recovery. It further emphasizes the best medical ideas and methodologies from the past and the present—from the wisdom of everyday people to the advanced knowledge of the best-trained TCM physicians and other healing arts practitioners. For these reasons and more, actual treatment with TCM, including acupressure, requires the expertise of a trained and licensed clinician. However, simple, everyday ailments respond well to acupressure performed as self-therapy.

In the United States, licensed physicians, acupuncturists, and massage therapists practice acupressure. Practitioners can be found by contacting state licensing boards and such national groups as the American Academy of Medical Acupuncture, the American Association of Acupuncture and Oriental Medicine, and the American Massage Therapy Association.

SAFETY ISSUES

Acupressure is an exceptionally safe modality because of its noninvasive nature. Contraindications (that is, conditions for which acupressure is not recommended) typically include acute illness (such as hypertensive urgency and tachycardia), serious illness (such as cancer), pregnancy, bleeding (such as with open wounds), and skin diseases and lesions (such as infections and ulcers). The largest concern with acupressure is people seeking a potentially ineffective treatment while delaying a potentially efficacious one.

—*George D. Zgourides, Michael A. Buratovich*

Further Reading

Adams, Angela, et al. "Acupressure for Chronic Low Back Pain: a Single System Study." *Journal of Physical Therapy Science*, vol. 29, no. 8, 2017, pp. 1416-20, doi:10.1589/jpts.29.1416.

Bleecker, Deborah. *Acupuncture Points Handbook: A Patient's Guide to the Locations and Functions of Over 400 Acupuncture Points.* Draycott Design Books, 2017.

Mafetoni, Reginaldo Roque, and Antonieta Keiko Kakuda Shimo. "The Effects of Acupressure on Labor Pains during Child Birth: Randomized Clinical Trial." *Revista Latino-Americana De Enfermagem*, vol. 24, no. 8, 2016, doi:10.1590/1518-8345.0739.2738.

Mehta, Piyush, et al. "Contemporary Acupressure Therapy: Adroit Cure for Painless Recovery of Therapeutic Ailments." *Journal of Traditional and*

Complementary Medicine, vol. 7, no. 2, 2017, pp. 251-63, doi:10.1016/j.jtcme.2016.06.004.

Noll, Eric, et al. "Efficacy of Acupressure on Quality of Recovery After Surgery: Randomised Controlled Trial." *European Journal of Anaesthesiology*, vol. 36, no. 8, 2019, pp. 557-65, doi:10.1097/EJA.0000000000001001.

Ogal, Hans P., and Wolfram Stor. *Pictorial Atlas of Acupuncture: An Illustrated Manual of Acupuncture Points*. H. F. Ullman Publishing, 2012.

Singh, Simon, and Ernst, Edzard. *Trick or Treatment: The Undeniable Facts about Alternative Medicine*. W. W. Norton and Company, 2008.

ACUPUNCTURE

Category: Treatment

Specialties and related fields: Alternative medicine, anesthesiology, preventive medicine

Definition: an ancient therapy developed in China in which designated points on the skin are stimulated by the insertion of needles, the application of heat, massage, or a combination of these techniques to treat impaired body functions or to induce anesthesia

KEY TERMS

Ch'i: Chinese concept of the vital essence; when Ch'i is unbalanced, disease results

meridians: designated pathways in the body with points that react to acupuncture stimulation

yang: Chinese concept of the positive, male element of the universe

yin: Chinese concept of the negative, female element of the universe

INDICATIONS AND PROCEDURES

The theory and practice of acupuncture are rooted in the Chinese concept of life—the *Chi* or *qi* (both are pronounced "chee"). The belief is that all things, animate and inanimate, have an internal source of energy, the Chi. This energy stabilizes the chemical composition of matter, and when this matter is broken down, energy is released. The practice of acupuncture is thought to stimulate this energy to relieve pain and speed healing.

According to the ancient Chinese system of medicine, two categories of organs are associated with the Chi: the Tsang and the Fou. The Fou is the group of organs that absorb food, digest it, and expel waste. They are all hollow organs such as the stomach, the large and small intestines, the bladder, and the gallbladder. Tsang organs are all associated with the blood-the heart, which circulates the blood around the body; the lungs, which oxygenate the blood; the spleen, which controls the red corpuscles; and the liver and the kidneys. For the energy flow to remain steady, it must pass unimpeded from one organ to another. If the organ is weak, the resultant energy passed on to the next organ is weakened. Acupuncture stimulates specifically designated points found on pathways in the body (called "meridians") to correct the problem.

According to the Chinese system, the human "circuit" of energy comprises twelve meridians, which stretch along with the limbs from the toes and the fingers to the face and chest. There are six meridians in the upper limbs and six in the lower. Ten meridians are connected to the main organ by the sympathetic nervous system branches. Each of these meridians contains the Chi, which varies in strength and is governed by the nerve impulses arising from the organs. The meridians and their attendant vessels contain the flow of energy that enables the body to function efficiently.

Later, the meridian line concept was hypothesized to explain the effectiveness of the points. Acupuncturists selected these meridian points by observing the effects of stimulation on particular signs and symptoms. The meridian points that proved effective for certain ailments were organized, and acupuncture practitioners gave specific names to each.

According to modern medical concepts, some of these points are thought to be relating points at which a specific visceral disorder stimulates the autonomic nervous system. Anatomically, some of the meridian points appear to correspond to areas where a nerve appears to surface from a muscle or areas where vessels and nerves are located relatively superficially, such as areas between a muscle and a bone or a bone and a joint. These areas are generally composed of connective tissue. No contemporary anatomical or physiological research has confirmed the presence or existence of Ch'i.

The insertion of needles allegedly stimulates the meridians. The commonly used needles range in size from the diameter of a hair to that of a sewing needle. In China, round and cutting needles are commonly used. In Europe, the needles are slightly shorter and slightly wider in diameter.

Acupuncture is an ancient Chinese medical practice based on the concept of meridians, channels in the body through which flows the life force called Ch'i; acupuncture involves the insertion and manipulation of tiny needles along these meridians.

The needles are gold, silver, iron, platinum, or stainless steel. Stainless steel needles are most used. Infection caused by needle puncture is said to be extremely rare. It is routine to wipe the skin with alcohol before inserting the sterilized needle. Acupuncturists usually wipe the needle with alcohol sponges before each insertion on the same patient. Needles are discarded after being used in patients with a history of jaundice or hepatitis.

Insertion of a needle requires great skill and much practice. There are three different angles of penetration into the skin: perpendicular, oblique, and horizontal. These angles correspond to 90 degrees, 45 degrees, and a minimum angle, respectively. The angles may be chosen based on the thickness of the skin and the proximity to muscle or bone at the desired puncture point. The depth of penetration will vary.

Tapping (the tube method) is one method of insertion: When the diameter of the needle is small, this method is extremely effective. The needle is placed into the tube from either direction. This tube is shorter than the needle. The tube is removed gently with the right index finger and thumb. Gentle tapping of the needle handle with the right index finger introduces the needle easily. The acupuncturist must immediately remove the tapping finger from the needle head; otherwise, it causes pain.

In the twirling method (the freehand method), the left thumb and index finger make contact at the acupuncture point. The left hand is called the "pushing hand." Next, the skin is cut with the needle tip, after which the needle is inserted by pushing and twirling it with the right hand.

The goal of advancing the needle and the needle motion is to create a needle feeling in the patient. The patient usually feels a dull, aching, paralyzing, or compressing sensation that radiates to a distal or proximal portion of the body. When the patient notices the needle feeling, the operator increases the feeling by using various needle motions. Numerous motions are available, such as the single-stick, twirling, vibration, intermittent, and retention motions.

Light skin and muscle massage are recommended to prepare the body to accept needle stimulation. Prepuncture massage makes skin cutting easier and helps the patient relax. In addition to these advantages, massage may make it possible to detect pathologies such as nodules, spasms, pain, and depression. Postpuncture massage helps confirm muscle hypersensitivity and the disappearance of pain or hard nodules that existed before the acupuncture was performed.

The amount of stimulation equals the strength of stimulation multiplied by the number of treatments; this depends on the patient's sensitivity. Gradual increases in stimulation are essential. For acute disease, treatment is usually given once a day for ten days and then terminated for three to seven days.

Treatment is administered once every two to three days for ten treatments and then terminated for seven days for chronic ailments. The patient is placed in a supine, sitting, prone, or side position-the most convenient position for the patient and physician. However, the patient may need a special position to relax the painful area.

One of the most important factors for effective acupuncture treatment is the accurate selection of acupuncture points. These points must be selected according to the specific ailment. The precise location of acupuncture points is crucial for obtaining the maximum therapeutic effect. This is difficult because of the different sizes and shapes of patients' bodies. Each acupuncture point is only about three millimeters in diameter.

USES AND COMPLICATIONS
Stimulation treatments such as hot soaks and the management of certain pain problems with physical therapy have long been in existence. Acupuncture, which is one mode of stimulation therapy, works by changing the pattern of the passage of stimulation from the peripheral nerves to the central nervous system. Acupuncture has been studied for decades, but the evidence that provides clinical benefits is weak and inconsistent.

The basic approach of modern medicine involves removing the causal factor of disease. However, in this approach, the pain associated with a disease or a surgical procedure may not be eradicated instantaneously. The management of pain becomes an issue until the disease is cured or until the surgery and healing are complete. Controlling chemical receptors and reducing the sensitivity of those receptors is one way of treating pain. Intensive studies of the stimulation that causes pain have indicated that intrinsic chemical substances (polypeptides) such as histamine and serotonin, which stimulate the receptors, are essential for pain. Therefore, an antagonistic drug for these chemicals is often effective in controlling pain.

Although acupuncture is used to treat conditions as diverse as allergies, circulatory disorders, dermatologic disorders, gastrointestinal disorders, genital disorders, musculoskeletal disorders, neurologic disorders, and psychiatric and emotional disorders, the use of acupuncture for pain control (analgesia) can be described as the most basic level of treatment.

The English words "anesthesia" and "analgesia" are misleading when used to describe the freedom from surgical or obstetrical pain produced by acupuncture. Suppose "analgesia" is described as insensibility to pain without loss of consciousness. In that case, it is a more appropriate word than "anesthesia," which is described as an insensibility, general or local, induced by anesthetic agents and a loss of sensation of neurogenic or psychogenic origin.

Acupuncture can produce partial numbness in any part of the body. The patient under acupuncture analgesia remains able to converse and cooperate with the surgical or obstetrical team. Obstetric patients recognize uterine contractions and can use their muscles to bring forth the fetus. Surgical patients can tell when incisions are made but not perceive them as painful. There is no memory loss, as in hypnosis or general anesthesia, and no paresthesia (abnormal sensations) comparable to the sensations following local anesthesia. However, acupuncture is not a substitute for general anesthesia during surgery.

Acupuncture is contraindicated for children under the age of seven, hemophiliacs, pregnant women, and people who fear needles. Because of heart, liver, or kidney disease, patients with anesthetic risks tolerate acupuncture analgesia well. Most operating room deaths and cases of cardiac arrest in the United States are caused by chemical anesthesia rather than by surgery.

Acupuncture can induce a feeling of well-being and calmness to allay the fear and apprehension most patients feel before surgery. It also appears to reduce both bleeding during surgical procedures and the incidence of shock. Postoperative acupuncture analgesia patients are spared nausea and the difficulties with urinating and defecating that frequently follow chemical anesthesia. Acupuncture analgesia does not mask symptoms as chemical anesthetics and analgesics do. The patient remains aware of their symptoms, but acupuncture diminishes them to a tolerable level.

Postoperative pain does not usually occur for several hours after the termination of acupuncture analgesia. When it does occur, acupuncture can be used again instead of narcotics, and the treatment seldom needs to be repeated more than once or twice. Some acupuncturists leave small needles superficially inserted for several days to relieve postoperative pain. Others give regular acupuncture treatments, leaving the needles in place for twenty minutes per day for as many days as necessary.

The main disadvantage of acupuncture analgesia is that it is less reliable than chemical analgesia or anesthesia. In some cases, acupuncture analgesia cannot be induced or becomes inadequate during a surgical procedure. It may not produce the relaxation desirable for some abdominal surgeries. For this reason, backup chemical anesthetics and analgesics are also available in most cases.

The actual induction of acupuncture analgesia takes about twenty minutes—slightly longer than chemical anesthesia. The more skilled the acupuncturist is, the fewer needles are required. In most cases, electroacupuncture instruments must remain attached to all acupuncture needles during the entire procedure. Still, these can usually be kept away from the surgical field. According to news reports, major surgical procedures in China have been performed with only one acupuncture needle as analgesia and without electric supplementation. However, these news reports are probably bogus.

The same thin (usually 30-gauge) stainless steel needles used for acupuncture treatments are used for acupuncture analgesia. In general, the points used to relieve chronic pain in a specific area are the points of choice for analgesia. To obtain sufficient analgesia for surgery, it is usually necessary to heighten the effect of the acupuncture needles by twirling them continually or by attaching electronic instruments to them to deliver a current of about two hundred microamperes, with a pulsating wave at a frequency of two hundred per minute during the entire procedure. Electronic instruments will usually increase the depth of analgesia or prolong an analgesic effect that is beginning to wear off.

Besides the acupuncture points for analgesia of specific areas of the body, points are often used to relieve anxiety and promote well-being. Needles are usually inserted for twenty minutes the evening before surgery and for at least twenty minutes before the actual surgery begins.

The theoretical principles of vital energy transmission determine which acupuncture points should be effective for the anticipated surgery. Acupuncture points on meridians passing directly through or in the vicinity of the surgical area are usually selected. An attempt is made to use points on these meridians as far away from the surgical field as possible.

PERSPECTIVE AND PROSPECTS

According to most reports, acupuncture appears to have been developed in the northernmost area of the middle region of China around 300 BCE. People in this area were primarily nomads, moving from one area to another.

Chinese high priests, who also often served as physicians, observed that men wounded in combat often reported the sudden disappearance of illnesses from which they had suffered for years. For example, a wound in a specific foot area would reduce blood pressure or relieve a headache or toothache, or an injury on the dorsal aspect of the knee joint would cure a migraine. Over the years, the high priests recorded numerous observations of the phenomenon of a wound in one part of the body curing a long-standing complaint at another point. They discovered that it was the location of the wound that was significant. A pinprick in the correct location was enough to effect relief. It was noted that certain body points responded more noticeably to stimulation than other points and that frequently there was a direct correlation between the responsive points and a particular ailment. They were subsequently named meridian points.

Later, when metal was introduced to the culture, needles were used as an irritant at meridian points. It was thought that pain from a specific ailment was diverted linearly through the meridian points to the body's surface. Thus, the "meridian line" concept was developed, and thus acupuncture was discovered.

At first, the surgeon-priests used fish bones and sharpened bamboo splinters to affect the pricks. Later came finely honed needles. Warlords and nobles were treated with needles forged from gold and silver. As the science of acupuncture developed, it was discovered that the needles needed only to be inserted in a point of skin measuring about one-tenth of an inch.

The earliest book describing acupuncture was written in 50 BCE. It described the clinical applications of acupuncture with anatomical and physiological references based principally on the concept of the body's meridian lines.

In 1912, Yüan Shih-K'ai, who had trained in modern Western culture, took office as president of the Republic of China. Under his rule, old Chinese medicine—including acupuncture—that had developed from tradition and experience was unable to survive except in outlying areas of China. In 1949, however, when Mao Zedong formed the People's Republic of China, he tried to repopularize the old Chinese medicine methods, which had been helpful to him. In the 1930s, when Mao and his followers were retreating to the north, he was forced to depend mainly on these traditional methods for medical treatment.

In 1955, Shyuken, a follower of Mao, stated his belief that acupuncture was effective in managing illness. He wished to study the ancient Chinese way of medicine more systematically, comparing it to Western medicine, which he believed too analytical. Thus, a new medical movement began that united Western and Chinese medical practices.

Stimulation therapy using local heat, massage, and pressure has been known since ancient times. Long periods of observations and analysis by Chinese physicians of the effects of irritation of varying degrees at particular points on the body surface made it possible to relate specific points on the body (meridian points) to specific conditions.

According to ancient Chinese clinical concepts, the meridian points are peepholes into the body and pass holes for energy. The total number of meridian points was believed to be 365. Each was named according to its effect, anatomical location, appearance, and relation to the meridian line. These meridian points were selected initially according to measurements based on the patient's unique anatomical standard (using the length between certain anatomical points, for example, between the shoulders). The examiner then selected the exact location of a meridian point, felt the areas chosen by the initial measurement, and observed the patient's response with their fingertips.

Acupuncture's popularity, like that of most techniques and discoveries, has waxed and waned throughout the years; for the most part, however, the Chinese have remained faithful to the five-thousand-year-old practice. The laws and acupuncture methods have endured, although these methods have been increasingly combined with Western medical techniques. Gradually, acupuncture has spread throughout the world, particularly in France, Russia, Japan, Switzerland, Germany, and the United States.

In 1997, the US National Institutes of Health (NIH) concluded that the efficacy of acupuncture is highly promising and a worthwhile research endeavor, especially in treating postoperative chemotherapy nausea and dental pain. Some studies showed that acupuncture might be useful in treating asthma and addiction and stroke rehabilitation. Other research has identified many of the mechanisms of action in acupuncture, most notably the release of opioids and other peptides and the corresponding changes in neuroendocrine functioning. However, the quality of acupuncture studies varies wildly, and some claims regarding acupuncture's healing potential have been terrifically overblown.

In 2002, the National Health Interview Survey found that 8.2 million adults in the United States had used acupuncture and that 2.1 million had used it within the last year. Although the number of people who use acupuncture is significant, the Food and Drug Administration (FDA) reports exceedingly few complications.

A review of government-funded research studies on acupuncture found numerous uses being evaluated, including labor stimulation, postsurgical wound healing, control of chemotherapy-induced vomiting, and the treatment of substance abuse, incontinence, autism, cerebral palsy, and depression.

—*Genevieve Slomski, LeAnna DeAngelo*

Further Reading

"Acupuncture." *Mayo Clinic*, 30 Apr. 2022, www.mayoclinic.org/tests-procedures/acupuncture/about/pac-20392763. Accessed 26 May 2022.

"Acupuncture: An Introduction." *National Center for Complementary and Alternative Medicine*. US Department of Health and Human Services, 2012.

Cassidy, Claire Monod. *Contemporary Chinese Medicine and Acupuncture*. Churchill Livingstone, 2002.

Ernst, Edzard, and Adrian White, editors. *Acupuncture: A Scientific Appraisal*. Butterworth-Heinemann, 2000.

Kidson, Ruth. *Acupuncture for Everyone: What It Is, Why It Works, and How It Can Help You*. Inner Traditions International, 2001.

Manaka, Yoshio, Kazuko Itaya, and Stephen Birch. *Chasing the Dragon's Tail: The Theory and Practice of Acupuncture in the Work of Yoshio Manaka*. Paradigm, 1997.

Mann, Felix. *Reinventing Acupuncture: A New Concept of Ancient Medicine*. Butterworth-Heinemann, 2000.

Molassiotis, A., et al. "A Randomized, Controlled Trial of Acupuncture Self-Needling as Maintenance Therapy for Cancer-Related Fatigue after Therapist-Delivered Acupuncture." *Annals of Oncology*, vol. 24, no. 6, 2013, pp. 1645-52.

Stux, Gabriel, and Bruce Pomeranz. *Basics of Acupuncture*. 5th ed., Springer, 2003.

Applied Kinesiology

Category: Therapy or technique

Also known as: Contact reflex analysis, functional neurologic assessment, kinesitherapy, kinesiology

Specialties and related fields: Alternative health practitioner, chiropractor

Definition: using techniques such as muscle testing to identify health problems

KEY TERMS

kinesiology: the study of the mechanics of body movements

muscle testing: an alternative medical technique that purports to diagnose illness or select treatments by testing muscles for strength and weakness

OVERVIEW

The modern practice of applied kinesiology (AK) began in 1964 when chiropractor George J. Goodheart Jr., observed that poor posture is often associated with weak muscles. Through his work, he linked specific diseases to the strength or weakness

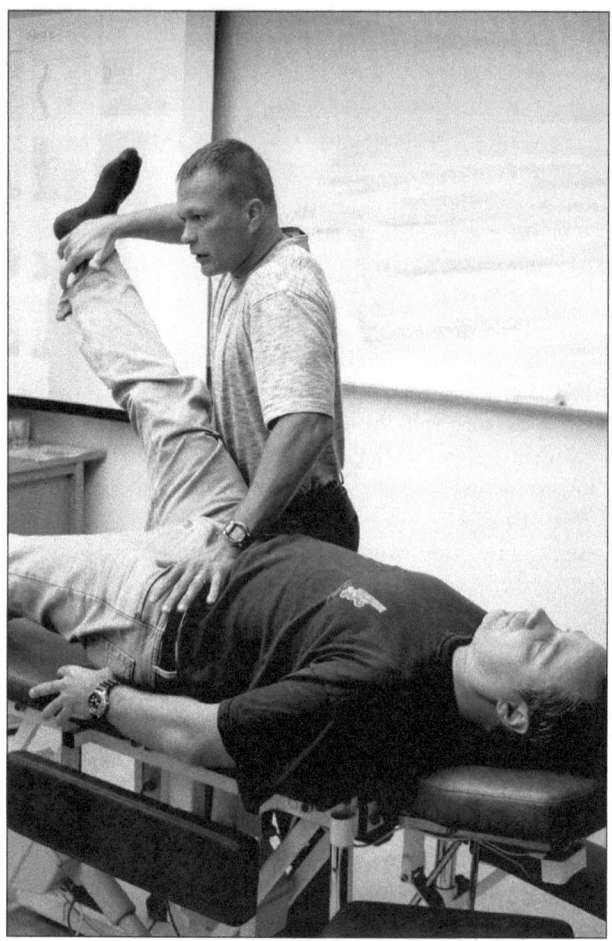

A chiropractor and a professional applied kinesiologist demonstrating a manual muscle test MMT of Psoas major and Iliacus muscles. Photo by Macpw, via Wikimedia Commons.

of muscles. Although many practitioners of AK refer to their work as kinesiology, AK should not be confused with standard kinesiology, which is the scientific study of the principles of mechanics and anatomy in relation to human movement.

MECHANISM OF ACTION
The fundamental idea of AK is that every organ dysfunction in the body is accompanied by specific muscle weakness. Particular disease states in the body can then be tied directly to the corresponding internal organs by determining what factor weakened a previously strong muscle.

USES AND APPLICATIONS
Applied kinesiology believes that practitioners can use muscle-testing procedures to diagnose whatever illness might be afflicting a person. Treatment with appropriate nutrients, special diets, acupressure, various reflex procedures, and spinal or joint manipulation may be used to improve health.

SCIENTIFIC EVIDENCE
Although there is little doubt that muscle movements detected by AK are unconsciously triggered, no published scientific studies establish specific links between muscle responses and diseases that affect organs. Researchers who have conducted elaborate double-blind trials have concluded that connections between muscle weakness and particular diseases are random phenomena. Diagnoses of nutritional deficiencies by AK are not verified by the nutrient levels determined by blood serum analysis.

Other studies demonstrate that the power of suggestion and distractions, variations in the amount of force or leverage applied to muscles, and muscle fatigue play a significant role in muscle-testing outcomes. Results from the scientific review of twenty research papers published by the International College of Applied Kinesiology concluded that none included statistical analyses rigorous enough to confer validity on their findings.

Although AK has been suggested to treat many conditions, high-quality scientific research and findings are very limited. Applied kinesiology has not been shown to diagnose or treat any disease effectively. Controlled studies using nutrient substances versus placebos failed to demonstrate statistically significant differences.

SAFETY ISSUES
Applied kinesiology techniques are generally safe but can produce temporary pain. Sole AK use could delay the time it takes for a person to see a qualified health-care provider about a potentially life-threat-

ening condition. Also, persons using AK could find that their illness has been left undetected and untreated. One should not rely solely on AK for diagnosis; instead, AK should be used to enhance standard medical diagnosis and therapy.

—*Alvin K. Benson*

Further Reading

Barrett, Stephen. "Applied Kinesiology: Phony Muscle-Testing for 'Allergies' and 'Nutrient Deficiencies.'" *Quackwatch*, 23 Aug., www.quackwatch.com/01quackeryrelatedtopics/tests/ak.html. Accessed 27 May 2022.

Frost, Robert. *Applied Kinesiology: A Training Manual and Reference Book of Basic Principles and Practices*. North Atlantic Books, 2002.

Neumann, Donald A. *Kinesiology of the Musculoskeletal System: Foundations for Rehabilitation*. 2nd ed., Mosby/Elsevier, 2010.

Walther, David S. *Applied Kinesiology: Synopsis*. 2nd ed., Systems DC, 2000.

"The World of Applied Kinesiology." *International College of Applied Kinesiology*, 2022, www.icak.com. Accessed 27 May 2022.

CUPPING

Category: Therapy or technique
Related terms: Baguanfa, body vacuuming, dijiufa fire cupping, hijama horn technique, jiaofa
Specialties and related fields: Alternative medical practitioners, athletic training, physical therapy
Definition: a skin-surface therapy involving cupped vessels under vacuum to suction the skin and relieve local congestion

KEY TERMS

moxibustion: a traditional Chinese medicine therapy that consists of burning dried mugwort at particular points on the body.
traditional Chinese medicine: an alternative medical practice drawn from traditional medicine in China

OVERVIEW

Cupping, typically associated with traditional Chinese medicine (TCM), is one of the oldest known therapeutic practices in the world. Cupping involves attaching a hollow cupped vessel to the skin's surface by heat or air suction. Once a vacuum is created, the underlying tissue is lifted, and blood is drawn to the area. The number, size, type, and movement of the cup and the degree and duration of suction can be varied according to the ailment being treated. The degree of skin discoloration indicates the nature of the congestion.

MECHANISM OF ACTION

Cupping is thought to stimulate the body's natural healing mechanisms by reducing "stagnant" blood, activating the immune system, improving circulation, and helping the body detoxify. The exact healing mechanism of cupping is unknown. Another possible explanation is the placebo effect.

USES AND APPLICATIONS

Cupping therapy is primarily used to relieve pain, gastrointestinal disorders such as abdominal pain and indigestion, respiratory problems such as chronic cough and asthma, menstrual disturbances, and skin conditions. Cupping is most commonly used with acupuncture, acupressure, bleeding treatments, and moxibustion.

SCIENTIFIC EVIDENCE

Most evidence supporting cupping as a cure for illness is anecdotal. Cupping has existed for hundreds of years, and many researchers have investigated its benefits. Still, it is a new area of study in Western medicine.

Various studies have suggested that cupping treatments effectively temporarily alleviate chronic pain. None, however, were double-blind, placebo-controlled trials, and most proved to be inconclusive because of low enrollment, poor study design, inade-

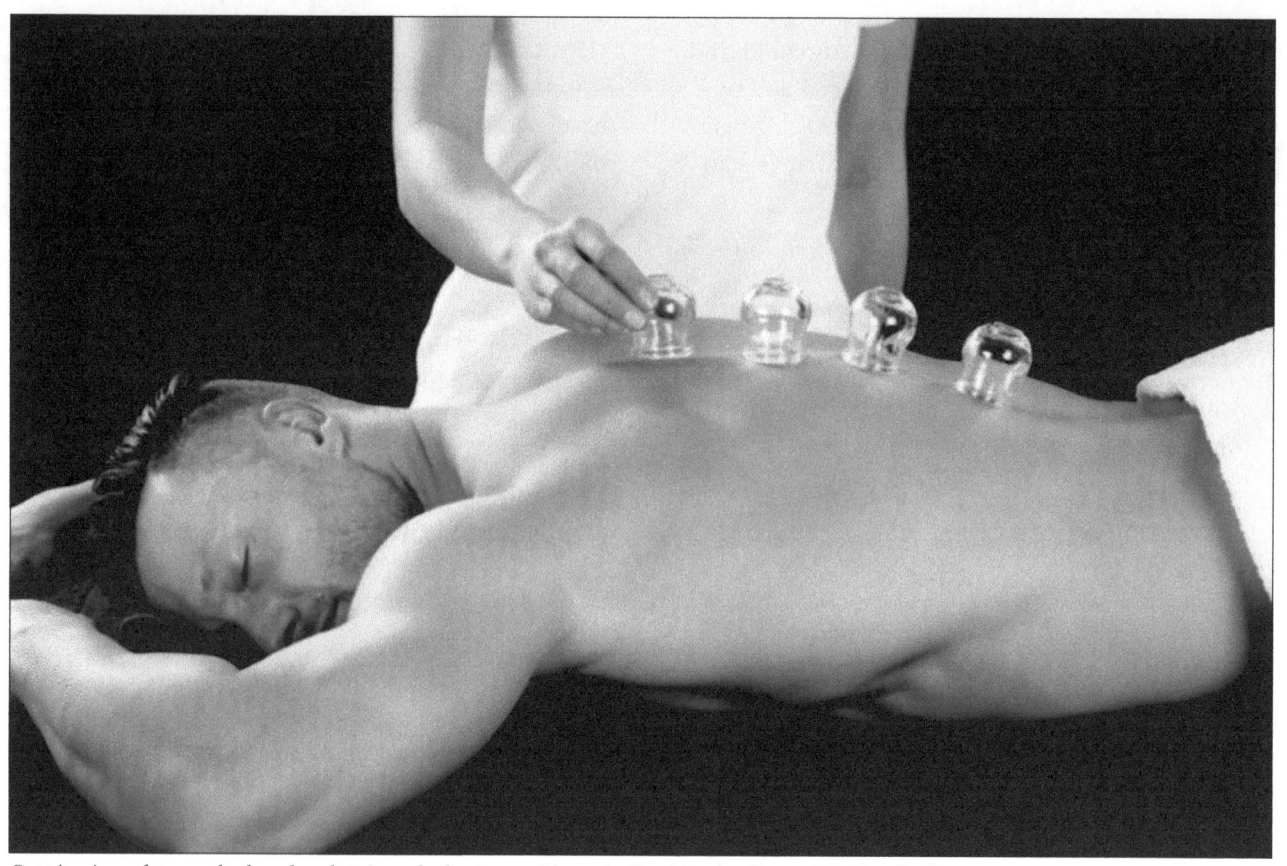

Cupping is used to ease back and neck pain and other issues. Photo via iStock/AndreyPopov. [Used under license.]

quate blinding procedures, and a lack of appropriate scientific control groups. Several studies indicate that cupping treatments combined with other therapies, such as acupuncture, may improve clinical outcomes, but scientific evidence is limited. A systematic review of cupping studies in 2011 concluded that: "Based on evidence from the currently available SRs (systematic reviews), the effectiveness of cupping has been demonstrated only as a treatment for pain, and even for this indication doubts remain." The quality of the evidence for cupping has changed little since 2011.

In 2021, Brazilian researchers designed a sham cupping technique and compared the efficacy of their sham cupping procedure to dry cupping and observed a significant difference. This sham cupping technique should help researchers perform more double-blinded, placebo-controlled cupping trials.

Cupping is an appealing natural treatment option for various illnesses because it is convenient and relatively safe. However, substantial bruising occurs at the site of cupping. A report of cupping a newborn infant in Istanbul, Turkey, generated immense outrage in the medical community. Cupping may be beneficial for various conditions because of its relaxation effect. However, more rigorous research studies are needed to assess the clinical value of cupping in Western medicine properly.

CHOOSING A PRACTITIONER

Cupping therapy is a relatively unregulated field. Skilled practitioners should perform treatments to avoid injury.

SAFETY ISSUES

Cupping therapy, which is considered safe with minimal side effects, may cause marks or bruising. The appearance of blisters, blood spots, or burns indicates an abnormally harsh treatment.

Cupping should be performed only on areas of soft muscle tissue. It should not be performed on young children, persons with skin ulcers, high fever, convulsions, cramps, bleeding disorders, cardiovascular disease, or women who are pregnant.

—*Rose Ciulla-Bohling, Michael A. Buratovich*

Further Reading

Chirali, Ilkay Z. *Traditional Chinese Medicine: Cupping Therapy*. 2nd ed., Churchill Livingstone/Elsevier, 2007.

Dharmananda, Subhuti. "Cupping." *Institute for Traditional Medicine Online*, Mar. 1999. Accessed 27 Jan. 2016.

Lee, Myeong Soo, et al. "Is Cupping an Effective Treatment? An Overview of Systematic Reviews." *Journal of Acupuncture and Meridian Studies*, vol. 4, no. 1, 2011, pp. 1-4, doi:10.1016/S2005-2901(11)60001-0.

Pringle, Michael. "Some Thoughts on Fire Cupping." *Journal of Chinese Medicine*, vol. 83, 2007, pp. 46-51.

Pritchard, Sarah, and Andrew Croysdale. *Tui Na: A Manual of Chinese Massage Therapy*. Singing Dragon, 2015, eBook Collection (EBSCOhost). Accessed 27 Jan. 2016.

Shixi, Huang, and Cao Yu. "Cupping Therapy." *Journal of Chinese Medicine*, vol. 82, 2006, pp. 52-57.

DIET-BASED THERAPIES

Category: Therapy
Specialties and related fields: Dietetics, cardiology, nutrition, personal trainers
Definition: therapies involving special dietary interventions to improve health, increase longevity, and prevent and treat specific health conditions and diseases

KEY TERMS

blood pressure: the pressure in the circulatory system, often measured for diagnosis since it is closely related to the force and rate of the heartbeat and the diameter and elasticity of the arterial walls

cardiovascular disease: circulatory conditions that include diseased vessels, heart and blood vessel structural problems, and blood clots

DASH diet: a low-sodium diet promoted by the US-based National Heart, Lung, and Blood Institute to prevent and control hypertension

sodium: a mineral found in many foods, required by the human body for normal muscle and nerve functions

OVERVIEW

Diet-based therapy uses specialized dietary regimens to promote wellness and prevent and treat specific diseases. A healthy eating plan includes vegetables, fruits, whole grains, fat-free or reduced-fat dairy, lean meats, poultry, and fish and limits saturated and trans fats, sodium, and added sugars. No single food can prevent cancer; however, a diverse and healthy diet may reduce cancer risk. Reducing obesity may prevent heart and other diseases. A healthy diet provides energy to stay active and nutrients for the growth and repair of cells. Diet therapies are more likely to be effective if practiced as a preventive measure against disease or started early after the onset of disease. A poor diet may raise the risk of dying from heart disease, stroke, and type 2 diabetes.

Humans need a balanced diet to be healthy. As a component of disease treatment, physicians may prescribe a special diet that their patients must carefully follow. Working closely with the doctor, staff, and the patient, they provide an individualized diet plan, counseling, and education to meet their dietary needs. While nurses often answer diet-related questions, an important part of the health-care team is the Registered Clinical Dietitian, who assesses the patient's therapeutic nutritional needs, develops and implements nutrition programs, and may even teach healthy cooking classes.

MECHANISM OF ACTION
Individuals may react differently to dietary interventions based on a variety of factors. Genetic factors, other health behaviors such as smoking, and physical activity levels must all be factored in to determine the results of dietary therapies. Before undertaking any diet therapy, the patient should discuss the plan with the physician. Physicians may recommend specific diets or recommend that the person see a registered clinical dietitian. Extreme diets that omit whole food classes are not always safe and should be undertaken only in consultation with the physician. Diet information must be critically evaluated before undertaking any specific diet. A healthy diet, appropriate exercise, and maintaining an appropriate body weight are always good ideas.

USES AND APPLICATIONS
Diets have been an important part of health-care management over the years. Diets have been used to treat various diseases, for example, hypertension. One of the most important science-based diets designed to control blood pressure is the Dietary Approaches to Stop Hypertension (DASH) diet, which is promoted by the National Heart, Lung, and Blood Institute, part of the National Institutes of Health (NIH).

The DASH diet is a plan that is low in saturated fats, cholesterol, and total fat. It emphasizes the intake of fruits, vegetables, fat-free or low-fat milk and milk products, whole grain products, fish, poultry, and nuts. The diet is low in lean red meat, sweets, added sugars, and sugar-containing beverages. It is rich in potassium, magnesium, calcium, protein, and fiber.

Type 2 diabetes is another chronic disease that diet can partially control. The ideal diabetic meal consists of bread, high-fat products, dairy items that provide protein, and starchy vegetables. Most of the protein in a diabetic diet comes from chicken, fish, lean beef, or dairy. Servings and portions in diabetic diets depend on a person's level of physical activity.

Cardiovascular diseases can also be prevented and controlled by diet. Histological studies show that vascular injury accumulates from adolescence, making it extremely important to monitor one's lifestyle and diet from childhood to prevent a heart condition in the future. Any diet designed to control or prevent cardiovascular disease must be low in saturated fats (less than 7 percent of the daily diet) and low in cholesterol (less than 0.06 teaspoon [300 milligrams]) per day for healthy adults and less than 0.04 teaspoon [200 milligrams]) per day for adults with high levels of low-density lipoprotein (LDL), or bad, cholesterol).

The American Cancer Society recommends that people with cancer not undertake a dietary program as an exclusive or primary means of treatment. Before beginning any changes, the cancer patient should discuss any dietary changes with the physician or medical oncologist.

SCIENTIFIC EVIDENCE
Multiple studies support the use of diet therapies in disease management. NIH studies have demonstrated that a low level of salt combined with the DASH diet effectively lowers blood pressure. The effect of this combination (at a sodium level of 0.3 teaspoon [1,500 milligrams]) was an average blood pressure reduction of 8.9/4.5 millimeters of mercury (systolic/diastolic) in normal subjects. Persons in the studies who were hypertensive experienced an average reduction of 11.5/5.7 millimeters of mercury.

A low intake of saturated fats will reduce LDL (bad) cholesterol and triglycerides in the blood. Studies have shown higher rates of heart disease in people who eat more saturated fats. The Diabetes Prevention Program demonstrated that losing weight and increasing exercise decreased the risk of diabetes by 58 percent, even more than a prescription drug. The American Cancer Society states staying at a healthy weight, staying active throughout life, following a healthy eating plan, and minimizing alcohol intake may greatly reduce a person's risk of developing or dying from cancer.

CHOOSING A PRACTITIONER

Registered clinical dietitians are educated and qualified to diagnose eating disorders and design diets to treat specific medical conditions and diseases with physicians and nurses. For example, dietitians recommend diet restrictions related to diabetes and address poor eating habits or loss of appetite from cancer. Dietitians most often practice in hospitals and formal health settings. Most states require licensure to practice as a registered clinical dietitian. Nutritionists are most likely found in schools, hospitals, cafeterias, long-term care facilities, and athletic organizations to deal with general nutritional aims and behaviors. The educational program is more rigorous for Registered Clinical Dietitians often requiring a grade point average (GPA) of 3.0 to enter the program. A nutritionist takes courses at the college level related to science and nutrition. However, anyone giving nutrition advice often may choose to call themselves a nutritionist because they are giving dietary advice. A registered dietitian nutritionist must have a master's degree and 1,200 hours of supervised practice.

SAFETY ISSUES

When beginning a therapeutic diet that involves a dramatically different way of eating, people should receive expert supervision to avoid nutritional deficiencies. Discussing diet changes with the physician is very important. The physician may recommend a consultation with a registered clinical dietitian or nutritionist before undertaking any diet modifications.

The human body, which needs carbohydrates, fats, and proteins for healthy function, burns its energy reserves in the absence of calorie intake. Fasting for extended periods leads to starvation, dehydration, and eventual death. Diets based on one type of food, such as those based solely on fruits, can cause protein deficiencies, which inhibit growth and development in children. Fruit-based diets can also cause deficiencies in vitamin D, vitamin B_{12}, calcium, iron, zinc, and essential fatty acids.

—*Fernando J. Ferrer, Patricia Stanfill Edens*

Further Reading

"American Cancer Society Updates Guideline for Diet and Physical Activity." *American Cancer Society*, 9 June 2020, www.cancer.org/latest-news/american-cancer-society-updates-guideline-for-diet-and-physical-activity.html.

"DASH Diet: Healthy Eating to Lower Your Blood Pressure." *Mayo Clinic*, 25 June 2021, www.mayoclinic.org/healthy-lifestyle/nutrition-and-healthy-eating/in-depth/dash-diet/art-20048456. Accessed 24 Aug. 2020.

"DASH Ranked Best Diet Overall for Eighth Year in a Row by U.S. News and World Report." *National Institutes of Health*, 3 Jan. 2018, www.nih.gov/news-events/news-releases/dash-ranked-best-diet-overall-eighth-year-row-us-news-world-report. Accessed 24 Aug. 2020.

"Food and Nutrition Information Center." *US Department of Agriculture. National Agricultural Library*, n.d., www.nal.usda.gov/fnic. Accessed 24 Aug. 2020.

"How Dietary Factors Influence Disease Risk." *National Institutes of Health*, 14 Mar. 2017, www.nih.gov/news-events/nih-research-matters/how-dietary-factors-influence-disease-risk. Accessed 24 Aug. 2020.

Rock, C. L., and C. Thomson, et al. "American Cancer Society Guideline for Diet and Physical Activity for Cancer Prevention." *CA: A Cancer Journal for Clinicians*, 9 June 2020, acsjournals.onlinelibrary.wiley.com/doi/full/103322/caac.21591. Accessed 24 Aug. 2020.

Homeopathic Remedies for Sports-Related Injuries

Category: Alternative and complementary medicines
Specialties and related fields: Alternative and complementary medicine
Definition: the use of highly diluted remedies to treat injuries from sports and exercise

KEY TERMS

double-blinded: a test or trial, especially of a drug, in which any information that may influence the tester's behavior or subject is withheld until after the test

homeopathy: the treatment of disease by minute doses of natural substances that in a healthy person would produce symptoms of the disease

placebo: a substance with no therapeutic effect, used as a control in testing new drugs

STUDIED HOMEOPATHIC REMEDIES

Topical combination homeopathic remedy: Preparation containing Arnica montana, Calendula, Hamamelis, aconite, belladonna, Bellis perennis, Chamomilla, Echinacea angustifolia, E. purperea, millefolium, Hepar sulphuris calcareum, Mercurius solubilis, Symphytum, and Hypericum

Oral homeopathic remedies: Arnica; combination of Arnica, Rhus toxicodendron, and sarcolactic acid

Traditional homeopathic remedies: Arnica, belladonna, Hypericum, Rhus tox, Symphyrum

INTRODUCTION

Although vigorous exercise is one of the most important steps toward good health, it can also have side effects, ranging from muscle soreness to injury. While these adverse consequences of exercise can be minimized by graduated training and careful activity, problems may develop anyway. Homeopathic treatments (especially topical creams) are quite popular for sports-related conditions, and they have shown some promise in studies.

SCIENTIFIC EVALUATIONS OF HOMEOPATHIC REMEDIES

There is some evidence to support the use of homeopathic creams to treat sports injuries. However, studies of oral homeopathic remedies for exercise-induced muscle soreness have not been promising.

Topical combination homeopathic treatments for sports injuries. Investigators performed a double-blind, placebo-controlled study of sixty-nine people with sports-related ankle sprains to test the efficacy of a combination homeopathic ointment. The product tested contains a combination of fourteen homeopathic preparations: Arnica montana, Calendula, Hamamelis, aconite, belladonna, Bellis perennis, Chamomilla, Echinacea angustifolia, E. purperea, millefolium, Hepar sulphuris calcareum, Mercurius solubilis, Symphytum, and Hypericum.

During the two-week trial, all of the participants received electrical muscle stimulation. The investigators also applied cream, either the treatment cream or placebo cream, seven times during the study. The results showed that people given the real treatment recovered more rapidly than those given a placebo.

In another double-blind, placebo-controlled study, researchers evaluated the effectiveness of the same homeopathic ointment and a modified version for the treatment of various mild to moderate sports injuries, including sprains. All the approximately one hundred participants in the trial had slight to moderate sports-induced injuries that had occurred in the past four days. The investigators applied the first ointment (and a bandage) on day one of treatment. Then the participants applied the ointment, twice daily for fourteen more days. The results were promising. By the end of the trial, participants who used either form of the ointment experienced significantly superior improvement, compared with those taking placebo, according to some but not all measures.

Oral homeopathic remedies for sports-related muscle soreness. A double-blind, placebo-controlled study tested homeopathic Arnica (30x) in 519 long-distance runners but did not find positive results. Participants took five pills twice daily, beginning the evening before a race and continuing for four successive days. Evaluation after the race showed that Arnica was no more effective than a placebo for reducing soreness or speeding recovery after a race. Earlier, much smaller studies had found some suggestions of benefit for long-distance runners. Still, the results were, in general, not statistically significant.

A double-blind, placebo-controlled study conducted in the physiotherapy department of a homeopathic hospital in England evaluated the efficacy of an oral homeopathic preparation in treating muscle soreness caused by stepping exercise. The remedy was a combination of Arnica, Rhus tox, and sarcolactic acid. The results showed no statistical difference between the treatment and control groups.

TRADITIONAL HOMEOPATHIC TREATMENTS

Classical homeopathy offers many possible homeopathic treatments for sports injuries. These therapies are chosen based on various specific details of the person seeking treatment.

For injuries that are sensitive to touch and have shooting, violent, tingling, or cutting pain, and if the injured person feels worse at night and in the cold, that person may match the symptom picture for homeopathic Hypericum. An injury with symptoms like these suggests nerve involvement, indicating an urgent need for physician examination.

If the affected person feels worse when exposed to motion, drafts, and heat, and during the afternoon, and if the person experiences spasms, shooting pains, tearing sensations, jerking, trembling, swelling, redness, and heat, possibly with cold extremities, then they may fit the classic symptom picture for homeopathic belladonna. Suppose one has a sprain with a great deal of swelling and inflammation of the soft tissue around a joint. In that case, the homeopathic remedy Arnica might be recommended. Arnica is also commonly used as a remedy for exercise-induced muscle soreness.

A person with an injury to a bone, cartilage, or tendon aggravated by touch, motion, and pressure (while warmth helps) may fit the symptom picture for homeopathic Symphytum. Many homeopathic practitioners use Symphytum after Arnica if deep pain or soreness remains after the initial soreness has cleared. A person with stiff, painful muscles brought on by straining, overlifting, or getting wet when already hot and perspiring, and a person whose muscles seize up with rest but loosen with exercise and heat, may fit the traditional homeopathic indications for Rhus tox.

—*EBSCO CAM Review Board*

Further Reading

Plezbert, J. A., and J. R. Burke. "Effects of the Homeopathic Remedy Arnica on Attenuating Symptoms of Exercise-Induced Muscle Soreness." *Journal of Chiropractic Medicine*, vol. 4, 2005, pp. 152-61.

Tveiten, D., and S. Bruset. "Effect of Arnica D30 in Marathon Runners." *Homeopathy*, vol. 92, 2003, pp. 187-89.

Vickers, A. J., et al. "Homeopathic Arnica 30x Is Ineffective for Muscle Soreness After Long-Distance Running." *Clinical Journal of Pain*, vol. 14, 1998, pp. 227-31.

———. "Homeopathy for Delayed Onset Muscle Soreness." *British Journal of Sports Medicine*, vol. 31, 1997, pp. 304-7.

Magnet Therapy

Category: Therapy or technique

Specialties and related fields: Alternative and complementary medicine

Definition: an alternative medicine practice involving the weak static magnetic field produced by a permanent magnet

KEY TERMS

alternating pole devices: magnets that expose the skin to both north and south magnetic fields

pulsed electromagnetic field therapy: uses electromagnetic fields in an attempt to heal nonunion fractures and depression

repetitive transcranial magnet therapy: a form of brain stimulation therapy used to treat depression and anxiety

static magnets: a magnet that retains its magnetism after being removed from a magnetic field

unipolar magnets: magnets with north on one side and south on the other; the north (or negative) side is typically applied to the skin

OVERVIEW

Long popular in Japan, magnet therapy has entered public awareness in the United States, stimulated by golfers and tennis players extolling the virtues of magnets in treating sports-related injuries. Magnetic knee, shoulder, and ankle pads, insoles, and mattress pads are widely available and are thought to provide myriad healing benefits.

Despite this enthusiasm, there is little scientific evidence to support using magnets for any medical condition. However, some small studies suggest that various forms of magnet therapy might have a therapeutic effect in certain conditions.

HISTORY OF MAGNET THERAPY

Magnet therapy has a long history in traditional folk medicine. Reliable documentation indicates that Chinese doctors have believed in the therapeutic value of magnets for two thousand years or more. In sixteenth-century Europe, Paracelsus used magnets to treat a variety of ailments. Two centuries later, Franz Mesmer became famous for treating various disorders with magnets.

In the middle decades of the twentieth century, scientists in various parts of the world began performing studies on the therapeutic use of magnets. From the 1940s on, magnets became increasingly popular in Japan. Yoshio Manaka, one of the influential Japanese acupuncturists of the twentieth century, used magnets in conjunction with acupuncture. Magnet therapy also became a commonly used technique of self-administered medicine in Japan. For example, a type of plaster containing a small magnet became popular for treating aches and pains, especially among the elderly. Magnetic mattress pads, bracelets, and necklaces also became popular, mainly among the elderly. During the 1970s, magnets and electromagnetic machines became popular among athletes in many countries for treating sports-related injuries.

These developments led to a rapidly growing industry creating magnetic products for various conditions. However, the development of this industry preceded any reliable scientific evidence that static magnets work for the purposes intended. In the United States, it was only in 1997 that properly designed clinical trials of magnets began to be reported. Subsequently, several preliminary studies suggested that both static magnets and electromagnetic therapy may offer therapeutic benefits for several disorders. These findings have escalated research interest in magnet therapy.

TYPES OF MAGNET THERAPY AND THEIR USES

The term "magnet therapy" usually refers to static magnets placed directly on the body, generally over regions of pain. Static magnets are either attached to the body by tape or encapsulated in specially designed products such as belts, wraps, or mattress pads. Static magnets are also sometimes known as "permanent magnets."

Static magnets come in various strengths. The units of measuring magnet strength are gauss (G) and tesla (T); 1 tesla equals 10,000 G. A refrigerator magnet, for example, is around 200 G. Therapeutic magnets measure anywhere from 200 to 10,000 G, but the most commonly used measure from 400 to 800 G.

Therapeutic magnets come in two types of polarity arrangements: unipolar magnets and alternating-pole devices. Magnets that have north on one side and south on the other are known, rather confusingly, as unipolar magnets. Bipolar or alternating-pole magnets are made from a sheet of magnetic material with north and south magnets arranged in an alternating pattern so that both north and south face the skin. This type of magnet exerts a weaker magnetic field because the alternating magnets tend to oppose each other. Each type of magnet has its own recommended uses and enthusiasts. There are many heated opinions on this matter, with no supporting evidence.

More complex magnetic devices have also been studied, not for home use but use in physicians' offices and hospitals. A special form of electromagnetic therapy, repetitive transcranial magnetic stimulation (rTMS), is particularly closely studied. Repetitive transcranial magnetic stimulation is designed specifically to treat the brain with low-frequency magnetic pulses. A large body of small studies suggests that rTMS might be beneficial for

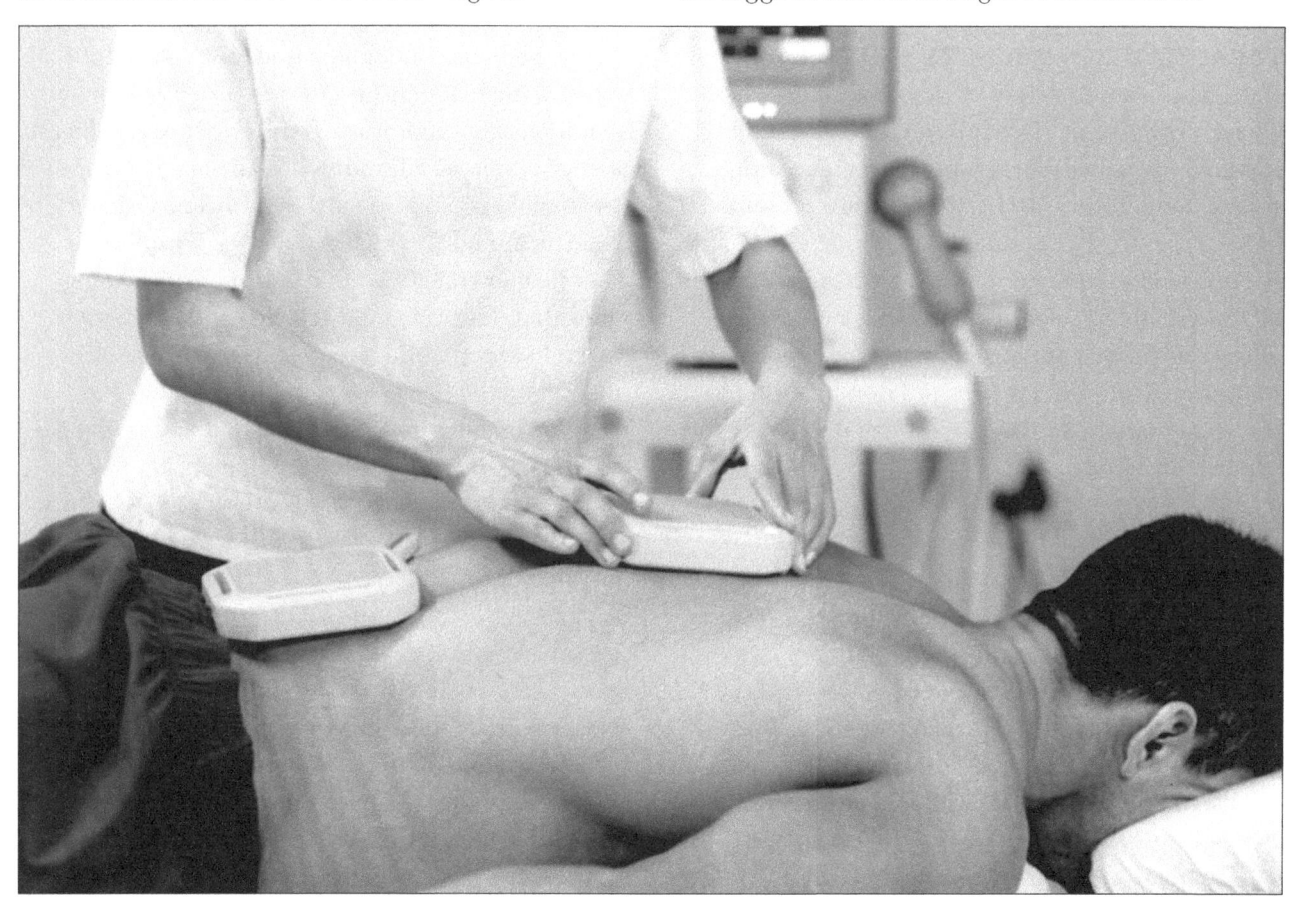

Magnet therapy involves placing different kinds of magnets on the body to increase overall health. Photo via iStock/microgen. [Used under license.]

depression. It is also being studied for the treatment of amyotrophic lateral sclerosis (ALS), Parkinson's disease, epilepsy, schizophrenia, and obsessive-compulsive disorder.

MECHANISM OF ACTION

Many commercial magnets have such a weak field that it is hard to believe they could affect the body. Some, however, are quite powerful and could conceivably cause effects at some depth. Nonetheless, biophysicists are skeptical that static magnets could significantly affect the body. The moving magnetic fields of rTMS and pulsed electromagnetic therapy, or PEMF, act differently. There is little doubt that they can affect nerve tissue and possibly other body parts.

PARACELSUS ON MAGNETS AND DISEASE

Physician-botanist-alchemist Paracelsus (1493-1541), an early proponent of what is now called "magnet therapy," discusses the use of magnets in treating disease in humans. Two perspectives are presented here.

Fortified by experience, which is the mistress of all things, and by mature theory, based on experience, I affirm that the Magnet is a stone which not only undeniably attracts steel and iron but also has the same power over the matter of all diseases in the whole body of man.

By the attractive power of a magnet acting upon the diseased aura of the blood in an affected part, that aura may be made to return into the center from which it originated and be absorbed therein, and thereby we may destroy the herd of the virus and cure the patient, and we need not wait idly to see what Nature will do. The magnet is therefore useful in all inflammations, in fluxes and ulcerations, in diseases of the bowels and uterus, in internal and external disease.

A commonly held misconception is that magnets attract the iron in blood cells, thus moving the blood and stimulating circulation. However, the iron in the blood is not in a magnetic form. Static magnets could affect charged particles in the blood, nerves, and cell membranes or subtly alter biochemical reactions. However, whether the effect is strong enough to make a difference remains to be shown. Some research results suggest that static magnets affect local blood circulation. Still, a rigorously designed double-blind trial found that commercially available static magnets do not affect blood flow. Another well-designed trial also failed to find effects on blood circulation. However, some weak evidence shows that static magnets may affect muscle metabolism. Further research will be necessary to sort out these possibilities.

SCIENTIFIC EVIDENCE

Static magnets. In double-blind, placebo-controlled trials, static magnets have shown promise for some conditions, but in no case is the evidence reliable. In a 2007 review of all studies of static magnets as a treatment for pain, researchers concluded that there is no meaningful evidence that they are effective; they further concluded that current evidence suggests that, for some pain-related conditions, static magnets are not effective (a much stronger statement than the first).

Some magnet proponents claim that it is impossible to carry out a truly double-blinded study on magnets because participants can simply use a metal pin or a similar object to discover whether they have a real magnet or not. Some researchers have gotten around this by using a weak magnet as the placebo treatment. Other researchers have designed more complicated placebo devices that participants have been found unable to identify as fake treatments.

Rheumatoid arthritis. A double-blind, controlled trial of sixty-four people with rheumatoid arthritis of the knee compared the effects of strong alternating polarity magnets with the effects of a weak unipolar magnet. Researchers used the weakened magnet as a control group so that participants would not find it easy to break the blind by testing the magnetism of their treatment.

After one week of therapy, 68 percent of the participants using the strong magnets (the treatment group) reported relief, compared with 27 percent in the control group. This difference was statistically significant. Two of four other subjective measurements of disease severity also showed statistically significant improvements. However, no significant improvements were seen in objective evaluations of the condition, such as blood tests for inflammation severity or physician's assessment of joint tenderness, swelling, or range of motion. This study suggests that magnet therapy may reduce the pain of rheumatoid arthritis without altering actual inflammation. However, the mixture of statistically significant and insignificant results indicates that a larger trial is necessary to factor out "statistical noise."

Postpolio syndrome. A double-blind, placebo-controlled study of fifty people with post-polio syndrome found evidence that magnets effectively relieve pain. For forty-five minutes, the magnets or placebo magnets were placed on previously determined trigger points (one per person). Trigger points are sore areas within a muscle that, when pressed, cause relief in other areas of the muscle and, conversely, when inflamed, cause pain in other parts of the muscle. In the treatment group, 76 percent of the participants reported improvement, compared with 19 percent in the placebo group.

Fibromyalgia. A six-month, double-blind, placebo-controlled trial of 119 people with fibromyalgia compared two commercially available magnetic mattress pads with sham and no treatment. Group 1 used a mattress pad designed to create a uniform magnetic field of negative polarity. Group 2 used a mattress pad that varied in polarity. In both groups, the researchers followed the manufacturer's instructions. Groups 3 and 4 used sham treatments designed to match in appearance the magnets used in groups 1 and 2. Group 5 received no treatment.

On average, participants in all groups showed improvement in the six months of the study. Participants in the treatment groups, especially group 1, showed a trend toward greater improvement; however, the differences between real treatment and sham or no treatment failed to reach statistical significance in most measures. This outcome suggests that magnetic mattress pads might be helpful for fibromyalgia. Still, a larger study would be necessary to identify the benefits.

An earlier double-blind, placebo-controlled study of thirty women with fibromyalgia did find significant improvement with magnets compared with placebo. The women slept on magnetic mattress pads (or sham pads for the control group) for four months. Of the twenty-five women who completed the trial, participants sleeping on the experimental mattress pads experienced a significant decrease in pain and fatigue compared with the placebo group, along with significant improvement in sleep and physical functioning.

A single-blind study of somewhat intricate design provides weak evidence that a gown made from a special "electromagnetic shielding fabric" can reduce fibromyalgia symptoms. The rationale for using this fabric is, however, somewhat scientifically implausible.

Peripheral neuropathy. A four-month, double-blind, placebo-controlled, crossover study of nineteen people with peripheral neuropathy found a significant reduction in symptoms compared with placebo. Participants wore magnetic foot insoles during the day throughout the trial period. Reduction in burning, numbness, and tingling symptoms was especially marked in those cases of neuropathy associated with diabetes.

Based on these results, the same researchers performed a far larger randomized, placebo-controlled follow-up study. This trial enrolled 375 people with peripheral neuropathy caused by diabetes. It tested the effectiveness of four months of treatment with magnetic insoles. The results indicated that the insoles produced benefits beyond the placebo effect, reducing symptoms such as burning pain, numbness, tingling, and exercise-induced pain.

Surgery support. A double-blind, placebo-controlled study looked at the effect of magnets on healing after plastic surgery. The study examined the use of magnets on twenty persons who had suction lipectomy (liposuction). Magnets in patches were placed over the operative region immediately after surgery and left in place for fourteen days. The treatment group experienced a statistically significant reduction of pain and swelling on postoperative days one through four and discoloration on days one through three, compared with the control group. However, another study of 165 people failed to find that using static magnets over the surgical incision reduced postsurgical pain. Furthermore, the positioning of static magnets at the acupuncture/acupressure point P6 in persons undergoing ear, nose, and throat or gynecological surgeries reduced nausea and vomiting no better than placebo in a randomized trial.

Low back pain and other forms of chronic musculoskeletal pain. A double-blind, placebo-controlled, crossover trial of fifty-four people with knee or back pain compared a complex static magnet array with a sham magnet array. Participants used either the real or the sham device for twenty-four hours; after a seven-day rest period, they used the opposite therapy for another twenty-four hours. Evaluations showed that using the real magnet was associated with greater improvements than the sham treatment.

Benefits were also seen in a double-blind, placebo-controlled trial of forty-three people with chronic knee pain who continuously used high-power but otherwise ordinary static magnets for two weeks. In another placebo-controlled trial, using a magnetic knee wrap for twelve weeks was associated with a significant increase in quadriceps (thigh muscle) strength in persons with knee osteoarthritis.

A double-blind, placebo-controlled, crossover study of twenty people who had chronic low back pain for a minimum of six months failed to find any evidence of benefit. However, this study's alternating-pole magnet produced a weak magnetic field. Another study found some benefits that failed to reach statistical significance.

In a double-blind study of 101 people with chronic neck and shoulder pain, using a magnetic necklace failed to prove more effective than the placebo treatment. Another study failed to find magnetic insoles helpful for heel pain.

Osteoarthritis. A widely publicized twelve-week study of 194 people reportedly found that using magnetic bracelets reduced osteoarthritis pain in the hip and knee. However, the study found statistically similar benefits among participants given placebo treatment. The researchers suggest that this failure to show superior effects may have been caused, in part, by an error: The study utilized weak magnets as the placebo treatments, but thirty-four persons in the placebo group accidentally received strong magnets instead. This would tend to decrease the difference in outcome seen between the treatment and the placebo group and could therefore hide a real treatment benefit. Nonetheless, this study does not provide evidence that magnetic bracelets offer any benefit for osteoarthritis beyond the placebo effect.

A much smaller study also failed to find statistically significant benefits. Still, it was too small to produce statistically meaningful results. Rather, it was designed to evaluate a special placebo magnet device. After the study, researchers polled the participants to see if they could correctly identify whether they had been given the real treatment or the placebo: They could not.

Pelvic pain. A double-blind, placebo-controlled study of fourteen women with chronic pelvic pain (from endometriosis or other causes) found no significant benefit when magnets were applied to abdominal trigger points for two weeks. However, statistical analysis showed that it would have been necessary to enroll a larger number of participants to detect an effect. A larger study did find some evidence of benefit after four weeks of treatment. Still, a high dropout rate and other design problems compromise the meaningfulness of the results. Another small study found possible evidence of benefits in menstrual pain.

Carpal tunnel syndrome. A double-blind, placebo-controlled study of thirty people with carpal tunnel syndrome found that a single treatment with a static magnet produced dramatic and long-lasting benefits. However, identical dramatic benefits were seen in the placebo group. In two more small, randomized trials, researchers again found no differences between the treatment and the placebo groups. Both groups experienced similar improvements in symptoms.

In a small study involving thirty-one people with long-standing carpal tunnel syndrome, a combination of static magnet and pulsed electromagnetic field therapy modestly improved deep pain but had no significant effect on overall pain in two months.

Sports performance. People who undergo intense exercise often experience muscle soreness afterward. One study tested magnet therapy for reducing this symptom. However, while the use of magnets did reduce muscle soreness, so did placebo treatment, and there was no significant difference between the effectiveness of magnets and placebo. Another study of more complex design also failed to find benefits.

Magnetic insoles have been advocated for increasing sports performance. However, a study of fourteen college athletes failed to find that magnetic insoles improved vertical jump, bench squat, forty-yard dash, or performance of a soccer-specific fitness test.

Pulsed electromagnetic field therapy. Pulsed electromagnetic field therapy (PEMF) is quite distinct from magnet therapy. (The term "electromagnetic field" does not, in this case, refer to magnetism in the ordinary sense.) For historical reasons, PEMF is often classified with true magnetic therapies.

Bone has a remarkable capacity to heal from injury. In some cases, though, the broken ends do not join, leading to what are called "nonunion fractures." Pulsed electromagnetic field therapy has been used to stimulate bone repair in union and other fractures since the 1970s; this is a relatively accepted use. This therapy has shown promise for osteoarthritis, stress incontinence, and possibly other conditions.

Osteoarthritis. Three double-blind, placebo-controlled studies enrolling more than 350 people suggest that PEMF therapy can improve symptoms of osteoarthritis. For example, a double-blind, placebo-controlled study tested PEMF in eighty-six people, with osteoarthritis of the knee and eighty-one with osteoarthritis of the cervical spine. Participants received eighteen half-hour sessions with either a PEMF machine or a sham device. The treated participants showed significantly greater improvements in disease severity than those given a placebo. For both osteoarthritis conditions, benefits lasted for a minimum of one month after treatment was stopped.

A later double-blind trial evaluated low-power, extremely low-frequency PEMF for the treatment of knee osteoarthritis. A total of 176 people received eight sessions of either sham or real treatment for two weeks. The results showed significantly greater pain reduction in the treated group.

Urinary incontinence. Many women experience stress incontinence, the leakage of urine following any action that puts pressure on the bladder. Laughter, physical exercise, and coughing can all trigger this unpleasant occurrence. A recent study suggests that PEMF treatment might be helpful. In this placebo-controlled study, researchers applied high-intensity pulsating magnetic fields to sixty-two women with stress incontinence. The intention was to stimulate the nerves that control the pelvic muscles.

The high-intensity magnetic field used in this treatment created electrical currents in the pelvic muscles and nerves. The results showed that one session of magnetic stimulation significantly reduced episodes of urinary leakage over the following week compared with a placebo. In the treated group, 74 percent experienced significant improvement, compared with only 32 percent in the placebo group. This was confirmed by an objective examination of thirteen participants, which found that magnetic stimulation increased the strength of closure at the exit from the bladder. However, there was one serious flaw in this study: It does not appear to have been double-blind. Researchers knew which participants were getting real treatment and which were not and, therefore, might have unconsciously biased their observations to conform to their expectations. Thus, the promise of electromagnetic therapy for stress incontinence still needs to be validated in properly designed trials.

Similarly, magnetic stimulation has been studied to treat bed-wetting (nocturnal enuresis). In a small preliminary study, using PEMF day and night for two months was helpful in girls.

Multiple sclerosis. A two-month, double-blind, placebo-controlled study of thirty people with multiple sclerosis was conducted using a PEMF device. Participants were instructed to tape the device to one of three acupuncture points on the shoulder, back, or hip. The study found statistically significant improvements in the treatment group, most notably in bladder control, hand function, and muscle spasticity. Benefits were seen in another small study too.

Erectile dysfunction. In a three-week, double-blind, placebo-controlled trial, twenty men with erectile dysfunction received PEMF therapy or a placebo. The magnetic therapy was administered through a small box worn near the genital area and kept in place as continuously as possible during the study period; neither participants nor observers knew whether the device was activated or not. The results showed that using PEMF significantly improved sexual function compared with a placebo.

Migraines. In a double-blind trial, forty-two people with migraine headaches were given treatment with real or placebo PEMF therapy to the inner thighs for one hour, five times per week for two weeks. The results showed benefits in headache frequency and severity. However, the study design was rather convoluted and nonstandard, so the results are difficult to interpret.

Postoperative pain. In a small, randomized trial, eighty women undergoing breast augmentation surgery were divided into three groups. The first group received PEMF therapy seven days after surgery on both breasts, the second group received fake PEMF therapy for both breasts as a control, and the third group received real and fake PEMF therapy for either breast. Compared to the control, women receiving PEMF therapy reported significantly less discomfort. They used fewer pain medications by the third postoperative day.

HOW MAGNET THERAPY MIGHT WORK

No scientific theory or manufacturer claim about how magnet therapy might work has been proven. Although some preliminary research has been conducted in animals and small clinical trials, the mechanisms by which magnets might affect the human body are unknown. Scientific researchers and magnet manufacturers have proposed that magnets might work by:

- Changing how nerve cells function and blocking pain signals to the brain

- Restoring the balance between cell death and growth
- Increasing the flow of blood and the delivery of oxygen and nutrients to tissues
- Increasing the temperature of the area of the body being treated

Electromagnetic therapy. Unlike PEMF, repetitive transcranial magnetic stimulation (rTMS) involves magnetic fields and is more closely related to standard magnet therapy. Repetitive transcranial magnetic stimulation, which involves applying low-frequency magnetic pulses to the brain, has been investigated for treating emotional illnesses and other conditions that originate in the brain. The results of preliminary studies have been generally promising.

Depression. About twenty small studies have evaluated rTMS for the treatment of depression, including severe depression that does not respond to standard treatment and the depressive phase of bipolar illness, and most found it effective. In one of these studies, seventy people with major depression were given rTMS or sham rTMS in a double-blind setting of two weeks. The results showed that participants who received actual treatment experienced significantly greater improvement than those receiving sham treatment. In a far larger study involving 301 depressed persons, none of whom were being treated with antidepressant medications, real rTMS was significantly more effective than fake rTMS after four to six weeks.

In another trial involving ninety-two elderly persons whose depression had been linked to poor blood flow to the brain (vascular depression), actual rTMS was significantly more effective than sham rTMS. Benefits were more notable in younger participants. In a particularly persuasive piece of evidence, researchers pooled the results of thirty double-blind trials involving 1,164 depressed persons. They determined that real rTMS was significantly more effective than sham rTMS.

Two separate studies suggest that rTMS may be an effective additional treatment for the 20 to 30 percent of depressed people for whom conventional drug therapy is not successful. Electroconvulsive therapy (shock treatment) is often used for people in this category, but rTMS may be an equally effective alternative. Another group of researchers pooled the results of twenty-four studies involving 1,092 persons and found rTMS more effective than sham for treatment-resistant depression.

Epilepsy. In a double-blind, placebo-controlled trial, twenty-four people with epilepsy (technically, partial complex seizures or secondarily generalized seizures) not fully responsive to drug treatment were given treatment with rTMS or sham rTMS twice daily for one week. The results showed a mild reduction in seizures among the people given real rTMS. However, the benefits rapidly disappeared when treatment was stopped. Similarly, short-lived effects were seen in an open trial.

Schizophrenia. A double-blind, placebo-controlled, crossover trial looked at the use of low-frequency rTMS in twelve people diagnosed with schizophrenia and manifesting frequent and treatment-resistant auditory hallucinations (hearing voices). Participants received rTMS for four days, with the length of treatment building from four minutes on the first day to sixteen minutes on the fourth day. Active stimulation significantly reduced the incidence of auditory hallucinations compared with sham stimulation. The extent of the benefit varied widely, lasting from one day in one participant to two months in another. Possible benefits were seen in other small studies. Researchers pooling the results of six controlled trials, which involved 232 persons with schizophrenia resistant to conventional treatment, found that real, low-frequency rTMS was significantly better at reducing auditory hallucinations than sham rTMS.

Parkinson's disease. In a double-blind, placebo-controlled trial of ninety-nine people with Parkinson's disease, real rTMS was more effective than sham rTMS delivered in eight weekly treatments. Similar benefits were seen in three other small studies. Even more encouraging, the combined results of ten randomized trials in persons with Parkinson's indicated significant benefit for rTMS (using higher frequencies).

Chronic pain syndromes. Repetitive transcranial magnetic stimulation technology has also been applied to areas other than the brain. Myofascial pain syndrome is a condition similar to fibromyalgia but is more localized. Whereas fibromyalgia involves tender trigger points all over the body, myofascial pain syndrome only involves trigger points clustered in one portion of the body. One controlled trial found indications that repetitive magnetic stimulation applied to the painful area may be effective for myofascial pain syndrome of the trapezius muscle.

In a placebo controlled trial involving sixty-one people with long-standing diabetes, low-frequency repetitive magnetic stimulation failed to diminish the pain associated with diabetic peripheral neuropathy. However, in another study involving twenty-eight people with peripheral neuropathy, high-frequency rTMS applied to the brain was more effective at reducing pain and improving quality of life than was fake rTMS.

Tinnitus. One preliminary study found indications that rTMS may be helpful for tinnitus (ringing in the ear).

Post-traumatic stress disorder. A small, double-blind, placebo-controlled study found that the use of rTMS may be able to reduce symptoms of post-traumatic stress disorder.

Cigarette addiction. A small, double-blind, placebo-controlled study found evidence that rTMS may reduce cigarette craving in people attempting to quit smoking.

Obsessive-compulsive disorder. A double-blind, placebo-controlled study of eighteen people with obsessive-compulsive disorder found no evidence of benefit with rTMS.

Amyotrophic lateral sclerosis. Amyotrophic lateral sclerosis also called "Lou Gehrig's disease," is a nerve disorder that causes progressive muscle weakness. A small pilot study hinted that rTMS might be beneficial, at least temporarily.

HOW TO USE MAGNET THERAPY

The following is a brief description of the use of magnet therapy. However, one should remember that the ways that magnets are used have not been fully evaluated by long-term clinical testing. A full medical evaluation is advisable before using magnets. One should not treat a painful back with magnets if the underlying cause of pain is a fracture or a tumor.

Types of magnets. There are several theories on the best size and type of magnets to use and where to apply them, based on the treatment type and other factors. Because unipolar magnets have a greater magnetic field penetration depth, some researchers consider these more effective in treating deeper tissues. Conversely, it is considered that alternating-pole magnet devices might be more effective at stimulating surface tissue. Thus, it might be appropriate to use a unipolar high-gauss magnet for low back pain that originates deep in the tissue and an alternating-pole configuration for an injury closer to the surface, such as a wrist sprain. However, there is no meaningful scientific evidence to support these distinctions.

In addition, some practitioners hold that the north side of the magnet calms and the south side excites and that using the right side of the magnet is crucial. However, from a scientific perspective, it is difficult to see how there could be any difference between the two poles of the magnet in terms of the effect on body tissue.

There is a consensus that the magnet should be placed as close to the affected part of the body as possible. Taping the magnet to the skin, slipping the magnet inside a bandage over the affected area, or applying a wrap with embedded magnets mitigates this problem.

Taping magnets to the body might irritate the skin; some research scientists and practitioners also suspect that the body may accommodate the magnetic field over time, thus reducing the therapeutic effect. To prevent irritation and the accommodation, practitioners usually recommend intermittent use, such as five days on, two days off, or twelve hours on, twelve hours off.

Magnetic devices available. Manufacturers make a wide range of magnetic devices. For treating large areas of the body, wraps, and belts containing magnets are available. Wraps are designed for the wrist, elbow, knee, ankle, neck, shoulder, and back. They are often made from thermal material to have the added effect of warming the area. These wraps are often recommended in cases of injury and arthritis, where heat feels better. Proponents of magnet therapy often recommend using magnetic mattress pads and mattresses for people with problems affecting several areas of the body, such as fibromyalgia or arthritis; they also recommend magnetic mattress pads for insomnia and fatigue.

Proponents of magnet therapy recommend magnetic foot insoles for people with diabetic peripheral neuropathy, leg aches and pains, circulatory problems of the lower extremities, or foot injuries and problems, and for people who stand all day. Magnetic necklaces are believed to relieve neck and shoulder pain and generalized aches and pains, and magnetic bracelets are advocated for wrist pain and general problems. However, a 2007 systematic review of static magnet studies in the Canadian Medical Association Journal debunked this belief, stating: "The evidence does not support the use of static magnets for pain relief, and therefore magnets cannot be recommended as an effective treatment."

SAFETY ISSUES

In general, magnets appear safe; the biggest risk appears to be skin irritation from any tape that is used to hold them in place. Magnetic resonance imaging (MRI) machines, for example, expose the body to gigantic magnetic fields, and extensive investigation has found no evidence of harm. However, during the MRI, a person is subjected to a high level of magnetism for a short period. In contrast, people who use static magnets daily or sleep on them every night are subjected to a low level of magnetism over a long period. It is not known whether this type of exposure has any harmful effects. Nonetheless, one study in which participants slept on a magnetic mattress pad every night for four months found no side effects. In addition, a safety study of rTMS found no evidence of harm. No significant adverse effects were reported in a large study in which rTMS was administered to numerous people with depression, totaling more than ten thousand cumulative treatment sessions. Transient headache and scalp discomfort were the most frequent problems reported. There were no seizures or changes in hearing or cognition.

It was previously thought that persons with an implantable cardioverter-defibrillator (ICD) or a pacemaker should not use magnetic devices, but this recommendation has been adjusted. One study found that except for magnetic mattresses and mattress pads, most magnets sold for therapeutic purposes do not interfere with the magnetically activated switches in most pacemakers. Magnetic mattress pads can deactivate and alter the function of ICDs and pacemakers. Still, other therapeutic magnets are safe if kept six inches or farther from these devices.

There are theoretical concerns that magnets might be risky for people with epilepsy. Similarly, until the physiological effects of magnet treatments are better understood, pregnant women should avoid them.

—*EBSCO CAM Review Board*

Further Reading

Abdulla, Fuad A., et al. "Effects of Pulsed Low-Frequency Magnetic Field Therapy on Pain Intensity in Patients with Musculoskeletal Chronic Low Back Pain: Study Protocol for a Randomised Double-Blind Placebo-Controlled Trial." *BMJ Open*, vol. 9, no. 6, 9 June 2019, doi:10.1136/bmjopen-2018-024650.

Kulish, Peter. *Conquering Pain: The Art of Healing with BioMagnetism*. 6th ed., BioMag Science, 2016.

"Magnets for Pain." *National Center for Complementary and Integrative Health*. US Department of Health and Human Services, 27 Dec. 2017, nccih.nih.gov/Health/magnets-for-pain.

Palermo, Elizabeth. "Does Magnetic Therapy Work?" *LiveScience*. Future US, Inc., 12 Feb. 2015, www.livescience.com/40174-magnetic-therapy.html.

Pittler, Max H., et al. "Static Magnets for Reducing Pain: Systematic Review and Meta-Analysis of Randomized Trials." *CMAJ: Canadian Medical Association Journal = Journal de l'Association Medicale Canadienne*, vol. 177, no. 7, 2007, pp. 736-42, doi:10.1503/cmaj.061344.

Sandoiu, Ana. "Treating Pain with Magnetic Fields." *Medical News Today*. MediLexicon International, 9 Aug. 2018, www.medicalnewstoday.com/articles/322718.php#1.

Vadalà, Maria, et al. "Mechanisms and Therapeutic Effectiveness of Pulsed Electromagnetic Field Therapy in Oncology." *Cancer Medicine*, vol. 5, no. 11, 17 Oct. 2016, pp. 3128-39, doi:10.1002/cam4.861.

PROLOTHERAPY

Category: Therapies and techniques
Related term: Sclerotherapy
Specialties and related fields: Alternative and complementary medicine, athletic training, chiropractic, occupational therapy, physical therapy

Definition: treatment involving injections of chemical irritant solutions into the area around a loose ligament

KEY TERMS

ligaments: a short band of tough, flexible fibrous connective tissue that connects two bones or cartilages or holds together a joint

myofascial release: an alternative medicine therapy claimed to be useful for treating skeletal muscle immobility and pain by relaxing contracted muscles, improving blood and lymphatic circulation, and stimulating the stretch reflex in muscles

tendons: a flexible but inelastic cord of strong fibrous collagen tissue attaching a muscle to a bone

OVERVIEW

Invented in the 1950s by George Hackett, prolotherapy is based on the theory that chronic pain is often caused by the laxness of ligaments responsible for keeping a joint stable. When ligaments and associated tendons are loose, the body is said to compensate by using muscles to stabilize the joint. According to prolotherapy theory, the net result is muscle spasms and pain.

Prolotherapy treatment involves injecting chemical irritant solutions into the area around such ligaments. These solutions are believed to cause tissue to proliferate (grow), increasing the strength and thickness of ligaments. Increased strength and thickness of ligaments presumably tighten up the joint and relieve the burden on associated muscles, stopping muscle spasms. In the case of arthritic joints, increased ligament strength would allow the joint to function more efficiently, thus reducing pain.

Prolotherapy has not been widely accepted in conventional medicine. Prolotherapy practitioners use the technique to treat many conditions, including back pain, osteoarthritis, fibromyalgia, plantar fasciitis, sciatica, sports injuries, temporomandibular joint disorder, tendonitis, and tension headaches.

Most studies have focused on its use in back pain and osteoarthritis. Still, the evidence does not support its effectiveness.

How is prolotherapy performed? Prolotherapy is generally administered at four to six weeks intervals, although studies have used a more frequent schedule. The treatment involves the injection of a mixture containing an irritant and a local anesthetic. A total of four to six treatments is typical. When treating back pain, prolotherapy practitioners frequently use a form of manipulation similar to chiropractic. However, the manipulation is applied after a local anesthetic has been injected and is somewhat intense.

There are several irritant solutions used in prolotherapy. Concentrated dextrose or glucose has become increasingly popular because it is completely nontoxic. Phenol (a potentially toxic substance) and glycerin are also sometimes used. Other nonirritant substances may be added to the solution, such as vitamin B_{12}, corn extracts, cod liver oil extracts, zinc, and manganese; however, there is no evidence that these substances add any benefit.

SCIENTIFIC EVIDENCE
Some animal and human studies have found that prolotherapy injections increase the strength and thickness of ligaments. Six double-blind human trials of prolotherapy have been reported: four involving back pain (with mixed results) and the other two involving osteoarthritis (with positive results).

Back pain. Although two studies have suggested prolotherapy may be effective for low back pain, two more recent studies found prolotherapy to be ineffective. In a review of five studies, three found prolotherapy to be no more effective than control treatments for low back pain. The other two studies suggested that prolotherapy was more effective than control treatments when used with spinal manipulation and exercise therapies. Another review suggested that prolotherapy may be effective with other therapies but not when used alone.

When used alone, prolotherapy is probably no more effective than a placebo injection to treat low back pain. However, there is evidence that the technique may be beneficial when combined with other therapies.

Osteoarthritis. A double-blind, placebo-controlled study evaluated the effects of three prolotherapy injections (using a 10 percent dextrose solution) at two-month intervals in sixty-eight people with knee osteoarthritis. At the six-month follow-up, participants who had received prolotherapy showed significant improvements in pain at rest and while walking. These participants also showed reduced swelling and fewer episodes of "buckling" than those who had received placebo treatment.

The same research group performed a similar double-blind trial of twenty-seven people with osteoarthritis in the hands. The six-month follow-up results showed that range of motion and pain with movement improved significantly in the treated group compared with the placebo group.

SAFETY ISSUES
In studies, prolotherapy has not caused any serious, irreversible injury. After each injection, the discomfort usually lasts for a few minutes to several days, but this discomfort is seldom severe. More concerning is that severe headaches have been reported in treating low back pain in a minority of patients. Also, because phenol is potentially toxic, treatment with a dextrose solution alone is preferable.

CHOOSING A PRACTITIONER
Prolotherapy is practiced by a medical doctor or a doctor of osteopathy. Generally, physicians specializing in orthopedics or physical medicine and rehabilitation are most likely to practice prolotherapy.

—*EBSCO CAM Review Board*

Further Reading

Bauer, Brent A. "Prolotherapy: Solution to Low Back Pain?" *Mayo Clinic*, 25 May 2018, www.mayoclinic.org/prolotherapy/expert-answers/faq-20058347.

Delzell, Emily. "Prolotherapy for Osteoarthritis." *Arthritis Foundation*, www.arthritis.org/diseases/more-about/prolotherapy-for-osteoarthritis.

Fletcher, Jenna. "Prolotherapy: Uses, Side Effects, and Costs." *Medical News Today*, 17 Dec. 2017, www.medicalnewstoday.com/articles/320330.

Hackett, George Stuart, et al. *Ligament and Tendon Relaxation: Treated by Prolotherapy*. Institute in Basic Life Principles, 1993.

Sports and Fitness Recovery

Category: Condition

Specialties and related fields: Athletic training, dietetics, nutritionist, personal training, physical therapy, strength and conditioning

Definition: treatment to aid recovery from the side effects of intense exercise and physical training

KEY TERMS

collagen: the main structural protein found in skin and other connective tissues, widely used in purified form for cosmetic surgical treatments

exercise recovery: the period between the end of a bout of exercise and the subsequent return to a resting or recovered state

herb: a plant or plant part used for its scent, flavor, or therapeutic properties

supplement: a nutritional product, such as vitamin, mineral, herb, amino acid, or enzyme, taken orally that augments someone's diet to ensure that their nutritional needs are satisfactorily met

vitamin: a nutrient that the body needs in small amounts to function and stay healthy

INTRODUCTION

In the competitive world of sports, the smallest advantage can make an enormous difference in the hundredths of seconds that can determine the outcome of a contest. A dietary supplement that can improve an athlete's strength, speed, and endurance can make the difference between tenth place and first place in a world-class, competitive race.

Supplements may play another beneficial role for athletes: aiding recovery from the side effects of intense exercise. While exercise of moderate intensity is almost undoubtedly a purely positive activity, high-intensity endurance exercise, such as running marathons can cause respiratory infections and damage parts of the body. In addition, all forms of exercise, when carried to an extreme, can cause severe muscle soreness, which may, in turn, affect training. Herbs and supplements advocated for these problems are discussed here.

PRINCIPAL PROPOSED NATURAL TREATMENTS

Extremely intense exercise, such as training for and running a marathon, also may decrease immunity; endurance athletes frequently become ill after maximum exertion. Vitamin C might help prevent this, although not all studies agree.

According to a double-blind, placebo-controlled study involving ninety-two runners, taking 600 milligrams (mg) of vitamin C for twenty-one days before a race significantly reduced the incidence of sickness afterward. Within two weeks of the end of the race, 68 percent of the runners taking a placebo developed symptoms of a common cold. In contrast, only 33 percent of those taking a vitamin C supplement developed cold symptoms. As part of the same study, nonrunners of similar genders and ages were given vitamin C or a placebo. For this group, the supplement had no apparent effect on upper respiratory infections. Vitamin C seemed to be specifically effective in this capacity for those who exercised intensively.

Two other studies found that vitamin C could reduce the number of colds experienced by groups of people involved in a rigorous exercise in extremely cold environments. One study involved 139 children attending a skiing camp in the Swiss Alps. At the same time, the other enrolled fifty-six military men engaged in a training exercise in Northern Canada during the winter months. In both cases, the participants took either 1 gram (g) of vitamin C or a placebo daily when their training program began. Cold symptoms were monitored for one to two weeks following training, and researchers found significant differences in favor of vitamin C. However, one large study of 674 US Marine Corps recruits found no such benefit. The results showed no difference in colds between the treatment and placebo groups.

There are many possible explanations for this discrepancy. Perhaps basic training in the Marine Corps is significantly different from other forms of exercise studied. Another point to consider is that the recruits did not start taking vitamin C at the beginning of training but waited three weeks before doing so. The study also lasted a bit longer than the earlier positive studies. Perhaps vitamin C is more effective at preventing colds in the short term. Of course, another possibility may be that vitamin C does not work.

OTHER PROPOSED NATURAL TREATMENTS

Glutamine is an important fuel source for some immune system cells. Like vitamin C, the amino acid glutamine may help prevent the infections that may take place after strenuous exercise. Some evidence suggests that athletes who have trained very hard experience lower-than-usual glutamine levels in their blood. One double-blind clinical trial involving 151 athletes found that supplementation with 5 g of glutamine immediately after heavy exercise and another 5 g two hours later reduced the incidence of infections significantly. Only 19 percent of those taking glutamine reported infections, while 51 percent of the placebo group succumbed to illness.

Probiotics are healthy organisms found in the digestive tract. Not only can they help prevent intestinal infections, but they also appear to help prevent colds. In a double-blind, controlled trial involving twenty healthy, elite distance runners, researchers found that a probiotic supplement (Lactobacillus fermentum) given for four months during winter training significantly reduced the number and severity of respiratory symptoms compared with a placebo. Weaker evidence suggests that beta-sitosterol might also offer some promise for this purpose. However, thymus extract, another proposed immune booster for athletes, does not seem to work, according to a double-blind, placebo-controlled trial of sixty athletes.

Exercising increases the presence of free radicals, naturally occurring substances that can damage tissue. Some researchers have theorized that such damage may, in part, cause muscle soreness and perhaps muscle deterioration that can accompany a strenuous workout. Based on this theory, but with little direct evidence, various antioxidants have been proposed to help prevent muscle soreness or muscle damage. These antioxidants include astaxanthin plus lycopene, beta-carotene, cherry juice, coenzyme Q10, oligomeric proanthocyanidins, selenium, vitamin C, and vitamin E. One double-blind trial compared vitamin C, vitamin E, and placebo for muscle soreness in twenty-four male volunteers. Vitamin C relieved muscle soreness, but vitamin E did not. Two other studies failed to find C combined with E effective. Another study failed to find benefits with the algae-derived carotenoid astaxanthin.

One small double-blind study found that using a mixed amino acid reduced muscle soreness caused by endurance exercising of the arm. These researchers performed two studies. The first involved taking the amino acid thirty minutes before exercising; this study failed to observe any benefit. The second, more effective regimen added one dose immediately after exercise and two doses daily for the next four days. In addition, a specific family of amino acids, branched-chain amino acids, have shown some promise for reducing muscle damage after long-distance running.

The proteolytic enzyme supplement bromelain, used for sports injuries, has also been proposed to reduce muscle soreness after exercise. However, a double-blind, placebo-controlled trial that compared bromelain with placebo failed to find benefit. Another study using a mixed proteolytic enzyme supplement also failed to find benefits.

Collagen hydrolysate is a nutritional supplement that may benefit cartilage tissue in joints. In a randomized, placebo-controlled study involving healthy college athletes with joint pain, 10 g daily of collagen hydrolysate appeared to reduce the pain effectively over twenty-four weeks.

The supplement phosphatidylserine has also failed to prove effective for reducing muscle soreness after exercise, as have chondroitin and magnet therapy. In one study, the supplement glucosamine not only failed to prove effective for reducing exercise-induced muscle soreness; it increased soreness.

Athletes who train excessively may experience a condition called "overtraining syndrome." Symptoms include depression, fatigue, reduced performance, and physiologic signs of stress. Numerous supplements have been suggested as treatments for this condition, including glutamine and, most prominently, antioxidants, but none has been proven effective.

—*Bruce E. Johansen*

Further Reading

Arendt-Nielsen, L., et al. "A Double-Blind Randomized Placebo-Controlled Parallel-Group Study Evaluating the Effects of Ibuprofen and Glucosamine Sulfate on Exercise-Induced Muscle Soreness." *Journal of Musculoskeletal Pain*, vol. 15, 2007, pp. 21-28.

Avery, N. G., et al. "Effects of Vitamin E Supplementation on Recovery from Repeated Bouts of Resistance Exercise." *Journal of Strength and Conditioning Research*, vol. 17, 2003, pp. 801-9.

Beck, T. W., et al. "Effects of a Protease Supplement on Eccentric Exercise-Induced Markers of Delayed-Onset Muscle Soreness and Muscle Damage." *Journal of Strength and Conditioning Research*, vol. 21, 2007, pp. 661-67.

Bloomer, R. J., et al. "Astaxanthin Supplementation Does Not Attenuate Muscle Injury Following Eccentric Exercise in Resistance-Trained Men." *International Journal of Sport Nutrition and Exercise Metabolism*, vol. 15, 2005, pp. 401-12.

Braun, W. A., et al. "The Effects of Chondroitin Sulfate Supplementation on Indices of Muscle Damage Induced by Eccentric Arm Exercise." *Journal of Sports Medicine and Physical Fitness*, vol. 45, 2006, pp. 553-60.

Cox, A. J., et al. "Oral Administration of the Probiotic Lactobacillus Fermentum VRI-003 and Mucosal Immunity in Endurance Athletes." *British Journal of Sports Medicine*, vol. 44, 2010, pp. 222-26.

Koba, T., et al. "Branched-Chain Amino Acids Supplementation Attenuates the Accumulation of Blood Lactate Dehydrogenase During Distance Running." *Journal of Sports Medicine and Physical Fitness*, vol. 47, 2007, pp. 316-22.

Mastaloudis, A., et al. "Antioxidants Did Not Prevent Muscle Damage in Response to an Ultramarathon Run." *Medicine and Science in Sports and Exercise*, vol. 38, 2006, pp. 72-80.

Nosaka, K., et al. "Effects of Amino Acid Supplementation on Muscle Soreness and Damage." *International Journal of Sport Nutrition and Exercise Metabolism*, vol. 16, 2006, pp. 620-35.

Sports Injuries and Homeopathy

Category: Homeopathy

Specialties and related fields: Alternative and complementary medicine

Definition: the use of highly diluted remedies to treat injuries from sports and exercise

KEY TERMS

Arnica: a genus of perennial, herbaceous plants in the sunflower family that are used to make homeopathic preparations

belladonna: a drug prepared from the leaves and root of deadly nightshade, containing atropine

homeopathy: the treatment of disease by minute doses of natural substances that in a healthy person would produce symptoms of a disease

placebo: a harmless pill, medicine, or procedure prescribed more for the psychological benefit to the patient than for any physiological effect

Symphytum: a genus of flowering plants in the borage family, Boraginaceae, used to make homeopathic preparations

INTRODUCTION

Although vigorous exercise is one of the most important steps toward good health, it can also have side effects, ranging from muscle soreness to injury. While these adverse consequences of exercise can be minimized by graduated training and careful activity, problems may develop anyway. Homeopathic treatments (especially topical creams) are quite popular for sports-related conditions, and they have shown some promise in studies.

SCIENTIFIC EVALUATIONS OF HOMEOPATHIC REMEDIES

There is some evidence to support the use of homeopathic creams to treat sports injuries. However, studies of oral homeopathic remedies for exercise-induced muscle soreness have not been promising.

Topical combination of homeopathic treatments for sports injuries. Investigators performed a double-blind, placebo-controlled study of sixty-nine people with sports-related ankle sprains to test the efficacy of a combination homeopathic ointment. The product tested contains a combination of fourteen homeopathic preparations: Arnica montana, Calendula, Hamamelis, aconite, belladonna, Bellis perennis, Chamomilla, Echinacea angustifolia, E. purperea, millefolium, Hepar sulphuris calcareum, Mercurius solubilis, Symphytum, and Hypericum.

During the two-week trial, all of the participants received electrical muscle stimulation. The investigators also applied cream, either the treatment cream or placebo cream, seven times during the study. The results showed that people given the real treatment recovered more rapidly than those given a placebo.

In another double-blind, placebo-controlled study, researchers evaluated the effectiveness of the same homeopathic ointment and a modified version for the treatment of various mild to moderate sports injuries, including sprains. All the approximately one hundred participants in the trial had slight to moderate sports-induced injuries in the past four days. The investigators applied the first ointment (and a bandage) on day one of treatment. Then the participants applied the ointment twice daily for fourteen more days. The results were promising. By the end of the trial, participants who used either form of the ointment experienced significantly superior improvement, compared with those taking placebo, according to some but not all measures.

Oral homeopathic remedies for sports-related muscle soreness. A double-blind, placebo-controlled study tested homeopathic Arnica (30x) in 519 long-distance runners but did not find positive results. Participants took five pills twice daily, beginning the evening before a race and continuing for four successive days. Evaluation after the race showed that Arnica was no more effective than a placebo for reducing soreness or speeding recovery after a race. Earlier, much smaller studies had found some suggestions of benefit for long-distance runners. Still, the results were, in general, not statistically significant.

A double-blind, placebo-controlled study conducted in the physiotherapy department of a homeopathic hospital in England evaluated the efficacy of an oral homeopathic preparation in treating muscle soreness caused by stepping exercise. The remedy was a combination of *Arnica*, Rhus tox, and sarcolactic acid. The results showed no statistical difference between the treatment and control groups.

The homeopathic remedy *Hypericum* C200 is prepared from *Hypericum perforatum*. This preparation is used to relieve postsurgical pain. A randomized, double-blind, monocentric, placebo-controlled clinical trial examined the efficacy of *Hypericum* C200 in patients who had undergone lumbar sequestrectomy surgery. In this study, no significant differences between the experimental and placebo groups could be shown. However, those who took potentiated Hypericum in addition to usual pain management consumed lower amounts of analgesics.

TRADITIONAL HOMEOPATHIC TREATMENTS
Classical homeopathy offers many possible homeopathic treatments for sports injuries. These therapies are chosen based on various specific details of the person seeking treatment.

For injuries that are sensitive to touch and have shooting, violent, tingling, or cutting pain, and if the injured person feels worse at night and in the cold, that person may match the symptom picture for homeopathic Hypericum. An injury with symptoms like these suggests nerve involvement, indicating an urgent need for physician examination.

If the affected person feels worse when exposed to motion, drafts, and heat, and during the afternoon, and if the person experiences spasms, shooting pains, tearing sensations, jerking, trembling, swelling, redness, and heat, possibly with cold extremities, then they may fit the classic symptom picture for homeopathic belladonna. Suppose one has a sprain with a great deal of swelling and inflammation of the soft tissue around a joint. In that case, the homeopathic remedy *Arnica* might be recommended. *Arnica* is also commonly used as a remedy for exercise-induced muscle soreness.

A person with an injury to a bone, cartilage, or tendon aggravated by touch, motion, and pressure (while warmth helps) may fit the symptom picture for homeopathic *Symphytum*. Many homeopathic practitioners use *Symphytum* after *Arnica* if deep pain or soreness remains after the initial soreness has cleared. A person with stiff, painful muscles brought on by straining, overlifting, or getting wet when already hot and perspiring, and a person whose muscles seize up with rest but loosen with exercise and heat, may fit the traditional homeopathic indications for *Rhus tox*.

—*EBSCO CAM Review Board*

Further Reading
Plezbert, J. A., and J. R. Burke. "Effects of the Homeopathic Remedy Arnica on Attenuating Symptoms of Exercise-Induced Muscle Soreness." *Journal of Chiropractic Medicine*, vol. 4, 2005, pp. 152-61.

Raak, Christa K., et al. "*Hypericum perforatum* to Improve Postoperative Pain Outcome After Monosegmental Spinal Sequestrectomy (HYPOS): Results of a Randomized, Double-Blind, Placebo-Controlled Trial." *Journal of Integrative and Complementary Medicine*, vol. 28, no. 5, 2022, pp. 407-17, doi:10.1089/jicm.2021.0389.

Tveiten, D., and S. Bruset. "Effect of Arnica D30 in Marathon Runners." *Homeopathy*, vol. 92, 2003, pp. 187-89.

Vickers, A. J., et al. "Homeopathic Arnica 30x Is Ineffective for Muscle Soreness After Long-Distance Running." *Clinical Journal of Pain*, vol. 14, 1998, pp. 227-31.

———. "Homeopathy for Delayed Onset Muscle Soreness." *British Journal of Sports Medicine*, vol. 31, 1997, pp. 304-7.

TISSUE ENGINEERING

Category: Biology
Specialties and related fields: Cardiology, dermatology, gastroenterology, orthopedics, pulmonology, surgery, urology

Definition: an integrative technology that combines cells, tissue culture protocols, synthetic scaffolds, and engineering technologies to establish suitable biochemical and physiological conditions to grow tissues and organs under artificial conditions to improve or replace dead or dying tissues and organs

KEY TERMS

biodegradability: the artificial scaffold used to support the growth of bioengineered tissue should dissolve once the transplanted tissue takes hold

biological scaffold: made of polyester (plastic), collagen (protein), or other sources, is used as a structural framework for tissue engineering

biomaterials: replacements for body tissues, sometimes used as implants. Examples are engineered skin tissue, renal tissue, or cardiac implants; biomaterials can be made of metal alloys, plastic polymers, and living tissues like collagen

biomechanical considerations: environmental (space) considerations conducive to cellular growth and development; effective tissue engineering may occur when combined with a biological scaffold and a blend of growth factors

immune rejection: natural antibody response to foreign transplanted tissue; tissues engineered from the patient's own cells will not have this type of rejection

pluripotent stem cells: stem cells that can differentiate into any adult cell type

regenerative medicine: another term for tissue engineering, where biological properties are employed to maintain, repair, replace or enhance tissue function

INDICATIONS AND PROCEDURES

Cells are the basic units of biological life. When molecular, chemical, and electrical signals organize cells into functional groups, they become tissues. If tissues are damaged or nonfunctional, tissue engineers can apply the biological principles of tissue growth and development to produce replacement tissues. Tissue engineering, sometimes referred to as regenerative medicine, employs biological principles to repair, maintain, enhance, or replace tissue function.

Tissue engineers come from many science-related fields, applying life science and engineering principles to develop functional bioactive tissues that can be restorative. Biologists, scientists, and biomedical engineers can engineer tissue repair or produce new tissue if cellular responses to various extracellular and intercellular signals are comprehensively detailed and the biochemical properties involved with these events are understood. Effective understanding begins with proper intercellular communication from cells, tissues, and their surrounding environments. This communication and organization by groups of cells develop support structures that provide a matrix or scaffold.

Tissue development can occur within an environment conducive to growth and development, a blend of growth factors, and a biological scaffold. A building scaffold is used to support materials and work crews that aid in constructing, repairing, or maintaining structures like bridges or buildings. A biological scaffold made of plastic (polyester), protein, or other sources, is used for tissue engineering.

Biological scaffolds can be used for tissue engineering by stripping cells away from donor organs, leaving a collagen (protein) scaffold. Kidney, liver, lung, and heart tissue have been bioengineered using collagen scaffolds. A scaffold using human tissue or organs harvested from surgical techniques combined with an individual's cells could create bioengineered tissues or organs resistant to immunological rejection.

While cells fabricate a natural structural matrix, the engineered extracellular matrix (scaffold) provides structural integrity. An important biological

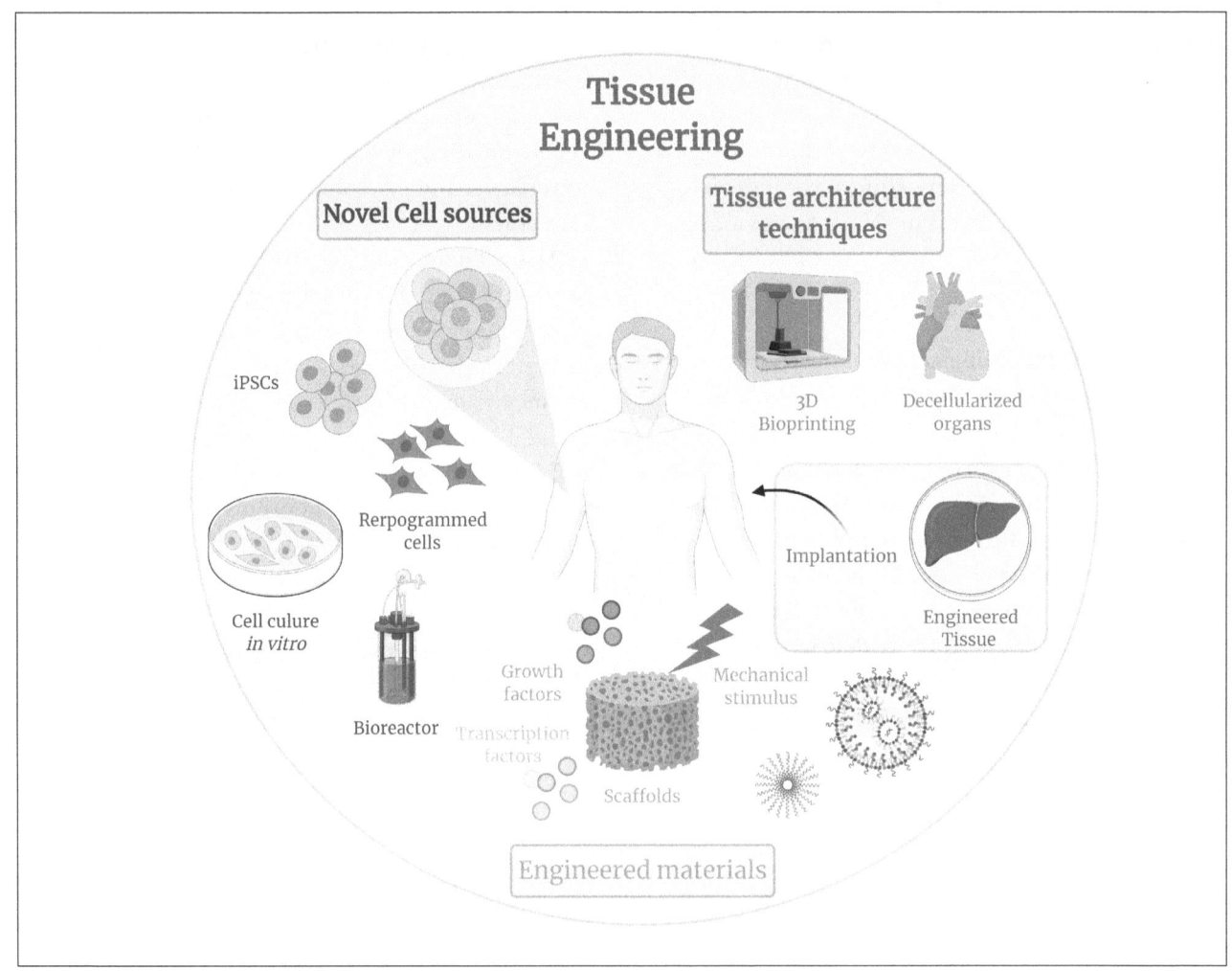

Throughout the past decade in the field of tissue engineering, novel cell sources, engineering materials, and tissue architecture techniques have provided engineering tissues that better restore, maintain, improve, or replace biological tissues. Image by Annaisasp, via Wikimedia Commons.

scaffolding characteristic is biodegradability—meaning the scaffold should dissolve once the transplanted tissues take hold. This concept of dissolving after ten days or two weeks in the body has been used in medicine when stitching with bioresorbable sutures for many decades. The degradation rate of the scaffold must coincide with the tissue formation rate. Surgical removal of the scaffold (often plastic or collagen) is not necessary if it dissolves after the cells produce their own supportive scaffolding, which can manage mechanical forces at play in their biological setting.

Transplantable human tissue built on a biodegradable scaffold can help with organ transplantation. The recipient's immune system attacks the transplanted tissue if the cell surface proteins on the donor tissue do not match the recipient's. Therefore, donor tissue works best if grown from the recipient's cells. Cells stripped from a kidney and functioning renal tissue bioengineered from the tissue scaffold created in this process have shown the promise of producing functioning organs/tissues created from the patient's cells, solving or minimizing immune rejection.

USES AND COMPLICATIONS

Although bioengineered tracheas, cartilage, skin grafts, bladders, and arteries have been implanted in humans, these procedures are in the experimental stage. Experimental protocols, personnel, laboratory, and health-related costs are expensive. Organ tissues, including liver, lung, and heart, have been laboratory-created. Still, surgical and medical procedures for successful patient implantation of bioengineered tissue ready to function in a human body effectively require much more experimentation and study. Some of these bioengineered tissues are used for research, including developing medications and producing biological tools for personalizing medicinal treatments. Using bioengineered tissue can reduce the need for animals in research and lower research costs.

Modified inkjet printers have been used to produce vascular networks in bioengineered tissue. Living tissue requires the nutrients and oxygen blood provides. Bioengineered tissue on a collagen scaffold will die without nourishment. A modified inkjet printer was used to "print" a lattice network made from a sugar solution, which then hardens. Bioengineered tissue is placed over the lattice, surrounding the lines of sugar. Blood added to the tissue/sugar mesh dissolves the sugar and leaves channels that serve as blood vessels.

PERSPECTIVE AND PROSPECTS

Current research related to tissue engineering includes developing new biological scaffolding materials and tools better enable the imaging, fabrication, and preservation of engineered tissues.

Stem cells have the potential to develop (differentiate) into a variety of cell types. Growing stem cells having the ability to develop into any cell type (known as "pluripotent stem cells") is an important part of current tissue engineering research. Pluripotent stem cells have been bioengineered from stem cells to bone grafts with potential human use.

Research using various combinations of growth factors has recently been supplemented by employing biomechanical elements, like different types of defined three-dimensional (3D) spaces, to help decipher how stem cells differentiate into distinct cell types. Subjecting growing stem cells to new spatial arrangements in addition to novel culture conditions, surfaces, and cocktails of growth factors influence the differentiation programs of pluripotent and adult stem cells. The creative uses of 3D culture systems also expand the number of cell types into which these stem cell populations can differentiate and increase their differentiation efficiency. Innovative approaches like the use of different spaces in addition to growth solutions can potentially help decipher the genetic, chemical, and structural factors related to tissue development and repair.

—*Richard P. Capriccioso*

Further Reading

Capriccioso, Richard P., and Capriccioso, Christina E. "Bionics and Biomedical Engineering." *Applied Science*, edited by Donald R. Franceschetti, Salem Press, 2012, pp. 228-33.

Fountain, Henry. "A First: Organs Tailor-Made with Body's Own Cells." *The New York Times*. 15 Sept. 2012, www.nytimes.com/2012/09/16/health/research/scientists-make-progress-in-tailor-made-organs.html?pagewanted=all&_r=0}.

"Introduction to Stem Cells." *NIH Stem Cell Information*. National Institutes of Health, 1 Feb. 2021, stemcells.nih.gov/info/basics.

Karcher, Susan J., and Richard P. Capriccioso. "Human Genetic Engineering." *Applied Science*, edited by Donald R. Franceschetti, Salem Press, 2012, pp. 987-95.

National Institute of Biomedical Imaging and Bioengineering. NIH US Department of Health and Human Services, www.nibib.nih.gov/.

Nerem, R. M., et al., editors. *Principles of tissue engineering*. 4th ed., Academic Press, 2013.

Vacanti, Joseph P., editor. *Tissue Engineering and Regenerative Medicine*. Cold Spring Harbor Laboratory Press, 2017.

MEDICATIONS

Several medicines help injured athletes rehabilitate without severe pain episodes and muscle spasms. While such medicines have their place, they have adverse effects. Some drugs, such as opioids, muscle relaxants, and anti-anxiety medicines, are addictive and have a high potential for abuse. This section lays down the good, the bad, and the ugly side of sports medicine medications. Baclofen, fentanyl, ketamine, morphine, NSAIDs, oxycodone, and valium are among the topics covered.

Anti-Inflammatory Drugs

Category: Drugs
Specialties and related fields: Dermatology, endocrinology, family medicine, internal medicine, ophthalmology, orthopedics, otorhinolaryngology, rheumatology, vascular medicine

KEY TERMS

arthritis: a painful condition that involves inflammation of one or more joints

bursitis: inflammation of the sac of lubricating fluid located between joints

hormone: a substance made by the body that travels through the bloodstream to reach its target organ and have its effect

inflammation: the body's response to injury that may include redness, pain, swelling, and warmth in the affected area

salicylates: a group of drugs (including aspirin) derived from salicylic acid, used to relieve pain, reduce inflammation, and lower fever

steroids: a class of hormones produced by the adrenal glands; can also be made synthetically

tendinitis: inflammation of a tendon, a tough band of tissue that connects muscle to bone

INDICATIONS

Nonsteroidal anti-inflammatory drugs (NSAIDs), such as aspirin, relieve painful conditions such as arthritis, bursitis, gout, menstrual cramps, tendonitis, sprains, and strains. Additionally, low-dose aspirin is commonly prescribed to reduce the risk of myocardial infarction (heart attack).

The NSAIDs inhibit the enzyme cyclooxygenase, which converts the fatty acid commonly found in cell membranes, arachidonic acid, to prostaglandin H (PGH). PGH is the starting molecule for synthesizing a host of pro-inflammatory molecules called "prostaglandins." By preventing prostaglandin synthesis, NSAIDs quell inflammation.

Nonsteroidal anti-inflammatory drugs come in two main forms, the salicylates and the classical NSAIDs. Salicylates include aspirin (acetylsalicylate), salsalate, and diflunisal. Some common classical NSAIDs, with their brand names in parentheses, are diclofenac (Voltaren), etodolac (Lodine), flurbiprofen (Ansaid), ibuprofen (Motrin, Advil, Rufen, Nuprin), nabumetone (Relafen), naproxen (Naprosyn or Aleve), meloxicam (Mobic, Vivlodex, Anjeso), and oxaprozin (Daypro). These drugs can come in capsules, caplets, tablets, liquids, and suppositories. While several NSAIDs require a prescription, many are sold over the counter.

Corticosteroids (synthetic glucocorticoids) make up the second group of anti-inflammatory drugs used to alleviate the symptoms associated with asthma, lupus, arthritis, and allergic reactions. Like NSAIDs, corticosteroids are available in various forms, including inhalants, creams, ointments, and oral (systemic) medications. Common corticosteroids are beclomethasone (Beconase, Vancensase, Vanceril), betamethasone (Diprolene, Lotrisone), hydrocortisone, mometasone (Elocon), prednisone (Deltasone, Orasone), and triamcinolone (Azmacort, Nasacort, Kenalog).

Synthetic glucocorticoids come as short-acting, intermediate-acting, or long-acting glucocorticoids. Short-acting glucocorticoids have a duration of action of eight to twelve hours and include cortisone and hydrocortisone. Cortisone comes in tablets that are taken orally. After ingestion, the liver converts cortisone to the active form, hydrocortisone. Consequently, cortisone has no activity if applied topically, but hydrocortisone does. Hydrocortisone or cortisol are also administered orally, intravenously, or injected intramuscularly. Because these drugs act quickly, they are the drugs of choice to treat adrenal insufficiency. Intermediate-acting glucocorticoids have a duration of action of twelve to thirty-six hours. This group includes prednisone, prednisolone, methylprednisolone, and triamcinolone. Prednisone comes in orally administered formulations, and prednisolone is available in oral, intravenous, and topical formulations. Methylprednisolone comes in oral, intravenous, intramuscular, or intra-articular formulations. Triamcinolone comes in inhaled, oral, topical, intramuscular, and intra-articular formulations. Intermediate-acting glucocorticoids are approximately four to five times more potent compared to short-acting glucocorticoids. Long-acting glucocorticoids are about twenty-five times more potent than short-acting glucocorticoids and have a duration of activity of thirty-six to seventy-two hours. Betamethasone and dexamethasone are two long-acting glucocorticoids given orally, intramuscularly, interarticularly, or intravenously.

Synthetic glucocorticoids help treat various autoimmune and inflammatory conditions, including rheumatoid arthritis, acute multiple sclerosis flares, Crohn disease, ulcerative colitis, idiopathic thrombocytopenic purpura, allergic rhinitis or conjunctivitis, or skin conditions like eczema. They also help treat hypersensitivity states like allergic reactions and prevent graft-versus-host disease in individuals who have received bone marrow transplants.

COMPLICATIONS

Although used across many medical specialties and for many reasons, NSAIDs are not without their dangers. There are two main cyclooxygenase enzymes,

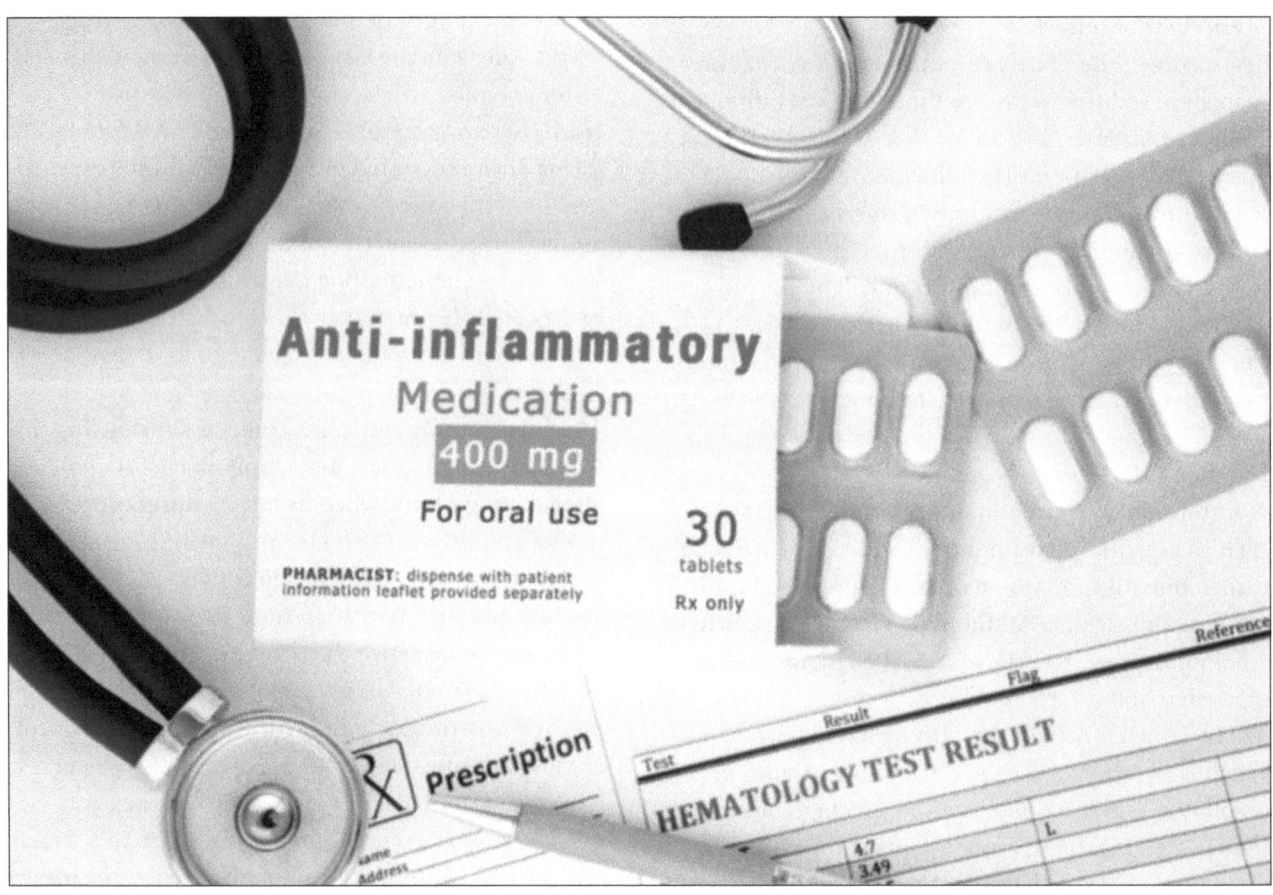

Photo via iStock/Shidlovski. [Used under license.]

cyclooxygenase-1 (COX-1) and cyclooxygenase-2 (COX-2). COX-2 is induced by events that cause inflammation, but COX-1 is a housekeeping enzyme that maintains the help of several tissues, specifically the stomach, kidneys, and blood vessels. COX-1 inhibition in the stomach diminishes the production of the protective mucus coating. Long-term NSAID use increases the risk of peptic ulcers and gastritis. The kidneys can also suffer damage from long-term NSAID use since COX enzymes increase renal blood flow. COX enzymes made by blood vessel cells (endothelial cells) decrease platelet adhesion and keep blood vessels clear.

Common NSAID side effects are mild and can include stomach pains or cramps, nausea, vomiting, indigestion, headache, and dizziness. Despite these relatively mild side effects, individuals currently taking other medications, women who are pregnant or who plan to become pregnant, breastfeeding women, and persons with stomach or intestinal problems, liver disease, heart disease, high blood pressure, bleeding diseases, diabetes, Parkinson's disease, or epilepsy should consult their physicians before taking NSAIDs. While side effects are rare, some can be life-threatening. Some NSAIDs can increase the risk of strokes and heart attacks. Any feelings of tightness in the chest, irregular heartbeat, swelling, or fainting are reasons to discontinue the use of NSAIDs and consult a physician. It is important to note that children should not be given aspirin if they are recovering from a viral infection. It can lead to Reye's syndrome—a potentially fatal condition that results in liver and brain swelling.

Corticosteroid therapy produces dramatic, immediate relief from pain, swelling, and inflammation due to arthritis. Small amounts of steroids may be injected directly into the inflamed joint, or they can be taken by mouth. However, the beneficial effects tend to be temporary. Long-term use can lead to cataracts, and increased blood sugar, which can worsen a person's diabetes, and reduce resistance to infections, gastrointestinal ulcers, and bleeding. The advent of other highly effective alternatives has led to less frequent use of steroids in the setting of arthritis.

Additionally, corticosteroids are a common treatment for persons suffering from more serious asthmatic conditions or when treatment with bronchodilators has not proven effective. Inhaled corticosteroids are not bronchodilators and do not open the airways. Instead, these medications reduce inflammation within the airways and allow the lungs to function properly. They should be used regularly and for the complete course as prescribed to achieve full benefits. Corticosteroids may be sprayed into the nose to relieve stuffy nose, irritation, hay fever, or other allergies. In contrast, oral corticosteroids are used primarily to prevent asthma attacks.

Ophthalmic anti-inflammatory medicines can reduce problems during or following eye surgery by alleviating eye inflammation. These can be obtained only with a doctor's prescription. Corticosteroids also relieve inflammation of the temporal arteries, the blood vessels that run along the temples. Inflammation here can disrupt the blood supply and result in blindness, partial vision loss, strokes, and even heart attacks.

Individuals who have medical conditions such as allergies, diabetes, pregnancy, osteoporosis, glaucoma, infections, thyroid problems, liver disease, kidney disease, heart disease, or high blood pressure should discuss these conditions with their physician before taking corticosteroids. If corticosteroids are used for a short time, the development of side effects is rare. However, breathing problems or tightness in the chest, pain, rash, swelling, extreme exhaustion, irregular heartbeat, or wounds that do not heal should be reported to a physician. Patients should not stop taking steroids abruptly without consulting a physician, especially if the steroids have been taken for a long time, as the body requires a weaning process to adapt.

PERSPECTIVE AND PROSPECTS

The bark of the willow tree, which contains salicylates, was known in eighteenth-century England to reduce fever and aches. In 1876, the first successful treatment of acute arthritis with sodium salicylate (aspirin) was reported. In the 1970s, pharmacologist John Vane amassed evidence of the effectiveness of NSAIDs.

The earliest demonstration of the importance of corticosteroids as anti-inflammatory agents occurred in the 1940s regarding rheumatoid arthritis. The challenge of corticosteroid therapy lies in achieving the desired results with minimum side effects.

—*Mary Hurd, Lillian Dominguez, Michael A. Buratovich*

Further Reading

Davis, Jennifer S., et al. "Use of Non-Steroidal Anti-Inflammatory Drugs in US Adults: Changes over Time and by Demographic." *Open Heart*, vol. 4, no. 1, 2017, doi:10.1136/openhrt-2016-000550.

Liska, Ken. *Drugs and the Human Body, with Implications for Society*. 8th ed., Pearson/Prentice Hall, 2009.

Shmerling, Robert H. "Are You Taking Too Much Anti-Inflammatory Medication?" *Harvard Health Blog*, 23 Mar. 2018, www.health.harvard.edu/blog/are-you-taking-too-much-anti-inflammatory-medication-2018040213540. Accessed 26 May 2022.

Szalay, Jessie. *What Is Inflammation?* LiveScience, 19 Oct. 2018, www.livescience.com/52344-inflammation.html. Accessed 26 May 2022.

Yaksh, Tony L., et al. "Development of New Analgesics: An Answer to Opioid Epidemic." *Trends in Pharmacological Sciences*, vol. 39, no. 12, 2018, pp. 1000-1002, doi:10.1016/j.tips.2018.10.003.

BACLOFEN

Category: Drugs (Muscle relaxant)
Also known as: Lioresal
Specialties and related fields: Athletic trainers, neurology, orthopedics, pharmacology, physical therapists, sports medicine

KEY TERMS

gamma-aminobutyric acid (GABA): the principal inhibitory neurotransmitter in the central nervous system that reduces neuronal excitability throughout the nervous system

muscle relaxant: a class of medications that reduce skeletal muscle function and decrease muscle tone, and treat muscle spasms, pain, and hyperreflexia

HISTORY OF USE

Baclofen was developed to control seizures in persons with epilepsy; however, its effectiveness for this treatment has been inadequate. Instead, baclofen has evolved into a treatment of choice for spasticity-related conditions.

Baclofen was introduced as a possible addiction treatment when physician Olivier Ameisen self-treated his alcohol addiction with high-dose baclofen. His results were published in a self-case study report in the journal *Alcohol and Alcoholism* in 2005, prompting the public and the medical community to evaluate the use of baclofen to treat addiction.

EFFECTIVENESS

Baclofen is a muscle relaxant that decreases painful muscle spasms. It is the first-line treatment for painful muscle spasms in individuals with multiple sclerosis or spinal cord injuries or diseases. Baclofen relieves flexor spasms, which include muscle spasms that involve the knee, ankle, or hip particularly well.

Baclofen also suppresses symptoms and cravings associated with alcohol dependence and reduces symptoms of alcohol withdrawal.

Baclofen's mode of action involves activating the gamma amino-butyric acid (GABA) B receptors in the central nervous system. Baclofen is safe and effective, even in persons with alcohol-related liver damage. However, patients with reduced kidney function must have their baclofen doses reduced.

Baclofen has few drug-drug interactions and causes fewer side effects than traditional medications used to treat alcohol dependence.

Baclofen possesses lower misuse potential than narcotics like opioids. However, baclofen is a psychotropic drug. The recreational use of baclofen among adolescents and young adults represents a serious problem that health-care professionals should consider. The medical literature reports several unfortunate cases of baclofen overdose resulting in death.

Baclofen is also being investigated to treat cocaine and opioid dependence and misuse disorders. Large-scale clinical trials are needed to prove the long-term safety and effectiveness of baclofen in treating substance misuse disorders.

PRECAUTIONS

High baclofen doses can cause excessive drowsiness, dizziness, psychiatric disturbances, and decreased muscle tone that may impair daily function. Overdoses of baclofen may precipitate seizures, slowed breathing, altered pupil size, and coma. Abrupt discontinuation of baclofen can result in withdrawal symptoms, including hallucinations, disorientation, anxiety, dizziness, memory impairments, and mood disturbances.

Owing to increased publicity regarding baclofen as a potential treatment for addictions, some people have turned to illegally buying baclofen over the internet to control their addictions. As with any medication, baclofen should be used only under the guidance and supervision of a trained medical professional.

—*Jennifer L. Gibson, Michael A. Buratovich*

Further Reading

Ameisen, Olivier, and Hilary Hinzmann. *The End of My Addiction: How One Man Cured Himself of Alcoholism.* Piatkus, 2010.

"Baclofen." *MedlinePlus.* US National Library of Medicine, 15 July 2017, medlineplus.gov/druginfo/meds/a682530.html.

Drevin, G., et al. "Baclofen Overdose Following Recreational Use in Adolescents and Young Adults: A Case Report and Review of the Literature." *Forensic Science International*, vol. 316, 2020, p. 110541, doi:10.1016/j.forsciint.2020.110541.

Ghanavatian, Shirin, and Armen Derian. "Baclofen." *StatPearls*, 1 Oct. 2019.

Muzyk, Andrew, et al. "Clinical Effectiveness of Baclofen for the Treatment of Alcohol Dependence: A Review." *Clinical Pharmacology: Advances and Applications*, vol. 5, 2013, p. 99, doi:10.2147/cpaa.s32434.

CARISOPRODOL

Category: Addiction risk; Muscle relaxant
Also known as: Carisoma; Soma, Sanoma; Sopradol; Vanadom
Specialties and related fields: Orthopedics, pharmacology, sports medicine
Definition: a muscle relaxant that can treat pain and stiffness from muscle spasms and is also a drug of abuse

KEY TERMS

addiction: a neuropsychological disorder characterized by persistent use of a drug, despite substantial harm and other negative consequence
anxiolytic: a drug used to reduce anxiety
muscle relaxant: a drug that affects skeletal muscle function and decreases the muscle tone

HISTORY OF USE

Since the mid-1950s, the North American market for tranquilizing medications has been enormous. Most tranquilizers developed at this time were designed to overcome specific problems apparent in earlier medications. For example, carisoprodol (brand name Soma) was developed because of problems with meprobamate. This older anxiolytic medication had a high potential for dependence and difficult withdrawals.

The brand name "Soma" refers both to the drink of the gods in Hindu religious literature and to a fictional medication in the dystopic novel *Brave New World* (1932) by Aldous Huxley. Since the late 1950s, the medical and scientific communities have recognized that although Soma is an effective skeletal-muscle relaxant, it also has a high potential for misuse, dependence, and illegal purchase.

EFFECTS AND POTENTIAL RISKS
How Soma works in the brain is not well understood. However, studies have suggested that it stimulates the receptors for gamma-aminobutyric acid, which prompts overall relaxation of skeletal muscles and then sedation. Because of these two effects, Soma has been frequently prescribed along with anti-inflammatory medications as an aid for muscle sprains.

However effective in the short term, Soma has significant potential risks. Like other tranquilizing medications, Soma can cause dependence; predictably, those who become dependent tend to take larger doses to achieve desired effects, which substantially increases the subsequent risk of cardiac problems, coma, and death. Some users have experienced anterograde amnesia after taking large doses. They have driven vehicles or engaged in other dangerous behaviors. Withdrawal from Soma also proves difficult. Its symptoms include increased sensitivity to pain and anxiety, jitteriness, hallucinations, memory loss, agitation, depression, and bizarre behavior.

In addition to the potential for dependency is the recreational use and misuse of Soma. More medical professionals have recently recognized the addictive properties of the drug and believe it to be more significant than originally anticipated: especially as a combination drug with alcohol, Xanax (alprazolam), and oxycodone (Soma combined with oxycodone and Xanax referred to the "Holy Trinity" among recreational drug users). Recreational users seek its muscle relaxing and euphoric effects. It is particularly popular with opioid users, who use Soma to combine with other narcotics for a more intense high and prevent withdrawals from opioid use.

—*Michael R. Meyers, Kelly Owen*

Further Reading
"Addiction to Muscle Relaxers: Carisoprodol (Soma)." *American Addiction Centers*, 17 Oct. 2019, americanaddictioncenters.org/prescription-drugs/soma-addiction.

"Carisoprodol." *MedlinePlus*, 15 Oct. 2018, medlineplus.gov/druginfo/meds/a682578.html.

Chou, Roger, et al. "Comparative Efficacy and Safety of Skeletal Muscle Relaxants for Spasticity and Musculoskeletal Conditions: A Systematic Review." *Journal of Pain and Symptom Management*, vol. 28, no. 2, 2004, pp. 140-75, doi:10.1016/j.jpainsymman.2004.05.002.

Horsfall, Joseph T., and Jon E. Sprague. "The Pharmacology and Toxicology of the 'Holy Trinity.'" *Basic & Clinical Pharmacology & Toxicology*, vol. 120, no. 2, 2016, pp. 115-19, doi:10.1111/bcpt.12655.

Paul, Gunchan, et al. "Carisoprodol Withdrawal Syndrome Resembling Neuroleptic Malignant Syndrome: Diagnostic Dilemma." *Journal of Anaesthesiology Clinical Pharmacology*, vol. 32, no. 3, 2016, p. 387, doi:10.4103/0970-9185.173346.

Reeves, Roy R., et al. "Carisoprodol." *Southern Medical Journal*, vol. 105, no. 11, 2012, pp. 619-23, doi:10.1097/smj.0b013e31826f5310.

CODEINE

Category: Addiction risk; Opioid
Also known as: Methylmorphine; Morphine methyl ester; 3-methylmorphine
Specialties and related fields: Oncology, orthopedics, pain management, pharmacology, sports medicine

Definition: a sleep-inducing and analgesic drug derived from morphine

KEY TERMS

analgesic: a drug that relieves pain

opiate: a substance derived from opium that relieves pain and induces sleep

opioid: compounds that resemble opium in their pain-relieving and sleep-inducing properties

HISTORY OF USE

Codeine was isolated from opium by French chemist Pierre-Jean Robiquet in 1832. It was used in the nineteenth century for pain relief and diabetes control. Near the end of the nineteenth century, codeine was used to replace morphine, another substance found in the opium poppy, because of the highly addictive properties of morphine. Codeine has effects similar to, albeit weaker than morphine, and was not thought to be addictive. Codeine was subsequently used in treatment for withdrawal from morphine.

A spoonful of promethazine/codeine syrup showing the characteristic purple color. "Purple drank" is a recreational drug created by combining prescription-grade cough syrup with a soft drink and hard candy. Effects include mild euphoric side effects and lethargy, drowsiness, and dissociative feelings. The first detailed report of codeine addiction is thought to be from 1905, and reports by others followed. In the 1930s, concern over the widespread misuse of codeine in Canada was noted. Codeine misuse in the United States was evaluated more fully in the 1960s, leading to the inclusion of codeine as a Schedule II controlled substance. Schedule II drugs have a high potential for misuse.

Subsequently, among substance misusers, prescription cough syrups containing codeine began to be mixed with soft drinks and candy (in a combination known as "lean syrup," "sizzurp," or "purple drank"). The combination remains a substance of concern.

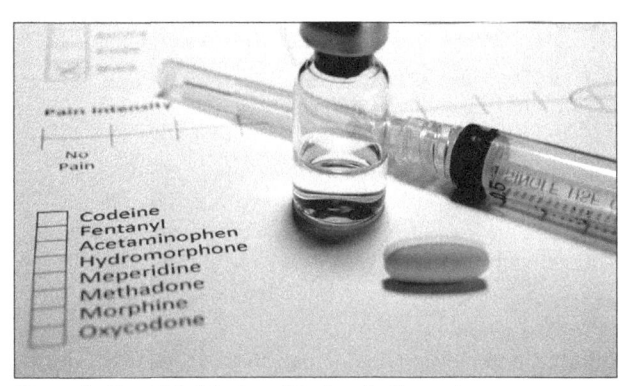

Photo via iStock/Hailshadow. [Used under license.]

EFFECTS AND POTENTIAL RISKS

Codeine primarily exerts its medicinal effects by being metabolized by liver enzymes to morphine, which binds to specific receptors in the central and peripheral nervous systems. Morphine effectively blocks the transmission of pain signals to the brain and inhibits the cough reflex. The metabolites also contribute to the usefulness of codeine in treating diarrhea by affecting, among other things, the contraction of gastrointestinal tract muscles.

Short-term use of codeine provides pain relief and euphoric effects. Some of the more common side effects of codeine ingestion include itching, constipation, dizziness, sedation, flushing, sweating, nausea, vomiting, and hives.

Long-term use of codeine can lead to tolerance, necessitating higher doses to achieve the same euphoric effect. Endorphin (natural painkiller) production may be slowed or stopped, causing increased sensitivity to pain if codeine is not used. More serious side effects include respiratory depression, central nervous system depression, seizures, and cardiac arrest.

—*Jason J. Schwartz*

Further Reading

Benini, Franca, and Egidio Barbi. "Doing without Codeine: Why and What Are the Alternatives?" *Italian Journal of Pediatrics*, vol. 40, no. 1, 2014, doi:10.1186/1824-7288-40-16.

Bhandari, Monika, et al. "Recent Updates on Codeine." *Pharmaceutical Methods*, vol. 2, no. 1, 2011, pp. 3-8, doi:10.4103/2229-4708.81082.

Carney, Tara, et al. "A Comparative Analysis of Pharmacists' Perspectives on Codeine Use and Misuse—A Three Country Survey." *Substance Abuse Treatment, Prevention, and Policy*, vol. 13, no. 1, 2018, doi:10.1186/s13011-018-0149-2.

"Codeine." *MedlinePlus*, 15 Mar. 2018, medlineplus.gov/druginfo/meds/a682065.html.

Smith, Cooper. "Codeine: Drug Effects, Addiction, Abuse and Treatment-Rehab Spot." *RehabSpot*, 9 July 2019, www.rehabspot.com/opioids/codeine/.

Fentanyl

Category: Addiction risk; Opioid

Also known as: Apache, the bomb, China girl, China white, dance fever, friend, goodfella, jackpot, murder 8, perc-a-pop, poison, tango and cash, TNT

Definition: a potent synthetic opioid, which, like morphine, produces analgesia but to a greater extent

KEY TERMS

analgesic: a drug that relieves pain

opioid: substances that act on opioid receptors to relieve pain relief, suppress diarrhea, suppress coughs, and augment anesthesia

INTRODUCTION

Fentanyl is a potent synthetic opioid used to relieve pain. It is 50 to 100 times more potent than morphine. One hundred micrograms of fentanyl produce the same pain relief as 10 mg of morphine. Fentanyl, unlike morphine, has strong sedative properties. In hospitals, health-care workers use fentanyl as a sedative in intubated patients. Because fentanyl is eliminated from the body by the liver and not the kidneys, it serves as an excellent pain reliever for people with renal failure.

The other indications for fentanyl include (1) preoperative analgesia; (2) supplementary anesthesia (anesthesia adjunct); (3) regional anesthesia supplement; (4) general anesthesia; and (5) postoperative pain relief; moderate to severe pain.

MECHANISM OF ACTION

Like other opioids, fentanyl binds to opioid receptors in the central nervous system, activating them. There are several distinct opioid receptor subtypes. The dominant opioid receptor subtype is the Mu receptor. Fentanyl selectively activates the Mu receptor and is termed a "Mu-selective opioid agonist."

When fentanyl activates the Mu opioid receptor, it secondarily increases the neurotransmitter dopamine concentration in the brain's reward areas. Increased dopamine neurotransmission in the brain's mesolimbic system causes the exhilaration and relaxation effects associated with the addiction to the drug.

HISTORY OF USE

Fentanyl was first synthesized in a medical drug research laboratory in Belgium in the late 1950s. The original formulation had an analgesic potency of about eighty times that of morphine. Fentanyl was introduced into medical practice in the 1960s as an intravenous anesthetic. Subsequently, two other fentanyl analogs were developed for medical applications: alfentanil, an ultrashort-acting analgesic (5-10 minutes), and sufentanil, an exceptionally potent analgesic (five to ten times more potent than fentanyl) for use in heart surgery. Fentanyl is used now for anesthesia and analgesia. The most widely used formulation is a transdermal patch to relieve chronic pain.

Illicit use of fentanyl first occurred within the medical community in the mid-1970s. Among anesthesiologists, anesthetists, nurses, and other workers in anesthesiology settings, fentanyl and sufentanil are the two agents most frequently misused. Poten-

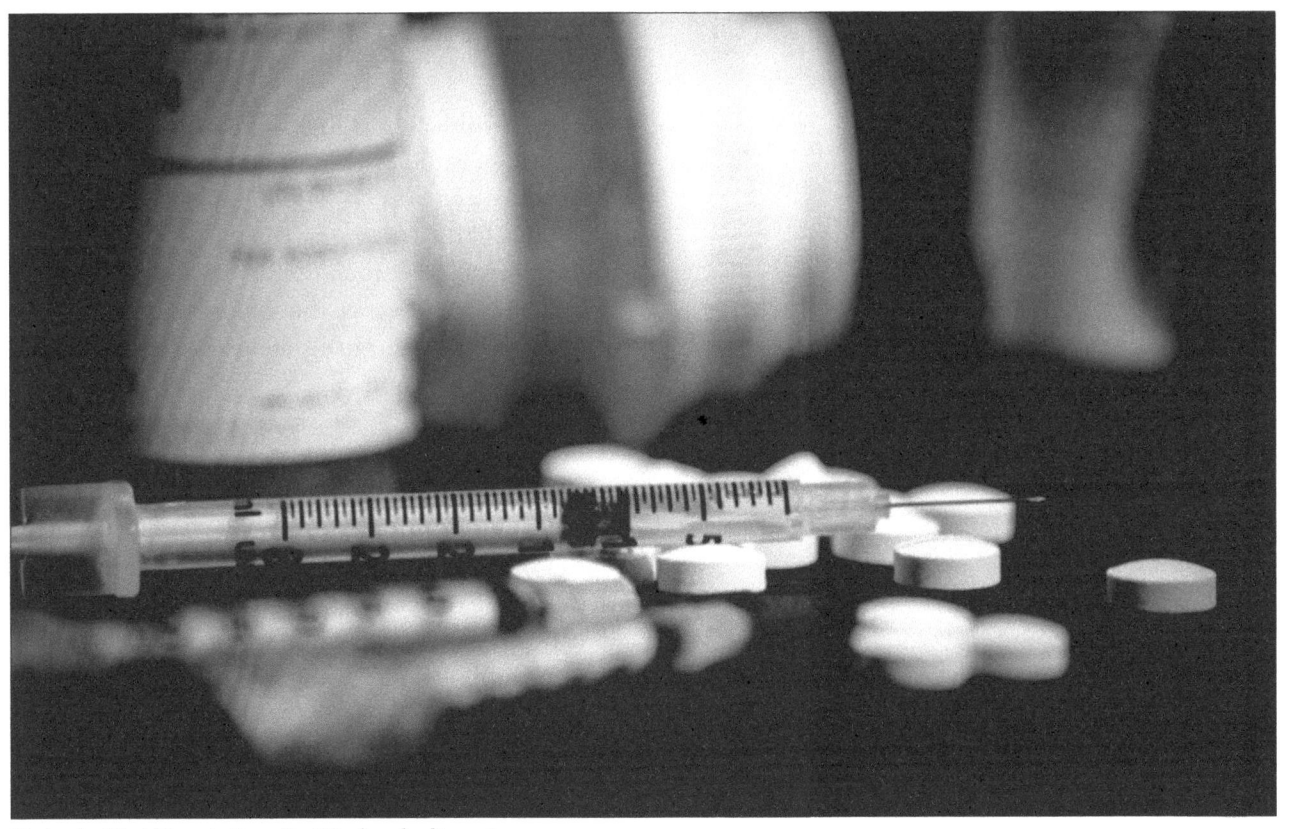

Photo via iStock/Darwin Brandis. [Used under license]

tial misusers have ready access to these agents in liquid formulations for injection. They can divert small quantities with relative ease. Drug abusers cannot readily adapt transdermal patches for misuse. The fentanyl lozenge has been diverted to illegal use. On the street, the lozenge is known as "perc-a-pop."

Since the mid-2000s, fentanyl misuse has emerged as a serious public health problem. More than one dozen analogs of fentanyl have been produced clandestinely for illegal use outside the medical setting. Fentanyl-laced heroin or cocaine powders have become the drugs of choice for some addicts. In the 2010s, fentanyl played a major part in the drastic spike in overdose deaths due to opioid misuse. The drug was often mixed with heroin or cocaine. Its potency means that users unaware of the mixture can easily overdose. Beginning around 2013 and accelerating in 2014 and 2015, the sharp rise of fentanyl-related overdose deaths contributed to the growing opioid crisis. In 2016 the National Institute on Drug Abuse (NIDA) estimated that overdoses of fentanyl analogs caused over 20,000 deaths.

EFFECTS AND POTENTIAL RISKS

The biological effects of fentanyl are indistinguishable from those of heroin, except that illicit fentanyl analogs may be hundreds of times more potent. Short-term effects of fentanyl misuse include mood changes, euphoria, dysphoria, and hallucinations. Anxiety, confusion, and depression also may occur. High doses or long-term use may impair or interrupt breathing due to respiratory depression. Unconsciousness and even death can occur.

The 2000s and 2010s have seen a sharp increase in fentanyl use and related overdoses and deaths. For example, in 2014, twenty-eight people died over two months in Philadelphia due to fentanyl-laced heroin. Police seizure of illegal drugs containing fentanyl tripled between 2013 and 2014; there were 942 fentanyl-related cases in 2013, compared with 3,344 in 2014. In 2015 the Drug Enforcement Administration (DEA) issued an alert about the spike in fentanyl-laced heroin. The problem was originally thought to be concentrated on the East Coast. Still, in April 2016, a spate of overdoses in the Sacramento area of California (thirty-six overdoses with nine deaths in a single week) showed that the problem was nationwide and growing. Notably, the drug used as a painkiller was responsible for the April 2016 death of the musician Prince.

With the rise of the opioid crisis, law enforcement and health-care organizations began to press for wider availability of the overdose medication naloxone, also known as "Narcan." The medication effectively reverses the effects of an overdose. However, some critics claim it encourages drug users to use more recklessly, as they know they can be revived in case of overdose.

—*Ernest Kohlmetz, Michael A. Buratovich*

Further Reading

Dima, Delia, et al. "The Use of Rotation to Fentanyl in Cancer-Related Pain." *Journal of Pain Research*, vol. 10, 2017, pp. 341-48, doi:10.2147/jpr.s121920.

"Fentanyl." *MedlinePlus*, 15 Oct. 2019, medlineplus.gov/druginfo/meds/a605043.html.

NIDA. "Fentanyl." *National Institute on Drug Abuse*, 6 June 2016, www.drugabuse.gov/drugs-abuse/fentanyl.

Ramos-Matos, et al. "Fentanyl." *StatPearls*, 8 May 2022, https://www.ncbi.nlm.nih.gov/books/NBK459275/. Accessed 8 June 2022.

Stanley, Theodore H. "The Fentanyl Story." *The Journal of Pain*, vol. 15, no. 12, 2014, pp. 1215-26, doi:10.1016/j.jpain.2014.08.010.

Westhoff, Ben. *Fentanyl, Inc.: How Rogue Chemists Are Creating the Deadliest Wave of the Opioid Epidemic*. Atlantic Monthly Press, 2019.

Ketamine

Category: Addiction risk; Anesthetic; Antidepressant
Also known as: K, Special K, Vitamin K
Specialties and related fields: Addiction, anesthesiology, pharmacology, psychiatry
Definition: a medication used for anesthetic induction and maintenance that induces dissociative anesthesia, a trancelike state providing pain relief, sedation, and amnesia

KEY TERMS

anesthetic: medicines that induce an anesthetic state
antidepressant: medications that alleviate depression
dissociative states: mental disorders that involve experiencing a disconnection and lack of continuity between thoughts, memories, surroundings, actions, and identity
N-methyl-D-aspartate (NMDA) receptors: a glutamate receptor and ion channel found in neurons

HISTORY OF USE

Ketamine was first synthesized in 1962 in the laboratories of the Parke-Davis pharmaceutical company. It was developed as an alternative to phencyclidine (PCP) for use as an anesthetic. Anesthesiologists initiated clinical use in short-term surgery in humans in 1975.

The anesthetic state is a condition that makes surgery tolerable for the patient and manageable for the surgeon. Anesthetics promote the anesthetic state by inducing: (1) unconsciousness, so the patient is not aware of their surroundings; (2) sedation to prevent patients from responding to painful stimuli; (3) amnesia, so the patient does not remember the procedure; and (4) analgesia to prevent the patient from feeling pain due to the procedure.

Anesthetics induce the anesthetic state by modulating the stimulatory and inhibitory processes in the brain. The neurotransmitter gamma-aminobutyric acid (GABA) mediates most of the inhibitory signals within the brain. Many anesthetics (e.g., propofol, midazolam) induce the anesthetic state by potentiating GABAergic processes in the brain. Other anesthetics induce the anesthetic state by inhibiting stimulatory processes in the brain. The primary stimulatory neurotransmitter in the brain is glutamate. Some anesthetics (e.g., ketamine, nitrous oxide) inhibit major glutamate receptors to induce the anesthetic state.

Anesthesia has two main phases, induction and maintenance. Induction brings the patient into the anesthetic state. Maintenance keeps the patient in the anesthetic state for the duration of the surgery.

Ketamine is a useful anesthetic that induces the anesthetic state and maintains it. It is given intravenously or as an intramuscular injection. Ketamine inhibits N-methyl-D-aspartate (NMDA) receptors, one of the main glutamate receptors in the central nervous system.

Ketamine has a rapid onset and longer duration of action than other anesthetics. It is also an excellent analgesic; anesthesiologists may use ketamine without other pain relievers like opioids. Ketamine also increases blood flow to the brain, making it dangerous for people who have suffered a head injury and have increased intracranial pressure. Because ketamine dilates airways in the lungs, it is a suitable anesthetic for patients with asthma. Ketamine also does not lower blood pressure, making it advantageous for patients at risk of abnormally low blood pressure. Ketamine causes "dissociative anesthesia," in which patients can breathe, swallow, open their eyes, and move involuntarily even though they neither feel pain nor will remember anything. Unfortunately, patients who awaken after ketamine anesthesia may hallucinate or experience delusions for a short time.

In 2019, the US Food and Drug Administration (FDA) approved an intranasal preparation of the S-isomer of ketamine (Spravato, esketamine) for adults with treatment-resistant depression (TRD). In 2020, FDA extended the approval of esketamine for depressive symptoms in adults with major depressive disorder (MDD) and acute suicidal ideation or behavior. Spravato was the first drug approved to treat this condition.

Predictably, many patients began reporting hallucinations while under ketamine influence. The drug was soon diverted from hospitals, medical offices, and supply houses. It became a popular drug for recreational use among teenagers and young adults in the club scene. Ketamine use is now limited in humans, but it has more widespread applications in veterinary medicine. The US Drug Enforcement Administration (DEA) added ketamine to its list of emerging drugs of misuse in the mid-1990s. It was classified as a schedule III-controlled substance in 1999.

Since the early 2000s, various institutions have studied ketamine as an antidepressant and mood stabilizer. The first small studies at the National Institutes of Health (NIH) and larger studies at Yale University and Mount Sinai Hospital determined that ketamine relieves depression within hours. It relieves depression in patients for whom other medications have not worked. Its antidepressant effects linger long after the drug is eliminated from the body.

EFFECTS AND POTENTIAL RISKS
Primary side effects of ketamine in medical settings include increased heart rate and blood pressure, impaired motor function and memory, numbness, nausea, and vomiting. While sedated, patients are unable to move or feel pain. Once the drug wears off, patients do not remember what occurred during sedation.

In unmonitored situations, ketamine produces a dose-related progression of serious adverse effects from a state of dreamy intoxication to hallucinations and delirium. A "trip" on ketamine has been described as being cut off from reality—"going down into a K hole"—and like an out-of-body or near-death experience. Users may be unable to interact with others or even see or hear them. Ketamine has been used as a date rape agent because the victim does not remember what occurred.

Because misusers feel no pain, they may injure themselves without realizing they are doing so. Chronic use can lead to panic attacks, rage, and paranoia. High doses or prolonged dosing can lead to respiratory depression, arrest, and even death. Ketamine is often mixed with heroin, cocaine, or ecstasy. Any of these combinations can be lethal.

—*Ernest Kohlmetz, Michael A. Buratovich*

Further Reading

Bell, Rae Frances, and Eija Anneli Kalso. "Ketamine for Pain Management." *Pain Reports*, vol. 3, no. 5, 2018, doi:10.1097/pr9.0000000000000674.

"Esketamine Nasal Spray (*Spravato*) for Treatment-Resistant Depression." *Medical Letter on Drugs and Therapeutics*, vol. 61, no. 1569, 2019, pp. 54-56.

Gass, Natalia, et al. "Differences between Ketamine's Short-Term and Long-Term Effects on Brain Circuitry in Depression." *Translational Psychiatry*, vol. 9, no. 1, 2019, doi:10.1038/s41398-019-0506-6.

Grady, Sarah E., et al. "Ketamine for the Treatment of Major Depressive Disorder and Bipolar Depression: A Review of the Literature." *Mental Health Clinician*, vol. 7, no. 1, 2017, pp. 16-23, doi:10.9740/mhc.2017.01.016.

Jonkman, Kelly, et al. "Ketamine for Pain." *F1000Research*, vol. 6, 20 Sept. 2017, p. 1711, doi:10.12688/f1000research.11372.1.

Meisner, Robert C. "Ketamine for Major Depression: New Tool, New Questions." *Harvard Health Blog*. Harvard Medical School, 20 May 2019, www.health.harvard.edu/blog/ketamine-for-major-depression-new-tool-new-questions-2019052216673.

Orhurhu, Vwaire, et al. "Ketamine Infusions for Chronic Pain." *Anesthesia & Analgesia*, vol. 129, no. 1, 2019, pp. 241-54, doi:10.1213/ane.0000000000004185.

Parsaik, Ajay K., et al. "Efficacy of Ketamine in Bipolar Depression." *Journal of Psychiatric Practice*, vol. 21, no. 6, 2015, pp. 427-35, doi:10.1097/pra.0000000000000106.

Serafini, Gianluca, et al. "The Role of Ketamine in Treatment-Resistant Depression: A Systematic Review." *Current Neuropharmacology*, vol. 12, no. 5, 12 Sept. 2014, pp. 444-61, doi:10.2174/1570159x12666140619204251.

Wadehra, Sunali, and Charles F. van Gunten. "Ketamine for Chronic Pain Management." *Practical Pain Management*, 4 Dec. 2018, www.practicalpainmanagement.com/patient/treatments/medications/ketamine-chronic-pain-management-current-role-future-directions.

Morphine

Category: Addiction risk; Opioid; Treatment

Also known as: Dreamer, Emsel, First Line, God's Drug, Hows, MS, Mister Blue, Morpho, Unkie

Specialties and related fields: Oncology, orthopedics, pain specialists, pharmacology

Definition: an analgesic and narcotic drug obtained from opium and used medicinally to relieve pain

KEY TERMS

euphoria: a feeling or state of intense excitement and happiness

opioid: substances that act on opioid receptors to relieve pain, including anesthesia, suppress diarrhea, reverse opioid overdose, and suppress coughs

HISTORY OF USE

The word "morphine" is derived from the term *morphium*, for Morpheus, the Greek god of dreams. Morphine was first isolated in the early nineteenth century by Friedrich Sertürner in Germany. Within twenty years, morphine was available across Europe as an agent for treating pain and for many other uses, including treating alcohol misuse.

In the United States, morphine became a controlled substance in 1914 under the Harrison Narcotics Tax Act. Morphine is now the gold standard by which other analgesics are measured. The drug is used for treating moderate and severe pain, both acute and chronic. Many available painkillers, such as codeine, are chemically related to morphine.

Illicit opioid use, including morphine, is more common now than cocaine, heroin, or methamphetamine (as reported by the 2008 National Survey of Drug Use and Health). Studies have shown that up to 40 percent of people who report misusing opioids have tried intravenous injections of opioids. The intravenous injection produces the fastest onset both of euphoric and negative effects, including respiratory depression and central nervous system (CNS) effects. Frequently these prescription opiates are legally prescribed for a friend or family member and then obtained by the drug misuser. Because of the legitimate pain-relieving properties of morphine, the drug is highly prescribed and used. This high level of use increases opportunities for diversion and misuse.

EFFECTS AND POTENTIAL RISKS

Decreased respiratory rate and sedation are two common adverse effects of morphine; effects experienced even in patients treated with normal doses and dosing regimens. However, these normal adverse effects can become extremely problematic and even fatal in acute morphine overdoses or chronic administration. Respiratory depression occurs more commonly in elderly patients and patients with underlying respiratory conditions. It occurs to a greater extent with intravenous administration. Respiratory complications and sedative effects are also much more common in patients who are opioid naïve.

Like other mu (μ) opioid agonists (such as oxycodone and hydrocodone), morphine causes a feeling of euphoria, which can lead to psychological dependence. Following intravenous administration, euphoria can occur within five minutes. Although the physiological effects can last for greater than six hours, the feeling of euphoria generally dissipates sooner. The waning of euphoria can lead a misuser to re-inject the medication at a time when their body is still reacting to the respiratory and CNS effects of the initial dose of morphine; this can lead to death. The intravenous injection also increases the risk of infection and vessel occlusion, which can have serious and fatal consequences.

Chronic morphine users who abruptly stop using can experience withdrawal. Signs and symptoms of withdrawal include nausea and diarrhea, profuse sweating, twitching muscles, and temperature disturbances, all of which can persist for up to two weeks in some persons.

—*Allison C. Bennett*

Further Reading

Gulur, Padma, et al. "Morphine versus Hydromorphone: Does Choice of Opioid Influence Outcomes?" *Pain Research and Treatment*, vol. 2015, Article ID 482081, 6 pages, 2015, doi.org/10.1155/2015/482081.

Jeurgens, Jeffrey, and Theresa Parisi. "Morphine Addiction and Abuse." *Addiction Center*, 12 Sept. 2019, www.addictioncenter.com/opiates/morphine/.

Kuebler, Karen M. "Using Morphine in End-of-Life Care." *Nursing*, vol. 44, no. 4, 2014, p. 69, doi:10.1097/01.nurse.0000444548.72595.ac.

"Morphine." *MedlinePlus*, 15 Oct. 2019, medlineplus.gov/druginfo/meds/a682133.html.

Nonsteroidal Anti-inflammatory Drugs (NSAIDs)

Category: Drugs
Specialties and related fields: Orthopedics, pain management, rheumatology, sports medicine
Definition: members of a therapeutic drug class that reduce pain and decrease inflammation and fever

KEY TERMS

colorectal: refers to cancers of the lower digestive tract consisting of the colon and the rectum

cyclooxygenase: an enzyme that is responsible for the formation of prostanoids, including thromboxane and prostaglandins such as prostacyclin, from arachidonic acid

diuretics: drugs that increase urine production

ductus arteriosus: a bypass vessel in fetal circulation connecting the pulmonary artery with the aorta that allows blood to skip circulating through the lungs

expression: the action of cell biochemistry to produce and release a particular hormone in response to a stimulus

patent ductus arteriosus: a persistent connection between two major blood vessels, the aorta, and the pulmonary artery, that lead from the heart

prostaglandins: a large group of biologically active unsaturated, twenty-carbon fatty acids that represent some of the metabolites of arachidonic acid

thromboxanes: a fat-soluble hormone of the prostacyclin type released from blood platelets that induces platelet aggregation and arterial constriction

HOW COX INHIBITORS WORK

The cyclooxygenase, or COX, enzymes catalyze the conversion of a fatty acid found in cell membranes, arachidonic acid, into prostaglandin H_2. Prostaglandin H_2 is the precursor for two families of signaling molecules called "prostaglandins" and "thromboxanes" (Fig. 1). Prostaglandins and thromboxanes regulate many inflammatory, pain, and fever-related processes and housekeeping functions in various tissues. Thromboxanes activate platelets and induce blood vessels to constrict when damaged.

There are two types of cyclooxygenases, COX-1, and COX-2. COX-1 is constantly expressed at low levels in many tissues and provides housekeeping functions. Several tissues express COX-2 at low levels, including the brain, kidneys, and blood vessel-based endothelial cells. Still, inflammation highly induces COX-2 expression, especially in the immune system.

In the stomach, prostaglandin synthesis inhibits gastric acid production and increases gastric blood flow and the production of gastric mucous and bicarbonate. Therefore, COX-1 protects the stomach lining from damage caused by acid and enzymes. Long-term COX inhibition causes peptic ulcers and gastritis.

Cyclooxygenase increases renal blood flow, filtration rates, and water and salt secretion in the kidney. COX inhibition in the kidney decreases renal blood flow and filtration rates. It further promotes water and salt retention, leading to hypertension and potential kidney damage.

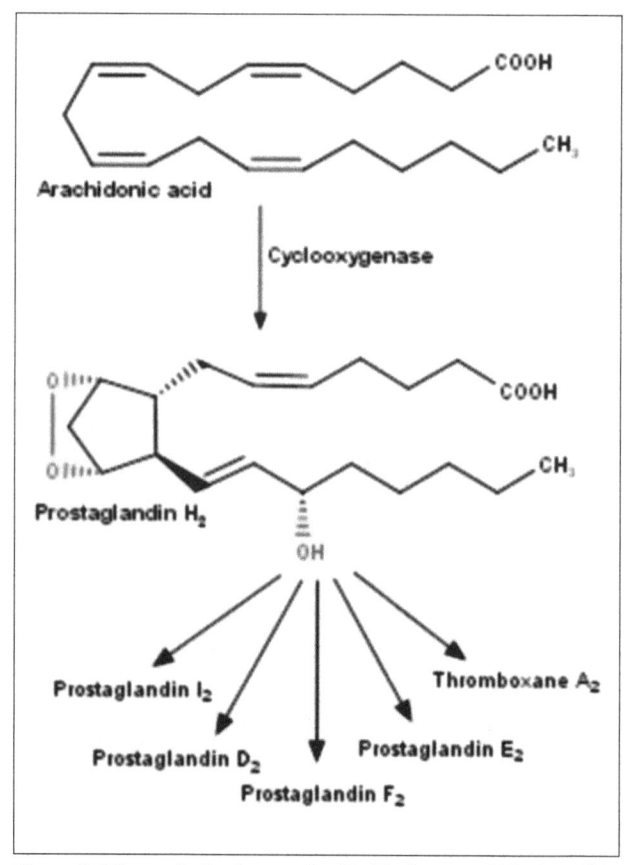

Figure 1. The synthesis of prostaglandin H_2 from arachidonic acid in a two-step reaction catalyzed by cyclooxygenase. Arachidonic acid is liberated from membrane phospholipids by the enzyme phospholipase A_2. This enzyme is activated by cell damage, inflammation, or other disease states. Various tissue-specific synthetases convert prostaglandin H_2 into the various prostaglandins. Image by M. Buratovich.

Prostaglandins play integral roles in the regulation of the cardiovascular system. Platelets express COX-1 and only make thromboxane A_2. Thromboxane A_2 promotes blood vessel constriction and platelet aggregation. However, the endothelial cells that line blood vessels express COX-1 and COX-2 and make prostaglandin I_2, which promotes blood vessel dilation and inhibits platelet aggregation. Blood vessel health depends on the thromboxane A_2/prostaglandin I_2 balance. Inhibiting thromboxane A_2 synthesis, for example, with low-dose aspirin, prevents blood clots from forming in blood vessels and prevents heart attacks and strokes. Inhibition of prostaglandin I_2 synthesis causes blood vessel constriction, leading to hypertension, platelet aggregation, causing thrombosis, and increased risk of heart attack and stroke.

Several cancers overexpress COX-2. Colorectal carcinomas and endometrial cancers overexpress COX-2, and aspirin is used as a supplementary treatment. Other studies have established that increased COX-2 expression tightly correlates with increased tumor invasiveness.

COX INHIBITORS

There are three types of COX inhibitors, salicylates, traditional nonsteroidal anti-inflammatory drugs (NSAIDs), and COX-2 specific inhibitors. The salicylates include acetylsalicylate, better known as "aspirin," "salsalate," and "diflunisal." All salicylates are derivatives of salicylic acid (Fig. 2). Aspirin is unusual among COX inhibitors because it irreversibly inhibits COX enzymes. All other COX inhibitors are competitive inhibitors of COX enzymes. Salicylates treat mild to moderate pain, inflammatory diseases, fevers, heart attack, stroke, and colon cancer prevention (low-dose aspirin). Diflunisal is unusual because it does not cross the blood-brain barrier and cannot treat fever.

Other COX inhibitors include the "traditional NSAIDs." NSAIDs, nonsteroidal anti-inflammatory drugs, treat arthritis and gout pain, and musculoskeletal pain. Some traditional NSAIDs, like ibuprofen and naproxen, are available over the counter. All others require a prescription. Traditional NSAIDs are listed in the table on the following page.

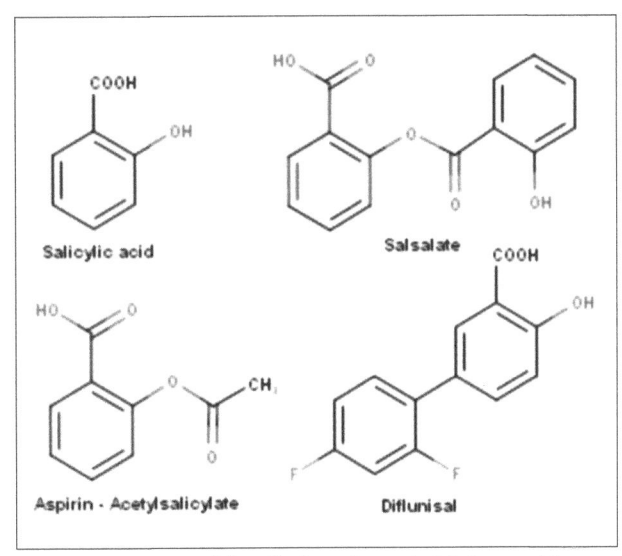

Figure 2. Structures of the salicylates. Image by M. Buratovich.

Ibuprofen has a rapid onset of action and is an ideal treatment for fever and acute pain. Naproxen also has a rapid onset of action and a long duration of action (~14 hours). Indomethacin is a potent anti-inflammatory drug with a high risk of gastrointestinal side effects. It should not be given to anyone to treat mild to moderate pain. Diclofenac comes in various forms ranging from orally administered capsules and powders to topical cremes and patches. Diclofenac inhibits COX-2 more robustly than COX-1. Therefore, it is associated with an increased heart attack and stroke risk. Ketorolac has opioid properties and is given intravenously to replace opioid analgesics.

COX-2-specific inhibitors inhibit COX-2 only. Previous members of this group, rofecoxib (Vioxx) and valdecoxib (Bextra), significantly increased the risk of heart attacks and were pulled from the market. The remaining COX-2-specific inhibitor,

NSAID	Preparations/Generic	Comments
Diclofenac	Generic; Cambia; Zipsor; Zorvolex	Comparable to aspirin with a longer duration
Diclofenac topical	Generic; Pennisaid; Solaraze; Voltaren Arthritis Pain; Aspercreme Arthritis Pain; Flector; Licart	
Diclofenac ophthalmic	Generic	For ocular inflammation after cataract surgery
Etodolac	Generic and extended-release generic	200 milligrams (mg) comparable to 400 mg ibuprofen
Fenoprofen	Generic; Nalfon	
Flurbiprofen	Generic	
Ibuprofen	Generic; Caldolor (Time to pain relief: 15–30 minutes)	200 mg equal to 650 mg of aspirin or acetaminophen; 400 mg comparable to acetaminophen/codeine
Indomethacin	Generic (capsules, extended-release capsules, submicronized capsules, and suppository); Indocin (liquid only); Tivorbex (submicronized)	High potency NSAID, high toxicity, used to close patent ductus arteriosus
Ketoprofen	Generic; Extended-release generic	25 mg comparable to ibuprofen 400 mg and superior to aspirin 650 mg; 50 mg superior to acetaminophen/codeine
Ketorolac	Generic (tablets and injectable); Sprix (nasal spray)	10 mg comparable to ibuprofen 400 or 800 mg or naproxen 500–550 mg Injected form comparable to 12 mg IM morphine with longer duration; time to pain relief: 30 minutes
Meclofenamate	Generic	
Mefenamic acid	Generic	Comparable to aspirin but more effective than aspirin in dysmenorrhea
Meloxicam	Generic; Mobic; submicronized–generic Anjeso–liquid	Appears to be more selective for COX-2 than COX-1 at low doses (7.5 mg)
Nabumetone	Generic	
Naproxen	Generic; Naprosyn; EC-Naprosyn	250 mg probably comparable to aspirin 650 mg with longer duration; 500 mg superior to aspirin 650 mg
Naproxen sodium	Generic; Anaprox DX	275 mg comparable to aspirin 650 mg with longer duration; 550 mg comparable to 400 mg ibuprofen with longer duration
Naproxen sodium OTC	Generic; Aleve	

celecoxib (Celebrex), treats migraine headaches and pain associated with arthritis, gout, and cancer.

Acetaminophen is an important drug that treats mild to moderate pain and fever. This drug does not inhibit peripheral COX-1 or COX-2. Instead, acetaminophen is metabolized in the brain to an active metabolite, AM404, that inhibits brain-specific COX enzymes. AM404 also acts on the brain's cannabinoid system in the pain and thermoregulatory centers of the brain. Therefore, acetaminophen treats fever and pain but has no anti-inflammatory activity and no effects on platelets.

SIDE EFFECTS

All NSAIDs can cause upset stomach (dyspepsia) and peptic ulcers. Severe side effects include stomach perforation and bleeding. Even intravenous NSAID preparations can cause gastrointestinal side effects. People who take high NSAID doses for prolonged periods have had previous peptic ulcer disease, take oral corticosteroids or aspirin (even 81 mg/day), drink excessive amounts of alcohol, or are elderly have heightened risks of gastrointestinal complications. Celecoxib causes less gastrointestinal adverse effects than other nonselective NSAIDs. Acetaminophen does not cause peptic ulcers. Ketorolac use is limited to five days because of its high risk of adverse effects, particularly gastrointestinal toxicity. Taking NSAIDs with a proton pump inhibitor such as omeprazole (Prilosec OTC and generics) can decrease gastrointestinal side effects.

Most NSAIDs interfere with platelet function. Consequently, they decrease the ability of the blood to form clots and prolong bleeding time. Exceptions include celecoxib and, to a lesser extent, meloxicam and nabumetone. The antiplatelet effect wears off when the NSAID is cleared from the body. However, because aspirin irreversibly inhibits COX enzymes, the body must remake all its platelets. Patients must wait up to two weeks before their platelet function returns to normal.

All NSAIDs, including celecoxib, inhibit renal prostaglandins and decrease renal blood flow. Decreased blood flow through the kidney causes fluid and salt retention. It leads to hypertension, leading to renal failure, particularly in elderly patients. People who take diuretic drugs, have diminished liver function, or have heart failure have an increased risk of NSAID-induced renal toxicity.

All NSAIDs, especially COX-2-selective NSAIDs such as celecoxib, may promote blood clots within blood vessels and increase the risk of a heart attack or stroke. Among nonselective NSAIDs, cardiovascular risk is highest with diclofenac and lowest with naproxen.

Children who might have a viral infection should not take NSAIDs. During a viral infection, stress on the liver causes NSAIDs to affect liver cell mitochondria. Without functional mitochondria, the liver cells die. Liver cell loss prevents ammonium processing, and blood ammonium levels rise. Ammonium can cross the blood-brain barrier, where it interferes with neurotransmitter synthesis. Encephalopathy results from higher brain ammonium levels, leading to declining brain function and brain swelling (edema). This condition is called "Reye syndrome" Salicylates are the most likely to cause Reye syndrome. Children with Reye syndrome are quiet, lethargic, sleepy, and may have vomiting. The next stage is characterized by stupor and seizures, followed by coma and death.

Most healthy people can take 4 grams (gm) of acetaminophen per day with no adverse effects. However, repeated consumption of 4 gm of acetaminophen daily can cause low-level liver damage. Acetaminophen overdosage causes serious or fatal liver damage. People who are fasting, are heavy alcohol users, or concurrently taking an interacting drug or herbal supplement, hepatotoxicity can develop after moderate acetaminophen overdosage or even with high therapeutic doses. Acute kidney injury can also occur with acetaminophen overdosage. A regular daily intake of 4 gm of acetaminophen modestly increases blood pressure in patients with hypertension. Long-term use of acetaminophen might increase the risk of renal cell cancer.

DRUG-DRUG INTERACTIONS

Because of their physiological effects in the kidneys, NSAIDs decrease the effectiveness of diuretics. Nonsteriodal anti-inflammatory drugs also decrease the clearance of other drugs, particularly lithium, which is given to treat bipolar disorder, methotrexate, an anti-inflammatory medicine, and aminoglycoside antibiotics. NSAIDs should never be used with these medications.

Since NSAIDs raise blood pressure, they antagonize the effects of antihypertensive medications given to lower blood pressure. Nonsteroidal anti-inflammatory drugs also increase the anticoagulant effects of anticoagulant and antiplatelet drugs. People who take anticoagulant or antiplatelet medicines should consult their physician before taking an NSAID with these other medications.

Salicylates are contraindicated in gout patients, but traditional NSAIDs are the first-line treatment for gout pain. Salicylates increase the blood concentration of uric acid and can cause gout flare-ups. Salicylates also amplify the hypoglycemic effects of sulfonylureas, which are prescribed to type 2 diabetics. People with type 2 diabetes using sulfonylureas should not use salicylates.

PREGNANCY AND BREASTFEEDING

In 2020, the US Food and Drug Administration (FDA) required drug manufacturers to include a new warning on all NSAID and NSAID-containing medications. This warning specified that pregnant women should not use NSAIDs during the final twenty weeks of their pregnancies. NSAID use during this period can cause fetal kidney dysfunction. At approximately twenty weeks gestation, most amniotic fluid is produced by the baby's kidneys as fetal urine. Maternal NSAID use decreases fetal renal function and diminishes amniotic fluid production. Fetal renal dysfunction leads to low amniotic fluid levels (oligohydramnios). Oligohydramnios impairs pulmonary, digestive, and muscular development and causes developmental malformations, growth restriction, and preterm birth.

The fetus does not yet use its lungs and relies on oxygenated blood from the placenta. Fetal circulation includes a bypass between the aorta and the pulmonary artery called the "ductus arteriosus." Oxygenated blood from the placenta flows into the right atrium, and most of the blood flows through a hole in the atrial septum called the "foramen ovale" into the left atrium. Blood that does not flow through the foramen ovale is pumped from the right ventricle into the pulmonary artery. Most of the blood flows through the ductus arteriosus to the aorta from the pulmonary artery. The ductus arteriosus remains open during fetal life because of high concentrations of prostaglandin E_2, made by the placenta and the ductus arteriosus. At birth, the removal of the placenta causes the ductus arteriosus to wither and becomes the ligamentum arteriosum.

Taking NSAIDs at thirty weeks' gestation may cause persistent neonatal pulmonary hypertension. Inhibiting prostaglandin E_2 biosynthesis prematurely closes the ductus arteriosus, resulting in congestion of the fetal pulmonary circulation. Any pregnant women taking NSAIDs should cease taking them six to eight weeks before delivery.

Some infants suffer from "patent ductus arteriosus," in which the ductus arteriosus remains open after birth. Maternal infection with Rubella virus is associated with patent ductus arteriosus. Such infants have blood routing from the aorta to the right pulmonary artery and taking multiple passes through the lungs. This condition causes no symptoms, but babies will have a "machinelike" murmur caused by blood moving from the aorta to the pulmonary artery. Later, as the baby gets older, their increased pulmonary blood volumes may cause pulmonary hypertension. Intravenous indomethacin is the treatment of choice to force closure of the ductus arteriosus.

Unfortunately, there is little safety data on NSAID use during breastfeeding. Low-dose aspirin is safe during breastfeeding, as is ibuprofen. None of the other NSAIDs have enough data to establish their safety and should be avoided.

—*Michael A. Buratovich*

Further Reading

"FDA Recommends Avoiding Use of NSAIDs in Pregnancy at 20 Weeks or Later Because They Can Result in Low Amniotic Fluid." *US Food and Drug Administration*, 15 Oct. 2020, www.fda.gov/drugs/drug-safety-and-availability/fda-recommends-avoiding-use-nsaids-pregnancy-20-weeks-or-later-because-they-can-result-low-amniotic. Accessed 7 June 2022.

"Nonopioid Drugs for Pain." *Medical Letter on Drugs and Therapeutics*, vol. 64, no. 1645, 2022, pp. 33-40.

"Non-Steroidal Anti-Inflammatory Drugs (NSAIDs)." *Cleveland Clinic*, 25 Jan. 2020, my.clevelandclinic.org/health/drugs/11086-non-steroidal-anti-inflammatory-medicines-nsaids. Accessed 7 June 2022.

"NSAIDs." *National Health Service (UK)*, 27 Feb. 2019, www.nhs.uk/conditions/nsaids/. Accessed 7 June 2022.

"NSAIDs: Do They Increase My Risk of Heart Attack and Stroke?" *Mayo Clinic*, 10 Dec. 2020, www.mayoclinic.org/diseases-conditions/heart-attack/expert-answers/nsaids-heart-attack-stroke/faq-20147557. Accessed 7 June 2022.

Solomon, Daniel H. "Non-Steroidal Anti-Inflammatory Drugs (NSAIDs) (Beyond the Basics)." *UpToDate*, 8 Mar. 2022, www-uptodate-com.arbor.idm.oclc.org/contents/nonsteroidal-antiinflammatory-drugs-nsaids-beyond-the-basics?search=NSAIDs&topicRef=7989&source=see_link. Accessed 7 June 2022.

Watson, James C. "Evaluation of Pain." *Merck Manual Consumer Version*, Apr. 2020, www.merckmanuals.com/home/brain,-spinal-cord,-and-nerve-disorders/pain/evaluation-of-pain. Accessed 7 June 2022.

OXYCODONE

Category: Addiction risk; Opioid
Also known as: Blue, hillbilly heroin, kicker; OC, OX, oxy, oxycotton, Perc, Roxy
Specialties and related fields: Addiction counseling, pain specialty, pharmacology, psychiatry, psychology

KEY TERMS

abuse-deterrent formulations: drug preparation intended to prevent, impede, or discourage physical and chemical tampering (e.g., crushing, chewing, extraction, smoking, snorting, injecting) while still being able to provide safe and accurate delivery of the opioid for therapeutic benefit

addiction: a neuropsychological disorder characterized by persistent use of a drug, despite substantial harm and other negative consequences

opioid: substances that act on opioid receptors to relieve pain, augment sedation, suppress diarrhea and coughs

HISTORY OF USE

Oxycodone is a semisynthetic opioid. In the United States, oxycodone comes in oral preparation only. Oxycodone is frequently combined with acetaminophen (Percocet) and is prescribed for acute pain. Long-acting formulations are commonly prescribed for chronic cancer pain. Oxycodone formulations are listed in the table below.

Drug name	Formulations
Oxycodone—generic	5 mg capsules, 5, 10, 15, 20, 30 mg tablets, 1, 100 mg/5 mL solution
Oxaydo	5, 7,5 mg tablets
Roxybond—extended-release, abuse-deterrent formulation	5, 15, 30 tablets
Oxycontin—extended-release, abuse-deterrent formulation	10, 15, 20, 30, 40, 60, 80, mg ER tablets
Xtampza ER—extended-release, abuse-deterrent formulation	5, 10 mg tablets
Generic, extended-release formation	5, 7.5, 10, 15, 20, 30, 40 mg ER tablets

Oxycodone is also available in fixed-dose combinations with acetaminophen (Percocet), aspirin (Percodan), and ibuprofen (Combunox).

Oxycodone was first synthesized in 1916 at the University of Frankfurt in Germany. It was developed as a nonaddictive substitute for opioids, including morphine, heroin, and codeine. Oxycodone became available in the United States in 1939. However, its misuse potential was not recognized until the 1950s, when Percodan, an oxycodone/aspirin combination, was introduced. As a result, all oxycodone-containing products are classified as schedule II-controlled substances, the strictest classification for legal medications. Schedule II drugs have a high misuse potential and legitimate medical use.

The illicit misuse of oxycodone dramatically increased in 1996 in the United States after the marketing by Purdue Pharma of OxyContin, the controlled-release prescription form of oxycodone. OxyContin, consumed for its relaxing and euphoric effects, became the best-selling narcotic pain reliever on the market.

Although oxycodone is not as potent as heroin, it remains one of the most highly addictive and widely misused prescription drugs. It has served as a gateway for many to heroin addiction. Despite numerous efforts to curb the illegal use of oxycodone-containing products, its misuse remains a major concern in the United States.

EFFECTS AND POTENTIAL RISKS

Oxycodone is structurally similar to codeine and hydrocodone but pharmacologically resembles morphine. It acts through opioid receptors to alter the brain's response to pain, lessening pain sensations. Like other opiates, oxycodone elevates dopamine levels, the neurotransmitter linked to pleasurable experiences. Oxycodone's short-term effects include a rush of euphoria and joy, leading to a dreamy, relaxed state. Negative short-term effects include nausea, vomiting, constipation, dizziness, and sedation. Physiological effects include pain relief, respiratory depression, sedation, constipation, cough suppression, and in combination with acetaminophen, may cause liver damage.

Many people use oxycodone to achieve an opiate-like high. In contrast, others use it to minimize withdrawal symptoms of morphine and heroin addiction. Oxycodone users achieve the greatest high by bypassing OxyContin's controlled-release mechanism, consuming the entire dose at once. Pills are typically chewed, crushed, snorted, mixed with a liquid, and injected.

Oxycodone, like other opioids, comes in abuse-deterrent formulations that turn into insoluble gels when mixed with liquids. This property presumably discourages low-tech methods for abusing these drugs. Unfortunately, no studies have compared the safety of abuse-deterrent formulations with other formulations. Additionally, although opioid manufacturers invested substantial time, money, and research into developing abuse-deterrent formulations, whether they discourage opioid abuse remains uncertain. No drug formulation prevents people from taking many pills at once, which is the most common abuse method.

Oxycodone leads to dependency and addiction and must be used with extreme caution and supervision. Individuals with a history of alcohol or drug addiction are more likely to become addicted to oxycodone. Long-term misuse may affect brain functioning because of hypoxia (low blood-oxygen levels) in the brain that results from repeated respiratory depression. Oxycodone addiction often requires professional intervention and treatment to help individuals overcome addiction. Greater emphasis is being placed on the illegal use of oxycodone, including physicians' legal prosecution of overprescribing.

—*Rose Ciulla-Bohling, Patricia Stanfill Edens, Michael A. Buratovich*

Further Reading

Jeurgens, Jeffrey, and Theresa Parisi. "Oxycodone Addiction and Abuse." *Addiction Center*, 16 July 2019, www.addictioncenter.com/opiates/oxycodone/.

Joseph, Andrew. "New Details Revealed about Purdue's Marketing of OxyContin." *STAT*, 18 Jan. 2019, www.statnews.com/2019/01/15/massachusetts-purdue-lawsuit-new-details/.

Moradi, Mohammad, et al. "Use of Oxycodone in Pain Management." *Anesthesiology and Pain Medicine*, vol. 1, no. 4, 2012, pp. 262-64, doi:10.5812/aapm.4529.

"Opioids for Pain." *Medical Letter on Drugs and Therapeutics*, vol. 60, no. 1544, 2018, pp. 57-64.

"Oxycodone." *MedlinePlus*, US National Library of Medicine, 15 Oct. 2019, medlineplus.gov/druginfo/meds/a682132.html.

Raffa, R. B., et al. "Oxycodone Combinations for Pain Relief." *Drugs of Today*, vol. 46, no. 6, 2010, p. 379, doi:10.1358/dot.2010.46.6.1470106.

Raleigh, M. D., et al. "Safety and Efficacy of an Oxycodone Vaccine: Addressing Some of the Unique Considerations Posed by Opioid Abuse." *PLOS One*, vol. 12, no. 12, 2017, doi:10.1371/journal.pone.0184876.

Schmidt-Hansen, Mia, et al. "Oxycodone for Cancer-Related Pain." *Cochrane Database of Systematic Reviews*, 2017, doi:10.1002/14651858.cd003870.pub6.

Pain Management

Category: Treatment

Specialties and related fields: Alternative medicine, anesthesiology, critical care, emergency medicine, geriatrics and gerontology, oncology, pharmacology, physical therapy, psychiatry, psychology

Definition: any treatment or management technique to lessen or eliminate pain or make it more tolerable

KEY TERMS

narcotics: psychoactive compounds with numbing or paralyzing properties

neuropathic pain: pain caused by a lesion or disease of the somatosensory nervous system

opioids: drugs that activate opioid receptors to relieve pain, augment anesthesia, suppress diarrhea, and quell coughing

pain: physical suffering or discomfort caused by illness or injury

pain relief: alleviation of pain, typically through medication

INDICATIONS AND PROCEDURES

Pain is experienced as an unpleasant reaction to either an external stimulus (e.g., a burn) or an internal process (e.g., a disease). The initial evaluation of pain is aimed at determining the cause. A good description by the patient aids diagnosis. The person experiencing the pain must communicate the intensity, location, pattern (throbbing, steady, or intermittent), and type (crushing, burning, sharp, or dull). In addition, factors that make the pain better or worse must be known and communicated. Duration is important; recent onset is called "acute" pain, while long-standing pain or pain that returns periodically is called "chronic."

Generally, the best way to treat pain is to prevent its occurrence. If pain avoidance fails, several different interventions should be used together. Whatever treatment is used, the health-care provider must tailor the therapy both to the patient and to the nature and severity of the pain. When medications are used, a review of some important principles is essential, such as the pharmacology, duration of effectiveness, and optimal dose of a certain medication. Health-care providers must consider even the route of administration in every case.

Treatment may include combinations of simple analgesics, narcotics, and other treatments. Combinations take advantage of the additive pain relief while sparing the patient potential side effects. When choosing pain medications, a stepwise approach is often used. It starts with simple analgesics: aspirin, acetaminophen, and nonsteroidal anti-inflammatory drugs (NSAIDs). These medications are generally well-tolerated, although aspirin and NSAIDs can produce gastrointestinal distress ranging from mild heartburn to bleeding ulcers. Additionally, adjuncts to these medications might be icing or heat, depending on the nature of the problem.

For more severe pain, the second step often includes a narcotic analgesic with or without the simple analgesics. Narcotics are very potent and have the potential for addiction. Furthermore, they may produce problems such as confusion, nausea and vomiting, constipation, and drowsiness. Suppose the pain has a significant inflammation component that does not resolve easily with milder analgesic approaches or narcotics. In that case, corticosteroids may be used to alleviate the pain. Corticosteroid use does not lend itself well to longer-term pain management, however, because of side effects such as fluid retention, stomach irritation, thrush, muscle weakness, weight gain, bone loss, suppressed adrenal function, and increased risk of infections, among others.

The third step in pain control involves alternative methods of pain control. Treatments here include physical therapy, nerve-blocking injections, transcutaneous electrical nerve stimulation (TENS), and behavioral approaches. The latter method seeks to identify the causes of preventable pain (physical or mental) and takes steps to minimize pain.

Medical research is leading to interesting discoveries about the management of pain. In 2002, researchers announced that they had identified a key protein that controls severe pain, a discovery that could lead to better pain management for patients who suffer from chronic pain or pain associated with terminal cancer. The protein, known by the acronym DREAM (downstream regulatory element antagonistic modulator), protects the neural reflex critical to survival, allowing individuals to feel pain and quickly pull away from its source. Still, DREAM seems to help sharp pain fade over time as the protein becomes disabled. Moreover, while there are many types of pain, disabling the DREAM protein appears to reduce its severity. The next step in this research will be to examine ways to disable the protein; a task scientists deem difficult because of its location deep within individual cells. Additional research in this area recognizes that pain has different causes and that it may be more productive to examine pain mechanisms rather than a disease-based approach.

—*Misa Hyakutake*

Further Reading

Ballantyne, Jane C., et al., editors. *Bonica's Management of Pain*. 5th ed., Lippincott Williams & Wilkins, 2018.

Cousins, Michael J., and P. O. Bridenbaugh, editors. *Cousins and Bridenbaugh's Neural Blockade in Clinical Anesthesia and Management of Pain*. 4th ed., Lippincott Williams & Wilkins, 2009.

Dillard, James M. *The Chronic Pain Solution: The Comprehensive, Step-by-Step Guide to Choosing the Best of Alternative and Conventional Medicine*. Bantam Books, 2002.

"DREAM Repression & Dynorphin Expression." *Protein Lounge*, n.d., proteinlounge.com/dream-repression-and-dynorphin-expression-pg-299.html.

Fenske J. N., et al. *Pain Management.* Michigan Medicine University of Michigan, 2021, www.ncbi.nlm.nih.gov/books/NBK572296/.

Ferrari, Lynne R., editor. *Anesthesia and Pain Management for the Pediatrician*. Johns Hopkins UP, 1999.

Fishman, Scott, with Lisa Berger. *The War on Pain: How Breakthroughs in the New Field of Pain Medicine Are Turning the Tide Against Suffering*. HarperCollins, 2001.

Hoppenfeld, J. D. *Fundamentals of Pain Medicine: How to Diagnose and Treat Your Patients*. Lippincott Williams & Wilkin, 2014.

"Pain Management Programs." *American Chronic Pain Association*, 2021, www.theacpa.org/pain-management-programs/.

"Pain Treatment." *Leukemia and Lymphoma Society*, n.d., www.lls.org/treatment/managing-side-effects/pain/pain-treatment.

Rosenfeld, Arthur. *The Truth About Chronic Pain: Patients and Professionals on How to Face It, Understand It, Overcome It*. Rev. ed., Basic Books, 2005.

Prescription NSAIDs

Category: NSAID, Anti-Inflammatory
Specialties and related fields: Orthopedics, pain medicine, pharmacology, rheumatology
Definition: a therapeutic drug class that reduces pain, decreases inflammation, decreases fever, and may prevent blood clots

KEY TERMS

cyclooxygenase: enzymes that catalyze the initial reactions that culminate in the synthesis of prostaglandins

NSAID: nonsteroidal anti-inflammatory drugs

platelets: blood cells that help your body form clots to stop bleeding

INTRODUCTION

Many people worldwide deal with pain caused by chronic inflammatory conditions like arthritis or musculoskeletal problems and receive significant benefits from Nonsteroidal anti-inflammatory drugs (NSAIDs) to manage their pain. NSAIDs are anti-inflammatory analgesic medications that treat mild to moderate pain, which can be short- or long-term. People can also take them to bring down a fever. NSAIDs are not opioids and do not have addictive properties. They are relatively inexpensive and accessible, but it is crucial to understand how to use them properly. Over twenty different brands of NSAIDs can be purchased over the counter, such as aspirin, Advil or Motrin (ibuprofen), and Aleve (naproxen sodium). Many other NSAIDs are prescription medications prescribed by health-care providers. Examples of prescription NSAIDs include Mobic (meloxicam) and Celebrex (celecoxib). Health care providers prescribe NSAIDs to patients with chronic pain to help them manage their pain more effectively. Patients differ in response to different NSAIDs for unknown reasons, so if one isn't working, another in the same class may work much better.

HOW NSAIDS WORK

Oral NSAIDs work within one hour of taking the medication, and their effects usually last from four to twelve hours, depending on whether they are short- or long-acting. Patients typically experience the maximum anti-inflammatory effects of NSAIDs after taking them for about two weeks.

NSAIDs inhibit cyclooxygenase enzymes (or COX enzymes) from working inside the body. These enzymes catalyze the formation of small molecules called "prostaglandins," which activate pain receptor nerve endings, thus causing a sensation of pain and mediating tissue inflammation. Prostaglandins also protect the gastrointestinal mucosa, regulate blood flow to the kidneys, and help with platelet aggregation. NSAIDs inhibit COX enzyme activity, which relieves pain. There are two subtypes of COX enzymes, COX-1 and COX-2. Most NSAIDs block the action of both COX-1 and COX-2, but usually, specific NSAIDs inhibit one type of COX enzyme more than the other. The reduction of COX-1 enzymatic activity concomitantly reduces pain and inflammation. Unfortunately, blocking COX-1 also diminishes the gastric protective properties of prostaglandins and, therefore, causes damage to the mucosa of the gastrointestinal tract and increases the risk of gastrointestinal bleeding. Celebrex is the FDA-approved medication that specifically inhibits COX-2. Pharmaceutical companies developed new NSAIDs targeting COX-2 to squelch inflammation and pain without the undesired gastrointestinal and bleeding effects. However, blocking COX-2 causes a greater risk of forming blood clots and having a heart attack or stroke.

USES AND APPLICATIONS

Nonsteroidal anti-inflammatory drugs are used for many types of pain, including toothaches, strains and sprains, joint pain, muscle pain, earaches, headaches, and menstrual cramps, to name a few. Providers can prescribe NSAIDs as pills, gels, or creams. Gels and creams are applied directly on the skin over the area of pain and provide similar benefits as the pill forms for arthritis and back pain. For some, the topical form may be safer than pill forms. The doses of prescription NSAIDs are higher than their over-the-counter versions.

SIDE EFFECTS
In general, NSAIDs are relatively safe medications and benefit many individuals. Nonsteroidal anti-inflammatory drugs' common side effects may include dizziness, heartburn, constipation, epigastric pain, nausea, rash, tinnitus, edema, fluid retention, headache, or vomiting.

Side-effect profiles of specific NSAIDs depend on their selectivity for COX-1 or COX-2. Those already at higher risk for gastrointestinal, cardiovascular, or renal adverse effects will have an increased risk for adverse effects. Those NSAIDs that are relatively nonselective for COX-1 or COX-2, such as aspirin, have more gastrointestinal side effects such as nausea, heartburn, indigestion, and potentially peptic ulcers. However, at low doses, aspirin is cardioprotective. Nonsteroidal anti-inflammatory drugs that are slightly more selective for COX-2 than COX-1, such as ibuprofen and naproxen, have a low risk of cardiovascular events but a higher risk of gastrointestinal side effects, though not as high as aspirin. Those NSAIDs that are even more selective for COX-2, such as meloxicam, diclofenac, etodolac, indomethacin, piroxicam, nabumetone, and sulindac, should be used with caution in patients with increased risk for cardiovascular side effects, but have a lower risk for gastrointestinal side effects. Celecoxib, marketed as Celebrex, is entirely selective for COX-2 and carries the lowest low risk of gastrointestinal side effects but the highest risk of blood clots, heart attacks, or stroke (in rare cases).

Patients on NSAIDs should take the lowest dose that achieves the desired effects. Such a strategy reduces the risk of adverse effects. Long-term NSAID use has serious side effects when taking high doses. Patients can prevent NSAIDs' gastrointestinal adverse effects by taking medications such as proton pump inhibitors (PPIs) with the NSAID. Those with high blood pressure need to use caution when taking NSAIDs, as they can further increase their blood pressure. Patients with cardiovascular disease should exercise care when taking NSAIDs since they may increase the risk of cardiac events. Likewise, patients with chronic renal failure should also avoid NSAIDs since they can harm the kidneys. Pregnant women should not use NSAIDs during the last three months of pregnancy. As with any drug, there is also a risk of an allergic reaction.

—*Jodi L. Guy*

Further Reading
Gorczyca, Pamela, et al. "NSAIDs: Balancing the Risks and Benefits." *US Pharmacist*, vol. 41, no. 3, 2016, pp. 24-26.
Hecht, Marjorie. "Side Effects from NSAIDs." *Healthline*, 23 July 2019, www.healthline.com/health/side-effects-from-nsaids#7-side-effects
Perry, Laura, et al. "Cardiovascular Risks Associated with NSAIDs and COX-2 Inhibitors." *US Pharmacist*, vol. 39, no. 3, 2014, pp. 35-38.
Prescribers Digital Reference, www.pdr.net. A resource to look up specific drugs.
Shah, Seema, and Vivek Mehta. "Controversies and Advances in Non-Steroidal Anti-Inflammatory Drug (NSAID) Analgesia in Chronic Pain Management." *Postgraduate Medical Journal*, vol. 88, no. 1036, 2012, pp. 73-78.
Underwood, M., et al. "Advice to Use Topical or Oral Ibuprofen for Chronic Knee Pain in Older People: Randomized Control Trial and Patient Preference Study." *British Medical Journal*, vol. 336, no. 138, 2007, pp. 1-12, doi:10.1136/bmj.39399.656331.25.

Tramadol

Category: Addiction risk; Opioid
Also known as: ConZip, Ultram
Specialties and related fields: Oncology, orthopedics, pain medicine, pharmacology, sports medicine
Definition: a centrally acting μ-opioid receptor agonist and SNRI (serotonin/norepinephrine reuptake-inhibitor) structurally related to codeine and morphine

KEY TERMS

analgesic: drugs used to relieve pain

opioid: substances that activate opioid receptors to relieve pain, augment anesthesia, suppress diarrhea and coughs

HISTORY OF USE

Tramadol was first synthesized in 1962 by the German pharmaceutical company Grünenthal. Tramadol has been in clinical use in Germany since 1977. Originally marketed as a safe painkiller with a low risk of misuse, tramadol became the most prescribed opioid on the European market. It was introduced to the prescription drug market in the United States in 1995 as Ultram, a nontraditional, centrally acting analgesic. Tramadol has a nonscheduled status, meaning it has a low potential for misuse.

Tramadol produces pleasurable sensations and relaxation without increased drowsiness, enabling people to remain productive while managing pain. It is an easily available opiate and can be habit-forming because of its morphine-like properties. Because of reports of increased tramadol misuse, it has been labeled a drug of concern by the US Food and Drug Administration and thus requires additional label warnings. Some US states have classified tramadol as a controlled substance.

EFFECTS AND POTENTIAL RISKS

Tramadol is a nontraditional, centrally acting opioid analgesic with morphine-like pain-relieving activity. It has a dual mechanism of pain relief because it includes a mixture of enantiomers.

Studies suggest that opioid and non-opioid or monoaminergic mechanisms mediate tramadol activity. Monoaminergic activity is displayed by inhibiting the reuptake of norepinephrine and serotonin, neurotransmitters responsible for altering pain response in the brain. It exhibits opioid activity by binding to specific opioid receptors in the brain that decrease pain perception.

The short-term effects of tramadol include feelings of euphoria, mood elevation, and relaxation. Tramadol is usually well tolerated but can be associated with negative short-term effects, including nausea, vomiting, constipation, drowsiness, dizziness, vertigo, weakness, and headache.

Long-term use of tramadol can be associated with drug dependence and possible addiction. Abruptly stopping tramadol may generate opiate-like withdrawal symptoms such as anxiety, agitation, sweating, abdominal upset, and hallucinations.

—Rose Ciulla-Bohling

Further Reading

Hassamal, Sameer, et al. "Tramadol: Understanding the Risk of Serotonin Syndrome and Seizures." *The American Journal of Medicine*, vol. 131, no. 11, 2018, doi:10.1016/j.amjmed.2018.04.025.

Jeurgens, Jeffrey, and Theresa Parisi. "Tramadol Addiction and Abuse." *Addiction Center*, 16 July 2019, www.addictioncenter.com/opiates/tramadol/.

Mayo Clinic. "Historically 'Safer' Tramadol More Likely than Other Opioids to Result in Prolonged Use." *ScienceDaily*, 14 May 2019, www.sciencedaily.com/releases/2019/05/190514090953.htm.

Shmerling, Robert H. "Is Tramadol a Risky Pain Medication?" *Harvard Health Blog*. Harvard Medical School, 16 Aug. 2019, www.health.harvard.edu/blog/is-tramadol-a-risky-pain-medication-2019061416844.

Subedi, Muna, et al. "An Overview of Tramadol and Its Usage in Pain Management and Future Perspective." *Biomedicine & Pharmacotherapy*, vol. 111, 2019, pp. 443-51, doi:10.1016/j.biopha.2018.12.085.

Thiels, Cornelius A., et al. "Chronic Use of Tramadol after Acute Pain Episode: Cohort Study." *BMJ*, vol. 365, 2019, doi:10.1136/bmj.l1849.

"Tramadol." *MedlinePlus*, 15 Jan. 2019, medlineplus.gov/druginfo/meds/a695011.html.

Valium (diazepam)

Category: Addiction risk; Anxiolytic; Muscle relaxant; Sedative

Also known as: Diazepam, 7-Chloro-1,3-dihydro-1-methyl-5-phenyl-2H-1,4-benzodiazepine-2-one, and by other various brand names internationally

Specialties and related fields: Addiction, orthopedics, pharmacology, physical medicine and rehabilitation, psychiatry, sports medicine

Definition: a tranquilizing muscle-relaxant drug used chiefly to relieve anxiety

KEY TERMS

anticonvulsants: a diverse group of pharmacological agents used to treat epileptic seizures

benzodiazepine: a class of psychoactive drugs whose core chemical structure is the fusion of a benzene ring and a diazepine ring that lower brain activity and are prescribed to treat conditions such as anxiety, insomnia, and seizures

gamma-aminobutyric acid (GABA): the chief inhibitory neurotransmitter in the mammalian central nervous system; its principal role is reducing neuronal excitability throughout the nervous system

muscle relaxant: a drug that affects skeletal muscle function and decreases muscle tone. It may be used to alleviate symptoms such as muscle spasms, pain, and hyperreflexia

HISTORY OF USE

Valium, a brand name of diazepam, was synthesized by chemist Leo Sternbach in 1963 while working at Hoffman-La Roche. It was the second benzodiazepine marketed by the company, the first being Librium (chlordiazepoxide) in 1960. *Valium*'s name is based on the Latin *valere* (meaning "be strong"). Valium is indicated to treat anxiety (including preoperative anxiety), seizures, agitation, tremor and impending acute delirium tremens in acute alcohol withdrawal, and skeletal muscle spasm or spasticity caused by various disorders, including cerebral palsy, paraplegia, and stiff-man syndrome.

Valium, Librium, and other benzodiazepines became a popular alternative to the drugs used at the time to treat nervous and mental disorders, including chloral hydrate, reserpine, barbiturates, and meprobamate, as such drugs had serious side effects and were habit-forming. Conversely, Valium, along with Librium, was less toxic and initially appeared to cause less dependence and side effects.

As a result of these desirable drug properties, enthusiasm in the medical community, and marketing campaigns, benzodiazepines became the most frequently prescribed drugs. Consequently, Americans consumed 2.3 billion tablets of Valium in 1978. Valium's prevalence in society was so great that the Rolling Stones wrote a song called "Mother's Little Helper" in 1966, which related to housewives' use of Valium to get through their busy and stressful days. The song's title became a nickname for Valium and other similar benzodiazepine drugs. Valium was referred to in best-selling books of the time, including Jacqueline Susann's *Valley of the Dolls*.

During this period of popularity, reports of misuse and dependence were published. These misuse/dependence concerns subsequently increased, especially when Valium was combined with other drugs, leading to various recommendations limiting the use of Valium. Even though newer generations of drugs have been developed to treat anxiety, Valium is still prescribed today to manage the various conditions described above effectively.

EFFECTS AND POTENTIAL RISKS

Neurotransmitters are chemical messengers which allow communication between nerve cells. Neurotransmitters regulate most systems in the human body, including breathing, brain activity, movement, and heart rate. Neurotransmitters typically exert their influence by binding to receptor proteins at the end of nerve cells, which, in turn, cause one or more various cellular events to occur. Valium exerts its effects by binding to the receptor for the neurotransmitter gamma-aminobutyric acid (GABA). GABA is an inhibitory neurotransmitter whose effects are increased upon Valium binding to the GABA receptor.

Some common side effects of Valium, which typically disappear after prolonged use, include fatigue, drowsiness, muscle weakness, and ataxia. Other adverse reactions include leucopenia, jaundice, hypersensitivity, irritability, aggression, restlessness, delusion, nightmares, hallucinations, psychoses, anterograde amnesia, and physical dependence. Many of these side effects are more likely to occur in children and the elderly, so extra care is recommended in such cases.

—*Lenela Glass-Godwin, Jason J. Schwartz*

Further Reading

Calcaterra, Nicholas E., and James C. Barrow. "Classics in Chemical Neuroscience: Diazepam (*Valium*)." *ACS Chemical Neuroscience*, vol. 5, no. 4, 2014, pp. 253-60, doi:10.1021/cn5000056.

Cheng, Tianze, et al. "*Valium* without Dependence? Individual GABAA Receptor Subtype Contribution toward Benzodiazepine Addiction, Tolerance, and Therapeutic Effects." *Neuropsychiatric Disease and Treatment*, vol. 14, 2018, pp. 1351-61, doi:10.2147/ndt.s164307.

"Diazepam." *MedlinePlus*, US National Library of Medicine, 15 July 2019, medlineplus.gov/druginfo/meds/a682047.html.

Pringle, A., et al. "Cognitive Mechanisms of Diazepam Administration: A Healthy Volunteer Model of Emotional Processing." *Psychopharmacology*, vol. 233, no. 12, 6 May 2016, pp. 2221-28, doi:10.1007/s00213-016-4269-y.

"Valium: Side Effects, Addiction, Symptoms & Treatment: What Is Valium?" *American Addiction Centers*, 14 Nov. 2019, americanaddictioncenters.org/valium-treatment.

DRUG DOPING

Cheating in sports is as old as humanity. From Gaylord Perry's spitballs to the Houston Astros banging on a garbage can to broadcast what pitch was to be thrown, professional athletes have done what they can to secure a competitive advantage. Anabolic steroids and other drugs illegitimately boost an athlete's strength and performance and have been banned. This section explores these substances, how they work, and why they are so bad for athletes in the long run. Some of the athletes who have been involved in scandals are discussed, including Lance Armstrong, Diego Maradonae, Marion Jones, and Andreea Raducan.

ATHLETE DRUG TESTING

Category: Testing
Specialties and related fields: Biochemistry, laboratory tests, medicinal chemistry
Definition: analyses conducted on athletes to determine if they have taken banned substances

KEY TERMS

gas chromatography: a common laboratory procedure used in analytical chemistry for separating and analyzing compounds that can be vaporized without decomposition

hormones: a regulatory substance produced in an organism and transported in tissue fluids such as blood to stimulate specific cells or tissues into action

performance-enhancing substances: substances that improve any form of activity performance in humans

SIGNIFICANCE

Athletes competing at high levels seek to gain advantages over their opponents. Some do so by using substances that they believe can improve athletic performance or the body's physical work capacity. Many of these substances are drugs, and many are banned by various organizations that regulate sports, such as the National Collegiate Athletic Association and the International Olympic Committee. Some athletes still use these substances despite such bans, making drug testing necessary to keep competition fair. Athletes who fail drug tests may be ruled ineligible for competition or have their previously awarded medals or titles revoked.

The use of particular substances to improve athletic performance dates back to the ancient Greeks. It was not until 1928 that the International Amateur Athletic Federation became the first sports organization to ban athletes' use of certain substances. The federation, however, had no way to detect whether athletes were breaking the rules, and the use of performance-enhancing substances continued to increase. Drug testing of athletes for banned substances was first used in 1966 by the international federations governing the sports of soccer and cycling. By the 1970s, the widespread use of anabolic steroids among athletes forced the introduction of drug testing by most international sports organizations. The National Collegiate Athletic Association (NCAA) implemented a drug-testing program in the fall of 1986 for all athletes participating in NCAA bowl games and national championships. By 1990, the NCAA had adopted year-round testing of athletes on teams within the association. In November 2007, the World Anti-Doping Code was approved and now guides testing worldwide.

DRUG-TESTING TECHNIQUES

Common methods used to detect illicit drug use include testing blood, urine, hair, and saliva samples. The method chosen for a particular purpose must consider the accuracy level provided by the test, the ease of obtaining the sample, and the period for which the test can detect drugs in the sample. Urine testing is most commonly used for athletes because it is accurate, no cutting or piercing of the skin is involved, and it can detect drug use for the previous seven days or longer. To complete a urine test, an athlete must provide a fresh sample of urine collected in a clean vessel under supervision. Although this may be awkward for some, the tester must be certain that the vessel contains that particular athlete's actual urine. After the vessel is appropriately labeled, it is sent to a laboratory for analysis.

The techniques used to examine urine for the presence of drugs include gas chromatography, mass spectrometry, and immunoassay. In gas chromatography, the urine sample is vaporized in the presence of a gaseous solvent as it travels through a machine called a "gas chromatograph." Because the various substances in the urine dissolve in the solvent at different rates. They come out of the solvent at different times, leaving a pattern on a liquid or solid material. A detector analyzes the pattern, and a chromatogram is produced. Because different drugs produce different chromatograms, the analyst can compare the urine sample output with known drug outputs to identify specific drugs in the urine. A mass spectrometer is a machine with a long magnetic tube with a detector at its end. An electron beam blasts the urine sample and sends it down the tube to the detector. Every substance has a unique mass spectrometer output. By comparing the outputs of known drugs with the urine output, the analyst can identify any specific drugs present in the urine. Immunoassay tests are used to detect the presence of hormonelike drugs in urine. A specific antibody (a protein that binds to particular substances) is tagged with a fluorescent dye or a radioactive marker and then mixed with the urine sample. The antibody binds to the drug (hormone). The analyst measures the amount of fluorescent light or radioactivity in the sample to determine the amount of the drug or hormone present. Because this test also measures naturally occurring hormones in the urine. The analyst must know the athlete's natural hormone level to determine whether the athlete has taken a hormonelike drug. Despite precautions, false-positive tests do occur. Therefore, appropriate follow-up testing and appeals processes must be in place.

CHALLENGES TO DRUG TESTING

The ongoing challenge for athletic drug testing is the constant development of new drugs that existing methods and technologies cannot detect. Athletes are continually looking for new advantages, and manufacturers are developing new drugs to improve athletic performance. After a new performance-enhancing substance becomes available, it often takes months or years for it to become popular enough to warrant the attention of sports officials. Then months or even years may elapse before scientists develop new tests to determine whether athletes have used these drugs. During this lag of up to several years before a given drug is detectable, more drugs are developed, and the process begins again. This cycle creates a perpetual challenge to those who seek to keep sports competitions free from the use of banned performance-enhancing substances. To combat this problem and discourage athletes from trying to beat the current tests, some agencies are testing and then preserving samples so laboratories can analyze them later with new test procedures.

—*Bradley R. A. Wilson*

Further Reading

Cooper, Chris. *Run, Swim, Throw, Cheat: The Science Behind Drugs in Sport*. Oxford UP, 2012.

Cotten, Doyice J., and John T. Wolohan. *Law for Recreation and Sport Managers*. 6th ed., Kendall/Hunt, 2013.

Gardiner, Simon, et al. *Sports Law*. 4th ed., Routledge, 2012.

Henne, Kathryn E. *Testing for Athlete Citizenship: Regulating Doping and Sex in Sport*. Rutgers UP, 2015.

Ray, Richard, and Konin, Jeff. *Management Strategies in Athletic Training*. 4th ed., Human Kinetics, 2011.

BLOOD DOPING

Category: Training

Specialties and related fields: Athletic training, hematology

Definition: the injection of oxygenated blood into an athlete before an event to enhance athletic performance

KEY TERMS

erythropoietin: a peptide hormone secreted by the kidneys that increases the rate of production of red blood cells in response to falling levels of oxygen in the tissues

HIF-1: hypoxia-inducible factor; a transcription factor that responds to decreases in available oxygen in the cellular environment, or hypoxia

polycythemia: an abnormally increased concentration of hemoglobin in the blood, through either reduction of plasma volume or increase in red cell numbers; it may be a primary disease of unknown cause or a secondary condition linked to respiratory or circulatory disorder or cancer

INTRODUCTION

Engineering the increase of red blood cells carried in the bloodstream is known as "blood doping." Red blood cells distribute oxygen to organ systems as well as muscle tissues. Higher levels of red blood cells elevate the ability of an athlete to perform in a given sport—more oxygen in the blood results in increased endurance, speed, and strength. The practice of blood doping existed under the radar of sports governing bodies until 1985. In professional sports, the practice is now illegal and is considered dangerous. The blood doping methods are varied and complex and can require intervention from health care professionals. Health risks associated with blood doping include heart attack, stroke, pulmonary embolism, and contamination. Blood contamination can also lead to sepsis, a systematic bacterial infection of the blood and organs that is often fatal. Pharmaceuticals used to increase blood oxygen levels can decrease the function of the liver and cause permanent damage to this organ.

BACKGROUND

Though various dates are recorded, blood doping was developed and practiced in the middle part of the nineteenth century. Before the practice was declared illegal, Kaarlo Maaninika received blood before winning two gold medals in track at the 1980 Olympics. Champion cyclist Joop Zoetmemelk in 1976 and many in the US cycling team in 1984 received transfusions preceding their wins. The International Olympic Committee ruled blood doping illegal in 1985. However, there was no test for it.

In 1993, the US Army began procedures to develop a strategy to give soldiers extended stamina, alertness, and persistence. It was named blood loading. Red blood cells were collected, stored, and administered just before the battle. The Australian and Canadian military adopted the same procedure after scientific testing proved blood loading preferable to other performance-enhancing approaches.

A wide array of methods increases red blood cells before a competition. Manipulating the messages sent to the body's bone marrow is a common pharmaceutical method. Erythropoietin (EPO) is a hormone created for managing the effects of cancer treatments such as radiation and chemotherapy. Erythropoietin signals increase the production of oxygen-carrying capacity as blood cells are built.

Related to EPO is another approach that involves hypoxia inducible factor (HIF) stabilizer. Hypoxia inducible factor recalibrates the body's natural ability to produce EPO and manipulates proteins in the body to elicit a natural increase in EPO is achieved. Pharmaceutical companies created this medicine for patients with chronic and terminal kidney disease.

A blood transfusion is a nonpharmaceutical approach. The blood of another person, who is typed and crossed to match the recipient, can provide red blood cells for transfusion. However, the athlete's blood, also known as an "autologous donation," can be used. Transfusing requires substantial assistance from medical staff to ensure patient safety in the various stages of this procedure. As with all blood doping methods, Timing is perhaps the most important aspect of the procedure. The donor's blood must be taken out weeks before a high-endurance competition to rebuild the loss of blood. Similarly, at least three days must pass between consecutive donations. Blood is frozen to preserve the quality of the red blood cells until the time of transfusion.

The synthetic compounds of perfluorocarbons and hemoglobin-based oxygen carriers can perform the work of blood elements. These compounds are engineered oxygen carriers that can increase blood oxygen at greater levels than EPO and HIF pharmaceuticals.

There are as many testing procedures for blood doping as methods to achieve it. Just as blood doping methods have been elastic and creative, so are the testing processes developed to monitor and track them. Transfusions from a donor can be identified by studying blood cell surfaces. Donor plasma will show a variance within a drawn sample. Identifying autologous donation requires that the athlete breathe a gas mixture for several minutes, and CO measures are then taken. Blood testing for synthetic elements to stimulate bone marrow production is also available, though highly complex and costly.

IMPACT

In 2000, the first cyclist to test positive for EPO was Niklas Axelson of Sweden. American cyclist Tyler Hamilton tested positive for the presence of other genetic blood cells in his system in 2004. He appealed the finding and was able to keep his Olympic gold medal because of errors revealed in the drug testing procedures, but eventually admitted to doping and returned the medal in 2011. Hundreds of Spanish professional athletes were implicated in blood doping in 2006. Alex Cherepanov, a Russian hockey player, died during a game in 2008. He frequently engaged in blood doping during the year before his death.

Cycling has endured the most coverage and is most responsible for educating the public about blood doping. The most winning cyclist in the history of the sport, Lance Armstrong, was banned for life from cycling and lost all seven of his Tour de France medals. The US Anti-Doping Agency revealed a programmatic doping system employed throughout the trajectory of the cyclist's career. Hamilton, a long-time racing team member with Armstrong, details the systematic training approach he endured in The Secret Race: Inside the Hidden World of the Tour de France (2013). While Armstrong's is the highest-profile case, blood doping was widespread in the sport in the 1990s and the first decade of the twenty-first century, and cycling has struggled to rid itself of this reputation. Though the sport avoided any major doping scandals for most of the 2010s, in 2017, Giro d'Italia winner Danilo Di Luca was banned after testing positive for EPO. André Cardoso, a Portuguese cyclist, scheduled to compete in the Tour de France, was also banned that year for blood doping.

In 2018, a minor blood doping scandal occurred in the lead-up to the Pyeongchang Olympics when the British newspaper *The Times* announced that it had been given "secret data" showing that hundreds of endurance skiers, including more than fifty who would be participating in the Olympics, had recorded abnormal blood test scores, yet had not been banned. The secretary-general of the International Ski Federation (FIS) denied this allegation.

Recent history has demonstrated the continual reinvention of pathways for achieving higher oxygen blood levels for athletic performance. Blood doping as a practice continues to evolve in response to the testing mechanisms for identifying unfair bioengineered advantages in athletic competition.

—*Joy Goldsmith*

Further Reading

"The Amateur's Complete Guide to Blood Doping." *Men's Health*, 3 Aug. 2017, www.menshealth.co.uk/fitness/blood-doping-in-sport. Accessed 27 Feb. 2018.

"At Tour de France, Doping Is Always Part of the Story." *USA Today*, 30 June 2017, www.usatoday.com/story/sports/cycling/2017/06/30/at-tour-de-france-doping-is-always-part-of-the-story/103308480/. Accessed 27 Feb. 2018.

Butler, Nick. "FIS Deny Blood Doping Allegations about Cross-Country Skiers at Pyeongchang 2018." *Inside the*

Games, 4 Feb. 2018, www.insidethegames.biz/articles/1061044/fis-deny-blood-doping-allegations-about-cross-country-skiers-at-pyeongchang-2018. Accessed 27 Feb. 2018.

deOliveira, Carolina Dizioli Rodriguez, Andre Valle de Bairros, and Mauricio Yonamine. "Blood Doping: Risks to Athlete's' Health and Strategies for Detection." *Substance Abuse and Misuse,* vol. 49, no. 4, 2014, pp. 1168-82.

Hamilton, Tyler, and Daniel Coyle. *The Secret Race: Inside the Hidden World of the Tour De France.* Bantam, 2013.

Jelkman, Wolfgang, and Carsten Lundby. "Blood Doping and Its Detection." *Blood Journal,* vol. 118, no. 9, 2013, pp. 2395-402.

Lentillon-Kaestner, V. "The Development of Doping Use in High-Level Cycling: From Team-Organized Doping to Advances in the Fight against Doping." *Scandinavian Journal of the Medical Sciences in Sports,* vol. 23, 2013, pp. 189-97.

Nelson, M., et al. "Proof of Homologous Blood Transfusion through Quantification of Blood Group Antigens." *Heamatologica,* vol. 88, no. 11, 2003, pp. 1284-95.

Vasic, Goran, et al. "Blood Doping and Risks." *Sports Montreal,* vol. 43, 2015, pp. 189-94.

Lance Armstrong Stripped of Tour de France Titles

Category: Doping
Specialties and related fields: Cycling, doping, performance-enhancing drugs
Definition: an American former professional road racing cyclist; regarded as a sports icon for winning the Tour de France seven consecutive times from 1999 to 2005, Armstrong's reputation was tarnished by a doping scandal that led to him being stripped of his Tour de France titles

KEY TERMS

doping: drug administration to inhibit or enhance sporting performance

performance-enhancing drugs: substances used to improve any form of activity performance in humans

triathlete: an athlete who competes in a multisport race that involves swimming, biking, and running across long distances

EARLY LIFE

Lance Edward Gunderson was born in Plano, Texas, on September 18, 1971. His father, Eddie Charles Gunderson, worked as a route manager for the *Dallas Morning News*. Linda Gayle, his mother, worked as a secretary. In 1973, they were divorced. His mother would later marry Terry Keith Armstrong. Terry Armstrong, who worked as a salesman, adopted Lance the same year as the marriage, 1974.

The young Lance showed an athletic aptitude at an early age. When he was twelve, he began swimming with the City of Plano Swim Club and finished fourth in Texas state 1,500-meter freestyle. Shortly after, he became interested in a junior triathlon called the Iron Kids Triathlon. He trained for this and won the event at the age of thirteen.

Lance continued to compete in events throughout his teen years. He was ranked the number one triathlete in the 1987-88 Tri-Fed/Texas. When he was only sixteen, Lance Armstrong became a professional triathlete.

LIFE'S WORK

In the early 1990s, Lance Armstrong emerged as the US national amateur cycling champion, winning the Thrift Drug Classic and the First Union Grand Prix. By the late 1990s, he was ranked among the top ten international cyclists. He won the Tour du Pont in 1995 and again in 1996 for an unprecedented second time while establishing records for the fastest average time-trial speed and the largest margin of victory.

In October 1996, Armstrong was diagnosed with advanced testicular cancer. When doctors discovered that the tumors had spread to his lungs, lymph nodes, and brain, they gave him a 40 percent chance of survival. He began an aggressive chemotherapy regimen and after a series of successful surgical procedures, was declared cancer-free in the early weeks of 1997. Unable to remain idle in the months following his diagnosis, he created the Lance Armstrong Foundation, also known as the Livestrong Foundation, an international organization dedicated to promoting cancer research, awareness, and early detection.

Armstrong returned to racing in 1998, competing in many international events. In May of that year, he married Kristin Richard, whom he had met the previous year at a charity function for his foundation. With a new contract with the United States Postal Service Pro Cycling team, Armstrong was ready to resume his place among the world's best cyclists. He returned to the Tour de France in the summer of 1999, garnering media attention for his plans to compete in the prestigious race soon after his cancer ordeal. After dominating most of the race, Armstrong became the first American to win the event since Greg LeMond in 1990, finishing with a margin of more than seven minutes over his closest competitor. Firmly denying the French media's accusations that he had used illegal performance-enhancing drugs to win the race, Lance returned the following year to a second Tour de France victory, once again joining LeMond as the only American to repeat as champion. In 2000, Armstrong competed at the Summer Olympics in Sydney, Australia, earning a bronze medal for road cycling in the men's individual time trial.

Armstrong continued to make cycling history by winning the Tour de France seven consecutive times, from 1999 to 2005. In 2002, he was named "Sportsman of the Year" by *Sports Illustrated* magazine, and from 2002 through 2005, the Associated Press named Armstrong "Male Athlete of the Year." However, Armstrong's professional accomplishments took a toll on his personal life. Lance and Kristin Armstrong filed for divorce in September 2003. Following his 2005 Tour De France victory, Armstrong retired from cycling, saying he wanted to focus his efforts on the work of his charitable foundation. In 2007, he joined a large contingent of other well-known sports figures in the founding of Athletes for Hope. This nonprofit organization coordinates and supports the philanthropic efforts of professional athletes.

In September 2008, Armstrong announced that he would return to cycling and said he hoped to earn another Tour de France victory in 2009. While competing in a race in Spain in March 2009, however, Armstrong fell and broke his collarbone. This injury would eventually require surgery. Nonetheless, Armstrong would go on to compete in the 2009

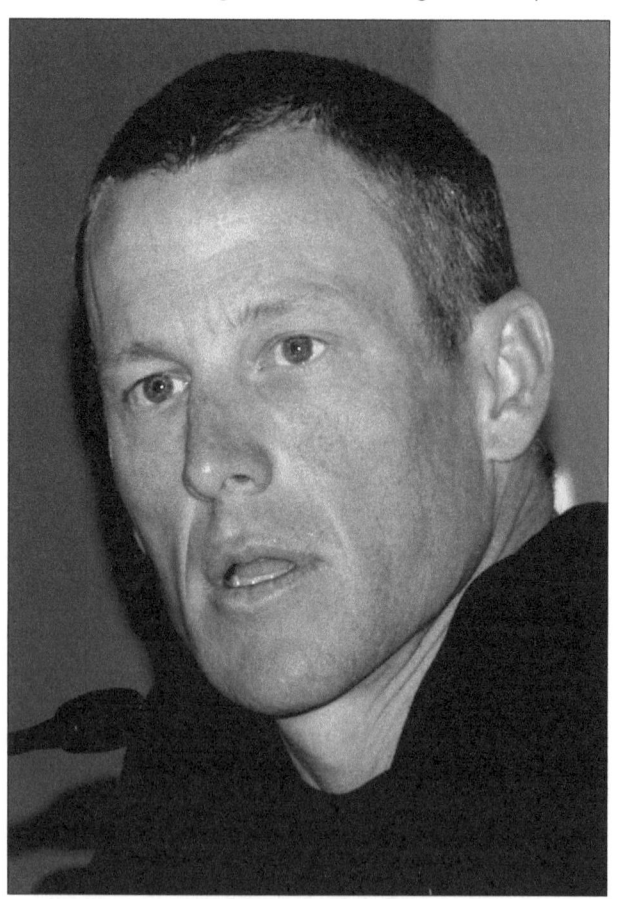

Photo by Paul Coster, via Wikimedia Commons.

Tour de France, finishing in third place. In 2010, Armstrong again competed in the Tour de France, this time on a racing team sponsored by electronics retailer RadioShack. However, his effort was thwarted by another injury after a crash, and he completed his final Tour in twenty-third place.

For years, Armstrong was dogged by accusations that he had used performance-enhancing drugs throughout his career. In June 2012, the US Anti-Doping Agency (USADA) formally charged Armstrong and several other team members with doping. At first, Armstrong denied the charges and filed a lawsuit to block the USADA's proposed punishment. When a federal judge dismissed the suit, Armstrong announced he would no longer contest the charges against him. In late August, the USADA stripped Armstrong of all competitive results from August 1998 to August 2012. Union Cycliste Internationale, the international governing body of professional cycling, quickly ratified the USADA's sanctions against Armstrong, ultimately stripping Armstrong of all his Tour de France titles and banning him from professional cycling for life. Armstrong was also later stripped of his 2000 Olympic bronze medal.

SIGNIFICANCE

After vehemently denying all allegations for years, Armstrong admitted to using performance-enhancing drugs in an Oprah Winfrey interview in early 2013. While the fate of Armstrong's legacy remains uncertain, his nearly unrivaled dominance during the height of his career will be hard to forget. He raised professional cycling's profile in the United States to unprecedented levels, and his trademark Livestrong bracelets have become a ubiquitous symbol of solidarity with the fight against cancer.

—*James Ryan*

Further Reading
Albergotti, Reed, and Vanessa O'Connell. *Wheelmen: Lance Armstrong, the Tour de France, and the Greatest Sports Conspiracy Ever*. Penguin, 2013.
Bissinger, Buzz. "Winning." *Newsweek*, vol. 160, no. 10, 2012, pp. 26-33.
Edwards, Elizabeth. "Lance Armstrong." *Time*, vol. 171, no. 19, 2008, pp. 66-67.
Osborne, Sue. "It's Not About the Bike: A Critique of Themes Identified in Lance Armstrong's Narrative." *Urologic Nursing*, vol. 29, no. 6, 2009, pp. 415-43.

ERYTHROPOIETIN

Category: Treatment
Specialties and related fields: Hematology, oncology
Definition: a glycoprotein cytokine secreted by the kidneys that increases the rate of production of red blood cells in response to falling levels of oxygen in the tissues

KEY TERMS

anemia: a condition in which the blood doesn't have enough healthy red blood cells
bone marrow: the soft, spongy tissue with many blood vessels found in the center of most bones
cytokine: a broad category of small, secreted proteins and glycoproteins, such as interferon, interleukin, and growth factors, secreted by certain cells of the immune system and other tissues that influence other cells
drug doping: the use of prohibited medications, drugs, or treatments by athletes to improve athletic performance

INTRODUCTION

Erythropoietin, also known as EPO, is a cytokine manufactured in the kidneys and can also be produced synthetically. It helps to stimulate the bone marrow to grow red blood cells, which help carry oxygen throughout the body. Erythropoietin is important in several ways. Measuring the level of erythropoietin in the body can help diagnose some illnesses. Erythropoietin can be administered to help increase the number of red blood cells a person's body produces. Erythropoietin treatment can help treat anemia, or low red blood cell levels, resulting from several causes. While EPO is used for many important and life-sustaining reasons, some athletes have inappropriately used it to improve their performance.

BACKGROUND

About 40 percent of the blood volume in the human body is made up of red blood cells, also called "erythrocytes." Red blood cells carry oxygen from the lungs to the rest of the body and transport waste products, including carbon dioxide, away from cells and tissue in the body. When there are not enough red blood cells, the body is deprived of its oxygen to generate energy. As a result, the person often becomes tired, pale, and possibly short of breath. This condition is known as "anemia."

Anemia is caused in one of two ways. First, anemia may result if the body does not produce enough erythrocytes. Certain medications, such as those used for chemotherapy, can impair the body's ability to make red blood cells. Illnesses or insufficient dietary iron or vitamin B12 can cause anemia since both are needed to produce red blood cells. The second cause is the loss or damage of blood cells. Prolonged bleeding, such as from an injury or illnesses such as infections, cancer, or kidney disease, can secondarily cause anemia.

Red blood cells generally live for about one hundred twenty days before they need to be replaced. The body is continuously replenishing its supply. Some cells located in healthy kidneys can detect the reduction in oxygen in the blood as the red blood cell level drops and release erythropoietin to trigger the bone marrow to produce new cells. The kidneys produce about 90 percent of the erythropoietin the body needs; the remainder comes from the liver.

In 1906, French physician Paul Carnot and his assistant, C. Deflandre, discovered that if they took blood from an anemic rabbit and injected it into a healthy rabbit, it made more red blood cells. They deduced that something in the anemic blood triggered the production of new cells. When it proved difficult to replicate their results, some doubted their hypothesis. However, in the middle of the twentieth century, researchers were finally able to confirm the results of Carnot and Deflandre. Additional experiments that connected the circulatory systems of two living rats determined that if one was exposed to low oxygen conditions, both developed new red blood cells. This experiment confirmed the existence of erythropoietin. Between 1964 and 1977, American biochemist Eugene Goldwasser was able to isolate and purify erythropoietin. Goldwasser's landmark discovery was followed in 1983 by the development of a synthetic or manufactured version of erythropoietin.

OVERVIEW

For many years, frequent blood transfusions and the addition of iron and B_{12}-rich foods to the diet were the only practical ways physicians treated anemia. The discovery of erythropoietin and the production of synthetic versions radically improved anemia treatment. It also made it possible to improve treatments for those undergoing treatment for serious diseases that deplete red blood cells, such as cancer, acquired immune deficiency syndrome (AIDS), and human immunodeficiency virus (HIV).

Patients who need treatment with erythropoietin receive it by injection into a vein (intravenously) or under the skin (subcutaneously). The drug requires a physician's order. The three forms are erythropoietin alfa, sold under the brand names Procrit, Epogen, and Retacrit, and darbepoetin alfa, sold under the brand name Aranesp. Darbepoetin alfa requires less frequent administration but has a mode of action identical to erythropoietin alfa. The third, very long-acting form of epoetin beta (Mircera) has methoxy polyethylene glycol (PEG) butanoic acid groups attached to erythropoietin. These attached groups decrease the molecule's elimination from the body and its activation of erythropoietin receptors. Consequently, patients only need one Mircera injection every two to four weeks.

Blood tests determine the effectiveness of erythropoietin. Since it takes several weeks for new red cells to form, these tests will be done two to four weeks after starting therapy with erythropoietin and may be repeated. A physician may adjust the dosages of the drug based on the results of the blood tests.

While these drugs can significantly improve anemia and help prevent it in patients with other conditions that lead to anemia, erythropoietin does have potentially serious side effects. It can cause blood clots, particularly in patients prone to them, who are idle because of prolonged bed rest, who have had surgery, or who are taking certain other medications, including several chemotherapy drugs. Patients at a higher risk of developing clots may take blood thinners while on erythropoietin to minimize the chance of clot formation. Cancer patients may experience increased progression of their cancers while on erythropoietin. For these reasons, erythropoietin products carry "Black Box Warnings" from the US Food and Drug Administration for these adverse effects. Erythropoietin formulations increase blood volume and can significantly raise blood pressure.

MISUSE

For decades, athletes have known that increasing the body's ability to use oxygen can improve athletic performance. For this reason, athletes do wind sprints and similar exercises to build the lungs' capacity to provide as much oxygen as possible. When erythropoietin became readily available in the late 1980s, professional athletes were quick to see its potential to artificially boost their oxygen capacity by building an abundance of oxygen-carrying red blood cells.

The use of "bootleg" synthetic erythropoietin led to "blood doping," in which athletes take drugs as a shortcut to improving their performance. Many professional sports leagues and associations banned the use of erythropoietin beginning in the 1990s. Erythropoietin was one of several performance-enhancing drugs used by cyclist Lance Armstrong. The revelation that he was using these drugs led to Armstrong being stripped of seven Tour de France titles and an Olympic medal in 2012. Other athletes also faced penalties after being caught misusing erythropoietin.

—*Janine Ungvarsky, Michael A. Buratovich*

Further Reading

Balentine, Jerry R., and Siamak N. Nabili. "Anemia." *Medicine Net*, 11 Oct. 2016, www.medicinenet.com/anemia/article.htm. Accessed 11 Mar. 2017.

Bunn, H. Franklin. "Erythropoietin." *Cold Spring Harbor Perspectives in Medicine*, Mar. 2013, www.ncbi.nlm.nih.gov/pmc/articles/PMC3579209/. Accessed 11 Mar. 2017.

Easton, John. "Eugene Goldwasser, Biochemist Behind Blockbuster Anemia Drug, 1922-2010." *University of Chicago*, 22 Dec. 2010, news.uchicago.edu/article/2010/12/22/eugene-goldwasser-biochemist-behind-blockbuster-anemia-drug-1922-2010. Accessed 11 Mar. 2017.

"History of Anaemia." *Renal Med*, 26 Aug. 2016, www.renalmed.co.uk/history-of/anaemia. Accessed 11 Mar. 2017.

Lichtin, Alan E. "Components of Human Blood." *Merck Manuals*, www.merckmanuals.com/home/blood-disorders/biology-of-blood/components-of-blood. Accessed 11 Mar. 2017.

Nabili, Siamak N. "Erythropoietin (EPO, the EPO test)." *Medicine Net*, 1 Sept. 2016, www.medicinenet.com/erythropoietin/page3.htm. Accessed 11 Mar. 2017.

"The Story of Erythropoietin." *American Society of Hematology*, www.hematology.org/About/History/50-Years/1532.aspx. Accessed 11 Mar. 2017.

Wilson, Jacque. "Lance Armstrong's Doping Drugs." *CNN*, 18 Jan. 2013, www.cnn.com/2013/01/15/health/armstrong-ped-explainer/. Accessed 11 Mar. 2017.

Mark McGwire Evades Congressional Questions on Steroid Use

Category: Drugs

Specialties and related fields: Drug abuse, government, medicine and health care, performance-enhancing drugs, sports

Definition: after being identified as a steroid user by former teammate José Canseco, Mark McGwire was asked to testify at a US House of Representatives hearing on steroid use in Major League Baseball; at the hearing, McGwire refused to answer questions about his history with performance-enhancing drugs or their use by baseball players in general

KEY TERMS

andro: short for androstenedione; a steroidal hormone produced in male and female gonads and the adrenal glands. It is known for its key role in the production of estrogen and testosterone; it is sold as an oral supplement to increase testosterone levels

creatine: a nitrogenous compound that recycles adenosine triphosphate, primarily in muscle and brain tissue, and is used as a weight training supplement to enhance exercise recovery

Major League Baseball (MLB): a professional baseball organization and the oldest major professional sports league in the world

Major League Baseball Players Association (MLBPA): the collective bargaining representative for all current MLB players

SUMMARY OF EVENT

On March 17, 2005, Mark McGwire appeared before the Government Reform Committee of the US House of Representatives to testify on steroid use in Major League Baseball (MLB). Also present at the hearing MLB commissioner Bud Selig, representatives from the Major League Baseball Players Association (MLBPA), and players José Canseco, Rafael Palmeiro, Curt Schilling, and Sammy Sosa. Player Frank Thomas appeared through videoconferencing. Also testifying were medical experts and the families of young amateur baseball players who had suffered physically and emotionally from steroid use.

McGwire's testimony became the lasting symbol of the hearings, broadcast on national television. After choking up while reading a written statement expressing his regret that younger players had suffered from steroid abuse, McGwire refused to answer questions asked by the committee. McGwire was asked about his use of performance-enhancing drugs, the integrity of the game of baseball, and whether steroid use constituted cheating, among other topics. McGwire's responses rarely went beyond variations of his statement, "I'm not here to discuss the past." Although he did say that steroids were bad and that players should not use them, he would not answer the question of how he knew that to be true. In the end, McGwire left the hearings disgraced and ridiculed for his failure to make pertinent or revealing statements about steroid use in baseball.

McGwire was not the only casualty of the hearings. Sosa, a native of the Dominican Republic, was criticized for using a translator, which many journalists claimed was a ruse by the veteran player. Palmeiro testified that he had never used steroids, but he failed a drug test within six months of the hearings and was forced to retire. Neither player could shake the shame of having used performance-enhancing drugs.

Canseco and Schilling were also disparaged for their testimony as they recanted previous statements. Canseco renounced the pro-steroid rhetoric he had used in previous interviews and writings. Schilling, a vocal critic of steroid use, said that he did not know much about the steroid problem in baseball, despite having earlier estimated that many players were users. Officials for both MLB and MLBPA also had a poor showing at the hearings. Members of Congress harshly condemned the weak drug-testing program that MLB and the player's union had put in place two weeks before the hearings.

McGwire had been one of the most popular Major League Baseball players of the late 1980s and 1990s. In 1987, he set the rookie record for most home runs in a season with forty-nine and won the American League Rookie of the Year Award. With Oakland A's teammate Canseco, McGwire was part of one of the most productive offensive tandems of the era. Playing for Oakland until 1997 and then with the St. Louis Cardinals until his retirement in 2001, McGwire was the most prolific home-run hitter in baseball from his debut in 1986 to 2001. During those sixteen seasons, only eleven of which he played more than one hundred games, he hit 583 home runs. As spectators became infatuated with homerun hitting during the 1990s, McGwire quickly became a fan favorite. His popularity only increased in 1998, when he and Chicago Cubs slugger Sosa pursued the single-season home-run record. With seventy home runs in the 1998 season, McGwire eclipsed the previous record of sixty-one, set in 1961 by Roger Maris. The excitement surrounding the home-run race between McGwire and Sosa helped baseball recover from the damage done to its popularity by the strike of 1994-95.

Although McGwire had always been a prodigious home-run hitter, the enormous totals he and others produced during the 1990s led to public suspicion that they were using performance-enhancing drugs, particularly anabolic steroids. As early as 1988, press

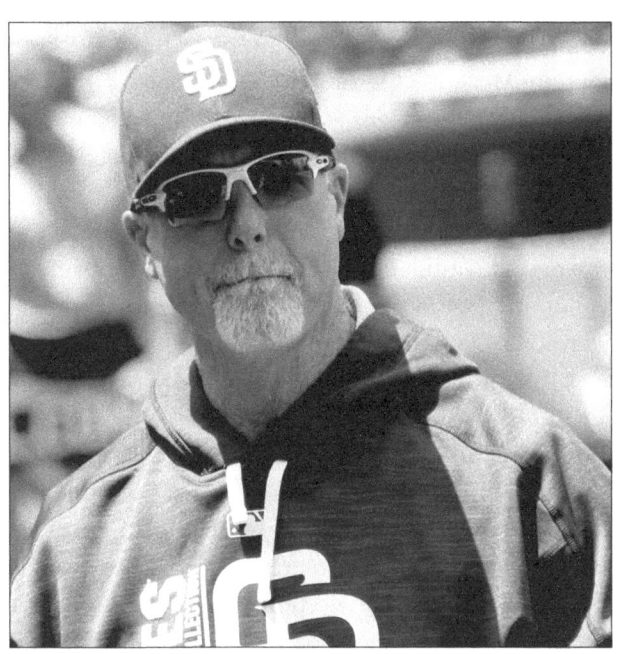

Photo by EricEnfermero, via Wikimedia Commons.

members alleged that Canseco was a steroid user, and he reportedly bragged of that use around his teammates and coaches. Although Canseco later claimed that he and McGwire used steroids together during their time in Oakland, McGwire was not generally suspected by the public of using the drug. During 1998's home-run race, a journalist revealed that McGwire's locker contained an androstenedione (andro) bottle, a legal, muscle-building supplement. When McGwire and Sosa later revealed that they also used creatine, another legal supplement, many fans and sportswriters wondered if the two players had also used illegal substances. Although the story was widely reported at first, it soon lost momentum as many fans accepted that andro and creatine were allowed by MLB and easily purchased over the counter.

In 2005, McGwire was at the center of the steroid maelstrom that prompted the congressional hearings. Early that year, Canseco published his tell-all memoir, *Juiced: Wild Times, Rampant 'Roids, Smash Hits, and How Baseball Got Big*. In the book, he named numerous steroid-using baseball players, including McGwire. Despite the extraordinary and damaging claims Canseco made, MLB declined to investigate the issue. The press, however, delved deeper into Canseco's allegations and found evidence to support some of his claims. In response to the press investigations, the Government Reform Committee announced it would hold hearings on steroid use in baseball.

IMPACT

McGwire's refusal to "discuss the past" at the congressional hearing destroyed his credibility with baseball fans. He had been one of baseball's most beloved stars only seven years earlier. In 2007, when he became eligible for election to the Hall of Fame, many voters and other sportswriters identified suspected steroid use and his testimony at the hearing as reasons they would not support his candidacy. Although McGwire had played at a level that justified his induction into the Hall of Fame, he only received support from 23.5 percent of voters, far short of the 75 percent necessary for inclusion. McGwire became the only eligible player with over 500 home runs not to be elected to the Hall of Fame.

The attention the hearings brought to steroid use in baseball forced MLB to become more proactive in preventing the use of performance-enhancing drugs. Although drug testing began three years before the hearings, the House Government Reform Committee criticized the lenient penalties. At the end of the season, MLB toughened its steroid policy. In a plan proposed shortly before the hearings, players who failed tests would be suspended ten games for the first failure. A fifth failed test was required before a lifetime suspension was even possible. Under the policy instituted in November 2005, a first-time offender received a fifty-game suspension, and a third failed test resulted in a mandatory lifetime ban from baseball. However, many continued to criticize MLB for having a drug policy that is lax when compared to that of the International Olympic Committee and other organizations.

On December 13, 2007, former US senator George J. Mitchell, acting as special counsel to the commissioner of baseball, issued his report on MLB steroid use, naming McGwire and nearly ninety other players (those active in 2007 and former players) as suspected steroid users. In the wake of the Mitchell Report, Major League Baseball commissioner Selig announced his intention once again to strengthen MLB's testing program.

—*Jacob F. Lee*

Further Reading

Bryant, Howard. *Juicing the Game: Drugs, Power, and the Fight for the Soul of Major League Baseball*. Viking Press, 2005.

Canseco, José. *Juiced: Wild Times, Rampant 'Roids, Smash Hits, and How Baseball Got Big*. Regan Books, 2005.

———. *Vindicated: Big Names, Big Liars, and the Battle to Save Baseball*. Simon Spotlight Entertainment, 2008.

Carroll, Will, with William L. Carroll. *The Juice: The Real Story of Baseball's Drug Problems*. Ivan R. Dee, 2005.

Fainaru-Wada, Mark, and Lance Williams. *Game of Shadows: Barry Bonds, BALCO, and the Steroids Scandal That Rocked Professional Sports*. Gotham Books, 2006.

Mitchell, George. *Report to the Commissioner of Baseball of an Independent Investigation into the Illegal Use of Steroids and Other Performance Enhancing Substances by Players in Major League Baseball*. Office of the Commissioner of Baseball, 2007.

GENETIC ENGINEERING

Category: Procedure
Also known as: Biotechnology, gene splicing, recombinant DNA technology
Specialties and related fields: Alternative medicine, biochemistry, biotechnology, dermatology, embryology, ethics, forensic medicine, genetics, pharmacology, preventive medicine

Definition: a wide array of techniques that alter the genetic constitution of cells or individuals by selective removal, insertion, or modification of individual genes or gene sets

KEY TERMS

gene cloning: the development of a line of genetically identical organisms that contain identical copies of the same gene or deoxyribonucleic acid (DNA) fragments

gene therapy: the insertion of a functional gene or genes into a cell, tissue, or organ to correct a genetic abnormality

polymerase chain reaction (PCR): an in vitro process by which specific parts of a DNA molecule or a gene can be made into millions or billions of copies within a short time

recombinant DNA: a hybrid DNA molecule created in the test tube by joining a DNA fragment of interest with a carrier DNA

Southern blot: a procedure used to transfer DNA from a gel to a nylon membrane, which in turn allows the finding of genes that are complementary to particular DNA sequences called "probes"

GENETIC ENGINEERING AND HUMAN HEALTH

Genetic engineering, recombinant deoxyribonucleic acid (DNA) technology and biotechnology constitute a set of techniques used to achieve one or more of three goals: to reveal the complex processes of how genes are inherited and expressed; to provide better understanding and effective treatment for various diseases (particularly genetic disorders); and to generate economic benefits, which include improved plants and animals for agriculture and the efficient production of valuable biopharmaceuticals. The characteristics of genetic engineering possess both vast promise and potential threats to humankind. It is an understatement to say that genetic engineering has revolutionized medicine and agriculture in the twenty-first century. As this technology unleashes its power to impact daily life, it has also brought challenges to ethical systems and religious beliefs.

Soon after the publication of the short essay by Francis Crick and James Watson on DNA structure in 1953, research began to uncover the way by which DNA molecules can be cut and spliced back together. With the discovery of the first restriction endonuclease by Hamilton Smith and colleagues in 1970, the real story of genetic engineering began to unfold. The creation of the first engineered DNA molecule through the splicing together of DNA fragments from two unrelated species was made public in 1972. What soon followed was an array of recombinant DNA molecules and genetically modified bacteria, viruses, fungi, plants, and animals. The debate over the issues of "tinkering with God" heated up, and public outcry over genetic engineering was widespread. In 1996, the birth of Dolly, a ewe that was the first mammal cloned from an adult body cell, elevated the debate over the impact of biological research to a new level. Furthermore, several genetically modified organisms (GMOs) have been released commercially since 1996. In 2006, it was estimated that more than 75 percent of food products in the United States contained some ingredients from GMOs.

Genetic engineering holds tremendous promise for medicine and human well-being. Medical applications of genetic engineering include diagnosing genetic and other diseases, treatment for genetic disorders, regenerative medicine using pluripotent (stem) cells, the production of safer and more effective vaccines and pharmaceuticals, and the prospect of curing genetic disorders through gene therapy. Many human diseases such as cystic fibrosis, Down syndrome, fragile X syndrome, Huntington's disease, muscular dystrophy, sickle cell anemia, and Tay-Sachs disease are inherited. There are no conventional treatments for these disorders because they do not respond to antibiotics or other conventional drugs. Genetic engineering is currently used successfully to treat chronic lymphocytic leukemia (CLL), Parkinson's disease, and X-linked severe combined immunodeficiency (SCID). Another area in which genetic engineering is commonly used is the commercial production of vaccines and pharmaceuticals through genetic engineering, which has emerged as a rapidly developing field. The potential of embryonic stem cells to become any cell, tissue, or organ under adequate conditions holds enormous promise for regenerative medicine. Particularly large studies have focused on animal models, mostly mice, to serve as human models for genetic modifications. Also, pig to human organ transplantation is a field that is rapidly growing due to inadequate human organ availability.

Prevention of genetic disorders. Although prevention may be achieved by avoiding any environmental factors that cause an abnormality, the most effective prevention, when possible, is to reduce the frequency of or eliminate the harmful genes (mutations) from the general population. As more precise tools and procedures for manipulating individual genes are optimized, this will become more commonly used. As of 2013, take-home kits for under $100 that assess individual DNA are available to the public, allowing people to understand the genetic diseases they may have or carry. However, the prevention of genetic disorders at present is usually achieved by ascertaining those individuals in the population who are at risk for passing a serious genetic disorder to their offspring and then offering them genetic counseling and prenatal screening, followed (in some serious cases) by the option of selective abortion of affected fetuses.

Genetic counseling is the process of communicating information gained through classic genetic studies and contemporary research to those individuals who are themselves at risk or have a high likelihood of passing defects to their offspring. During counseling, information about the disease's severity and prognosis, whether effective therapies exist, and the risk of recurrence are generally presented. For those couples who find the risks unacceptably high, counseling may also include discussions of contraceptive methods, adoption, prenatal diagnosis, possible abortion, and artificial insemination by a donor. The final decision must still rest with the couple themselves. Still, the significant increase in the accuracy of risk assessment through genetic technology has made it easier for parents to make well-informed decisions.

For those couples who find the burden of having an affected child unbearable, prenatal diagnosis may solve their dilemma. Prenatal screening could be performed for a variety of genetic disorders. It requires samples, acquired through either amniocentesis or chorionic villus sampling, of fetal cells or chemicals produced by the fetus. After sampling, several analyses can be performed. First, biochemical analysis determines the concentration of chemicals in the sample and, therefore, to diagnose whether a particular fetus is deficient or low in enzymes that facilitate specific biological reactions. Next, analysis of the chromosomes of the fetal cells can show if all the chromosomes are present and whether there are structural abnormalities in any of them. Finally, the most effective means of detecting the defective genes is through recombinant DNA techniques. This has become possible with the rapid increase of DNA copies through a technique called polymerase chain reaction (PCR), which can produce virtually unlimited copies of a specific gene or DNA fragment, starting with as little as a single copy. Perinatologists can perform routine prenatal diagnosis to screen a fetus for Down syndrome, Huntington's disease, sickle cell anemia, and Tay-Sachs disease.

TREATMENT OF DISEASES AND GENETIC DISORDERS

Genetic engineering may be used for direct treatments of diseases or genetic disorders through various means, including the production of possible vaccines for acquired immunodeficiency syndrome (AIDS), the treatment of various cancers, and the synthesis of biopharmaceuticals for a variety of metabolic, growth, and development diseases. In general, biosynthesis is a process in which the gene coding for a particular product is isolated, cloned into another organism (mostly bacteria), and later expressed in that organism (the host). By cultivating the host organism, large quantities of the gene products can be harvested and purified. A few examples can illustrate the useful features of biosynthesis.

Insulin is essential for treating insulin-dependent diabetes mellitus, the most severe form of diabetes. Historically, insulin was obtained from a cow or pig pancreas. Two problems exist with this traditional supply of insulin. First, large quantities of the pancreas are needed to extract enough insulin for continuous treatment of one patient. Second, insulin isolated from animals is not chemically identical to human insulin; some patients may produce antibodies that can seriously interfere with treatment. Human insulin produced through genetic engineering is quite effective yet without side effects. It has been produced commercially and made available to patients since 1982.

Another successful story in biosynthesis is the production of human growth hormone (HGH), which is used in the treatment of children with growth retardation called "pituitary dwarfism." The successful biosynthesis of HGH is important for several reasons. The conventional source of HGH was human pituitary glands removed at autopsy. Each child afflicted with pituitary dwarfism needs twice-a-week injections until the age of twenty. Such a treatment regime requires more than a thousand pituitary glands. The autopsy supply could hardly keep up with the demand. Furthermore, due to a small amount of virus contamination in the extracted HGH, many children receiving this treatment developed virus-related diseases.

Another gene therapy treatment recently approved in Europe is alipogene tiparvovec, used for people with a lipoprotein lipase deficiency (LPLD). This is a condition that results in high-fat concentration in the bloodstream and increases the risk of pancreatitis. Alipogene tiparvovec has been shown to greatly reduce the incidence of pancreatitis and decrease fat concentrations in the blood in a few weeks. Biopharmaceuticals under development in preclinical or clinical trials through genetic engineering include anticancer drugs, antiaging agents, and possible vaccines for AIDS and malaria.

Genetic engineering can include the concept of modifying or using portions of the genetic system, like messenger ribonucleic acid (mRNA), to obtain a desired therapeutic result. mRNA gene therapies use a component of the genetic system, mRNA, to cause cellular production of specific proteins impacting illness and disease, including (severe acute respiratory syndrome) SARS-CoV-2 viral infections. Messenger RNA vaccines induce cells to produce protein molecules prompting an immune response. These vaccines are currently widely used as a vaccine against Covid infections. This same technology has the potential for treating or preventing influenza, autoimmune diseases, and cancer. Messenger ribonucleic acid therapies are currently researched or in clinical trials for infectious diseases, including herpes simplex 2, malaria, rabies, influenza, human immunodeficiency virus (HIV), and hepatitis C. Some allergies, cancers, and autoimmune diseases are in research for mRNA-induced production of therapeutic proteins.

Researchers at Tel Aviv University have genetically engineered human spinal cord tissue and implanted the engineered tissue in a laboratory setting involving muscle tissue with chronic paralysis. Walking ability was reportedly restored at an 80 percent success rate. Clinical trials in human patients are anticipated. Genetically engineered fat cells were reprogrammed to resemble embryonic stem cells. The stem cells were then processed in a manner mimicking the embryonic spinal cord development of the spinal cord. These cells became implants of neuronal networks containing motor neurons. There are three types of gene therapy: germ line therapy, enhancement gene therapy, and somatic gene therapy. All gene therapy trials currently underway or in the pipeline are restricted to the somatic cells as targets for gene transfer. Germ line therapy involves the introduction of novel genes into germ cells, such as eggs or in early embryos. Although it has the potential for correcting defective genes completely, germ line therapy is highly controversial. Enhancement gene therapy raises an even greater ethical dilemma through which human potential might be enhanced for some desired traits. Both germline and enhancement gene therapies have been banned based on the unresolved ethical issues.

Somatic gene therapy is designed to introduce functional genes into body cells, thus enabling the body to perform normal functions and temporarily correct genetic abnormalities. The cloned human gene is first transferred into a viral vector, used to infect white blood cells removed from the patient. The transferred normal gene is then inserted into a chromosome and becomes active. After growth to enhance their numbers under sterile conditions, the cells are reimplanted into the patient. They produce a missing gene product in the untreated patient, allowing the individual to function normally. Several disorders are currently being treated with this technique, including SCID. Individuals with SCID have no functional immune system and usually die from infections that would be minor in normal people. While several young boys with SCID remarkably showed almost complete recovery following gene therapy, a high percentage of them have subsequently developed leukemia following the introduction of genetically engineered bone marrow stem cells. Gene therapy is also being used or tested to treat cystic fibrosis, skin cancer, breast cancer, brain cancer, and AIDS.

Most of these treatments are only partially successful, and prohibitively expensive. Over ten years, from 1990 to 2000, more than four thousand people were treated through gene therapy. Unfortunately, most of these trials were failures that led to some loss of confidence in gene therapy. These failures have been attributed to inefficient vectors and the inability to specifically target the required host tissues in many cases. In the future, as more efficient vectors are engineered, gene therapy is expected to be a common method for treating many genetic disorders.

GENETIC ENGINEERING IN AGRICULTURE, FORENSICS, AND ENVIRONMENTAL SCIENCE

As genetic engineering expands rapidly, it is difficult to generate an exhaustive list of all possible applications. Still, three other areas are worth noting: forensic, environmental, and agricultural applications. Although these areas are not directly related to medicine, they certainly profoundly impact human well-being. There are numerous ways that genetic engineering may be used to benefit agriculture and food production. First, the production of vaccines and applying methods for transferring genes are likely to benefit animal husbandry, as scientists can alter commercially important traits such as milk yield, butterfat, and the proportion of lean meat. For example, the bovine growth hormone produced through genetic engineering has been used since the late 1980s to boost milk production by cows. A mutant form of the myostatin gene has been identified and found to cause heavy muscling after this gene was introduced first into a mouse and later into the Belgian Blue bull. This technique marks the first step toward breeding cows and meat animals with lower fat and a higher proportion of lean meat.

Other examples of using genetic engineering in animal husbandry include hormones for a faster growth rate in poultry and the production of recombinant human proteins in livestock milk.

Second, genetic engineering is expected to alter dramatically the conventional approaches to developing new strains of crops through breeding. The technology allows the transferring of genes for nitrogen fixation; the improvement of photosynthesis (and therefore yield); the promotion of resistance to pests, pathogens, and herbicides; tolerance to frost, drought, and increased salinity; and the improvement of nutritional value and consumer acceptability. Genetically engineered tobacco plants have been grown to produce the protein phaseolin, naturally synthesized by soybeans and other legume crops. The first genetically engineered potato was approved for human consumption by the US government in 1995 and Canada in 1996. This NewLeaf potato, developed by corporate giant Monsanto, carries a gene from the bacterium *Bacillus thuringiensis*. This gene produces a protein toxic to the Colorado potato beetle. This insect causes substantial loss of the crop if left uncontrolled. The production of this protein by potato plants equips them with resistance to beetles, hence alleviating crop loss, saving on the cost of pesticides, and reducing the risk of environmental contamination.

Antiviral genes have been successfully transferred and expressed into cotton. The release of new cotton strains with resistance to multiple viruses is a matter of time. At least five transgenic corn strains with resistance to herbicides or pathogens had been developed and commercially produced by US farmers by 2002. Some genes coding tolerance to drought and subfreezing temperatures have been cloned and transferred into or among crop plants, some of which have already greatly impacted agriculture in developing countries. Initial effort has been made to replace chemical fertilizers with more environment-friendly biofertilizers. Secondary metabolites produced naturally by plants have also been purified and used as biopesticides. Genetically enhanced vitamin-enriched food is on the rise as well. A prime example is "golden rice," rice that has been engineered to have a higher content of vitamin A. Currently, many grains, produce, milk, and meat produced by animals or plants have been genetically engineered.

Genetic engineering is also useful in forensics. The DNA fingerprints from samples collected at crime scenes provide strong evidence in trials, thus helping to solve many violent crimes. It can be isolated easily from tissue left at a crime scene, a splattering of blood, a hair sample, or even skin left under a victim's fingernails. Various techniques can be used routinely to determine the probability of matching between sample DNA and that of a suspect. Those fingerprints are also useful in paternity and property disputes and the study of the genealogy of various species.

The growth rate and metabolic capabilities of microorganisms offer great potential for coping with some environmental problems. The metabolism of micro-organisms can be altered through genetic engineering, which enables them to absorb and degrade waste and hazardous material from the environment. Sewage plants can use engineered bacteria to degrade many organic compounds into nontoxic substances. Microbes may be engineered to detoxify specific substances in waste dumps or oil spills. Many bacteria can extract heavy metals (such as lead and copper) from their surroundings and incorporate them into recoverable compounds, thus cleaning them from the environment. Many more such applications have yet to be tested or discovered.

PERSPECTIVE AND PROSPECTS

Since the discovery of the double-helical structure of DNA by Francis Crick and James Watson in 1953, human curiosity regarding this amazing molecule has propelled the advancement of biological sciences in an unprecedented fashion. The first successful experiment in genetic engineering was described in 1972 when DNA fragments from two different organisms were joined together to produce a biologically functional hybrid DNA molecule. The next milestone came in 1975, when Edward Southern introduced "Southern blotting," a technique with many applications and proved invaluable for the subsequent development of genetic engineering. This technique identifies a particular gene or DNA fragment from a mixture of thousands of different genes or DNA fragments. Later, the automated DNA sequencers, which can rapidly churn out letter sequences from DNA fragments, and the discovery of reverse transcriptase and PCR further improved the capabilities of scientists in studying and manipulating DNA molecules and the genes that they carry.

The first prenatal diagnosis of a genetic disease was made in 1976 for alpha-thalassemia, a genetic disorder caused by the absence of globin genes, using these techniques. This represented a monumental step forward in using genetic tools in the medical field. It paved the way for later developments in which mutations in many genes could be detected in early pregnancy. Three years later, insulin was first synthesized through genetic engineering. In 1982, the commercial production of genetically engineered human insulin became a reality.

Gene therapy trials began in 1990, first with SCID. The first complete human genetic map was published in 1993. Various new techniques in DNA fingerprinting and the isolation of specific genes were developed. Also, an increasing number of pharmaceuticals have been produced through genetic engineering. Two versions of the draft copy of the human genome were published in 2001, launching the genomic revolution, and by 2006 complete DNA sequences of the genomes of over two hundred model research organisms, from bacteria to mice, were publicly available for researchers. In the twenty-first century, genetic engineering will continue to offer more medicine and agriculture benefits in undreamed ways.

In retrospect, genetic engineering presents a mixed blessing of invaluable benefits and dilemmas that science and technology have always offered humankind. Some would like to restrict the uses of genetic engineering and who might prefer that such technology had never been developed. Others believe that the benefits far outweigh the possible risks. Any potential threat can be overcome easily through government regulation or legislation. Others do not take sides in the debate but are greatly concerned with some specific applications.

The power of genetic engineering demands a new set of decisions, both ethical and economical, by individuals, government, and society. Considerable concern has been expressed by both scientists and the general public regarding possible biohazards from genetic engineering. What if engineered organisms prove resistant to all known antibiotics or carry cancer genes that might spread throughout the community? What if a genetically engineered plant becomes an uncontrollable superweed? Would these kinds of risks outweigh the potential benefits? Others argue that the risk has been exaggerated and therefore do not want to impose limits on research. Genetic engineering has also generated legal issues concerning intellectual properties and patents for different aspects of the technology.

Even more controversial are the many ethical issues. Perhaps the most obvious ethical issue surrounding genetic engineering is the objection to some applications that are considered socially undesirable and morally wrong. One example is bovine growth hormone. Some vigorously opposed its use in boosting milk production for two main reasons. First, the recombinant hormone could change the composition of the milk. However, this view was dismissed by experts from the National Institutes of

Health (NIH) and the Food and Drug Administration (FDA) after a thorough study. Second, many dairy farmers feared that greater milk production per cow would drive prices further and put some small farmers out of business.

Numerous aspects of the application of genetic engineering to humans also present ethical challenges. In some couples, both people carry a defective gene and have an appreciable chance of having an affected child. Should they refrain entirely from having children of their own? For genetic disorders caused by chromosomal abnormalities, such as Tay-Sachs disease, prenatal diagnosis can detect the defect in a fetus with great precision. Should the fetus be aborted if the screening result is positive? Should screening tests of infants for genetic disorders be required? If so, would such a requirement infringe on the individual's rights by the government? Perhaps the greatest concern of all is the possibility of designing or cloning a human being through genetic engineering. The debate over the ethical, legal, and social implications of genetic engineering should help formulate and optimize public policy and laws regarding this technology, and genetic engineering research and its applications should proceed with caution.

—*Richard P. Capriccioso*

Further Reading

Brungs, Robert S. J., and R. S. M. Postiglione, editors. *The Genome: Plant, Animal, Human.* ITEST Faith/Science Press, 2000.

Daniell, H., S. J. Streatfield, and K. Wycoff. "Medical Molecular Farming: Production of Antibodies, Biopharmaceuticals, and Edible Vaccines in Plants." *Trends in Plant Science*, vol. 6, 2001, pp. 219-26.

Frankel, M. S., and A. Teich, editors. *The Genetic Frontier.* American Association for the Advancement of Science, 1994.

"Genetic Engineering & Biotechnology News." *Mary Ann Lieber Inc.*, 2013 www.genengnews.com.

Gerdes, Louise I., editor. *Genetic Engineering: Opposing Viewpoints.* Greenhaven Press, 2004.

Haddley, K. "Alipogene Tiparvovec for the Treatment of Lipoprotein Lipase Deficiency." *Drugs of Today*, vol. 49, no. 3, 2013, p. 161, journals.prous.com/journals/servlet/xmlxsl/pk_journals.xml_summaryn_pr?p_JournaIId=4&p_RefId=1937398#.

Holland, Suzanne, Karen Lebacqz, and Laurie Zoloth, editors. *The Human Embryonic Stem Cell Debate: Science, Ethics, and Public Policy.* MIT Press, 2001.

Kilner, John F., R. D. Pentz, and F. E. Young, editors. *Genetic Ethics: Do the Ends Justify the Genes?* Wm. B. Eerdmans, 1997.

Merino, Noël. *Genetic Engineering: Opposing Viewpoints.* Greenhaven Press, 2013.

Panno, Joseph. *Gene Therapy: Treating Disease by Repairing Genes.* Facts On File, 2005.

Pasternak, Jack J. *An Introduction to Human Molecular Genetics.* 2nd ed., Wiley-Liss, 2005.

Primrose, S. B., R. M. Twyman, and R. W. Old. *Principles of Genetic Manipulation: An Introduction to Genetic Engineering.* 6th ed., Blackwell Science, 2001.

Tal, J. "Adeno-Associated Virus-Based Vectors in Gene Therapy." *Journal of Biomedical Science*, vol. 7, 2000, pp. 279-91.

Gymnast Andreea Raducan Loses Her Olympic Gold Medal

Category: Drugs and Doping

Specialties and related fields: Biochemistry, International Olympic Committee, medical laboratory testing, pharmacology, sports medicine

Definition: sixteen-year-old Romanian gymnast Andreea Raducan was stripped of her gold medal in the women's individual all-around competition at the 2000 Summer Olympics in Sydney, Australia, after testing positive for the banned stimulant pseudoephedrine; the substance is a common ingredient in cold medicines, which she had been given by a team physician the night before her competition

KEY TERMS

doping: drug administration to enhance sporting performance

pseudoephedrine: a drug obtained from plants of the genus *Ephedra* (or prepared synthetically) and used as a nasal decongestant

stimulant: a substance that raises levels of physiological or nervous activity in the body

SUMMARY OF EVENT

Andreea Raducan was born in Barlad, Romania, in 1983. She showed promise in gymnastics from an early age and was a top gymnast on the Romanian national team by the late 1990s. She lived and trained at the national training center in Deva. She became known for her high energy, skills, dance ability, and artistry, receiving comparisons to legendary Romanian gymnast Nadia Comaneci.

Raducan's specialties were the floor exercise, vault, and balance beam. She won the gold medal in the floor exercise finals. She placed fifth in the individual all-around finals at the 1999 World Championships. She was one of the top gymnasts in the world leading up to the 2000 Summer Olympic Games in Sydney, Australia.

At the 2000 Games, Raducan helped the Romanian women's gymnastics team earn the gold medal in the team competition, the first gold medal for Romania since the 1984 Summer Olympics in Los Angeles. Her scores in the team competition also qualified her for the individual all-around, floor exercise, and vault finals. She finished the preliminary round of the all-around finals with the second-highest total score, just behind gold-medal favorite Svetlana Khorkina of Russia. Raducan went on to win the individual all-around gold medal in the controversial final round of the competition.

Halfway through the event, the vaulting apparatus was found to have been set to an incorrect height, a mistake that led several competitors to "crash"; however, there were few injuries. Khorkina had been among those who vaulted at the incorrect height and crashed. Raducan also vaulted at the incorrect height, but she completed the vault without serious error. Those who had competed at the incorrect height had the option of vaulting again, but Raducan chose not to. She became the first Romanian gymnast to win the Olympic individual all-around title since Comaneci at the 1976 Olympics. Romanian teammates Simona Amanar and Maria Olaru took the silver and bronze medals, respectively.

On September 26, a few days after the all-around competition, the Romanian team was notified that Raducan had tested positive for the stimulant

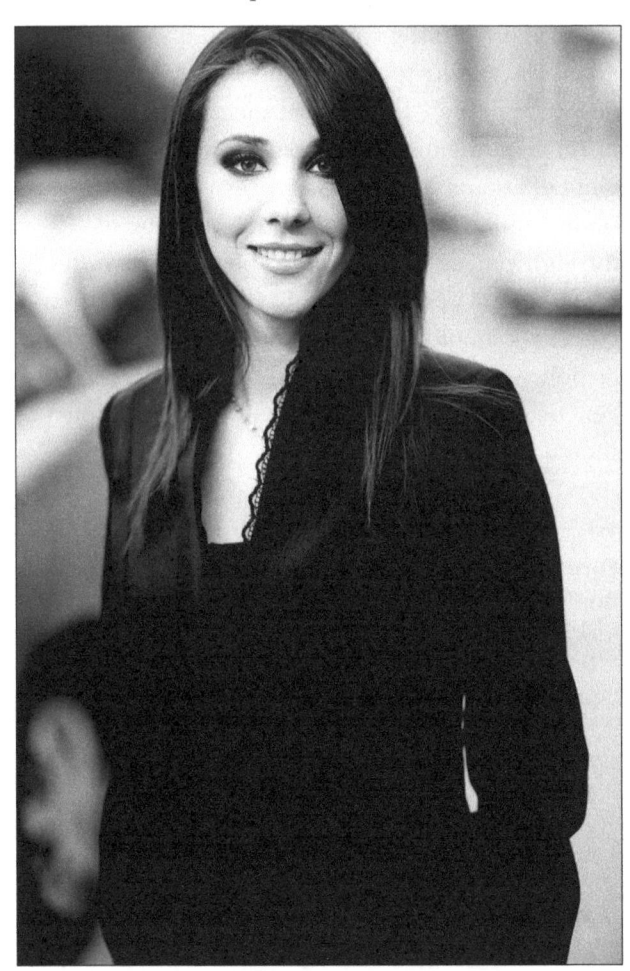

Photo by AdySarbus at English Wikipedia, via Wikimedia Commons.

pseudoephedrine, which was on the International Olympic Committee's (IOC) list of banned substances. She was stripped of her gold medal in the individual all-around event but was allowed to compete in the event finals, where she won the silver medal on the vault but faltered on her usually solid floor exercise to finish seventh of eight competitors. Raducan, her coaches, and Romanian Olympic Committee president Ion Tiriac protested the IOC's withdrawal of her gold medal, claiming that the pseudoephedrine had been in two tablets of *Nurofen*, a commonly available, over-the-counter cold medicine given to her by Romanian team physician Ioachim Oana to treat her fever and cough. The IOC rejected the protests, stating that although they believed Raducan did not knowingly ingest the substance and did not receive a performance benefit, they must enforce rules violations regardless of the circumstances.

As a result of the IOC decision, the individual all-around gold medal was awarded to second-place finisher Simona Amanar, who accepted it on behalf of Romania but qualified her acceptance by stating that Raducan was the rightful winner. Third-place finisher Olaru received the silver medal, and fourth-place finisher Liu Xuan of China received the bronze medal. Raducan was allowed to keep her gold medal from the team competition and her silver medal from the vault competition because she had not been tested for drugs after the team event and had passed a drug test after the event finals.

The decision to strip Raducan's medal created a wave of public sympathy for the young, petite Raducan, who did not meet the profile of an intentional doping violator. The same day her medal was stripped, Raducan and the Romanian Gymnastics Federation appealed the IOC's decision to the Court of Arbitration for Sport (CAS), the sporting world's highest court of appeal based in Lausanne, Switzerland. An ad hoc CAS group meeting in Sydney ruled on September 28 that Raducan was innocent of any wrongdoing and that she had not gained a competitive advantage from the pseudoephedrine. However, it rejected her appeal to reinstate her gold medal for the individual all-around event. The court agreed with the IOC's rationale that regardless of the emotions or circumstances of the case, the Olympic antidoping code must be upheld in fairness to all athletes. Romanian team physician Oana was expelled from his job for the remainder of the Sydney Games and also was banned from the 2002 Winter Games in Salt Lake City and the 2004 Summer Games in Athens.

Raducan remained a popular figure to many, both inside and outside gymnastics. The International Gymnastics Federation (IGF) also exonerated her of any wrongdoing. It imposed no further sanctions, stating that the loss of her medal was punishment enough. She continued to train with and compete for the Romanian team and won five medals at the 2001 World Championships before retiring from the sport in 2002. After her retirement, she became a sports announcer, television-show host, and model. She studied for a master's degree in journalism at the University of Bucharest. Oana kept his medical license but received a four-year ban from the European championships and all IGF-sponsored events in addition to his Olympic sanctions.

IMPACT

The withdrawal of Raducan's gold medal attracted worldwide media attention. It highlighted the tougher IOC position on violations of its antidoping code. Despite the public's sympathy for Raducan, many people believed that preserving the Games' fairness and integrity is more important for the integrity of the Olympics than any individual case.

At the time Raducan lost her medal, the IOC had been facing increasing public pressure to crack down on doping violators and uphold the Olympic movement's commitment to drug-free sport, which led to the more stringent antidoping policies. The uniqueness of Raducan's case, her proclaimed innocence, and her sympathetic nature would test the IOC's determination to enforce those policies. Its decision to follow its own rule and automatically disqualify an athlete regardless of the circumstances of the charges sent a message that accidental violations would not be tolerated or defensible.

Oana's suspension also sent the message that team physicians and other medical personnel working with athletes must know the ingredients of all medications they prescribe or otherwise supply and that all persons affiliated with a team, not just athletes, could face sanctions for their carelessness.

—*Marcella Bush Trevino*

Further Reading

Begley, Sharon, and Devin Gordon. "Under the Shadow of Drugs: Doping—Tainted by Scandals, the IOC Starts to Crack Down." *Newsweek*, October 9, 2000, p. 56.

Birchard, Karen. "Olympic Committee Bans Doctor After Doping Case." *The Lancet*, vol. 356, 2000, p. 1171.

Pound, Richard W. *Inside the Olympics: A Behind-the-Scenes Look at the Politics, the Scandals, and the Glory of the Games*. John Wiley & Sons Canada, 2004.

"Raducan Tests Positive for Stimulant." *Associated Press*, 26 Sept. 2000, assets.espn.go.com/oly/summer00/news/2000/0925/776388.html. Accessed 8 Jun. 2022.

"Request Denied: Arbitrators Uphold Decision to Strip Raducan of Gold." *CNN Sports Illustrated*, 13 Nov. 2000, web.archive.org/web/20040928011117/http://sportsillustrated.cnn.com/olympics/2000/gymnastics/news/2000/09/27/raducan_decision_ap/. Accessed 8 Jun. 2022.

Wilson, Wayne, and Ed Derse. *Doping in Elite Sport: The Politics of Drugs in the Olympic Movement*. Human Kinetics, 2001.

OLYMPIC ATHLETE MARION JONES ADMITS STEROID USE

Category: Doping
Specialties and related fields: Biochemistry, International Olympic Committee, medical laboratory testing, pharmacology, sports medicine

Definition: Olympic track star Marion Jones admitted in court to having lied to federal investigators in 2003 about her use of performance-enhancing drugs and about her knowledge of the involvement of a former boyfriend and former coach in a scheme to cash millions of dollars' worth of stolen and forged checks; Jones was jailed and ordered to forfeit her Olympic medals

KEY TERMS

anabolic steroids: a synthetic steroid hormone that resembles testosterone in promoting muscle growth; such hormones are used medicinally to treat some forms of weight loss and (illegally) by some athletes and others to enhance physical performance

doping: administration of drugs to inhibit or enhance sporting performance.

performance-enhancing drugs: substances that are used to improve any form of activity performance in humans

SUMMARY OF EVENT

Marion Jones was the premier female runner of her generation. In 1997, after a four-year absence from track-and-field competition and after only a few months of serious training, she won the US championship in the 100-meter sprint. That victory earned her instant recognition as the fastest woman in the world. During the next season, she participated in an unprecedented world tour for its ambition. She entered meets at a furious pace, returning home just long enough to become the first woman in fifty years to win three events at the US championships in New Orleans, Louisiana.

In 1998, Jones participated in thirty-seven different running and long-jumping events and won thirty-six of them. By the time the year ended, she had held the number one position in the world in the 100 meters, 200 meters, and long jump. She capped off the year by marrying shot put champion C. J. Hunter, a future Olympic athlete.

A charismatic and attractive woman, Jones quickly became a media favorite and one of the most famous female athletes in the world. Reporters and fans speculated that she would win five gold medals—more than any other woman ever in track and field—at the 2000 Sydney Olympics. Jones came close, winning the 100-meter race by the second-widest margin in Olympic history—among men and women. She won the 200-meter race by the largest margin since Wilma Rudolph's victory in Rome in 1960. Jones took a third gold medal as part of the US 1,600-meter relay team. In the 400-meter relay, the US team botched the baton handoff between the second and third legs. Jones made up some ground, but the Americans took the bronze for third place. The long jump, traditionally Jones's weakest event, left her with a fifth medal, a second bronze. In recognition of her achievements, Jones was named the Associated Press Female Athlete of the Year.

As with other sports, the track-and-field world had long been dogged by allegations that athletes use performance-enhancing drugs. Jones repeatedly stated throughout her career that she wanted a drug-free sport and never used illegal drugs. However, there were persistent rumors that she used drugs. On September 26, 2000, her husband, Hunter, tested positive for steroid use. He was suspended for two years, and then he retired. The couple divorced in 2002. In the autumn of 2003, Jones testified before a federal grand jury in San Francisco, California, investigating athlete steroid use and those athletes' possible connections with a local company, Bay Area Laboratory Co-operative (Balco). The grand jury found a calendar at Balco with the initials "MJ" written on it, seeming to indicate a schedule for steroid use by Marion Jones ("MJ") in 2001. Hunter also reportedly told investigators that he had injected Jones with banned substances and witnessed her doing the same.

On May 16, 2004, Jones insisted that she was drug-free and stated her intent to sue if the US

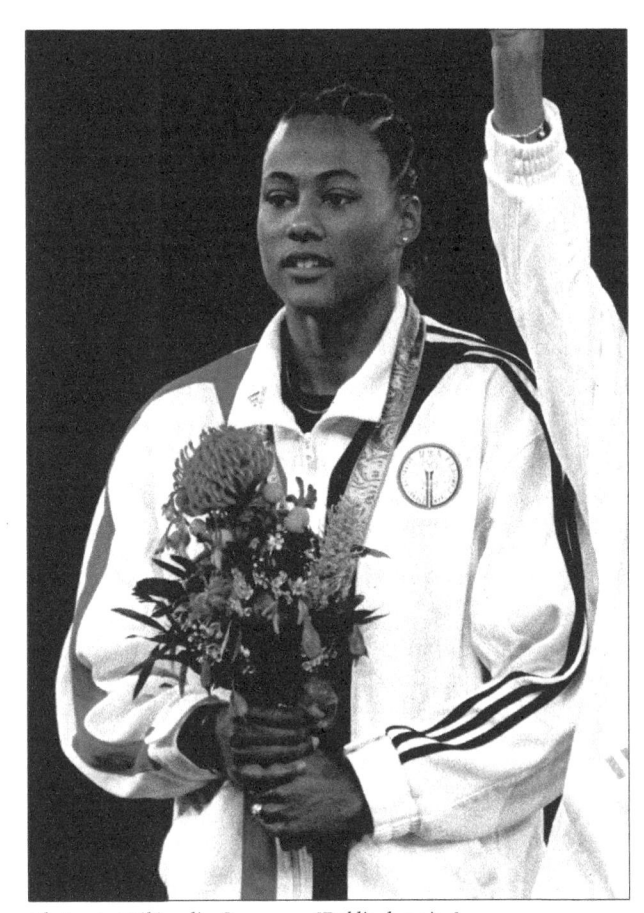

Photo via Wikimedia Commons. [Public domain.]

Anti-Doping Agency barred her from competing in that year's Athens Olympics without a positive drug test. In August at Athens, Jones finished fifth in the long jump, and her 4 x 100 relay team failed to finish after a bad baton handoff. By this time, sponsors had begun to drop Jones because of the rumors of drug use.

On December 7, the International Olympic Committee (IOC) opened an investigation into doping allegations against Jones after Balco founder Victor Conte alleged that he supplied her with an array of banned drugs before and after the Sydney Olympics. One year later, on December 13, 2005, an American Olympic sprinter and former boyfriend of Jones, Tim Montgomery, received a two-year ban from the sport based on evidence gathered in the Balco investigation. Jones was now linked to a second athlete convicted of using steroids. (Montgomery and Jones had a son together in 2003.)

Nevertheless, Jones remained adamant that she was drug-free. On February 5, 2006, she settled a $25 million federal defamation lawsuit against Conte for damaging her reputation by declaring on ABC's *20/20* that he supplied her and Montgomery with performance-enhancing drugs. Five days later, the IOC announced that it would continue investigating whether Jones took illegal substances at the 2000 Sydney Games. On June 23, Jones's "A" sample from the US Track and Field Championships tested positive for the banned endurance-boosting hormone erythropoietin (EPO). This lab result could lead to a possible two-year ban from the sport. However, on September 6, Jones's backup, or "B," sample came back from the lab negative. She was therefore cleared of any wrongdoing and allowed to return to competition. Observers later noted that it is very rare for a "B" sample to fail to confirm the "A" sample and speculated that any EPO in the "B" sample could have deteriorated beyond recognition.

While she had once planned to compete until she was in her forties, Jones soon declared that she had grown weary of defending herself. She married Barbadian sprinter Obadele Thompson in 2007 and retired to raise a family. However, the steroid scandal would not go away. On October 5, Jones tearfully admitted in federal court that she had used the performance-enhancing drug known as "the clear" from September 2000 through July 2001 and asked for forgiveness. She was on trial for providing false statements to federal investigators in the Balco case and a check fraud case involving Montgomery and her former coach, Steven Riddick. Montgomery cashed stolen and forged checks, and Jones had received one of those checks, which was deposited into her checking account but never cleared. Jones pleaded guilty to lying to investigators at the October 5 trial.

In January 2008, Jones received a six-month jail sentence and was ordered to perform four hundred hours of community service in each of the two years following her release. On March 7, Jones began her sentence at the Federal Medical Center Carswell, located at the Naval Air Station, Joint Reserve Base, in Fort Worth, Texas. Although the facility specializes in medical and mental health services, it also has inmates (including Jones) who do not require such care. She was released on September 5.

IMPACT

On April 10, after Jones was sentenced, the women who won Olympic medals in 2000 by running relays with Jones were ordered by Olympic officials to forfeit their victories and return their medals. The IOC stripped gold medals from Jearl-Miles Clark, Monique Hennagan, LaTasha Colander-Richardson, and Andrea Anderson. Runners Chryste Gaines, Torri Edwards, Nanceen Perry, and Passion Richardson were ordered to forfeit their bronze medals. The women were not accused of any wrongdoing, but the Jones scandal tainted their victories. However, they refused to surrender their medals, arguing it would be unfair to punish them for Jones's actions, and challenged the IOC through the Court of Arbitration for Sport.

Jones asked US President George W. Bush to commute her sentence in July. A commutation reduces or eliminates a sentence but does not remove civil liabilities stemming from a criminal conviction. Doug Logan, the chief executive officer of US Track and Field, publicly opposed commutation because to do so would send a terrible message to youths. Logan added that a commutation would also send the wrong message to the international community. By cheating and lying, Jones violated the principles of track and field and international Olympic competition. Logan was especially angry that Jones had challenged anyone who doubted her purity, talent, and work ethic and that she had successfully duped many people into giving her the benefit of the doubt.

Bush did not commute Jones's sentence, leading some observers to wonder if the harshness of Jones's sentence, her not receiving a commutation, and the demonizing of her in the media had more to do with race than justice, given that champion black athletes have historically been targets of suspicion and doubt.

—*Caryn E. Neumann*

Further Reading

Cazeneuve, Brian. "Running on Empty: With Funds and Friends in Short Supply, Marion Jones May Face Prison." *Sports Illustrated*, 2008, vault.si.com/vault/2008/01/14/running-on-empty.

Gutman, Bill. *Marion Jones*. Simon Pulse, 2004.

Jones, Marion, and Kate Sekules. *Marion Jones: Life in the Fast Lane*. Warner Books, 2004.

Rapoport, Ron. *See How She Runs: Marion Jones and the Making of a Champion*. Algonquin Books, 2000.

Smith, Stephen A. "Falls from Grace: What Young Black Athletes Should Learn from the Michael Vick and Marion Jones Dramas." *Ebony*, vol. 63, no. 3, 2008, p. 40.

Olympic Champion Lasse Virén Is Accused of Blood Doping

Category: Sport, track and field (long-distance runs)
Specialties and related fields: Endurance fitness, long-distance running, track and field competition
Definition: a Finnish former long-distance runner, winner of four gold medals at the 1972 and 1976 Summer Olympics

KEY TERMS

Olympics: a major international multisport event normally held once every four years

Rolf Haikkola: Finnish long-distance runner and middle-distance runner who coached the celebrated Finnish long-distance runner Lasse Virén

EARLY LIFE

Lasse Artturi Virén was born on July 22, 1949, in Myrskylä, Finland. *Myrskylä* means "stormy village." His parents, Elvi and Illmarie Virén, had three other sons, Erkki, Nisse, and Heikki. Lasse grew up on the family farm. He went to elementary school for eight years and helped his father drive and repair trucks. Lasse began running as a teenager and had initial success by winning the Finnish Junior Championships in the 3,000-meter run. He ran regularly, even when he worked late with his father. Lasse ran for the local club Myrskylän Myrsky, which means "the storm of the stormy village."

THE ROAD TO EXCELLENCE

Haikkola was a former world-class 5,000-meter runner whose training philosophy was influenced by the great New Zealand coach Arthur Lydiard. At eighteen, Lasse quit attending mechanical trade school to train more. He began serious long-distance training in 1969 when he was nineteen. Lasse was coached by Rolf Haikkola from Myrskylä.

Generally, under Haikkola's direction, Lasse ran long distances mixed with speed work conducted on forest trails or dirt roads. Haikkola was interested in Lasse's development as a runner and focused primarily on peaking him for only a few key races each year. Lasse trained hard during the long Finnish winter months and used the short summer season for peaking. Early in his career, Lasse worked to support himself as a country police officer. This job allowed him valuable time off for travel and training.

By 1971, Lasse had improved substantially in his training and racing. He excelled at the 5,000- and 10,000-meter distances. Lasse was not known well at the international level of competition because Coach Haikkola limited his exposure to racing. Before the 1972 Munich Olympics, Lasse set a world record in the 2-mile run. He qualified in 5,000 and 10,000 meters to represent Finland at Munich.

THE EMERGING CHAMPION

At the Munich Olympics, Lasse qualified for the finals of the 10,000 meters. The final field was one of the fastest groups of distance runners ever assembled. Midway into the final, Lasse was involved in some jostling back in the pack of runners and fell to the track. He had lost 10 meters to the pack by the time he recovered. Appearing unfazed by his fall, Lasse gained the lead by the last lap of the race and sprinted away to victory in world-record time. Lasse's win was the first Olympic victory for Finnish distance runners since 1936. It made him a national hero, marking the resurgence of distance running enthusiasm in Finland.

By the Olympic 5,000-meter race, Lasse had become the clear favorite to win based on his 10,000-meter performance. That placed tremendous pressure on Lasse to live up to the world's expectations. He won his preliminary round of the 5,000 meters. In the final, the pace was slow until the last mile of the race. At that point, the pace rapidly increased, and it was a five-man race going into the last lap. Once again, Lasse displayed a powerful kick and won in Olympic-record time. He covered his last mile in 4 minutes and 1 second, an outstanding feat.

CONTINUING THE STORY

Following the Munich Olympics, Lasse was besieged with business opportunities and speaking engagements. His schedule became hectic, and he got little rest. The disruptions in his personal life had a negative influence on his training. Haikkola encouraged Lasse to commit to prepare for the defense of his Olympic titles at Montreal in 1976.

Lasse struggled in the off years between the Olympics because of illness and injuries. There were also rumors that he had used "blood doping"—a method of increasing the oxygen-carrying capacity of the blood—to improve his performance. Some track experts thought this might explain how Lasse had improved at the elite level so quickly. The rumors were unsettling because blood doping was illegal. An athlete could be banned from competition if the charges were substantiated.

Lasse and Haikkola denied the doping charges. They pointed out that their well-planned training program was responsible for the remarkable peaking ability that Lasse had displayed.

In 1976, Lasse qualified for the 5,000- and 10,000-meter runs at the Montreal Olympics. He had trained as much as 150 miles per week in preparation. Once again, he beat all his rivals to claim the gold medals in both races. His accomplishments were unprecedented in Olympic history. If that was not remarkable enough, he entered the marathon

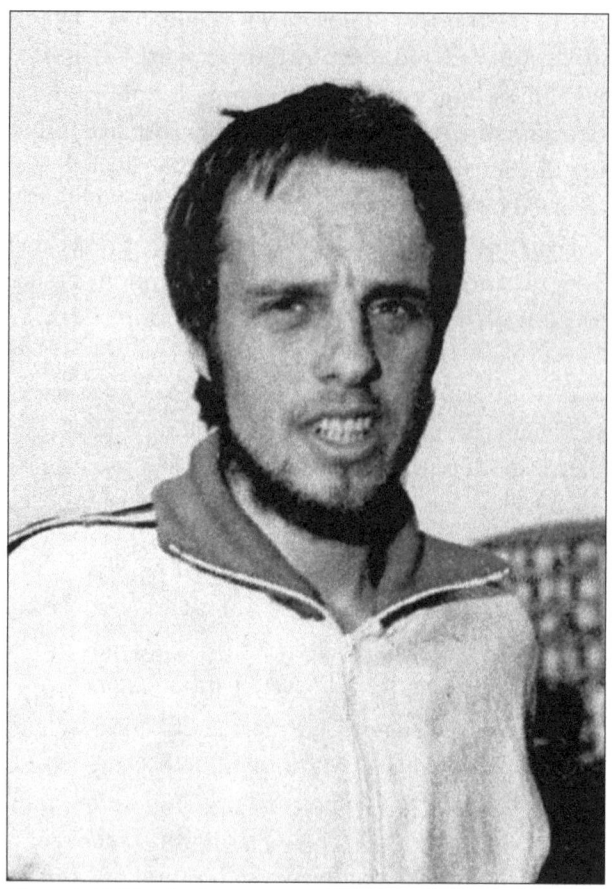

Photo via Wikimedia Commons. [Public domain.]

following the 5,000-meter race and finished in fifth place.

SUMMARY

Following the Montreal Olympics, Lasse Virén returned to the privacy of Myrskylä. Rumors continued to fly concerning his possible involvement with blood doping. Lasse and his coach blamed the rumors on misunderstandings with the media and jealous rivals.

In 1980, at the Moscow Olympics, Lasse participated in his third Olympics and finished fifth in the 10,000-meter run. He also started the marathon but had to drop out before finishing. Based on his Olympic performances, Lasse ranks as one of the best 5,000- and 10,000-meter runners ever. He was a legend in the world of Finnish distance running. In 1999, his reputation helped earn him a seat in the Finnish parliament.

—*Tinker D. Murray*

Further Reading

Bloom, Marc. "Greatest Olympic Moments." *Runner's World*, vol. 39, no. 7, 2004, pp. 70-77.
Sandrock, Michael. *Running with the Legends*. Human Kinetics, 1996.
Virén, Lasse, et al. *Lasse Virén: Olympic Champion*. Continental, 1978.
Wilner, Barry, and Ken Rappoport. *Harvard Beats Yale 29-29, and Other Great Comebacks from the Annals of Sports*. Taylor Trade, 2008.

PERFORMANCE-ENHANCING DRUGS

Category: Doping
Specialties and related fields: Biochemistry, biotechnology, medical biotechnology
Definition: substances that are used to improve any form of activity performance in humans

KEY TERMS

anabolic steroids: synthetic steroid hormones that resemble testosterone and promote muscle growth; they are used to treat some forms of weight loss and, illegally, by some athletes and others to enhance physical performance

blood doping: the injection of oxygenated blood into an athlete before an event in an attempt to enhance athletic performance

erythropoietin: a hormone secreted by the kidneys that increases the rate of production of red blood cells in response to falling levels of oxygen in the tissues

human growth hormone: a peptide hormone that stimulates growth, cell reproduction, and cell regeneration in humans and other animals

stimulants: substances that increase physiological or nervous activity in the body

INTRODUCTION

As the level of athletic competition continues to rise worldwide, athletes are always looking for ways to get a competitive edge. Superior nutrition and training programs are not enough for some athletes; many choose to use performance-enhancing drugs even though such substances are banned by sports federations and illegal unless prescribed for medical purposes. Law enforcement agencies expend significant resources to address such drugs' illegal sale and use.

BACKGROUND

Athletes' use of particular substances to improve their physical performance dates back to ancient Greece. Competitors in the ancient Olympics took stimulants such as strychnine and extracts from cola plants, cacti, and fungi to improve their performance. Although the beneficial effects of these substances are questionable, many believe that their widespread use was one of the elements that led to the termination of the Olympic Games and other sporting competitions in about 400 CE.

HOW IT WORKS

Competitive sports did not gain great popularity again until the time of the second phase of the Industrial Revolution, around 1850. With competition, the use of performance-enhancing drugs also returned. In particular, competitive swimmers, runners, and cyclists used caffeine, strychnine, codeine, cocaine, heroin, and nitroglycerin to stimulate their bodies to perform. Numerous athletes died from taking these drugs, but their deaths did deter many others from using such drugs. After World War II and throughout the Cold War period, the use of performance-enhancing drugs escalated, particularly the use of anabolic steroids.

Bodybuilding supplements. The most widely known class of performance-enhancing drugs used since the 1930s is anabolic steroids (also known as "anabolic-androgenic steroids"). These are testosterone-like substances that augment male sex characteristics and muscle building. Anabolic steroids were first developed in Nazi Germany and were used to increase the aggressiveness of troops in battle.

Many studies have shown that anabolic steroids increase muscle mass and strength, which has made them popular among many different kinds of athletes, from football players to track-and-field athletes who participate in throwing events. Athletes use two strategies to maximize strength and muscle mass with anabolic steroids: stacking and pyramiding. Stacking is blending different types of drugs in oral and injectable forms to maximize their effects. Pyramiding is the continual increase in dosage over time to maximize its benefit. However, taking large doses of anabolic steroids have many dangerous side effects. Because the liver is responsible for breaking down and removing excess chemicals from the body, anabolic steroids can cause severe liver damage. These substances have also been linked to high blood pressure, adult-onset diabetes mellitus, increased blood clotting factors, and decreased high-density lipoproteins (good cholesterol) in the blood, all of which increase the risk of cardiovascular disease.

Human growth hormone (HGH) is another substance that has been reported to increase muscle mass and strength is human growth hormone (HGH). With the advances made in genetic engineering during the 1980s, HGH became increasingly widely available and hit the black market, where athletes could access it. However, research on the effects of HGH has been very limited, and any actual benefits of the substance for athletes have not been identified conclusively. Athletes at the 2012 Summer Olympics were tested for HGH. Still, the unreliability of one of the test's constituent assays was taken off the market, rendering the tests invalid.

Two other substances that have been promoted as useful in increasing muscle mass and strength are dehydroepiandrosterone (DHEA) and androstenedione. Both are precursors to testosterone that are converted to testosterone by the body. Research has not found either substance to be effective for enhancing athletic abilities, and both decrease the high-density lipoproteins in the blood, increasing the risk of cardiovascular disease.

One supplement that is effective in improving performance in high-intensity exercise is creatine. Research indicates that ingesting creatine in high doses helps the muscles work harder and increases the body's ability to gain muscle and strength. Although creatine is not regulated by the US Food and Drug Administration (FDA), it is banned by most sports federations. The long-term side effects of this substance have not been identified.

Stimulants. The primary stimulant substances used by athletes for much of recent history are amphetamines. Athletes take these drugs to decrease fatigue, increase alertness, and decrease reaction time. Most research has found, however, that these drugs do not improve athletes' quickness; rather, the athletes only perceive themselves as being quicker under the influence of the drugs. In addition, amphetamines offer only a short-term reduction of fatigue; thus, in using amphetamines, athletes gain no real performance benefits while exposing themselves to dangerous side effects: amphetamines are highly addictive, and those who take them experience increased metabolism, loss of appetite, and weight loss.

Athletes also use stimulants that are not regulated drugs: caffeine and ephedrine. Endurance athletes use caffeine to increase their bodies' use of fat for energy and to conserve carbohydrates for later stages of their competitive events. Research has found such use to be effective and have limited side effects, including increased urine output and blood vessel spasms. The sports federations have not banned caffeine, but most place limits on the amount allowed in a competing athlete's body. Ephedrine is a naturally occurring stimulant similar to amphetamines. Like amphetamines, it has not been shown to have performance-enhancing benefits, and it has similar side effects. Most sports federations ban ephedrine.

Blood doping. Many athletes in the past have improved their performance through blood doping—that is, by increasing the number of red blood cells that carry oxygen in their blood. Increased red blood cells increase the oxygen available to muscles and improve athletic performance in endurance events.

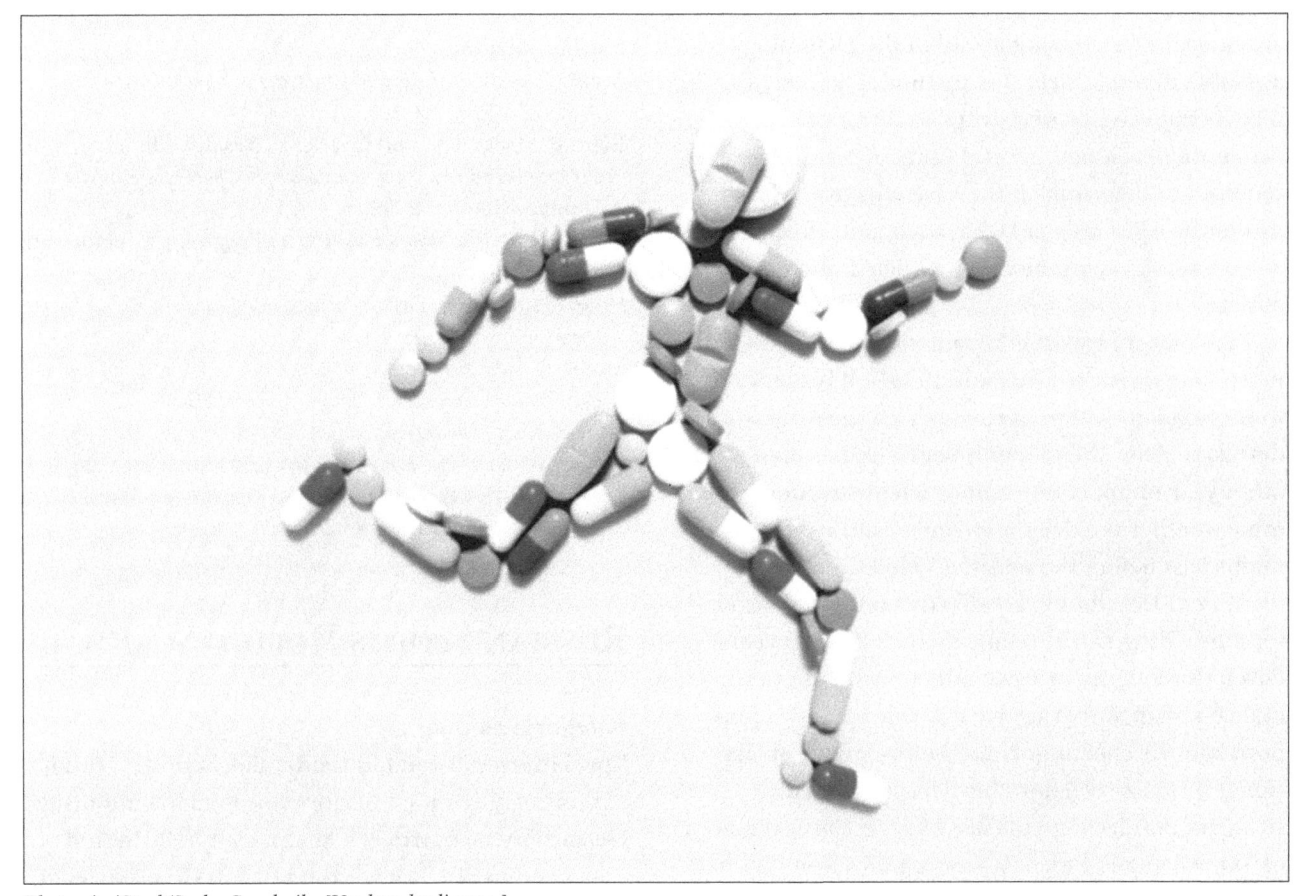

Photo via iStock/Sasha Brazhnik. [Used under license.]

Historically, athletes who practiced blood doping would have several units of their blood drawn and placed in storage six to eight weeks before the competition. Their bodies would produce more red blood cells in the intervening time. Then, before the competition, the athletes would reinfuse their stored blood to increase their red blood cells. This process has generally been replaced by the use of the hormone erythropoietin, which causes the body to increase the production of red blood cells. Sports federations ban all methods of blood doping.

IMPORTANT ISSUES

A major concern related to performance-enhancing drugs is the lack of available information. New drugs and variations on older drugs are continually being developed, largely because manufacturers and users are interested in staying ahead of the technology available to test athletes for the use of banned and illegal drugs. When new drugs or forms of older drugs are developed, several years of research are required to determine if they are effective, what the proper dosages are, and what their side effects are, as well as to develop new tests to detect their use by athletes.

Typically, a new drug formulation is available for more than a year before awareness of it becomes widespread enough that research on the drug is undertaken. After the research begins, more than another year might elapse before scientists can determine whether the drug is effective, and many years might pass before the negative side effects can be identified. Developing an effective testing method for a new drug can also take months or even years. Given this lengthy process, athletes who use performance-enhancing drugs have a wide window of opportunity for cheating. Nonetheless, major professional sports associations have implemented stringent antidoping policies. Most, including that of Major League Baseball—an organization that has had well-documented problems with its athletes taking performance-enhancing drugs—have successfully deterred athletes from using illegal substances.

Another serious concern raised by using performance-enhancing drugs is the effect of such substances on athletes' health. Many athletes take very high doses, whether taking FDA-approved drugs or nontested substances. Many take higher doses than what researchers can ethically test. Thus, the true benefits and side effects of these substances are not known. Given that many known side effects have negative health implications, athletes who use illegal and banned substances to enhance their performance are not only breaking the rules but also risking serious health problems.

—*Bradley R. A. Wilson*

Further Reading

Aretha, David. *Steroids and Other Performance-Enhancing Drugs*. Enslow, 2005.

Bahrke, Michael S., and Charles E. Yesalis, editors. *Performance-Enhancing Substances in Sport and Exercise*. Human Kinetics, 2002.

Espejo, Roman. *Performance-Enhancing Drugs*. Greenhaven, 2015.

Haley, James, and Tamara Roleff. *Performance-Enhancing Drugs*. Greenhaven, 2003.

Monroe, Judy. *Steroids, Sports, and Body Image: The Risks of Performance-Enhancing Drugs*. Enslow, 2004.

Scott, Celicia. *Doping: Human Growth Hormone, Steroids, and Other Performance-Enhancing Drugs*. Mason Crest, 2015.

Yesalis, Charles E. *Anabolic Steroids in Sport and Exercise*. 2nd ed., Human Kinetics, 2000.

Russian Sports Doping Scandal

Category: Doping

Specialties and related fields: Biochemistry, drug, doping, Olympics, performance-enhancing drugs

Definition: a controversy that began in 2014 and peaked in 2018, when the Russian Olympic team was banned from the 2018 Winter Olympics in South Korea for taking banned performance-enhancing drugs

KEY TERMS

anabolic steroids: synthetic steroid hormones that resemble testosterone and promote muscle growth, used medicinally to treat some forms of weight loss and illegally by some athletes and others to enhance physical performance

doping: drug administration to inhibit or enhance sporting performance

human growth hormone (HGH): a peptide hormone that stimulates growth, cell reproduction, and cell regeneration in humans and other animals. It is thus important in human development

performance-enhancing drugs (PEDs): substances used to improve any form of activity performance in humans

KEY EVENTS

December 2014: German broadcaster ARD (Association of Public Broadcasting Corporations in the Federal Republic of Germany), airs a documentary alleging widespread, state-sponsored doping in Russian athletics, prompting investigations into the matter.

November 4, 2015: Former International Association of Athletics Federations (IAAF) president Lamine Diack is accused of taking bribes to cover-up several Russian athletes' positive drug tests.

November 9, 2015: The World Anti-Doping Agency's (WADA) independent commission publishes a report alleging widespread bribery, corruption, and state-sponsored doping in Russian track and field.

July 18, 2016: Richard McLaren published his first WADA-commissioned report on doping in Russian athletics, focusing particularly on the 2014 Winter Olympics in Sochi, Russia, claiming that Russia's Ministry of Sport and the Federal Security Service (FSB) had engaged in a cover-up to hide doping.

December 9, 2016: Second McLaren report provides strong evidence of expansive state-supported doping orchestrations.

December 5, 2017: The International Olympic Committee (IOC) announces that Russia is banned from competing in the 2018 Winter Olympics but agrees to allow athletes from the country with no known doping history to compete neutrally.

February 28, 2018: The IOC announces that Russia's Olympic membership has been reinstated following the end of the Winter Olympics.

KEY FIGURES

Lamine Diack: Former IAAF president accused of corruption.

Richard McLaren: Canadian attorney hired by WADA to independently investigate allegations of Russian doping.

Denis Oswald: Swiss sports official in charge of the IOC's disciplinary commission regarding the Russian doping scandal.

Grigory Rodchenkov: Former head of Russia's antidoping laboratory.

SUMMARY

The Russian sports doping scandal is a controversy that began in 2014 and peaked in 2018 when the Russian Olympic team was banned from the 2018 Winter Olympics in South Korea. Investigative journalism and official investigations exposed a widespread, state-sponsored doping program in Russian athletics, particularly Olympic events, with many Russian athletes implicated. The size and scale of the operation have generated further debates over the effectiveness of antidoping efforts, the credibility of sports governing authorities, and the responses to abuses of performance-enhancing substances.

STATUS

On February 1, 2018, following appeals, the Court of Arbitration for Sport (CAS) announced that it was lifting the lifetime bans formerly placed on twenty-eight Russian athletes, a decision met with criticism from numerous Olympic officials; the CAS argued that the evidence against the athletes in question was insufficient to prove doping. Despite two of the Russian athletes allowed to compete in the 2018 Winter Olympics in South Korea being disqualified after testing irregularities indicated that they had been using performance-enhancing substances, not long after the closing ceremony later that month, the IOC announced that Russia's Olympic committee had been formally reinstated, enabling Russian athletes to again participate in future Olympic Games.

IN-DEPTH OVERVIEW

The Russian sports doping scandal began in earnest with a December 2014 report from German broadcaster ARD alleging the existence of a secret doping program in Russian athletics that was being systematically covered up and backed by state and possibly international officials. Within days, the WADA announced it would organize an independent commission to investigate the allegations in the report. By early November 2015, Lamine Diack, who had stepped down as president of the IAAF, which had come under fire in the report as having been neglectful in its antidoping efforts, was being detained and investigated by French prosecutors on suspicion that he had taken bribes to cover up positive doping tests. The WADA commission's initial report, issued days later, confirmed, mainly through a consideration of the sport of track and field, the allegations made in the ARD documentary and suggested significant evidence existed to indicate a state-sponsored doping program in Russian athletics. The IAAF temporarily suspended Russia's membership, prohibiting the country from further international competitions, as the committee determined how to proceed.

In May 2016, Grigory Rodchenkov, the former head of Russia's antidoping laboratory who had defected to the United States after losing his job, gave an interview with the *New York Times* in which he detailed a state-run doping system that he participated in, including developing a special blend of banned substances that was given to many Russian athletes at the 2014 Sochi Olympics before their samples of urine were covertly substituted with clean ones. WADA subsequently commissioned an independent investigation into the issue, led by Canadian attorney Richard McLaren. The first part of McLaren's report, released in July 2016, focused on confirming that systematic doping was orchestrated at Sochi and provided sufficient evidence to indicate a reasonable belief that widespread doping in Russian competitive sports had been occurring for years, covered-up, and supported by Russian officials; the findings indicated interference by the country's Ministry of Sport and FSB. Regardless, the controversial decision was made not to completely ban Russia from competing in that year's Summer Olympics in Rio de Janeiro, Brazil; prospective competitors did have to meet especially strict criteria to qualify. A second part of the McLaren report was published in December, providing what he described as incontrovertible proof of state-sponsored doping in the Olympics and other competitive sporting events across a range of sports. Though top Russian officials continued to deny the findings, the report implicated more than one thousand athletes.

The IOC set up a disciplinary commission known as the "Oswald Commission," headed by IOC member Denis Oswald, to investigate the situation and issue penalties. Following the reanalysis of urine samples, the Oswald Commission began issuing sanctions in November 2017. Russia was stripped of several of the medals awarded to its athletes during the Sochi Olympics. In December 2017, it was also announced that Russia would be banned from competing as a nation in the 2018 Winter Olympics in South Korea. Vitaly Mutko, Russia's minister of sport, was banned from the Olympics for life. However, to avoid punishing the athletes themselves for the actions of other athletes and officials, it was agreed that athletes without any known history of doping would still be allowed to compete as Olympic Athletes from Russia (OAR), but that any medals won would not count toward Russia's totals, and the athletes would not be allowed to display the Russian flag.

—Micah L. Issitt

Further Reading

Ingle, S. "Russia Banned from Winter Olympics Over State-Sponsored Doping." *The Guardian,* 5 Dec. 2017, www.theguardian.com/sport/2017/dec/05/russian-olympic-committee-banned-winter-games-doping.

"Majority of Russian Athletes Doping, Alleges German Documentary." *CNN,* 5 Dec. 2014, www.cnn.com/2014/12/05/sport/russia-doping-allegations/index.html.

Masters, J., and E. McKirdy. "Olympic Doping Ban Overturned for 28 Russian Athletes." *CNN,* 1 Feb. 2018, www.cnn.com/2018/02/01/europe/russia-doping-ban-lifted-on-28-athletes-intl/index.html.

Ruiz, R. R. "Report Shows Vast Reach of Russian Doping: 1,000 Athletes, 30 Sports." *The New York Times,* 9 Dec. 2016, www.nytimes.com/2016/12/09/sports/russia-doping-mclaren-report.html.

Ruiz, R. R., and M. Schwirtz. "Russian Insider Says State-Run Doping Fueled Olympic Gold." *The New York Times,* 12 May 2016, www.nytimes.com/2016/05/13/sports/russia-doping-sochi-olympics-2014.html.

Soccer Star Diego Maradona Is Expelled from World Cup

Category: Doping
Specialties and related fields: Biochemistry, performance-enhancing drugs, soccer

Definition: Diego Maradona, generally regarded as one of the greatest soccer players of the modern era, tested positive for ephedrine doping and was sent home from the 1994 World Cup competition

KEY TERMS

anabolic steroids: synthetic steroid hormones that resemble testosterone and promote muscle growth, used medicinally to treat some forms of weight loss and illegally by some athletes and others to enhance physical performance

doping: drug administration to inhibit or enhance sporting performance

human growth hormone (HGH): a peptide hormone that stimulates growth, cell reproduction, and cell regeneration in humans and other animals. It is thus important in human development

performance-enhancing drugs (PEDs): substances used to improve any form of activity performance in humans

KEY FIGURES

Diego Maradona: Argentine soccer star.
Daniel Cerrini: Argentine body builder and weight-loss trainer.
Carlos Menem: president of Argentina, 1989-99.

SUMMARY OF EVENT

Even among the greatest modern soccer players—Pelé, Franz Beckenbauer, Johann Cruiff, Roberto Baggio, Alfredo Di Stéfano, and Zico—Diego Maradona was a unique presence. His skill at the world's most popular sport was unrivaled. Like these other great offensive players, he rose to his best in the World Cup final matches, held every four years and watched by hundreds of millions of fans.

Likewise, Maradona's play so dominated his national team that he became inextricably associated with Argentina's image and was the most famous Argentine in the world. However, unlike his peers, who felt a certain obligation to represent their nations in

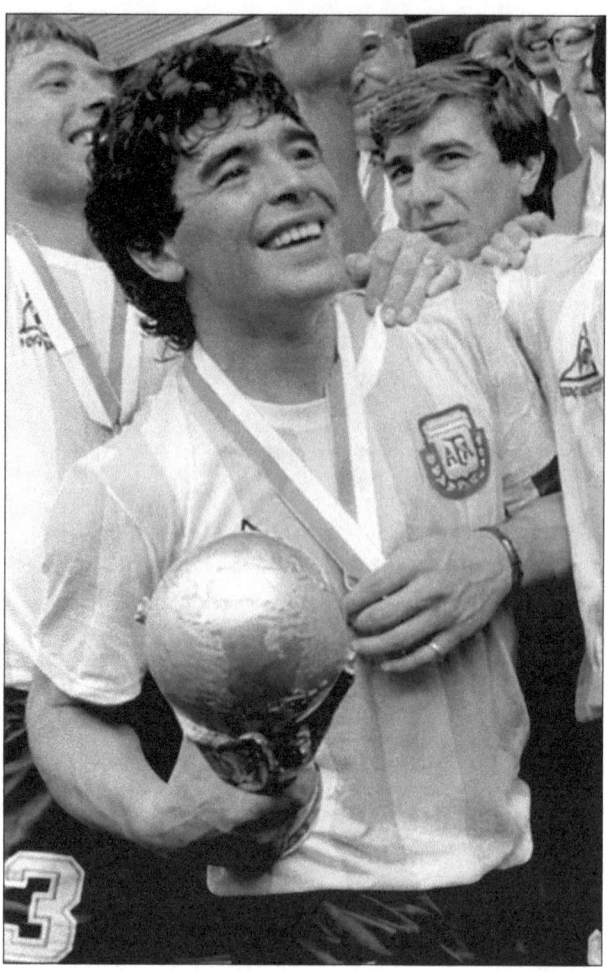

Photo via Wikimedia Commons. [Public domain.]

a dignified manner, Maradona sometimes said that he believed that international soccer existed for his benefit. Off the field—and sometimes on as well—he was often embroiled in controversy and seemed but one step from scandal.

Maradona was born on October 30, 1960, in a shanty town outside Buenos Aires. He began playing soccer at the age of three. By age twelve, he was already well-known for his soccer skills and tricks. Starring for several professional soccer clubs, Maradona played in his first World Cup competition in 1982. In 1986, as team captain, he led Argentina to victory at the Mexico World Cup with a brilliant tournament.

The most memorable game of the 1986 cup was the June 22 quarterfinal match between Argentina and England. These two countries had been at war over the Falkland Islands off the coast of Argentina. The two goals Maradona scored in Argentina's 2-1 victory are among the most famous in World Cup history. The first goal was the infamous hand of God goal, in which Maradona was accused of illegally knocking the ball into the English net with his hand (the "hand of God," Maradona claimed). The second goal is considered by many fans to be the greatest in soccer history and has been dubbed the goal of the century. Maradona dribbled the ball 55 yards (50 meters) past five of England's fabled defenders before shooting it past the superb goalkeeper Peter Shilton. In 1990, Argentina lost the final-round World Cup match to the champion Italian team.

By the 1990s, however, Maradona struggled with cocaine addiction and a tendency to gain weight. Playing for a Naples, Italy, soccer club, he was under the spotlight of European tabloids for his unruly personal life and under investigation by the Italian police for drug use and Mafia connections. On March 17, 1991, a random drug test revealed the presence of cocaine in his body. He was banned from professional soccer for fifteen months. When Maradona returned to professional soccer in 1992, he was overweight, depressed, and had a diminished presence on the soccer field. His fans—and he himself—saw the 1994 World Cup, to be played over the summer in the United States, as an opportunity for Maradona to restore his tarnished reputation, both on and off-field.

In the summer of 1993, Maradona had begun training with Argentine personal trainer and body builder Daniel Cerrini, who prescribed intense exercise, rigorous dieting, supplements of vitamins and minerals, and energy-boosting drugs. Soon, Maradona had lost 33 pounds (15 kilograms) and felt ready for the World Cup. He arrived in the United States during the summer of 1994. Cerrini joined Maradona's longtime fitness trainer, Fernando Signorini, for the trip as well. During the first two qualifying games, Maradona performed well. He led his team to a 4-0 victory over Greece on June 21 and a well-played 2-1 win against Nigeria four days later. One of the few players of international renown, he was cheered by the American fans in Boston.

Cerrini and Signorini were still disputing Maradona's ideal weight. Maradona weighed 169 pounds (76.8 kilograms) at the start of the tournament, which was acceptable to Signorini. Still, Cerrini wanted him at 154 pounds (70 kilograms) and continued to prescribe him diet supplements. The team physician, Ernesto Ubalde, was not involved in the diet regimen.

On June 25, during half-time in the Argentina-Nigeria match, two urine samples were collected from Maradona, according to the new random drug-testing policy of the Fédération Internationale de Football Association (FIFA), which called for testing players during the qualifying rounds. On July 1, the World Cup organizing committee announced that Maradona's urine test revealed the presence of the stimulant ephedrine and four other substances prohibited by FIFA doping control regulations. Maradona, waiting in Dallas for Argentina's game against Bulgaria, was immediately suspended from further play. In addition, an investigation was launched into his use of drugs. After his suspension, he took a lucrative position as a commentator on the games for Argentine television.

On August 24, the organizing committee announced the results of the investigation. Although Maradona was found not to have taken drugs to enhance his performance and was, in fact, not even aware of the contents of the drug, he nevertheless was in breach of FIFA regulations. Cerrini was assigned ultimate responsibility for the infraction. Still, FIFA did take into account Maradona's previous history of drug abuse in holding him partly responsible. Both Maradona and Cerrini were banned from participation in all soccer events for fifteen months and fined twenty thousand Swiss francs. With Maradona off the team, Argentina was soon eliminated from the 1994 World Cup tournament.

The outcry in response to Maradona's suspension was worldwide. In Dhaka, more than twenty thousand Bangladeshis demonstrated in protest. American newspapers, many sympathetic to Maradona, compared the scandal to the one seared in the consciousness of American sports fans—the Black Sox baseball scandal of 1919. In Argentina, fans were devastated. Argentine President Carlos Menem wrote FIFA a five-page letter pleading for clemency for Maradona. Nevertheless, the committee affirmed its decision, recommending that in the future, all players' medical treatments should be under the exclusive supervision of the team physician.

IMPACT

Maradona garnered much sympathy because of his heroic training regimen for the World Cup. By all accounts, his conditioning level was the best in years, and he recovered his playing skills. When told of his suspension, he said, "They have sawed off my legs."

Moreover, there is little reason to doubt Maradona's contention—confirmed by the organizing committee—that the drug infraction was the byproduct of his attempt to stabilize his weight, not enhance his performance. In his 2000 autobiography, published in English in 2007, Maradona claimed that Cerrini had made an innocent mistake. Maradona had run out of his usual supplement, Ripped Fast. Cerrini had substituted the over-the-counter product Ripped Fuel, not knowing that it contained a small amount of ephedrine.

Fédération Internationale de Football Association was required to act on the matter. By expelling Maradona, FIFA took overdue measures against the proliferation of stimulants in soccer. This problem was increasingly plaguing all sports. While

Maradona's explanation for the accidental presence of ephedrine was plausible, there is no denying its potential for stimulating athletic energy.

The 1994 games would be tragically marred as well by the combination of illegal drug money and the importance of soccer in Latin American culture. When the Colombian defender Andres Escobar returned home after making a well-publicized mistake in the game with the United States, he was gunned down on the crime- and drug-plagued streets of Medellín, Colombia.

Maradona retired from soccer a few years after the doping affair. His drug addiction continued, and he eventually had a heart attack in 2004 following a cocaine overdose. Maradona appeared to change after this, becoming free of weight concerns and cocaine addiction.

—Howard Bromberg

Further Reading
Burns, Jimmy. *Hand of God: The Life of Diego Maradona.* Lyons Press, 2003.
Lisi, Clemente Angelo. *A History of the World Cup: 1930-2006.* Scarecrow Press, 2007.
Maradona, Diego, et al. *Maradona: The Autobiography of Soccer's Greatest and Most Controversial Star.* Skyhorse, 2007.
Radnedge, Keir. *The Complete Encyclopedia of Soccer.* Carlton Books, 2007.

STEROID ABUSE

Category: Disease/Disorder
Specialties and related fields: Exercise physiology, psychiatry, psychology, sports medicine
Definition: the use of illegal anabolic steroids to increase athletic performance, with negative side effects on physical and psychological health

KEY TERMS
anabolic steroids: synthetic steroid hormones that resemble testosterone and promote muscle growth; they treat some forms of weight loss and, illegally, by some athletes and others to enhance physical performance
performance-enhancing drugs: substances used to improve any form of activity performance in humans

CAUSES AND SYMPTOMS
Steroids provide many valuable medical benefits for various conditions ranging from asthma, infections, and delayed puberty to spastic colon. Unfortunately, steroid abuse has become an increasingly prevalent issue. Steroid abuse has gained attention in the past few years mainly due to its relation to professional sports. Numerous well-known athletes have admitted to using steroids to increase their athletic edge. A lack of social acceptability around steroid use has resulted from the more than seventy side effects associated with steroid use, including such immediate problems as rage, depression, and highly aggressive behavior. Reports have included findings of teenagers committing acts as brutal as murder, without any history of criminal or aggressive behavior, while under the influence of steroids. While such acts are rare, the connection between steroids and out-of-control rage is well known. In addition, steroid abuse has been linked with long-term problems like heart attacks, strokes, and changes in the reproductive system. Increasing attention will likely be focused on these long-term effects, both in research and in terms of problem reporting. Increases in access to anabolic steroids are also partly responsible for increasing visibility and attention to such problems.

Social research also has demonstrated important findings related to steroid use in college students and athletes. One study, for example, demonstrated that college students consistently rated anabolic steroid-using athletes more negatively than drug-free athletes. Students tended to evaluate anabolic steroid-using athletes just as negatively as they would an athlete who was using cocaine. In another study, researchers demonstrated that steroid use is not only physically reinforcing but also psychologically reinforcing. Specifically, in interviews with thirty-five male self-reported anabolic steroid users, males with a positive perception of their physique had lower anxiety levels and higher levels of satisfaction with their upper body than the control subjects. A psychological gain associated with steroid use was directly related to the shorter-term physical benefits of their use.

PERSPECTIVE AND PROSPECTS

Recent estimates suggest that about 1.4 percent of college athletes use anabolic steroids. A 2001 report by the National Collegiate Athletic Association (NCAA) demonstrated that this decreased from the 4.9 percent of student-athletes who reported using steroids in 1985. Nationwide, according to the NCAA, collegiate football players had the highest use rate, at 3.0 percent. The survey suggested, however, that this lowered rate may reflect underreporting. Factors such as the illegality of drug use or a lack of social acceptability in acknowledging such personal behavior may be responsible. Such underreporting assertions are also based on other reports that 2.6 percent of male high school students and 0.4 percent of female high school students have used anabolic steroids. Furthermore, among athletes not in college, reported rates are much higher. Weightlifters, powerlifters, track-and-field athletes, football players, and sprinters had the highest reported usage rates. Major League Baseball banned steroids in 2002 and instituted a testing program after several top players admitted to steroid use. Future work in this area will likely explore these psychological factors and focus on how to intervene effectively.

> **INFORMATION ON STEROID ABUSE**
>
> **Causes**: Psychological and emotional factors, competitive sports
>
> **Symptoms**: Relatively rapid gain in muscle tone, increased aggressiveness, violent temper, increased acne, premature balding, abnormal breast development
>
> **Duration**: Temporary to long-term
>
> **Treatments**: Cessation of drug use, counseling

Additionally, social interventions will likely be explored. Athletics remain competitive and financially lucrative, so special attention will need to be paid to the social context in which steroid abuse occurs. There is little research or studies on the treatment of steroid abuse. Most knowledge on treatment comes from the experience of a small number of physicians who have treated steroid withdrawal themselves. The most effective treatment is prevention.

—*Roman J. Miller, Nancy A. Piotrowski, Samar Aslam*

Further Reading

"Anabolic Steroid Drug Facts." *National Institutes on Drug Abuse*, Aug. 2018, www.drugabuse.gov/publications/drugfacts/anabolic-steroids

Craig, Charles R., and Robert E. Stitzel, editors. *Modern Pharmacology with Clinical Applications*. 6th ed., Lippincott, 2004.

Melmed, Shlomo, et al., editors. *Williams Textbook of Endocrinology*. 14th ed., Elsevier, 2019.

Taylor, William N. *Anabolic Steroids and the Athlete*. 2nd ed., McFarland, 2002.

Yesalis, Charles E., editor. *Anabolic Steroids in Sport and Exercise*. 2nd ed., Human Kinetics, 2000.

Yesalis, Charles E., and Michael S. Bahrke. "Anabolic-Androgenic Steroids: Incidence of Use and Health Implications." *President's Council on Physical Fitness and Sports Research Digest*, vol. 5, no. 5, 2005, pp. 1-8.

Steroids: HGH and PEDs

Category: Doping
Specialties and related fields: Biochemistry, sports medicine, strength and conditioning
Definition: substances taken to improve strength, speed, endurance, or mental focus

KEY TERMS

anabolic steroids: synthetic steroid hormones that resemble testosterone and promote muscle growth, used medicinally to treat some forms of weight loss and illegally by some athletes and others to enhance physical performance

doping: drug administration to inhibit or enhance sporting performance

human growth hormone (HGH): a peptide hormone that stimulates growth, cell reproduction, and cell regeneration in humans and other animals. It is thus important in human development

performance-enhancing drugs (PEDs): substances used to improve any form of activity performance in humans

INTRODUCTION

Trying to gain an edge in athletic competitions is nothing new. The first recorded use of a performance-enhancing drug (PED) in the Olympic Games occurred in 1904 when a marathon runner injected himself with strychnine, a poison that acts as a muscle stimulant. Before 1935, almost all PEDs were stimulants similar to amphetamines and cocaine. That changed in the 1940s after a chemist learned how to make the male hormone testosterone in the laboratory.

Testosterone is a type of anabolic-androgenic steroid (AAS). Steroids are a class of compounds that include both male and female sex hormones. Anabolic refers to the muscle-building properties of the hormone. Androgenic indicates that the hormone increases male sexual characteristics. Other steroid hormones include estrogen, progesterone, and cortisol, but only AASs increase muscle mass. In athletic circles, AAS drugs are commonly just called "steroids," or 'roids.

By 1960, chemists had figured out how to synthesize several synthetic AASs not normally produced by the body, but that had an effect similar to testosterone. Competitive athletes and bodybuilders embraced these drugs. Anabolic-androgenic steroids were banned by the International Olympic Committee in 1975. As drug-testing technology improved, many competitors were stripped of their medals for abusing these drugs. The United States added AASs to the list of controlled substances in 1990. This legislation made providing steroids for nonmedical uses a felony. However, even down to the high school level, athletes continued using them. Today illicit laboratories and unethical physicians work to provide a constantly changing stream of synthetic AASs that either mimics the actions of testosterone or stimulate the body to produce excess amounts of the hormone. Makers of these drugs are always looking for ways to stay one step ahead of drug testing agencies such as the World Anti-Doping Agency (WADA).

The use of human growth hormone (HGH) has a much shorter history. In the body, it is made by the pituitary gland. Chemists were able to synthesize HGH in the laboratory in the 1980s and used it to treat children with genetic defects who failed to produce enough of the hormone naturally. Later, HGH was embraced by healthy adult athletes in the belief that it would increase strength and slow aging. HGH is especially attractive to illegal users because it cannot be detected in urine tests; a blood test must document its presence. As of 2015, there is little evidence that HGH affects adults.

HOW ANABOLIC-ANDROGENIC STEROIDS WORK

Testosterone is in the class of hormones called "androgens" that includes several related compounds sold with names such as Androstenedione, Oxandrin, Dianabol, Winstrol, Deca-Durabolin, and Equipoise. Street names include gym candy, pumpers, halo, stackers, var, drol, the clear, and primo. The testes naturally produce testosterone in men. It stimulates increased protein production. Levels of the hormone normally increase at puberty, leading to the development of male sexual characteristics such as growth in muscle mass, development of denser bones, body hair, thickening of the vocal cords leading to a lower-pitched voice, the distinctive male profile of broad shoulders and a narrow waist, and an increased sex drive.

Testosterone production peaks in the early twenties and decreases gradually with age. However, despite advertisements to the contrary, low testosterone, or low T, is not a common disorder among healthy men. Legitimate medical uses of the hormone include treatment for delayed puberty and muscle wasting in diseases such as cancer and acquired immunodeficiency syndrome (AIDS). Bodybuilders and athletes abuse testosterone and related AASs to become larger, stronger and have better-defined muscles.

EFFECTS OF ANABOLIC-ANDROGENIC STEROIDS

Anabolic-androgenic steroids increase muscle mass and bone density, but to achieve this, individuals must take levels of the drug ten to one hundred times greater than the therapeutic dose. Testosterone and its relatives can be taken as an injection, a pill, or as a gel applied to the skin. HGH is given as an injection.

Using AASs excessively and over time can cause serious negative health effects. Men who use AASs can become sterile. The testes atrophy (shrivel), and sperm fail to mature. These side effects occur because the testes stop producing testosterone when high levels of artificial testosterone are circulating in the body. In addition, excess testosterone in men may be converted into estrogen, a female sex hormone. Excessive estrogen causes men to develop breasts; a condition called "gynecomastia." Other side effects of AAS abuse include acne and baldness.

Because the heart is a muscle, it increases in size when stimulated by AASs. As the heart enlarges, its pumping capacity decreases, and heart rhythm irregularities can develop, leading to a heart attack, even in young people. Other side effects include an increased risk of liver damage or liver cancer, kidney failure, high blood pressure, and high cholesterol levels. HGH abusers can develop abnormal hearts and thin, weak bones (osteoporosis). Women who abuse AASs often develop male characteristics such as a deepened voice, broad shoulders, facial hair, a disrupted menstrual cycle, and the internal effects on the heart, liver, and kidney seen in men.

Anabolic-androgenic steroids also affect mood and behavior. Continued use can lead to aggression, temper explosions, and violence often called "roid rage." Extended use can also cause paranoia, irritability, and impaired judgment. These behavioral changes tend to interfere with normal social relationships.

To minimize side effects, many athletes practice cycling or taking AASs for a set period and then quitting for a period. Stopping often leads to depression, mood swings, restlessness, insomnia, loss of appetite, decreased sex drive, and drug cravings.

Along with AAS drugs, abusers often take excessive quantities of dietary supplements. This practice is called "stacking." Dietary supplements include vitamins, minerals, herbs, amino acids, and enzymes. Supplements are not regulated with the same rigor and do not require testing as pharmaceutical drugs. Multiple studies have found that many dietary supplements, especially those sold over the internet, do not conform to their labeling. Either they fail to contain the advertised ingredient in the specified amount or unlisted ingredients. Some of these supplements contain banned substances, while others can enhance the side effects of AASs.

In recent years, testing for PEDs has increased and improved. Many professional athletes such as Barry Bonds, Mark McGwire, Bill Romanowski, and Lyle Alzado have been involved in steroid-use scandals. Cyclist Lance Armstrong was stripped of his seven Tour-de-France titles and banned for life from professional cycling after an investigation revealed his PED use.

—*Tish Davidson*

Further Reading

"Anabolic Steroids." *United States National Library of Medicine*, 18 Sept. 2014, www.nlm.nih.gov/medlineplus/anabolicsteroids.html.

"Effects of PEDs." *United States Anti-Doping Agency (USADA)*, 13 May 2015, www.usada.org/substances/effects-of-performance-enhancing-drugs.

Kille, L. W. "Performance-enhancing Drugs in Athletics: Research Roundup." *The Journalist's Resource*, 9 May 2013, journalistsresource.org/studies/society/culture/athletic-academic-performance-enhancing-drugs-research-roundup.

Wedro, B. "Steroids Types, Side Effects, and Treatment." *emedicinehealth*, 29 July 2014, www.emedicinehealth.com/steroids/article_em.htm.

Woolston, C. "Human Growth Hormone." *HealthDay*, 11 Mar. 2015, consumer.healthday.com/encyclopedia/substance-abuse-38/illicit-drugs-news-217/human-growth-hormone-647257.html.

STEROIDS IN BASEBALL

Category: Doping
Specialties and related fields: Biochemistry, personal training, sports medicine, strength and conditioning

Definition: an ongoing issue for Major League Baseball (MLB); several players have suggested that drug use is rampant in baseball

KEY TERMS

anabolic steroids: synthetic steroid hormones that resemble testosterone and promote muscle growth; they treat some forms of weight loss and, illegally, by some athletes and others to enhance physical performance

performance-enhancing drugs (PEDs): substances used to improve any form of activity performance in humans

INTRODUCTION

In 2003, Major League Baseball (MLB) implemented a policy to test players for performance-enhancing drugs (PEDs) such as steroids. Following a raid on a laboratory believed to be supplying illegal steroids to players, several of the league's biggest stars were accused of taking steroids. Throughout the decade, federal investigations and a league-wide review of steroid use in baseball implicated nearly ninety players. The fallout from using steroids in baseball sullied the league's reputation. It threatened the legacies of some of baseball's most revered players.

The steroid era of baseball had a major impact on the sport and its fans during the 2000s. At the end of the 1990s and the beginning of the 2000s, some of MLB's biggest stars—Mark McGwire, Barry Bonds, and Sammy Sosa—were celebrated for surpassing the single-season home-run record. However, at the start of the 2000s, news reports revealed that the league, which banned PEDs but did not have a testing program, had a PED-use problem that likely included these superstars.

THE BALCO RAID

In September 2003, federal investigators raided the Bay Area Laboratory Co-Operative (BALCO) in

Burlingame, California, on suspicion that the company was supplying undetectable steroids and other PEDs to professional athletes. Following the raid, a grand jury convened to investigate BALCO. Among the BALCO figures under scrutiny was Greg Anderson. He was a trainer for San Francisco Giants player Bonds, one of the players subpoenaed to testify before the grand jury about his connections to BALCO. Another player, Jason Giambi, admitted to using BALCO-supplied PEDs. In contrast, Bonds admitted that Anderson gave him a topical balm and a cream that he did not realize contained steroids.

The BALCO raid and investigation sent shock waves through the league. Commissioner Bud Selig called upon the players union to work with him to rid baseball of PEDs. However, this mandate, along with many teams' reactions to the BALCO revelations, appeared to analysts as somewhat hypocritical since most felt that virtually everyone involved in the sport either knew or should have known that allegations of PED use were not only attached to some of the biggest names in baseball but also that steroid use was rampant.

The BALCO raid and investigation led to the indictments of BALCO officials, plea deals, and jail terms for coaches and trainers connected to professional baseball and track and field events. In March 2005, several current and former baseball players testified before the House Government Reform Committee regarding steroid use in baseball. Although subpoenaed, Mark McGwire evaded the congressional questions and essentially refused to answer questions posed to him. He responded primarily with a statement that he was not there to "discuss the past."

THE MITCHELL REPORT

To better understand the breadth of steroid use in baseball, MLB officials turned to former senator George Mitchell. In 2006, Mitchell was asked to investigate steroid use among players since the beginning of the 2000s (although he was given license to look back further in some cases). Mitchell's panel interviewed hundreds of people associated with MLB, such as general managers, coaches, and trainers (although, with a few exceptions, players refused to cooperate with his inquiry).

Mitchell's final report was damning for the entire league. The panel took to task both the commissioner's office and the players union for failing at least to acknowledge the use of PEDs if not creating an environment in which such behavior was acceptable. The report also named nearly ninety players who, the panel was told, used steroids. Among them were Bonds, former Cy Young Award-winning pitcher Éric Gagné, 2002 Most Valuable Player Miguel Tejada, and pitching superstar Roger Clemens.

The Mitchell report was considered an eye-opener for professional sports in general. However, it was not without controversy. Players, in particular, argued that the report was based on hearsay rather than facts. Players and their agents and attorneys argued that since the players themselves did not cooperate, the others were not in a position to make such accusations. To be sure, when Mitchell reached out to the players and the players union, the athletes flatly refused, citing their concern that any information uncovered about the players would somehow make it to the public eye. With Mitchell's panel unable to guarantee confidentiality, the information provided in the report was derived from apparent witnesses, not the players themselves.

FEDERAL INVESTIGATIONS

As the revelations about BALCO and the Mitchell Report came to light, players named in either of the proceedings were quick to defend themselves. One player, in particular, Bonds, was targeted by the grand jury and the Mitchell Report and the investigation by the House Government Reform Committee. Bonds had told the BALCO grand jury that his trainer unknowingly gave him steroids. Others involved in the Mitchell Report and the BALCO grand jury investigation refuted Bonds's claim, stating that Bonds knew precisely what he was using and had used other steroids repeatedly throughout the latter part of his career.

The contradictory stories surrounding Bonds led to a formal federal investigation determining whether Bonds perjured himself before that grand jury. Anderson refused to cooperate with the Bonds investigation and was jailed for a lengthy-term. Meanwhile, another of Bonds's associates, Steve Hoskins (a longtime friend and business partner), told the grand jury that Bonds complained to him of soreness from his frequent steroid injections. Hoskins also secretly recorded Anderson in 2003, when Anderson stated that he injected Bonds on many occasions. According to Bond's defense, this evidence was sullied by the fact that Hoskins and Bonds had a falling out after Bonds reported to federal agents that Hoskins had stolen from their business venture.

Meanwhile, Clemens was also targeted but instead was accused of perjury. Clemens, who had testified at a congressional committee in 2007 with other baseball stars named in the Mitchell Report, told the committee that he never knowingly took steroids or other PEDs. Congress turned the case over to the Justice Department, believing that evidence (such as Brian McNamee's claims in the Mitchell Report that he had personally injected Clemens) indicated Clemens lied to the legislative committee. Clemens maintained his innocence throughout the affair, as investigators and detractors continued to accuse him of drug use. By the end of the 2000s, the Clemens case remained unresolved, and Clemens retired from professional baseball to deal with the ongoing case. (He was acquitted on all charges in 2012.)

The Bonds and Clemens cases provided illustrations of the zeal with which investigators and others wished to hold athletes responsible for their alleged use of PEDs. Many, including supporters of these and other players, argued that these cases amounted to a witch hunt, with prosecutors fighting with unnecessary vigor to make an example of these players. Many believed prosecutors continued to push for convictions despite the lack of hard or reliable evidence, stretching the cases out for years.

DRUG TESTING

The revelation that PED use was widespread in baseball (and that MLB had failed to address the issue) damaged the league's reputation. Baseball needed to repair the disastrous public image this issue cre-

Prominent Players Listed in the Mitchell Report

Players	Career Batting Average (as of 2012)
Bonds, Barry	.298
Canseco, José	.266
Dykstra, Lenny	.285
Giambi, Jason	.281
Justice, David	.279
Knoblauch, Chuck	.289
Lo Duca, Paul	.286
Roberts, Brian	.280
Sheffield, Gary	.292
Tejada, Miguel	.285
Vaughn, Mo	.293
Williams, Matt	.268

Pitchers	Career Earned Run Average (as of 2012)
Brown, Kevin	3.28
Clemens, Roger	3.12
Gagné, Éric	3.47
Neagle, Denny	4.24
Pettitte, Andy	3.85
Rocker, John	3.42
Stanton, Mike	3.92

ated for the sport by making some statement that seemed genuinely apologetic—a difficult undertaking, considering the prevailing perception that baseball could have policed itself years prior. League officials also had to look to the future by installing a new steroid testing policy that would result in serious punishments for those caught using PEDs. This task for the league was seemingly as daunting as repairing its image; in fact, the two seemed to go hand in hand.

After the BALCO case and the Mitchell Report came to bear, the players union and league officials began to discuss a new testing policy that was mutually agreeable to both parties, and that would show a league-wide desire to curb steroid use. The final policy, agreed upon in 2005, involved random testing of players (even during the off-season), with lengthy suspensions for those caught using steroids for the first time. These punishments would also be made public, a point that Commissioner Bud Selig argued would further deter steroid use.

In the minds of many onlookers and analysts, parts of the testing policy seemed strict. Still, overall, the policy did not go far enough to prevent further steroid use in baseball. For example, the tests looked for steroids, not human growth hormone or amphetamines. Furthermore, the policy did not seem to account for the ever-evolving nature of the PED industry—BALCO and other steroid-producing laboratories were consistently working to develop new, undetectable, and more effective steroids for professional athletes. Some experts argued that the policy had too many loopholes and lacked any external oversight to make a difference. Meanwhile, as the decade's end approached, several superstars, many of whom were likely Baseball Hall of Fame inductees, were linked to PED use. These players included Manny Ramirez, who was suspended for fifty games in 2009 for testing positive for human chorionic gonadotropin (a testosterone-increasing hormone), and Alex Rodriguez, who admitted in 2009 that he had used steroids for three seasons at the beginning of the decade.

IMPACT

The raid of the BALCO facility and the subsequent federal investigation made public what many people within professional baseball had known for years: steroid use was rampant, particularly during the 1990s. The Mitchell Report that followed went even further, humiliating not only the players but also the league, which it suggested ignored the drug use of its players. Only a few years earlier, fans and the league celebrated the record-setting accomplishments of players like McGwire, Sosa, and Bonds. Still, by the early 2000s, these players were thrust into the spotlight, and their careers and reputations were tarnished as representatives of the steroid era.

The revelation of steroid use in baseball had strong implications for all US professional sports, which were called upon to ensure the implementation of strict testing standards governing steroids, human growth hormone, and other PEDs. Professional baseball put such a program in place that resulted in several high-profile suspensions and the marring of accomplishments.

—*Michael Auerbach*

Further Reading

Comarow, Avery, and Lisa Stein. "Baseball's Iffy Steroid Test." *U.S. News and World Report*, vol. 136, no. 8, 2004.

Elfrink, Tim, and Gus Garcia-Roberts. *Blood Sport: A-Rod and the Quest to End Baseball's Steroid Era*. Plume, 2015.

Fainaru-Wada, Mark, and Lance Williams. *Game of Shadows: Barry Bonds, BALCO, and the Steroids Scandal That Rocked Professional Sports*. Gotham, 2007.

Kimball, Bob, and Beau Dure. "BALCO Investigation Timeline." *USAToday.com*, 27 Nov. 2007, usatoday30.usatoday.com/sports/balco-timeline.htm.

Mitchell, George J. *The Negotiator: A Memoir*. Simon & Schuster, 2015.

Radomski, Kirk. *Bases Loaded: The Inside Story of the Steroid Era in Baseball by the Central Figure in the Mitchell Report*. Hudson, 2009.

Ryan, Dennis J., and Arthur Remillard. "From Purity to Pollution: The Transformation of Baseball in the Steroid Era." *Journal of Student Research at Saint Francis University*, vol. 5, no. 1, 2014, p. 4.

Schmotzer, Brian, et al. "'The Natural'? The Effects of Steroids on Offensive Performance in Baseball." *Chance*, vol. 22, no. 2, 2009, pp. 21-32.

Verducci, Tom. "Reason to Believe." *Sports Illustrated*, vol. 102, no. 8, 2005, pp. 39-45.

TRACK-AND-FIELD CHAMPION HEIKE DRESCHLER DOPING SCANDAL

Category: Sport, track and field (long jump)

Specialties and related fields: Athletic training, personal training, strength and conditioning, track and field

Definition: a German former track and field athlete who represented East Germany and later Germany and was one of the most successful long jumpers of all-time

KEY TERMS

East Germany: officially the German Democratic Republic, was a state that existed from 1949 to 1990 in middle Germany as part of the Eastern Bloc in the Cold War

long jump: a track and field event in which athletes combine speed, strength, and agility in an attempt to leap as far as possible from a takeoff point

EARLY LIFE

Heike Dreschler was born Heike Gabriela Daute on December 16, 1964, in Gera, East Germany (now in Germany). She lost her father in an untimely accident at a fairground when he was only thirty-one. Her mother, a shift worker, was left to raise Heike and three other children.

Heike was groomed for greatness as a part of the old East German sports system. Throughout her lengthy and successful career as a long jumper, sprinter, and heptathlete, she seldom failed to live up to her country's expectations.

Behind the Iron Curtain, success in sports translated into money, privilege, and power. Knowing that Heike's family encouraged her to pursue sports. Tall, agile, and strong for her age, Heike was spotted by German coaches when she was a schoolgirl and was recruited for track and field. She quickly established herself as an international star and became one of the premier female long jumpers of all time.

As a teen, Heike was involved in the Free German Youth, an official organization of the German Democratic Republic that attempted to indoctrinate young athletes in Marxist-Leninist Communist philosophy. As allegedly revealed in documents found after the fall of the Berlin Wall, by 1983, she had become an informer for the East German secret police unit nicknamed the "Stasi." Heike, whose code name was *Springen* (Jump), regularly reported to the authorities on the activities of her teammates.

THE ROAD TO EXCELLENCE

In 1981, at seventeen, Heike made her international debut by setting a world junior record in the heptathlon with 5,812 points. Then she set two records in the long jump. As of 2008, the last record of 23.43 feet (7.14 meters) still stood. At the time, she was 5 feet 11 inches, and her slim athletic build and world-class speed made her an immediate threat in the senior ranks.

After moving up to face elite competition at her first World Track and Field Championships in 1983, Heike won her first world title in the long jump. She became the youngest athlete at nineteen to win a gold medal. In the process, she also upset the reigning world-record holder Ani oara Cu mir-Stanciu of Romania. As an East German heroine, Heike was elected as a representative to the *Volkshammer* (The

People's Chamber) of the bicameral East German legislature in 1984.

THE EMERGING CHAMPION

Heike continued her winning streak by compiling more titles and places in the record books in long jumping and sprinting. In 1986, she won the indoor 100-meter title at East Germany's national championships and equaled countrywoman Marita Koch's world-record time of 21.71 seconds in the 200 meters. From 1982 through 1996, Heike won 206 of 245 long-jump competitions, including her one-hundredth victory at the 1992 Olympic Games in Barcelona, Spain.

One of Heike's major claims to fame as an athlete was her spirited rivalry with some of the best American track athletes. In competitions with Jackie Joyner-Kersee, she tallied five of the top ten all-time best jumps, while Joyner-Kersee garnered three. Joyner-Kersee won their head-to-head contest at the 1988 Olympic Games in Seoul, South Korea; however, with a record-breaking performance, Heike had to settle for the silver medal.

Heike continued her competitive streak in the long jump against American Marion Jones. In 1999, she beat Jones with a jump of 22.41 feet to 22.24 feet and was the only woman to defeat Jones at any event during the 1998 season. At the World Cup in Athletics in Johannesburg, South Africa, Heike ended Jones's winning streak of thirty-six competitions, beating her by 2.76 inches with a jump of 23.20 feet.

CONTINUING THE STORY

Few athletes enjoyed Heike's longevity and domination. However, she continued to perform for more than fifteen years after joining the elite level at thirty-five. In 1999, Heike competed in her seventh consecutive World Track and Field Championships in Seville, Spain. Only German discus thrower Jürgen Schult and Jamaican sprinter Merlene Ottey have equaled Heike's streak.

In 2000, competing for Germany, Heike won her second Olympic gold medal in the long jump, eight years after her first. Her jump beat those of Jones and Italian Fiona May. She never expected to win the gold and stated that the 2000 Olympics was her last.

Heike's success in sports was remarkable, considering she took time out to start a family. She married soccer player Andreas Dreschler and petitioned the German sports federation for permission to have a baby in the prime of her competitive career. After much debate, German officials relented, and Heike gave birth to her first child, daughter Toni, on No-

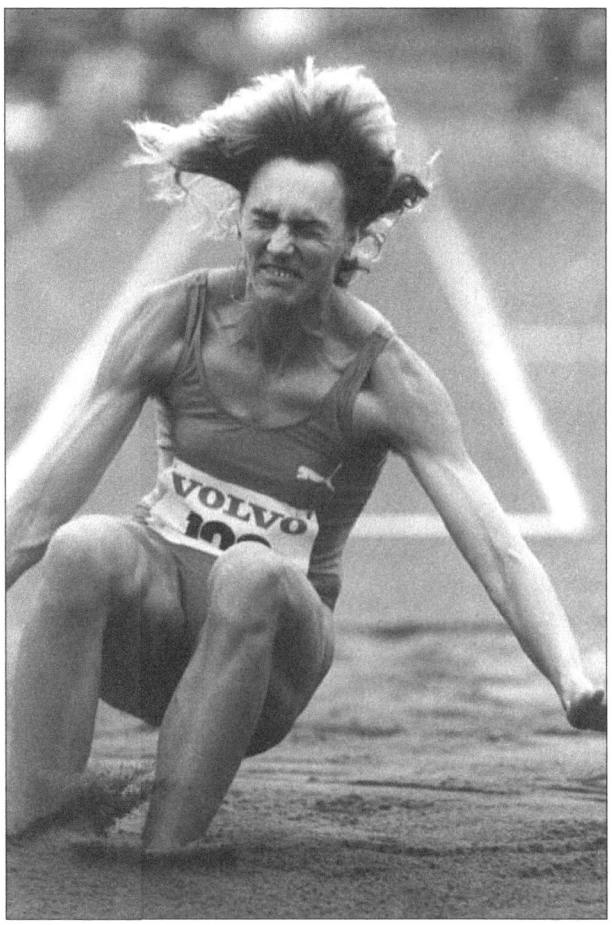

Photo by Bundesarchiv, via Wikimedia Commons.

vember 1, 1989, just eight days before the fall of the Berlin Wall. Divorced from Dreschler, Heike moved with her son to Karlsruhe, Germany, with French decathlete and former European champion Alain Blondel. However, she continued to train with her former father-in-law, Erich Dreschler.

Once the Iron Curtain fell, Heike capitalized on her fame by signing lucrative endorsement deals. At the start of 1995, she left Jena, her club of fifteen years, for an attractive offer at Chemnitz, which included a deal to be a spokeswoman for a health insurance company. In 1999, she was among those considered for the International Association of Athletic Federation's (IAAF's) female athlete of the century. However, the honor went to Fanny Blankers-Koen, a Dutch sprinter who flourished between the late 1930s and the early 1950s. Heike was nominated for the IAAF's women's committee and, in 2007, was elected as the German representative.

SUMMARY

Heike Dreschler stood out as a superior athlete years after her affiliation with an East German athletic regime that employed systematic doping. Her long jumping earned her three world titles, two Olympic gold medals, four European titles, and three world records. She was the first woman to jump beyond 25 feet (7.62 meters) and cleared 22.96 feet (7 meters) more than four hundred times during her career, setting a record. Equally skilled as a sprinter, Heike won bronze medals in the 100 meters and 200 meters at the Seoul Olympics, a silver medal in the 100 meters at the 1987 Rome World Track and Field Championships, a bronze medal in the 4x100-meter relay at Tokyo in 1991, a gold medal in the 200 meters at the 1986 European Championships in Athletics, and a silver medal in the 200 meters at the 1990 European Championships in Athletics.

—*Jack Ewing*

Further Reading

Barber, Gary. *Getting Started in Track and Field Athletics: Advice and Ideas for Children, Parents, and Teachers.* Trafford, 2006.

Dreschler, Heike. *Absprung: An Autobiography.* Central Books, 2001.

Layden, Tim. "Running Amok." *Sports Illustrated*, vol. 93, no. 14, 2000, pp. 39-45.

Wallechinsky, David, and Jaime Loucky. *The Complete Book of the Olympics: 2008 Edition.* Aurum Press, 2008.

SPORTS IN GENERAL

Sports are fun. Have you ever asked yourself why? Competition is a fantastic rush. Do you know why? This section looks at the benefits and risks of sports participation and other aspects of sports from a psychological and sociological perspective. Exercise addiction, mental health benefits, overtraining, sports engineering, and sports psychology are offered for discussion.

Benefits of Playing Sports

Category: Sports participation
Specialties and related fields: Athletes, athletic coaches, athletic coordinators, youth athletes
Definition: the tendency of sports to help reach fitness goals, maintain a healthy weight, encourage healthy decision-making, good mental health, and lower the osteoporosis risk and breast cancer later in life

KEY TERMS

athletic competition: a contest between athletes
mental health: a person's condition regarding their psychological and emotional well-being
sports: an activity involving physical exertion and skill in which an individual or team competes against another or others for entertainment
youth sports: any sports event where competitors are younger than adult age, whether children or adolescents

INTRODUCTION

In the United States, schools and other organizations initiated organized sports for boys in the early 1920s. Business leaders realized that young boys needed to develop character and skills. Sports were a good way to accomplish it. Over time this led to business funding and support for sports leagues such as Pop Warner Football, Little League Baseball, and the American Youth Soccer Association. By the 1970s, the Women's Movement began to address gender inequities and advocated for similar sports programs for girls. Title IX legislation expanded the sports opportunities for females.

All types of sports participation can help youth develop important life skills. Currently, girls and boys have many opportunities to play competitive sports at various levels, from recreation to elite programs. Whatever level is chosen, athletes can develop many skills that will benefit them later in life, whether in their career, family, or community. In addition to physical well-being, the potential benefits are many and include social, behavioral, and intellectual growth. Not everyone has to play at the highest levels. For example, an athlete playing at a high level may not have the opportunity to develop as many leadership skills when spending more time on the bench than playing at a lower level and spending more time on the field.

SOCIAL BENEFITS

Participation in sports, particularly team sports, helps develop the social skills needed later in life. Most young people will eventually have to work in an organization with other workers. Some will become involved in the community and civic programs. Others may become coaches. In all these situations, people must work together toward a common goal. Whether a sports team or a work organization, the members must have the social skills for the group to be successful.

Teamwork is one of the fundamental skills developed in sports participation. Several people, each with specific responsibilities, must do their part for the whole to be successful. In sports, success is generally winning. At work, success may be completing a project and getting a contract. Either way, the skills required for success are the same, and those learned as a child playing sports also benefit the worker later in life. An important part of teamwork is accepting individual responsibilities, being accountable for them, and doing one's best to complete them effectively and unselfishly.

Sports and life are competitive, and participants must be humble in success and accept defeat. There should be respect for the rules, authority, and others involved on both sides. No one is successful all the time and learning to handle failure is an important life lesson.

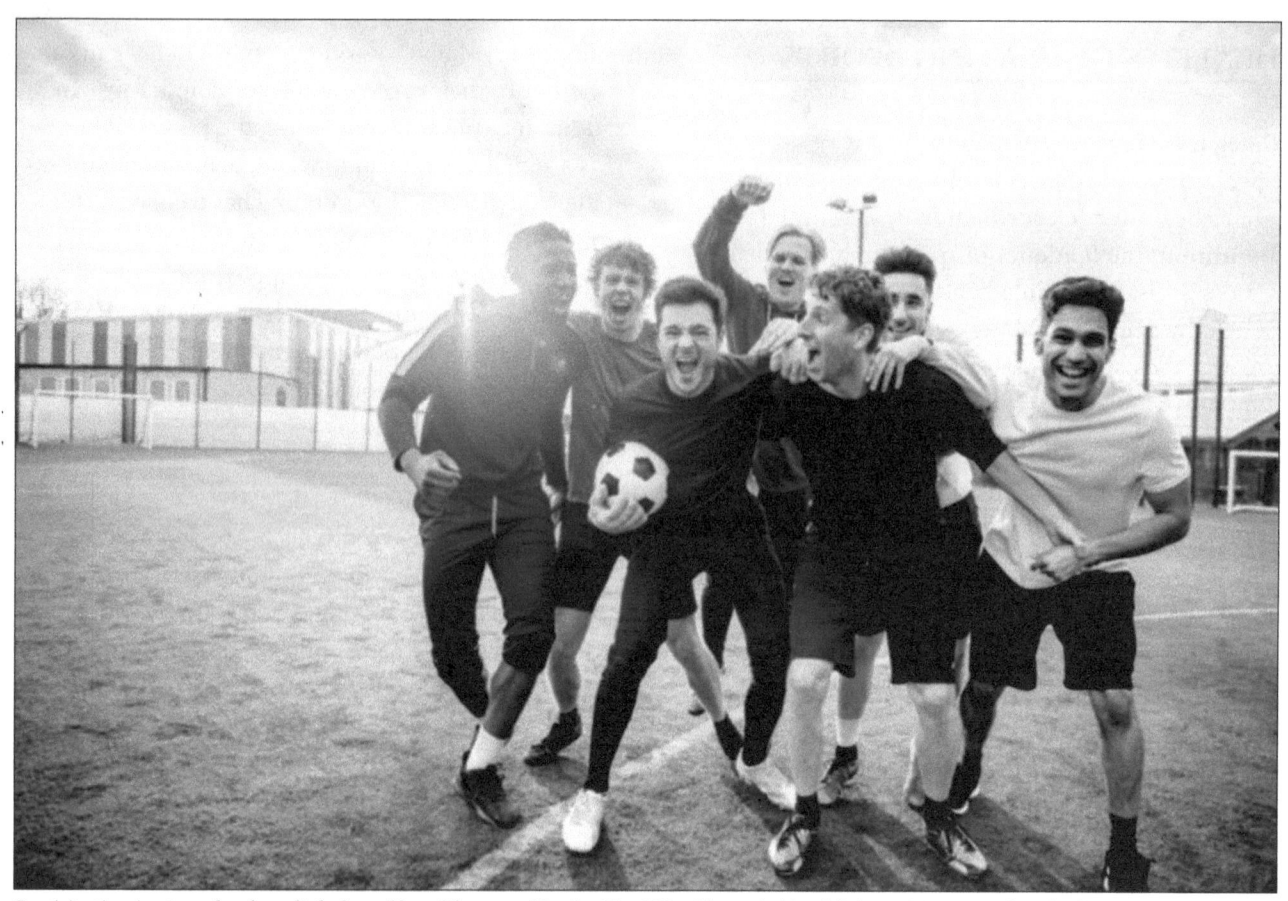

Participating in sports has been linked to self-confidence and leadership skills. Photo via iStock/JohnnyGrieg. [Used under license.]

One common desire in sports and life is to have fun. Most athletes play sports because they have fun playing them. Not all parts of sports training are fun, but athletes learn to work through the hard times because they enjoy the competition. Like later in life, people must work hard at responsibilities they do not enjoy experiencing the successes that the hard work produces. This is often called "delayed gratification."

BEHAVIORAL BENEFITS
Being an effective team member requires many individual skills. Communication is the transfer of information among the team members. Playing sports help members learn, through action, how to effectively disseminate information to team members and listen to interpret the information from others accurately. Developing communication skills will help young athletes in future interactions at work, with family, and in the community.

Discipline, motivation, dedication, and sacrifice are needed when playing sports. Regularly attending organized practices and training sessions helps athletes develop discipline. Having training rules and following them consistently teaches athletes to meet the expectations of others now and in the future. To be disciplined requires motivation or the desire to do well in the sport and make continual improvements. This develops dedication or a commitment to the sport. However, these traits are not developed without sacrifice. Discipline, motivation, and dedication require athletes to give up time that could be spent doing something else fun. However, sacrifice for a sport can develop behavioral skills that will prepare them for future challenges in work, family, and life. It helps to form a positive work ethic.

Playing sports also provides the opportunity to develop leadership skills. Although some athletes will develop better leadership skills than others, those that do will benefit from the sports experience in the future. There are many types of leaders. Not all are formal, obvious leaders. Even learning subtle leadership skills can be beneficial later in life.

A major benefit of playing sports is the development of self-esteem or having a positive impression of oneself. Certainly, sports can negatively affect self-esteem if the athlete is unsuccessful and does not meet individual expectations of performance. Those who have realistic goals and see consistent development in sports skills and performance can benefit from improvements in self-esteem. This will help build confidence to meet other challenges in life.

INTELLECTUAL BENEFITS
All sports have different strategies that must be understood to win. Although playing sports is a very physical activity, successful athletes also must understand how to play the game. Therefore, playing sports can also develop cognitive skills. Athletes must learn to analyze the competitive situation and make good strategic decisions quickly. This requires focus, concentration, and confidence. These are also skills needed to be successful in life. Sports participation can also improve math skills as athletes calculate in their minds how far the team is ahead or behind and then use that information to make appropriate adjustments in strategy.

HEALTH BENEFITS
Since there is physical activity involved in most sports, playing can have health benefits—training or working the body to perform well causes many physiological changes that can benefit health over time. Muscles, heart, lungs, and bones become stronger, which can have lifelong benefits when reinforced with continued regular exercise. Serious athletes tend to eat healthier diets to help improve training and performance. Fewer athletes are overweight compared with nonathletes.

Other health benefits include the ability to handle stress. Although competition can be very stressful for some, athletes have less stress and depression than nonathletes. One reason is regular exercise helps to reduce stress and depression. Athletes also have better mood states. These noted benefits may be in part since athletes sleep better. The recovery provided by sleep is instrumental in managing stress.

By developing healthy habits of exercise, good nutrition, and stress management, athletes get a better start toward a lifetime of healthy living. It is easier to develop healthy habits during the younger years than change bad habits later in life.

CONCLUSION
As people go through life, they develop new skills and improve on others. Getting an early start on developing life skills can be facilitated by playing sports. While many youths play sports, it should be noted that there are many other ways to develop skills for the future. Adult supervised activities such as music, art, theater, and debate, to name a few, can also develop many of the important skills needed for a successful career and life.

—*Bradley R. A. Wilson*

Further Reading
"The Benefit of Youth Sports." *President's Council on Sports, Fitness & Nutrition Science Board*, 17 Sept. 2020, health.gov/sites/default/files/2020-09/YSS_Report_OnePager_2020-08-31_web.pdf. Accessed 28 May 2022.

Coakley, J. *Sports in Society: Issues and Controversies*. 11th ed., McGraw Hill Higher Education, 2014.

Lumpkin, A., et al. *Practical Ethics in Sport Management.* McFarland and Company, 2012.

Price-Mitchell, M. "The Psychology of Youth Sports." *Psychology Today,* 8 Jan. 2012, www.psychologytoday.com/us/blog/the-moment-youth/201201/the-psychology-youth-sports. Accessed 28 May 2022.

Exercise Addiction

Category: Condition
Specialties and related fields: Addiction counseling, psychiatry, psychology. sports psychology
Definition: an unhealthy obsession with physical fitness and exercise

KEY TERMS

disorder: an illness that disrupts normal physical and mental functions

dysmorphia: deformity or abnormality in the shape or size of a specified part of the body

physical fitness: a state of health and well-being through proper nutrition, moderate-vigorous physical exercise, and sufficient rest, along with a formal recovery plan so that someone can perform aspects of sports, occupations, and daily activities

thinspiration addiction: an obsession with a thin physique

INTRODUCTION

Regular exercise is a healthy way for people to stay in shape and decrease the risk for many life-threatening diseases. However, in today's thin-obsessed society, people are becoming addicted to working out more than ever. The Centers for Disease Control and Prevention (CDC) has recommendations for adults between eighteen and sixty-four. Many people in today's society exceed these recommendations, becoming addicted to working out.

While exercise addiction is not explicitly included in the new *Diagnostic and Statistical Manual of Mental Disorders* (*DSM-5*), it can be found under behavior addiction in the addictive disorder section. In the *DSM-5*, a behavior addiction is loosely defined as a person's behavior becoming obsessive, compulsive, or dysfunctional in a person's life. In today's world, the media is obsessed with body image, which puts pressure on both males and females to obtain often unrealistic standards. When people decide they want to lose weight, they often look to popular diets or fad fitness classes to get the results they want in the fastest way possible. Often, these trends are not the safest or healthiest ways to lose weight because people will plateau or get bored; however, some people become consumed with the idea of having the "perfect" figure that these fitness trends promote. While working out consistently may not appear to be a bad thing, when it interferes with a person's daily life because they feel the need to work out for more than two hours every day, it becomes a problem. Another issue with exercise addiction is that people often cut calories while working out, leading to many physical issues. Finally, one of the biggest and arguably scariest parts of exercise addiction is that working out is seen as a healthy lifestyle choice, and many people do not realize it is a problem.

SOCIETAL EXPECTATIONS AND WEIGHT LOSS

In the past decade, weight loss shows have taken television by storm. Whether it is *The Biggest Loser* or *Extreme Weight Loss*, many shows encourage people to lose weight and demonstrate safe and effective ways to achieve weight loss goals. Along with television shows, the media is generally obsessed with body image. From the covers of celebrity gossip magazines showing perfect "bikini bodies" to news shows discussing whether or not women should lose baby weight immediately, we are constantly saturated with the idea of being thin. While the internet is a great source of inspiration for losing weight and researching effective diet and fitness plans, it can also cause people to form unrealistic body goals. "Thinspo" or "thinspiration" was created to inspire other women to lose weight and become thin. Often, these pictures show women who have body mass indexes lower than what is in the normal range. By promoting images of unhealthy women, thinspiration further perpetuates the unobtainable ideal of being skinny rather than healthy, which can lead to exercise addiction.

EXERCISE ADDICTION

Typical exercise guidelines. According to the CDC, the average eighteen- to sixty-four-year-old should use the following guidelines for living a healthy, active lifestyle: two hours and thirty minutes of moderate-intensity aerobic activity every week and two or more days of muscle-strengthening activities. Or, adults can do one hour and fifteen minutes of vigorous-intensity aerobic activity every week and muscle-strengthening activities on two or more days. Or, adults in that age range can do an equivalent mix of moderate and vigorous-intensity aerobic activity and muscle-strengthening activities on two or more days a week.

Exercise addiction. While this seems like a lot to do during a given work week, people who have an addiction to exercise often work out to a much greater extent than CDC guidelines and allow working out to dictate their lives. Their exercise typically interferes with social, work, and family activities. Because exercise is seen as positive and can work out

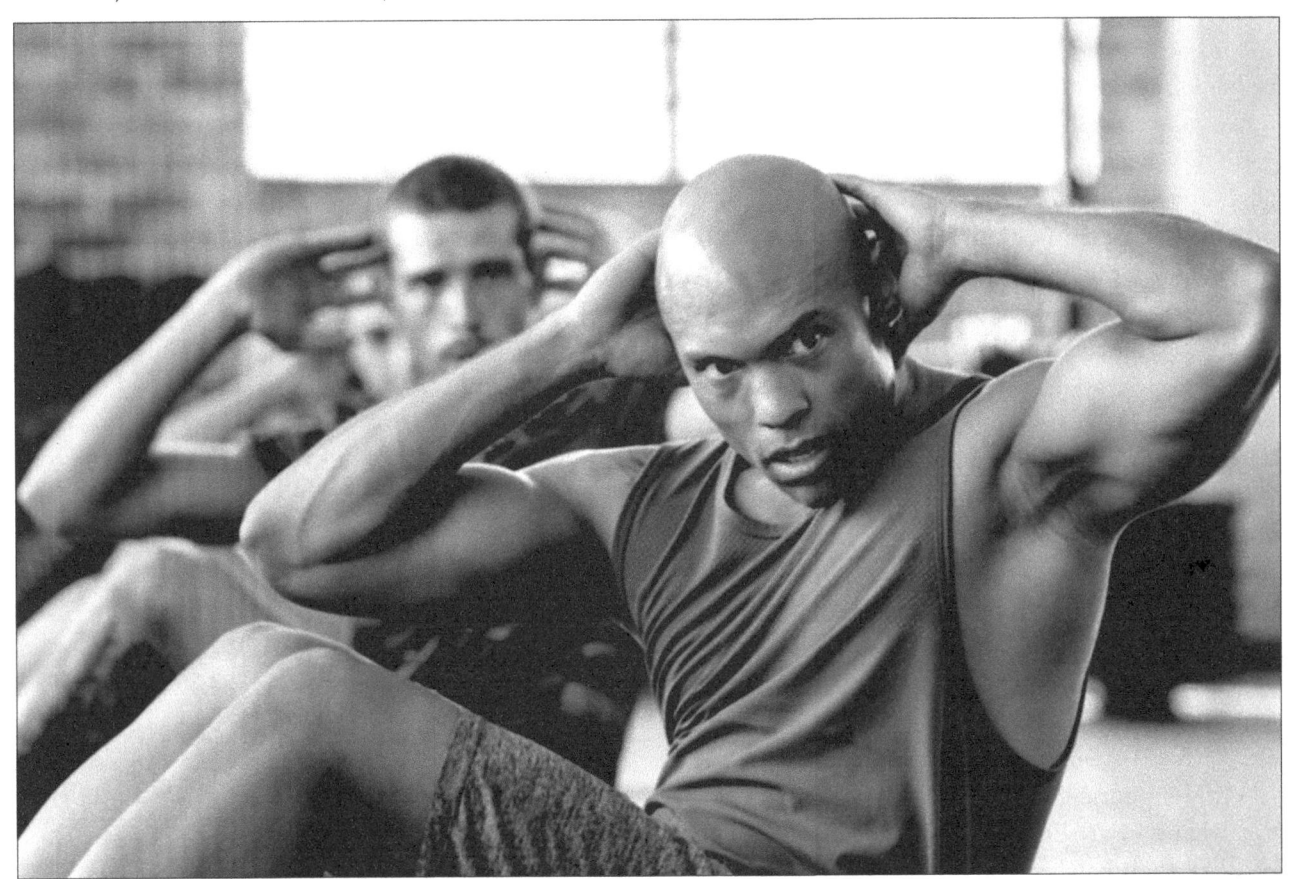

Although there is no specific amount of time that demarcates addiction, other areas of an individual's life being affected could indicate an unhealthy obsession with exercise. Photo via iStock/Ridofranz. [Used under license.]

more than the CDC suggests without becoming addicted, it is often difficult to diagnose exercise addiction. While it is difficult to diagnose, a few signs signal when exercising moves from a healthy habit to the realm of addiction.

Signs of exercise addiction. One of the first signs is that the amount of exercise is harmful to an individual. For example, suppose a person is working out four hours a day and is not consuming enough calories to provide enough fuel for their body. In that case, the caloric deficit can lead to stress fractures or another injury. Another sign of exercise addiction is that the person seems in a bad mood if they do not work out. Suppose a person relies on the euphoric feeling after a workout to be happy. In that case, the chances are high that they have an exercise addiction. One of the biggest red flags for people should be if a person is exercising through an injury or medical condition. While people may do some forms of exercise while injured, others raise concerns. For example, if a person has had major surgery and is out the next day trying to go for a run or lift weights, it would be safe to suggest talking to them about a potential addiction to exercise.

CAUSES OF EXERCISE ADDICTION

While exercise addiction can occur due to several factors, one of the most held beliefs is that people become addicted to the euphoric feeling after a workout. When a person pushes him or herself hard at the gym, endorphins are released, causing a euphoric feeling. Like drug addiction, people want to continue to feel this good which leads to them working out more to experience euphoria. Again, mirroring drug addiction, people who work out and are in good shape will have to work out harder and increase the frequency and length of their workouts to feel this euphoric feeling. Because people believe that what they are doing is healthy, many do not consider their behavior as being an addiction. Rather they perceive it as something healthy.

Another important component of exercise addiction is body dysmorphia. People suffering from exercise addiction often struggle with seeing a distorted vision of their bodies when they look in the mirror. People who suffer from body dysmorphic disorder usually see themselves as being fat or larger than they are, which leads to excessive exercise. It is important to note that people who suffer from both body dysmorphic disorder and exercise addiction often become angry, hostile, or defensive when someone suggests they have a problem.

SOURCES OF SUPPORT

Because exercise addiction is identified as similar to any other kind of substance abuse disorder, the treatment is also similar. In treatment, issues surrounding body image are discussed and explored, helping the client find ways to deal with their insecurities healthily. Group therapy, individual counseling, and, in severe cases, inpatient facilities are used to help treat the addiction. Along with professional help, it is important that the person suffering from an exercise addiction feels supported by their friends, family, and other loved ones.

—*Lauren Ruvo*

Further Reading

"How Much Physical Activity Do Adults Need?" *Centers for Disease Control and Prevention*, 2 Jun. 2022, www.cdc.gov/physicalactivity/basics/adults/index.htm. Accessed 6 Jun. 2022.

Landolfi, E. "Exercise Addiction." *Sports Medicine*, vol. 43, 2012, pp. 111-19.

Wichmann, S., and D. R. Martin. "Exercise Excess: Treating Patients Addicted to Fitness." *Physiological Sports Medicine*, vol. 20, 1992, pp. 193-200.

Exercise and Mental Health

Category: Exercise benefits

Definition: exercise can significantly improve mood, alertness, and overall feelings of well-being while simultaneously decreasing fatigue, tension, stress, and depressed mood

KEY TERMS
anorexia nervosa: an eating disorder characterized by abnormally low body weight, an intense fear of gaining weight, and a distorted perception of weight

bulimia nervosa: an emotional disorder involving distortion of body image and an obsessive desire to lose weight, in which bouts of extreme overeating are followed by depression and self-induced vomiting, purging, or fasting

mental health: a person's condition concerning their psychological and emotional well-being

INTRODUCTION
Physical exercise affects mental health by releasing endorphins, or hormones that place the body in a pleasurable state. Exercise may be naturally reinforcing because endorphins may serve as a positive reinforcer.

Often, doctors and specialists recommend an exercise regimen as part of a treatment program for conditions related to anxiety, depression, and stress reduction. Additionally, regular exercise can also positively impact conditions exacerbated by stress by helping to reduce stress. Headaches, pain disorders, fibromyalgia, chronic fatigue, and conditions such as diabetes may benefit from stress-reduction in this regard. Stress reduction may also result from the social bonding associated with exercise, including pairs or team sports, or simply walking or running with a friend. Additionally, the combined direct effects on body fat, blood pressure, weight, and flexibility, among other physical aspects of health, make exercise beneficial for these conditions.

Mental health and exercise are also primary topics of sports psychology, which focuses on how men-

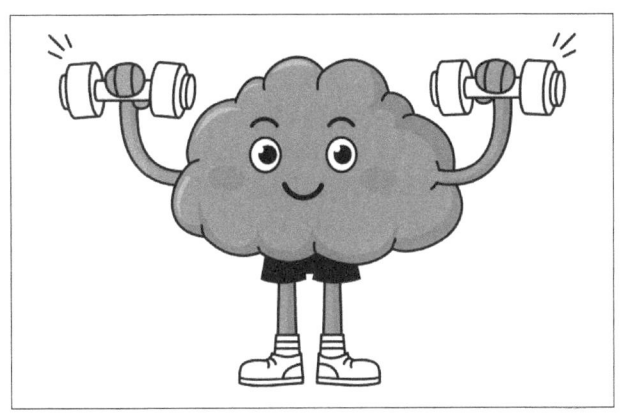

Regular exercise has been shown to reduce anxiety and depression and to improve cognitive function. Image via iStock/zoljo. [Used under license.]

tal state can affect athletic performance. Practitioners of sports psychology use numerous techniques to facilitate improved performance and persistence. Using visual imagery to see oneself successfully performing is one example of a sports psychology technique. Another method involves using positive self-statements to facilitate expectations of successful performance. Often, athletes and fitness enthusiasts may experience reductions in performance that may be accompanied by thoughts or beliefs that can cause or exacerbate poor performance. Therefore, approaches encouraging positive self-statements and ways of reshaping beliefs to support performance improvement can be extraordinarily beneficial.

DISORDERS RELATED TO EXERCISE
Although exercise has many physical and mental health benefits, it can also be associated with varying mental health problems. Some individuals may have extreme concerns about their weight, as found in anorexia nervosa, and may engage in excessive exercise. Suppose fears of obesity drive a person. In that case, exercise may function as a compulsion and behavior to reduce fear and anxiety. Unfortunately, reducing these uncomfortable feelings about excessive weight can be negatively reinforcing, meaning that the reduction in anxiety serves as a benefit to en-

courage more and more exercise. Unlike positive reinforcement or stimuli that increase behaviors, negative reinforcement works via the removal of stimuli, in this case, reducing the fear and reinforcing the exercise. These compulsive patterns may develop into rituals. When the ritual is pathological, its interruption can further prompt anxiety, which then may help to build further the compulsion to follow through with the exercise rituals.

Exercise is seen as a means of regaining control. Similarly, individuals with bulimia nervosa may engage in exercise as a compensatory behavior for other problematic behaviors, such as binge eating. Binge eating can trigger fears of losing control and excessive weight; people may use exercise to compensate for overeating.

Individuals with body dysmorphic disorder, a condition where a person has serious concerns about a physical flaw or how a body part appears, may also engage in excessive exercise. The desire to affect the body, such as to gain control over its appearance, may also be related to compulsive exercise.

Despite the harmful effects of excessive exercise, especially for those with low body-fat levels and a dysregulated hormone system, the individual will remarkably feel driven to exercise. These are conditions where the benefits of exercise do not objectively outweigh the risks; however, the individual cannot see this. In reality, individuals must recognize the value of moderation, even in exercise. Conversely, a healthy exercise that supports mental health is beneficial behavior that outweighs the negative effects of exercise.

—*Nancy A. Piotrowski*

Further Reading

Bassuk, Shari S., Timothy S. Church, and JoAnn E. Manson. "Why Exercise Works Magic." *Scientific American*, vol. 309, no. 2, 2013, pp. 74-79.

Bourne, Edmund J., and Lorna Garano. *Coping with Anxiety: Ten Simple Ways to Relieve Anxiety, Fear, and Worry*. New Harbinger, 2003.

Cox, Richard. *Sports Psychology: Concepts and Applications*. McGraw, 2006.

Friedman, Peachy. *Diary of an Exercise Addict*. Pequot, 2008.

Gregg, Jennifer A., Glenn M. Callaghan, and Steven C. Hayes. *Diabetes Lifestyle Book: Facing Your Fears and Making Changes for a Long and Healthy Life*. New Harbinger, 2008.

Malcolm, Estelle, et al. "The Impact of Exercise Projects to Promote Mental Wellbeing." *Journal of Mental Health*, vol. 22, no. 6, 2013, pp. 519-27.

Powers, Pauline S., and Ron Thompson. *The Exercise Balance: What's Too Much, What's Too Little, What's Just Right for You!* Gurze, 2008.

Szabo, Attila. "Acute Psychological Benefits of Exercise: Reconsideration of the Placebo Effect." *Journal of Mental Health*, vol. 22, no. 5, 2013, pp. 449-55.

Health Risks to Student Athletes

Category: Injuries
Specialties and related fields: Emergency medicine, neurology, physical medicine and rehabilitation, physical therapy, psychiatry, sports medicine, sports psychology
Definition: although sports increase strength, agility, confidence, motor skills, and team cooperation, sports participation comes with injury risks; risk management is an integral part of any athletic career and a vital task for parents of athletic children

KEY TERMS

athletic injury: injuries that occur when engaging in sports or exercise
concussion: temporary unconsciousness or confusion caused by a blow on the head
injury risk: a state in which a person has the potential for being physically harmed due to participation in certain athletic competitions or practices
risk management: the forecasting and evaluation of injury risks and the identification of procedures to avoid or minimize injury probability or impact

INTRODUCTION

While participating in athletics is a great way to build strength and speed, athletes also risk their health by participating in competitive sports. Concussions, back and knee injuries, and other medical problems are common in athletes of all ages. Many communities are now debating whether certain sports are appropriate for younger athletes. Controversially, colleges and universities often offer little assistance to injured players, which is one of the issues often cited by critics and reformers in the field.

HOW COMMON ARE SPORTS INJURIES?

According to a 2015 study published in the *Morbidity and Mortality Weekly Report* from the Centers for Disease Control and Prevention (CDC), there were 1,053,370 injuries among National Collegiate Athletic Association (NCAA) athletes for the 2013-14 season, out of 176.7 million exposures (meaning situations in which an athlete could potentially have been injured). The potential for injury varies widely among different sports. College football players, for instance, were most likely to get injured playing the game. Still, wrestling had the highest injury rate overall.

Other studies have found similar results, with as many as 20 percent of NCAA athletes experiencing injuries requiring a week or more to recover. In college football, more than 20,000 injuries are recorded each year, including 4,000 knee injuries and 1,000 spinal injuries. While injury rates for other sports are not well-known, injuries are also common in wrestling, baseball, hockey, and basketball. Overuse injuries were the most common type of injury recorded for college athletes. Most of these were recoverable and not considered severe. But even seemingly minor injuries can have serious consequences.

Activity intensity is the key factor in injury statistics. Division I athletes may need to dedicate thirty to forty hours per week to exercise. They may spend more than four hours per day engaged in practice, exercise, or other activities with the potential to cause injury. Added to this are the demands of academic commitment and the nature of college life. College athletes are less likely to dedicate sufficient time to sleep and recovery and often lack adequate nutrition. This combination puts college athletes at extremely high risk for certain injuries, especially those from overuse and muscular injuries.

CONCUSSIONS AND MOBILITY

By far, the most concerning and oft-debated kind of sports injury is concussion, a type of traumatic brain injury (TBI) that occurs when an individual receives a blow to the head or body that causes the brain to shift or twist within the skull rapidly. When this occurs, areas of the brain may be damaged, and chemical changes in the brain can also cause problems. People with concussions can experience various symptoms, including headaches, difficulty thinking or recalling information, loss of motor control, loss of consciousness, or mood and behavior changes. They may become nauseous, experience problems with balance or vision, or have difficulty adjusting to light or noise. Symptoms can immediately follow an injury or manifest several days later.

While a minor concussion may present little or no danger to an athlete, severe concussions can leave an injured person with lifelong symptoms. Individuals with severe concussions can have long-term problems with cognition and memory, learning, or managing emotions. Physically speaking, concussion sufferers may have long-lasting problems with speech, hearing, or vision. They may have difficulty with coordination and balance.

According to the CDC, 1.6 to 3.8 million sports-related concussions occur annually in the United States. CDC data also indicates that 10 percent of contact sports athletes experience a concussion yearly. Concussions are most common in boxing (where at least 87 percent of professionals have sustained lasting brain injuries) and in football, where data suggests at least one concussion for every five football games played. At least 10 percent of college football players and 20 percent of high school players will suffer a brain injury at some point while playing the game.

Concussions are among the most concerning sports injuries because many concussions are never diagnosed. Further, damage to the brain is cumulative. Studies indicate that a person who experiences one concussion is up to six times more likely to suffer another concussion. Each time an athlete's brain is injured, there is an increased chance of suffering long-lasting or severe injury; athletes who suffer multiple concussions are at high risk for developing problems later in life, such as chronic traumatic encephalopathy (CTE), a neurogenerative disorder. Repeated studies have shown that boxers and football players are at extremely high risk of developing CTE, which may not appear until much later. A 2017 study published in the *Journal of the American Medical Association* found evidence of CTE in 110 of 111 former NFL players and 48 of 53 former college football players.

The public debate over the risk of concussions and complications like CTE tends to focus on professional football players and high school players out of a concern for child welfare. Still, studies indicate that college players are also at extremely high risk. Greg Ploetz, who played football in college but did not enter a professional league, developed CTE in his sixties, which led to severe emotional and cognitive decline, a loss in motor control, and an inability to speak; Ploetz required twenty-four-hour nursing care. While Ploetz's CTE is among the worst diagnosed outside of professional sports, his experience raises serious questions about the welfare of college athletes over the longer term.

Concussion is only one of the many injuries frequently suffered by athletes. But the concussion controversy touches on the broader issue of student athletics and injury. Student athletes, to remain competitive, must dedicate significant time and effort to perfecting their sport, increasing their exposure to risk and injuries that can be, in extreme cases, fatal or life-changing. Critics argue that American culture must seriously discuss the value of student athletics in light of the risk to student athletes.

RISKS AND REWARDS
Research indicating that sports injuries are more common and have long-lasting effects has fueled public debates over health and welfare in professional and amateur athletics. Like professional athletes, college athletes are at elevated risk for injuries. Yet, unlike professional athletes, college athletes are not paid for playing and are not guaranteed medical coverage. While the NCAA requires that student athletes have medical coverage options available to them, the organization does not require colleges or universities to subsidize this coverage or to cover the costs of injuries and recovery. Further, many college athletes receive partial or full scholarships for playing on a sports team, but if they are injured and temporarily or permanently unable to continue performing, colleges and universities are not required to maintain scholarship assistance. An injured college athlete may face personal financial hardship, a loss of educational opportunities, and potentially lasting physical difficulties.

Some critics argue that because NCAA athletes bring in millions in revenue for colleges and universities and indirect revenue for cities and states, colleges and universities should provide medical coverage for those who experience injuries while playing for collegiate sports franchises. While the NCAA offers some programs to help cover the expenses of injuries, such as a Student-Athlete Disability Insurance program, programs like these are helpful only in a small minority of cases because they only cover athletes whose injuries are severe enough that they will never be able to play again. Further, this is an option that student athletes must purchase with their own money. An evaluation of disability insurance by Kevin Fixler published in *The Atlantic* found that the NCAA had only paid out about twelve claims under their disability insurance program in twenty years. In Fixler's assessment, disability insurance is hardly worth the cost for most athletes.

While serious injury is always a concern, many athletes each year suffer one of the more common types of injuries, like strains, fractures, pulled tendons, and overuse injuries. While these kinds of injuries might not be life-threatening, they can have a lasting effect on an individual's mobility and physical capabilities and still present student athletes with considerable cost. Repairing injured knees, for instance, costs an average of $11,000, though the cost can be substantially higher. Knee injuries are one of the most common injuries for football players, and the side effects of such an injury can be significant. Players with leg, back, or arm injuries may require years of expensive medical assistance or surgeries, and many suffer long-term impairment. None of these injuries is automatically covered for NCAA athletes, meaning that student athletes, especially those without significant resources, risk their health and welfare, and financial well-being each time they sign on to play.

As the United States, and the global community, faced the COVID-19 crisis, new questions arose about athletics. While college sports injuries have been a risk for young athletes for many years, 2020 and 2021 brought a new set of COVID-19-related risks. Playing professional sports typically means close contact, dramatically increasing the risk of transmitting an airborne illness. Athletes who continued to play also faced an increased risk of contracting the disease and then potentially spreading it to family and loved ones. As with the broader question about injury, the risk of COVID-19 raised questions about the degree to which educational institutions should be responsible for the health and welfare of players. An investigation at Clemson University found that insurance plans offered by the university for athletes would not cover COVID-related illness because the plans only covered injuries resulting directly from competitions or practice. Because athletes might contract COVID-19 outside of their participation in sports, Clemson's student-athlete insurance would not provide coverage.

Student athletes assume a substantial risk when facing COVID-19, concussion, or other injuries. In some cases, they assume this risk independently with little or no support from universities or the NCAA. Given the considerable revenues and global interest in college sports, and the rewards enjoyed by those who play at this level, there is more than enough incentive to maintain the industry. But can the industry be reformed to protect the athletes who risk their health and welfare to keep the college sports going?

—*Micah L. Issitt*

Further Reading

Billitz, Jess. "19 College Athlete Injury Statistics (The Risk of Sports)." *Noobgains*, 12 Nov. 2020, noobgains.com/college-athlete-injury-statistics/. Accessed 18 May 2021.

Fixler, Kevin. "The $5 Million Question: Should College Athletes Buy Disability Insurance?" *The Atlantic*, 11 Apr. 2013, www.theatlantic.com/entertainment/archive/2013/04/the-5-million-question-should-college-athletes-buy-disability-insurance/274915/. Accessed 20 May 2021.

"Heads Up." *CDC*, 12 Feb. 2019, www.cdc.gov/headsup/basics/concussion_symptoms.html. Accessed 18 May 2021.

Hruby, Patrick. "The NCAA Is Running Out of Excuses on Brain Injuries." *Deadspin*, 24 May 2018, deadspin.com/the-ncaa-is-running-out-of-excuses-on-brain-injuries-1819854361.

Kerr, Zachary Y., et al. "College Sports-Related Injuries United States, 2009-10 through 2013-14 Academic Years." *Morbidity and Mortality Weekly Report (MMWR)*, vol. 64, no. 48, 2015, pp. 1330-36, www.cdc.gov/mmwr/preview/mmwrhtml/mm6448a2.htm. Accessed 16 May 2021.

"Madness, Inc.: How College Sports Can Leave Athletes Broken and Abandoned." *Chris Murphy, US Senator for Connecticut*, 2019, www.murphy.senate.gov/imo/media/doc/Madness%203...pdf. Accessed 17 May 2021.

Mez, Jesse, et al. "Clinicopathological Evaluation of Chronic Traumatic Encephalopathy in Players of American Football." *JAMA*, vol. 318, no. 4, 2017, pp. 360-70, https://jamanetwork.com/journals/jama/fullarticle/2645104. Accessed 20 May 2021.

Spector, Jesse. "Will Colleges Cover Medical Bills for Athletes Who Get COVID-19? Don't Count on It." *Deadspin*, 2 July 2020, deadspin.com/will-colleges-cover-medical-bills-for-athletes-who-get-1844251705. Accessed 20 May 2021.

Walsh, Meghan. "'I Trusted 'Em': When NCAA Schools Abandon Their Injured Athletes." *The Atlantic*, 1 May 2013, www.theatlantic.com/entertainment/archive/2013/05/i-trusted-em-when-ncaa-schools-abandon-their-injured-athletes/275407/. Accessed 20 May 2021.

"What Is a Concussion?" *Brain Injury Research Institute*, 2021, www.protectthebrain.org/Brain-Injury-Research/What-is-a-Concussion-.aspx. Accessed 19 May 2021.

Intramural Sports

Category: Sports participation
Specialties and related fields: Physical education, physical fitness, sports administration, sports management
Definition: recreational sports organized within a particular institution, usually an educational institution, or a set geographic area

KEY TERMS

character development: the possession of those personal qualities or virtues that facilitate the consistent display of moral action or choosing the moral ideal over competing values

fair play: conformity to established rules, upright conduct, and equitable conditions in and around the playing field

intramural sports/activities: recreational sports or activities that primary and secondary schools provide and are held before or after the school day and, in some schools, during recess

leadership skills: set of skills that contribute to the ability to motivate, communicate with, and lead others effectively

mission statement: brief description of an organization's purpose

physical activity: physical exercise forces the body to undergo physiological adaptations related to an increase in cardiovascular and musculoskeletal health

physical fitness: the ability to perform physical activity

positive competition: competition that focuses on respecting the opponent and putting forth effort

self-esteem: the overall appraisal one has for oneself and includes self-confidence, self-respect, and self-worth

OVERVIEW TRADITIONAL BENEFITS OF INTRAMURAL SPORTS AND ACTIVITIES

Intramural sports and activities in primary and secondary schools offer students opportunities to participate in recreational sports and activities involving physical activity before or after the traditional school day and, in some schools, during recess. Scholastic intramural programs may include an array of traditional sports (e.g., basketball, volleyball, floor hockey) or may include creative modifications of traditional sports (e.g., basketball played with a rubber chicken or different type of ball) or new nontraditional sport-related activities (e.g., Harry Potter's Quidditch) all with the focus on students having fun. Intramural programs focus on intrascholastic contests with teams playing against other teams from within the school. Depending on the focus of the intramural program, these before and after school programs can complement a school's physical education program by making it a more broad-based and comprehensive program. The intramural programs extend the physical education curriculum to the intramural program, where students are afforded additional time to practice the skills learned in class, perform self-testing, and have opportunities to learn new and unique activities. Typically, intramural programs are managed and administered by one or more teachers (e.g., physical education teachers or classroom teachers) and, in some cases, in collaboration with a group of students. Financial backing for intramural programs may come in the form of school administration classifying intramural management as an extra duty for staff members and paying these teachers accordingly. Yet, these programs may also receive additional funding from the school district (e.g., equipment, officials, facility usage) or through fundraising and support from school groups such as the Parent-Teacher Association.

PHYSICAL BENEFITS OF INTRAMURAL SPORTS AND ACTIVITY PROGRAM

Intramural sport and activity programs offer the overall student population an opportunity to engage in physical activity and sports programming that is less competitive than regular team interscholastic athletic programs. The recreational focus of intramural programs provides many benefits to the student participants, including intellectual/academic, physical, social, and psychological benefits. Research has indicated that the academically related benefits of participation in physical activity include helping students improve their concentration, academic performance, and readiness for class. The physical benefits of intramural sports/activity participation include improved physical fitness and additional, structured opportunities for students to choose as a means to engage in physical activity. Intramural programs seek to provide opportunities for all students and not just the athletically gifted students, therefore providing all students the choice to participate in physical activity at a level of competition that is comfortable and appropriate for that student.

PSYCHOLOGICAL BENEFITS OF PARTICIPATION

The psychosocial benefits of intramural participation are numerous. Intramural activities offer students opportunities to socialize outside the structured classroom setting and develop and learn new social skills. Also, the social interaction during intramural programs helps students develop social harmony and social integration. The program may include students from various backgrounds, social groups, and with varying levels of athletic ability who are grouped to work toward a common goal. Participation in intramural programs may also foster character development in the students if the program focuses on effort, respect, and fair play. Intramural programs also provide school staff an occasion to allow students to take on leadership roles in helping administer, create, and develop the intramural programs. Through creating and developing leadership opportunities for the students, intramural programs can enhance students' leadership skills under the guidance and support of school staff.

The psychological benefits of intramural sport and activity participation are also abundant. Research has indicated that participation in physical activity that is considered fun by the participant can decrease anxiety and depression and improve their overall well-being. Research has also suggested that participants in physical activities experience a sense of joy or personal enjoyment, personal growth, and enhanced self-esteem due to being physically active. Effective intramural programs focus on providing fun activities for students, therefore suggesting that the student participants experience joy, less anxiety, depression, and an improved sense of well-being and self-esteem. Effective intramural programs can help students attain these psychosocial benefits if the program is well designed with a focus on fun, equal opportunity, and personal effort and improvement.

DEVELOPMENT OF PROGRAM MISSION & PHILOSOPHY

Based on research in physical activity and sport management, scholars have provided suggestions and guidelines to direct practitioners in developing effective scholastic intramural sports and activities programs. In developing an intramural program for a primary or secondary school setting, it is critical to determine where the program is headed in terms of its goals and orientation. Program administrators must determine the overall outcome goals of the program by asking themselves several questions, including:

- Why begin an intramural program?
- Who is the program targeting?
- What are the outcome goals of the program?
- How does the program need to be organized to achieve the identified goals?

Answering each of these questions helps the administration develop the program's philosophy and the mission statement that guides practice. Different goals and program foci may determine how the program is created regarding the types of activities, who may participate, how often the program will run, and so forth.

In developing a philosophy for an intramural program that seeks to reap all the student-focused benefits that have been described above, several suggestions have been made. Scholars suggest that the program should be student-centered and offer a wide variety of activities that focus on fun, promote physical activity, and promote character development. Each of these qualities can be achieved by considering and implementing several factors that affect programming.

WAYS OF ENCOURAGEMENT

Fun can be encouraged in several ways, including:

- It provides a variety of activities. By providing a wide variety of activities, the intramural program is more likely to appeal to a wider variety of students, particularly those who do not already participate in organized athletics within or outside the school.
- It provides all students with equal opportunities to participate. By including programming that includes activities with modified game rules (e.g., change in the type of ball used, substituting the ball with a silly object), the students are placed on a more equal "playing field" as variations in skill competency are not as readily apparent in these types of game situations. These modified activities are the foundation of intramural programs that meet the needs of the entire school population, not just the athletically gifted students.
- It provides activities that are developmentally appropriate for the target student population.
- It provides guidelines for team selection that do not ostracize students but focus on fairness and equal opportunity.
- They are providing a welcoming environment for all students. Programs can facilitate positive experiences to increase student self-esteem and self-confidence.
- It focuses on effort and positive competition rather than enforced competition.

Engagement in physical activity can be encouraged in intramural programs by providing various fun activities that appeal to a wide array of students, including those who are athletically gifted and those who are not. By providing programming that meets the needs of many students, more students will become engaged in physical activity, enhance their physical fitness, and continue participating in physical activity.

NUMEROUS WAYS OF CHARACTER DEVELOPMENT

Character development may also be promoted in a variety of ways. These include the following:

- Providing students with leadership opportunities. Students may be involved in leading the intramural program through the establishment of an "intramural council." The intramural council provides students with opportunities to serve and take on leadership roles while developing leadership skills through playing a part in the creation and development of the intramural program.
- It provides a framework for the intramural program to promote fair play.
- It emphasizes respect in all aspects of the program. The mission and philosophy of the intramural program should emphasize respect for the rules of the game, the officials and their decisions, and respect for the opponents.

Effective intramural programs are guided by an approach that emphasizes fun for all participants, physical activity engagement, and character development promotion. Program mission, philosophy, and structure set the stage for the program's outcomes, indicating that strict attention must be paid to the program foundation to meet the program goals. How the program is administered also plays a part in the overall success of the intramural program.

ADMINISTRATION OF THE INTRAMURAL PROGRAM

The administration of the intramural program supports and enforces the program's mission, philosophy, and goals. The school staff that oversees the program's administration provides the overall leadership and guides the direction in which the program will be managed. Scholars have recommended several guidelines for program administrators, including the development of an intramural handbook, the assessment of available facilities, safety precautions, and opportunities for student leadership.

An intramural handbook outlines the procedures related to the administration of the intramural program. The handbook reduces the chances that misinformation and miscommunication will occur among the program stakeholders (i.e., supervisors, teachers, students, administration, and parents. The handbook should outline all aspects of the policies and procedures related to the intramural program and include a description of each of the following:

A list of possible sports and activities that should be offered in the intramural program:

- The expectations for all student participants.
- Description of procedures for the overall program (including clothing requirements, guidelines for afternoon rides, changing clothes, and signing into the program).
- Guidelines for student behavior.
- Guidelines for the organization of teams.
- How student attendance and participation will be counted.
- Guidelines for the training of officials.
- Listing of all safety rules and procedures.
- Outline of program administration organization (e.g., professional staffing).
- Description of student leadership opportunities.
- How intramural activities will be scheduled.

FACTORS RESPONSIBLE TO ENSURE SUCCESSFUL PROGRAM

A few other factors must be considered to ensure a successful program. First, school or district administrators should set some form of recognition for all teachers and staff involved. Recognition of these individuals displays school support for teachers and staff involved in this extracurricular activity. It encourages their continued involvement in the program. As mentioned previously, it has been suggested that the school administration consider working with the intramural program as an extra duty and appropriately compensate the teachers and staff members.

Second, the administrators of the intramural program should assess the school's facilities and determine how to use these facilities for the intramural program most effectively. Suppose the school is challenged with a small gymnasium or competes for time to use the facility with other programs. In that case, intramural leaders should consider creative alternatives and community facilities that may be appropriate to host certain intramural activities. While competing for space or having limited space may initially present a roadblock in program development, teachers and staff who think creatively can still run a successful program that may even provide a more diverse variety of activities for the students to enjoy.

Lastly, program administrators should strongly consider incorporating student leadership opportunities into the administrative structure of the intramural program: teachers and staff guide student leaders in intramural programs. One way to integrate students into the decision-making and leadership of the program is to create an intramural council. Positions on this council may be elected, volunteers, or nominated, with these individuals guiding the program's direction with the guidance of the professional staff members. Once a program is created and the mission, philosophy, and administration are intact, the intramural program must be promoted to recruit participants.

PROGRAM PROMOTION

The promotion of the intramural program is critical to generating student interest. Byl suggested that program promotion be creative and implemented using simple methods such as fun posters and public address announcements. Program promotion is an opportunity for more teachers and staff to get involved by utilizing staff strengths in creating promotional materials (e.g., art teachers may create posters, and computer teachers may create material for posting on the school or district website). Program promotion also provides another outlet for professional staff to promote the program's mission. By incorporating the program mission into promotional materials, the purpose and foci of the program are clearly communicated to all students, faculty, and staff members. Once the program begins, it will become important for the program administrators to conduct an assessment of the program.

PROGRAM ASSESSMENT

Conducting a program assessment will provide the professional staff information on how successful the program is in terms of the number of participants, which activities are popular and which are not, and the general student response or interest in the program. The program administrators should track monthly participation in all intramural activities. Tracking monthly participation provides a picture of who is participating, what programs are popular, and what is the actual workload for the professional staff members who are involved. This type of assessment provides feedback to the staff and intramural council for consideration in the continued development of the intramural program. Also, assessing the workload for the professional staff may lend support for making the position an "extra duty" if it is not already considered one or serves as a work record for compensation.

Program assessment is an important factor in the continued development and improvement of the intramural sports and activities program. Another means of assessment is creating and administering a survey that evaluates the student's interest and enjoyment of the intramural program. This assessment provides further information about the specific activities that students enjoy and what other activities they would like to participate in that are not offered. It may also provide evidence to school or district administrators about the program's success that may be considered for future funding.

CONCLUSION

Intramural sports and activity programs allow students to engage in fun-focused physical activity in a welcoming, smaller-scale environment compared to interscholastic athletics. Successful and effective programs must be developed considering several developmental and psychosocial factors that directly impact the intramural program's mission, philosophy, and administration. Effective and successful programs emphasize fun and enjoyment, character development, and equal opportunities for all students to participate regardless of athletic ability.

—*Shelby L. Hinkle Smith*

Further Reading

Byl, J. "Organizing Effective Elementary and High School Intramural Programs." *Physical and Health Education*, vol. 70, 2004, pp. 22-24.

Casperson, C. J., et al. "Physical Activity, Exercise, and Physical Fitness: Definitions and Distinctions for Health-Related Research." *Public Health Reports*, vol. 100, 1985, pp. 126-31.

Forrester, S., and B. Beggs. "Gender and Self-Esteem in Intramural Sports." *Physical and Health Education Journal*, vol. 70, no. 4, Winter 2004/2005, pp. 12-19.

Fuller, D., et al. "School Sports Opportunities Influence Physical Activity in Secondary School and Beyond." *Journal of School Health*, vol. 81, 2011, pp. 449-54.

Holt, N. L., et al. "Physical Education and Sport Programs at an Inner-City School: Exploring Possibilities for Positive Youth Development." *Physical Education & Sport Pedagogy*, vol. 17, 2012, pp. 97-113.

Shields, D. L., and B. J. Bredemeier. *Character Development and Physical Activity*. Human Kinetics, 1995.

Tenoschok, M. "The Intramural Handbook." *Teaching Elementary Physical Education*, vol. 14, 2003, p. 32.

Tenoschok, M., et al. "How Good Is Your Intramural Program?" *Teaching Elementary Physical Education*, vol. 13, 2002, pp. 30-31.

Todorovich, John, editor. "Influence of Sports and Physical Activity Programs on the Activity of High School Youths and Young Adults." *JOPERD: The Journal of Physical Education, Recreation & Dance*, vol. 83, no. 4, 2012, p. 49.

Overtraining Syndrome

Category: Disease/Disorder
Specialties and related fields: Exercise physiology, psychology, sports medicine
Definition: perceptible and lasting decrease in athletic performance, often coupled with mood changes, which do not quickly resolve following a normal period of rest

KEY TERMS

muscle soreness: muscle pain commencing after a workout
overexertion: any case in which a person works or exerts themselves beyond their physical capabilities
recovery: the period between the end of a bout of exercise and the subsequent return to a resting or recovered state

CAUSES AND SYMPTOMS

To achieve peak athletic performance, increased effort in training, sometimes to the point of overexertion, is required. Initial periods of overexertion followed by a temporary decrease in performance are often referred to as "overreaching." This is distinguishable from overtraining syndrome by the desired increase in performance following a brief period of rest. Overtraining syndrome appears to develop from an overload of training, psychosocial stressors, and performance without adequate recovery or rest periods.

Diagnosing this syndrome can be complicated because a single diagnostic test or tool has yet to be developed. Symptoms may vary depending on the individual athlete or the sport, so other possible causes for a long-term decrease in performance, such as diet or disease, should be ruled out first. More than eighty-four symptoms or markers have been attributed to overtraining syndrome. Most often noted in diagnosis are impaired performance, variations in heart rate, variations in blood pressure, loss of coordination, elevated basal metabolic rate, decreased body fat, weight loss, chronic fatigue, sleep disturbances, increased thirst, headaches, nausea, elevated C-reactive protein (CRP), hormone changes, excessive production of cytokines, mood changes, depression, increased susceptibility to colds, difficulty concentrating, restlessness, increased aches and pains, and muscle soreness. Sport-specific stress tests conducted to the point of exhaustion may aid the diagnosis.

TREATMENT AND THERAPY

Rest from training, performance, or competition is needed. The recovery period may take anywhere from several weeks to years. Prevention is seen as the better option as the rest period needed to recover from overtraining syndrome fully may vary greatly from one athlete to the next. A training schedule alternating high and low training intensities with at least one day of rest is suggested to reduce the risk of developing this condition. Other possible preventive measures include managing stress and maintaining a log to track training intensities, diet, and sleep.

PERSPECTIVE AND PROSPECTS

Research on the characteristics of overtraining syndrome, such as how it affects men and women differently or athletes from various sports, continues to offer new insight. Several physiological tests to aid in detecting overtraining syndrome, including hormone levels, enzyme levels, and blood plasma changes, have been implemented. Still, none thus far have proved to be a valid measure for diagnosing this condition. More research, especially longitudinal research, is needed to understand the condition better, including its diagnosis, prevention, and treatment.

—*Susan E. Thomas*

> **INFORMATION ON OVERTRAINING SYNDROME**
>
> **Causes**: Training overload, stress, inadequate recovery or rest periods
>
> **Symptoms**: Impaired performance, loss of coordination, elevated metabolism, body fat loss, chronic fatigue, sleep disturbances, increased thirst, headaches, nausea, depression, muscle soreness
>
> **Duration**: Chronic
>
> **Treatments**: None; prevention through rest periods, stress management

Further Reading

Brooks, K. A., and J. G. Carter. "Overtraining, Exercise, and Adrenal Insufficiency." *Journal of Novel Physiotherapies*, vol. 3, no. 125, 2013, p. 11717, doi:10.4172/2165-7025.1000125.

Hausswirth, Christophe, and Iñigo Mujika. *Recovery for Performance in Sport*. Human Kinetics, 2012.

Kerksick, Chad M., editor. *Nutrient Timing: Metabolic Optimization for Health, Performance, and Recovery*. CRC Press, 2012

Kreider, Richard B., et al., editors. *Overtraining in Sport*. Human Kinetics, 1998.

McDuff, David R. *Sports Psychiatry: Strategies for Life Balance and Peak Performance*. American Psychiatric Publishing, 2012.

Romain, Meeusen, et al. "Prevention, Diagnosis, and Treatment of the Overtraining Syndrome." *European Journal of Sport Science*, vol. 6, no. 1, 2006, pp. 1-14.

Urhausen, Axel, and Wilfried Kindermann. "Diagnosis of Overtraining: What Tools Do We Have?" *Sports Medicine*, vol. 32, no. 2, 2002, pp. 95-102.

Wyatt, Frank B., Alissa Donaldson, and Elise Brown. "The Overtraining Syndrome: A Meta-Analytic Review." *Journal of Exercise Physiology*, vol. 16, no. 2, 2013, pp. 12-23.

Sociology of Sport

Category: Sports
Specialties and related fields: Sociology
Definition: a branch of social science that analyzes the social dynamics of sport and the roles sporting activities serve in the social and cultural lives of athletes, fans, and society

KEY TERMS

classism: social inequalities based on class that favor or privilege wealthier or more affluent individuals or families over those less affluent; also refers to elitist attitudes that disparage or devalue the poor and working class

conflict theory: a theoretical framework within sociology that envisions tensions, divisions, and inequalities as a basic feature of society due to unequal access to education, wealth, and other valuable social resources

ethnocentrism: a biased perspective in which one assumes that the social or cultural understandings that are familiar to them are inherently "natural," "normal," "best," or "right"

feminist theory: a set of various social theories that critically examined how ideas regarding gender are defined and socially constructed within society; during its early years, feminist theories focused primarily on the experiences of females, but contemporary feminist scholarship also examines men as gendered beings

functionalist theory: a sociology theory that envisions society as a living organism, with its institutions serving as the organs, each of which has its niche to perform to ensure the maintenance and survival of society; functionalist theory seeks to explain how unity and cohesion are maintained within society

homophobia: feelings of prejudice or acts of discrimination against gays and lesbians solely based on their sexual orientation

symbolic interaction theory: a theoretical approach within sociology that examines the shared symbolic meanings that members of a society attach to certain objects, behaviors, or cultural phenomena, as well as how these meanings shape individuals' and collective groups' behaviors

INTRODUCTION

The sociology of sport is a growing field within sociology that analyzes the social dynamics of sport, and the roles sporting activities serve in the social and cultural lives of athletes, fans, and society. Sports sociology differs from sports journalism and sports management in several important ways. Sociologists who study sports as a social institution must be careful to do so in an unbiased or nonethnocentric manner. Sociologists studying sports utilize various theoretical approaches in their research, such as functionalist, conflict, symbolic interaction, and feminist theories. A growing number of professional academic societies and peer-reviewed journals geared towards the field have emerged.

OVERVIEW

Also referred to as "sports sociology," the field uses sociological perspectives, theoretical frameworks, analysis, and research methods to examine sports as a social institution critically. In short, the sociology of sport examines the relationship between sports and the larger society. Sports sociology often examines topics that are frequently studied within the larger, broad field of sociology—such as race/ethnicity, gender, sexuality, social class, religion, age, crime, drug use, and domestic violence—and investigates how these social variables manifest themselves, are influenced by, or are reinforced or challenged through sports. The sociology of sports often incorporates research and findings from other academic disciplines, such as physical and cultural anthropology, psychology, history, physical education, and ethnic and women's studies, into its analyses of the relationship between sports and society. This cross-disciplinary collaboration and influence reflect a broader trend within academia since the late 1970s that has somewhat blurred the boundaries between what was previously viewed as completely distinct and discrete academic subjects.

Sports sociology differs considerably from sports journalism and sports management. Sports journalism centers on media coverage of the results of sporting events (e.g., sports scores, winners and losers, updates on injuries to athletes) and key developments among coaches, athletes, and sports teams that either do or may have a bearing on the outcomes of games or matches. In contrast, sports management focuses on the administrative aspects of sports, such as coaching philosophies, marketing, and other business-related dimensions of sports. Sports sociology is much less concerned with the win-loss outcomes of particular sporting events or the statistics accumulated by athletes; its focus instead is on a critical examination of sports as an aspect of social and cultural life, as a key institution of society, and as the ramifications of sports on society as a whole, as well as in the lives of individual athletes and fans. This involves thinking critically and analytically about sports to understand the social and cultural dynamics at play in all levels of sport (e.g., recreational, scholastic, collegiate, amateur, professional) and in all dimensions of sport (e.g., preparation, performance, coaching, fandom, celebrity). Such an approach requires examining sports from an intellectual, as opposed to an emotional,

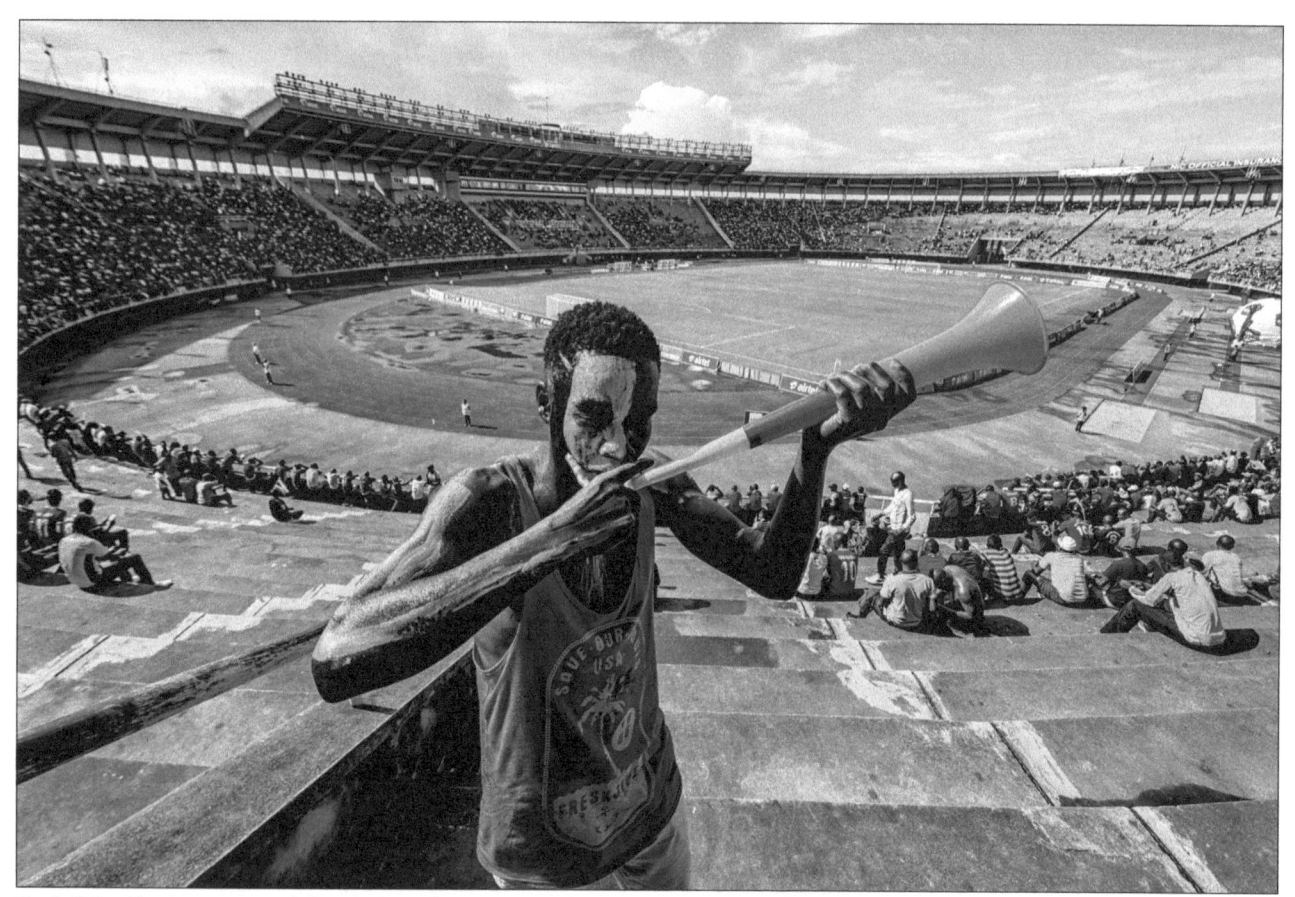

Football fan blowing a trumpet before the Uganda vs. Cape Verde game. Photo by Museruka Emmanuel, via Wikimedia Commons.

perspective—not always an easy task for students and researchers, given the intense devotion that die-hard sports fans may have toward their favorite sports, teams, and players. Such partisanship can easily stem from value judgments, ethnocentric and culture-bound assumptions regarding sports (such as an American asserting that football or baseball are "better" than soccer or cricket), discrediting or dismissing as unimportant the sports that one is unfamiliar with, or uncritically assuming that the social dynamics that characterize a certain sport (in terms of the racial/ethnic, gender, or social class demographics of the athletes who comprise a sport) are "natural" or "just the way things are." As part of their academic training, sociologists are taught to become aware of their own ethnocentric biases to avoid allowing them to study society intellectually and critically.

Individuals unfamiliar with sociology may assume that sports, as a form of exercise and recreation, are a trivial or unimportant topic of social analysis. However, there are several compelling reasons for critically examining sports. Sports are a central part of many people's lives, both in the United States and worldwide, either as athletes or as fans and spectators. Sports are also connected to other key social intuitions in various ways. Schools, colleges, and universities typically offer several sports programs for student participation. Interscholastic and intercollegiate sporting contests are a major aspect of social life at both the scholastic and collegiate levels. Many churches often sponsor baseball, basketball, and football programs, and even several police departments in large urban metropolitan regions sponsor midnight basketball leagues or youth amateur boxing programs as part of their crime prevention and gang deterrent efforts. Sports also heavily influence the larger culture of a society. For example, professional athletes worldwide are often major celebrities whose popularity rivals that of musicians and movie stars, and athletes often serve as role models for children and teenagers. Furthermore, sports serve as an important source of national, local, ethnic, or collegiate pride in many people's lives, making sports a key part of the collective identity in the lives of millions of individuals.

The matter of just who participates in which sport(s) is not solely a question of individual talent and skill, as strong racial/ethnic, social class, gender, and national underpinnings influence that social group(s) get drawn into which particular sporting venues. Even the most casual of sports fans probably are aware that certain sports tend to feature athletes predominantly of one social background or another. Furthermore, sports are not as egalitarian or equally accessible as many people initially assume because some sports are much more expensive to participate in than others. Consequently, strong social class dimensions affect who is capable of partaking in several sports. Golf, tennis, swimming, skiing, skating, gymnastics, rowing, and equestrian events are some sports that tend to be confined to members of the middle and upper classes because of the high costs of equipment and private training they entail.

Since the 1960s, a growing number of professional academic societies and peer-reviewed journals have emerged to promote the continuing growth of sports as a major focus of research among sociologists. Some of these academic societies include the International Sociology of Sport Association, the North America Society for the Sociology of Sport, the Sports Studies Caucus of the American Studies Association, the Japan Society of Sport Sociology, and the European Association for Sociology of Sport. At present, however, the American Sociological Association (the largest national professional network of sociologists in the United States) does not have a specific members' section or chapter devoted exclusively to sports sociology. Major peer-reviewed journals devoted to studying sports sociology include *Sporting Cultures and Identities, Sport and Society: Annual Review, Journal of Sport & Social Issues, Sport* in *Society, Sociology of Sport Journal*, and *International Review for the Sociology of Sport*.

VIEWPOINTS

Sociologists who study sports differ in the theoretical frameworks from which they approach their research and analysis. Major sociological theories include functionalist theory, conflict theory, symbolic interaction theory, and a variety of feminist theoretical frameworks. Functionalist theory is a classic sociological theory that dates to the discipline's early years in the nineteenth century and is sometimes known as the "organic analogy" because it envisions society as a metaphorical organism. Just as an organism consists of many different organs, each of which most properly performs its function to ensure the body's health, well-being, and overall survival, functionalist theory likewise envisions society as consisting of a variety of social institutions. Each of these institutions contributes to the overall structure and survival of a society. Under a functionalist theoretical approach, sports and athletics are analyzed to determine how they serve to maintain social cohesion and unity among citizens within the larger society.

Conflict theory is also one of the earliest theories in sociology. It stems from Karl Marx's nineteenth-century ideas of how capitalism fosters economic inequalities, resulting in competition for limited employment opportunities, financial resources, and social mobility. Conflict theory is almost directly opposed to functionalist theory, which examines how society promotes or reinforces social divisions, from basic inequalities to discriminatory attitudes, to social protest movements, to violent conflicts between various factions within society. On the other hand, symbolic interaction theory, one of the most influential theories in contemporary sociology, examines the role that shared symbolic meanings and understandings regarding social behaviors and phenomena play in shaping people's behaviors, both as individuals and as collective members of groups. In other words, the power of shared subjective understandings or attitudes about certain social phenomena shapes individuals' behaviors within a group context.

Feminist theoretical approaches seek to highlight the social construction of gender and the social experiences of females as a focus of academic study. Traditionally, various academic disciplines, ranging from the social sciences to the arts and humanities, overlooked the life experiences, social realities, and contributions of females by heavily limiting their focus to analyses of men, masculinity, and male experiences. There is not one singular form of feminist theory; rather, feminism encompasses a variety of theoretical approaches that seek to examine gender from different angles. During the 1960s and 1970s (the era of "second-wave feminism"), feminist scholars focused primarily on sexist discrimination against women and societal inequalities between males and females. Since the 1980s, however, feminist scholars (known as "third-wave feminists") have begun to emphasize that neither women nor men are homogenous or monolithic. Feminist scholars examine how other social factors, such as race/ethnicity, class, age, and sexual orientation, play important roles in shaping a person's societal experiences. Furthermore, contrary to popular opinion, feminist scholars study men and socially defined ideals of masculinity as part of their analysis of gender.

Each of these theoretical approaches has a contribution to make toward the sociology of sports. For example, functionalist analyses study the role that sports and athletic participation play in building a sense of national unity and identity. For example, in the immediate aftermath of 9/11, the New York Yankees baseball team experienced a temporary surge of nationwide popularity, given that they represent the city most devastated by the terrorist attacks. Another vivid example is the historic 1980 Winter Olympics ice hockey game between the underdog United States and the hockey powerhouse Soviet

Union in Lake Placid, New York. The American team upset the Soviets in a game now popularly referred to as the "Miracle on Ice," and the game's outcome produced a surge of patriotic sentiments—along with the now-common "U-S-A!, U-S-A!" that American sports fans still chant during international competitions. However, many sociologists criticize a purely functionalist analysis of society because it overlooks divisions and inequalities by focusing excessively on social cohesion. Conflict theorists would examine how various social inequalities, such as racism or sexism, affect sports or how the world of sports contributes to the perpetuation of inequalities, such as the stereotype that blacks are naturally athletically gifted or the homophobic prejudices that athletes or sports fans exhibit. Meanwhile, a symbolic interactionist approach would examine, for example, how high school students may feel compelled to join the football, wrestling, or cheerleading teams to be seen as "cool" by their peers. Finally, feminist approaches to sports may examine the lower prestige and spectator support that women's athletics generally hold compared with their male counterparts or how female athletes are often discussed more regarding their physical appearance than their athletic talents.

Journalist Dave Zirin, the sports editor for *The Nation*, who is known for his publications analyzing the social and political dynamics of sports in both American society and the global context, has praised and criticized the sociology of sport. Zirin's praise for the sociology of sport stems from his belief that a critical, systematic examination of sport sheds light on the social inequalities, such as sexism, racism, homophobia, and social class oppression, often reflected in the world of sports. However, he criticizes the sociology of sport because the field is dominated by scholars who produce books and articles that are written in dense, academic jargon that the average layperson or sports fan would find very difficult or impossible to understand; as such, the publications produced by sports sociologists largely remain confined to academic journals with no mass, public circulation or appeal. Because of this, sports sociologists tend to reach only an academic, scholarly audience with their works. The general public (including passionate sports fans), whom Zirin feels would benefit tremendously from sociological analysis of sports, do not learn to approach sports from a more critical and theoretically informed standpoint. Zirin has called for several reforms to make sports sociology more practical and relevant, including the establishment of a "sports and society" column authored by sociologists in each college newspaper and major sports publication, the appearance of sports sociologists on sports talk radio and television to share their knowledge with sports fans, and the publication of books by sports sociologists that target the general public and sports spectators, as opposed to the scholarly community.

—*Justin D. García*

Further Reading

Butryn, T. M., et al. "We Walk the Line: An Analysis of the Problems and Possibilities of Work at the Sport Psychology-Sport Sociology Nexus." *Sociology of Sport Journal*, vol. 31, no. 2, 2014, pp. 162-84.

Coakley, J. *Sports in Society: Issues and Controversies*. 11th ed., McGraw-Hill, 2014.

Crossman, A. "Symbolic Interaction Theory." *About.com*, 14 June 2015, sociology.about.com/od/Sociological-Theory/a/Symbolic-Interaction-Theory.htm.

Gregory, S. "U.S. Ranks Worst in Sports Homophobia Study." *Time*, 9 May 2015, time.com/3852611/sports-homophobia-study/.

Millington, B., and R. Millington. "'The Datafication of Everything': Toward a Sociology of Sport and Big Data." *Sociology of Sport Journal*, vol. 32, no. 2, 2015, pp. 140-60.

Rader, B. *American Sports: From the Age of Folk Games to the Age of Televised Sports*. Prentice-Hall, 2009.

Sage, G., and D. S. Eitzen. *Sociology of North American Sport*. 10th ed., Oxford UP, 2015.

"Sociology of Sport." *UNI.edu*. Dec. 1998, www.uni.edu/greenr/soc/sportsoc.htm.

Thorpe, H., et al. "Toward New Conversations Between Sociology and Psychology." *Sociology of Sport Journal*, vol. 31, no. 2, 2014, pp. 131-38.

"What Is Sociology?" *Department of Sociology*. University of North Carolina at Chapel Hill, 2015, sociology.unc.edu/undergraduateprogram/sociology-major/what-is-sociology/.

Zirin, D. "Calling Sports Sociology Off the Bench." *Contexts.org*, 1 July 2008, contexts.org/articles/calling-sports-sociology-offthe-bench/.

Sports Engineering

Category: Sports equipment
Specialties and related fields: Clothing design, engineering, materials science, sports medicine
Definition: the study of how sports equipment affects performance and safety

KEY TERMS

aerodynamics: the study of the properties of moving air and the interaction between the air and solid bodies moving through it

computational fluid dynamics: a branch of fluid mechanics that uses numerical analysis and data structures to analyze and solve problems that involve fluid flows

computer-aided design (CAD): the use of computers to aid in the creation, modification, analysis, or optimization of a design

friction: the force resisting the relative motion of solid surfaces, fluid layers, and material elements sliding against each other

traction-test devices: measures the length of time that rats can keep their front paws on a horizontally suspended bar

DEFINITION AND BASIC PRINCIPLES

Sports engineering is the application of engineering principles to the study of sports equipment and sports venues. This field most closely resembles mechanical engineering. Mechanical engineering uses physics and mathematics to study and design physical processes and mechanical systems and uses various computer-based tools, including computer-aided design (CAD) and simulation software. Sports engineering uses the same techniques to study and design sport-specific equipment and venues. Since the 1990s, sports engineers have been involved in sports as varied as golf, hockey, speed skating, and tennis.

BACKGROUND AND HISTORY

Sports engineering is a relatively new field formed as a subdiscipline of mechanical engineering. Although the specific field of sports engineering is new, the fundamentals that make up this subdiscipline are based on centuries of study. The best-known sports engineering program is at the University of Sheffield in the United Kingdom. The University of Sheffield program, founded in 1998, divides the discipline into the areas of aerodynamics, sports surfaces, impact, and friction.

The earliest recorded Olympic competition dates back to ancient Greece. As technology improves, it has been applied to virtually all sports. Advances in sports clothing provide sports-specific advantages such as improved aerodynamics, breathable fabric, thinner insulating fabrics, and superior waterproofing. Sports engineers also work with the governing bodies of sports organizations to meet the regulations of those specific sports.

The fields of engineering evolved from physics and mathematics. The first societies were formed in the nineteenth century. As the specific field of mechanical engineering evolved, the principles of physics and mathematics were already being applied to sports equipment. Biomechanics and kinesiology developed as specialized fields in the subject of human movement; however, these fields did not specifically address sports equipment. There are now a handful of universities around the world that offer degrees in sports engineering and other mechanical engineer-

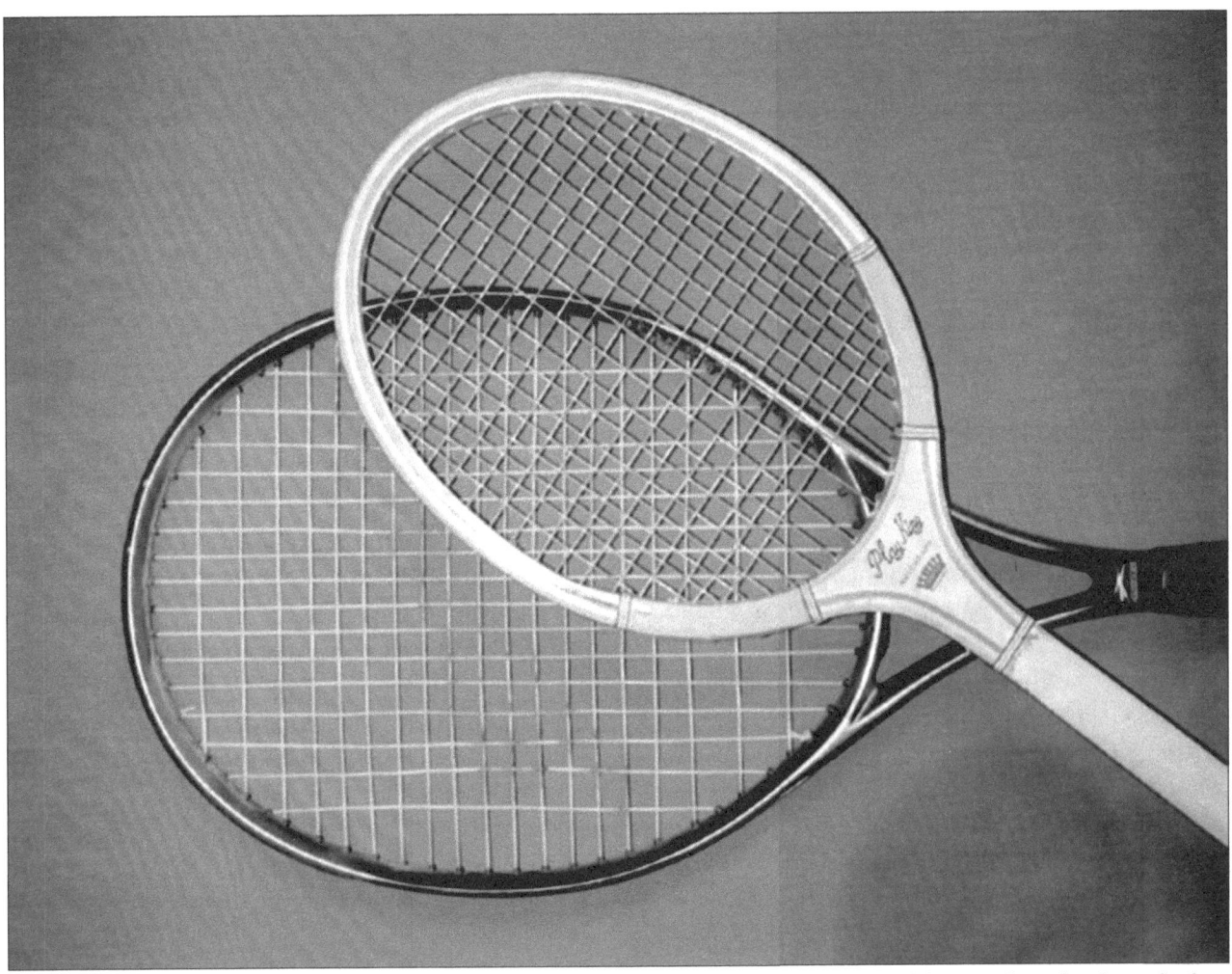

A tennis racket made of an advanced material such as carbon fiber reinforced plastic can have a larger head than a traditional racket made of wood. Photo by CORE-Materials, via Wikimedia Commons.

ing programs that offer classes in sports engineering. The University of Sheffield provides a focused area of study in sports equipment and venues by founding the sports engineering program and the Sports Engineering Research Group (SERG). The International Sports Engineering Association (ISEA) was founded to provide a forum for engineers interested in this subject.

HOW IT WORKS

Mechanical engineering applies mathematics and physics to designing and studying physical and mechanical processes. Sports engineering uses mechanical engineering knowledge to focus on studying and designing sports equipment and venues. Refinements in equipment lead to improved performance by athletes and safety for participants. Regulations of various sports have been modified to accommodate new forms of equipment while maintaining fairness between competitors and improving sports safety. It is useful to use the University of Sheffield's divisions of aerodynamics, sports surfaces, impact, and friction to understand the areas of study that makeup sports engineering.

Aerodynamics. Aerodynamics uses mathematics and physics to describe and model the airflow around objects. For any sport that uses balls, it is helpful to understand the trajectories that may result under different circumstances to develop techniques for improved accuracy and speed. Aerodynamics also applies to any sports that involve speed. Skeleton, speed skating, bobsledding, sprinting, downhill skiing, and many other sports use specialized equipment and clothing to reduce the effects of airflow on performance.

There are a variety of techniques that can be employed to study the aerodynamics of sports equipment. Wind-tunnel tests and laser scanners are used in studying sports aerodynamics along with sophisticated mathematical techniques such as computational fluid dynamics (CFD). Forces such as lift and drag can be calculated using these methods. Variations in the surface roughness of a ball or clothing, spin on a ball, or other factors will change how an object moves through space. The most familiar example of this is the variation in the behavior of a baseball, depending on the pitch.

Sports surfaces. The interactions between athletic shoes or equipment and the sports surface play a large role in performance and can result in injuries. Surfaces may vary even within a sport, such as tennis and soccer. Shoe manufacturers and other manufacturers use information about these interactions to design equipment that will reduce injuries and optimize performance. Traction-test devices are used to simulate conditions in some cases. A traction-test device is a shoe surface mounted on a plate that evaluates shoe interaction with various surfaces.

Each sport has different materials and requirements for movements on the surface, with inter-athlete differences. There are numerous variables involved in the interactions of surfaces. The mathematic models needed to study these interactions are so complex that SERG researchers have turned to neural-network modeling to generate information that engineers can use to design better equipment.

Impacts. One of the most-studied sports has been tennis. The variables of racquet design, swing technique, ball design, and area of the strings used will all change the trajectory and speed of the tennis ball in play. Sports engineers can study numerous other sports in terms of impacts, including baseball, squash, hockey, field hockey, and cricket.

Sports engineers can use three-dimensional (3D) ideography and high-speed photography to study the effects of different variables in the impact stage and the resulting trajectory of the ball. This information can then be used to refine the athlete's technique and to design more effective equipment.

Friction. Surface characteristics of balls, fields and other sports equipment will affect sports performance. The interactions between the athlete's skin and grip must be considered in addition to environmental conditions such as moisture in these circumstances. The effects of sports surfaces on human skin are also studied to reduce injuries.

This area of sports engineering overlaps with biomechanics since it involves the interaction of the skin and other tissues with the sports equipment or sports surface.

Special considerations. There are areas where these SERG divisions will overlap or where specialized knowledge is required. For speed skaters, the interaction of the skate blade and the ice surface creates a melting effect that must be understood to design faster skates. Experts in this specific interaction are working to improve the skate-blade design. For changing conditions, such as outdoor skiing or biking, different types of equipment are designed for specific conditions. One example is the powder ski, which has different shape and design characteristics compared to slalom or downhill skis. The varied requirements for each sport result in various specializations for sports engineers.

APPLICATIONS AND PRODUCTS

Engineering techniques have been used to improve sports equipment of all types, even before a designation called "sports engineering." There are many examples of this in sporting history. The pole vault record increased to 6.14 meters due to improvements in materials and design during the twentieth century, a 53 percent increase from the first official competition. Sports engineering has resulted in improvements in areas as diverse as fly-fishing rods and Frisbees. Amateur, professional, and Olympic competitors have all benefited from improvements in equipment and venues.

Olympic sports. Sports engineering has increasingly been used to improve Olympic-athlete performance. Researchers at the University of Sheffield were credited with helping the British cycling team win four gold medals at the 2004 Summer Olympic Games in Athens. Researchers then turned to study the skeleton and used complex modeling and digital shape sampling and processing to improve performances in the 2006 Winter Olympic Games in Turin, Italy. Sports engineering can be particularly helpful in those sports where one-hundredth of a second might be the difference between a gold and silver medal.

Amateur sports. Well-known sports manufacturers hire sports engineers to improve existing products continually. These improvements have benefited casual athletes as well as more serious amateurs. Sporting-equipment manufacturers use designers and engineers to produce better-performing shoes, skis, racquets, and other products for the general public.

For example, lighter materials and the development of the oversize tennis racquet in the 1970s made it easier for beginners. Improved materials have increased racquet stiffness, allowing a more efficient transfer of force to the ball, leading to faster speeds.

In mountain biking, the addition of front and rear shock absorbers, lightweight frames, improved gearing, and step-in-toe clips have made it easier for the less experienced riders to navigate difficult terrain. Similarly, skis and snowboards have evolved to increase ease of turning, which helps beginner and intermediate skiers and snowboarders.

Lightweight helmets are now worn by most bikers and skiers, which improves safety. Many ski helmets have improved features such as removable inserts for warmth and vents that can be opened or closed for cooling. Wearable water backpacks are now commonplace among many athletes and are more convenient than the standard water bottle.

As of 2021, virtually every sport has benefitted from sports engineering.

Professional sports. Improvements in sports equipment are driven by the demand for increased performance by Olympians and professional athletes. Advances in technology, such as the larger tennis racquet head and increased racquet stiffness that have benefited amateur tennis players have also benefited professional tennis players. The larger head allows highly skilled professionals to achieve more topspin and higher speeds.

Professional golfers use advanced golf clubs and ball designs. Differences in weighting and shaft construction influence performance. Golf balls are also evolving with the introduction of solid cores, which lead to longer drives. The dimpling on the golf balls is designed to give maximum flight. These dimples are modified in some newer balls to optimize flights. Equipment improvements have benefited professional sports of all types, and professional organizations continue pushing for the technological edge to make them more competitive.

Sports venues. Sports engineers are also involved in designing and studying sports venues. An example of this is the development by SERG engineers of a trueness meter for greens evaluation. Trueness meters help greens keepers evaluate the smoothness of turf. This information improves the ability of the greenkeeper to achieve optimum conditions for best performance.

Throughout the first decades of the twenty-first century, the National Hockey League (NHL) discussed the need for improved safety to reduce concussions in players. Discussions included possible changes to the glass surrounding the rinks. This type of design change to improve the safety of a sporting venue is an area in which sports engineers may get involved.

Sports safety. Sports-equipment engineering has had an impact on injury prevention at all levels. Helmets have become commonplace for sports such as downhill skiing and bicycling. In sports such as hockey, a helmet is required at both the amateur and professional levels. Baseball is another sport in which a helmet is required for certain positions. In some jurisdictions, bicycle helmets are required by law to be worn by riders under eighteen. Many amateur participants will wear helmets to reduce the chance of injury, even if they are not mandatory. There is evidence in the peer-reviewed medical literature that helmet use for sports such as bicycling and hockey does reduce injury. Full facial protection has also been shown to reduce injury in hockey players. In football, another high-contact sport, the first decades of the twenty-first century have seen an increased effort to find a helmet design that can protect players against not only the worst injuries but also the types of injuries that have become of increasing concern for the long-term health of players. The biggest issue facing designers is the prevalence of concussions, which research, sparked by several high-profile deaths and suicides of football players, has increasingly shown can cause long-term brain damage and related psychological trauma.

For venues, sports engineering can be used to modify existing venues or to design newer, safer venues. In the 2010 Winter Olympic Games in Vancouver, the death of twenty-one-year-old Georgian luge athlete Nodar Kumaritashvili during a skeleton run sparked a public debate about track safety. Mechanical engineers made some modifications shortly after the accident to improve safety. However, the debate continued about the role of inexperience versus track design as a cause for the accident.

Safety considerations include the durability of equipment and risk of sudden equipment failure, and impact the choice of materials that sports engineers consider when they design sports equipment. These considerations affect athletes at all levels, organizations, governing bodies, and manufacturers.

Clothing. Clothing for high-speed sports has been improved to reduce the drag from airflow. High-tech clothing has been credited with improvements in sprinters, speed skaters, and downhill skiers. Shoes are another area of innovation, with improvements in material durability and performance characteristics. Weight, durability, cushioning, spikes, and flexibility are engineered to provide the best attributes for each sport.

CAREERS AND COURSEWORK

Sports engineering is a newer field compared with other engineering disciplines. Some university programs offer a sports engineering degree, and others have sports engineering courses within their mechanical engineering degree program. Bachelor of engineering degrees will usually require three to five years to complete. A strong background in mathematics and physics is needed. Advanced degrees such as a master's or doctorate may be required for some career paths, such as teaching. Specific jobs may require some knowledge of biomechanics, kinesiology, or anatomy.

An interest in sports or a particular skill in sports can be helpful in sports engineering. In some cases, athletes will go on to become sports engineers. For example, British aerospace engineer and Olympic skeleton competitor Kristan Bromley has researched sled design to optimize performance.

The applications of sports engineering are wide-ranging, so there are several paths an individual career might take. Additional expertise or training in materials, architecture, physiology, kinesiology, or biomechanics may be needed for some applications. This specialization might come with an advanced degree or work experience.

SOCIAL CONTEXT AND FUTURE PROSPECTS

As sports engineers become more commonplace and sports engineering degree programs are created, this discipline is likely to be more widely recognized as a field separate from mechanical engineering. It is similar to the field of geomatics engineering, which was a branch of civil engineering and is now recognized as a separate field of engineering.

Since the middle of the twentieth century, new sports have evolved through material and design changes. The Frisbee and in-line skates were invented, and snowboarding was created. In Nordic skiing, a new technique called "skate skiing" became popular due to technique and equipment changes. This invention changed how many Nordic trails are prepared, such that the classic ski tracks are to one side, and a larger flat area of packed snow is created for the skate skiers. Skateboarding and skateboard parks are other examples of a sport and venues that have become popular as a result of improvements in equipment. These innovations will continue to occur in the future with modifications to existing sports and inventions of new sports.

Athletes, amateur, and leisure, reap benefits and experience enhanced comfort, performance, and safety as manufacturers continually improve their products. Entrepreneurs will create new products with the help of sports engineers, who will likely play an important role in the evolution of sports going forward.

—*Ellen E. Anderson Penno*

Further Reading

Baine, Celeste. *High Tech Hot Shots: Careers in Sports Engineering*. National Society of Professional Engineers, 2004.

Cho, Adrian. "Engineering Peak Performance." *Science*, vol. 305, no. 5684, 2004, pp. 643-44.

Estivalet, Margaret, and Pierre Brisson, editors. *The Engineering of Sport 7*. Vol. 2. Springer, 2009.

Farish, Mike. "Bottoms Up." *Engineering*, vol. 248, no. 3, 2007, pp. 45-47.

Hamilton, Tracy Brown. *Dream Jobs in Sports Equipment Design*. Rosen Publishing Group, 2018.

James, David. "Design Engineering—Managing Technology: Slight Advantage." *Engineer*, 5 May 2008, p. 34.

Moore, Jack. "The Limits of Football Helmets." *The Atlantic*, 5 Feb. 2016, www.theatlantic.com/health/archive/2016/02/super-bowl-football-helmet-concussion/460092/. Accessed 28 Nov. 2021.

Moritz, Eckehard Fozzy, and Steve Haake, editors. *The Engineering of Sport 6: Developments for Disciplines*. Vol. 2. Springer, 2006.

"A Powerful Duo; HPC and Graphene Paving the Way for Cutting-Edge Sports Gear Design." *NIMBIX*, 21 Sept. 2021, www.nimbix.net/blog-graphene-hpc-sports-gear. Accessed 28 Nov. 2021.

Romeo, Jim. "Using 3D Printing to Improve Sports Equipment." *GrabCAD*, 6 July 2020, blog.grabcad.com/blog/2020/07/06/3d-printing-sports-equipment/. Accessed 28 Nov. 2021.

Sports Psychology

Category: Sports and exercise science

Specialties and related fields: Cognition, emotion, learning, motivation, neurology, personality, psychiatry, psychology, social psychology, stress

Definition: involvement in sports as a participant or spectator serves similar psychological functions for individuals: both help people create and maintain a positive self-concept, allow them to feel a sense of membership in social groups, and provide pleasant stimulation

KEY TERMS

attribution: how the social perceiver uses information to arrive at causal explanations for events

eustress: a positive response one has to a stressor, which can depend on one's current feelings of control, desirability, location, and timing of the stressor

motivation: the study of understanding what drives a person to work towards a particular goal or outcome

participant: a person who takes part in an investigation, study, or experiment

self-esteem: confidence in one's own worth or abilities; self-respect

social identity: the qualities, beliefs, personality traits, appearance, and expressions that characterize a person or group

spectator: the effect on performance when a task is carried out in the presence of others

INTRODUCTION

Sports psychology, also called "sport psychology," studies the relationship between psychological or mental factors and sports participation and appreciation. Practitioners study how athletes' psychology affects their sports performance and how fans' identification with a team affects their well-being. For athletes, sports psychology involves understanding skills such as relaxation, visualization, concentration, and goal setting. Sports psychology assumes that people's motivational level is a critical determinant of their involvement in sports, either as participants or spectators. Involvement in sports by both participants and spectators is a result of similar motivational factors: the desire to maintain a positive self-concept, the need to affiliate with or belong to influential social groups, and the need for positive stress levels.

POSITIVE SELF-CONCEPT

As illustrated by the work of social psychologists such as Henri Tajfel, John Turner, and Jennifer Crocker, who have tested aspects of social identity theory, humans tend to maintain a positive view of themselves. Therefore, evaluations that people make of the groups they belong to affect their social identity. For many people, the goal of feeling positive about themselves can be accomplished, at least in part, through involvement with athletics—either actively as participants or passively as spectators.

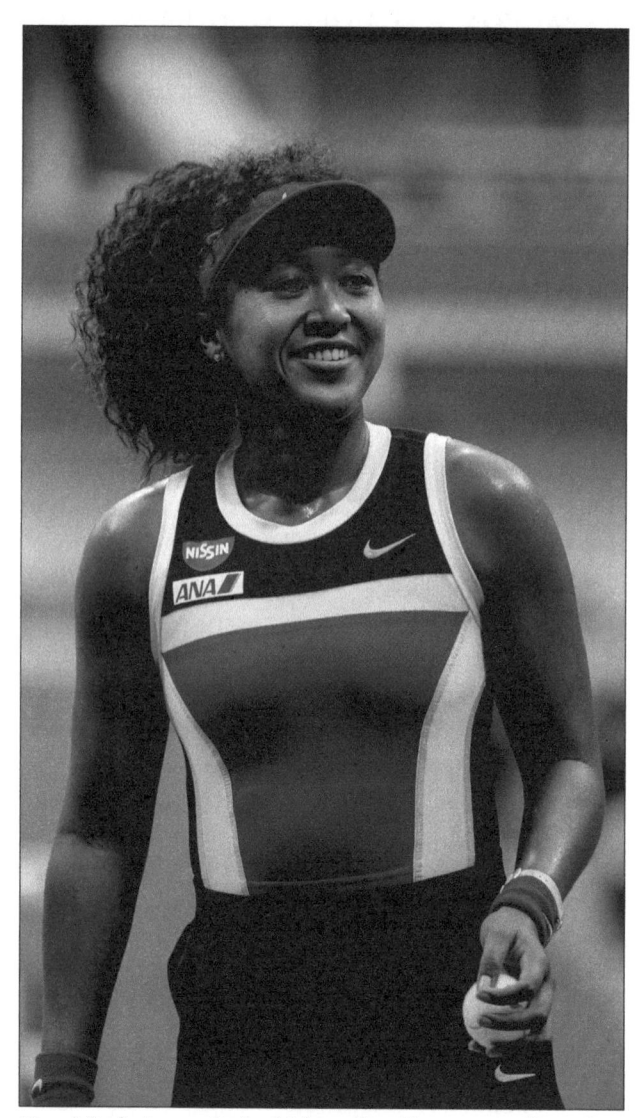

Naomi Osaka is one of a few high-profile athletes to go public with her struggles with depression, and she has become an advocate for destigmatizing mental health issues in sport. Photo by Andrew Henkelman, via Wikimedia Commons.

For the athlete, self-esteem plays an important motivational role in early childhood. Children tend to choose activities in which they are successful, allowing them to feel proud of their accomplishments. Children who find success in athletic games begin to prefer them to other recreational or intellectual activities. In short, those with the most skill (presumably a genetic predisposition) tend to show the most enthusiasm for sports participation. Success and its subsequent self-esteem benefits fuel their desire to continue or increase their participation in athletics.

When studying children's motivation, it is important to distinguish between intrinsic and extrinsic motivation. When an individual is intrinsically motivated to complete a task, that person is moved by internal factors such as feelings of competence or an interest in the task itself. Extrinsically motivated persons are driven by external rewards, such as money, trophies, or praise from coaches and parents. Ideally, children should become involved in sports for intrinsic reasons, and most do become involved due to such motives. When intrinsically motivated children are given external rewards for their performance, however, the result can be a reduced overall motivation to participate in sports; that is, they tend to become less interested. The findings on the intrinsic-extrinsic motivational dichotomy have been used to help people trying to establish youth sports leagues. In the early stages of a league, intrinsic motives should be emphasized. Increases in extrinsic motivation via rewards and trophies will probably result in reduced intrinsic motivation and decreased interest in the activity. Simply having children come to expect their parents' praise can reduce intrinsic motivation. Unexpected praise and rewards are less likely to reduce intrinsic motivation. Generally, it is probably best to take a hands-off approach to children's athletic games.

Coaches often try to increase the motivation of athletes to increase their performance; however, increasing the player's motivation is only one method of enhancing performance. Another popular technique, referred to as using mental imagery (what many call visualization), involves having the athlete mentally rehearse game situations. Before shooting a free throw, a basketball player might form a mental image of lining up their body correctly with the basket, bending at the knees when ready to release the ball, and following through with the fingertips and wrist after release. For example, L. Verdelle Clark had varsity and junior varsity high school basketball players practice their free-throw shooting through mental imagery and physical practice. The results indicated that mental practice was almost as effective as physical practice.

SELF-ESTEEM

The desire to maintain positive levels of self-esteem continues to be a primary motivational force for adolescent and adult athletes. Participation in athletics allows them the opportunity to feel good about themselves by helping fulfill their need for achievement and status. Successful athletic performance provides them with a feeling of accomplishment and mastery.

Self-esteem also serves as a motivational force for sports spectators. Although spectators do not personally accomplish performance goals, they can experience satisfaction and accomplishment with their team members. Sports fans report elation following their team's victory and sorrow after their team's defeat, with levels of intensity similar to those of the players. The success of a fan's favorite team produces feelings of pride and increased self-esteem. Thus, spectators can improve their self-concept without any special athletic skills.

In general, fans of the local team, regardless of the team's success, tend to have higher self-esteem, experience fewer negative emotions, and report greater life satisfaction than those who are not fans of the team. Such high self-esteem seems to be caused by the social support gained through interactions with other fans. Nyla Branscombe and Daniel Wann performed a series of studies showing that spectators may experience increases in self-esteem even if their favorite team is not of championship-caliber, as team identification provides a buffer from the feelings of isolation and alienation damaging to a society that values mobility.

The desire to affiliate with and belong to certain groups motivates sports participants. As adolescents begin to detach themselves from their families, social groups involving their peers become increasingly important, and a primary source of peer-group membership is belonging to sports teams. Membership in such teams permits adolescents to be accepted by their peers, extends their social network, gives them a sense of belonging, and helps establish their social identity. Adults also may satisfy their need for affiliation and belonging by playing in recreational sports leagues.

POSITIVE STRESS

Another factor shown to motivate both athletes and spectators is a desire for positive stress levels. Unlike the negative stress that often accompanies academic or work endeavors, positive stress, called "eustress," reflects people's desire to find stimulation in life. For participants and spectators, an athletic event involving their chosen team can be very stimulating. Hearts begin to race, people may feel nervous, and generally, the event can be quite arousing—much like a roller-coaster ride. Many people actively seek this stimulation, and involvement in sports is an easy way to obtain it.

ATTRIBUTION

The motivational forces described earlier help explain a wide variety of the behaviors exhibited by athletic participants and spectators. For example, the importance of maintaining a positive self-concept has been used to explain players' and fans' self-serving attributions—the explanations people give when explaining why certain events occur. Attributions can be either external (the "A" grade attributable to luck or easy questions) or internal (the "A" on a test attributable to intelligence or intensive studying). Because of the desire for a positive self-concept, people tend to use external attributions to explain their failures (thereby protecting their self-concept) while forming internal attributions concerning their successes (thereby enhancing their self-concept). This self-serving attributional bias can be found in many areas, including athletics. Research has demonstrated that when a participant or a spectator's team has failed a competition, people tend to form external attributions to explain the defeat. For example, when asked to explain why they lost, athletes often blame the officials, bad luck, or the opponents' dirty play. They do not perceive the failure to be internal (attributable to a lack of skill or ability on their part); hence, their self-concept is protected. Conversely, when victorious, athletes tend to assign internal causes for their success. When they win the contest, it is attributed to their skill rather than luck.

This pattern of self-serving attributions is also found among sports spectators. When their favorite team is successful, sports fans tend to give internal attributions similar to the players. When their team loses, spectators choose external attributions to explain the defeat. This bias, used most frequently by highly allegiant or identified fans, is driven by a desire to maintain the belief that the groups with which they are associated are good. Spectators can increase their self-esteem through a related process called "basking in reflected glory" by Robert Cialdini and his colleagues. Cialdini found that spectators enhance their self-esteem by increasing their association with successful teams and protect their self-esteem by decreasing their association with failing teams. In one study, students at a large university were telephoned and asked to describe the most recent game of the university's football team.

When the team had won, people tended to give statements such as "We won" or "We were victorious." When the team had lost, however, the typical reply was "They lost" or "They were defeated." In a second study, the day after their college team played, more students wore clothing that identified their university affiliation following a victory than after a defeat. The most allegiant fans, however, continued showing support for their team even when it lost over long periods.

MOTIVATION RESEARCH

The topic of motivation is one of the major areas of emphasis within the discipline of sports psychology, and it has attracted considerable research and theoretical attention. Since the 1990s, sports psychologists have been increasingly researching sports participation and spectatorship. Increased interest in the factors underlying the motivation of sports participants and spectators has been driven by the fact that sports are among the most popular leisure-time activities. Satisfaction with leisure-time activities greatly influences other areas of an individual's life, such as school or work.

Understanding the motivations of sports spectators and participants is important for several reasons. First, most individuals begin their involvement with sports at a young age, usually by early adolescence. Because of the impact of peer relations on the psychological development of youth, insight into these relationships is important, and some comprehension can be gained by studying athletic team formation and cohesion. Second, because self-esteem plays a critical role in determining whether individuals will become involved in sports, the positive emotional impact of athletics may be used for therapeutic purposes. Third, professional sports is a very big business with millions of dollars at stake. Suppose an individual's performance could be increased by increasing motivation. In that case, the result could be profitable for team owners and the professionals involved.

DEVELOPMENT OF THE FIELD

Sports psychology is a relatively young specialty area within psychology. Pioneers, such as Coleman R. Griffith of the University of Illinois's Athletic Research Laboratory, expressed interest in sports psychology in the early twentieth century. Griffith published *Psychology of Coaching* (1926) and *Psychology of Athletics* (1928). The field, however, did not develop at that time. Most national and international professional organizations designed to examine issues in sports psychology were founded no earlier than the 1970s. It was not until 1986 that the American Psychological Association (APA) recognized sports psychology as a separate academic division. Organizations promoting professionalism include the North American Society for the Psychology of Sport and Physical Activity and the International Society of Sport Psychology.

Sports psychologists can receive certification from the Association for the Advancement of Applied Sport Psychology or by completing continuing education courses offered by the American Board of Sport Psychology. Individual sports psychologists train athletes differently and use various treatment methods. Some analyze how social environments influence the behavior of athletes, while others focus on cognitive aspects, such as how mental processes shape athletic behavior. Others focus on psychophysiology, which correlates with how brain chemistry affects behavior. The concept of motor development interests many sports psychologists. In addition to traditional forms of counseling, sports psychologists use biofeedback, hypnosis, and neurofeedback. Certified sports psychologists can register with the United States Olympic Committee and National Collegiate Athletic Association to assist elite and student athletes in fine-tuning their performances and developing coping and psychological skills to deal with demanding high-profile lives.

SPECIALTIES AND APPLICATIONS

Sports psychology research has expanded as psychologists develop specialties within the field to explore both familiar and emerging concerns. Research topics include self-determination theory, emotional intelligence, and mood states, especially how anxiety and catastrophe theory affect athletes. Technological developments offer sports psychologists new tools such as real-time online surveying and the ability to study athletic performance via virtual reality. The internet provides sports psychology resources for experts, athletes, and related personnel worldwide to network and share insights to advance research on universal issues.

Some sports psychologists focus on individual athletes, while others study the dynamics of teams and how members communicate to achieve effective cohesiveness. Investigators collect data concerning athletes' perceptions of sports psychology and subsequent acceptance of or resistance to such efforts to improve their performances.

Sports psychologists and physicians study athletes' psychological responses to injuries and illnesses, particularly those medical conditions that halt high-profile athletic careers. They also examine psychological factors involved in rehabilitation and how athletes endure pain, deal with their temporary inability to compete, and commit to physical therapy. Health professionals are also interested in learning more about athletes who engage in substance abuse, have eating disorders, or develop mental illnesses.

Many therapists address aging-related concerns, especially as professional athletes attempt to lengthen their careers and amateur athletes seek recreational exercise during retirement. Some researchers evaluate how athletes' age, gender, and ethnicity affect the development of the psychological skills that aid athletic performances. They also study how grief and terrorism affect athletes and how exercise psychologically benefits casual exercisers.

Some sports psychologists apply techniques used for athletes to situations outside sports. Sports psychologists can improve employees' performance as consultants to corporations by teaching them cognitive restructuring and visualization methods to cope with stressful situations such as presentations. Private patients benefit from learning to focus on the process instead of the outcome and to relax with breathing methods to achieve better job performances on and off athletic fields.

—*Nyla R. Branscombe, Daniel L. Wann, Elizabeth D. Schafer, Anthony J. Fonseca*

Further Reading

Gallucci, Nicholas T. *Sport Psychology: Performance Enhancement, Performance Inhibition, Individuals, and Teams*. Psychology, 2013.

Jarvis, Matt. *Sport Psychology: A Student's Handbook*. Rev. ed., Routledge, 2006.

Lane, Andrew M., editor. *Mood and Human Performance: Conceptual, Measurement, and Applied Issues*. Nova, 2007.

Mohiyeddini, Changiz. *Contemporary Topics and Trends in the Psychology of Sports*. Nova Science, 2013.

Moran, Aidan P. *Sport and Exercise Psychology: A Critical Introduction*. Routledge, 2004.

Papaioannou, Athanasios G., and Dieter Hackfort. *Routledge Companion to Sport and Exercise Psychology: Global Perspectives and Fundamental Concepts*. Taylor, 2014.

Schinke, Robert J. *Innovative Writings in Sport and Exercise Psychology*. Nova Science, 2014.

Silva, John M., and Diane E. Stevens, editors. *Psychological Foundations of Sport*. 2nd ed., Allyn, 2002.

Singer, Robert N., et al., editors. *Handbook of Sport Psychology*. 2nd ed., Wiley, 2001.

Taylor, Jim, and Gregory S. Wilson, editors. *Applying Sport Psychology: Four Perspectives*. Human Kinetics, 2005.

Van Raalte, Judy L., and Britton W. Brewer, editors. *Exploring Sport and Exercise Psychology*. 3rd ed., APA, 2014.

Wann, Daniel L. *Sport Fans: The Psychology and Social Impact of Spectators*. Routledge, 2001.

Weinberg, Robert S., and Daniel Gould. *Foundations of Sport and Exercise Psychology*. 4th ed., Human Kinetics, 2007.

Williams, Jean M., editor. *Applied Sport Psychology: Personal Growth to Peak Performance*. 5th ed., McGraw, 2006.

Transgender Athletes: Overview

Category: Sports
Specialties and related fields: Endocrinology, general surgery, pediatrics, sports medicine
Definition: athletes with a gender identity that differs from the sex one was assigned at birth

KEY TERMS

cisgender: having a gender identity corresponding to the sex one was assigned at birth; may be shortened to "cis"

gender identity: one's inner conception of their gender, whether female, male or something else

International Association of Athletics Federation (IAAF): the organization that sets rules and regulations for international track-and-field events

International Olympic Committee (IOC): the organization that sets the rules and regulations that govern, among other things, the criteria for participation in the Olympic Games

intersex: a broad term used to describe natural variations in which individuals have sex characteristics that are not typically male or female; chromosomal differences or unusual hormone levels may cause intersex variations

sex: refers to a person's reproductive characteristics, including chromosomes, hormones, and internal and external organs

testosterone: a sex hormone, a type of androgen, an anabolic steroid that affects sexual characteristics and physical strength; typically produced in greater quantities by male bodies, testosterone can be used for hormone therapy and as a performance-enhancing drug

transgender: having a gender identity that differs from the sex one was assigned at birth; often shortened to "trans"

INTRODUCTION

For years, many international sports organizations prohibited transgender women athletes from participating in the women's divisions of elite athletic competitions. Then, in 2004 the International Olympic Committee (IOC) changed its rules to allow transgender women to compete in women's divisions for the first time. Initially, the rules required athletes to complete full surgical transition, which raised significant human rights concerns. In 2015, the IOC lifted the surgery requirement in favor of allowing hormone-only transition, further intensifying the controversy.

Some welcomed the IOC's new policy for being more inclusive of athletes across the gender spectrum. In contrast, others criticize the change because it is unfair to cisgender women, as trans women often have higher testosterone levels, which can affect strength and endurance. Both sides agree that more research is needed to understand the impact of transition on athletic performance. However, one side believes transgender athletes should be allowed to compete until it is proven that they have an unfair competitive advantage. In contrast, the other side believes they should be barred from competition until proven they do not have such an advantage.

HISTORY

Historically, professional athletics associations and elite sporting events prohibited transgender athletes from competition, particularly in women's sports divisions. The organization's stated goals were to ensure that men disguised as women did not gain an unfair advantage. However, the rules prevented transgender athletes from competing as their identified gender and caused traumatic situations for intersex athletes or those with hormonal differences.

These rules frequently involved invasive practices such as genital inspection and chromosome testing. Olympic officials at the 1936 Berlin Games requested that US runner Helen Stephens be physically examined after her record-setting performance in the 100-meter race aroused suspicion. Following World War II, the International Association of Athletics Federation (IAAF) instituted a policy requiring a physician's letter confirming the sex of all-female track-and-field athletes. The IOC followed suit in 1948. Later, anatomical checks were required to avoid the possibility of forged doctors' notes, and chromosome tests were instituted starting in the 1960s. Protests from both athletes and the medical community, based on the difficulty of clearly identifying sex in all cases, led to the discontinuation of mandatory sex testing by the end of the twentieth century; however, both the IAAF and the IOC still allowed testing in cases of reasonable suspicion.

The IOC updated its regulations in 2003 to allow transgender athletes to compete in the 2004 Olympics in Athens, Greece. However, athletes needed to have undergone genital surgery, two years of postoperative hormone therapy, and changed their gender legally to qualify. The surgical requirement, in particular, generated human rights concerns, which led the IOC to revise its policy in 2015. The new rule eliminated the legal and surgical requirements, allowing athletes to compete in women's divisions as long as their testosterone level was under a threshold value of 10 nanomoles per liter (nmol/L), near the low end of what is considered normal for a man. In theory, this allowed for more representation of transgender women in the 2016 Summer Olympics in Rio de Janeiro; in practice, no openly transgender women competed that year. The IOC's decision to remove the surgical requirement was partly motivated by the case of Chris Mosier, an American transgender man who qualified for a place on the men's national duathlon (running/biking) team in 2015.

The IOC's new policy generated mixed reactions. Many felt the change was a step in the right direction for elite transgender athletes. At the same time, some advocated for an even more inclusive policy by noting that testosterone concentration limits still exclude many athletes who identify as women. By contrast, those who criticized the new policy argued that physiological differences gave transgender women an unfair advantage, particularly for those who transitioned later and spent years training at an elite level as men, with high testosterone levels.

The biggest criticism of the IOC's policy, however, was the lack of scientific support for the 10 nmol/L threshold. A 2017 *British Journal of Sports Medicine* study conducted by Drs. Stephane Bermon and Pierre-Yves Garnier suggested that higher testosterone levels can provide performance advantages in cer-

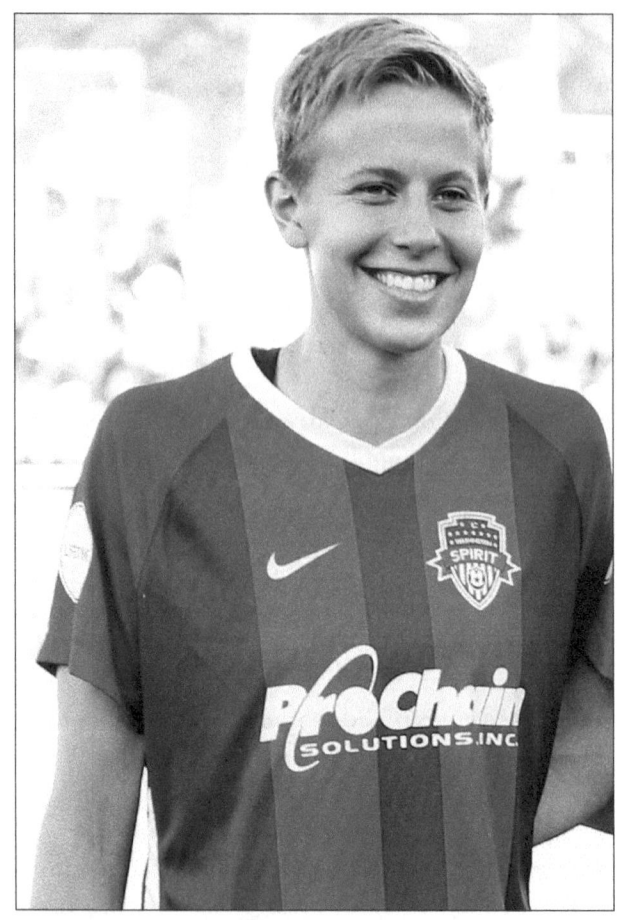

In 2021, at the 2020 Tokyo Olympics, Quinn became the first out, transgender, nonbinary athlete to compete at the Olympics, the first to medal, and the first to earn a gold medal. Photo by Jamie Smed, via Wikimedia Commons.

tain sports, particularly those involving speed and strength. Such studies bolster the argument of those who want the IOC to reduce its testosterone threshold for women still further, to 5 nmol/L. However, no decision had been made by the end of 2019.

Very few studies exist comparing elite athletes' performance before and after transition. IOC-affiliated researcher Dr. Joanna Harper noted that the most significant study so far found that the race times of trans women runners slowed significantly after transitioning. However, the study only reviewed data for eight runners and did not address any strength-related sports such as weightlifting. She believes further study is needed before making any definitive rulings.

TRANSGENDER ATHLETES TODAY

Controversy continues to build regarding the inclusion of transgender athletes—particularly trans women—in athletic events at all levels. One such controversy is USA Powerlifting's ban on transgender women athletes competing in its events at any level. This ban affected powerlifter JayCee Cooper, a trans woman who was banned from competing in USA Powerlifting events despite being qualified to compete in women's division athletics under the IOC rules. After unsuccessfully lobbying USA Powerlifting to bring its rules into line with other governing bodies' transgender policies, Cooper filed a discrimination lawsuit with the Minnesota Department of Human Rights in June 2019. By November 2019, Cooper and USA Powerlifting had agreed to mediation in hopes of resolving the case without litigation.

On the opposite side of the debate, the conservative Christian group Alliance Defending Freedom filed a legal complaint in Connecticut on behalf of three cisgender female high school runners. The June 2019 complaint challenges Connecticut's policy that high school athletes may compete in the category of the gender with which they identify without further requirement and alleges that because of this policy, nearly all the state's running titles are held by two transgender girls. In August, the US Department of Education's office for civil rights began investigating the case.

As athletes enter the qualification period for the 2020 Summer Olympics in Tokyo, Japan, debate continues over the IOC's existing and proposed rules for inclusion. The IOC rules state that male-to-female transgender athletes must undergo hormone therapy, have testosterone levels below 10 nmol/L in the year before and throughout the competition, and have declared their gender identity at least four years before the start of the competition. The IOC has been reviewing this policy and may decrease the allowed testosterone level to 5 nmol/L, which would align with the more restrictive limit maintained by the IAAF. However, September 2019 media coverage of draft proposals suggested that the IOC might keep its existing rules in place due to a lack of clear scientific support for lowering the limit and the sensitive nature of the issue.

On the national, state, and local levels, each sport's governing body has the power to establish its own rules as long as they do not run afoul of antidiscrimination laws. However, many follow the IOC's lead, so a change in the IOC's policy could impact even those transgender athletes who do not compete at the elite or international level.

—*Tracey M. DiLascio-Martinuk*

Further Reading

Fessler, Leah. "The First Transgender Athlete on Team USA Reveals How He Combats Sexism in Sports." *Quartz*, 30 Oct. 2018, qz.com/work/1408533/the-first-transgender-athlete-on-team-usa-reveals-how-he-combats-sexism-in-sports/. Accessed 27 Nov. 2019.

Harper, Joanna. "Transgender Olympians." *HuffPost*, 1 Sept. 2016, www.huffpost.com/entry/transgender-olympians_b_57c5c596e4b004ff0420e1af. Accessed 27 Nov. 2019.

Ingle, Sean. "IOC Delays New Transgender Guidelines after Scientists Fail to Agree." *The Guardian*, 24 Sept. 2019, www.theguardian.com/sport/2019/sep/24/ioc-delays-new-transgender-guidelines-2020-olympics. Accessed 27 Nov. 2019.

Megan, Kathleen. "Transgender Sports Debate Polarizes Women's Advocates." *The CT Mirror*, 22 July 2019, ctmirror.org/2019/07/22/transgender-issues-polarizes-womens-advocates-a-conundrum/. Accessed 27 Nov. 2019.

"Naturally Produced Testosterone Gives Female Athletes 'Significant' Competitive Edge." *BMJ*, 7 July 2018, www.bmj.com/company/newsroom/naturally-produced-testosterone-gives-female-athletes-significant-competitive-edge. Accessed 21 Nov. 2019.

Rogol, Alan D., and Lindsay Parks Pieper. "Genes, Gender, Hormones, and Doping in Sport: A Convoluted Tale." *Frontiers in Endocrinology*, 12 Oct. 2017, doi:10.3389/fendo.2017.00251. Accessed 27 Nov. 2019.

Sosin, Kate. "USA Powerlifting Agrees to Meditate Dispute with Trans Athlete." *NewNowNext*. Viacom International, 1 Nov. 2019, www.newnownext.com/usa-powerlifting-to-mediate-lawsuit-jaycee-cooper-trans-athlete/11/2019/. Accessed 18 Nov. 2019.

Transgender College Athletes

Category: Sports
Specialties and related fields: Endocrinology, general surgery, pediatrics, sports medicine
Definition: collegiate athletes with a gender identity that differs from the sex one was assigned at birth

KEY TERMS

cisgender: a person whose gender identity matches the sex assigned to them at birth; contrast with transgender

intersex: a person born with physical sex characteristics that do not conform to the binary male-female distinction, especially those with rare sexual phenotype-chromosome combinations or ambiguous genitalia

LGBTQ: lesbian, gay, bisexual, transgender, and queer, an initialism in use since the 1990s to refer to the nonheterosexual or noncisgender community, expanding "LGBT," which itself replaced the older and more limited term "gay community"

NCAA: the National Collegiate Athletic Association, the regulatory body for intercollegiate athletics for over 1,200 participating institutions (divided into three divisions)

Title IX: the portion of federal education law that forbids discrimination based on gender in education programs that receive federal funding

transgender: a person whose gender identity differs from the sex assigned to them at birth; a trans man was born female and has transitioned to male; a trans woman was born male and has transitioned to female

INTRODUCTION

In the twenty-first century, the first openly transgender athletes began competing in intercollegiate sports, prompting new discussions about transgender rights and their treatment in athletics, several decades after that discussion began in professional and Olympic sports. The National Collegiate Athletic Association (NCAA) adopted its first formal policy on transgender athletes in 2011. While it left out many young transgender athletes, it was a step towards greater inclusiveness, accompanied by a resource guide carefully articulating the association's commitment to diversity and explaining transgender issues.

OVERVIEW

Historically, not just in the United States but in many other countries, most school athletic competitions (and sometimes even noncompetitive programs such as gym classes) have been divided into two categories, into which participants are sorted according to their biological sex. Except for intersex individuals, biological sex is a fixed trait. In contrast,

The Transgender Pride Flag was created by American trans woman Monica Helms in 1999. Photo via iStock/Aleksei Maznychenko. [Used under license]

gender identity is neither fixed nor necessarily mapped to biological sex. Not all cisgender people—people who identify with their biological sex—easily accept this. Until the twenty-first century, popular awareness of transgender issues outside of the lesbian, gay, bisexual, transgender, and queer (LGBTQ) community was low.

Transgender college athletes have faced unique challenges in their personal lives and student-athlete careers and raised new issues for their institutions and communities. The use of tests to determine the biological sex of athletes in professional and Olympic-qualifying competitions (beginning with the International Olympic Committee [IOC] in the 1960s)—an issue on which relevant governing bodies have had shifting policies—has raised significant ethical concerns about discrimination and inclusiveness. The nature of the tests raises questions, as do the underlying assumptions about the necessity of sex-segregated athletic competition. In the twenty-first century, transgender acceptance spread enough for transgender college athletes to feel safe outing themselves and participating in sports. In contrast, a general push for better treatment of transgender individuals led to a new NCAA policy acknowledging their rights.

The first openly transgender athlete to compete in the NCAA's Division I was Kye Allums, a trans man who played for the George Washington Colonials women's basketball team at George Washington University in Washington, DC. He played for the Colonials for three seasons from 2008 through 2011, coming out as a trans man in 2010. As discussed below, the 2011 NCAA policy required trans men receiving hormone therapy to compete on men's teams. Though previously receiving testosterone treatments, Allums suspended therapy to remain on the women's team. Since graduating, Allums has been a transgender activist, visiting schools to discuss transgender rights and awareness, bullying issues, transgender athletics, and his own story. Profiled on ESPN and in Laverne Cox's documentary *The T Word*, he later revealed that the publicity from the ESPN profile contributed to stress that motivated his suicide attempt.

Another early transgender athlete competing in Division I was Schuyler Bailar, recruited by Harvard for their women's swim team in 2013. After transitioning during a post-high school gap year and coming out as a trans man, Bailar initially competed on the women's team while living as a man outside of athletic life. After experiencing stress attributed to the disconnect, on the advice of his coaches, he tried out for and was offered a spot on the men's team instead, swimming for them beginning in 2015.

FURTHER INSIGHTS

Transgender awareness has grown in the twenty-first century, but misunderstanding remains widespread. Transgender is not a sexual orientation, nor is it synonymous with cross-dressing or drag, which are activities centered on dressing as the opposite sex, but not necessarily because that sex conforms to the person's gender identity. The transgender community's association with the LGB community has more to do with common ground and common interest because of shared experiences of discrimination and exclusion and because historically, the LGB community was a welcoming subculture for transgender people when medical transitioning was impossible. (Medical transitioning remains unavailable or unaffordable for many transgender people in the twenty-first century.) Transgender is also not synonymous with intersex, a person born with physical sex characteristics that do not conform to the male/female binary. Still, transgender and intersex people face many of the same challenges in dealing with a society whose institutions traditionally enforce cisgender norms. Furthermore, intersex athletes have faced many of the same specific challenges as transgender athletes, with the burden of proving their eligibility to compete often shifted to them.

The psychiatric term for the distress, anxiety, and depression experienced by identifying with a gender other than the one assigned at birth is "gender dysphoria." Though a diagnosis of gender dysphoria is often necessary to obtain a prescription for hormone therapy to transition to the preferred gender, many people oppose the term because it contributes to the stigmatization of transgender people and the misconception that transgenderism is a mental illness. While clinical depression can, in some cases, be explained chemically—with reference purely to the patient's biology—there is an argument that gender dysphoria is simply the transgender patient's response to how society treats them and to the confusion and distress they feel from being excluded.

Because birth certificates in the United States usually list biological sex, transgender people face unique legal challenges. In some states, they cannot obtain legal identification reflecting their gender identity or even the name they have chosen for themselves. This not only presents practical day-to-day difficulties in activities other Americans take for granted (traveling, voting, banking, applying for a mortgage or a job) but also can make it impossible for them to hide their transgender status in circumstances where they must present identification. Only in the 2010s has legislation slowly begun to change in this area, and no federal law designates transgender as a protected class for the purposes of federal discrimination legislation. Less than half of US states prohibit discrimination based on gender identity.

Transgender students face significant threats of harassment and fears for their safety. According to national surveys, transgender students, staff, and faculty experience more frequent harassment on campus than LGB students, and many transgender students report fearing for their safety. Furthermore, transgender people of color report the highest levels of harassment and safety concerns.

While suicide is a concern for adolescents overall, it is of serious concern to transgender youth. A 2016 study found that thirty percent of transgender students (age twelve to twenty-two) had attempted suicide. The same study revealed that nearly two-thirds had experienced bullying, and 17 percent had repeated a grade in school. A separate study of transgender students in college found an elevated risk of suicide attempts among transgender students who are denied access to bathroom facilities or gender-segregated housing that matches their gender identity. The underlying sources of stress are a complex topic, but many transgender students describe such circumstances, and similar ones such as being addressed by the wrong pronouns, as ones that deny their identity and contribute to feelings of isolation and alienation. Further, these stresses increase the stress of gender dysphoria. One of the bases for transgender inclusion in college athletics, and specifically inclusion based on gender identity, is the belief that exclusion similarly contributes to these stresses.

ISSUES

The NCAA did not adopt a formal policy on transgender athlete participation until 2011, several years after the first-out transgender college athletes began competing. Under that policy, transgender student athletes may compete on the team of the gender with which they identify, but only if they receive hormone treatments. Furthermore, that is the only team on which they may compete. While a significant limitation, as many transgender people do not receive hormone treatments, the policy also marked a step forward by no longer deferring gender definition to participating institutions and state laws. The resource book explaining the policy to member institutions included a policy statement of transgender inclusiveness and an appendix of transgender-related terminology, signaling the association's good intentions.

While the NCAA's policy is criticized as unfairly exclusive for its emphasis on hormone treatment, it is nevertheless more inclusive and less invasive than some of the policy frameworks young athletes face. Some individual schools and states, for example, require legal documentation. Some high school athletic associations leave the decision up to a committee that investigates the petitioning student's gender before making a decision. In theory, this is meant to allow for a certain kind of flexibility rather than specifying the kind of "evidence" needed to prove gender identity, but subjects young transgender athletes to intense scrutiny at one of the most vulnerable times in their lives.

The National Intramural-Recreational Sports Association (NIRSA), which supports collegiate recreational sports, issued guidelines for transgender athletes in 2014. These guidelines were significantly more inclusive than the NCAA's. Unlike the NCAA's, NIRSA's did not use hormone treatments as the determining factor or any legal change of identity as in some states, but simply self-defined gender identity: students identifying as women are eligible to play on women's or mixed teams, and students identifying as men are eligible to play on men's or mixed teams. The policy, designed to put the least burden on transgender students, explicitly states that a student athlete's transgender status should never be disclosed without the student's permission. In further contrast with the NCAA and many other policies, the NIRSA policy acknowledges that gender identity may be fluid over time, permitting students to change the gender they identify with throughout their college career. The new NIRSA "best practices" for facilities also call for private, enclosed changing areas, showers, and toilets, and for transgender athletes to be allowed to use whichever facilities accord to their gender identity. However, in this case, best practices are suggestions, not a requirement for an institution to host a competition or exhibition associated with NIRSA.

The NCAA and NIRSA both participated in developing the Campus Pride Sports Index (hereafter "the Index"), which is maintained online at CampusSportsPrideIndex.org. The Index is a national listing of LGBTQ-friendly colleges and universities with sports programs. Launched in 2007 after six years of development, the Index intends to provide prospective students and families with an online tool for finding LGBTQ-friendly campuses while establishing national benchmarks of LGBTQ inclusiveness and supporting campus recruitment and retention efforts. The Index has since extended these original goals to address inclusion and campus safety. Institutions' profiles are based on school officials' responses to self-assessment questions in eight categories, including student and academic life, housing, campus safety, counseling and health, recruitment and retention efforts, inclusion policies, and institution commitment.

The National Association of Intercollegiate Athletics (NAIA) organizes athletic programs and competitions for small to mid-size American colleges and universities (and three Canadian members), sponsoring 25 national championships in various sports. It serves a similar function as the NCAA for smaller programs. The NAIA adopted a transgender student-athlete policy that is scheduled to go into effect as of the 2016-17 school year, mirroring the NCAA policy: trans women must complete one year of hormone treatment before competing on a women's team, while trans men taking testosterone must not compete on a women's team and may compete on the men's team only after receiving a medical exception from the NAIA's drug testing committee. Transgender athletes not taking hormone treatments are limited to the athletic teams according to their assigned birth gender.

In November 2016, the NAIA Cross Country Championships, originally scheduled to take place in Charlotte, North Carolina, were relocated in response to an ongoing boycott of North Carolina businesses in response to North Carolina House Bill 2, known as the "bathroom bill" because of its ban on transgender people using the bathroom that accords to their gender identity. The NCAA had similarly relocated championships scheduled to take place in North Carolina, and the National Basketball Association had relocated the 2016 All-Star Game, which would have been held in Charlotte.

Though Title IX protections against sex discrimination could always have been read to include protections for transgender students, this reading was made explicit by a sexual assault-specific declaration by the US Department of Education's Office of Civil Rights in 2014, which further accelerated the process of colleges and universities modifying their policies for better Title IX compliance.

The chief concern raised in opposition to the participation of transgender athletes in events according to their gender identity has been the perception that male-to-female athletes have a physical advantage over athletes born female, a concern raised at least as early as trans woman Renee Richards' successful 1977 discrimination lawsuit against the Women's Tennis Association. This concern is based on the supposition that being born male confers a greater athletic advantage, carried through to adulthood, than being born female. As the NCAA resource book and numerous authorities point out, the natural variation among both men and women is so great that it is unreasonable to expect to find such an advantage when talking about a group of highly trained and devoted athletes.

—*Bill Kte'pi*

Further Reading
Cronn-Mills, K., and A. N. Nelson. *LGBTQ+ Athletes Claim the Field: Striving for Equality*. Twenty-First Century Books, 2016.
DeWitt, P. M. *Dignity for All: Safeguarding LGBT Students*. Corwin Press, 2012.

Gleaves, J., and T. Lehrbach. "Beyond Fairness: The Ethics of Inclusion for Transgender and Intersex Athletes." *Journal of the Philosophy of Sport*, vol. 43, no. 2, 2016, pp. 311-26.

Krane, V., and K. S. Barak. "Current Events and Teachable Moments: Creating Dialog About Transgender and Intersex Athletes." *JOPERD: The Journal of Physical Education, Recreation & Dance*, vol. 83, no. 4, 2012, pp. 38-43.

Mahoney, T. Q., et al. "Progress for Transgender Athletes: Analysis of the School Success and Opportunity Act." *JOPERD: The Journal of Physical Education, Recreation & Dance*, vol. 86, no. 6, 2015, pp. 45-47.

Mayo, Cris. *LGBTQ Youth and Education: Policies and Practices*. Teachers College Press, 2013.

Michel, S. "Not Quite a First Place Finish: An Argument That Recent Title IX Policy Clarification from the United States Department of Education Does Not Adequately Protect Transgender Interscholastic Athletes." *Law & Sexuality: A Review of Lesbian, Gay, Bisexual & Transgender Legal Issues*, vol 25, 2016, pp. 145-69.

Skinner-Thompson, S., and I. M. Turner. "Title IX's Protections for Transgender Student-Athletes." *Wisconsin Journal of Law, Gender & Society*, vol. 28, no. 3, 2013, pp. 271-300.

Sparks, S. D. "Suicidality, Self-Harm, and Body Dissatisfaction in Transgender Adolescents and Emerging Adults with Gender Dysphoria." *Education Week*, vol. 36, no. 3, 2016, p. 5.

Sutton, H. "Transgender College Students More at Risk for Suicide When Denied Bathroom, Housing Rights." *Campus Security Report*, vol. 13, no. 2, 2016, p. 9.

Wahlert, L., and A. Fiester. "Gender Transports: Privileging the 'Natural' in Gender Testing Debates for Intersex and Transgender Athletes." *American Journal of Bioethics*, vol. 12, no. 7, 2012, pp. 19-21.

Zeigler, C. *Fair Play: How LGBT Athletes Are Claiming Their Rightful Place in Sports*. Akashic Books, 2016.

Ziegler, E. M., and T. I. Huntley. "'It Got Too Tough to Not Be Me': Accommodating Transgender Athletes in Sport." *Journal of College & University Law*, vol. 39, no. 2, 2013, pp. 467-509.

CAREERS

Loving both sports and science can be a great way to focus on a career that combines both. Sports is the subject of various scientific studies, university departments, and scientific journals. Careers in sports medicine and ancillary professions are examined in this section. Also highlighted is the training it takes to get into these careers. Topics include: neuroscience, cardiology, exercise science, and athletic training.

Athletic Training

Category: Careers
Specialties and related fields: Athletic trainers, life coaches, strength and conditioning coaches
Definition: an allied health-care profession recognized by the American Medical Association that encompasses the prevention, examination, diagnosis, treatment, and rehabilitation of emergent, acute, or chronic injuries and medical conditions

KEY TERMS

accreditation: the process of review and certification for athletic training programs

athletic trainer: an allied health professional who provides health care in the areas of physical medicine and rehabilitation services by preventing, assessing, and treating injuries

athletic training programs (ATEPs): collegiate education programs professionally and academically preparing athletic trainers

cognitive sequential: a learning style that prefers structured, physical hands-on tasks

Commission on Accreditation of Athletic Training Education (CAATE): the organization responsible for accrediting athletic training preparation programs and curricula

Gregorc mind styles: theory of learning styles that focuses on the cognitive skills of perception and organization

learning style: differences in how individuals successfully acquire knowledge, that is, visual, tactile, auditory

National Athletic Trainers Association (NATA): professional association for members who are certified athletic trainers and other individuals who are interested in the athletic training career

peer-assisted learning: learning which takes place by way of experiences and instruction led by or done in conjunction with students who are at the same or nearly the same academic or experiential level

reflective journaling/learning log: provides students an opportunity to ponder and reflect on an experience and to give meaning to that incident

OVERVIEW

According to the National Athletic Trainers Association (NATA), the athletic training profession is a part of the allied health field. Athletic trainers provide health care in physical medicine and rehabilitation services by helping prevent, assess, treat, and rehabilitate injuries. Athletic trainers also coordinate health care with physicians and similar health professionals like physical therapists, occupational therapists, and physicians' assistants. They typically work in high schools, colleges, professional sports, hospitals, corporations, clinics, and the military. Approximately 50 percent of certified athletic trainers are employed outside the traditional 'school' setting. Still, common employment sites are the athletic programs in colleges, universities, and secondary schools.

In the secondary school or collegiate setting, athletic trainers are often the first health professional that treats an injured athlete. Within the secondary school setting, certified athletic trainers provide important support to the athletic programs as important members of the allied health-care team since team physicians are not typically on staff for all athletic events. Athletic trainers working in a secondary school setting may be responsible for nutritional counseling, aspects of athletes' rehabilitation programs, strength and conditioning, and injury prevention and treatment (taping, bracing, etc.) pregame and prepractice.

During games and practices, athletic trainers evaluate injuries and determine whether the athlete should see a physician or if the injury can be treated and managed by the athletic training staff. The secondary school athletic trainer may be employed full-time by the school as the certified athletic trainer, they may also be a teacher in the school (e.g., physical education or health teacher), or they may be contracted to work for the high school's athletic program through a private sports medicine clinic or corporation.

The NATA, founded in 1950, is a membership association for certified athletic trainers and individuals interested in an athletic training career. The association serves to set standards and guidelines for the athletic training profession. A very active professional organization, the NATA also provides up-to-date guidelines for the treatment of frequently occurring illnesses and injuries (e.g., heat-related illness, head injuries), professional conferences, continuing education opportunities, position papers on controversial topics, information on the profession, promotion of research, legislation/political activism that will impact health care and the field of athletic training, and information targeting individuals who engage in physical activity.

Certified athletic trainers are required to earn a bachelor's degree in athletic training, have successfully passed a rigorous three-part certification examination, engage in continuing education, and adhere to the guidelines and policies set forth by the NATA. The undergraduate curriculum for athletic training education includes classroom and clinical-based education. The coursework includes the following foundation courses/subject areas: "human anatomy and physiology, kinesiology/biomechanics, nutrition, statistics, research design, strength training and reconditioning, and acute injury and illness."

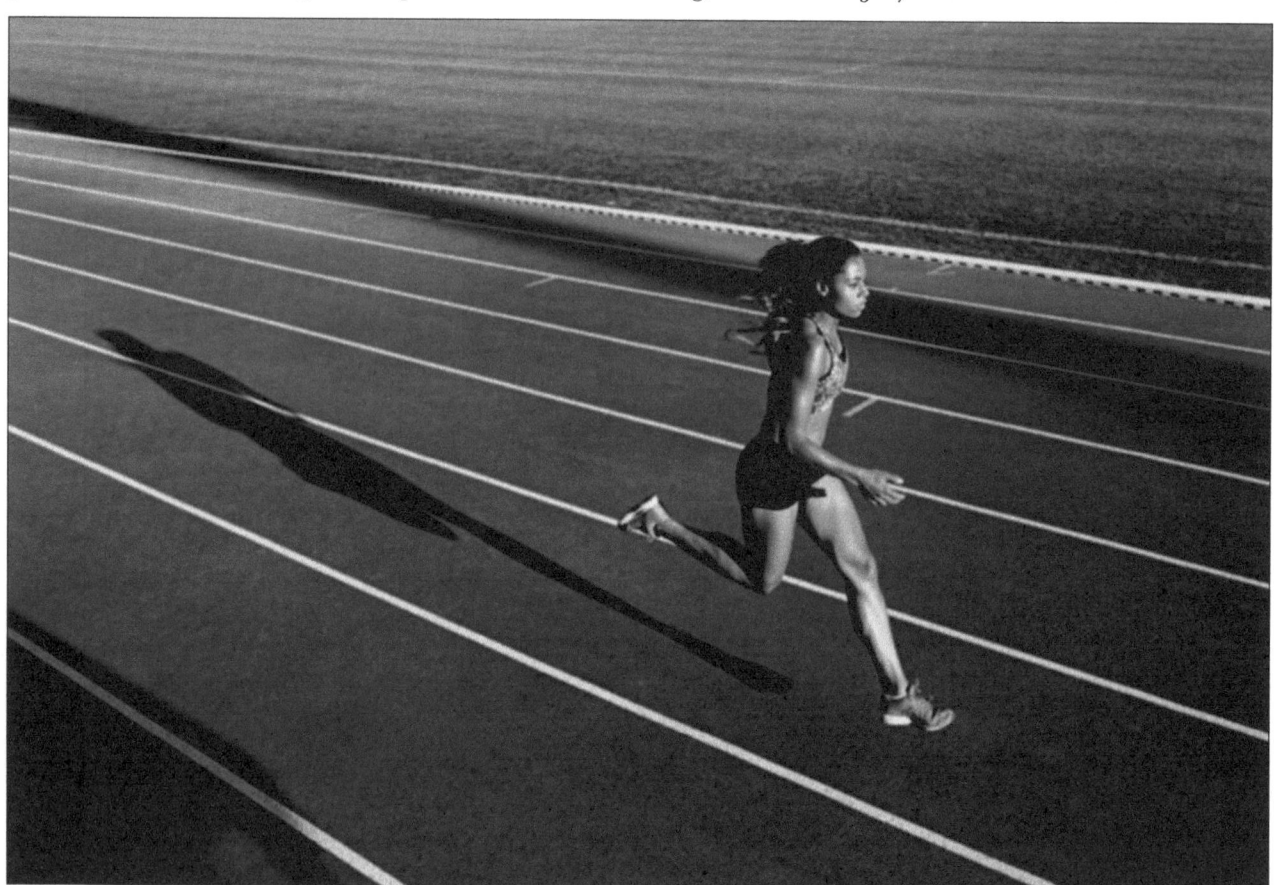

Photo via iStock/jacoblund. [Used under license.]

Students are also required to complete coursework in the professional areas of: risk management of injury/illness prevention, pathology of injury/illness, assessment of injury/illness, general medical conditions and disabilities, therapeutic modalities, therapeutic exercise and rehabilitation, health care administration, weight management and body composition, psychosocial intervention and referral, medical ethics and legal issues, pharmacology, and professional development and responsibilities.

Athletic training education programs (ATEPs) require two years of clinical setting education that includes attending to patients with general medical ailments. After students have completed their initial entry-level athletic training education through an accredited program, they may sit for the Board of Certification, Inc. Examination to become an Athletic Trainer, Certified (ATC). The examination process ensures that students are educated and trained in "prevention, recognition, evaluation, and assessment, immediate care, treatment, rehabilitation, and reconditioning, organization and administration, and professional development."

While the NATA and Board of Certification, Inc. both provide professional preparation and ethical guidelines for the profession of athletic training, the Commission on Accreditation of Athletic Training Education (CAATE) is an independent organization that is responsible for accrediting and monitoring athletic training education/preparation programs and their curricula. The CAATE aims to "develop, maintain, and promote appropriate minimum quality standards of entry-level Athletic Training education programs."

For an institution's athletic training program to become accredited, the institution must successfully meet a rigorous set of standards including, but not limited to, institutional sponsorship, appropriate and sufficient staffing (including program director and clinical instruction staff), a physician who acts as a consultant to the program, sufficient support and administrative staff, financial resources, physical resources (i.e., facilities, equipment, clinic), operational plan and policies, and curriculum design and course development. These standards are to be met and documented in the comprehensive review process, including an extensive self-study report and on-site visit to verify the self-study report and decide how well the program meets the standards set by the CAATE.

After the on-site visit, a report of the findings from the visit is submitted to the program. They must submit a rejoinder outlining and responding to each point of deficiency noted by the initial visit report. Once accreditation application materials are submitted, the application review process takes approximately one year. Athletic training education programs may or may not be fully accredited. Accreditation is valid for five years, and continuing accreditation for seven years. The CAATE may place programs on "probation, withholding, withdrawing accreditation, and [allowing] voluntary accreditation withdrawal."

Many departments may house undergraduate and graduate athletic training programs, including exercise science, kinesiology, sports science, sports medicine, physical education, or health science. Athletic training education programs demand students' time and commitment due to the extended hours days students must complete once in the clinical setting.

Undergraduate students typically complete foundation coursework and must meet set standards (e.g., a specific grade point average minimum, letters of recommendation) to advance to the clinical site portion of their academic preparation. Students may, for example, complete clinical work with the college or university's athletic teams, with local high school athletic programs, or in physical therapy/sports medicine clinics under the supervision of physicians and certified athletic trainers. While the athletic training education program focuses on the foundation and professional coursework and the clinical education components, the profession and its professional preparation programs are still faced with challenges in promoting professional and ethical development, different student learning styles, and effective teaching methods.

PROFESSIONAL DEVELOPMENT
Once an athletic training student has completed the academic preparation, they sit for the Board of Certification examination and start their first professional position; it is of the utmost importance that the athletic trainer is competent and confident enough to make ethical and professional decisions. The professional leap between working in a clinical setting with faculty and mentor supervision to being a certified athletic trainer in the "real world" can challenge new athletic trainers.

To assist the transition, athletic training education program directors and faculty can set forth guidelines and policies to assist student professional development. Faculty and advisors should act as role models for their students by displaying appropriate ethical and professional behavior. Some formal experiences that colleges and universities can also implement into an athletic training program include:

- *Athletic training student organization*: By creating an athletic training student organization, the program faculty can promote students' responsibility, management, and organization skills by maintaining the student organization. These student organizations may be designed to meet the needs and goals of the student group, which may be attained through community volunteering opportunities, sponsoring workshops, fund-raising events, maintaining a budget, and assisting and encouraging students to attend professional conferences.
- *A "professional-points" program*: This program sets a requirement for the minimum number of points athletic training students must earn through volunteering and working at various athletic training-related events and requires students to maintain current membership in the NATA each year. Awards are given to students who exceed the minimum requirements. Students who do not meet the minimum requirements are penalized by having all course grades lowered by one level.
- *Student-mentor program*: Student-mentor programs provide mentorship to beginning athletic training students from junior and senior students who serve as mentors. The mentors assist newer students in their clinical observations, signing off on their clinical hours, guiding students through the educational process, and evaluating their professional behavior. The new athletic training students are provided with the opportunity to observe appropriate professional behavior and have another student serve as an athletic training program "guide."
- *Journal club*: Faculty encourages students to continue this practice after graduation by providing them with the tools, confidence, and interest in continuing their education through staying current in the field. These suggestions for student professional development illustrate how faculty can successfully and effectively incorporate professional development into the curriculum.

STUDENT LEARNING STYLES AND TEACHING METHODS
An important topic in athletic training education is how students learn concepts, theories, and practices essential to the academic preparation of athletic trainers. Scientific research in these areas is increasing as research is being conducted to identify the learning styles of athletic training students, and what learning methods are effective and provide new insights into traditional teaching methods. Athletic training programs have incorporated the clinical portion of the education program to provide stu-

dents with hands-on practice and learning in their chosen field of study. Scientific research has lent support to the inclusion of the clinical learning environment; however, more recently, scholars have suggested the need for athletic training educators to consider student learning styles and how these impact teaching methods in all areas of the professional preparation process. Listed below is a selection of learning and teaching research and methods.

Peer-assisted learning is a practice that athletic training educators have used in a clinical setting that houses students who learn how to work together to learn, practice, or teach. Research in allied health fields has shown that students experience a lower level of anxiety and stress when working with their fellow students rather than clinical instructors, improved organizational skills, increased confidence in their ability to make decisions, improved proficiency test scores, and improved leadership skills. However, this type of research has been limited in the athletic training field.

Henning, Weidner, and Jones researched the effects of peer-assisted learning in the athletic training clinical setting. This research indicated that students reported that they enhanced and refined their understanding of their clinical skills based on interactions with their peers. These interactions included working with peers on clinical skills and receiving feedback on skill demonstrations.

This feedback appeared beneficial because faculty and mentors provided it immediately in the learning environment. Yet, the results indicated that the athletic training students did not view this feedback as more effective or helpful than clinical instructors' feedback. Students also reported a decrease in anxiety and stress when working with their peers on practicing skills than when they were required to practice skills in the company of their clinical instructors. This research supports the implementation or continuation of peer-assisted learning in the athletic training education program.

In the clinical setting, athletic training students must practice and learn clinical skills that they will eventually have to recall and perform independently. By practicing with peers, students can gain confidence in their abilities to execute the clinical skills before testing for proficiency under the direction of their instructor. Henning and her colleagues also suggest that peer-assisted learning provides a unique opportunity for the more experienced or advanced students to teach clinical skills to newer students. This exercise requires the advanced students to demonstrate their ability to synthesize the information needed for the skill and articulate that information to the learner. Peer-assisted learning in the clinical setting can complement instruction being provided in a manner that is effective for the learning styles of each student.

Gould & Caswell researched what learning styles athletic training students prefer based on Gregorc mind styles. This research indicated that these students prefer a cognitive sequential learning style. As defined by the Gregorc mind style model utilized by the researchers, the cognitive sequential style of learning indicates that the athletic training students prefer a structured environment that involves hands-on activities.

Given the nature of the athletic training profession, this finding is not astonishing. Yet, due to the limited amount of research conducted on learning styles, this finding supports the continuation and extension of this type of research. Based on their findings, Gould and Caswell suggest that athletic training educators should focus on providing opportunities for hands-on activities through simulations and breakout sessions. This finding also suggests that peer-assisted learning in the clinical setting should be accompanied by well-prepared and structured instruction.

The use of reflective journaling/learning logs in clinical athletic training allows students to reflect on an experience outside of the moment in which the situation occurred. By reflective journaling after the moment has passed, students can analyze and comment on a situation and the decisions that were made or not made without the emotion of the moment clouding the critical evaluation and thought process. This reflective opportunity extends the learning situation beyond the moment of the situation to maximize learning. Reflective journaling in athletic training education helps students develop their critical thinking and problem-solving skills while deepening their level of understanding.

Kaiser noted that reflective journals/learning logs serve as documentation of student progression. Students can learn from mistakes and how to empathize, observe, and identify those incidents that are critical to their learning and the field of athletic training. Through self-expression, athletic training students develop personally and reduce stress by allowing themselves an opportunity to relieve tension or frustration. Clinical instructors can evaluate reflective journals through a pass/fail system by skimming and responding to select passages and peer-reviewing with instructor criteria.

Athletic training has become an allied health-care profession through the field's professionalization. The creation of the NATA in 1950 provided professional support and guidance to athletic trainers and those groups or individuals interested in the field. Through the accreditation process, undergraduate and graduate-level athletic training programs are required to develop curricula that align with the standards set forth by the CAATE. Research on the teaching methods and learning techniques of athletic training students can provide faculty and staff insight into how to more effectively deliver the course material to meet the needs of the students in the classroom and clinical setting.

—*Shelby L. Hinkle Smith*

Further Reading

"2020 Standards for Accreditation of Professional Athletic Training Programs." *Commission on Accreditation of Athletic Training Education,* Jan. 2018, caate.net/wp-content/uploads/2018/09/2020-Standards-for-Professional-Programs-copyedited-clean.pdf. Accessed 27 May 2022.

"Accreditation Application Process." *Commission on Accreditation of Athletic Training Education*, 2022, caate.net/accreditation-application-process/. Accessed 27 May 2022.

"Athletic Training." *National Athletic Trainers Association (NATA)*, 2022, www.nata.org/about/athletic-training. Accessed 27 May 2022.

"Athletic Training." *Troy University*, 2022, www.troy.edu/academics/academic-programs/graduate/athletic-training.html. Accessed 27 May 2022.

"Education Overview." *National Athletic Trainers Association (NATA)*, 2022, www.nata.org/about/athletic-training/education-overview. Accessed 27 May 2022.

Gardiner, A., and J. M. Mensch. "Promoting Professional Development in Athletic Training." *Athletic Therapy Today*, vol. 9, 2004, pp. 30-31.

Gould, T. E., and S. V. Caswell. "Stylistic Learning Differences between Undergraduate Athletic Training Students and Educators: Gregorc Mind Styles." *Journal of Athletic Training*, vol. 41, 2006, pp. 109-16.

Henning, J. M., et al. "Peer-Assisted Learning in the Athletic Training Clinical Setting." *Journal of Athletic Training*, vol. 41, 2006, pp. 102-8.

Kaiser, D. A. "Using Reflective Journals in Athletic Training Clinical Education." *Athletic Therapy Today*, vol. 9, 2004, pp. 41.

Mestre, L. S. "Matching Up Learning Styles with Learning Objects: What's Effective?" *Journal of Library Administration*, vol. 50, no. 7/8, 2010, pp. 808-29.

"Physical Education." *Play and Playground Encyclopedia*, 2022, www.pgpedia.com/p/physical-education. Accessed 27 May 2022.

Robles, J., et al. "The Impact of Preceptor and Student Learning Styles on Experiential Performance Measures." *American Journal of Pharmaceutical Education*, vol. 76, 2012, pp. 1-7.

Wilson, M. L. "Learning Styles, Instructional Strategies, and the Question of Matching: A Literature Review." *International Journal of Education*, vol. 4, 2012, pp. 67-87.

Cardiology

Category: Specialty
Specialties and related fields: Emergency medicine, preventive medicine, vascular medicine
Definition: the branch of medicine concerned with the diagnosis and treatment of diseases of the heart and the coronary arteries, including arteriosclerosis, hypertension, and congenital disabilities

KEY TERMS

acute: referring to the onset of a disease process
chronic: referring to a lingering disease process
coronary arteries: the two arteries that surround the heart and supply the heart muscle with oxygen and nutrients
heart attack: the common term for a myocardial infarction
heart failure: a condition in which the heart pumps inefficiently, allowing fluid to back up into the lungs or body tissue
sudden cardiac death: a situation in which the heart stops beating or beats irregularly, stopping blood flow

SCIENCE AND PROFESSION

Cardiology is the study of the heart and its various diseases: inflammation of the heart muscle, diseases of the heart valves, atherosclerosis, and arteriosclerosis (*athero* meaning "deposits of soft material," *arterio* meaning "pertaining to the arteries," and *sclerosis* meaning "hardening"), and congenital disabilities. This field also concerns related diseases, such as hypertension (high blood pressure) and certain renal, endocrine, and lung disorders.

The heart contains four chambers, the right and left atria on top and the right and left ventricles below. The heart walls are three layers of tissue: the outer layer, the epicardium; the middle layer, the myocardium; and an inner layer, the endocardium, which includes the heart valves. The heart is contained in a protective sac, the pericardium.

The pumping of the heart is a coordinated contraction. The right atrium receives blood from the veins and contracts, pumping blood through the tricuspid valve into the right ventricle. The right ventricle then contracts, pumping blood through the pulmonary valve into the lungs, where it gives up carbon dioxide and receives oxygen. Blood enters the left atrium and travels through the mitral valve to the left ventricle. The blood then enters the venous system into the venules (tiny veins that lead to larger veins) and finally to one of the two branches of the vena cava: the superior vena cava from the upper part of the body and the inferior vena cava from the lower. They connect outside the heart and bring blood back into the right atrium.

The heartbeat, the rhythmic contraction of the heart muscle, is controlled by the conduction system. Electrochemical impulses cause muscle fibers to contract, pumping blood through the chambers and relax, letting the chambers fill again. The contractions are initiated by specialized "pacemaker" tissues in the sinoatrial (S-A) or sinus node, in the junction of the superior vena cava and the right atrium. The pacemaker signal travels to the atrioventricular (A-V) node near the tricuspid valve. The impulse crosses the A-V node and travels to the bundle of His, specialized fibers that carry it to the ventricles.

Virtually every part of the heart is subject to disease: each layer of the heart muscle, each valve, each chamber, and the coronary arteries. The coronary arteries are quite small and are subject to plaque accumulation on their inner walls, a condition known as "atherosclerosis." This plaque can be cholesterol, scar tissue, clotted blood, or calcium. As the plaque accumulates, the artery narrows, reducing blood flow into the heart muscle. The reduction in blood flow reduces the heart's oxygen supply, causing myocardial ischemia (lack of blood). There is usually a signal of pain called "angina pectoris" (*angina*

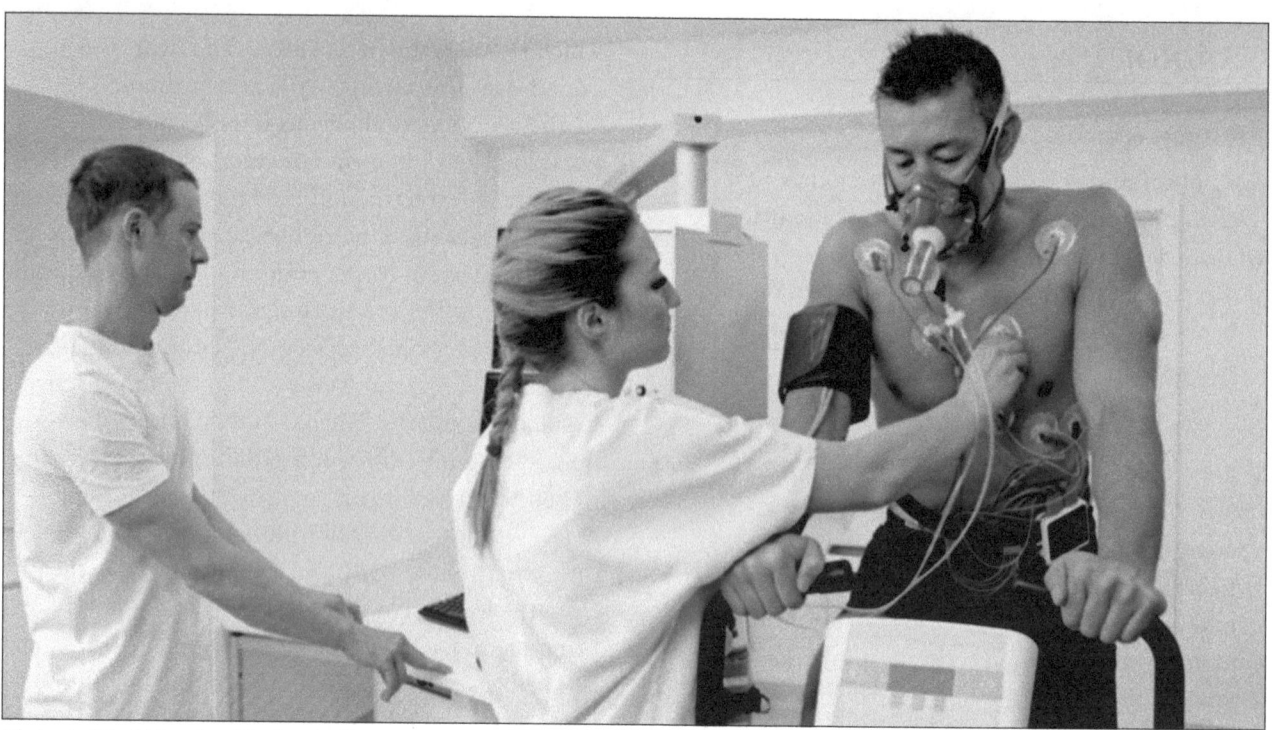

Photo via iStock/simonkr. [Used under license.]

meaning "choking pain" and *pectoris* meaning "of the chest"). Often, the patient feels a tightening in the chest with a sharp pain behind the sternum. The pain can radiate into either arm or the jaw. It is usually caused by overexertion, exposure to cold, stress, or overeating.

As a rule, an attack of angina pectoris lasts only a few minutes and is relieved by rest. Still, it can signal the beginning of a heart attack. In addition, coronary arteries contain muscle fibers that can go into spasms and tighten, reducing blood flow into the heart. This condition, too, can cause anginal pain, heart attack, and death. Some patients who have myocardial ischemia do not have anginal pain. This event is known as "silent ischemia." It is usually discovered only with an electrocardiogram (ECG) or exercise stress test.

There are four major classes of angina pectoris: stable angina, in which pain begins when the heart's need for oxygen exceeds the amount that it receives; unstable angina, which is significantly more serious than stable angina; variant angina, which is characterized by chest pain at rest and may be caused by spasm of the coronary arteries; and postinfarction angina, unstable angina that appears after acute myocardial infarction.

When atherosclerotic plaque builds up in the coronary arteries, the vessel's inner lining becomes rough. As a result, a blood clot (thrombus) can form on the plaque, narrowing the vessel or clogging it completely (coronary thrombosis). When this occurs, blood flow to parts of the heart is stopped, and heart cells die from lack of oxygen. This condition is medically known as "myocardial infarction" (from *infarct*, meaning "an area of dead cells"). It is commonly known as a "heart attack."

The prognosis for patients who survive a heart attack is variable. In two-thirds of patients, spontaneous thrombolysis (the dissolution of the blood clot) starts to occur within twenty-four hours. However, about half of heart attack patients will develop postinfarction angina, which usually indicates severe, multivessel coronary artery disease.

Diseases of the conduction system can result in arrhythmias or disturbances in the regularity of the heartbeat. Arrhythmias can be relatively benign or severely restrict the patient's physical activity. They can also cause sudden cardiac death. The most common arrhythmias are bradycardia, an excessively slow heartbeat, and tachycardia, an unduly fast heartbeat.

Normally, the chambers beat in synchronization with each other. In some arrhythmias, the chambers of the heart beat out of synchronization. These arrhythmias include atrial fibrillation, paroxysmal atrial tachycardia, ventricular tachycardia, and ventricular fibrillation. In atrial fibrillation, the atria beat very rapidly (three hundred beats per minute), out of synchronization with the ventricles. When the condition is prolonged, blood clots may form in the atria and may be carried to the cerebral vessels, where they cause a stroke or the stoppage of blood flow in a blood vessel. With paroxysmal atrial tachycardia, a disturbance in the conduction of the A-V node causes the heart to beat up to two hundred fifty times a minute. The condition is usually not serious, but fainting or heart failure could develop if it persists. Ventricular tachycardia exists when ectopic, or irregular, beats develop in the ventricular muscle; if they go on, blood pressure falls. In ventricular fibrillation, the leading cause of sudden cardiac death, ventricular contractions are weak, ineffective, and uncoordinated. Blood flow stops, and the patient faints. If the condition is not corrected, the patient can die in minutes.

Heart block can be another consequence of conduction disease. If for various reasons, all the impulses from the sinus node do not pass through the A-V node and the bundle of His, the result is one of three degrees of heart block. First-degree heart block, which is not apparent to the patient, appears on the ECG as a delay in the impulse from the atria to the ventricles. Second-degree heart block occurs when some of the impulses from the atria fail to reach the ventricles. Often, the result is an irregular pulse. This condition can be attributable to a certain heart drug and may disappear when the drug is discontinued. In third-degree heart block, impulses from the pacemaker tissues fail to reach the ventricles. A lower pacemaker assumes the function of stimulating contractions of the ventricles in an "escape rhythm." When this occurs in third-degree heart block, the heart rate often slows down so precipitously that blood flow to the brain and other organs are severely restricted. Dizziness and loss of consciousness may follow. Heart block can also result from a congenital disability, inflammation, myocardial infarction, or other causes.

Disorders in the valves of the heart are most often caused by congenital disabilities or the effects of rheumatic fever. Streptococcal bacteria cause rheumatic fever, which usually begins with a throat infection. Rheumatic fever may develop if this "strep throat" is not treated soon. Acute rheumatic fever is associated with mitral or aortic valve insufficiency (leakage). Chronic rheumatic heart disease can include mitral or aortic stenosis (narrowing). Valves are scarred with fibrous tissue or calcific (calcium-containing) deposits that cause the valve openings to become narrower.

Mitral stenosis usually develops slowly. Ten to twenty years after rheumatic fever, the valve narrows so much that blood flow from the atrium into the ventricle is impeded. As blood accumulates in the left atrium, the pressure within the atrium increases, and the chamber becomes enlarged. Blood is forced back into the lungs, resulting in pulmonary edema (fluid in the lungs). Blood vessels in the lungs become engorged; the increased pressure forces fluid into the air sacs. Symptoms of mitral stenosis include shortness of breath, fatigue, feelings of suffocation, wheezing, agitation, and anxiety. In severe cases, fluid may also accumulate in the lower extremities. Mitral stenosis can also cause atrial fibrillation, generating potentially lethal blood clots.

Mitral "regurgitation" (or insufficiency), another mitral valve disorder, can be due to rheumatic fever or other causes. The valve fails to close completely during left ventricle contraction. Blood leaks back into the left atrium, and blood flow into the aorta is reduced. The heart has to work harder to pump blood into the body. Mitral regurgitation may lead to enlargement of the left atrium and left ventricle. Pulmonary edema, shortness of breath, fatigue, and palpitations are late symptoms of severe disease.

Still another disorder is mitral valve prolapse, which can also result in mitral regurgitation. The mitral valve consists of two leaflets of tissue that fall apart to open and come together to close. Prolapse occurs when either or both of these leaflets bulge into the left atrium, as occurs in a significant percentage of the population whose valves consist of "floppy" (myxomatous) tissue. The condition is usually of little clinical significance. Still, some patients experience palpitations and chest pain, and some have a heart murmur. In rare cases, significant valve leakage occurs, requiring surgery.

The aortic valve consists of three leaflets or "cusps" that can become fused, calcified, or otherwise compromised because of rheumatic fever or a congenital heart defect. The opening narrows, and blood flow into the aorta is reduced. Pressure increases inside the left ventricle, causing it to pump harder. The wall of the left ventricle thickens, a condition called "ventricular hypertrophy." Symptoms include heart murmur, weakness, fatigue, anginal pain, breathlessness, and fainting. Aortic stenosis may not be evident until it is quite advanced.

Tricuspid stenosis and regurgitation are relatively rare, as is pulmonary regurgitation. However, pulmonary or pulmonic valve stenosis is a common congenital heart defect. There is a characteristic heart murmur produced by turbulence of blood through the narrow pulmonary valve—pressure increases in the right ventricle. Fainting and heart failure are possible in severe cases.

In congestive heart failure, the heart pumps inefficiently, failing to deliver blood to the body and allowing blood to back up into the veins. It may occur on the left or the right side, or both. If the left side of the heart is pumping inefficiently, blood flows back into the lungs, causing pulmonary edema. Suppose the right side of the heart is inefficient. In that case, blood seeps back into the legs, resulting in edema of the extremities. Blood can also back up into the liver and the kidneys, resulting in engorgement and reduced arterial flow that prevent these organs from getting the nutrition and oxygen they need. The most common cause of heart failure is ischemic cardiomyopathy due to coronary artery disease, other cardiomyopathies, and valvular disease.

Cardiomyopathy refers to diseases of the myocardium. There are many possible causes, including "end-stage" coronary artery disease; infectious agents such as fungi, viruses, and parasites; overconsumption of alcohol; or genetic defects. The three main classes of cardiomyopathy are dilated congestive cardiomyopathy, hypertrophic cardiomyopathy, and restrictive cardiomyopathy. In dilated congestive cardiomyopathy, all the heart chambers (diffuse) or some but not all chambers are involved (nondiffuse). The cause of this class of cardiomyopathy is usually ischemia. Still, viral infection (myocarditis), drugs, alcohol, and nonviral diseases may be responsible. The heart pumps inefficiently, causing fatigue, breathlessness, and edema in the lower extremities. The heart chambers may enlarge, and blood clots may form. With hypertrophic cardiomyopathy, the myocardium thickens and reduces the left ventricle cavity, so blood flow into the aorta is reduced. The condition is usually chronic, with fainting, fatigue, and breathlessness symptoms. Restrictive cardiomyopathy is rare. The heart muscle loses elasticity and cannot expand to fill with blood between contractions. Symptoms include edema, breathlessness, and atrial and ventricular arrhythmias.

The endocardium and the pericardium can inflate because of infection or injury, resulting in endocarditis or pericarditis. Bacterial endocarditis usually affects abnormal valves and heart structures that have been damaged by rheumatic fever or congenital disabilities. Fulminant (sudden and severe) infections can destroy normal heart valves, especially with intravenous drug abuse. The symptoms of bacterial endocarditis are fever, weight loss, malaise, night sweats, fatigue, and heart murmurs. The condition can be fatal if the invading organism is not eradicated. Nonbacterial thrombotic endocarditis or noninfective endocarditis arises from the formation of thrombi on cardiac valves and endocardium caused by trauma, immune complexes, or vascular disease. Pericarditis often occurs concomitantly with, or due to, viral respiratory infection. The inflamed pericardium rubs against the epicardium, causing acute pain. Large amounts of fluid may develop and press on the heart in "cardiac tamponade." This condition can impede heart action and blood flow and can be life-threatening. In constrictive pericarditis, the pericardium becomes thicker and contracts. This action prevents the heart chambers from filling, decreasing the amount of blood drawn into the heart and pumped out to the body.

Primary cardiac tumors, those originating in the heart, are rare. While usually benign, they can have fatal complications. Malignant tumors also occur, and metastasis (movement of cancer cells throughout the body) may bring malignancies to the heart.

Congenital heart defects occur in approximately eight in every 1,000 live births. The most common is a ventricular septal defect, a hole in the wall between the ventricles. A loud murmur upon auscultation helps detect it. An atrial septal defect is common but rarely leads to symptoms until the third decade of life.

DIAGNOSTIC AND TREATMENT TECHNIQUES

The stethoscope, ECGs, and X-rays are basic tools that the cardiologist uses to diagnose heart conditions. By listening to heart sounds through the stethoscope, the physician can learn much about the status of heart function, particularly heart rhythm, congenital disabilities, and valve dysfunction.

Electrocardiogram patterns of electrical impulses help the physician discover chamber enlargement and other cardiac abnormalities. The ECG is attached to a patient running on a treadmill or riding an apparatus similar to a bicycle in a stress test. The test assesses the exercise tolerance of patients with coronary artery disease and other conditions.

The chest X-ray provides a picture of the size and configuration of the heart, the aorta, the pulmonary arteries, and related structures. It can detect enlarged chambers and vessels and other disorders. In some cases, radioactive isotopes are injected into the patient. A scanner reads the patterns they form in the heart and surrounding arteries to help the physician diagnose. The echocardiogram uses ultrasound to outline heart chambers and detect abnormalities within them and the myocardium. It is also used to analyze patterns of blood flow.

The cardiologist's more sophisticated instruments include fast-computed tomography, called "cine-CT," allowing the physician to visualize heart activity. Magnetic resonance imaging (MRI), MR spectroscopy, and positron emission tomography (PET) scanning help cardiologists investigate heart function and anatomy.

These techniques and procedures are conducted outside the body. Sometimes it is necessary, however, to go into the body. One such technique is diagnostic catheterization with angiography. A thin, flexible tube (catheter) is inserted into a blood vessel in the groin or arm and threaded into a coronary artery or the heart. Pressures and blood oxygen are measured in the heart chambers. A radiopaque dye is then injected through the catheter. The inside of the artery or the heart becomes visible to the X-ray. It is recorded on film (a process sometimes called "cineangiography"). Angiography can also be used with radioactive isotopes. The radiation detected by a scanner can help the physician discover abnormalities in the coronary arteries and the heart.

Diagnosis of angina pectoris is usually based upon the patient's complaint of chest pain. An ECG can help confirm the diagnosis. Yet many patients with coronary artery disease have normal ECGs at rest, so stress testing with the ECG is more reliable. Patients may be given pharmacologic stress tests if they cannot do physical exercise.

Drug therapy for coronary artery disease and angina pectoris aims to keep the coronary arteries open and avoid myocardial ischemia. Primary among the drugs used is nitroglycerin, taken under the tongue or in a transdermal (through-the-skin) patch or, in emergencies, intravenously. Many nitrate compounds fulfill similar functions. Beta-adrenergic blocking agents, or beta-blockers, decrease heart rate and blood pressure, reducing the heart's oxygen requirement and workload, thus reducing the incidence of angina. Some serious arrhythmias are also suppressed. Calcium-channel blockers dilate coronary arteries and maintain coronary blood flow while decreasing blood pressure, reducing heart work, and stabilizing heart rhythm. Angiotensin-converting enzyme (ACE) inhibitors help relax the blood vessels, reducing blood pressure. Cholesterol-lowering medications help reduce the amount of cholesterol in the blood, thereby reducing plaque deposits and helping to prevent atherosclerosis. Low-dose aspirin and other blood thinners can also help reduce the risk of obstruction of the coronary arteries by blood clots.

If coronary artery disease progresses to the point where there is a risk of myocardial infarction, various catheter and surgical procedures may be considered. Coronary angioplasty is used to open a clogged artery mechanically. The cardiologist threads a catheter with a tiny balloon into the clogged artery and inflates the balloon at the site of the blockage. This procedure is repeated until the vessel is open. A stent may be inserted into the artery to help prevent future blockages. Coronary artery bypass surgery is another procedure used when coronary arteries are blocked. The surgeon takes sections of vein or artery from another part of the body and implants them between the aorta and the heart, creating new coronary arteries and bypassing clogged ones.

When clogged coronary arteries cause a myocardial infarction, the patient should be treated in a special medical facility, preferably in a coronary care unit (CCU). Heart attacks rarely begin in the hospital, so the medical team must keep the patient alive during their trip to the CCU. Primary ventricular fibrillation is the greatest danger, and it must be corrected immediately by medication or electrical defibrillation. Sometimes heart block and profound bradycardia occur, which could cause a drop in blood pressure that could, in turn, cause cardiac arrest.

Emergency myocardial infarction treatment aims to ease discomfort, minimize the mass of infarcted myocardial tissue, reduce heart work, stabilize heart rhythm, and maintain oxygen perfusion throughout the body by regulating blood pressure. The CCU's treatment and medications include continuous ECG monitoring (both during and after the heart attack), oxygen, nitroglycerin, antiarrhythmic agents, analgesics for pain, and thrombolytic agents to dissolve clots, diuretics, agents to treat shock, and sedatives. Cardiologists may also use beta-blockers, calcium-channel blockers, anticoagulants, and antianxiety drugs.

About 60 percent of patients who have suffered from myocardial infarction develop congestive heart failure. The cardiologist uses dietary instruction and medication to treat congestive heart failure from heart attacks or other causes. The three most commonly prescribed drugs are diuretics to reduce edema, digitalis (digoxin or digitoxin) to increase the force of the heart's contraction, and vasodilators to reduce the resistance of blood vessel walls to facilitate blood flow and reduce heart work. Salt restriction is recommended to reduce edema. Intractable congestive heart failure may be a reason for a heart transplant.

The main goals of therapy for cardiac arrhythmias are to improve heart function and prevent sudden cardiac death. Drug therapy must be individualized to correct the particular arrhythmia. Digitalis, procainamide, amiodarone, and atropine are often used. Beta-blockers and calcium-channel blockers are also helpful in stabilizing heart rhythm. If a heart block becomes severe, an artificial pacemaker is implanted in the chest to regulate the heartbeat.

Disorders of the heart valves are not usually treated with drugs. While awaiting surgery, it may be necessary to treat heart failure or the effects of valve disease in other parts of the body. For example, diuretics may be required to reduce edema, an antiarrhythmic agent may be needed to control atrial fibrillation, or anticoagulants may be used to prevent blood clots. Some stenotic valves can be opened using a modification of the balloon catheter technique, or surgical reconstruction may be possible. Often, it is necessary to replace the valve with a new one made of human or porcine tissue or with a mechanical valve.

Pulmonary edema is a severe form of heart failure and is life-threatening. Medications are given to relieve pulmonary congestion. In emergencies, oxygen is given, in severe cases, by inserting a breathing tube into the patient's trachea. If the heart's pumping action is compromised, digitalis or another medication can strengthen the contractility of the heart.

In treating dilated cardiomyopathy, the cardiologist uses appropriate medications, including diuretics, vasodilators, antiarrhythmic agents, and digitalis. Alcohol restriction is required.

Patients with congenital or valvular heart disease are at high risk for cardiac and valve infection. They are given preventive antibiotic therapy before undergoing surgical or dental procedures. If bacteria or other microorganisms are involved, appropriate antibiotic therapy must be instituted to eradicate the cause.

In acute pericarditis, if excessive fluid builds up, pericardiocentesis may be performed to drain the fluid between the pericardium and the heart wall. In cardiac tamponade, pericardiocentesis may be lifesaving. In chronic constrictive pericarditis, an operation may be necessary to remove tissue that has stiffened and strangled the heart.

PERSPECTIVE AND PROSPECTS
Cardiology is a major medical specialty because heart disease is the leading cause of death worldwide. Today's cardiologist turns increasingly to preventive medicine to reduce morbidity (the relative incidence of a disease) and mortality. These measures include programs against smoking and programs advocating cholesterol reduction, stress reduction, increased exercise, and other measures that have been found useful in preventing heart disease.

Ongoing studies continue to accumulate data on increasingly large populations in more and more countries. Links between behavior, habits, nutrition, and ecology may be found to give a clearer picture of how to prevent and treat heart disease. Increased knowledge will improve diagnosis and treatment, improving patient care and the quality of life for heart disease sufferers.

—*C. Richard Falcon*

Further Reading

Baum, Seth J. *The Total Guide to a Healthy Heart: Integrative Strategies for Preventing and Reversing Heart Disease.* Kensington, 2000.

Bonow, Robert O., et al., editors. *Braunwald's Heart Disease: A Textbook of Cardiovascular Medicine.* 9th ed., Elsevier-Saunders, 2011.

"Coronary Artery Disease—Coronary Heart Disease." *American Heart Association*, 31 July 2015, www.heart.org/en/health-topics/consumer-healthcare/what-is-cardiovascular-disease/coronary-artery-disease. Accessed 2 June 2022.

Crawford, Michael H., editor. *Current Diagnosis and Treatment-Cardiology.* 4th ed., McGraw-Hill Medical, 2013.

Eagle, Kim A., and Ragavendra R. Baliga, editors. *Practical Cardiology: Evaluation and Treatment of Common Cardiovascular Disorders.* 2nd ed., Lippincott Williams & Wilkins, 2008.

"Heart Surgery Overview." *Texas Heart Institute*, n.d., www.texasheart.org/heart-health/heart-information-center/topics/a-heart-surgery-overview/. Accessed 2 June 2022.

Litin, Scott C., editor. *Mayo Clinic Family Health Book.* 4th ed., HarperResource, 2009.

Murphy, Joseph G., and Margaret A. Lloyd. *Mayo Clinic Cardiology: Concise Textbook.* 4th ed., Mayo Clinic Scientific Press, 2012.

Piscatella, Joseph, and Barry Franklin. *Prevent, Halt & Reverse Heart Disease: 109 Things You Can Do.* Rev. ed., Workman, 2011.

Swanton, R. H. *Cardiology.* 6th ed., Blackwell Science, 2008.

"Your Guide to Living Well with Heart Disease." *National Heart, Lung, and Blood Institute*, Nov. 2015, www.nhlbi.nih.gov/files/docs/public/heart/living_well.pdf.

Zaret, Barry L., et al., editors. *Yale University School of Medicine Heart Book.* William Morrow, 1992.

EXERCISE SCIENCE

Category: Specialty

Specialties and related fields: Occupational therapy, personal training, physical therapy, sports medicine, strength and conditioning

Definition: a discipline that studies movement and the associated functional responses and adaptations

KEY TERMS

Achievement Goal Theory: a theory of motivation that considers the individual's concept of ability as well as personal and situational factors that influences the meaning that is attached to successful or unsuccessful experiences

biomechanics: the study of the anatomical principles of human movement

body composition: proportion of lean muscle mass to fat mass

ego/performance-orientation/oriented/involved: goal orientation that is centered on performance, other-reference assessment of ability, and competitive-based rewards

fundamental motor skills: motor skills that are the building blocks of movement, including, for example, skipping, running, catching, throwing, bending and swaying

kinesiology: the scientific study of human movement

motivation: choice, effort and persistence to engage in a particular activity or task

motivational climate: the psychological climate in a learning environment that addresses what goal-reward structure (i.e., mastery of goals—individual rewards or performance goals—competitive rewards) is emphasized

motor development: the study of changes in motor behavior which reflects the interaction of maturation and the environment

motor learning: the study of practice in acquiring and perfecting motor skills

muscular endurance: the ability for a muscle group to perform, or contract, repeatedly at resistance below the maximum resistance the muscle can move

muscular strength: the force that a muscle can produce or exert in a maximal effort one time, in other words, the greatest amount of weight or resistance a muscle can move or lift for one repetition only; this measure of strength is also known as the "one rep max" or 1 rm

National Standards: content standards for physical education curricula set forth by the National Association of Sport and Physical Education (NASPE)

overload: the body must undergo a level of stress that is greater than the norm in order for the body to undergo physiological adaptations that increase muscular strength, muscular endurance, and aerobic endurance

physical fitness: the ability to perform physical activity

skill variations: different movement patterns or action characteristics that can be produced from the same movement pattern

sport & exercise psychology: the study of the psychological aspects of human movement

task/mastery-orientation/oriented/involved: goal orientation that is centered on learning, self-referenced assessment of ability, and individual-based rewards

OVERVIEW

Exercise science has been defined by the National Institutes of Health as "the scientific study of human movement performed to maintain or improve physical fitness" and by the American Society of Exercise Physiologists as "a diverse field of study that may include sport psychologists, exercise physiologists, bio-mechanics, physical educators, and kinesiologists." Each of these areas of exercise science, with the addition of motor learning and development, inform the fundamental components of physical education teacher preparation, pedagogy, and curricula. One of these components, kinesiology, is generally defined as the study of human movement and is sometimes used interchangeably with the term "exercise science" as it encompasses all aspects of exercise science including anatomy, physiology, psychology, motor learning and development, but also includes sociology, and the history and philosophy of sport and exercise. Each of the components of exercise science can also be specifically applied to physical education and the achievement of the National Standards for Physical Education. The National Standards for Physical Education as set forth by National Association of Sport and Physical Education (NASPE) provide a set of guidelines for what physical education should focus on in order to achieve a learning environment in which students are developing skills to keep them physically active over a lifetime. These six National Standards state that a physically educated person:

- Demonstrates competency in motor skills and movement patterns needed to perform a variety of physical activities;
- Demonstrates understanding of movement concepts, principles, strategies, and tactics as they apply to the learning and performance of physical activities;
- Participates regularly in physical activity;
- Achieves and maintains a health-enhancing level of physical fitness;
- Exhibits responsible personal and social behavior that respects self and others in physical activity settings; and
- Values physical activity for health, enjoyment, challenge, self-expression, and/or social interaction.

For physical education teachers to help their students achieve these standards, it is vital for professional preparation programs to include all aspects of exercise science. The first component of exercise science is sport and exercise psychology, which is defined as "the study of the psychological aspects of human movement." Sport psychology, within the context of physical education, involves the application of psychological principles to the learning and teaching methods that are employed in the classroom to help motivate students to participate in the

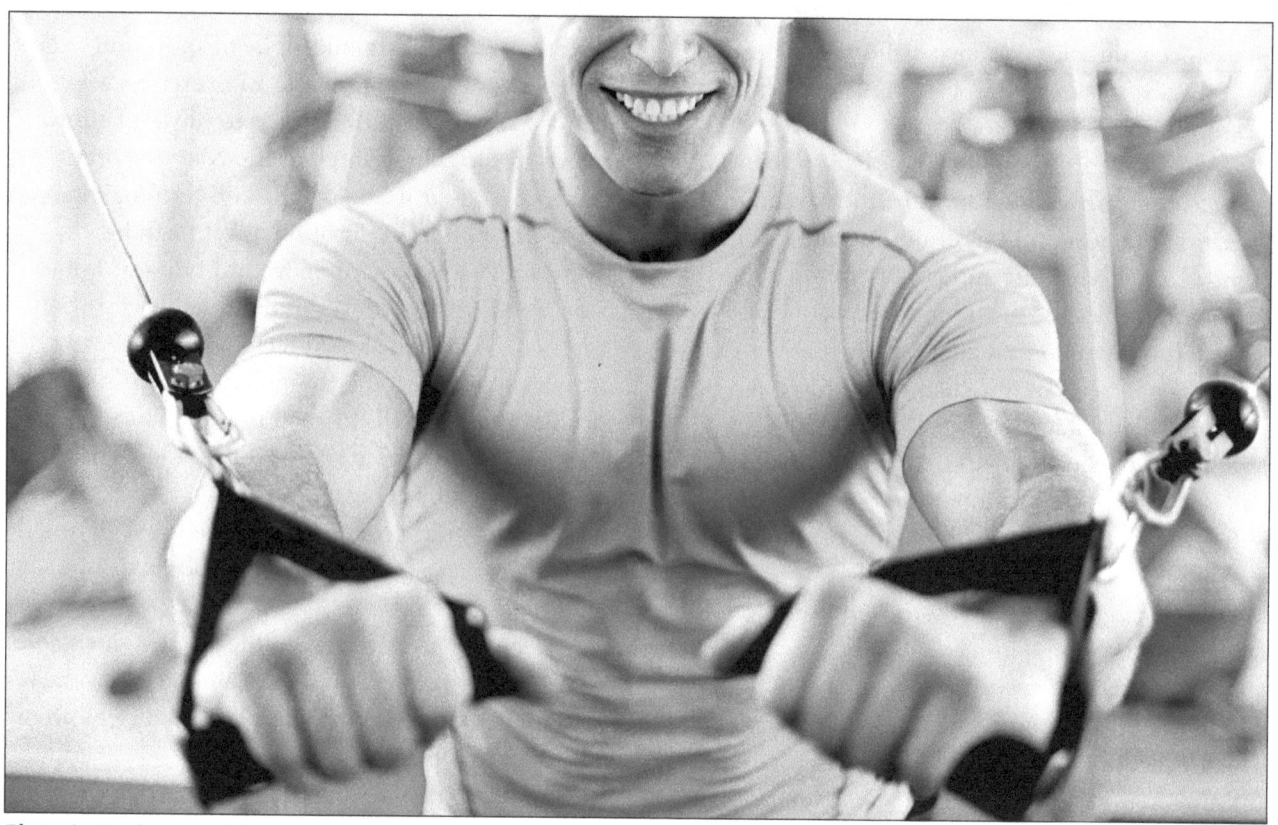

Photo via iStock/gilaxia. [Used under license.]

physical activities and to utilize these skills to engage in healthy behaviors outside of the classroom setting. Four of these six National Standards can be directly encouraged by the application of sport psychology theories and techniques to teaching. These four standards address students' (1) Regular engagement in physical activity, (2) Achievement and maintenance of physical fitness that enhances health, (3) Responsible social and personal behavior, and (4) An understanding of the value of physical activity. Motivational theory and application and character and moral development are areas of sport psychology that are applied to the physical education setting in an effort to improve and foster student development both physically and psychologically. Through the implementation of sport psychology theory and methods, teachers can foster students' motivation to maintain the activity over a life span.

The second component of exercise science is exercise physiology, which is defined as "the identification of physiological mechanisms underlying physical activity, the comprehensive delivery of treatment services concerned with the analysis, improvement, and maintenance of health and fitness, rehabilitation of heart disease and other chronic diseases and/or disabilities, and the professional guidance and counsel of athletes and others interested in athletics, sports training, and human adaptability to acute and chronic exercise." The subdiscipline of exercise physiology, within the context of physical education, involves the application of physiological principles and an understanding of how the human body responds to physical activity to provide activities that enhance students' fitness levels in a safe manner. Standard four of the NASPE National Standards addresses student development and maintenance of a level of fitness that enhances health. For physical education teachers to achieve this standard with their students it is necessary for physical education teachers to have a solid understanding of the physiological mechanisms that underlie physical activity and how to design activities to challenge the students in a manner by which their bodies adapt physiologically, leading to improved cardiovascular and muscular fitness.

The third component of exercise science is biomechanics, which is defined as the study of the anatomical principles of human movement. Biomechanics in the field of exercise science also examines inanimate structures that influence performance, such as sports equipment, athletic footwear and playing surfaces. Within the context of physical education, biomechanics focuses on the instruction of proper technique when engaging in physical activity to avoid or reduce the chances of injury. Biomechanics is more typically applied to sport in assisting athletes to develop efficient technique or products and equipment to improve performance.

Motor learning is the study and practice of acquiring and perfecting motor skills. Motor development is the study of changes in motor behavior which reflect the interaction of maturation and the environment over a life span. Components of exercise science are central to physical education as they are the foundation for the learning and development of skill. Motor learning and development concepts provide the foundation of knowledge for physical education teachers to provide classroom experiences for the students to meet the first two NASPE National Standards for Physical Education. To develop students who are competent in motor skills and movement patterns, as well as developing an understanding of movement concepts, principles, strategies, and tactics as they apply to learning, physical educators need to provide developmentally appropriate learning activities for their students.

APPLICATIONS

Sport and exercise psychology. Sport and exercise psychology, within physical education, focuses on the motivation of the students as it is a key component necessary for a student to be an active and engaged participant in physical education classes and invested in committing to a physically active lifestyle. Within the physical education context, motivation can be defined as why an individual participates in and persists at engaging in an activity or set of behaviors. One theory of motivation that is applied and frequently explored in the physical education context is Achievement Goal Theory. Achievement Goal Theory addresses the relationship between effort and ability in an achievement setting. This relationship is specific to each individual and determines if the student adopts a task/mastery-orientation or ego/performance-orientation.

A student who is task/mastery-oriented judges his or her ability through self-referenced evaluation and feels successful when he or she puts forth more effort. Conversely, ego/performance-oriented students focus on ability and view success as displaying superior ability (as compared to others). The task-oriented student will choose challenging tasks and display greater persistence than those students who are ego/performance-oriented. These differing goal orientations are attributed to individual differences and situational factors. The application of this theory to the classroom setting is addressed through the concept and application of motivational climate as the classroom learning environment is the situational factor affecting goal orientation. The motivational climate, as it relates to the classroom setting, can be defined as the social climate that is created by important social factors (e.g., the teacher) as it relates to perspectives on achievement. Researchers have suggested that a student's dispositional goal orientation or goal involvement (i.e., task/mastery or ego/performance) in combination with the social climate will determine the meaning of achievement and influence behavioral patterns in the educational setting.

Sport psychology goes beyond motivation in that its concepts and application to physical education can also be used in the development of students who meet the national standard of becoming socially and personally responsible. This opportunity for students to develop character and become socially and personally responsible through their physical education experiences can be structured and built into the class environment. Compassion, fairness, sportspersonship, and integrity are four components of character that can become a part of moral/character education through physical education. Compassion can be learned through the process of role-taking, perspective-taking, and empathy in physical education. Fairness can be developed through the introduction to hypothetical and actual moral dilemmas into the structured class environment. Sportspersonship can also be addressed through a task-oriented motivational climate where emphasis is placed on self-reference improvement and success. Integrity is another component of character education that can be promoted through physical education. Integrity can be promoted by providing students with a sense of autonomy and opportunities to use problem-solving skills within the social context.

Exercise physiology. The application of physiological principles and the understanding of the body's response to stress is essential knowledge which enhances the students' level of physical fitness in a safe manner. Physical fitness is defined as the ability to perform physical activity, while health-related fitness is a term that is used to indicate physical activity that aims to promote good health and wellness. Health-related fitness, which is applicable to the physical education setting, encompasses five components: (1) muscular strength, (2) muscular endurance, (3) aerobic endurance, (4) flexibility, and (5) body composition. Physiological mechanisms underlie the development of each of the health-related fitness components. To increase muscular endurance, muscular strength, and aerobic endurance, the physiological principle of overload requires that the body must undergo a level of stress that is greater than the norm for the body to undergo physiological adaptations that increase muscular strength and endurance.

Physical educators design class activities to challenge the students to work at a harder than normal rate or intensity so that their bodies begin to adapt physiologically to increase muscle strength, muscle resistance, aerobic endurance, and to change body composition with physical activity designed to target these fitness components. Resistance training is a method which develops muscular strength and muscular endurance as well as change body composition by progressively overloading the muscles. Aerobic endurance improves by regularly overloading the cardiorespiratory system. The body begins to make physiological adaptations and increases its capacity to engage in prolonged and more intense activity. These adaptations are evident in the increased efficiency of the heart and lungs to pump oxygen to the muscles for the muscles to sustain the activity level. The efficiency and any improvement in efficiency of the heart and lungs can be assessed by taking and recording heart rates and monitoring the rate of breathing. When an individual engages in regular physical activity, he or she begins to train the heart and lungs to become more efficient through the process of overloading the heart muscle and respiratory system, which results in a decreased heart rate and breathing rate.

Motor learning and motor development. The application of motor learning and development concepts are important to physical educators as it is essential to understand how different factors may affect the learning process to make appropriate decisions. Learning occurs when the teacher creates a learning environment for the students that effectively integrates knowledge about the processes and factors of learning and when students are engaged in developmentally appropriate activities. This presents physical educators with the challenge of creating a learning environment and situations in which each student in the class is challenged at the appropriate level for motor development to occur for each student. This is essential in the development of fundamental motor skills. Fundamental motor skills are considered the building blocks of movement and include such skills as running, skipping, catching, throwing, and bending. These fundamental skills do not simply emerge during childhood, rather the child must sequentially move through series of movements leading up to mature motor patterns and eventually skill variations and sport specific skills.

Magill cites three different aspects of motor learning research that are applicable to the physical educator, including feedback, practice time, and teaching skill variations. Physical education teachers should have an understanding of not only what is appropriate feedback, but also how much is helpful for the student to make the changes necessary to learn the skill. It is suggested that teachers provide feedback about the critical aspect of the movement since research has indicated that correcting one aspect of a skill can oftentimes correct the remaining skill features. Another aspect of motor learning that is important to skill acquisition is time on task. For example, it is important for a teacher to know how much practice is enough in one class session. Research has indicated that short amounts of practice time per class period or practice session are effective, yet if the practice times are short then practice needs to be spread out over a longer period or more sessions. The third aspect of motor learning that is important to physical education is how a teacher should organize practice sessions to teach skill variations. It is suggested that, based on findings from research, skill variations should be taught during every class session throughout the whole instructional unit. The physical educator must understand these concepts of motor learning that are then complemented by their understanding of motor development. Both motor learning and motor development must be considered when planning class activities and units.

Environmental engineering, which is defined as "designing environments to provide individualized motor development," is an important strategy to consider when teaching fundamental motor skills. The environment in which a motor skill is practiced is an important piece of the development of motor skills. Physical education teachers are faced with the challenge of having students in the same class who are not on the same developmental level. This could be due to previous practice and experience with a motor skill or gender of the student. To provide skill practice sessions that are developmentally appropriate, the teacher must provide students with skill variations, opportunities to assess themselves and choose their task, and provide the appropriate amount of time on the tasks. This may include, for example, allowing students to have multiple practice stations in the class, a choice in how difficult the task is, and the amount of time they would feel is necessary to practice a skill. These choices provide students an opportunity to take responsibility for their learning and have a sense of autonomy over that process, as well as learn in an environment that allows them to practice at a level that is appropriate for their personal level of development.

Exercise science is a broad field that includes several subdisciplines that are important for the physical educator to understand to provide physical education curricula that can be successful in achieving the National Standards for Physical Education. The challenge for physical educators and those responsible for their professional preparation is how to successfully integrate each of these subdisciplines in a manner that is appropriate and effective for aspiring physical educators in order for them to apply the multitude of scientific principles to their physical education classroom.

—*Shelby L. Hinkle Smith*

Further Reading

American Society of Exercise Physiologists, 2022, www.asep.org/.

Bulger, S., et al. "Preparing Prospective Physical Educators in Exercise Physiology." *QUEST*, vol. 52, 2000, pp. 166-85.

Feltz, D. L., and A. P. Konos. "The Nature of Sport Psychology." *Advances in Sport Psychology*, edited by T. Horn, Human Kinetics, 2002, pp. 3-20.

Goodway, J. D., and H. Savage. "Environmental Engineering in Elementary Physical Education." *Teaching Elementary Physical Education*, vol. 12, 2001, pp. 12-14.

Graser, S., et al. "Children's Perceptions of Fitness Self-Testing, the Purpose of Fitness Testing, and Personal Health." *Physical Educator*, vol. 68, 2011, pp. 175-87.

Magill, R. A. "Motor Learning is Meaningful for Physical Educators." *QUEST*, vol. 42, 1990, pp. 126-33.

Maina, M. P., et al. "Muscle Building Activities for Elementary and Middle School Children." *Teaching Elementary Physical Education*, vol. 12, 2001, pp. 13-18.

Ntoumanis, N., and S. J. H. Biddle. "A Review of Motivational Climate in Physical Activity." *Journal of Sport Sciences*, vol. 17, 1999, pp. 643-65.

Papaionnou, A. G., et al. "Motivational Climate and Achievement Goals at the Situational Level of Generality." *Journal of Applied Sport Psychology*, vol. 19, 2007, pp. 16-37.

"Play and Playground Encyclopedia." *National Association for Sport and Physical Education*, 2022, www.pgpedia.com/n/national-association-sport-and-physical-education.

Santiago, J. A., et al. "Elementary Physical Education Teachers' Content Knowledge of Physical Activity and Health-Related Fitness." *Physical Educator*, vol. 69, 2012, pp. 395-412.

Shields, D. L., and B. J. Bredemeier. *Character Development and Physical Activity*. Human Kinetics, 1995.

Silverman, S. "Thinking Long Term: Physical Education's Role in Movement and Mobility." *QUEST*, vol. 57, 2005, pp. 138-47.

Todorovich, J. R., and E. D. Model. "The TARGET Approach to Motivating Students." *Teaching Elementary Physical Education*, vol. 16, 2005, pp. 8-10.

Treasure, D. C., and G. C. Roberts. "Applications of Achievement Goal Theory to Physical Education: Implications for Enhancing Motivation." *QUEST*, vol. 47, 1995, pp. 475-89.

Van Dusen, Duncan P. "Associations of Physical Fitness and Academic Performance Among Schoolchildren." *Journal of School Health*, vol. 81, no. 12, 2011, pp. 733-40.

Weiss, M. R., and E. Ferrer-Caja. "Motivational Orientations in Sport Behavior." *Advances in Sport Psychology*, edited by T. Horn, Human Kinetics, 2002, pp. 101-84.

Kinesiology

Category: Careers

Specialties and related fields: Anatomy, biochemistry, biomechanics, chemistry, coaching, ergonomics, exercise physiology, motor behavior, sport psychology, sport sociology, physiology, physics

Definition: a multidisciplinary field that specializes in the science of human movement

KEY TERMS

action: type of movement made by a muscle contraction

adenosine triphosphate: a form of stored energy that can be used directly by muscle cells for contraction

aerobic exercise: physical activity that is vigorous, continuous, and rhythmical

alveoli: lung structure in which oxygen is transferred from air to the blood

antagonist: a muscle that has an opposite action from its paired muscle and limits its action

applied kinesiology: a dubious diagnostic technique used in chiropractic medicine

hemoglobin: component in blood that attaches to and transfers oxygen *insertion*: point of muscle attachment on the bone that moves

isokinetic machine: an instrument that measures the strength of muscles through the joint's full range of motion

metabolism: the sum of all chemical reactions in a living organism

motor: relating to or involving movements of a muscle

origin: point of muscle attachment on the bone that remains stationary

BASIC PRINCIPLES

Kinesiology is the study of human movement. Although it technically is not limited to humans, as an applied science, it almost always is. Kinesiology is primarily concerned with all physical activity, including competitive sports and activities designed to maintain and improve health. It is a major part of physical rehabilitation and injury prevention. It can be used to design ergonomic workstations and minimize hazards.

A key component of kinesiology is understanding which muscles are involved in specific movements. Each major joint in the human body has identifiable planes of movement. Each movement in the plane is named according to its direction, with certain muscles contributing to it. Muscles can be primary movers at the joint or can assist in the movement. Using this information, kinesiologists can observe movement patterns, identify which joints are involved, determine the movement at each joint, and ascertain which muscles contribute to the movement. Furthermore, they can develop training programs to work the appropriate muscles to improve the joint's strength, movement, and muscle balance. The field of kinesiology should not be confused with applied kinesiology, a diagnostic technique used in chiropractic medicine. The clinician applies a force to a muscle or muscle group, and the patient resists the force. The clinician makes a diagnosis based on the patient's response to the force. This is not a generally accepted practice in medicine and is not related to kinesiology.

Summary of long-term adaptations to regular aerobic and anaerobic exercise. Adaptations include an increase in stroke volume (SV) and maximal aerobic capacity (VO2$_{max}$), as well as a decrease in resting heart rate (RHR). Long-term adaptations to resistance training include muscular hypertrophy, an increase in the physiological cross-sectional area (PCSA) of muscle(s), and an increase in neural drive, both leading to increased muscular strength. Neural adaptations begin more quickly and plateau before the hypertrophic response.

BACKGROUND

The term "kinesiology" comes from the Greek words *kinein* meaning "to move," and *logos* meaning "discourse." The field of kinesiology is believed to have begun in ancient Greece. Aristotle is considered the father of kinesiology for his work using geometry to describe the movement of humans. It was not until the fifteenth century that Leonardo da Vinci helped expand the knowledge of human movement by studying the mechanics of standing, walking, and jumping.

One of the greatest contributors to kinesiology, Sir Isaac Newton, did not study human movement. In the late 1600s and early 1700s, Newton developed three laws of rest and movement that laid the foundation for the analysis of human movement in the following years. The development of photography in the 1800s enabled researchers to study how animals moved by taking several pictures in rapid succession. They first studied horses, then humans. Cinematography further enabled researchers to understand human movement.

In 1990, the American Academy of Physical Education (later the American Academy of Kinesiology and Physical Education) recommended that programs of study involving human movement be

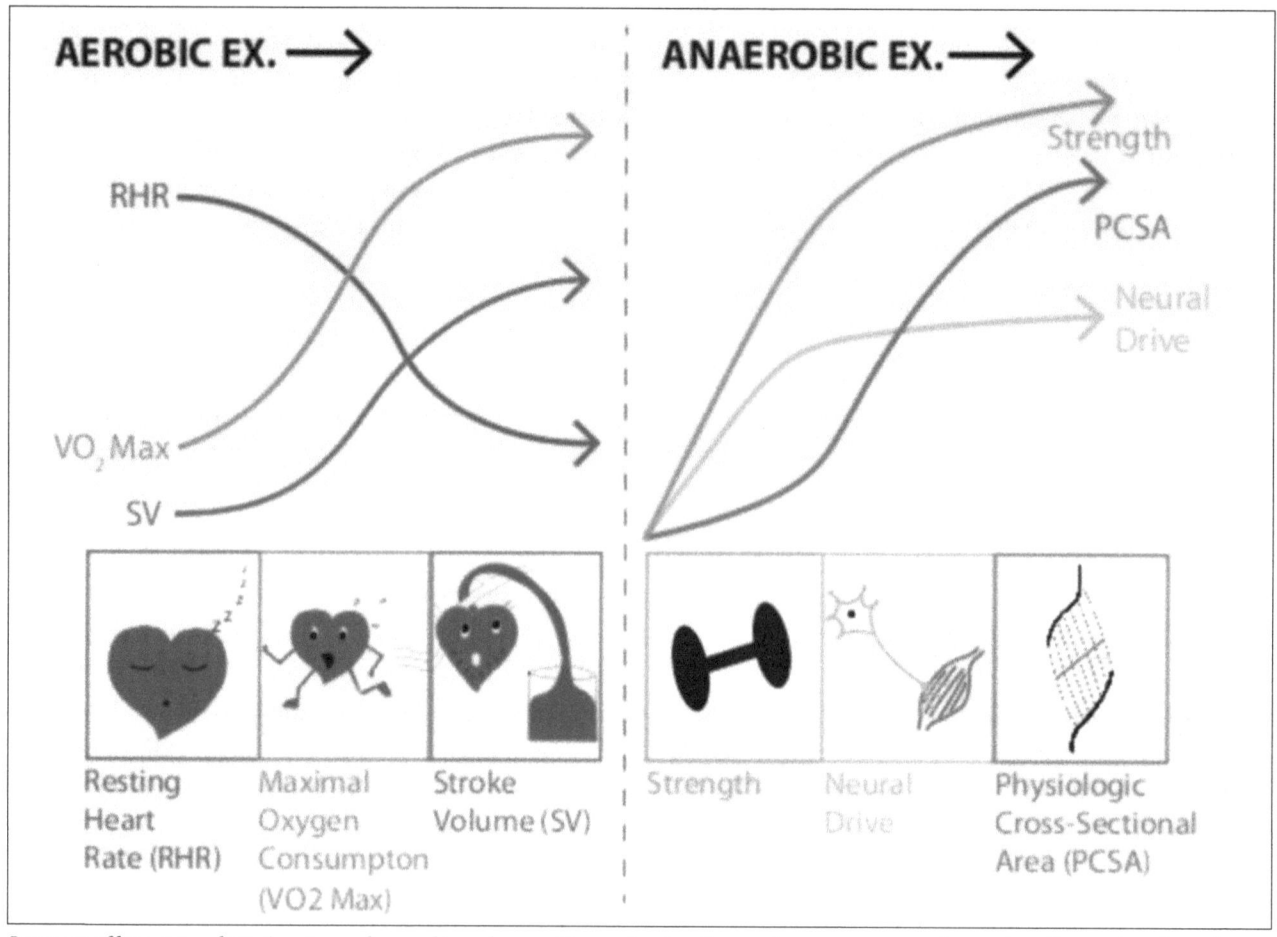

Summary of long-term adaptations to regular aerobic and anaerobic exercise. Aerobic exercise can cause several central cardiovascular adaptations, including an increase in stroke volume (SV) and maximal aerobic capacity (VO2 max), as well as a decrease in resting heart rate (RHR). Long-term adaptations to resistance training, the most common form of anaerobic exercise, include muscular hypertrophy, an increase in the physiological cross-sectional area (PCSA) of muscle(s), and an increase in neural drive, both of which lead to increased muscular strength. Neural adaptations begin more quickly and plateau prior to the hypertrophic response. Image by Plin7 at English Wikipedia, via Wikimedia Commons.

called "kinesiology." This idea gained wide acceptance, and kinesiology as a field came to include many other specialized fields beyond the traditional anatomy and biomechanics. Kinesiology can include any area related to human movements, such as history, sociology, psychology, physiology, philosophy, and motor behavior.

HOW IT WORKS

Movement analysis. Traditionally, courses in kinesiology focused on the anatomy and mechanics of human movement. Although more advanced courses sometimes take the same approach, introductory courses tend to be an overview of the broader field of kinesiology.

A thorough understanding of muscle and skeletal anatomy is required to understand movement. This includes the names of the bones and the names, origins, insertions, and actions of the major muscles of the human body. The origin and insertion of a muscle are where it attaches to bones. These locations determine the action of the muscle based on the angle of pull on the bones. This knowledge is important in understanding which muscles are involved in specific movements.

Bodily movements are described by the planes and rotations at the various joints. These movements include flexion, extension, adduction, abduction, internal rotation, and external rotation. Kinesiologists watch a specific movement and determine the actions at the joint or joints being evaluated. They can also evaluate movements to determine if they are completed properly. Slow-motion cinematography is helpful when analyzing the very fast movements often found in sports.

After determining the movement at a joint, kinesiologists can use their knowledge of anatomy to determine which muscles are involved. Additionally, they can use this information to develop strength training programs for the specific muscles used in the activity. It is important to note that muscles that generate a movement (agonist muscles) have antagonist muscles that stop the movement. Therefore, strengthening an antagonist muscle is just as important as strengthening the muscle that initiates the movement.

Physiological function. Human movement requires oxygen and energy beyond the levels needed to survive. Exercise physiology includes studying how the body gets food and oxygen from the environment to the working muscles. Oxygen is crucial for sustaining activity during intense exercise, during which the cardiovascular, respiratory, and muscular systems are primarily involved. The respiratory system transfers oxygen from the atmosphere into the blood. Air, about 21 percent oxygen, is inhaled into the lungs, and much of it enters the alveoli at the ends of the airways. Oxygen diffuses from the alveoli into the blood, which binds with the hemoglobin. The pumping action of the heart carries the blood to the muscles. When the oxygenated blood gets near muscle cells that are low in oxygen, the hemoglobin releases the oxygen, which goes into the cell. A strong, healthy heart and blood with normal amounts of hemoglobin can deliver sufficient amounts of oxygen to support high levels of muscle movement and activity. When oxygen enters the muscle cell, it is metabolized. It goes through a series of chemical reactions in which oxygen and energy are converted into adenosine triphosphate (ATP). The muscle can use only ATP to make the fibers contract and the body move. When highly trained people exercise at very high intensity, the amount of oxygen consumed can increase more than twenty times. The muscle cells' ability to use oxygen to produce ATP limits high-intensity human movement. The oxygen consumed and several other measures can be determined with a metabolic cart, a piece of important testing equipment used in exercise physiology.

Behavioral control. The areas of kinesiology that involve the brain and nervous system are motor development, sport psychology, and sport sociology. Motor development involves skills that take stored movement patterns in the brain and communicate them to the muscles. Most skilled movements are an organized, synchronous set of smaller movements. Therefore, the muscle contractions needed to perform the skill must be stored and retrieved often. Practicing the movement patterns regularly is required to refine the skills. Sport psychology and sociology are the segments of kinesiology that relate to the mental aspects of human movement and performance. One of the largest fields is clinical sport psychology, in which psychologists assist athletes with aggression, stress, motivation, mood, adherence, leadership, and several other related issues. Sport sociology is a smaller element of kinesiology that focuses on social relationships in sports and how sports affect different segments of society and organizational structures.

APPLICATIONS

Rehabilitation. Kinesiology is a very important component of muscular and skeletal rehabilitation.

Kinesiology techniques, especially those regarding the muscular and skeletal systems, are used daily in physical rehabilitation. Physicians, chiropractors, physical therapists, and athletic trainers use their knowledge of muscle origins, insertions, and actions to diagnose injuries and determine exercises that will help people recover from them. Isokinetic machines can determine the muscular strength at any joint through the entire range of motion. Identifying points of weakness during movement helps determine which muscles need to be strengthened. A muscle and its antagonist can be tested to see if one is weaker than the other. Good muscle balance is needed to prevent injuries and reinjury. Limbs (arms and legs) are tested to see if the left and right sides are equally strong or if one side, usually the injured side, is weaker.

Cardiovascular rehabilitation focuses on kinesiology, including the cardiovascular and respiratory systems. In this area, exercise is used to strengthen the heart muscle. When a person has a heart attack, some heart tissue dies and is replaced by connective tissue. With some of the muscle gone and unable to pump blood, the heart is weaker. In cardiac rehabilitation, patients perform aerobic exercises to increase the strength of the remaining heart muscle. Through kinesiology applications, patients can strengthen their hearts and improve their ability to engage in daily living activities.

Health promotion and injury prevention. The principles of kinesiology are used to maintain good health and prevent injuries. For many years, exercise has been recognized as an important component of health promotion. Kinesiology studies have involved developing and researching the best types of exercise to improve health. Exercise specialists such as physical education instructors, fitness trainers, and sports coaches rely on kinesiology to help people exercise safely and efficiently. They create exercise programs or develop exercise sessions based on kinesiology principles. Exercise can take the form of group classes or individual instruction (personal training). Cardiovascular exercise is very important for health and fitness. Exercise specialists are often charged with helping a person develop the endurance to engage in physical activity for extended periods. Exercise specialists use exercise physiology principles to prescribe activities based on an assessment of the person's health and fitness. The prescription, or exercise plan, is often based on heart rate so that the individual can use their pulse to gauge whether the right level of effort is being attained. Another important type of exercise for health and fitness is strength training. Exercise specialists use kinesiology principles to demonstrate proper lifting techniques and help clients get stronger. Attention is paid to balancing muscle strength across the body. Movement mechanics are also used to improve flexibility. A stretching program is designed to improve or maintain flexibility throughout the body and help clients move more freely. A good training program will help clients stay healthier throughout their lives and enable them to perform the activities of daily living more easily and longer.

An overriding factor in exercise for health is adherence to the program. Health benefits are obtained only with regular participation. The psychological area of kinesiology studies provides information about getting and keeping exercisers motivated.

Coaching. Coaches use kinesiology in many of their activities. Sports skill development requires regular evaluation of movement to determine if the sports skill is being performed properly, which maximizes performance and reduces the chances of injuries. Coaches must consider all the involved joints, the type of muscle contractions, and the planes of movements. Of great importance is the synchronization of the movements around the involved joints. Energy transfer from one joint to the next is critical for superior performance. Coaches use their knowledge of kinesiology to teach proper sport skills.

Coaches also must use kinesiology for strength and conditioning. Athletes must employ proper mechanics while weight-lifting and engaging in other exercises. The variety of available equipment makes a basic understanding of kinesiology imperative for teaching athletes effectively. Additionally, coaches must determine which exercises should be performed and which muscles should be strengthened.

Coaches also use sport psychology to motivate athletes to perform their best and develop the leadership skills important for success. Athletic competition can be stressful, especially as most athletes must deal with demands on their time and concentration that stem from their social and academic or work-related obligation. Coaches often teach athletes stress management techniques to help them cope.

Ergonomics. Kinesiology can be applied at the workplace in the area of ergonomics, in which science uses body mechanics concepts to design more comfortable workstations and minimize overuse injuries from repetitive movements. Any workstation can be analyzed and appropriately modified. Ergonomic solutions for people in desk jobs are relatively simple, but finding answers for people in jobs that require lifting and carrying requires more kinesiology principles. After the proper techniques for lifting and carrying have been determined, the worker must be trained to perform the movements properly.

FUTURE PROSPECTS

Kinesiology continues to be a growing field. The participants have traditionally paid for programs that use kinesiology professionals. Kinesiology benefited those who could pay for good sport trainers, health and fitness clubs, and sports medicine. More programs, including youth sports programs, are emerging to provide access to exercise facilities and sports training to those who cannot afford to pay. Some insurance plans provide free or discounted gym membership, and many companies offer employee gyms or discounted gym memberships. Professional sports remain popular worldwide, and the emergence of new competitive sports such as extreme sports results in more research and more need for people trained in kinesiology. Also, more people are interested in maintaining good health, and positions in fitness training are likely to increase to meet the demands of these exercisers. With more people exercising and participating in sports, the number of sports-related injuries is likely to grow. Kinesiology education will be needed to train rehabilitation professionals to research injuries, educate the public about injuries, and rehabilitate those injured.

—Bradley R. A. Wilson

Further Reading

Floyd, R. T., and Clem Thompson. *Manual of Structural Kinesiology*. 21st ed., McGraw-Hill, 2020.

Hoffman, Shirl J., and Duane V. Knudson, editors. *Introduction to Kinesiology: Studying Physical Activity*. 5th ed., Human Kinetics, 2017.

Klavora, P. *Foundations of Kinesiology: Studying Human Movement and Health*. Sport Books, 2007.

———. *Introduction to Kinesiology: A Biophysical Perspective*. Sport Books, 2009.

Kornspan, Alan S. *Fundamentals of Sport and Exercise Psychology*. Human Kinetics, 2009.

Lippert, Lynn S. *Clinical Kinesiology and Anatomy*. 6th ed., F. A. Davis Company, 2017.

Muscolino, Joseph E. *Kinesiology: The Skeletal System and Muscle Function*. 4th ed., Elsevier, 2022.

Oatis, Carol A. *Kinesiology: The Mechanics of Human Movement*. 3rd ed., Lippincott Williams & Wilkins, 2016.

NEUROSCIENCE

Category: Specialty

Specialties and related fields: Neurology, psychiatry, pediatrics, pharmacology, geriatrics, toxicology, neuropsychology

Definition: the scientific study of nerves, the nervous system, and associated behaviors

KEY TERMS

axon: the part of a neuron responsible for sending information to other neurons

dendrite: the part of a neuron responsible for receiving information from other neurons through the binding of neurotransmitters

electroencephalograph: a physiological instrument used to record electrical activity from the scalp

electrophysiology: the study of the electrical properties of cells

excitation: one consequence of the binding of neurotransmitters to the dendrite of a neuron; when the neuron receives enough excitation in its dendrite, the cell will release the neurotransmitter from its axon onto other cells

neuron: the basic cell of the nervous system; commonly referred to as a "brain cell"

neurotransmitter: any of several chemicals that facilitate communication between neurons

plasticity: a characteristic of brain cells that allows them to change as a result of stimulation or changes in activity

synapse: the space between the axon of one neuron and the dendrite of another where communication between cells takes place

SCIENCE AND PROFESSION

Neuroscience is a broad, interdisciplinary field that spans many disciplines, including medicine, psychology, biology, chemistry, physics, computer science, mathematics, economics, education, ethics, and law. The term "neuroscience" replaced several earlier labels for the field, including psychobiology, biopsychology, and biological psychology. Neuroscience is closely related to neurology and neurobiology. However, the former focuses on clinical and medical phenomena, and the latter is concerned more with biology than behavior. Most neuroscientists have earned PhDs, though some will also hold MDs (in contrast, all neurologists are physicians).

There are many subdisciplines within neuroscience, such as behavioral neuroscience (which examines the relationship between the brain and behavior using animal models), cellular and molecular neuroscience (explores chemical and electrical events at the cellular level), cognitive neuroscience (uses neuroimaging to study the brain's role in thinking, feeling, and behaving in humans), computational neuroscience (uses computer modeling to understand how neurons and neuronal networks work), and developmental neuroscience (examines how the nervous system changes throughout a lifetime).

PERSPECTIVE AND PROSPECTS

Though the heart was seen as the seat of intellect in the ancient world, the Greek Hippocrates and later the Roman Galen theorized that the brain might be responsible for complex behaviors. Despite the accuracy of these early thinkers, it would be hundreds of years before neuroscience advanced beyond the gross anatomical studies that existed during the Middle Ages and early Renaissance. It was only after several notable discoveries about the physics of electrical conduction that neuroscientific progress resumed, this time with advances in electrophysiology.

Around the turn of the twentieth century, the two great neuroanatomists, Camillo Golgi and Santiago Ramon y Cajal, debated whether the structure of the nervous system was a "reticulum" (Golgi) or a discontinuous series of "connections" between neurons (Cajal). Though neither anatomist possessed a microscope powerful enough to determine who was correct at the time, over fifty years later, Palade and Palay used electron microscopy to verify the existence of synapses and show that it was Cajal who was correct. This demonstration, along with the work of Nobel Laureates John Eccles and Bernard Katz, among others, solidified a modern understanding of the typical structure and workings of the nervous system. Namely, although communication within individual neurons is electrical, communication be-

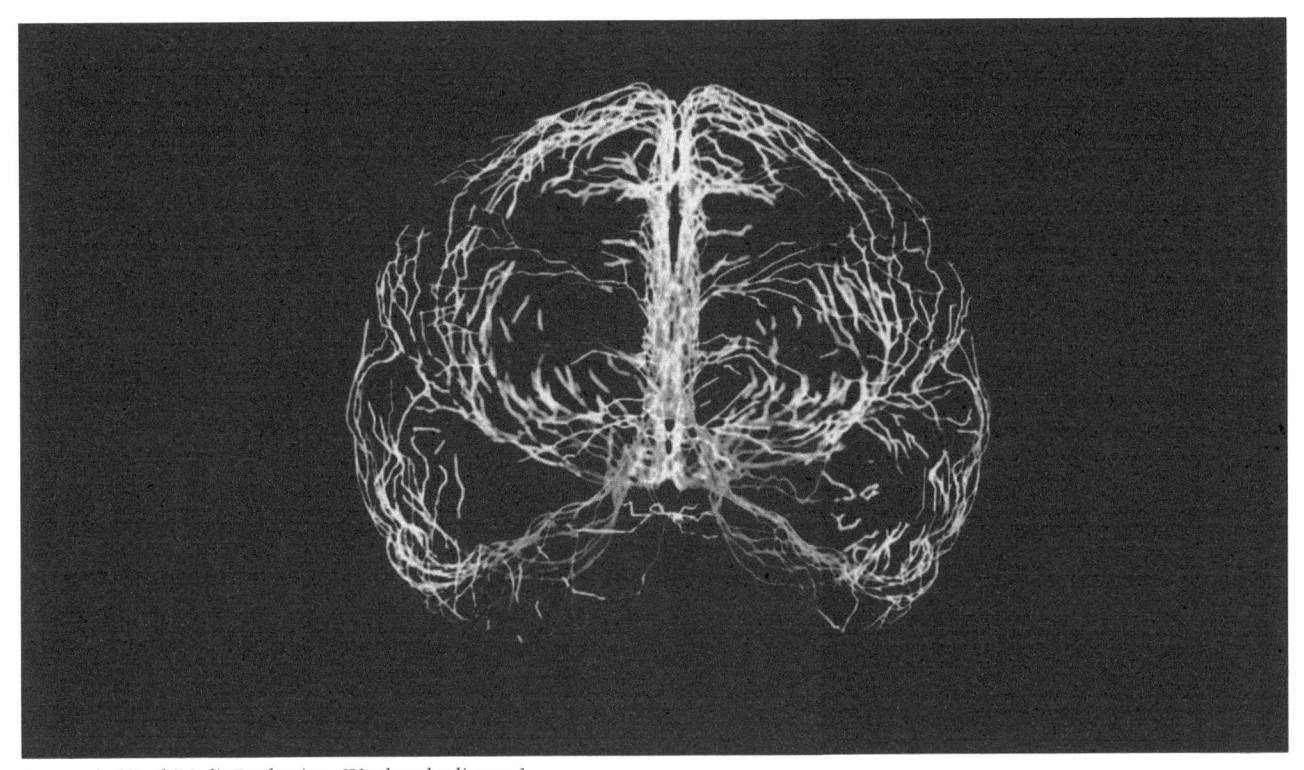

Image via iStock/MediaProduction. [Used under license.]

tween neurons is chemical. It occurs by releasing a neurotransmitter from an axon into the synapse. Once in the synapse, the neurotransmitter then binds to the dendrite of a different neuron, thus creating a change in the electrical potential within that neuron.

While neuroanatomists and neurophysiologists were unraveling where and how messages are sent in the nervous system, the Canadian psychologist, Donald Hebb, theorized how information could be retained. In his 1949 book, *On the Organization of Behavior*, Hebb outlined the parameters via which the nervous system could be modified in response to activity, the phenomenon now known as "plasticity." His book, one of the most influential texts in all of neuroscience, laid the foundation for everything from the visual system's development to learning and memory.

Before the 1950s, most neuroscientific research was conducted using animal models. The advent of modern neuroimaging techniques, such as functional magnetic resonance imaging, or fMRI, revolutionized the study of the brain and behavior in humans. Unlike brain wave recordings collected using an electroencephalograph (EEG), which had been used for decades, fMRI allowed neuroscientists to see exactly where the brain activity was taking place when a human was thinking or behaving.

Continuing technological advances now allow neuroscientists to peer into the brain with greater resolution and detail. Because of this enhanced ability to see what happens within the brain when a human engages in complex reasoning, these advances have facilitated the integration of neuroscience with seemingly unrelated fields such as economics and education.

—*Jerome L. Rekart*

Further Reading

"BrainFacts.org." *Society for Neuroscience*, www.brainfacts.org.
Carter, Rita. *Mapping the Mind*. U of California P, 2010.
Gazzaniga, Michael S. *The Cognitive Neurosciences*. MIT Press, 2009.
Gross, Charles G. *A Hole in the Head: More Tales in the History of Neuroscience*. MIT Press, 2012.
Hebb, Donald O. *The Organization of Behavior: A Neuropsychological Theory*. Wiley, 1949.
Kalat, James W. *Biological Psychology*. 11th ed., Wadsworth, 2013.
Kandel, Eric, et al. *Principles of Neural Science*. 5th ed., McGraw Hill Professional, 2012.
LeDoux, Joseph. *Synaptic Self: How Our Brains Become Who We Are*. 2nd ed., Penguin Books, 2003.
Satel, Sally, and Scott O. Lilienfield. *Brainwashed: The Seductive Appeal of Mindless Neuroscience*. Basic Books, 2013.
"The Brain from Top to Bottom." *McGill University*, thebrain.mcgill.ca.

Occupational Therapist

Category: Careers

Specialties and related fields: Occupational therapy

Definition: a form of therapy for those recuperating from physical or mental illness that encourages rehabilitation through the performance of activities required in daily life

KEY TERMS

American Occupational Therapy Association (AOTA): the national professional association was established in 1917 to represent the interests and concerns of occupational therapy practitioners and students and improve the quality of occupational therapy service

National Board for Certification in Occupational Therapy (NBCOT): a professional organization that administers the national exam for occupational therapy certification

occupational therapy programs: certified training programs at high learning institutes that train students to work as licensed occupational therapists

physical ailment: a physical disorder or illness, especially of a minor or chronic nature

therapeutic treatments: therapeutics, treatment, and care of a patient for both preventing and combating disease or alleviating pain or injury

OVERVIEW

Sphere of work. Occupational therapists provide therapeutic services aimed at helping variously disabled people perform everyday tasks in their life and work. Occupational therapists treat people with temporary and chronic motor function impairments caused by mental, physical, developmental, or emotional issues. An occupational therapist may help patients with skills such as self-care (dressing, eating), household care (cleaning, cooking), communication devices such as telephones and computers, and basic activities such as writing, problem-solving, memory, and coordination. Occupational therapists develop patient treatment plans that attempt to maintain, develop, or recover a patient's daily functioning, productivity, and quality of life.

Work environment. Occupational therapists work in rehabilitation facilities, hospitals, nursing homes, occupational therapy clinics, and schools. In medical environments, occupational therapists generally partner with medical and social service professionals, such as doctors and social workers, to increase patients' physical and mental abilities and overall independence. In school settings, occupational therapists partner with educational professionals such as

Profile

- **Working Conditions**: Work Indoors
- **Physical Strength**: Medium Work
- **Education Needs**: Master's Degree
- **Licensure/Certification**: Required
- **Physical Abilities Not Required**: No Heavy Labor

teachers and special education coordinators to address the physical or mental issues of students with special needs. Occupational therapy is a common component of a special needs child's individualized education plan (IEP). Occupational therapists generally work a standard forty-hour week, and scheduled appointments are the norm.

Occupation interest. Individuals attracted to occupational therapy tend to be physically capable people who enjoy hands-on work and close interaction with others. Individuals who excel as occupational therapists exhibit intellectual curiosity, problem-solving, a desire to help, patience, and caring. Occupational therapists must be good at science and able to work as part of a team to meet patient needs.

A DAY IN THE LIFE—DUTIES AND RESPONSIBILITIES

An occupational therapist's daily duties and responsibilities include full days of hands-on patient interaction and treatment and administrative duties. Patients seen by occupational therapists include those experiencing physical limitations caused by accident or injury, stroke, or congenital conditions such as cerebral palsy or muscular dystrophy; other patients may require services due to developmental delays, learning disabilities, or mental retardation.

Occupational therapists interact with patients or clients daily as medical or therapeutic professionals. Daily work responsibilities may include conducting patient assessments; developing patient treatment plans; providing patients with special instruction in life skills; advising patients on the use of adaptive equipment such as wheelchairs or orthopedic aids; providing early intervention services to young children with physical and social delays and limitations; building adaptive equipment for patients with special needs not met by existing options; providing instruction in self-care such as dressing and eating; counseling patients on technical or physical adaptations that will allow the patient to continue to work

> **DUTIES AND RESPONSIBILITIES**
> - Testing and evaluating patients' physical and mental abilities
> - Designing special equipment to aid disabled patients
> - Instructing and informing patients how to adjust to home, work, and social environments
> - Evaluating patients' progress, attitudes, and behavior

at their chosen occupation; and meeting with patient treatment team or patient families.

An occupational therapist's daily administrative responsibilities include record-keeping with patient evaluation and treatment. Occupational therapists must draft treatment plans, record notes following patient treatment sessions, provide written updates to patient treatment teams, and provide insurance companies with patient records and progress notes as required. Independent occupational therapists working outside a school or medical clinic may also be responsible for patient appointment scheduling and billing.

OCCUPATION SPECIALTIES

Directors of occupational therapy. Directors of occupational therapy plan, direct, and coordinate occupational therapy programs in hospitals, institutions, and community settings to facilitate the rehabilitation of those who are physically, mentally, or emotionally disabled.

Industrial therapists. Industrial therapists arrange salaried, productive employment in an actual work environment for disabled patients to enable them to perform medically prescribed work activities and to prepare them to resume employment outside of the hospital environment.

WORK ENVIRONMENT

Physical environment. Occupational therapists work in rehabilitation facilities, hospitals, nursing homes, therapy clinics, and schools. Therapeutic office settings used by occupational therapists may be shared with other therapeutic professionals such as physical, recreational, or speech and language therapists.

Human environment. Examples of patients needing occupational therapy to increase their independence and quality of life include people suffering balance and strength issues caused by cerebral palsy, spinal cord injuries, or muscular dystrophy; stroke victims experiencing memory loss or coordination problems; people experiencing mental health problems; and children or adults with developmental disabilities. Occupational therapists usually work as part of a patient treatment team that includes patient families, social workers, teachers, doctors, and other therapists. As a treatment team member, occupational therapists participate in frequent team meetings. They are responsible for communicating patient progress to fellow team members.

Technological environment. Occupational therapists use a wide variety of technology in their work. Computers and internet communication tools are a ubiquitous part of occupational therapy work. Occupational therapists often introduce specialized computer programs to patients that need help with their reasoning, problem-solving, memory, and sequencing. In addition, occupational therapists generally learn how to use and teach adaptive devices such as wheelchairs, orthopedic aids, eating aids, and dressing aids.

EDUCATION, TRAINING, AND ADVANCEMENT

High school/secondary. High school students interested in pursuing the profession of occupational therapy in the future should pursue coursework in biology, psychology, anatomy, sociology, and mathematics to prepare for college-level studies. Students interested in the occupational therapy field will benefit from seeking internships or part-time work with occupational therapists or people with physical, developmental, or social problems that have an impact on their daily lives.

> **RELEVANT SKILLS AND ABILITIES**
>
> **Interpersonal/social skills**
> - Being able to remain calm
> - Cooperating with others
> - Teaching others
> - Working as a member of a team
>
> **Organization and management skills**
> - Coordinating tasks
> - Demonstrating leadership
> - Making decisions
> - Managing people/groups
> - Meeting goals and deadlines
> - Paying attention to and handling details
> - Performing duties that change frequently
>
> **Research and planning skills**
> - Creating ideas

Suggested High School Subjects
- Algebra
- Applied Biology/Chemistry
- Applied Communication
- Arts
- Biology
- Chemistry
- College Preparatory
- Composition
- Crafts
- English
- Health Science Technology
- Physical Education
- Physical Science
- Physiology
- Psychology
- Science
- Sociology

College/postsecondary. Occupational therapists typically have a master's degree or higher in their field. Interested college students should complete coursework in occupational therapy if offered by their school and courses in physical therapy, special education, biology, psychology, anatomy, sociology, and mathematics. Students interested in attending graduate school in occupational therapy will benefit from seeking internships or working with occupational therapists, people with impaired functioning, or as occupational therapy assistants or special education aides. Student membership in the American Occupational Therapy Association (AOTA) may provide networking opportunities and connections.

Related College Majors
- Anatomy
- Exercise Science/Physiology/Movement Studies
- Human and Animal Physiology
- Occupational Therapy
- Adult Job Seekers

Adult job seekers in the occupational therapy field should generally have completed master's or doctoral training in occupational therapy from an accredited university (as determined by the Accreditation Council for Occupational Therapy Education [ACOTE]) and earned the necessary professional licensure. Occupational therapists seeking employment will benefit from the networking opportunities, job workshops, and job lists offered by professional occupational therapy associations such as the AOTA.

PROFESSIONAL CERTIFICATION AND LICENSURE

Occupational therapists must have a professional occupational therapy license before beginning their professional practice. Upon completing an accredited master's or doctoral program in occupational therapy, candidates take a national occupational therapy licensing exam and, if successful, earn the Occupational Therapist Registered (OTR) title. In addition to national licensing, occupational therapists must register with their state health board and engage in continuing education as a condition of their license. State licensing boards generally have additional requirements for occupational therapists specializing in early education, mental health, or gerontological occupational therapy.

ADDITIONAL REQUIREMENTS

Occupational therapists enjoy helping other people achieve greater freedom and independence in their daily lives. They find satisfaction working in health care or educational environments with special needs populations. Occupational therapists require high levels of integrity and ethics, as they work with confidential and personal patient information. Successful occupational therapists engage in ongoing professional development. Membership in professional occupational therapy associations is encouraged among junior and senior occupational therapists as a means of building status within a professional community and networking.

SELECTED SCHOOLS

Many colleges and universities have bachelor's degree programs in counseling and rehabilitation therapy, often specializing in occupational therapy. The student may also gain an initial grounding in the field at a technical or community college. Consult with your school guidance counselor or research area postsecondary programs to find the right fit for you.

According to *U.S. News and World Report*, the twenty best occupational therapy programs are:
- Boston University
- University of Southern California
- University of Illinois, Chicago
- University of Pittsburgh
- Washington University in St. Louis
- Thomas Jefferson University
- Colorado State University
- Columbia University
- New York University
- Tufts University
- University of Florida

- University of North Carolina, Chapel Hill
- Medical University of South Carolina
- Ohio State University
- Creighton University
- Virginia Commonwealth University
- Quinnipiac University
- St. Catherine University
- Texas Women's University
- University of Kansas Medical Center

—*Simone Isadora Flynn*

Further Reading

"About Occupational Therapy." *American Occupational Therapy Association*, 2022, www.aota.org/about/for-the-media/about-occupational-therapy. Accessed 13 June 2022.

"About Occupational Therapy." *WFOT*, 2022, wfot.org/about/about-occupational-therapy. Accessed 13 June 2022.

"Best Occupational Therapy Programs." *U.S. News and World Report*, 2020, www.usnews.com/best-graduate-schools/top-health-schools/occupational-therapy-rankings. Accessed 13 June 2022.

Finlan, Timothy. "Occupational Therapy." *Nemours KidsHealth*, Jan. 2020, kidshealth.org/en/parents/occupational-therapy.html. Accessed 13 June 2022.

"What Occupational Therapists (OTs) Do." *College of Occupational Therapists of Ontario*, 2017, www.coto.org/you-and-your-ot/what-occupational-therapists-do. Accessed 13 June 2022.

ORTHOPEDICS

Category: Specialty

Specialties and related fields: Physical therapy, podiatry, rheumatology, sports medicine

Definition: the field of medicine concerned with the prevention and treatment of disorders, either developmental or caused by injury or disease, that are associated with the skeleton, joints, muscles, and connective tissues

KEY TERMS

articulation: a joint between two bones of the skeleton; also called an "arthrosis"

bursa: a connective tissue sac filled with fluid that reduces friction at joints

collagen: a fibrous protein found in skin, bone, ligaments, tendons, and cartilage

inflammation: the reaction of tissue to injury, with its corresponding redness, heat, swelling, and pain

ligament: a structure of tough connective tissue that attaches one bone to another bone

synovial: referring to the lubricating fluid in the joints or the membrane surrounding the joints

tendon: a structure of tough connective tissue that attaches a muscle to a bone

SCIENCE AND PROFESSION

Orthopedics is the branch of medicine primarily concerned with the movement of the human body and its parts and disorders that affect its function. Such activities as maintaining posture, walking, doing manual work, and exercising involve a complex relationship between the nervous, muscular, and skeletal systems. While orthopedists must be familiar with the nervous system, they focus primarily on preventing and treating disorders of the skeleton and muscles. They also have expertise in properly developing these systems in childhood and the changes that occur because of aging.

The brain sends signals to the muscles when a person decides to move. The muscles contract by pulling on the bones to which they are attached, causing that body part to move. The anchor point for the muscle is the origin, and the attachment point to the bone being moved is the insertion. Muscles work in groups to perform a movement. The principal muscle involved is the prime mover or agonist. The muscles that help the prime mover are called "synergists." When a prime mover contracts, the muscle on the opposite side of the bone, termed the antagonist, must relax. An illustration of this would be the muscle and bone interaction involved in arm flexing. The biceps muscle, anchored to the bone in the shoulder, contracts, pulling on the bone in the lower arm to which it is attached by a tendon. Its synergist, the brachialis, also contracts. On the back of the upper arm, its antagonist, the triceps muscle, relaxes to allow the arm to bend. When the arm is extended, the triceps becomes the prime mover for that action, and the biceps is the antagonist.

The skeletal system is made of bone and cartilage. Bone cells, called "osteocytes," take in nutrients from the blood and constantly renew the bony matrix. The chemical composition of bone includes calcium and phosphorus salts, which provide stiffness. The fibrous protein collagen gives bones some flexibility. Cartilage cells, called "chondrocytes," manufacture cartilage, a mass of collagen and elastic fibers embedded in a gelatin-like substance. The nature of this structure gives cartilage more flexibility than bone, making it an ideal substitute for bone in certain areas. The ribs, for example, are attached by cartilage to the sternum or breastbone. This arrangement allows for the expansion of the chest during breathing.

Tendons, ligaments, and bursas are also part of the skeletal and muscular systems. Tendons attach muscles to bones. They are made of fibrous tissue so strong that, under stress, the muscle will tear or the bone will break before the tendon is damaged. Ligaments, also made of fibrous tissue, attach bones to other bones and provide stability at the joints. Bursas are fluid-filled connective tissue sacs between muscle and bone, tendon and bone, or other areas around joints. They reduce the damage to the softer tissue as it rubs against the bone with each movement. Because of their close interdependence, the skeleton, attached muscles, and other associated structures are often referred to as the musculoskeletal system.

The health of the musculoskeletal system during childhood is of primary importance to an individual in attaining full growth and physical function as an adult. A cartilage skeleton is formed in the early developmental stages of the embryo and fetus. This structure is replaced with bone in an ossification process that continues for years after birth. Good nutrition is vital to this process. In particular, the body requires adequate amounts of protein, calcium, and vitamin D. The ends of a long bone are separated from the shaft of the bone by cartilage until the child reaches full growth. Care should be taken when participating in sports since damage to these areas could affect the growth of that limb. Hormonal production influences the development of the skeleton. Adequate amounts of growth hormone are needed to ensure proper growth. At puberty, sex hormones, especially testosterone, stimulate the adult skeleton's final growth spurts and completion.

A woman of childbearing age must eat a healthy diet if she is to nourish a fetus that, in turn, is developing its skeleton.

Young adults have attained full growth, but the skeleton must continually renew itself to remain strong and maintain its ability to repair an injury. Both men and women must take care to exercise since the stress of activity builds muscle and sends messages to the bone to maintain its strength. Calcium and vitamin D intake must continue, or the bones may begin to dissolve some of their calcium matrices. Automobile accidents, work injuries, and sports injuries are more likely to occur at this stage of life.

As adults age, metabolic and other cellular processes become less efficient. Care must be taken to maintain functions and prevent further losses. At one time, disorders such as osteoarthritis and osteoporosis were considered an inevitable part of the aging process. While heredity is certainly a risk factor in these conditions, substantial evidence has been accumulated showing that some degenerative processes can be traced to lifestyle and diet. Osteoarthritis is the type of joint tissue degeneration associated with wear and tear on the joints. A person who is obese puts excessive pressure on the skeletal system, especially the hips, knees, and ankles. This pressure increases the damage to the joints. A person who fails to exercise begins to lose flexibility in the joints, and muscles become weaker.

Osteoporosis occurs as bones become porous and brittle. As osteocytes age, they become less efficient at calcium absorption and renewal of the bony matrix. At a time in life when more calcium is needed to make up for this inefficiency, most people consume fewer dairy products, either because of lactose intolerance or because of the ingestion of other beverages. Older women are at particular risk because

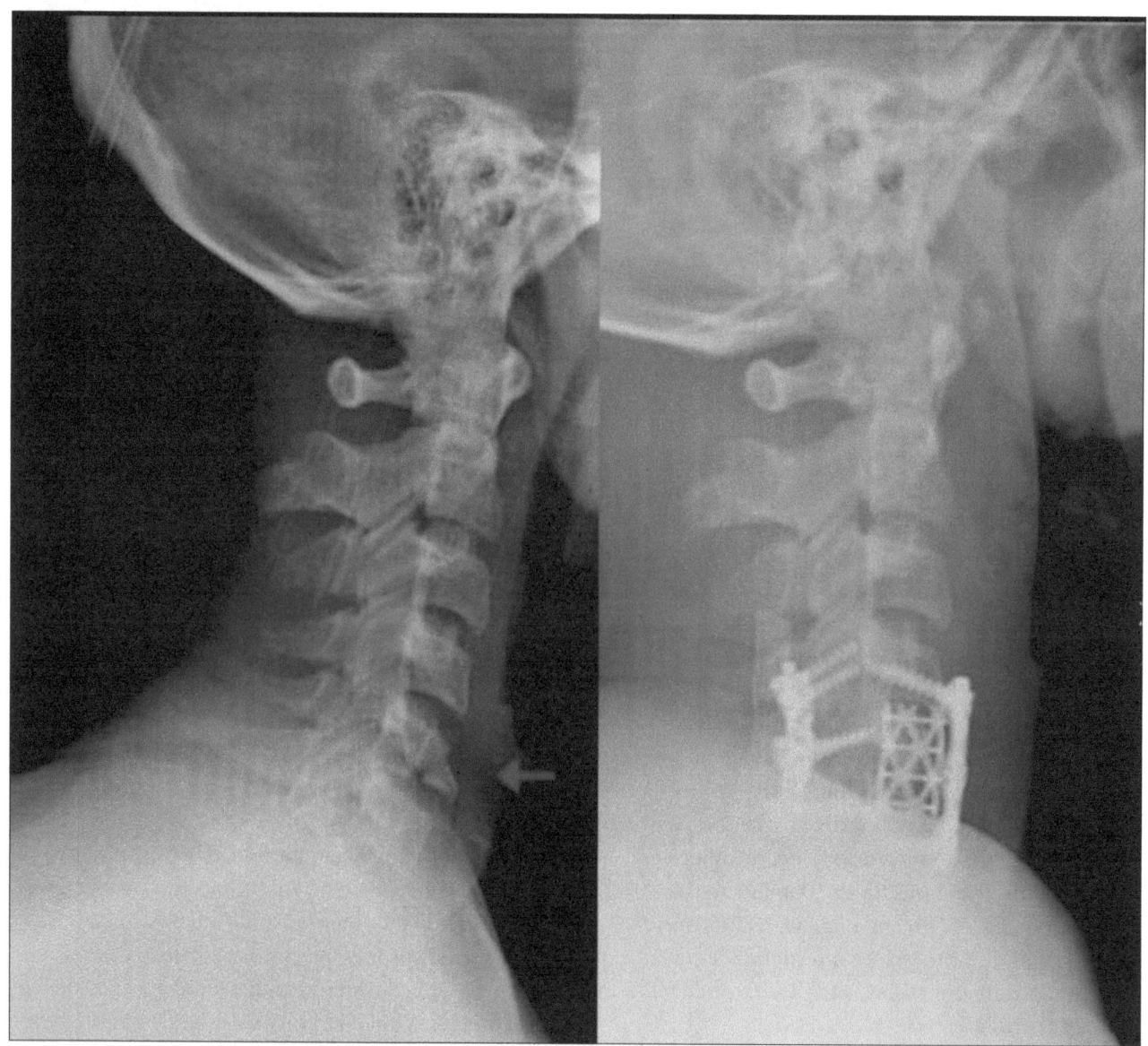

This fracture of the lower cervical vertebrae is one of the conditions treated by orthopedic surgeons and neurosurgeons. Photo by Moquito 17 at the English-language Wikipedia, via Wikimedia Commons.

their bones are lighter than men's. After menopause, women lose some of the protection that estrogen provides by stimulating the absorption of calcium and thus bone renewal. Suppose older people lose the ability to move as surely as before, and their reflexes slow down. In that case, injuries are more likely to occur due to falls. These injuries are much more serious if the bones are brittle. Even if osteoporosis is not a factor, fractures and other injuries in an older individual do not heal as quickly as in a younger person.

Because of their knowledge of developmental processes, orthopedists and pediatricians can advise parents concerned about their growing children and the appropriate precautions for sports activities. Orthopedists make recommendations about the design and utilization of safety equipment to prevent or reduce injury. Physicians may also advise on nutrition and exercise for adults to reduce the incidence of problems as a person ages, allowing the continuation of an active, independent life.

DIAGNOSTIC AND TREATMENT TECHNIQUES

In nonemergency situations, patients with some pain or disorder of the muscles, bones, or joints are usually referred to an orthopedic surgeon. The first office visit begins with a review of the condition. The physician will take a general medical history and obtain a history of the current complaint. This history will include the time frame from the onset, any action that may have initiated the condition, and a description of any movement difficulty the patient has. A physician will then perform a physical examination to determine the areas affected and observe range-of-motion exercises to determine if function has been lost.

X-rays or other imaging methods are ordered to see whether any structural defect can be seen. The physician may order blood tests if a disease process is suspected. Once a diagnosis has been made, a physician may prescribe medication, order physical therapy or home exercises, schedule surgery, or take other therapeutic measures to correct the condition. The abnormalities treated by orthopedists generally fall into one of three categories: injuries caused by accidents, repetitive motion disorders, and diseases affecting the skeleton, skeletal muscles, or joints.

The most common situation in which a patient sees an orthopedist is after an accidental injury. The patient may be transported to a hospital emergency room if the injury is severe. Care is taken to keep the injury site immobilized until a physician can see the patient. The type of treatment needed will be determined by the type and severity of the injury. In a closed or simple fracture, the skin is unbroken; the bones are manipulated back in line and then immobilized with a plaster cast or brace. An open or compound fracture occurs when the ends or fragments of the bone protrude through the skin. In this case, or if surgery is needed to align the bones properly, there is a higher risk of infection. Sometimes, the orthopedic surgeon must use pins or wires to hold the bone in position. Fractures of the skull or vertebrae are of special concern because of the possibility of permanent damage to the brain or spinal cord; a neurologist (a physician with specialty training in the nervous system) is usually called to assist an orthopedic surgeon.

Because of twisting movements, injuries that affect one or more joints are common. A dislocation occurs when the bones at a joint are separated. An orthopedist must realign the bones as closely as possible to the original positions and immobilize the joint to allow healing. Joint sprains result from severe twisting of a joint without dislocation. The severity of joint injury and recovery time depend on the extent of the damage to surrounding ligaments, tendons, cartilage, and other tissues. The orthopedist may schedule an arthroscopy procedure since damage to soft tissue may not be revealed in an X-ray. An orthopedic surgeon inserts a flexible tube, called an "arthroscope," into the injury site. This tube, combined with lights and a camera, allows the surgeon to view the joint cavity to see if any abnormality is present and, if possible, repair it.

Some damage to the musculoskeletal system is not the result of a single accident but actions repeated over a long period as a part of work duties or recreational activities. These are termed "repetitive motion disorders". For example, bursitis, or inflammation of the bursas, may arise in a baseball pitcher's shoulder or a tennis player's elbow. Because the same motion is repeated over and over, the rub of the bursa and other soft tissue over bone causes irritation and inflammation, resulting in pain each time the movement is attempted. Treatment consists of reducing the inflammation by using cortisone or other similar drugs, usually by injection at the affected site, coupled with rest. Resumption of the activity may occur following recommendations from an orthopedist or therapist on a change in technique to reduce the trauma. Sometimes, the condition becomes chronic, and the patient may have to discontinue the activity altogether.

Many occupations arising in the mid-twentieth century involved small movements of the hands and wrists. A worker on an assembly line who installs a specific part and an employee who uses a computer keyboard all day are examples of people at high risk for repetitive motion disorders. An understanding of the structure of the wrist leads to a better understanding of the problem involved. The median nerve leads from the spinal cord through a tunnel in the wrist's carpal bones and then branches out to the fingers. It is encircled, together with tendons leading to the fingers, by the transverse carpal ligament. When constant friction causes swelling of the tendons and tissues adjacent to the nerve, the nerve is pinched, resulting in pain, tingling, and weakness in the hand and fingers. This condition is termed carpal tunnel syndrome. Therapy may include changing work positions, wearing a splint to hold the wrist straight, using medications to reduce inflammation, and injecting cortisone at the injury site. If the problem continues, the patient may need surgery. In this procedure, the orthopedic surgeon makes an incision in the wrist and cuts the transverse carpal ligament, thus releasing the pressure on the nerve and tendons. If the motion or activity that initially caused carpal tunnel syndrome is not stopped, the condition is likely to recur.

Diseases can affect the bones and joints. Congenital disabilities and inheritance may result in deformities that can be treated by orthopedic devices or surgery. A physician may use hormone therapy to help a child attain full growth. Nutritional disorders, such as rickets, may cause the softening of the bones, with the corresponding bowed-leg deformity. Rickets is caused by vitamin D deficiency and must be treated with vitamin therapy and braces to keep the legs straight while the bones harden. Multiple myeloma is a form of cancer that invades the bone and bone marrow and must be treated with chemotherapy and surgery to remove the tumor. Infections such as gangrene affect the limbs and, if not treated in time, may necessitate amputation by the orthopedic surgeon.

Of all the musculoskeletal system diseases, arthritis and related disorders are the most common. "Arthritis" is a general term referring to inflammation of a joint. Osteoarthritis is a degenerative disease resulting to some extent from aging. However, it can be exacerbated by obesity, lifestyle, or injury. Arthritis can also be caused by infection or deposits of uric acid crystals; a condition called "gout." The most serious form of joint disease is "rheumatoid arthritis." This term is sometimes used to encompass a group of related disorders. These diseases are classified as autoimmune conditions because the body is making antibodies against itself—in this case, against the tissues associated with the joints. A specialist often treats the disease process itself called a "rheumatologist," who tries various medications to alleviate the condition. A referring physician may call an orthopedic surgeon to help correct the deformities resulting from the disease or replace defective joints with artificial ones. Special care must be taken in cases of juvenile rheumatoid arthritis since the growth process may also be affected. Systemic lupus erythematosus (SLE), ankylosing spondylitis, and scleroderma are some other autoimmune diseases that affect the musculoskeletal system.

PERSPECTIVE AND PROSPECTS

In the study of prehistoric humans, a major source of information is their skeletal remains. Archaeologists have found evidence of broken bones that were set and healed, indicating some rudimentary attempts at treating injuries. Examination of hieroglyphs shows that ancient Egyptians set bones and used wooden splints held in place by the same gum and bandages used to wrap mummies. There were no medical specialties and the treatment of wounds and fractures as part of the duties of any medical practitioner.

The branch of medicine known as orthopedics had its start in the eighteenth century. The term "orthopedics" is a combination of two Greek words: *orthos*, meaning "straight" or "correct," and *pais*, meaning "child." A physician named Jean André Venel (1740-91) opened an institute in Switzerland to correct skeletal deformities in children. Treatment of congenital deformities such as clubfoot and defects caused by rickets or injury was the primary function of this type of clinic.

In the nineteenth century, the development of quick-setting plaster for casts aided physicians in immobilizing broken bones after they were set. The development of anesthesia and antiseptic techniques to prevent infection allowed the practice of orthopedic surgery to expand. Research using the microscope added to the understanding of the structure and function of bone as living tissue.

In 1895, Wilhelm Conrad Röntgen (1845-1923) discovered that radiation from a cathode-ray tube would produce a photographic image of the bones of his hand. By the early twentieth century, the medical X-ray became widespread, providing an invaluable diagnostic tool for orthopedists. In the 1940s and 1950s, a better understanding of radioactive phenomena allowed the development of safer X-ray equipment and techniques. In the 1970s and 1980s, other imaging techniques, such as computed tomography (CT) scanning and magnetic resonance imaging (MRI), increased the ability of orthopedic surgeons to diagnose and treat musculoskeletal disorders.

One of the greatest orthopedic surgical advances has been in the ability to treat badly damaged limbs. At one time, the best the orthopedic surgeon could do for some patients was to amputate the limb to prevent the spread of infection and the development of gangrene, then help the patient cope with the amputations by using artificial limbs. More sophisticated techniques, incorporating the microscope with computer-directed surgical instruments, allow the reattachment of limbs in many cases by enabling the surgeon to connect even the smallest blood vessels and nerves.

If amputation is necessary, artificial limbs or prostheses have become more sophisticated. Artificial hands have become functional because of computer technology that enables the patient to direct the movement of the fingers by contracting and relaxing arm muscles. New plastics and other materials are being developed and used for synthetic joint replacements, increasing mobility and decreasing pain for arthritic patients.

Joints are now routinely replaced. The most common replacements are hip and knee joints, although techniques have been developed to replace other joints. The surgery is performed in a hospital. Recipients are encouraged to use their replaced joints within twenty-four to forty-eight hours after surgery. Complete rehabilitation requires several months of increasingly intense physical activity and exercise.

Contemporary materials have an expected useful life of twenty or more years.

A better understanding of the natural healing process at the cellular level has also allowed advances in the treatment of fractures. It has been found that attaching a device that generates a weak electric current can increase the rate of healing in some patients. This current stimulates the multiplication of osteocytes and the growth of new bone in the area.

As the understanding of disease and degenerative processes increases, better treatments can also be devised. For example, osteoporosis is, in many cases, a preventable condition when a correct diet and sufficient physical exercise are maintained throughout life. After menopause in women, treatment with estrogen replacement therapy gives further protection against osteoporosis. New imaging devices allow osteoporosis to be detected earlier and more aggressive treatment measures to be applied. The genetic factor in diseases and conditions that trigger autoimmune disorders are other areas of research that are being pursued. While accidents will always occur, orthopedic research into the injury process can help devise methods of prevention, as well as new treatments for the orthopedic problems that arise.

—*Edith K. Wallace, L. Fleming Fallon Jr.*

Further Reading

American Academy of Orthopaedic Surgeons, www.aaos.org.
Cash, Mel. *Pocket Atlas of the Moving Body*. Crown, 2000.
Currey, John D. *Bones: Structures and Mechanics*. 2nd ed., Princeton UP, 2006.
Delforge, Gary. *Musculoskeletal Trauma: Implications for Sport Injury Management*. Human Kinetics, 2002.
Marcus, Robert, David Feldman, and Jennifer Kelsey, editors. *Osteoporosis*. 3rd ed., Academic Press/Elsevier, 2008.
Marieb, Elaine N., and Katja Hoehn. *Human Anatomy and Physiology*. 11th ed., Pearson, 2018.
"Orthopedic Services." *MedlinePlus*, n.d., medlineplus.gov/ency/article/007455.htm.
Rosen, Clifford J., Julie Glowacki, and John P. Bilezikian. *The Aging Skeleton*. Academic Press, 1999.
Salter, Robert Bruce. *Textbook of Disorders and Injuries of the Musculoskeletal System*. 3rd ed., Williams & Wilkins, 1999.
Slovik, David M. *Osteoporosis: A Guide to Prevention and Treatment*. Harvard Health Publishing, 2019.
Tortora, Gerard J., and Bryan Derrickson. *Principles of Anatomy and Physiology*. 16th ed., Wiley, 2020.

Personal Trainer

Category: Career
Specialties and related fields: Personal trainers, physical fitness, strength and conditioning
Definition: individuals who have earned a certification that demonstrates they have achieved a level of competency for creating and delivering safe and effective exercise programs for apparently healthy individuals and groups or those with medical clearance to exercise

KEY TERMS

conditioning: the process of training to become physically fit through a regimen of exercise, diet, and rest
exercise: activity requiring physical effort, carried out to sustain or improve health and fitness
physical fitness: activity requiring physical effort, carried out to sustain or improve health and fitness
strength: the measure of a human's exertion of force on physical objects; increasing physical strength is the goal of strength training

OVERVIEW

Sphere of work. Personal trainers design, organize, and lead exercise and sports programs that allow individuals to improve their health through cardiovascular activity, strength training, and stretching exercises. They usually offer private lessons as well as group instruction. They teach the fundamentals of fitness by presenting clients with various techniques,

> **PROFILE**
>
> - **Interests**: People, things
> - **Working conditions**: Work inside, work outside, work both inside and outside
> - **Physical Strength**: Medium Work
> - **Education Needs**: Bachelor's Degree
> - **Licensure/Certification**: Recommended
> - **Physical Abilities Not Required**: Not Climb
> - **Opportunities for Experience**: Internship, Volunteer Work

helping them set individually tailored fitness goals, and motivating them physically and mentally to reach those goals. Personal trainers often focus on multiple areas of fitness, such as aerobics, weightlifting, yoga, or Pilates.

Work environment. Personal trainers work in various settings, from health clubs and exercise studios to resorts and universities. Some travel to clients' homes to provide regular instruction, while others organize fitness programs for large businesses. Most personal trainers work indoors in cool climates; however, some offer instruction in pleasant outdoor environments. Most personal trainers work full time with irregular hours, as they must cater to their clients' schedules. They often work early in the morning, at night, on weekends, and during holidays. Personal trainers spend most of their time standing, walking, and participating in physical activities.

OCCUPATION INTEREST

Those looking to become personal trainers must be in excellent physical condition and have natural athletic ability. They should have a passion for instructing and motivating individuals. Sometimes clients are reluctant to participate in specified activities, so personal trainers should be firm, persuasive, and encouraging. Creativity and patience are also valuable traits. Personal trainers must have strong customer service skills to find and maintain their clientele.

A DAY IN THE LIFE—DUTIES AND RESPONSIBILITIES

A personal trainer works one-on-one with a client to create and follow a fitness training plan customized to the client's specific goal(s): strength training, weight loss, improved performance, disease management, or enhanced health. Trainers introduce individualized exercise plans and should always keep current with the latest trends and professional recommendations in fitness and nutrition.

Professional personal trainers have national certification and advanced knowledge of human anatomy and physiology, nutrition, and exercise science. They create and lead individual and group exercise sessions tailored to the health needs of their clients. Fitness trainers conduct client assessments to develop these plans, help establish healthy nutritional behaviors and motivate their clients to succeed.

> **DUTIES AND RESPONSIBILITIES**
>
> - Create and present fitness and exercise programs to clients
> - Motivate and guide clients through fitness routines
> - Evaluate and measure client progress using measurement tools.
> - Meet with new clients and discuss fitness and nutritional goals
> - Study new techniques and advances in fitness and nutrition
> - Practice new routines and exercises
> - Alter programs for clients to meet changing needs

EDUCATION, TRAINING, AND ADVANCEMENT

High school/secondary. Most national certification bodies require candidates to have a high school diploma or equivalent to sit for a certifying examination. Although postsecondary education, in the form of a certificate, training course, or formal degree, is highly recommended, completing the minimum educational requirement is important.

Vocational and technical schools typically offer either short-term personal training programs or courses that focus on a specific personal training certification program, such as the Certified Personal Trainer (CPT) examination from the National Academy of Sports Medicine (NASM). Vocational programs are career-focused, allowing students to concentrate their studies in an area of interest (e.g., aerobics) without completing the requirements for an entire degree.

Postsecondary. Community college programs are designed to be short, professionally oriented instruction that prepares graduates for direct entry into a career field. Community college students may select from several types of training, including stand-alone certificate programs, personal training programs, and formal associate degree programs in majors such as exercise science, kinesiology, and personal training. Each of these programs aims to prepare graduates for national certification examinations.

Four-year universities and colleges offer undergraduate (bachelor's) and graduate (master's and PhD) programs for individuals interested in expanding their knowledge of personal fitness, wellness, and health. These programs are much broader in scope, with a curriculum covering both general education and courses in specialized fields, such as exercise science.

Professional certification and licensure. Prospective trainers can select a specialization that matches their skill sets, personal interests, and professional goals, such as the following: group exercise, individualized personal training, and fitness programming. Once you decide on your path, you should review various fitness certifying bodies and the fitness certifications they offer to find the program that makes the most sense to prepare you for the career you envision for yourself.

Once you have determined the certification that is best for you, whether CPT from the American Council on Exercise (ACE) or the NASM, you can start to prepare for the certification examination by taking exam prep courses, multisession training classes, undergraduate degrees in exercise science, or even graduate degrees in kinesiology.

Certain certifying bodies, such as the American College of Sports Medicine (ACSM), offer personal training courses. These live clinics last one to three days in length, serving as exam preparation workshops that include lectures and practical instruction from experienced and certified trainers. At the conclusion, graduates are prepared to take national certification examinations.

Personal trainers must be ready to deal with physical emergencies when working with clients. They should complete cardiopulmonary resuscitation (CPR) and automated external defibrillator (AED) certification programs to be ready for them. Nearly every national personal training certification organization requires AED and CPR certifications. These programs teach trainers how to recognize a medical

---

RELEVANT SKILLS AND ABILITIES

Communication Skills
- Communicating with clients from a variety of backgrounds
- Creating simple instructions for clients

Interpersonal/Social Skills
- Engaging in frequent daily interactions with clients and other professionals
- Motivating and encouraging clients and giving constructive feedback

Organization & Management Skills
- Managing class and training schedules
- Helping to keep clients on track for meeting goals
- Creating fitness routines for new clients

Research & Planning Skills
- Researching and learning about new fitness techniques
- Practicing exercises and other fitness activities

Technical Skills
- Utilizing basic technology for communication and scheduling
- Using physical monitoring/measurement equipment

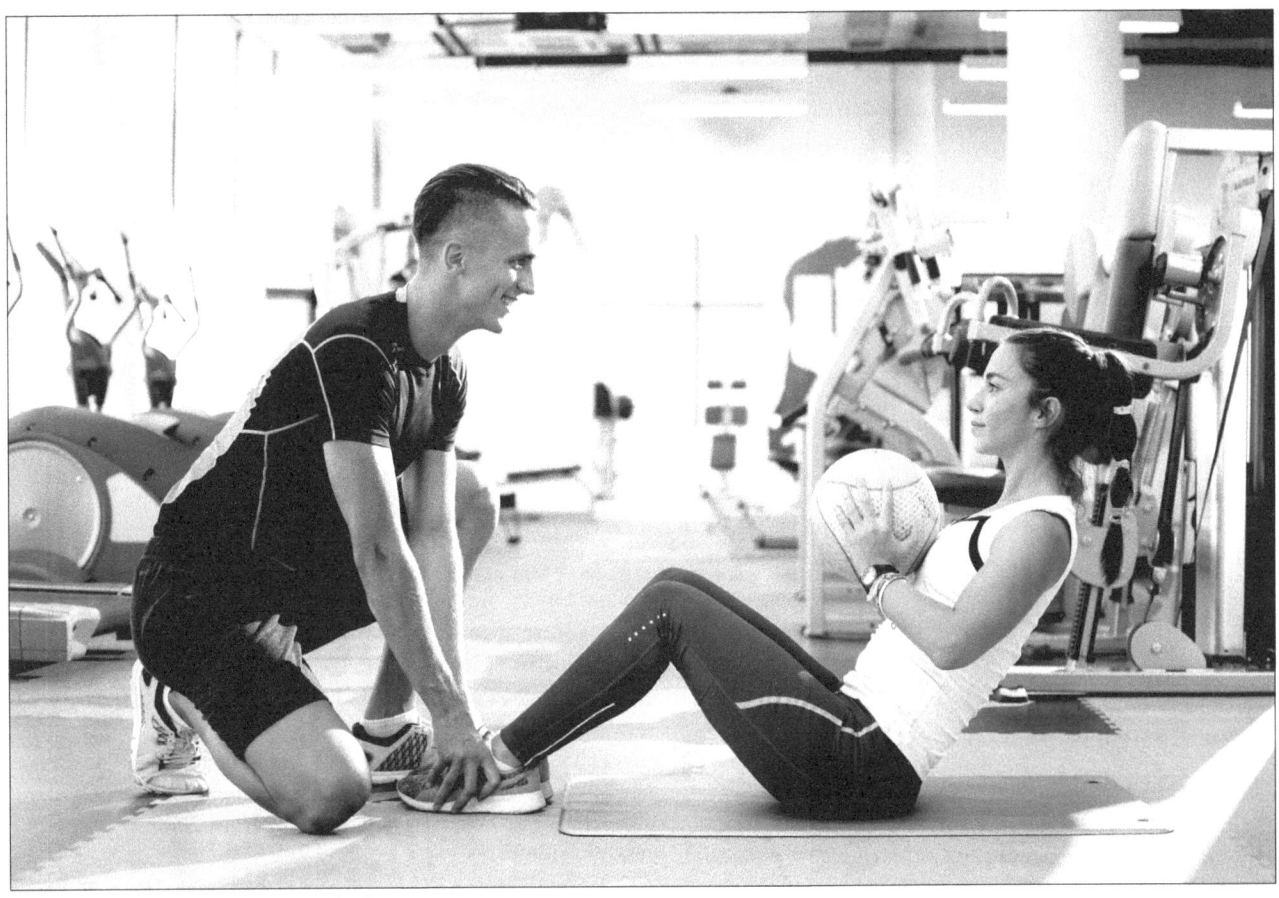

Photo via iStock/Bojan89. [Used under license.]

emergency, deal appropriately with cardiac or breathing emergencies, and act swiftly to help a client until professional first responders arrive.

You should register for the selected certification examination, which typically includes an application and fee. Most personal training certifications are computer-based tests that include 120 and 150 multiple-choice questions. For example, the CPT Certification from the NASM has questions across four sections: Program Planning; Client Consultation and Fitness Assessment; Exercise Techniques; and Safety/Emergency Issues.

The National Commission for Certifying Agencies (NCCA) is the primary accrediting body for personal training certifications. Individuals interested in personal trainer careers should ensure they select accredited programs as most employers prefer accredited candidates. The four major certifying bodies include the following:

- American College of Sports Medicine (ACSM)
- National Academy of Sports Medicine (NASM)
- American Council on Exercise (ACE)
- National Strength and Conditioning Association (NSCA)

THE FITNESS INDUSTRY

The fitness industry is large, with several different personal trainer careers in nutrition, conditioning, performance, sports medicine, and more. Below are five examples of potential career specializations for individuals seeking beyond personal training.

Exercise physiologist. Exercise physiologists work with diverse populations, ranging from world-class athletes to individuals with chronic diseases, to maintain, improve, or enhance their clients' overall fitness, health, and physical performance. An undergraduate degree in kinesiology or exercise science is usually required, along with national certification from the ACSM and a master's degree and board certification from the American Society of Exercise Physiologists for clinical positions.

Sports nutritionist. Sports nutritionists understand how the body uses food to fuel physical activity. They work with clients, including sports teams or as part of corporate wellness programs to develop nutritionally sound menus, implement education programs, and assist in one-on-one nutritional counseling. State educational requirements vary, but a bachelor's degree in nutrition, kinesiology, exercise science, or a related field is the typical minimum educational requirement. Certification from the American Dietetics Association or board certification from the Commission on Dietetic Registration is commonly required.

Group exercise instructor. Group exercise instructors design, develop, and lead group personal training sessions in specialty exercise modalities, including yoga, aerobics, cycling, Pilates, and more. Instructors lead the class, doing the exercises with their clients to provide motivation and teach and model proper technique. Professional certification from organizations such as the ACSM and the American Council on Fitness is typically required for employment.

Corrective exercise specialist. Corrective exercise specialists use their knowledge of posture and the mechanics of body movement to help clients deal with flexibility issues, joint pain, or muscle through individualized corrective exercise programs to restore full-body movement in clients. Professional experience and a CPT certification are generally required before earning a Corrective Exercise Specialist certification from the NASM.

Strength and conditioning coach. Strength and conditioning coaches generally have two goals for their clients: Improved athletic performance and fewer athletic injuries. They traditionally work with sports teams but may also work in physical therapy clinics, fitness clubs, and high schools. A bachelor's degree, previous fitness experience, and certification from the NSCA are typically required.

Further Reading

"Earn Your Personal Trainer Certification (NASM-CPT)." *The National Academy of Sports Medicine*, n.d., www.nasm.org/become-a-personal-trainer.

"Personal Trainer Job Description." Workable Technology Limited, n.d., resources.workable.com/personal-trainer-job-description.

"Scope of Practice for NFPT Personal Trainers." National Federation of Personal Trainers, n.d., www.nfpt.com/the-role-of-a-personal-trainer.

Trivium. *ACE Personal Trainer Exam Prep: Study Guide with Practice Test Questions for the American Council on Exercise CPT Examination.* Trivium Test Prep, 2020.

Physical Medicine and Rehabilitation (PM&R)

Category: Specialty
Specialties and related fields: Neurology, pain medicine, physical medicine and rehabilitation, physical therapy, sports medicine
Definition: a branch of medicine that aims to enhance and restore functional ability and quality of life to people with physical impairments or disabilities

KEY TERMS

injury: hurt, damage, or loss of function due to some event or illness *rehabilitation*: restoring someone to health or normal life through training and therapy after imprisonment, addiction, or illness

trigger point: a sensitive area of the body, stimulation or irritation of which causes a specific effect in another part, especially a tender area in a muscle that causes generalized musculoskeletal pain when overstimulated

INTRODUCTION

Physical medicine and rehabilitation (PM&R), also known as "physiatry", is a field of medicine that deals with healing a person as a whole. It treats patients who have incurable diseases, physical or cognitive impairments, or disabilities that can make performing day-to-day activities difficult. These conditions, which may be inherited or caused by medical conditions, surgery, or injury, can affect parts of the body, including the bones, brain, joints, ligaments, muscles, nerves, spinal cord, and tendons, causing loss of body functions. Physicians known as "physiatrists" are trained in PM&R to treat patients with these medical conditions. Physiatry not only treats patients' physical conditions but also considers illness-related functional, emotional, and psychosocial issues that may arise.

BACKGROUND

Physician Frank H. Krusen is credited with the founding of the field of PM&R. Motivated by his own treatment for tuberculosis in the 1920s, Krusen decided to devote his life to researching physical medicine. He studied physical agents of healing such as light, heat, and water to treat certain medical conditions. He helped begin a physical therapy program at Temple University in Philadelphia, Pennsylvania. He then went to work at the Mayo Clinic.

In 1936, Krusen and more than a dozen other physicians, known as "physical therapy physicians," began working on establishing the Department of Physical Medicine at the Mayo Clinic. The program eventually became a three-year residency, the first of its kind in the United States. The group then worked with the American Medical Association (AMA) to receive a specialty status for the branch.

Krusen came up with the term "physiatrist" for a doctor specializing in physical medicine in 1938. While the term was close to the word psychiatrist, he emphasized the third syllable of the word (pronounced *fizz-ee-AT-rist*) to avoid confusion between the two. In the years that followed, Krusen and the other physicians, now known as physiatrists, routinely met with the AMA and the American Board of Medical Specialties (ABMS). Although the groups agreed that the field should be certified, they disagreed on whether it should have its own specialty status or be grouped with another field of medicine. Krusen published the PM&R textbook *Handbook of Physical Medicine and Rehabilitation* in 1941.

Physiatry began to receive more attention after World War II (1939-45) when injured soldiers returned home and needed care to help them recover and regain their lives. The AMA eventually recognized the term physiatrist in 1946. A year later, Krusen and fellow physicians Walter Zeiter and John Coulter again presented their plans for an American Board of Physical Medicine and Rehabilitation (ABPMR). The AMA and ABMA finally recognized the field and the board and installed Krusen as the chairman. Nearly eighty doctors took the first board exams for physical medicine that year and became certified in the new field.

OVERVIEW

Physiatrists must complete medical school and four years of training in a PM&R residency. The ABPMR requires the passage of both written and oral examinations to become board certified in PM&R. Because of the large range of conditions physiatrists treat; many choose to complete training in additional fields such as pediatrics, internal medicine, and neurology. They may receive subfield certification, including brain injury medicine, hospice and palliative medicine, neuromuscular medicine, pain medicine, pediatric rehabilitation medicine, spinal cord injury medicine, or sports medicine.

Physical medicine and rehabilitation may be used to treat numerous conditions, such as neurological disorders caused by spinal cord injury, traumatic brain injury, stroke, multiple sclerosis, and Parkinson's disease; chronic pain issues, such as back and neck pain, joint and muscle pain, arthritis, and carpal tunnel syndrome; musculoskeletal problems, such as osteoarthritis, osteoporosis, rheumatoid arthritis, and fibromyalgia; sports-related injuries, such as tendonitis, stress fractures, and concussion; genetic conditions, including cerebral palsy, muscular dystrophy, spina bifida, and Down syndrome; organ transplants; amputations; cardiac/pulmonary disease; swallowing and speech disorders; bowel and bladder problems; cancers; and burns.

PM&R helps people live with their medical conditions. Some conditions, such as Down syndrome, are inherited, while others, such as broken bones, may be caused by accidents. Instead of focusing on a cure, many of these conditions can only be managed, not cured. Instead, the goal of PM&R is to treat the medical issue to enhance the patient's quality of life and restore their functional ability. The treatment not only helps people manage physical pain but also helps patients reach a point where they can perform daily living activities, such as eating, dressing, bathing, using the bathroom,

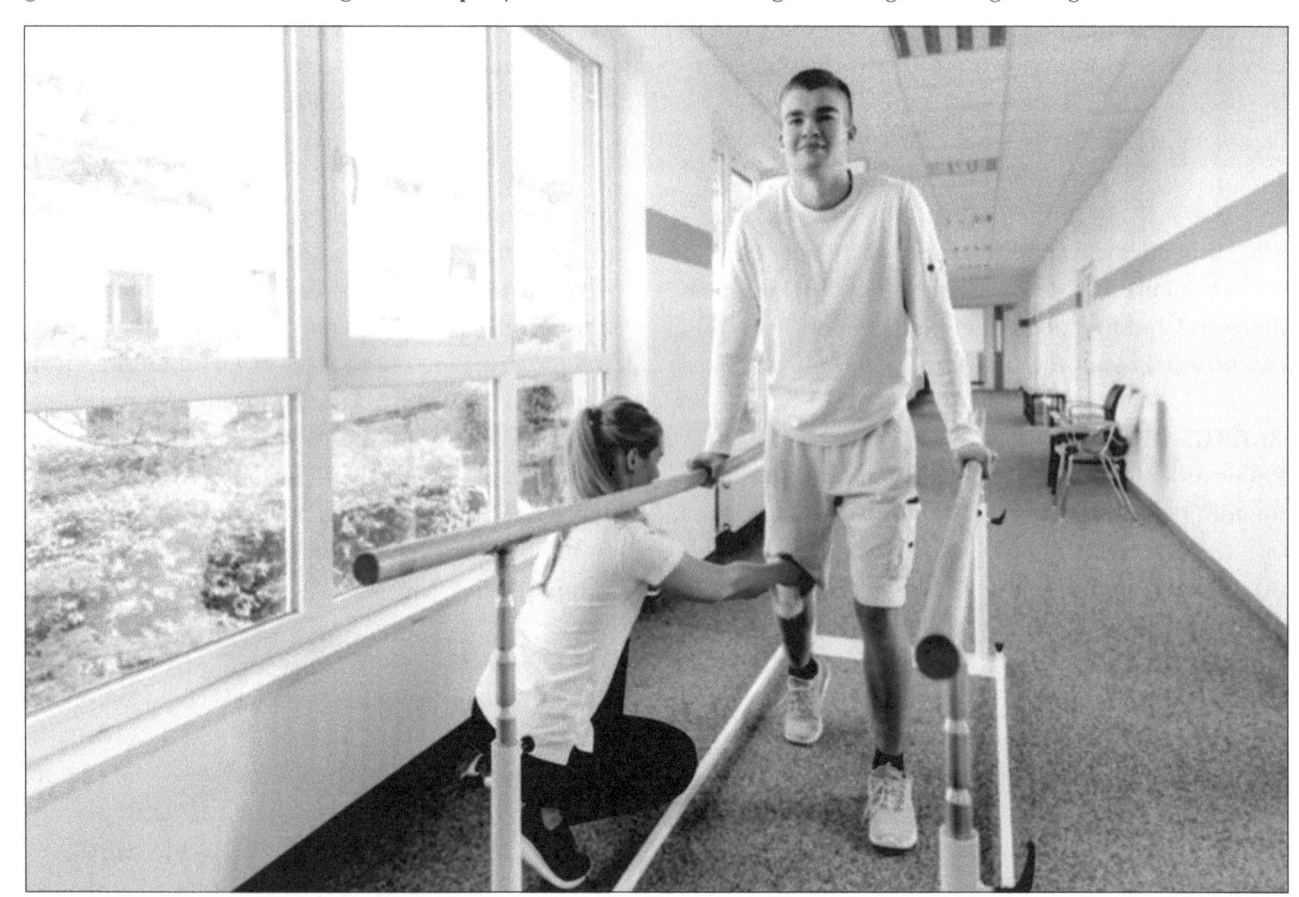

Photo via iStock/kzenon. [Used under license.]

or moving to and from a wheelchair independently.

Physiatrists design a specific patient-centered treatment plan to work on their needs exclusively. Such plans treat medical, physical, social, emotional, and work-related problems that may arise from a condition or an illness. In addition, physiatrists work with other physicians and specialists (neurologists, orthopedists, neurosurgeons, physical and occupational therapists, social services, psychiatrists, speech pathologists, etc.) to ensure that patients receive the care they need. For example, physiatrists may help amputees with fitting and using prostheses. They may plan to include pain management, physical therapy, and psychiatric care so the patient can deal with the physical and emotional issues associated with losing a limb.

Physiatrists perform and prescribe treatments such as injections, ultrasounds, discography, nerve stimulation, biopsies, and prosthetics and orthotics. For example, for muscular issues, they may use electromyography (EMG), which involves inserting tiny needles into muscles to assess movement and weakness. They use nerve conduction studies (NCS) to monitor motor and sensory responses. Peripheral joint injections can aid in bone and soft tissue disorders. Such injections may treat conditions such as orthopedic or sports-related injuries. Trigger point injections combined with physical therapy can treat chronic myofascial or soft tissue pain. Other treatments, such as acupuncture, platelet injections, and stem cell treatments, also may be used.

—Angela Harmon

Further Reading

"About Physical Medicine and Rehabilitation." *American Academy of Physical Medicine and Rehabilitation*, 2022, www.abpmr.org/consumers/pmr_definition.html. Accessed 14 Jun. 2022.

"Conditions and Treatments." *American Academy of Physical Medicine and Rehabilitation*, 2022, www.aapmr.org/about-physiatry/conditions-treatments.

"Dr. Frank Kriise of Mayo Clinic, 75." *New York Times*, 18 Sept. 1973, www.nytimes.com/1973/09/18/archives/dr-frank-krusen-of-mayo-clinic-75-rehabilitation-expert-diesled.html?_r=0. Accessed 21 Nov. 2016.

"History of the Specialty." *American Academy of Physical Medicine and Rehabilitation*, 2022, www.aapmr.org/about-physiatry/history-of-the-specialty. Accessed 21 Nov. 2016.

"Physiatry—Rehabilitation Medicine." *Johns Hopkins Medicine*, n.d., www.hopkinsmedicine.org/physical_medicine_rehabilitation/. Accessed 14 Jun. 2022.

"Physical Medicine and Rehabilitation." *Mayo Clinic*, 20 Nov. 2021, www.mayoclinic.org/departments-centers/physical-medicine-rehabilitation/overview. Accessed 21 Nov. 2016.

"Physical Medicine and Rehabilitation." *MedlinePlus*, 8 Oct. 2015, medlineplus.gov/ency/article/007448.htm. Accessed 21 Nov. 2016.

Staehler, Richard A. "What Is a Physiatrist?" *Spine-health.com*, 29 Sept. 2011, www.spine-health.com/treatment/spine-specialists/what-a-physiatrist. Accessed 21 Nov. 2016.

PHYSICAL THERAPIST

Category: Career

Specialties and related fields: Physical medicine and rehabilitation, physical therapy, physiotherapy

Definition: the treatment of disease, injury, or deformity by physical methods such as massage, heat treatment, and exercise rather than by drugs or surgery

KEY TERMS

ASTYM®: a tool used to break up scar tissue and damaged soft tissue to promote regeneration of healthy tissue to improve one's function

hydrotherapy: exercises in a pool as part of treatment for conditions such as arthritis or partial paralysis

therapeutic exercise: movement prescribed to correct impairments, restore muscular and skeletal function and maintain a state of well-being

therapeutic massage: the manipulation of the body's soft tissues to treat body stress or pain

ultrasound therapy: an ultrasonic procedure that uses ultrasound for therapeutic benefit

OVERVIEW

Sphere of work. Physical therapists (PTs) provide therapeutic services to patients with temporary and chronic physical conditions or illnesses that limit physical movements and mobility, thereby negatively affecting patients' life and work. Physical therapists develop treatment plans to help maintain or recover a patient's physical mobility, lessen pain, increase productivity and independence, and improve quality of life. When working with patients, a physical therapist may use therapeutic exercise, manual therapy techniques, assistive devices, adaptive devices, hydrotherapy, and electrotherapy.

Work environment. Physical therapists work in rehabilitation facilities, hospitals, nursing homes, physical therapy clinics, and schools. In medical environments, physical therapists work with a team of medical and social service professionals to increase a patient's physical abilities and overall independence. Physical therapists partner with educational professionals in school settings, such as teachers and special education coordinators, to address a student's physical issues. Physical therapists generally work a standard forty-hour workweek, and scheduled appointments are the norm.

PROFILE

- **Interests**: Data, People, Things
- **Working Conditions**: Work Inside
- **Physical Strength**: Medium Work, Heavy Work
- **Education Needs**: Bachelor's Degree, Master's Degree
- **Licensure/Certification**: Required
- **Physical Abilities Not Required**: Not Climb
- **Opportunities for Experience**: Internship, Military Service, Volunteer Work, Part-Time Work

---

OCCUPATION INTEREST

Individuals attracted to physical therapy tend to be physically strong people who enjoy hands-on work and close interaction with people from diverse backgrounds. Those who excel as physical therapists exhibit physical stamina, problem-solving, empathy, patience, and caring traits. Physical therapists should enjoy learning, stay knowledgeable about changes in therapeutic techniques, and expect to work as part of a team to address patient needs effectively.

A DAY IN THE LIFE—DUTIES AND RESPONSIBILITIES

A physical therapist's daily duties and responsibilities include full days of hands-on patient interaction and treatment and administrative duties. Physical therapists' patients include those experiencing physical limitations and effects from neck and spinal cord injuries; traumatic brain injury; arthritis; burns; cerebral palsy; muscular dystrophy; strokes; limb or digit amputation; or work- or sports-related injuries.

As medical or therapeutic professionals, physical therapists interact with patients or clients daily and strive to understand the particular challenges faced by each individual. Some of a physical therapist's daily responsibilities include conducting patient assessments, developing patient treatment plans, and providing physical treatment to patients with severe physical limitations. Treatment typically includes a blend of physical techniques and emotional encouragement since the patient may be adjusting to a major life change. Physical therapists frequently advise patients on using adaptive equipment, such as wheelchairs and orthopedic aids. Some provide early intervention services to young children experiencing physical delays and limitations. Others may offer consultation on or participate in building customized adaptive equipment for patients with special needs not met by existing options. Physical therapists also instruct individuals and groups on physical exercises to prevent injury, lead fitness, and

> **DUTIES AND RESPONSIBILITIES**
> - Recording patients' treatments, responses, and progress
> - Evaluating the physician's referral and the patient's medical records to determine the treatment required
> - Performing tests, measurements, and evaluations such as range-of-motion and manual-muscle tests, gait and functional analyses, and body-parts measurements
> - Administering manual therapeutic exercises to improve or maintain muscle function
> - Administering treatments involving the application of such agents as light, heat, water, and ice massage techniques

health classes and workshops, and counsel patients on physical adaptations that can help them continue working at their chosen occupation. They may also supervise the activities of physical therapy assistants and aides.

During the course of treatment, a physical therapist will consult with a team of physicians, educators, social workers, mental health professionals, occupational therapists, speech therapists, and other medical professionals to help ensure that each patient receives comprehensive care.

A physical therapist's administrative responsibilities include documenting treatment sessions and ongoing patient evaluation. Physical therapists must draft treatment plans, record notes following patient treatment sessions, provide written updates to the other members of a patient's treatment team, and provide insurance companies with patient records and progress notes as required. Independent physical therapists who do not work as part of a school or medical clinic may also be responsible for scheduling appointments and submitting bills to insurance companies or patients.

OCCUPATION SPECIALTIES
Directors of physical therapy. Directors of physical therapy plan, direct, and coordinate physical therapy programs and ensure the program complies with state requirements.

IMMEDIATE PHYSICAL ENVIRONMENT
Physical therapists work in rehabilitation facilities, hospitals, nursing homes, therapy clinics, and schools. Other professionals may share therapeutic office settings used by physical therapists, such as occupational, recreational, or speech and language therapists.

HUMAN ENVIRONMENT
Physical therapists work with patients who use physical therapy to improve their strength and mobility, as well as their independence and quality of life. Potential clients may include people experiencing balance and strength issues caused by cerebral palsy, spinal cord injuries, or muscular dystrophy; stroke victims experiencing coordination problems or paralysis; and children or adults suffering the physical effects of injuries, abuse, or accidents. Physical therapists usually work as part of a patient treatment team that includes families, social workers, teachers, doctors, and additional therapists.

TECHNOLOGICAL ENVIRONMENT
Physical therapists use a wide variety of technology in their work. Computers and internet communication tools are widely used in physical therapy work and practice. Specialized therapies, such as electrotherapy, hydrotherapy, and ultrasound therapy, require technical equipment and training. In addition, physical therapists must learn how to use and teach others how to use adaptive devices, such as wheelchairs and orthopedic aids.

EDUCATION, TRAINING, AND ADVANCEMENT
High school/secondary. High school students interested in pursuing the profession of physical therapy in the future should develop good study habits. High school biology, psychology, anatomy, sociol-

ogy, and mathematics courses will prepare students for college- and graduate-level studies. Students interested in the physical therapy field will benefit from seeking internships or part-time work with physical therapists or with people who have physical issues that affect their range of movement or daily life.

Suggested High School Subjects
- Algebra
- Applied Communication
- Applied Math
- Applied Physics
- Biology
- Chemistry
- College Preparatory
- English
- Geometry
- Health Science Technology
- Humanities
- Physical Education
- Physics
- Physiology
- Psychology
- Science
- Trigonometry

POSTSECONDARY EDUCATION

Postsecondary students interested in becoming physical therapists should complete coursework in physical therapy, as well as courses on occupational therapy, special education, biology, psychology, anatomy and physiology, sociology, and mathematics. Before graduation, college students interested in joining the physical therapy profession should apply to graduate-level physical therapy programs or secure physical therapy-related employment. Those who choose to pursue a master's degree tend to have better prospects for employment and advancement in the field. American Physical Therapy Association (APTA) membership may help provide postsecondary students with networking opportunities and connections.

Related College Majors
- Adapted Physical Education/Therapeutic Recreation
- Anatomy
- Art Therapy
- Exercise Science/Physiology/Movement Studies
- Health & Physical Education, General
- Human & Animal Physiology
- Physical Therapy
- Sports Medicine & Athletic Training

ADULT JOB SEEKERS

Adult job seekers in the physical therapy field should have a master's degree in physical therapy from a college or university accredited by the Commission on Accreditation in Physical Therapy Education. They must also earn the necessary professional licensure. Advancement in physical therapy often depends on the individual's education and specialty certification. Physical therapists seeking employment may benefit from the networking opportunities, job workshops, and job lists offered by professional physical therapy associations, such as the APTA and the American Board of Physical Therapy Specialties.

PROFESSIONAL CERTIFICATION AND LICENSURE

Physical therapists must have earned a professional physical therapy (PT) license before beginning their professional practice. Upon completion of an accredited master's or doctoral program in physical therapy, candidates take the National Physical Therapy Examination (NPTE) administered by the Federation of State Boards of Physical Therapy (FSBPT). In addition to passing the NPTE, physical therapists must register with their state health board, pass a state exam, and engage in continuing education as a condition of their PT license.

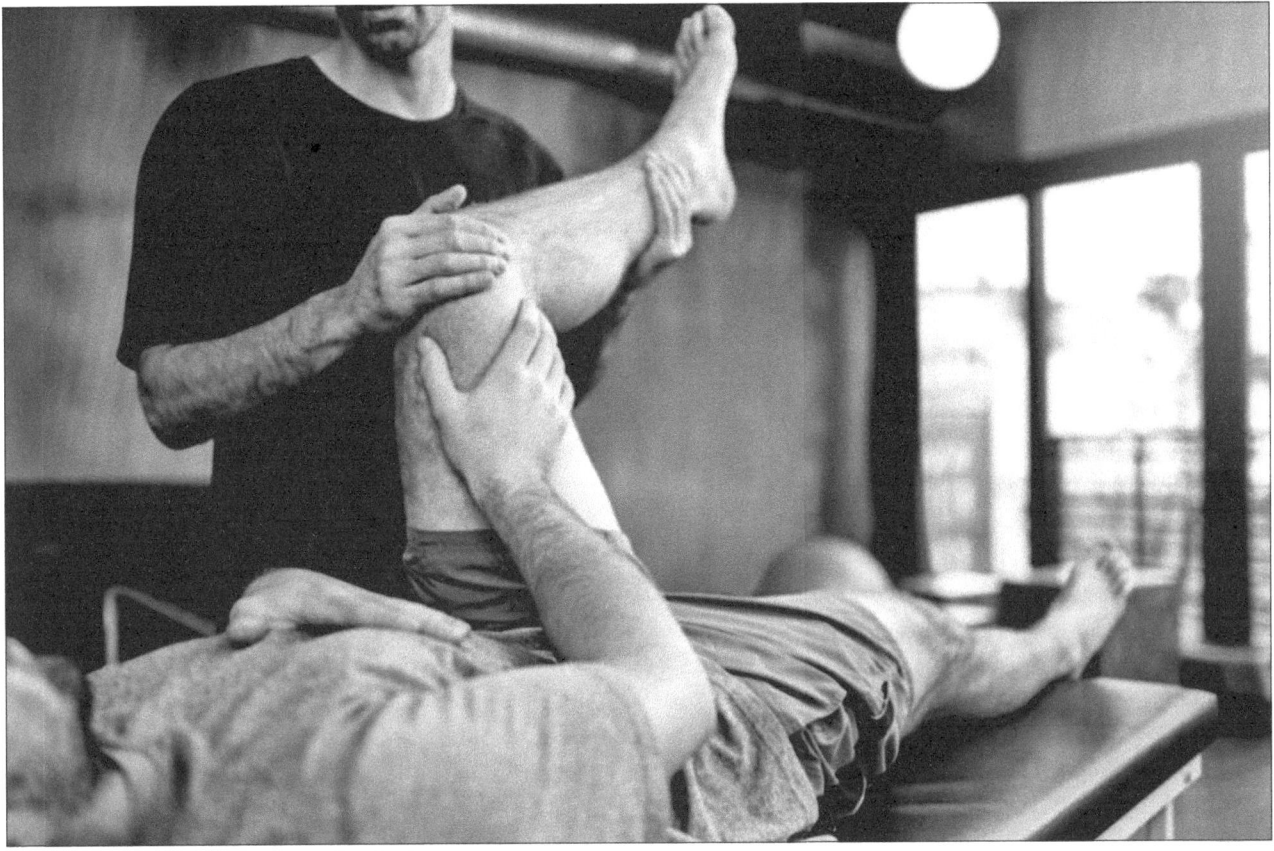

Photo via iStock/Cecilie_Arcurs. [Used under license.]

Physical therapists may pursue additional, specialized physical therapy certification from the American Board of Physical Therapy Specialties. Certification is available for the following specialties: cardiovascular and pulmonary, clinical electrophysiology, geriatrics, neurology, pediatrics, sports, and women's health.

ADDITIONAL REQUIREMENTS

Physical therapists who find satisfaction, success, and job security also are knowledgeable about their profession's requirements, responsibilities, and opportunities. Successful physical therapists engage in ongoing professional development related to changes in therapeutic techniques, ethical standards, and new technology. Because physical therapists work with vulnerable people and share confidential patient information with other medical professionals, adherence to strict professional and ethical standards is required. Both entry-level and senior-level physical therapists may find it beneficial to join professional associations to build professional community and networking.

—*Simone Isadora Flynn*

Further Reading

"Careers in Physical Therapy." American Physical Therapy Association, n.d., www.apta.org/your-career/careers-in-physical-therapy.

Myers, Betsy, and June Hanks. *Management of Common Orthopaedic Disorders: Physical Therapy Principles and Methods*. 5th ed., Lippincott Williams & Wilkins, 2022.

"Occupational Outlook Handbook: Physical Therapy." *US Bureau of Labor Statistics*, 18 Apr. 2022, www.bls.gov/ooh/healthcare/physical-therapists.htm.

Olson, Kenneth A. *Manual Physical Therapy of the Spine.* 3rd ed., Elsevier, 2021.

O'Sullivan, Susan B., et al., editors. *National Physical Therapy Examination Review and Study Guide, 2022.* 25th ed., TherapyEd, 2022.

Smith, Lori. "How Can Physical Therapy Help?" *Medical News Today*, 6 Jan. 2022, www.medicalnewstoday.com/articles/160645.

PODIATRY

Category: Specialty
Specialties and related fields: Dermatology, orthopedics, vascular medicine
Definition: the medical field that involves the diagnosis and treatment of diseases and abnormalities of the feet, ankles, and lower legs

KEY TERMS

corticosteroid: a fatlike molecule (or steroid), produced by the adrenal gland or made synthetically, that can be used to treat inflammation

dysfunction: the disordered or impaired function of a body system, organ, or tissue

orthopedics: the surgical or manipulative treatment of any disorder of the skeletal system and the associated motor organs

orthotic device: a podiatric appliance or prosthesis that is used to correct a foot deformity

pharmacology: the aspect of biomedical science that studies therapeutic drugs, their administration, and their bioproperties

SCIENCE AND PROFESSION

The human foot, a very complex structure, is located at the end of the lower leg and connected to the leg by the ankle. Feet are designed to optimize both balance and mobility. Each foot comprises twenty-six bones, ligaments that connect and articulate these bones, blood vessels that provide nutrients and oxygen, sensory nerves, and a thick covering of tough, strong skin. Heredity and a lack of proper foot care frequently result in painful calluses, corns, bunions, enlarged joints, and ingrown toenails. In addition, various diseases, such as diabetes mellitus and cardiovascular problems, can lead to many other serious foot dysfunctions.

Podiatrists—more correctly called "doctors of podiatric medicine"—examine, diagnose, and treat dysfunctions of the foot and related problems associated with the ankle and the lower leg. The first record of a process associated with podiatric medicine was the creation, in 100 BCE, of plasters that were used to treat corns in the Greek city of Smyrna. Although other records of podiatric treatments were found in antiquity and the Middle Ages, the modern science of podiatry arose from the activities of the fourteenth-century barber-surgeons of Europe.

In the United States, the first truly prominent modern podiatrist—then termed a chiropodist—was Isacher Zacharia. Zacharia, foot doctor to President Abraham Lincoln, published the first American podiatry text in 1862. Two other milestones in the history of American podiatry are the founding of the National Association of Chiropodists and the opening of the New York School of Chiropody. Both of these events occurred in 1912.

In 1958, the National Association of Chiropodists was renamed the American Podiatric Medical Association. From the New York School of Chiropody, whose first curriculum required only one year of chiropodic training, arose today's schools of podiatric medicine, which require a four-year study period and award graduates the doctor of podiatric medicine (DPM) degree. This degree derives from a uniform curriculum that all schools follow.

There are more than sixteen thousand licensed podiatrists in the United States. These podiatric practitioners serve patients in American hospitals, government health programs, and the armed forces. However, most of them are in private, individual practice. Furthermore, modern podiatric medicine is an accepted part of all major health insurance plans, including Medicare and Medicaid. Licensed DPM must complete a four-year course of postgraduate study at a school of podiatric medicine.

Admission to all American podiatry schools requires completing at least three years of a solid bachelor's degree program, including a year each of biology, inorganic chemistry, and organic chemistry. Most podiatry school entrants have completed a bachelor's degree. In addition, a solid grade-point average and good scores on the Medical College Admissions Test (MCAT) are required for admission.

The first two years of podiatric professional education inculcate the scientific background of podiatric medicine. The first two years of podiatry school include laboratory and lecture hall training in anatomy, biochemistry, physiology, pharmacology, diagnostic radiology, and numerous other biomedical sciences. The third and fourth years of training are dedicated to acquiring clinical expertise by practicing podiatric medicine in college or community clinics, hospitals, and the offices of experienced, well-established podiatrists.

Upon graduation, the new DPM usually completes a hospital residency encompassing three to four years. In the first year, clinical expertise is gained in podiatric orthopedics, biomechanics, and neurology. The first-year podiatry resident engages in supervised primary care, which involves observing, evaluating, and treating many dysfunctions of the feet, ankles, and lower legs. Minor podiatric surgery, such as hammertoe correction, is also carried out during this training period. In the remaining

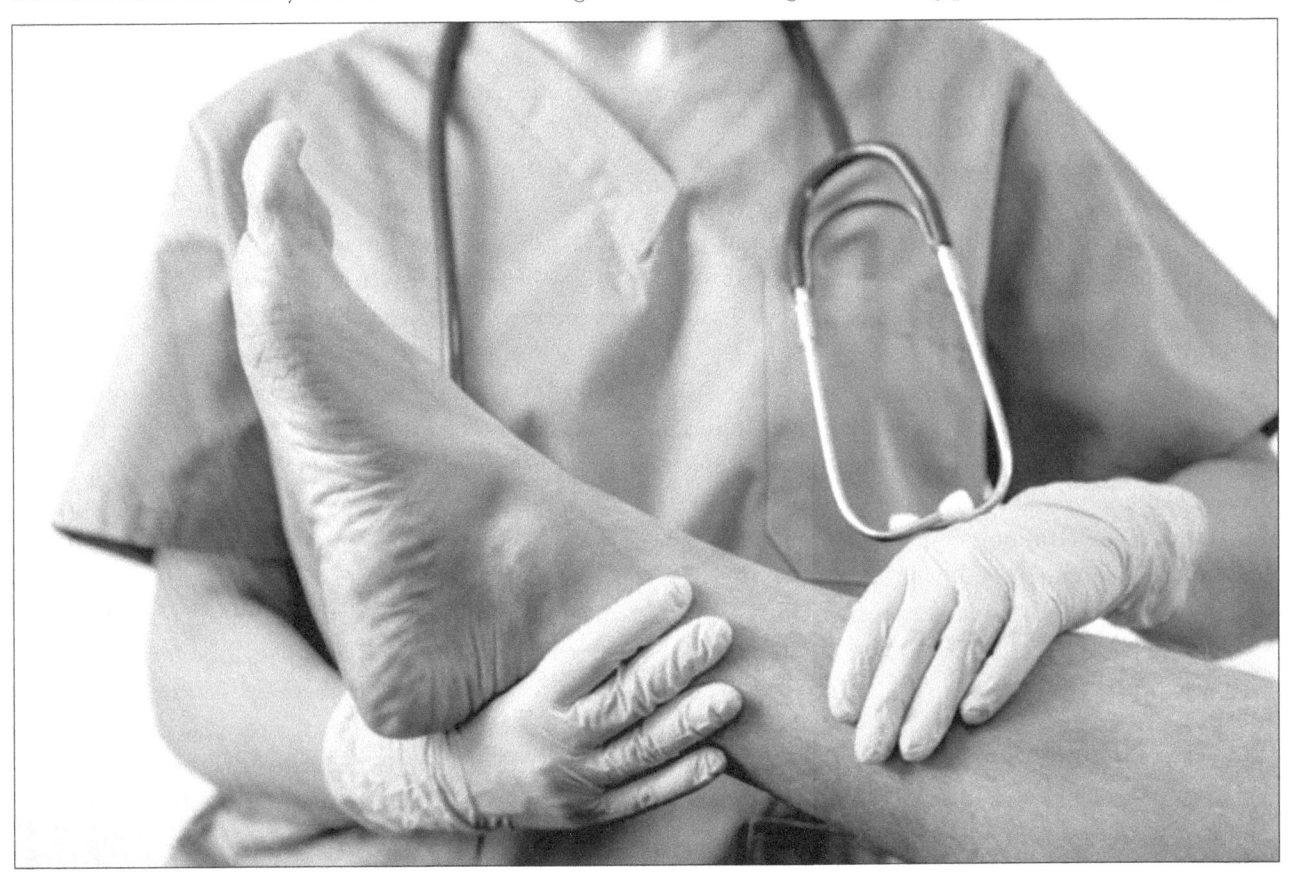

Photo via iStock/Igor Vershinsky. [Used under license.]

residency years, the resident learns to carry out the more demanding aspects of podiatric surgery on the foot, ankle, and leg. During this time, the podiatric resident becomes more independent and skilled.

Podiatric practitioners require licenses to practice. In the United States, these licenses are most often gained by passing state board examinations. Satisfactory scores on the separate tests given by the National Board of Podiatric Medical Examiners are also deemed satisfactory for podiatric licensing by many states. However, the renewal of podiatry licenses requires that podiatrists undergo extensive continuing education to keep them at the field's cutting edge.

Specialization is also possible for podiatrists. Podiatric specialists can be certified by the American Board of Podiatric Surgery, the American Board of Podiatric Medicine, or the American Board of Podiatric Public Health. Each of these podiatric specialty boards requires advanced clinical training, completion of written and oral examinations, and extensive experience in specific aspects of modern podiatric practice. Such board certification indicates that the individuals involved have met much higher standards than those required for licensing alone. Some podiatrists also belong to the American College of Foot and Ankle Surgery of the American Medical Association (AMA).

In modern practice, podiatric surgical procedures designed to prevent or correct podiatric deformities now supplant many more conventional methods that originally made up the expertise of most podiatric practitioners. In addition, numerous techniques that cause the improvement of the health and the function of the foot and the ankle to preclude foot deformities have become key aspects of the modern podiatric profession.

DIAGNOSTIC AND TREATMENT TECHNIQUES
A thorough podiatric examination begins with the complete medical history of the patient, inspection of the patient's gait, and careful examination of both feet, the ankles, and the lower legs. When these procedures point to diagnosing a particular podiatric problem, X-ray examination, muscle testing, and neurological consultation may be carried out to search for more subtle problems that the initial examination suggested but did not prove.

Once a clear, complete diagnosis has been obtained, a treatment regimen—including physical therapy, various surgical treatments, medications, and the use of podiatric (orthotic) appliances—is prescribed. Often, all aspects of treatment are carried out in the podiatrist's office. However, complex podiatric surgery may require the use of a hospital surgical suite or its equivalent.

Among the podiatric problems most often seen are athlete's foot, bunions, calluses, corns, ingrown toenails, hammertoes, heel spurs, traumatic injuries to the ankles or feet, and plantar warts, and complaints associated with arthritis, cardiovascular disease, or diabetes mellitus. In many cases—especially those engendered by athletics, diabetes, and cardiovascular problems—the podiatrist refers patients to other health practitioners, such as orthopedists, cardiologists, or endocrinologists. However, podiatrists and other specialists are increasingly working together as teams to solve such health problems.

Bunions are deformities of the big toes and their joints; they may or may not be painful, but they are almost always considered uncosmetic. When a bunion is not painful, it is usually treated by using an orthotic device that prevents further damage and pain. In cases where bunion pain is caused by inflammation, oral or injected anti-inflammatory drugs, such as corticosteroids, are often used for the shortest period needed to correct the problem. Such short-term treatment is necessary for the potential health risks caused by this therapy, such as cardiovascular problems. In the most severe cases, surgery is used to remove the bunion. An incision is made near the bunion site, and a surgical burr is used to trim away the region of excess bone causing the problem. In cases where manipulative examination or X-rays show that the bunion problem is in the joint, much more complex surgery is required.

Corns and hammertoes may be considered together, as hammertoes cause many corns. Corns are not restricted to occurrence along with hammertoes, however, as they also arise spontaneously on any toe subject to inappropriate biomechanical stress. A corn (or heloma) is a skin protrusion, or thickening, atop or on the side of a toe. Corns can occur wherever a toe has been bent out of shape by a biomechanical problem or by a tight shoe. They can be quite painful. Hammertoe, a contracture of one of the toe joints, produces a toe malformation that makes wearing shoes painful and can lead to corns. Corns may be trimmed periodically or removed surgically. The treatment used by podiatrists depends on the severity of the problem seen. Similarly, hammertoes are corrected surgically. After treatment of these problems, the patient needs to wear shoes that fit appropriately, use corrective orthotic devices that are prescribed, and follow closely the instructions given by the podiatrist. Failure to do so can counteract the results of the podiatric treatment.

Calluses, like corns, are buildups of tough, thickened skin. Unlike corns, however, they occur most often on the bottoms of the feet. Calluses form to protect the foot from undue stress resulting from uneven weight-bearing by the bottom of the foot. Therefore, they will form again after removal wherever the causative mechanical stress recurs. When a callus becomes painful, the appropriate treatment regimen varies greatly from case to case. Often, an orthotic device is used to produce evenness of weight-bearing by the foot. In other cases, the callus is trimmed. In the most severe instances, up to three months of diminished physical activity is required to enable complete healing of the trimmed metatarsal bones. In the most extreme cases, minor surgery is used to correct the anatomical defect in the metatarsal bone causing the problem. Again, success in callus treatment is optimized by carefully following the podiatrist's directions. Calluses may also occur at the back of the heel due to tight shoes and dermatologic problems. These calluses are usually handled by trimming and purchasing more appropriate shoes.

Heel spurs, Achilles tendonitis, ankle problems, dermatologic problems of the foot, and diabetic/cardiovascular complications may also be treated by podiatrists. Furthermore, it should be recognized that podiatrists will often repair damaged bones, muscles, and tendons surgically. They can also prescribe medications and treat fractures or sprains by applying casts and braces.

PERSPECTIVE AND PROSPECTS

Many advances in podiatric medicine have occurred in recent years. Most encouraging is the improved ability of podiatrists to handle severe foot problems. This improvement is largely attributable to advances in the field and more thorough training in professional school and postgraduate experiences. The increasing positive interaction of podiatrists and other health-care professionals in treating dermatologic, cardiovascular, and diabetic problems is another great step forward.

It is believed that the job prospects for podiatrists will expand rapidly in the next fifty years, and there will be even greater success in the podiatric treatment of problems that are presently difficult to handle. It is also expected that other podiatric medical schools will open to meet the need for more DPMs throughout the United States.

There are two main reasons for the excellent job prospects for podiatrists. First, is the increase in the population of senior citizens. Because these individuals have had more wear and tear on their lower legs and feet than younger people, they have foot ailments that require treatment more frequently. Second, is the increased interest in jogging and other sports in the general population, which will lead to more injuries that require podiatric intervention.

These factors are also expected to produce advances in the uses of orthotic appliances, generate sophisticated new diagnostic and surgical techniques, and lead to better cooperation between podiatrists and other health-care professionals.

—*Sanford S. Singer*

Further Reading

Alexander, Ivy L., editor. *Podiatry Sourcebook*. 2nd rev. ed., Omnigraphics, 2007.

Brennan, Todd, and Leslie Johnston. *The Foot Book: Everything You Need to Know to Take Care of Your Feet*. Cider Mill Press, 2022.

Copeland, Glenn. *The Foot Doctor: Lifetime Relief for Your Aching Feet*. Rev. ed., Macmillan Canada, 2000.

Farr, J. Michael, editor. *Enhanced Occupational Outlook Handbook*. 7th ed., JIST Works, 2009.

Fink, Brett Ryan, and Mark S. Mizel. *The Whole Foot*. Demos Medical, 2011.

Fox, Stuart I., and Krista Rompolski. *Human Physiology*. 16th ed., McGraw Hill, 2021.

Kelikian, Armen S., and Shahan K. Sarrafian. *Sarrafian's Anatomy of the Foot and Ankle: Descriptive, Topographic, Functional*. 4th ed., Lippincott Williams & Wilkins, 2022.

Lippert, Frederick G., and Sigvard T. Hansen. *Foot and Ankle Disorders: Tricks of the Trade*. Thieme, 2003.

Lorimer, Donald L., et al., editors. *Neale's Disorders of the Foot*. 7th ed., Churchill Livingstone/Elsevier, 2006.

Thordarson, David B., editor. *Foot and Ankle*. 2nd ed., Lippincott Williams & Wilkins, 2013.

Sports Medicine

Category: Specialty

Anatomy or system affected: Bones, circulatory system, feet, hands, head, heart, joints, knees, legs, ligaments, muscles, musculoskeletal system, nervous system, spine, tendons

Specialties and related fields: Cardiology, emergency medicine, exercise physiology, family medicine, internal medicine, nutrition, orthopedics, pharmacology, physical therapy, preventive medicine, psychology, rheumatology

Definition: a medical subspecialty concerned with the care and prevention of athletic injuries, primarily those related to the musculoskeletal system

KEY TERMS

joint: a specialized structure in the body where bones come together, and motion occurs

ligament: a tough, rubber-band-like structure that connects one bone to another and prevents the abnormal motion of these bones in relationship to each other

musculoskeletal: a term used to describe the relationship between bones and muscles within the framework of the body and how they provide stability and locomotion

musculotendinous unit: a structure that consists of a muscle that provides motion of a bone and its attachment to the bone, the tendon, which is a tough, inelastic fibrous structure

orthopedic surgery: the field of surgery that deals with the musculoskeletal system

SCIENCE AND PROFESSION

Sports medicine is a field that has become popular as the number of people who exercise has increased. More than 50 percent of people in the United States exercise daily. People all over the country are participating in sports, from recreational sports to professional competitive sports. There has been a growing trend of participation in exercise as more and more studies have proved that exercise is beneficial to health; however, exercise places people at risk for injuries that a sedentary person would not have. This fact has led to the emergence of sports medicine, with its specially trained health-care professionals. These professionals include physical therapists, athletic trainers, nutritionists, exercise physiologists, cardiologists, sports psychologists, family practitioners, internists, and orthopedic surgeons. They all contribute by bringing special knowledge and understanding to the care of athletes and athletic injuries. Such knowledge can relate to nutrition, strength training, cardiovascular conditioning, psychosocial issues, musculoskeletal care, or one or more of many other areas related to the health of athletes. Therefore, sports medicine is a very broad and diverse field that requires a team approach.

Athletic injuries occur regularly, but very few injuries are unique to sports. Yet treating an injured athlete does not necessarily require the same process as that used to treat an injured sedentary person. The athlete tends to have greater expectations than does the average sedentary person. These expectations usually increase proportionately with the competitive level of the athlete. For example, the athlete with an ankle sprain will spend ten to twelve hours per day performing treatment and rehabilitation supervised by a physical therapist or athletic trainer. However, the sedentary person might go to physical therapy three times per week. Although the treatment philosophy is the same, the number of treatments and the desired outcomes are completely different. Athletes also require extensive information regarding their injuries, treatment, and rehabilitation. Athletes are not afraid to ask questions regarding their injuries because they want to know when they will be able to return to competition.

Sports medicine is a challenging and rewarding profession. It is enjoyable working with patients with a high level of compliance and motivation. The reward of watching an athlete recover from an injury and compete is exceptional. The sports medicine physician must realize, however, that they will also be called upon by the athlete and the athlete's coach and parents to communicate the severity of the injury and its significance—a process that can be difficult at times, especially when what the physician has to say is not what anyone wants to hear. Nevertheless, it is the role of the physician to act in the athlete's best interest. For the physician to be prepared to handle this, they must fully understand the demands of each sport. Attendance at games is usually not enough to achieve this level of knowledge and experience. Observing practice sessions and workouts is often useful. Except for high-impact collision sports like hockey and football, most injuries occur during practice and workout sessions. Furthermore, such observation allows the physician to participate in education and injury prevention. Many athletic injuries are witnessed by an athletic trainer or physician who may be called upon to administer first aid in the field or provide treatment for injuries.

By attending practices or competitions, the physician may also have the opportunity to observe the actual mechanism of injury, which can be useful in evaluating the type and severity of the injury. Many physicians call the first twenty minutes after an injury has occurred, before the onset of swelling and spasm, the "golden period." At this time, the physician can perform an accurate and meaningful physical examination on the injured athlete. The recreational athlete usually arrives at the physician's office one to two days after the injury, when swelling and spasms are maximal. At this time, examining the injured body part is quite difficult. It may not be meaningful, resulting in diagnosis and definitive treatment delays. Such delays will probably not be significant for the sedentary person and the occasional athlete. However, the highly competitive athlete would be dissatisfied if an injury delayed their return to competition. Although most athletic injuries differ very little from other cases of musculoskeletal trauma, the finer points of managing them are unique.

Most athletic injuries affect one of three structures in the body: bones, ligaments, or musculotendinous units. These injuries may be acute or chronic in onset. Most acute injuries occur due to trauma, with the presentation soon after the incident. Chronic injuries, which are often insidious in onset, usually result from a change in the athlete or the athletic environment. Most acute injuries can be classified as sprains, strains, or fractures, and most chronic injuries can be classified as strains or stress fractures. Chronic injuries tend to be difficult to recognize and treat effectively. The best approach to chronic injuries is prevention.

Sprains are injuries to ligaments; strains are injuries to the musculotendinous unit. Sprains occur when there is excessive abnormal motion at a joint. This results in overstretching of the ligaments and produces local pain, swelling, limitation of motion, and a sense of instability. Such overstretching can result in partial tears (mild) or complete tears (severe) of the ligament. Strains are usually the result of an abrupt increase in the tension of the musculotendinous unit. For example, they may occur when one lifts weights that are too heavy. This increase may result in partial or complete tears of the muscle, the tendon, or the bone to which the tendon is attached. The most important principle is to realize that strains do not result from overstretching but occur well within the normal limits of motion. Strains are also graded from mild to severe. Often, there is an obvious deformity at the injury site because the muscle rolls up into a ball. Fractures are breaks in the bones of the body. Stress fractures occur when excessive demands are placed on the bone. Eventually, the bone fails to accommodate these demands, and microscopic breaks result.

DIAGNOSTIC AND TREATMENT TECHNIQUES

The initial management of acute injuries is the same in athletics as in other musculoskeletal trauma. Treatment should be directed at the prevention of bleeding and edema. These conditions usually lead to pain and decreased function of the injured body part, which requires the application of ice, compression, elevation, and rest. Other treatment methods used in the professional setting are also useful in preventing or reducing bleeding and edema. These include electric stimulation, contrast baths, ultrasound, and compression stockings. After the initial phase of bleeding and edema, therapy should be directed at restoring range of motion, strength, and, finally, functional tasks that will ultimately result in the athlete's return to competition. Chronic injuries, however, usually require the elimination of the precipitating factors as well as increased rest. At the same time, the injured body part is allowed to heal. This may require a special taping procedure, a brace, a change in footwear, the alteration of practice sessions, or simply refraining from that activity for a short period.

Chronic injuries and overuse injuries are usually caused by change. Change can occur in the athlete, the environment, or the activity. Identifying these changes can be helpful in injury prevention since the majority of injuries in athletics are chronic. In addition, the treatment requires elimination of the offending change and restoration of the proper condition. Strains to the musculotendinous unit can also occur chronically. They tend to result from muscle fatigue, too much training too fast, or poor training conditions. Many of these injuries are called "tendinitis," which means inflammation of the tendon. The most prominent aspect of such an injury is pain, which is almost always located in the region of the injured structure. Management is directed at avoiding painful activity, eliminating the offending factor, and symptomatic relief of pain with ice, ultrasound, injections, electric stimulation, and medications. Rehabilitation is aimed at restoring strength and flexibility and avoiding the initial cause.

Most sprains can be treated with routine physical therapy and rehabilitation, but many severe sprains require surgery. The average time lost from athletics ranges from seven days (e.g., for a mild ankle sprain) to one year (for a severe knee sprain with a reconstruction of ligaments). With strains, complete tears of the tendon usually require surgery, while injury to the muscle itself does not. Treatment is similar to sprains; rehabilitation should be directed at regaining strength and flexibility. The diagnosis of a fracture can be made through X-ray imaging. Treatment of fractures requires immobilization in a cast, special splint, or brace. Some fractures will require an orthopedic surgeon's placement of plates or screws. Rehabilitation of fractures involves restoring motion, strength, flexibility, and proprioception. Proprioception is the unconscious awareness of where a body part is in space (e.g., a person can tie their shoes with their eyes closed because the brain knows where the hands are in space). The treatment of stress fractures differs from other fractures in that immobilization is seldom necessary. Adaptation of activity and relative rest are usually all that are required. Return to competition averages three to six weeks but may be longer.

Sports medicine personnel also provide education and guidance to coaches, athletes, and parents. They make themselves available to provide the best and most efficient care possible. It is the responsibility of the sports medicine physician to coordinate this care. This all begins with the preseason screening history and physical exam.

The preseason screening also identifies athletes at risk for developing strains and sprains because their flexibility is lower than normal. Identifying these athletes allows the athletic trainer to work with them on a stretching program intended to reduce the number and severity of such injuries. During the preseason, the athletes are at the greatest risk for injury since the workouts are long and numerous and most athletes are not yet in shape. Injuries may occur at any time during practice or a game. However, most injuries occur during practice, especially at the end of the session, because athletes are tired and their concentration level is low.

Before the commencement of each athletic season, athletes are usually required to provide a medical history and undergo a physical examination. These examinations aim to identify athletes who may have potential problems in the sport in which they have chosen to compete. The requirements of such examinations vary from state to state, college to college, and professional league to professional league. Below are some example patient cases that show the role of preparticipation sports evaluations in keeping individuals healthy and safe.

Julian is a fifteen-year-old high school student who wants to try out for the football team. During his preparticipation sports evaluation, the doctor listens to his heart and hears a heart murmur. Julian's murmur intensity is worse with the Valsalva maneuver. This diagnostic technique may be used to evaluate a cardiac condition. The Valsalva maneuver decreases the cardiac preload, which is the force that stretches the heart before its contraction. Maneuvers that increase the amount of blood in the heart's ventricles, such as squatting and passive leg elevation, decrease the intensity of his heart murmur. Julian notes that his father and paternal uncle died suddenly during intense exercise at age thirty. The physician refers Julian to a cardiologist for further workup. Evaluation by the cardiologist reveals that Julian has hypertrophic cardiomyopathy. Hypertrophic cardiomyopathy is a genetic condition that results in enlargement and thickening of the walls of the left ventricle. The left ventricle is the part of the heart responsible for pumping blood into the circulation for the rest of the body. Hypertrophic cardiomyopathy may lead to ventricular stiffness and decreased outflow of blood into the systemic circulation. Patients with hypertrophic cardiomyopathy are at an increased risk for sudden death, especially in a state of high myocardial oxygen demand, such as during physical exertion. The cardiologist strongly advises Julian to avoid heavy lifting or strenuous exercise.

Hypertrophic cardiomyopathy is an important cause of sudden cardiac death in young patient populations, thus supporting the value of preparticipation sports evaluation.

An incoming first-year college student went to a family medicine physician to establish care and request a preparticipation physical examination for volleyball. Reviewing her medical history, she tells the physician that she has been healthy but has previously visited the hospital twice. The first time she went to the hospital was at age ten when she had retinal detachment after a ball hit her head. Two years ago, she was evaluated at an emergency room after a left shoulder dislocation. When asked about medical conditions in her family, she states that she has one healthy brother who plays basketball in high school. However, her mother passed away from a ruptured cerebral aneurysm when she was forty-nine. On physical exam, the patient is six feet one, has long extremities, and has slender fingers. The doctor asks the patient to place her thumbs in the palms of the same hand and form a fist. When the patient does this, in both hands, the tips of her thumbs protrude beyond the fifth digit. This is called a "positive thumb sign." After considering the information obtained from the medical history and the physical exam findings, the family medicine physician refers this patient for an ultrasound imaging of the heart called "echocardiography." The results of this test showed mild dilation of the aortic root. The patient is referred for genetic testing, which confirmed the family medicine physician's clinical suspicion of Marfan syndrome. Marfan syndrome is an inherited medical condition that causes a defect in the body's connective tissue. This disease results in various clinical manifestations, such as cardiovascular disorders, joint hypermobility, tall stature, and retinal detachment. Early diagnosis of this medical condition is especially important in athletes because sports activities that involve high levels of dynamic exercise can increase aortic wall stress, which could put an athlete with Marfan syndrome at a higher risk for aortic dissection. Aortic dissection occurs when blood enters between blood vessel layers to create a false lumen, leading to fatal consequences like cardiac tamponade. Cardiac tamponade is a compression of the heart by fluid, impairing the heart's ability to circulate blood throughout the body. This scenario demonstrates the importance of preparticipation sports history and physical exams. In this case, for example, confirming this patient's diagnosis may also benefit her brother. Suppose Marfan syndrome is diagnosed early and treated before developing fatal complications. In that case, athletes may be counseled appropriately about sports activities.

Dean is a twenty-year-old college soccer player who went to an urgent care center for one week of fever, malaise, and sore throat. He is diagnosed with infectious mononucleosis, an infection caused by the Epstein-Barr virus. His trainer advises him to follow up with the team physician for a sports evaluation. During his evaluation by the team physician, Dean is informed that he is at high risk for splenic rupture due to infectious mononucleosis. In infectious mononucleosis, the spleen, a small organ that filters the blood, enlarges due to the proliferation of immune cells in response to the viral infection. Splenic rupture from infectious mononucleosis is rare, but it is the most common cause of death in individuals with this infection. Splenic rupture is considered a medical emergency since it may cause massive intra-abdominal bleeding, leading to rapid clinical deterioration. Strenuous contact sports like soccer are associated with an increased risk of splenic rupture after infectious mononucleosis; thus, the team physician advises Dean to refrain from his sports activities for a minimum of four weeks. Dean recovers and returns gradually to his sports activities after six weeks. With the trainer's aid and prompt attention from the team physician, a potentially fatal medical emergency was prevented.

Mary is a fifteen-year-old high school all-state cross-country runner. She is now entering her junior year and is expected to compete nationally. Six weeks into the fall season, Mary's times begin to decrease slightly. When asked about her performance, she states that she has been experiencing pain in both her shins, particularly the one on the right, for two weeks. Her coach asks Mary to see her family doctor since the school does not have an athletic trainer or team physician. Mary's doctor tells her that she has shin splints and should rest. Mary does not accept this and continues to run against her doctor's advice. In the next race, Mary finishes last. The pain has become unbearable. Mary is referred to a sports medicine physician, who discovers several relevant facts. Mary is underweight and has not been eating well. She has been forcing herself to vomit for several days before each race. She has also not experienced her first menses. X-rays of Mary's right leg reveal severe stress fractures. Mary is referred to several specialists, including an orthopedic surgeon who places her in a cast, a nutritionist, a psychologist who evaluates and treats her eating disorder, and a gynecologist who proceeds with a workup for her late development. Mary is diagnosed with functional hypothalamic amenorrhea, which is a menstrual dysfunction in the setting of restrictive eating and excessive exercise. This condition is referred to as the female athlete triad of functional hypothalamic amenorrhea. It is characterized by strenuous physical activity or low intake of calories, low bone mineral density, and amenorrhea, a lack of menses. The pathophysiology of functional hypothalamic amenorrhea involves low energy availability (due to caloric restriction or excessive exercise) and elevated cortisol levels (secondary to stress or excessive exercise), which results in decreased hypothalamic gonadotropin-releasing hormone (GnRH) pulsatile secretion. Normally, GnRH from the hypothalamus stimulates the release of luteinizing hormone (LH) and follicle-stimulating hormone (FSH) from the anterior pituitary. In functional hypothalamic amenorrhea, the decreased GnRH pulsatile secretion results in decreased secretion of both LH and FSH, which consequently decreases estrogen levels. The reduced estrogen levels in individuals with functional hypothalamic amenorrhea lead to anovulation and amenorrhea. After several months of collaborative treatment by several health-care professionals, Mary begins retraining on a bicycle under the direction of an athletic trainer and a physical therapist. She moves on to compete in the spring track and field season and becomes a national champion. Without the collaborative care of the sports medicine team, Mary's condition could have progressed to serious complications or even death. This is a common scenario among adolescent athletes. The pressures placed upon them by friends, coaches, and parents can damage their emotional and physical well-being.

Henry is a fifty-five-year-old businessman who spends five days a week playing tennis at the local health club to stay in shape. After buying a new racket, he begins to experience pain in his right elbow. An orthopedic surgeon who specializes in sports medicine evaluates him. After speaking with Henry and examining his elbow, the doctor recommends anti-inflammatory medication, a special forearm strap, and the use of the old racket. Henry's condition, called "tennis elbow" or lateral epicondylitis, is quite common. Lateral epicondylitis is caused by excessive pronation, supination, and extension motions of the wrist, resulting in inflammation of the wrist extensor muscles. After several weeks of the initial treatment, Henry does not feel any better. His doctor, therefore, injects him with medication to ease the pain and calm the inflammation. Henry is instructed to rest his arm for a week before starting tennis again.

Henry follows the doctor's instructions carefully. He begins to play tennis again and feels fine for about a month, after which he begins to experience the same discomfort. This time, the doctor recommends surgery for Henry's elbow. Three months after the surgery, Henry is free of pain.

These examples have demonstrated how sports medicine can be beneficial to athletes. Each scenario differs in type of athlete, location, diagnosis, and treatment.

PERSPECTIVE AND PROSPECTS

Sports medicine is assuming a significant role in the medical profession today. Sports medicine was first recognized in the days of the early Olympics. It was not until the final decades of the twentieth century, however, that it emerged into a field of its own. Sports medicine training programs have been developing at an exponential rate. Interest in sports medicine can be pursued in various ways. Most sports medicine physicians undergo a one-year fellowship either after a five-year orthopedic residency training program or after completion of a family medicine residency, internal medicine, pediatrics, emergency medicine, or physical medicine and rehabilitation training program.

Athletic trainers must pass a national examination for certification. Most have master's degrees, and all have some form of bachelor's degree. Their expertise is in preventing, treating, and rehabilitating athletic injuries. These are the primary caregivers of the sports medicine world. Certified athletic trainers are being hired at all major universities, high schools, and health clubs across the country. Various types of sports medicine centers are continually being developed. These centers offer professional and amateur athletes a wide range of services. As more and more people begin to exercise, the need for sports medicine professionals will increase.

Athletes' needs and goals are different from those of most other people. Although the injuries they experience are not unique to sports, the rapidity with which they recover is of utmost importance. This identifies them as a distinct group of people with special demands for medical care. Because of this and the growing number of people who exercise daily, sports medicine has evolved into a viable medical field. Sports medicine will continue to grow and play an important role in preventing many injuries afflicting people in the United States.

—*Jason Pyon, Marichelle Pita*

Further Reading

Ahmad, Z., N. et al. "Lateral Epicondylitis: A Review of Pathology and Management." *Bone Joint Journal*, vol. 95-B, no. 9, Sept. 2013, pp. 1158-64, doi:10.1302/0301-620X.95B9.29285. PMID:23997125.

Auwaerter, P. G. "Infectious Mononucleosis: Return to Play." *Clinical Sports Medicine*, vol. 23, no. 3, July 2004, pp. xi, 485-97, doi:10.1016/j.csm.2004.02.005. PMID:15262384.

Blumenstein, Boris, Michael Bar-Eli, and Gershon Tenenbaum, editors. *Brain and Body in Sport and Exercise: Biofeedback Applications in Performance Enhancement.* John Wiley & Sons, 2002.

De Souza, M. J., A. Nattiv, E. Joy, et al. "Expert Panel: 2014 Female Athlete Triad Coalition Consensus Statement on Treatment and Return to Play of the Female Athlete Triad: 1st International Conference held in San Francisco, California, May 2012 and 2nd International Conference held in Indianapolis, Indiana, May 2013." *British Journal of Sports Medicine*, vol. 48, no. 4, Feb. 2014, p. 289, doi:10.1136/bjsports-2013-093218. PMID: 24463911.

Delforge, Gary. *Musculoskeletal Trauma: Implications for Sport Injury Management.* Human Kinetics, 2002.

Gordon, C. M., K. E. Ackerman, S. L. Berga, et al. "Functional Hypothalamic Amenorrhea: An Endocrine Society Clinical Practice Guideline." *The Journal of Clinical Endocrinology & Metabolism*, vol. 102, no. 5, 1 May 2017, pp. 1413-39, doi:10.1210/jc.2017-00131. PMID: 28368518.

Landry, Gregory L., and David T. Bernhardt. *Essentials of Primary Care Sports Medicine*. Human Kinetics, 2003.

Loeys, B. L., H. C. Dietz, A. C. Braverman, et al. "The Revised Ghent Nosology for the Marfan Syndrome." *Journal of Medical Genetics*, vol. 47, no. 7, pp. 476-85, doi:10.1136/jmg.2009.072785.

McArdle, William, Frank I. Katch, and Victor L. Katch. *Exercise Physiology: Energy, Nutrition, and Human Performance*. 7th ed., Lippincott Williams & Wilkins, 2010.

Nishimura, R. A., H. Seggewiss, and H. V. Schaff. "Hypertrophic Obstructive Cardiomyopathy." *Circulation Research*, vol. 121, no. 7, 2017, pp. 771-83, doi:10.1161/circresaha.116.309348.

O'Connor, T. E., L. J. Skinner, P. Kiely, and J. E. Fenton. "Return to Contact Sports Following Infectious Mononucleosis: The Role of Serial Ultrasonography." *Ear, Nose & Throat Journal*, vol. 90, no. 8, Aug. 2011, pp. E21-24, doi:10.1177/014556131109000819.

Pelliccia, A., F. M. Di Paolo, E. De Blasiis, et al. "Prevalence and Clinical Significance of Aortic Dilatation in Highly Trained Competitive Athletes." *Circulation*, vol. 122, 2010, pp. 698-706.

Scuderi, Giles R., and Peter D. McCann, editors. *Sports Medicine: A Comprehensive Approach*. 2nd ed., Mosby/Elsevier, 2005.

Small, Eric, et al. *Kids and Sports: Everything You and Your Child Need to Know About Sports, Physical Activity, and Good Health*. Newmarket Press, 2002.

Warren, M. P., and N. E. Perlroth. "The Effects of Intense Exercise on the Female Reproductive System." *Journal of Endocrinology*, vol. 170, July 2001, pp. 3-11, doi:10.1677/joe.0.1700003. PMID:11431132.

Won, A. C., and A. Ethell. "Spontaneous Splenic Rupture Resulted from Infectious Mononucleosis." *International Journal of Surgery Case Reports*, vol. 3, no. 3, 2012, pp. 97-99, doi.org/10.1016/j.ijscr.2011.08.012.

Bibliography

"8 Minute Stretching Routine for Women!" *YouTube*, uploaded by fabulous50s, 6 Sept. 2019, www.youtube.com/watch?v=6CfUWws9IYs.

"2020 Standards for Accreditation of Professional Athletic Training Programs." *Commission on Accreditation of Athletic Training Education*, Jan. 2018, caate.net/wp-content/uploads/2018/09/2020-Standards-for-Professional-Programs-copyedited-clean.pdf. Accessed 27 May 2022.

Abad-Jorge, Ana. "The Role of DHA and ARA in Infant Nutrition and Neurodevelopmental Outcomes." *Today's Dietitian*, vol. 10, no. 10, 2008, p. 66.

Abbott, Ryan, and Helen Lavretsky. "Tai Chi and Qigong for the Treatment and Prevention of Mental Disorders." *Psychiatric Clinics of North America*, vol. 36, no. 1, 2013, pp. 109-19, doi:10.1016/j.psc.2013.01.011.

Abdulla, Fuad A., et al. "Effects of Pulsed Low-Frequency Magnetic Field Therapy on Pain Intensity in Patients with Musculoskeletal Chronic Low Back Pain: Study Protocol for a Randomised Double-Blind Placebo-Controlled Trial." *BMJ Open*, vol. 9, no. 6, 9 June 2019, doi:10.1136/bmjopen-2018-024650.

"About Heart Valves." *American Heart Association*, 7 May 2020, www.heart.org/en/health-topics/heart-valve-problems-and-disease/about-heart-valves. Accessed 8 June 2022.

"About Occupational Therapy." *American Occupational Therapy Association*, 2022, www.aota.org/about/for-the-media/about-occupational-therapy. Accessed 13 June 2022

"About Occupational Therapy." *WFOT*, 2022, wfot.org/about/about-occupational-therapy. Accessed 13 June 2022.

"About Physical Medicine and Rehabilitation." *American Academy of Physical Medicine and Rehabilitation*, 2022, www.abpmr.org/consumers/pmr_definition.html. Accessed 14 Jun. 2022.

Abrahams, Peter H., Johannes M. Boon, and Jonathan D. Spratt. *McMinn's Color Atlas of Human Anatomy*. 6th ed., Mosby/Elsevier, 2008.

Abrams, Jonathan. "Phillip Adams Had Severe C.T.E. at the Time of Shootings." *New York Times*, 14 Dec. 2021, www.nytimes.com/2021/12/14/sports/football/phillip-adams-cte-shootings.html. Accessed 25 Jan. 2022.

"Accreditation Application Process." *Commission on Accreditation of Athletic Training Education*, 2022, caate.net/accreditation-application-process/. Accessed 27 May 2022.

"Acupuncture." *Mayo Clinic*, 30 Apr. 2022, www.mayoclinic.org/tests-procedures/acupuncture/about/pac-20392763. Accessed 26 May 2022.

"Acupuncture: An Introduction." *National Center for Complementary and Alternative Medicine*. US Department of Health and Human Services, 2012.

Adams, Angela, et al. "Acupressure for Chronic Low Back Pain: a Single System Study." *Journal of Physical Therapy Science*, vol. 29, no. 8, 2017, pp. 1416-20, doi:10.1589/jpts.29.1416.

"Addiction to Muscle Relaxers: Carisoprodol (Soma)." *American Addiction Centers*, 17 Oct. 2019, americanaddictioncenters.org/prescription-drugs/soma-addiction.

"Adult Forearm Fractures." *OrthoInfo*, Sept. 2021, orthoinfo.aaos.org/en/diseases—conditions/adult-forearm-fractures.

Agur, Anne M. R., and Arthur F. Dalley. *Grant's Atlas of Anatomy*. 15th ed., Lippincott Williams & Wilkins, 2020.

Ahmad, Moghis U., editor. *Fatty Acids: Chemistry, Synthesis, and Applications*. Academic Press and ACCS Press, 2017.

Ahmad, Z., N. et al. "Lateral Epicondylitis: A Review of Pathology and Management." *Bone Joint Journal*, vol. 95-B, no. 9, Sept. 2013, pp. 1158-64, doi:10.1302/0301-620X.95B9.29285. PMID:23997125.

Albergotti, Reed, and Vanessa O'Connell. *Wheelmen: Lance Armstrong, the Tour de France, and the Greatest Sports Conspiracy Ever*. Penguin, 2013.

Alexander, Ivy L., editor. *Podiatry Sourcebook*. 2nd rev. ed., Omnigraphics, 2007.

Ali, Naheed. *Arthritis and You: A Comprehensive Digest for Patients and Caregivers*. Rowman and Littlefield, 2013.

"The Amateur's Complete Guide to Blood Doping." *Men's Health*, 3 Aug. 2017, www.menshealth.co.uk/fitness/blood-doping-in-sport. Accessed 27 Feb. 2018.

Ameisen, Olivier, and Hilary Hinzmann. *The End of My Addiction: How One Man Cured Himself of Alcoholism*. Piatkus, 2010.

American Academy of Orthopaedic Surgeons, www.aaos.org.

"American Cancer Society Updates Guideline for Diet and Physical Activity." *American Cancer Society*, 9 June 2020, www.cancer.org/latest-news/american-cancer-society-updates-guideline-for-diet-and-physical-activity.html.

American College of Sports Medicine. *ACSM's Guidelines for Exercise Testing and Prescription*. 11th ed., Wolters Kluwer, 2022.

———. *ACSM's Resources for the Exercise Physiologist*. 3rd ed., Wolters Kluwer, 2022.

American Diabetes Association. *American Diabetes Association Complete Guide to Diabetes*. 4th Rev. ed., Bantam Books, 2006.

American Society of Exercise Physiologists, 2022, www.asep.org.

"Anabolic Steroid Drug Facts." *National Institutes on Drug Abuse*, Aug. 2018, www.drugabuse.gov/publications/drugfacts/anabolic-steroids

"Anabolic Steroids." *MedlinePlus*, 2 June 2021, medlineplus.gov/anabolicsteroids.html.

"Anabolic Steroids." *United States National Library of Medicine*, 18 Sept. 2014, www.nlm.nih.gov/medlineplus/anabolicsteroids.html.

Anderson, Jon R. "Kaatsu Training Is Blowing Fitness Researchers' Mind." *Military Times*, 6 Feb. 2015, www.militarytimes.com/2015/02/06/kaatsu-training-is-blowing-fitness-researchers-minds/. Accessed 22 Oct. 2018.

Anderson, Marcia K. *Foundations of Athletic Training: Prevention, Assessment, and Management*. Philadelphia: Lippincott Williams & Wilkins, 2012.

Andrews, James R., et al. "The Ulnar Collateral Ligament Procedure Revisited: The Procedure We Use." *Sports Health*, vol. 4, no. 5, 2012, pp. 438-41.

Antonio H. Lara, and Jonathan D. Wallis. "The Role of Prefrontal Cortex in Working Memory: A Mini Review." *Frontiers in Systems Neuroscience*, 18 Dec. 2015, www.frontiersin.org/articles/10.3389/fnsys.2015.00173/full. Accessed 4 May 2020.

Appleton Amber, et al. *Metabolism and Nutrition*. Mosby/Elsevier, 2013.

Arbogast, Kristy B., et al. "Cognitive Rest and School-Based Recommendations Following Pediatric Concussion: The Need for Primary Care Support Tools." *Clinical Pediatrics*, vol. 52, no. 5, 2013, pp. 397-402.

Archibald, John M. *Genomics: A Very Short Introduction*. Illustrated ed., Oxford UP, 2018.

Arendt-Nielsen, L., et al. "A Double-Blind Randomized Placebo-Controlled Parallel Group Study Evaluating the Effects of Ibuprofen and Glucosamine Sulfate on Exercise-Induced Muscle Soreness." *Journal of Musculoskeletal Pain*, vol. 15, 2007, pp. 21-28.

Aretha, David. *Steroids and Other Performance-Enhancing Drugs*. Enslow, 2005.

"Arm Injuries and Disorders." *MedlinePlus*, 3 Jan. 2017, medlineplus.gov/arminjuriesanddisorders.html.

Arnsten, Amy F. T. "Stress Signaling Pathways that Impair Prefrontal Cortex Structure and Function." *Nature Reviews Neuroscience*, vol. 10, no. 6, 2009, pp. 410-22.

Aronowitz, E. R., and J. P. Leddy. "Closed Tendon Injuries of the Hand and Wrist in Athletes." *Clinics in Sports Medicine*, vol. 17, no. 3, 1998, pp. 449-67.

Arribas Ayllon, M., et al. *Genetic Testing: Accounts of Autonomy, Responsibility, and Blame*. Routledge, 2011.

"Arthroplasty." *Johns Hopkins Medicine*, 2019, www.hopkinsmedicine.org/health/treatment-tests-and-therapies/arthroplasty.

"Assessment of Brain SPECT: Report of the Therapeutics and Technology Assessment Subcommittee of the American Academy of Neurology." *Neurology*, vol. 46, no. 1, 1996, pp. 278-85, doi:10.1212/wnl.46.1.278.

Astorino, T. A., et al. "Is Running Performance Enhanced with Creatine Serum Ingestion?" *Journal of Strength Conditioning Research*, vol. 19, 2005, pp. 730-34.

"At Tour de France, Doping Is Always Part of the Story." *USA Today*, 30 June 2017, www.usatoday.com/story/sports/cycling/2017/06/30/at-tour-de-france-doping-is-always-part-of-the-story/103308480/. Accessed 27 Feb. 2018.

"Athletic Training." *National Athletic Trainers Association (NATA)*, 2022, www.nata.org/about/athletic-training. Accessed 27 May 2022.

"Athletic Training." *Troy University*, 2022, www.troy.edu/academics/academic-programs/graduate/athletic-training.html. Accessed 27 May 2022.

Auwaerter, P. G. "Infectious Mononucleosis: Return to Play." *Clinical Sports Medicine*, vol. 23, no. 3, July 2004, pp. xi, 485-97, doi:10.1016/j.csm.2004.02.005. PMID:15262384.

Avery, N. G., et al. "Effects of Vitamin E Supplementation on Recovery from Repeated Bouts of Resistance Exercise." *Journal of Strength and Conditioning Research*, vol. 17, 2003, pp. 801-9.

"Baclofen." *MedlinePlus*. US National Library of Medicine, 15 July 2017, medlineplus.gov/druginfo/meds/a682530.html.

Bahrke, Michael S., and Charles E. Yesalis, editors. *Performance-Enhancing Substances in Sport and Exercise*. Human Kinetics, 2002.

Baine, Celeste. *High Tech Hot Shots: Careers in Sports Engineering*. National Society of Professional Engineers, 2004.

Balch, James F., and Phyllis A. Balch. *Prescription for Nutritional Healing: A Practical A to Z Reference to*

Drug-Free Remedies Using Vitamins, Minerals, Herbs, and Food Supplements. 4th rev. ed., Avery, 2008.

Balentine, Jerry R., and Siamak N. Nabili. "Anemia." *Medicine Net*, 11 Oct. 2016, www.medicinenet.com/anemia/article.htm. Accessed 11 Mar. 2017.

Ballantyne, Jane C., et al., editors. *Bonica's Management of Pain*. 5th ed., Lippincott Williams & Wilkins, 2018.

Ballard, Carol. *Bones*. Heinemann Library, 2002.

Bannuru, R. R., et al. "Comparative Effectiveness of Pharmacologic Interventions for Knee Osteoarthritis: A Systematic Review and Network Meta-Analysis." *Annals of Internal Medicine*, vol. 162, no. 1, 2015, pp. 46-54, doi:10.7326/M14-1231.

Barasi, Mary E. *Human Nutrition: A Health Perspective*. 2nd ed., Oxford UP, 2003.

Barber, Gary. *Getting Started in Track and Field Athletics: Advice and Ideas for Children, Parents, and Teachers*. Trafford, 2006.

Barresi, Michael J. F., and Scott F. Gilbert. *Developmental Biology*. 12th ed., Sinauer Associates, 2022.

Barrett, Stephen. "Applied Kinesiology: Phony Muscle-Testing for 'Allergies' and 'Nutrient Deficiencies.'" *Quackwatch*, 23 Aug., www.quackwatch.com/01quackeryrelatedtopics/tests/ak.html. Accessed 27 May 2022.

Barrett, Stephen, et al. *Consumer Health: A Guide to Intelligent Decisions*. 9th ed., McGraw-Hill Education, 2012.

Bassuk, Shari S., Timothy S. Church, and JoAnn E. Manson. "Why Exercise Works Magic." *Scientific American*, vol. 309, no. 2, 2013, pp. 74-79.

Baszanger, Isabelle. *Inventing Pain Medicine: From the Laboratory to the Clinic*. Rutgers UP, 1998.

Bates, Jane A. *Abdominal Ultrasound: How, Why, and When*. 3rd ed., Churchill Livingstone/Elsevier, 2011.

Bauer, Brent A. "Prolotherapy: Solution to Low Back Pain?" *Mayo Clinic*, 25 May 2018, www.mayoclinic.org/prolotherapy/expert-answers/faq-20058347.

Baum, Seth J. *The Total Guide to a Healthy Heart: Integrative Strategies for Preventing and Reversing Heart Disease*. Kensington, 2000.

Beam, Joel W. *Orthopedic Taping, Wrapping, Bracing, and Padding*. 4th ed., F. A. Davis Company, 2021.

Bear, Mark F., et al. *Neuroscience: Exploring the Brain*. 4th ed., Jones and Bartlett Learning, 2020.

Beck, T. W., et al. "Effects of a Protease Supplement on Eccentric Exercise-Induced Markers of Delayed-Onset Muscle Soreness and Muscle Damage." *Journal of Strength and Conditioning Research*, vol. 21, 2007, pp. 661-67.

Becker, Kenneth L., et al., editors. *Principles and Practice of Endocrinology and Metabolism*. 3rd ed., Lippincott Williams and Wilkins, 2001.

Beery, Theresa, et al. *Genetics and Genomics in Nursing and Health Care*. 2nd ed., F. A. Davis Company, 2018.

Begley, Sharon, and Devin Gordon. "Under the Shadow of Drugs: Doping-Tainted by Scandals, the IOC Starts to Crack Down." *Newsweek*, October 9, 2000, p. 56.

Bell, Rae Frances, and Eija Anneli Kalso. "Ketamine for Pain Management." *Pain Reports*, vol. 3, no. 5, 2018, doi:10.1097/pr9.0000000000000674.

Bellenir, Karen, editor. *Pain Sourcebook: Basic Consumer Health Information About Specific Forms of Acute and Chronic Pain*. 2nd ed., Omnigraphics, 2002.

Belson, Ken. "'It's Not the Ending He Wanted.'" *New York Times*, 16 Dec. 2021, www.nytimes.com/2021/12/16/sports/football/vincent-jackson-death-cte.html. Accessed 25 Jan. 2022.

Bemben, M. G., et al. "Creatine Supplementation During Resistance Training in College Football Athletes." *Medicine and Science in Sports and Exercise*, vol. 33, 2001, pp. 1667-73.

"The Benefit of Youth Sports." *President's Council on Sports, Fitness & Nutrition Science Board*, 17 Sept. 2020, health.gov/sites/default/files/2020-09/YSS_Report_One Pager_2020-08-31_web.pdf. Accessed 28 May 2022.

Benini, Franca, and Egidio Barbi. "Doing without Codeine: Why and What Are the Alternatives?" *Italian Journal of Pediatrics*, vol. 40, no. 1, 2014, doi:10.1186/1824-7288-40-16.

Berg, Jeremy M., et al. *Biochemistry*. 9th ed., W.H. Freeman, 2019.

Berk, Laura E. *Child Development*. 9th ed., Pearson/Allyn & Bacon, 2013.

Berkowitz, Aaron. *Lange Clinical Neurology and Neuroanatomy: A Localization-Based Approach*. McGraw Hill / Medical, 2016.

Bernstein, Eugene F., editor. *Vascular Diagnosis*. 4th ed., Mosby, 1993.

"Best Beginner Weight-Training Guide with Easy-to-Follow Workout!" *Bodybuilding.com*, 8 Sept. 2015, www.bodybuilding.com/fun/beginner_weight_training.htm.

"Best Occupational Therapy Programs." *U.S. News and World Report*, 2020, www.usnews.com/best-graduate-schools/top-health-schools/occupational-therapy-rankings. Accessed 13 June 2022.

Bhandari, Monika, et al. "Recent Updates on Codeine." *Pharmaceutical Methods*, vol. 2, no. 1, 2011, pp. 3-8, doi:10.4103/2229-4708.81082.

Bilezikian, John P. *Primer on the Metabolic Bone Diseases and Disorders of Mineral Metabolism*. 9th ed., Wiley-Blackwell, 2018.

Billitz, Jess. "19 College Athlete Injury Statistics (The Risk of Sports)." *Noobgains*, 12 Nov. 2020, noobgains.com/college-athlete-injury-statistics/. Accessed 18 May 2021.

Binkoski, A. E., et al. "Iron Supplementation Does Not Affect the Susceptibility of LDL to Oxidative Modification in Women with Low Iron Status." *Journal of Nutrition*, vol. 134, 2004, pp. 99-103.

"Biotin: Fact Sheet for Health Professionals." *NIH Office of Dietary Supplements*. US Department of Health and Human Services, 10 Jan. 2022, ods.od.nih.gov/factsheets/Biotin-HealthProfessional/. Accessed 28 May 2022.

Birchard, Karen. "Olympic Committee Bans Doctor After Doping Case." *The Lancet*, vol. 356, 2000, p. 1171.

Bishop, Jan Galen. *Fitness through Aerobics*. Cummings, 2013.

Bisset, L., et al. "A Systematic Review and Meta-analysis of Clinical Trials on Physical Interventions for Lateral Epicondylalgia." *British Journal of Sports Medicine*, vol. 39, 2005, pp. 411-22.

Bisset L. M., and B. Vicenzino. "Physiotherapy Management of Lateral Epicondylalgia." *Journal of Physiotherapy*, vol. 61, no. 4, 2015, pp. 174-81, doi:10.1016/j.jphys.2015.07.015.

Bissinger, Buzz. "Winning." *Newsweek*, vol. 160, no. 10, 2012, pp. 26-33.

Black, Jonathan. *Making the American Body: The Remarkable Saga of the Men and Women Whose Feats, Feuds, and Passions Shaped Fitness History*. U of Nebraska P, 2013.

Blahd, William. "Lactic Acidosis and Exercise: What You Need to Know." *WebMD*, 14 July 2017, www.webmd.com/fitness-exercise/guide/exercise-and-lactic-acidosis#1. Accessed 11 June 2019.

Blakey, Paul. *The Muscle Book*. Himalayan Institute, 2000.

Bleecker, Deborah. *Acupuncture Points Handbook: A Patient's Guide to the Locations and Functions of Over 400 Acupuncture Points*. Draycott Design Books, 2017.

Blessing, Jill. "The Chemical Reaction That Takes Place in the Body after Exercise." *Live Strong*, www.livestrong.com/article/375841-the-chemical-reaction-that-takes-place-in-the-body-after-exercise/. Accessed 11 June 2019.

"Blood Flow Restriction Training." *American Physical Therapy Association*, www.apta.org/PatientCare/BloodFlowRestrictionTraining/. Accessed 22 Oct. 2018.

Bloom, Floyd E., M. Flint Beal, and David J. Kupfer, editors. *The Dana Guide to Brain Health*. Dana Press, 2006.

Bloom, Marc. "Greatest Olympic Moments." *Runner's World*, vol. 39, no. 7, 2004, pp. 70-77.

Bloomer, R. J., et al. "Astaxanthin Supplementation Does Not Attenuate Muscle Injury Following Eccentric Exercise in Resistance-Trained Men." *International Journal of Sport Nutrition and Exercise Metabolism*, vol. 15, 2005, pp. 401-12.

Blumenstein, Boris, Michael Bar-Eli, and Gershon Tenenbaum, editors. *Brain and Body in Sport and Exercise: Biofeedback Applications in Performance Enhancement*. John Wiley & Sons, 2002.

"Body MRI." *RadiologyInfor.org: For patients*, 15 June 2020, www.radiologyinfo.org/en/info/bodymr.

Boelcke, Allison. "What Is Dynamic Stretching?" *Wise Geek*. Conjecture Corporation, 20 Mar. 2015, www.wisegeekhealth.com/what-is-dynamic-stretching.htm. Accessed 24 Mar. 2015.

Bohn, Amy Miller, Stephanie Betts, and Thomas L. Schwenk. "Creatine and Other Nonsteroidal Strength-Enhancing Aids." *Current Sports Medicine Reports*, vol. 1, no. 4, 2002, pp. 239-45.

"Bone Diseases." *MedlinePlus*, 15 Mar. 2016, medlineplus.gov/bonediseases.html. Accessed 28 May 2022.

"Bone Health for Life: Health Information Basics for You and Your Family." *NIH Osteoporosis and Related Bone Diseases National Resource Center*, Apr. 2018, www.bones.nih.gov/health-info/bone/bone-health/bone-health-life-health-information-basics-you-and-your-family. Accessed 29 May 2022.

"Bone Infections." *MedlinePlus*, 21 Mar. 2016, medlineplus.gov/boneinfections.html. Accessed 28 May 2022.

"Bones, Joints, and Muscles." *Healthdirect*, Sept. 2021, www.healthdirect.gov.au/bones-muscles-and-joints

"Bones, Muscles, and Joints." *KidsHealth*, Jan. 2019, kidshealth.org/en/parents/bones-muscles-joints.html. Accessed 29 May 2022.

Bongard, Frederick, et al., editors. *Current Diagnosis and Treatment: Critical Care*. 3rd ed., McGraw-Hill Medical, 2008.

Bonow, Robert O., et al., editors. *Braunwald's Heart Disease: A Textbook of Cardiovascular Medicine*. 9th ed., Elsevier-Saunders, 2011.

Bonza, John E., et al. "Shoulder Injuries Among United States High School Athletes During the 2005-2006 and 2006-2007 School Years." *Journal of Athletic Training*, vol.

44, no. 1, 2009, pp. 76-83, www.ncbi.nlm.nih.gov/pmc/articles/PMC2629044/.

Borenstein, David G., et al. *Low Back and Neck Pain: Comprehensive Diagnosis and Management*. 3rd ed., W. B. Saunders, 2004.

Boslaugh, Sarah. *Genetic Testing*. Greenwood, 2020.

Bourn, David. *Diagnostic Genetic Testing: Core Concepts and the Wider Context for Human DNA Analysis*. Springer, 2021.

Bourne, Edmund J., and Lorna Garano. *Coping with Anxiety: Ten Simple Ways to Relieve Anxiety, Fear, and Worry*. New Harbinger, 2003.

Bowman, Joe. "Post-Concussion Syndrome." *Healthline*, 28 Aug. 2019, www.healthline.com/health/post-concussion-syndrome#causes3. Accessed 30 Oct. 2017.

Braham, R., et al. "The Effect of Glucosamine Supplementation on People Experiencing Regular Knee Pain." *British Journal of Sports Medicine*, vol. 37, 2003, pp. 45-49.

"Brain Basics: Know Your Brain." *National Institute of Neurological Disorders and Stroke*, 2022, www.ninds.nih.gov/health-information/patient-caregiver-education/brain-basics-know-your-brain. Accessed 30 May 2022.

"Brain Diseases from A-Z." *American Brain Foundation*, 2022, www.americanbrainfoundation.org/diseases/. Accessed 30 May 2022.

"Brain Diseases." *MedlinePlus*, 28 June 2018, medlineplus.gov/braindiseases.html. Accessed 30 May 2022.

"The Brain from Top to Bottom." *McGill University*, thebrain.mcgill.ca.

"Brain Injury Diagnosis." *Brain Injury Association of America*, 2022, www.biausa.org/brain-injury/about-brain-injury/diagnosis. Accessed 30 May 2022.

"Brain Map Frontal Lobes." *Queensland Government*, 18 Apr. 2017, www.health.qld.gov.au/abios/asp/bfrontal. Accessed 4 May 2020.

"BrainFacts.org." *Society for Neuroscience*, www.brainfacts.org.

Brämberg, Elisabeth Björk, et al. "Effects of Yoga, Strength Training and Advice on Back Pain: A Randomized Controlled Trial." *BMC Musculoskeletal Disorders*, vol. 18, no. 1, 29 Mar. 2017, doi:10.1186/s12891-017-1497-1.

Braun, W. A., et al. "The Effects of Chondroitin Sulfate Supplementation on Indices of Muscle Damage Induced by Eccentric Arm Exercise." *Journal of Sports Medicine and Physical Fitness*, vol. 45, 2006, pp. 553-60.

Breene, Sophia. "13 Mental Health Benefits of Exercise." *Huffington Post*. TheHuffingtonPost.com, 27 Mar. 2013, www.huffingtonpost.com/2013/03/27/mental-health-benefits-exercise_n_2956099.html.

Brennan, Richard. *Back in Balance: Use the Alexander Technique to Combat Neck, Shoulder, and Back Pain*. Watkins, 2013.

Brennan, Todd, and Leslie Johnston. *The Foot Book: Everything You Need to Know to Take Care of Your Feet*. Cider Mill Press, 2022.

Brooks, K. A., and J. G. Carter. "Overtraining, Exercise, and Adrenal Insufficiency." *Journal of Novel Physiotherapies*, vol. 3, no. 125, 2013, p. 11717, doi:10.4172/2165-7025.1000125.

Brower, Anne C. *Arthritis in Black and White*. Elsevier Saunders, 2012.

Brown, H. C. "Common Injuries of the Athlete's Hand." *Canadian Medical Association Journal*, vol. 117, no. 6, 1977, pp. 621-25.

Brown, S. A., et al. "Oral Nutritional Supplementation Accelerates Skin Wound Healing." *Plastic and Reconstructive Surgery*, vol. 114, 2004, pp. 237-44.

"Bruise." *MedlinePlus*, 16 Nov. 2016, medlineplus.gov/bruises.html. Accessed 30 May 2022.

"Bruise: First Aid." *Mayo Clinic*, 12 Nov. 2020, www.mayoclinic.org/first-aid/first-aid-bruise/basics/art-20056663. Accessed 30 May 2022.

Brukner, Peter, and Karim Khan. *Brukner & Khan's Clinical Sports Medicine*. 4th ed., McGraw-Hill, 2010. Print.

Brummett, Chad M., and Steven P. Cohen. *Managing Pain: Essentials of Diagnosis and Treatment*. Oxford UP, 2013.

Brungs, Robert S. J., and R. S. M. Postiglione, editors. *The Genome: Plant, Animal, Human*. ITEST Faith/Science Press, 2000.

Brunicardi, F. Charles, et al., editors. *Schwartz's Principles of Surgery*. 9th ed., McGraw-Hill, 2010.

Bryant, Howard. *Juicing the Game: Drugs, Power, and the Fight for the Soul of Major League Baseball*. Viking Press, 2005.

Bulger, S., et al. "Preparing Prospective Physical Educators in Exercise Physiology." *QUEST*, vol. 52, 2000, pp. 166-85.

Bunn, H. Franklin. "Erythropoietin." *Cold Spring Harbor Perspectives in Medicine*, Mar. 2013, www.ncbi.nlm.nih.gov/pmc/articles/PMC3579209/. Accessed 11 Mar. 2017.

Bunta, Andrew D., and Joseph M. Lane. "Bone Health Lifetime Challenges." *AAOS*, 1 June 2016, www.aaos.org/aaosnow/2016/jun/clinical/clinical07/. Accessed 28 May 2022.

Burke, Edmund. *Optimal Muscle Performance and Recovery*. Rev. ed., Putnam, 2003.

Burn, Loic. *Back and Neck Pain: The Facts*. Oxford UP, 2006.

Burns, Jimmy. *Hand of God: The Life of Diego Maradona*. Lyons Press, 2003.

Bushong, Stewart C., and Geoffrey Clarke. *Magnetic Resonance Imaging: Physical and Biological Principles*. 4th ed., Mosby, 2014.

Butler, Nick. "FIS Deny Blood Doping Allegations about Cross-Country Skiers at Pyeongchang 2018." *Inside the Games*, 4 Feb. 2018, www.insidethegames.biz/articles/1061044/fis-deny-blood-doping-allegations-about-cross-country-skiers-at-pyeongchang-2018. Accessed 27 Feb. 2018.

Butryn, T. M., et al. "We Walk the Line: An Analysis of the Problems and Possibilities of Work at the Sport Psychology-Sport Sociology Nexus." *Sociology of Sport Journal*, vol. 31, no. 2, 2014, pp. 162-84.

Buxton, Richard B. *An Introduction to Functional Magnetic Resonance Imaging: Principles and Techniques*. 2nd ed., Cambridge UP, 2009.

Byl, J. "Organizing Effective Elementary and High School Intramural Programs." *Physical and Health Education*, vol. 70, 2004, pp. 22-24.

Cailliet, Rene. *Low Back Pain Syndrome: A Medical Enigma*. Lippincott Williams & Wilkins, 2003.

Calcaterra, Nicholas E., and James C. Barrow. "Classics in Chemical Neuroscience: Diazepam (*Valium*)." *ACS Chemical Neuroscience*, vol. 5, no. 4, 2014, pp. 253-60, doi:10.1021/cn5000056.

Campbell, A. Malcolm, and Laurie J. Heyer. *Discovering Genomics, Proteomics, and Bioinformatics*. 2nd ed., CSHL Press, 2009.

Campbell, Barbara, J., and Stuart J. Fischer. "Bone Health Basics." *OrthoInfo*, May 2020, orthoinfo.aaos.org/en/staying-healthy/bone-health-basics/. Accessed 29 May 2022.

Candow, Darren G., et al. "Effect of Whey and Soy Protein Supplementation Combined with Resistance Training in Young Adults." *International Journal of Sport Nutrition and Exercise Metabolism*, vol. 16, no. 3, 2006, pp. 233-44.

———. "Variables Influencing the Effectiveness of Creatine Supplementation as a Therapeutic Intervention for Sarcopenia." *Frontiers in nutrition*, vol. 6, 2019, doi:10.3389/fnut.2019.00124. Accessed 25 June 2020.

Canseco, José. *Juiced: Wild Times, Rampant 'Roids, Smash Hits, and How Baseball Got Big*. Regan Books, 2005.

———. *Vindicated: Big Names, Big Liars, and the Battle to Save Baseball*. Simon Spotlight Entertainment, 2008.

Capriccioso, Richard P., and Capriccioso, Christina E. "Bionics and Biomedical Engineering." *Applied Science*, edited by Donald R. Franceschetti, Salem Press, 2012, pp. 228-33.

"Carbohydrate Choice Lists." *Centers for Disease Control and Prevention*, 10 Aug. 2021, www.cdc.gov/diabetes/managing/eat-well/diabetes-and-carbs/carbohydrate-choice-lists.html. Accessed 2 Jun. 2022.

"Carbohydrates." *MedlinePlus*, 17 Jan. 2022, medlineplus.gov/carbohydrates.html. Accessed 2 Jun. 2022.

"Carbohydrates: How Carbs Fit into a Healthy Diet." *Mayo Clinic*, 22 Mar. 2022, www.mayoclinic.org/healthy-lifestyle/nutrition-and-healthy-eating/in-depth/carbohydrates/art-20045705. Accessed 2 Jun. 2022.

"Care of Casts and Splints." *OrthoInfo*, Mar. 2020, orthoinfo.aaos.org/en/recovery/care-of-casts-and-splints/.

"Careers in Physical Therapy." American Physical Therapy Association, n.d., www.apta.org/your-career/careers-in-physical-therapy.

"Carisoprodol." *MedlinePlus*, 15 Oct. 2018, medlineplus.gov/druginfo/meds/a682578.html.

Carney, Tara, et al. "A Comparative Analysis of Pharmacists' Perspectives on Codeine Use and Misuse—A Three Country Survey." *Substance Abuse Treatment, Prevention, and Policy*, vol. 13, no. 1, 2018, doi:10.1186/s13011-018-0149-2.

"Carpal Tunnel Syndrome." *Mayo Clinic*, 25 Feb. 2022, www.mayoclinic.org/diseases-conditions/carpal-tunnel-syndrome/symptoms-causes/syc-20355603. Accessed 8 June 2022.

Carpenter, K. C., et al. "Baker's Yeast Beta-Glucan Supplementation Increases Monocytes and Cytokines Post-Exercise: Implications for Infection Risk?" *The British Journal of Nutrition*, vol. 109, no. 3, 2013, pp. 478-86.

Carr, Kevin, and Mary Kate Feit. *Functional Training Anatomy*. Human Kinetics, 2021.

Carroll, Will, with William L. Carroll. *The Juice: The Real Story of Baseball's Drug Problems*. Ivan R. Dee, 2005.

Carter, Rita. *Mapping the Mind*. U of California P, 2010.

Cash, Mel. *Pocket Atlas of the Moving Body*. Crown, 2000.

Casperson, C. J., et al. "Physical Activity, Exercise, and Physical Fitness: Definitions and Distinctions for Health-Related Research." *Public Health Reports*, vol. 100, 1985, pp. 126-31.

Cassidy, Claire Monod. *Contemporary Chinese Medicine and Acupuncture*. Churchill Livingstone, 2002.

Cazeneuve, Brian. "Running on Empty: With Funds and Friends in Short Supply, Marion Jones May Face Prison." *Sports Illustrated*, 2008, vault.si.com/vault/2008/01/14/running-on-empty.

Centers for Disease Control. "Genomics & Health Impact Update: August 6, 2013." *CDC Public Health Genomics*, Aug. 1-8, 2013.

"Cetylated Fatty Acids Help Osteoarthritis Joints." *Health24*, 19 Jan. 2017, www.health24.com/Medical/Arthritis/Managing-pain/Cetylated-fatty-acids-help-joints-20120721.

Challem, Jack. *The Inflammation Syndrome: Your Nutritional Plan for Great Health, Weight Loss, and Pain-Free Living*. Rev. ed., Wiley-Blackwell, 2010.

Cheatham, S. W., et al. "The Efficacy of Instrument Assisted Soft Tissue Mobilization: A Systematic Review." *Journal of the Canadian Chiropractic Association*, vol. 60, no. 3, 2016, pp. 200-211.

Chen, N. C., J. B. Jupiter, et al. "Sports-Related Wrist Injuries in Adults." *Sports Health*, vol. 1, no. 6, 2009, pp. 469-77.

Cheng, Tianze, et al. "*Valium* without Dependence? Individual GABAA Receptor Subtype Contribution toward Benzodiazepine Addiction, Tolerance, and Therapeutic Effects." *Neuropsychiatric Disease and Treatment*, vol. 14, 2018, pp. 1351-61, doi:10.2147/ndt.s164307.

Chevan, Julia, and Phyllis A. Clapis. *Physical Therapy Management of Low Back Pain: A Case-Based Approach*. Jones Bartlett Learning, 2013.

Chilibeck, P. D., et al. "Effect of Creatine Ingestion After Exercise on Muscle Thickness in Males and Females." *Medicine and Science in Sports and Exercise*, vol. 36, 2004, pp. 1781-88.

Chirali, Ilkay Z. *Traditional Chinese Medicine: Cupping Therapy*. 2nd ed., Churchill Livingstone/Elsevier, 2007.

Cho, Adrian. "Engineering Peak Performance." *Science*, vol. 305, no. 5684, 2004, pp. 643-44.

Chou, Roger, et al. "Comparative Efficacy and Safety of Skeletal Muscle Relaxants for Spasticity and Musculoskeletal Conditions: A Systematic Review." *Journal of Pain and Symptom Management*, vol. 28, no. 2, 2004, pp. 140-75, doi:10.1016/j.jpainsymman.2004.05.002.

Chughtai, M., et al. "A Novel, Nonoperative Treatment Demonstrates Success for Stiff Total Knee Arthroplasty after Failure of Conventional Therapy." *Journal of Knee Surgery*, vol. 29, no. 3, 2016, pp. 188-93.

"CI Therapy Research Group." *University of Alabama at Birmingham Department of Psychology*, www.uab.edu/citherapy/. Accessed 29 Nov. 2017.

Cifu, David X. *Braddom's Physical Medicine and Rehabilitation*. 6th ed., Elsevier, 2020.

Clark, Luke, and D. Phil. "Cognitive Neuroscience and Brain Imaging in Bipolar Disorder." *Dialogues in Clinical Neuroscience*, vol. 10, no. 2, 2008, pp. 153-65.

Clarke, Sonya, and Julie Santy-Tomlinson. *Orthopaedic and Trauma Nursing: An Evidence-Based Approach to Musculoskeletal Care*. Wiley-Blackwell, 2014.

Clarkson, Hazel M. *Musculoskeletal Assessment: Joint Motion and Muscle Testing*. Wolters Kluwer Health/Lippincott Williams & Wilkins, 2013.

Coakley, J. *Sports in Society: Issues and Controversies*. 11th ed., McGraw Hill Higher Education, 2014.

Coakley, Sarah, and Kay Kaufman Shelemay, editors. *Pain and Its Transformations: The Interface of Biology and Culture*. Harvard UP, 2008.

"Codeine." *MedlinePlus*, 15 Mar. 2018, medlineplus.gov/druginfo/meds/a682065.html.

Codsi, Michael, and Chris R. Howe. "Shoulder Conditions: Diagnosis and Treatment Guideline." *Physical Medicine and Rehabilitation Clinics of North America*, vol. 26, no. 3, 2015, pp. 467-89, doi:10.1016/j.pmr.2015.04.007.

Collier, Mark. "Understanding Wound Inflammation." *Nursing Times*, vol. 99, no. 25, 2003, pp. 63-64.

Collins, A. *Strength Training Over 40: A 6-Week Program to Build Muscle and Agility*. Rockridge Press, 2020.

Comarow, Avery, and Lisa Stein. "Baseball's Iffy Steroid Test." *U.S. News and World Report*, vol. 136, no. 8, 2004.

"Common Shoulder Injuries." *OrthoInfo*, July 2009, orthoinfo.aaos.org/topic.cfm?topic=a00327.

"Concussion." *MedlinePlus*, n.d., medlineplus.gov/ency/article/000799.htm. Accessed 30 May 2022.

"Concussion (Traumatic Brain Injury)." *WebMD*, 25 Aug. 2020, www.webmd.com/brain/concussion-traumatic-brain-injury-symptoms-causes-treatments#1. Accessed 30 Oct. 2017.

"Conditions and Treatments." *American Academy of Physical Medicine and Rehabilitation*, 2022, www.aapmr.org/about-physiatry/conditions-treatments.

"Constraint Induced Movement Therapy." *Children's Hemiplegia and Stroke Association*, chasa.org/treatment/constraint-induced-movement-therapy/. Accessed 29 Nov. 2017.

"Constraint Induced Movement Therapy." *Physiopedia*, www.physio-pedia.com/Constraint_Induced_Movement_Therapy. Accessed 29 Nov. 2017.

Cooke, David, editor. *Microbiology: Concepts and Applications*. Callisto Reference, 2018.

Coombes, B. K., et al. "Management of Lateral Elbow Tendinopathy: One Size Does Not Fit All." *Journal of Orthopaedic & Sports Physical Therapy*, vol. 45, no. 11, 2015, pp. 938-49, doi:10.2519/jospt.2015.5841.

Cooper, Chris. *Run, Swim, Throw, Cheat: The Science Behind Drugs in Sport*. Oxford UP, 2012.

Cooper, Kenneth H. *Aerobics Program for Total Well-Being: Exercise, Diet and Emotional Balance*. Bantam, 2013.

———. *Regaining the Power of Youth at Any Age: Startling New Evidence from the Doctor Who Brought Us Aerobics, Controlling Cholesterol, and the Antioxidant Revolution*. Nelson, 2005.

Copeland, Glenn. *The Foot Doctor: Lifetime Relief for Your Aching Feet*. Rev. ed., Macmillan Canada, 2000.

Corbett, Christina, et al. "A Randomised Comparison of Two 'Stress Control' Programmes: Progressive Muscle Relaxation versus Mindfulness Body Scan." *Mental Health & Prevention*, vol. 15, 2019, p. 200163, doi:10.1016/j.mph.2019.200163.

"Coronary Artery Disease-Coronary Heart Disease." *American Heart Association*, 31 July 2015, www.heart.org/en/health-topics/consumer-healthcare/what-is-cardiovascular-disease/coronary-artery-disease. Accessed 2 June 2022.

Costandi, Moheb. *Neuroplasticity*. MIT Press, 2016.

Costanzo, Linda S. *Physiology: Cases and Problems*. 4th ed., Lippincott, 2012.

Cotten, Doyice J., and John T. Wolohan. *Law for Recreation and Sport Managers*. 6th ed., Kendall/Hunt, 2013.

Cousins, Michael J., and P. O. Bridenbaugh, editors. *Cousins and Bridenbaugh's Neural Blockade in Clinical Anesthesia and Management of Pain*. 4th ed., Lippincott Williams & Wilkins, 2009.

Cowan, Ruth Schwartz. *Heredity and Hope: The Case for Genetic Screening*. Harvard UP, 2008.

Cox, A. J., et al. "Oral Administration of the Probiotic Lactobacillus Fermentum VRI-003 and Mucosal Immunity in Endurance Athletes." *British Journal of Sports Medicine*, vol. 44, 2010, pp. 222-26.

Cox, Richard. *Sports Psychology: Concepts and Applications*. McGraw, 2006.

Craig, Charles R., and Robert E. Stitzel, editors. *Modern Pharmacology with Clinical Applications*. 6th ed., Lippincott, 2004.

Cramer, J. T., et al. "Effects of Creatine Supplementation and Three Days of Resistance Training on Muscle Strength, Power Output, and Neuromuscular Function." *Journal of Strength Conditioning Research*, vol. 21, 2007, pp. 668-77.

Crawford, Michael H., editor. *Current Diagnosis and Treatment-Cardiology*. 4th ed., McGraw-Hill Medical, 2013.

"Creatine." *MedlinePlus*, 26 Oct. 2021, medlineplus.gov/druginfo/natural/873.html.

Cronn-Mills, K., and A. N. Nelson. *LGBTQ+ Athletes Claim the Field: Striving for Equality*. Twenty-First Century Books, 2016.

Crossman, A. "Symbolic Interaction Theory." *About.com*, 14 June 2015, sociology.about.com/od/Sociological-Theory/a/Symbolic-Interaction-Theory.htm.

"Cross-training for Fun and Fitness." *American Council on Exercise (ACE)*, 2013, acewebcontent.azureedge.net/assets/education-resources/lifestyle/fitfacts/pdfs/fitfacts/itemid_2547.pdf.

Crouch, James E. *Functional Human Anatomy*. 4th ed., Lea & Febiger, 1985.

Cuncic, Arlin. "Chill Out: How to Use Progressive Muscle Relaxation to Quell Anxiety." *Verywell Mind*, 13 July 2019, www.verywellmind.com/how-do-i-practice-progressive-muscle-relaxation-3024400.

Currey, John D. *Bones: Structures and Mechanics*. 2nd ed., Princeton UP, 2006.

Cutting, K. F., and K. G. Harding. "Criteria for Identifying Wound Infection." *Journal of Wound Care*, vol. 3, no. 4, 1994, pp. 198-201.

Da Poian, Andrea T., and Miguel A. R. B. Castanho. *Integrative Human Biochemistry: A Textbook for Medical Biochemistry*. 2nd ed., Springer, 2021.

Daniell, H., S. J. Streatfield, and K. Wycoff. "Medical Molecular Farming: Production of Antibodies, Biopharmaceuticals, and Edible Vaccines in Plants." *Trends in Plant Science*, vol. 6, 2001, pp. 219-26.

Dartt, Darlene A. *Immunology, Inflammation and Diseases of the Eye*. Academic Press, 2011.

"DASH Diet: Healthy Eating to Lower Your Blood Pressure." *Mayo Clinic*, 25 June 2021, www.mayoclinic.org/healthy-lifestyle/nutrition-and-healthy-eating/in-depth/dash-diet/art-20048456. Accessed 24 Aug. 2020.

"DASH Ranked Best Diet Overall for Eighth Year in a Row by U.S. News and World Report." *National Institutes of Health*, 3 Jan. 2018, www.nih.gov/news-events/news-releases/dash-ranked-best-diet-overall-eighth-year-row-us-news-world-report. Accessed 24 Aug. 2020.

Daugherty, J., et al. "Traumatic Brain Injury-Related Deaths by Rae/Ethnicity, Sex, Intent, and Mechanism of Injury-United States, 2000-2017." *MMWR Morbidity and*

Mortality Weekly Report, vol. 68, 2019, pp. 1050-56, doi.http://dx.doi.org/10.15585/mmwr.mm6846a2.

Davies, C. C., D. Brockopp, and K. Moe. "Astym® Therapy Improves Function and Range of Motion Following Mastectomy." *Breast Cancer: Targets and Therapy*, vol. 8, 2016, pp. 39-45.

Davis, Jennifer S., et al. "Use of Non-Steroidal Anti-Inflammatory Drugs in US Adults: Changes over Time and by Demographic." *Open Heart*, vol. 4, no. 1, 2017, doi:10.1136/openhrt-2016-000550.

Davis, Joel. *Mapping the Mind: The Secrets of the Human Brain and How It Works*. Replica Books, 1999.

Davis, Martha, et al. *The Relaxation and Stress Reduction Workbook*. 5th ed., New Harbinger, 2000.

De Bock, K., et al. "Acute Rhodiola rosea Intake Can Improve Endurance Exercise Performance." *International Journal of Sport Nutrition and Exercise Metabolism*, vol. 14, no. 3, 2004, 298-307.

De Souza, M. J., A. Nattiv, E. Joy, et al. "Expert Panel: 2014 Female Athlete Triad Coalition Consensus Statement on Treatment and Return to Play of the Female Athlete Triad: 1st International Conference held in San Francisco, California, May 2012 and 2nd International Conference held in Indianapolis, Indiana, May 2013." *British Journal of Sports Medicine*, vol. 48, no. 4, Feb. 2014, p. 289, doi:10.1136/bjsports-2013-093218. PMID: 24463911.

Deacon, S. J., et al. "Randomized Controlled Trial of Dietary Creatine as an Adjunct Therapy to Physical Training in COPD." *American Journal of Respiratory and Critical Care Medicine*, vol. 178, 2008, pp. 133-39.

"Defining Adult Overweight and Obesity." *Overweight and Obesity, Centers for Disease Control*, 3 June 2022, www.cdc.gov/obesity/basics/adult-defining.html. Accessed 13 June 2022.

Delforge, Gary. *Musculoskeletal Trauma: Implications for Sport Injury Management*. Human Kinetics, 2002.

Delzell, Emily. "Prolotherapy for Osteoarthritis." *Arthritis Foundation*, www.arthritis.org/diseases/more-about/prolotherapy-for-osteoarthritis.

Denniston, Katherine, et al. *General, Organic, and Biochemistry*. 10th ed., McGraw-Hill Education, 2019.

deOliveira, Carolina Dizioli Rodriguez, Andre Valle de Bairros, and Mauricio Yonamine. "Blood Doping: Risks to Athlete's' Health and Strategies for Detection." *Substance Abuse and Misuse*, vol. 49, no. 4, 2014, pp. 1168-82.

Devlin, Thomas M., editor. *Textbook of Biochemistry: With Clinical Correlations*. 7th ed., Wiley-Liss, 2011.

Dewey, K. G., et al. "Iron Supplementation Affects Growth and Morbidity of Breast-Fed Infants: Results of a Randomized Trial in Sweden and Honduras." *Journal of Nutrition*, vol. 132, 2002, pp. 3249-55.

DeWitt, P. M. *Dignity for All: Safeguarding LGBT Students*. Corwin Press, 2012.

Dharmananda, Subhuti. "Cupping." *Institute for Traditional Medicine Online*, Mar. 1999. Accessed 27 Jan. 2016.

"Diazepam." *MedlinePlus*, US National Library of Medicine, 15 July 2019, medlineplus.gov/druginfo/meds/a682047.html.

"Dietary Fats." *American Heart Association*, 1 Nov. 2021, www.heart.org/en/healthy-living/healthy-eating/eat-smart/fats/dietary-fats. Accessed 13 June 2022.

"Dietary Proteins." *MedlinePlus*, 25 Mar. 2015, medlineplus.gov/dietaryproteins.html.

"Dietary Supplements for Exercise and Athletic Performance." *National Institutes of Health, Office of Dietary Supplements*, US Department of Health and Human Services, 4 Oct. 2017, ods.od.nih.gov/factsheets/ExerciseAndAthleticPerformance-Consumer/. Accessed 30 June 2020.

Dillard, James M. *The Chronic Pain Solution: The Comprehensive, Step-by-Step Guide to Choosing the Best of Alternative and Conventional Medicine*. Bantam Books, 2002.

Dima, Delia, et al. "The Use of Rotation to Fentanyl in Cancer-Related Pain." *Journal of Pain Research*, vol. 10, 2017, pp. 341-48, doi:10.2147/jpr.s121920.

Dingemanse, R., et al. "Evidence for the Effectiveness of Electrophysical Modalities for Treatment of Medial and Lateral Epicondylitis: A Systematic Review." *British Journal of Sports Medicine*, vol. 48, no. 12, 2014, pp. 957-65, doi:10.1136/bjsports-2012-091513.

The Doctors Book of Home Remedies. Rev. ed., Bantam Books, 2009.

Doherty, Gerard M., and Lawrence W. Way, editors. *Current Surgical Diagnosis and Treatment*. 13th ed., Lange Medical Books/McGraw-Hill, 2009.

Doidge, Norman. *The Brain's Way of Healing: Remarkable Discoveries and Recoveries from the Frontiers of Neuroplasticity*. Penguin Books, 2015.

Dolan, Eric W. "In Depressed People, the Medial Prefrontal Cortex Exerts More Control over Other Parts of the Brain." *PsyPost*, 19 June 2017, www.psypost.org/2017/06/depressed-people-medial-prefrontal-cortex-exerts-control-parts-brain-49168. Accessed 4 May 2020.

"Dr. Frank Kriise of Mayo Clinic, 75." *New York Times*, 18 Sept. 1973, www.nytimes.com/1973/09/18/archives/

dr-frank-krusen-of-mayo-clinic-75-rehabilitation-expert-diesled.html?_r=0. Accessed 21 Nov. 2016.

"DREAM Repression & Dynorphin Expression." *Protein Lounge*, n.d., proteinlounge.com/dream-repression-and-dynorphin-expression-pg-299.html.

Dreschler, Heike. *Absprung: An Autobiography*. Central Books, 2001.

Drevin, G., et al. "Baclofen Overdose Following Recreational Use in Adolescents and Young Adults: A Case Report and Review of the Literature." *Forensic Science International*, vol. 316, 2020, p. 110541, doi:10.1016/j.forsciint.2020.110541.

"Drugs for Postmenopausal Osteoporosis." *Medical Letter on Drugs and Therapeutics*, vol. 62, no. 1602, 2020, pp. 105-12.

Dunford, Emma, and Miles Thompson. "Relaxation and Mindfulness in Pain: A Review." *Reviews in Pain*, vol. 4, no. 1, 2010, pp. 18-22, doi:10.1177/204946371000400105.

Duyff, Roberta Larson. *American Dietetic Association Complete Food and Nutrition Guide*. 3rd ed., John Wiley & Sons, 2007.

Eagle, Kim A., and Ragavendra R. Baliga, editors. *Practical Cardiology: Evaluation and Treatment of Common Cardiovascular Disorders*. 2nd ed., Lippincott Williams & Wilkins, 2008.

"Earn Your Personal Trainer Certification (NASM-CPT)." *The National Academy of Sports Medicine*, n.d., www.nasm.org/become-a-personal-trainer.

Earnest, C. P., et al. "Low vs. High Glycemic Index Carbohydrate Gel Ingestion during Simulated 64-km Cycling Time Trial Performance." *The Journal of Strength and Conditioning Research*, vol. 18, no. 3, 2004, pp. 466-72.

Easton, John. "Eugene Goldwasser, Biochemist Behind Blockbuster Anemia Drug, 1922-2010." *University of Chicago*, 22 Dec. 2010, news.uchicago.edu/article/2010/12/22/eugene-goldwasser-biochemist-behind-blockbuster-anemia-drug-1922-2010. Accessed 11 Mar. 2017.

Eckerson, J. M., et al. "Effect of Creatine Phosphate Supplementation on Anaerobic Working Capacity and Body Weight After Two and Six Days of Loading in Men and Women." *Journal of Strength Conditioning Research*, vol. 19, 2005, pp. 756-63.

Edlin, Gordon, and Eric Golanty. *Health and Wellness*. 10th ed., Jones and Bartlett, 2010.

"Education Overview." *National Athletic Trainers Association (NATA)*, 2022, https://www.nata.org/about/athletic-training/education-overview. Accessed 27 May 2022.

"Edward Taub, PhD." *American Psychological Association*, www.apa.org/action/careers/health/edward-taub.aspx. Accessed 29 Nov. 2017.

Edwards, Christopher R., and Dennis W. Lincoln, editors. *Recent Advances in Endocrinology and Metabolism*. 4th ed., Churchill Livingstone, 1992.

Edwards, Elizabeth. "Lance Armstrong." *Time*, vol. 171, no. 19, 2008, pp. 66-67.

"Effects of PEDs." *United States Anti-Doping Agency (USADA)*, 13 May 2015, www.usada.org/substances/effects-of-performance-enhancing-drugs.

Egol, Kenneth, Kenneth J., et al., editors. *Handbook of Fractures*. 4th ed., Lippincott Williams and Wilkins, 2010.

Ehrman, Jonathan, et al. *Clinical Exercise Physiology*. 3rd ed., Human Kinetics, 2013.

El-Bogdadi, Daniel. "Tendinitis and Bursitis." *Arthritis and Rheumatism Associates, P.C.*, n.d., arapc.com/tendonitis-and-bursitis/.

"Elbow Fractures in Children." *OrthoInfo*, June 2019, orthoinfo.aaos.org/en/diseases—conditions/elbow-fractures-in-children/.

Elfrink, Tim, and Gus Garcia-Roberts. *Blood Sport: A-Rod and the Quest to End Baseball's Steroid Era*. Plume, 2015.

Ellis, Marie. "Heart Benefits Linked to Marathon Training, Researchers Say." *Medical News Today*, 28 Mar. 2014, www.medicalnewstoday.com/articles/274749.php.

Ellis-Christensen, Tricia. "What Is Static Stretching?" *Wise Geek*. Conjecture Corporation, 23 Mar. 2015, www.wisegeekhealth.com/what-is-static-stretching.htm. Accessed 24 Mar. 2015.

"Endurance Exercise (Aerobic)." *American Heart Association*, 24 Mar. 2015, www.heart.org/HEARTORG/Healthy Living/PhysicalActivity/FitnessBasics/Endurance-Exercise-Aerobic_UCM_464004_Article.jsp#.VtSlGubl9pA.

"Epidemiology of Osteoporosis and Fragility Fractures." *International Osteoporosis Foundation*, 2022, www.osteoporosis.foundation/facts-statistics/epidemiology-of-osteoporosis-and-fragility-fractures. Accessed 29 May 2022.

Ernst, Edzard, and Adrian White, editors. *Acupuncture: A Scientific Appraisal*. Butterworth-Heinemann, 2000.

"Esketamine Nasal Spray (*Spravato*) for Treatment-Resistant Depression." *Medical Letter on Drugs and Therapeutics*, vol. 61, no. 1569, 2019, pp. 54-56.

Espejo, Roman. *Performance-Enhancing Drugs*. Greenhaven, 2015.

Estivalet, Margaret, and Pierre Brisson, editors. *The Engineering of Sport 7*. Vol. 2. Springer, 2009.

Evans, Amanda, and Patricia Coccoma. *Trauma-Informed Care: How Neuroscience Influences Practice*. Routledge, 2014.

Evans, Randolph W., editor. *Neurology and Trauma*. 2nd ed., Oxford UP, 2006.

Fainaru-Wada, Mark, and Lance Williams. *Game of Shadows: Barry Bonds, BALCO, and the Steroids Scandal That Rocked Professional Sports*. Gotham, 2007.

Farish, Mike. "Bottoms Up." *Engineering*, vol. 248, no. 3, 2007, pp. 45-47.

Farr, J. Michael, editor. *Enhanced Occupational Outlook Handbook*. 7th ed., JIST Works, 2009.

"FDA Recommends Avoiding Use of NSAIDs in Pregnancy at 20 Weeks or Later Because They Can Result in Low Amniotic Fluid." *US Food and Drug Administration*, 15 Oct. 2020, www.fda.gov/drugs/drug-safety-and-availability/fda-recommends-avoiding-use-nsaids-pregnancy-20-weeks-or-later-because-they-can-result-low-amniotic. Accessed 7 June 2022.

Feek, Colin, and Christopher Edwards. *Endocrine and Metabolic Disease*. Springer, 1988.

Feldman, Robert S. *Development Across the Life Span*. 6th ed., Pearson/Prentice Hall, 2011.

Felten, D. L., et al. *Netter's Atlas of Neuroscience*. Elsevier Health Sciences, 2015.

Feltz, D. L., and A. P. Konos. "The Nature of Sport Psychology." *Advances in Sport Psychology*, edited by T. Horn, Human Kinetics, 2002, pp. 3-20.

Feng, James, et al. "Total Knee Arthroplasty: Improving Outcomes with a Multidisciplinary Approach." *Journal of Multidisciplinary Healthcare*, vol. 11, 2018, pp. 63-73, doi:10.2147/jmdh.s140550.

Fenske J. N., et al. *Pain Management*. Michigan Medicine University of Michigan, 2021, www.ncbi.nlm.nih.gov/books/NBK572296/.

"Fentanyl." *MedlinePlus*, 15 Oct. 2019, medlineplus.gov/druginfo/meds/a605043.html.

Ferrari, Lynne R., editor. *Anesthesia and Pain Management for the Pediatrician*. Johns Hopkins UP, 1999.

Fessler, Leah. "The First Transgender Athlete on Team USA Reveals How He Combats Sexism in Sports." *Quartz*, 30 Oct. 2018, qz.com/work/1408533/the-first-transgender-athlete-on-team-usa-reveals-how-he-combats-sexism-in-sports/. Accessed 27 Nov. 2019.

Fetterman, Anne, Joseph Campellone, and Raymond Kent Turley. "Understanding the Teen Brain." *University of Rochester Medical Center Rochester*, 2020, www.urmc.rochester.edu/encyclopedia/content.aspx?ContentTypeID=1&ContentID=3051. Accessed 4 May 2020.

"Fine Motor Control." *MedlinePlus*, n.d., medlineplus.gov/ency/article/002364.htm. Accessed 8 Jan. 2019.

Fink, Brett Ryan, and Mark S. Mizel. *The Whole Foot*. Demos Medical, 2011.

Finlan, Timothy. "Occupational Therapy." *Nemours KidsHealth*, Jan. 2020, kidshealth.org/en/parents/occupational-therapy.html. Accessed 13 June 2022.

Firestein, Gary S., et al., editors. *Kelley's Textbook of Rheumatology*. 8th ed., Elsevier, 2008.

Fishman, Scott, with Lisa Berger. *The War on Pain: How Breakthroughs in the New Field of Pain Medicine Are Turning the Tide Against Suffering*. HarperCollins, 2001.

Fixler, Kevin. "The $5 Million Question: Should College Athletes Buy Disability Insurance?" *The Atlantic*, 11 Apr. 2013, www.theatlantic.com/entertainment/archive/2013/04/the-5-million-question-should-college-athletes-buy-disability-insurance/274915/. Accessed 20 May 2021.

Fletcher, Jenna. *Anti-Inflammatory Diet: What to Know*. Medical News Today, MediLexicon International, 3 Jan. 2020, www.medicalnewstoday.com/articles/320233. Accessed 26 May 2022.

———. "Prolotherapy: Uses, Side Effects, and Costs." *Medical News Today*, 17 Dec. 2017, www.medicalnewstoday.com/articles/320330.

———. "What is a Doppler Ultrasound?" *MedicalNewsToday*, 28 Oct. 2019, www.medicalnewstoday.com/articles/326824.

"Flexor Tendon Injuries." *OrthoInfo*, Jan. 2022, orthoinfo.aaos.org/en/diseases—conditions/flexor-tendon-injuries/.

Flink, H., et al. "Effect of Oral Iron Supplementation on Unstimulated Salivary Flow Rate." *Journal of Oral Pathology and Medicine*, vol. 35, 2006, pp. 540-47.

Floyd, R. T., and Clem Thompson. *Manual of Structural Kinesiology*. 21st ed., McGraw-Hill, 2020.

"Food and Nutrition Information Center." *US Department of Agriculture. National Agricultural Library*, n.d., www.nal.usda.gov/fnic. Accessed 24 Aug. 2020.

"Foods That Fight Inflammation." *Harvard Health Publishing*, 7 Nov. 2018, www.health.harvard.edu/staying-healthy/foods-that-fight-inflammation. Accessed 26 May 2022.

Ford, Earl S. "Combined Television Viewing and Computer Use and Mortality from All-Causes and Diseases of the Circulatory System among Adults in the United States." *BMC Public Health*, vol. 12, no. 1, 2012, pp. 70-79.

"Forearm Fractures in Children." *OrthoInfo*, June 2019, orthoinfo.aaos.org/en/diseases—conditions/forearm-fractures-in-children/.

Forrester, S., and B. Beggs. "Gender and Self-Esteem in Intramural Sports." *Physical and Health Education Journal*, vol. 70, no. 4, Winter 2004/2005, pp. 12-19.

Forsyth, L. M., et al. "Therapeutic Effects of Oral NADH on the Symptoms of Patients with Chronic Fatigue Syndrome." *Annals of Allergy, Asthma, and Immunology*, vol. 82, 1999, pp. 185-91.

Foster, Zoë J., and Jeffrey A. Housner. "Anabolic-Androgenic Steroids and Testosterone Precursors: Ergogenic Aids and Sport." *Current Sports Medicine Reports*, vol. 3, no. 4, 2004, pp. 234-41.

Fountain, Henry. "A First: Organs Tailor-Made with Body's Own Cells." *The New York Times*. 15 Sept. 2012, www.nytimes.com/2012/09/16/health/research/scientists-make-progress-in-tailor-made-organs.html?pagewanted=all&_r=0}.

Fouré, Alexandre, and David Bendahan. "Is Branched-Chain Amino Acids Supplementation an Efficient Nutritional Strategy to Alleviate Skeletal Muscle Damage? A Systematic Review." *Nutrients*, vol. 9, no. 10, 2017, p. 1047.

Fox, Barry, and Nadine Taylor. *Arthritis for Dummies*. 3rd ed., For Dummies, 2022.

Fox, Stuart I., and Krista Rompolski. *Human Physiology*. 16th ed., McGraw Hill, 2021.

Frankel, M. S., and A. Teich, editors. *The Genetic Frontier*. American Association for the Advancement of Science, 1994.

Frankle, W. G., et al. "Neuroreceptor Imaging in Psychiatry: Theory and Applications." *International Review of Neurobiology*, vol. 67, 2005, pp. 385-440.

Friedman, Peachy. *Diary of an Exercise Addict*. Pequot, 2008.

Frontera, Walter R., et al., editors. *DeLisa's Physical Medicine and Rehabilitation: Principles and Practice*. 6th ed., Lippincott Williams & Wilkins, 2019.

Frost, H., et al. "Randomised Controlled Trial of Physiotherapy Compared with Advice for Low Back Pain." *British Medical Journal*, vol. 329, 2004, p. 708.

Frost, Robert. *Applied Kinesiology: A Training Manual and Reference Book of Basic Principles and Practices*. North Atlantic Books, 2002.

Fry, A. C., et al. "Effect of a Liquid Multivitamin/Mineral Supplement on Anaerobic Exercise Performance." *Research in Sports Medicine*, vol. 14, no. 1, 2006, pp. 53-64.

Fuchs, Eberhard, and Gabriele Flügge. "Adult Neuroplasticity: More than 40 Years of Research." *Neural Plasticity*, vol. 2014, 4 May 2014, www.hindawi.com/journals/np/2014/541870/. Accessed 11 Jan. 2017.

Fuller, D., et al. "School Sports Opportunities Influence Physical Activity in Secondary School and Beyond." *Journal of School Health*, vol. 81, 2011, pp. 449-54.

Gaddour, B. J. "The Fastest Way to Make Your Muscles Grow." *Men's Health*, 21 Dec. 2016, www.menshealth.com/fitness/a19534758/blood-flow-restriction-to-build-muscle/. Accessed 22 Oct. 2018.

Gallin, John I., and Ralph Snyderman, editors. *Inflammation: Basic Principles and Clinical Correlates*. 3rd ed., Raven Press, 1999.

Gallucci, Nicholas T. S*port Psychology: Performance Enhancement, Performance Inhibition, Individuals, and Teams*. Psychology, 2013.

Gardiner, A., and J. M. Mensch. "Promoting Professional Development in Athletic Training." *Athletic Therapy Today*, vol. 9, 2004, pp. 30-31.

Gardiner, Simon, et al. *Sports Law*. 4th ed., Routledge, 2012.

Garrick, James G., and David R. Webb. *Sports Injuries: Diagnosis and Management*. 2nd ed., W. B. Saunders, 1999.

Garrison, Cheryl. *The Iron Disorders Institute Guide to Anemia: Understanding the Causes, Symptoms, and Healing of Iron Deficiency and Other Anemias*. 2nd ed., Cumberland House, 2009.

Garrison, Susan J., editor. *Handbook of Physical Medicine and Rehabilitation: The Basics*. 2nd ed., Lippincott Williams & Wilkins, 2003.

Gass, Natalia, et al. "Differences between Ketamine's Short-Term and Long-Term Effects on Brain Circuitry in Depression." *Translational Psychiatry*, vol. 9, no. 1, 2019, doi:10.1038/s41398-019-0506-6.

Gazzaniga, Michael S. *The Cognitive Neurosciences*. MIT Press, 2009.

———. *The Consciousness Instinct: Unraveling the Mystery of How the Brain Makes the Mind*. Farrar, Straus and Giroux, 2018.

"Genetic Engineering & Biotechnology News." *Mary Ann Lieber Inc.*, 2013 www.genengnews.com.

Gerdes, Louise I., editor. *Genetic Engineering: Opposing Viewpoints*. Greenhaven Press, 2004.

Gersh, Bernard J. *The Mayo Clinic Heart Book: The Ultimate Guide to Heart Health*. 2nd ed., William Morrow, 2000.

"Get To Know Your Brain Series-The Frontal Lobe." *UPMC HealthBeat*, 1 Dec. 2014, share.upmc.com/2014/12/get-know-brain-series-frontal-lobe/. Accessed 4 May 2020.

Getz, Glen E. *Applied Biological Psychology*. Springer, 2014.

Ghanavatian, Shirin, and Armen Derian. "Baclofen." *StatPearls*, 1 Oct. 2019.

Ghosh, Asok Kumar. "Anaerobic Threshold: Its Concept and Role in Endurance Sport." *US National Library of Medicine*, 2004, www.ncbi.nlm.nih.gov/pmc/articles/PMC3438148/. Accessed 11 June 2019.

Gleaves, J., and T. Lehrbach. "Beyond Fairness: The Ethics of Inclusion for Transgender and Intersex Athletes." *Journal of the Philosophy of Sport*, vol. 43, no. 2, 2016, pp. 311-26.

Glycolysis. Physiopedia, n.d., www.physio-pedia.com/Glycolysis. Accessed 14 Apr. 2022.

"Glycolysis Pathway Made Simple!! Biochemistry Lecture on Glycolysis." *YouTube*, uploaded by MEDSimplified, 24 Nov. 2016, www.youtube.com/watch?v=8qij1m7XUhk.

Gogineni, Hrishikesh C., et al. "Transition to Outpatient Total Hip and Knee Arthroplasty: Experience at an Academic Tertiary Care Center." *Arthroplasty Today*, vol. 5, no. 1, 2019, pp. 100-105, doi:10.1016/j.artd.2018.10.008.

Goldberg, Stephen. *Clinical Neuroanatomy Made Ridiculously Simple*. 4th ed., MedMaster, 2010.

Gonzalez-Fernandez, Marlis, and Stephen Schaaf, editors. *Handbook of Physical Medicine and Rehabilitation*. Demos Medical, 2021.

Goodway, J. D., and H. Savage. "Environmental Engineering in Elementary Physical Education." *Teaching Elementary Physical Education*, vol. 12, 2001, pp. 12-14.

Gorczyca, Pamela, et al. "NSAIDs: Balancing the Risks and Benefits." *US Pharmacist*, vol. 41, no. 3, 2016, pp. 24-26.

Gordon, C. M., K. E. Ackerman, S. L. Berga, et al. "Functional Hypothalamic Amenorrhea: An Endocrine Society Clinical Practice Guideline." *The Journal of Clinical Endocrinology & Metabolism*, vol. 102, no. 5, 1 May 2017, pp. 1413-39, doi:10.1210/jc.2017-00131. PMID: 28368518.

Gordon, Caroline, and Wolfgang Gross. *Connective Tissue Diseases: An Atlas of Investigation and Management*. Clinical Publishing, 2011.

Górski, Andrzej, Hubert Krotkiewski, and Michal Zimecki, editors. *Inflammation*. Kluwer, 2001.

Gottlieb, William. *Alternative Cures: More than One Thousand of the Most Effective Natural Home Remedies*. Rodale, 2008.

Gould, T. E., and S. V. Caswell. "Stylistic Learning Differences between Undergraduate Athletic Training Students and Educators: Gregorc Mind Styles." *Journal of Athletic Training*, vol. 41, 2006, pp. 109-16.

Grady, Sarah E., et al. "Ketamine for the Treatment of Major Depressive Disorder and Bipolar Depression: A Review of the Literature." *Mental Health Clinician*, vol. 7, no. 1, 2017, pp. 16-23, doi:10.9740/mhc.2017.01.016.

Grafman, Jordan, and Andres M. Salazar. *Handbook of Clinical Neurology: Traumatic Brain Injury, Part 1*. Elsevier, 2015.

Graham, T. E. "Caffeine and Exercise: Metabolism, Endurance, and Performance." *Sports Medicine*, vol. 31, no. 11, 2001, pp. 785-807.

Graser, S., et al. "Children's Perceptions of Fitness Self-Testing, the Purpose of Fitness Testing, and Personal Health." *Physical Educator*, vol. 68, 2011, pp. 175-87.

Grassel, Susanne, and Attila Aszodi, editors. *Cartilage: Pathophysiology*. Springer, 2017.

Green, Robert J. *Green's Respiratory Therapy: A Practical and Essential Tutorial on the Core Concepts of Respiratory Care.* ? Aventine Press, 2017.

Greenfield Boyce, Nell. "DNA Blood Test Gives Women a New Option for Prenatal Screening." *NPR*. Shots, 24 Feb. 2015. Accessed 2 Feb. 2016.

Gregg, Jennifer A., Glenn M. Callaghan, and Steven C. Hayes. *Diabetes Lifestyle Book: Facing Your Fears and Making Changes for a Long and Healthy Life*. New Harbinger, 2008.

Gregory, S. "U.S. Ranks Worst in Sports Homophobia Study." *Time*, 9 May 2015, time.com/3852611/sports-homophobia-study/.

Griffin, Darren K., and Gary L. Harton, editors. *Preimplantation Genetic Testing: Recent Advances in Reproductive Medicine*. CRC Press, 2020.

Griffith, H. Winter, et al. *Complete Guide to Sports Injuries: How to Treat Fractures, Bruises, Sprains, Strains, Dislocations, Head Injuries*. 3rd ed., Body Press/Perigee, 2004.

———. *Complete Guide to Symptoms, Illness, and Surgery*. 6th Rev. ed., TarcherPerigee, 2012.

Groh, J. M. *Making Space: How the Brain Knows Where Things Are*. Harvard UP, 2014.

Gropper, Sareen S., and Jack L. Smith. *Advanced Nutrition and Human Metabolism*. 6th ed., Cengage Learning, 2013.

Gross, Charles G. *A Hole in the Head: More Tales in the History of Neuroscience*. MIT Press, 2012.

"Gross Motor Control." *MedlinePlus*, n.d., medlineplus.gov/ency/article/002368.htm. Accessed 8 Jan. 2019.

Guha, Sushovan, et al. *Inflammation, Lifestyle, and Chronic Disease: The Silent Link*. CRC Press, 2012.

Gulli, Benjamin, Les Chatelain, and Chris Stratford, editors. *American Academy of Orthopaedic Surgeons*.

Emergency Care and Transportation of the Sick and Injured. 9th ed., Jones and Bartlett, 2005.

Gulur, Padma, et al. "Morphine versus Hydromorphone: Does Choice of Opioid Influence Outcomes?" *Pain Research and Treatment*, vol. 2015, Article ID 482081, 6 pages, 2015, doi.org/10.1155/2015/482081.

Gutman, Bill. *Marion Jones.* Simon Pulse, 2004.

Guyton, Arthur C., and John E. Hall. *Human Physiology and Mechanisms of Disease.* 6th ed., B. Saunders, 1997.

Hackett, George Stuart, et al. *Ligament and Tendon Relaxation: Treated by Prolotherapy.* Institute in Basic Life Principles, 1993.

Haddley, K. "Alipogene Tiparvovec for the Treatment of Lipoprotein Lipase Deficiency." *Drugs of Today*, vol. 49, no. 3, 2013, p. 161, journals.prous.com/journals/servlet/xmlxsl/pk_journals.xml_summaryn_pr?p_JournalId=4&p_RefId=1937398#.

Haff, G. Gregory, and N. Travis Triplett. *Essentials of Strength Training and Conditioning.* 4th ed., Human Kinetics, 2016.

Hagan, Arthur D., and Anthony N. DeMaria. *Clinical Applications of Two-Dimensional Echocardiography and Cardiac Doppler.* 2nd ed., Little, Brown, 1989.

Hales, Dianne. *An Invitation to Health Brief.* Updated ed., Wadsworth/Cengage Learning, 2010.

Haley, James, and Tamara Roleff. *Performance-Enhancing Drugs.* Greenhaven, 2003.

Hall, John E., and Michael E. Hall. *Guyton and Hall Textbook of Medical Physiology.* 14th ed., Elsevier, 2020.

Hall, Thomas. *Ideas of Life and Matters.* Vol. 1. U of Chicago P, 1969.

Halpern, Brian. *The Knee Crisis Handbook: Understanding Pain, Preventing Trauma, Recovering from Knee Injury, and Building Healthy Knees for Life.* Rodale Books, 2003.

Hamilton, S. F., et al. "The Effect of Ingestion of Ferrous Sulfate on the Absorption of Oral Methotrexate in Patients with Rheumatoid Arthritis." *Journal of Rheumatology*, vol. 30, 2003, pp. 1948-50.

Hamilton, Tracy Brown. *Dream Jobs in Sports Equipment Design.* Rosen Publishing Group, 2018.

Hamilton, Tyler, and Daniel Coyle. *The Secret Race: Inside the Hidden World of the Tour De France.* Bantam, 2013.

Hampton, Debbie. "Neuroplasticity: The 10 Fundamentals of Rewiring Your Brain." *Reset.me*, 28 Oct. 2015, reset.me/story/neuroplasticity-the-10-fundamentals-of-rewiring-your-brain/. Accessed 11 Jan. 2017.

"Hand Fractures." *OrthoInfo*, May 2022, orthoinfo.aaos.org/en/diseases—conditions/hand-fractures.

"Hand Injuries and Disorders." *MedlinePlus*, 31 Aug. 2016, medlineplus.gov/handinjuriesanddisorders.html.

Handal, Kathleen A. *The American Red Cross First Aid and Safety Handbook.* Little, Brown, 1992.

Harper, Joanna. "Transgender Olympians." *HuffPost*, 1 Sept. 2016, www.huffpost.com/entry/transgender-olympians_b_57c5c596e4b004ff0420e1af. Accessed 27 Nov. 2019.

Hassamal, Sameer, et al. "Tramadol: Understanding the Risk of Serotonin Syndrome and Seizures." *The American Journal of Medicine*, vol. 131, no. 11, 2018, doi:10.1016/j.amjmed.2018.04.025.

Hausswirth, Christophe, and Iñigo Mujika. *Recovery for Performance in Sport.* Human Kinetics, 2012.

Hayden, J. A., et al. "Meta-analysis: Exercise Therapy for Nonspecific Low Back Pain." *Annals of Internal Medicine*, vol. 142, 2005, pp. 765-75.

Haywood, Kathleen, et al. *Advanced Analysis of Motor Development.* Human Kinetics, 2012.

"Heads Up." *CDC*, 12 Feb. 2019, www.cdc.gov/headsup/basics/concussion_symptoms.html. Accessed 18 May 2021.

"Healthy Eating: Vitamins and Minerals for Older Adults." *National Institute on Aging.* National Institutes of Health, 2 Jan. 2021, www.nia.nih.gov/health/vitamins-and-minerals-older-adults. Accessed 13 June 2022.

"Heart Diseases." *MedlinePlus*, 31 Dec. 2020, medlineplus.gov/heartdiseases.html. Accessed 8 July 2022.

"Heart Surgery Overview." *Texas Heart Institute*, n.d., www.texasheart.org/heart-health/heart-information-center/topics/a-heart-surgery-overview/. Accessed 2 June 2022.

"Heart Treatments." *NIH National Heart, Lung, and Blood Institute*, 24 Mar. 2022, www.nhlbi.nih.gov/health/heart-treatments-procedures. Accessed 8 June 2022.

"Heart Valves and Circulation." *American Heart Association*, 7 May 2020, www.heart.org/en/health-topics/heart-valve-problems-and-disease/about-heart-valves/heart-valves-and-circulation. Accessed 8 June 2022.

Hebb, Donald O. *The Organization of Behavior: A Neuropsychological Theory.* Wiley, 1949.

Hecht, Marjorie. "Side Effects from NSAIDs." *Healthline*, 23 July 2019, www.healthline.com/health/side-effects-from-nsaids#7-side-effects

———. "Understanding Tendinopathy." *Healthline*, 8 Nov. 2018, www.healthline.com/health/tendinopathy. Accessed 8 Jun. 2022.

Hendleman, Walter J. *Atlas of Functional Neuroanatomy*. 2nd ed., CRC, 2006.

Hendler, Sheldon Saul. *The Doctors' Vitamin and Mineral Encyclopedia*. Simon & Schuster, 1990.

Hendrickson, Mark. "Repetitive Stress Injury." *Cleveland Clinic*, 2018, my.clevelandclinic.org/health/diseases/17424-repetitive-stress-injury. Accessed 23 Feb. 2018.

Henne, Kathryn E. *Testing for Athlete Citizenship: Regulating Doping and Sex in Sport*. Rutgers UP, 2015.

Henning, J. M., et al. "Peer-Assisted Learning in the Athletic Training Clinical Setting." *Journal of Athletic Training*, vol. 41, 2006, pp. 102-8.

"Hereditary Connective Tissue Disorders." *University of Miami Health System*, 2022, umiamihealth.org/en/treatments-and-services/genetics/hereditary-connective-tissue-disorders.

Hernandez, Joe. "NFL Players Are 4 Times More Likely to Develop ALS, a New Study Shows." *NPR*, 16 Dec. 2021, www.npr.org/2021/12/16/1064850108/nfl-players-als-study. Accessed 25 Jan. 2022.

Herrero-Beaumont, G., et al. "Glucosamine Sulfate in the Treatment of Knee Osteoarthritis Symptoms: A Randomized, Double-Blind, Placebo-Controlled Study Using Acetaminophen as a Side Comparator." *Arthritis and Rheumatism*, vol. 56, no. 2, 2007, pp. 555-67.

Hespel, P., et al. "Oral Creatine Supplementation Facilitates the Rehabilitation of Disuse Atrophy and Alters the Expression of Muscle Myogenic Factors in Humans." *Journal of Physiology*, vol. 536, 2001, pp. 625-33.

Hickin, Sarah, et al. *Respiratory System*. 4th ed., Mosby, 2015.

Hill, Z. B. *Endurance and Cardio Training*. Mason Crest, 2015.

Hillier, Susan, and Anthea Worley. "The Effectiveness of the Feldenkrais Method: A Systematic Review of the Evidence." *Evidence-Based Complementary and Alternative Medicine*, 8 Apr. 2015, pp. 1-12, doi:10.1155/2015/752160.

"History of Anaemia." *Renal Med*, 26 Aug. 2016, www.renalmed.co.uk/history-of/anaemia. Accessed 11 Mar. 2017.

"History of the Specialty." *American Academy of Physical Medicine and Rehabilitation*, 2022, www.aapmr.org/about-physiatry/history-of-the-specialty. Accessed 21 Nov. 2016.

Hodges, Paul W., et al. *Spinal Control: The Rehabilitation of Back Pain-State of the Art and Science*. Churchill Livingstone/Elsevier, 2013.

Hoffman, Shirl J., and Duane V. Knudson, editors. *Introduction to Kinesiology: Studying Physical Activity*. 5th ed., Human Kinetics, 2017.

Hoffmann, Georg F., et al. *Inherited Metabolic Diseases*. Lippincott Williams & Wilkins, 2002.

Holecko, Catherine. "Motor Planning, Control, and Coordination." *VeryWell Family*, 26 Oct. 2018, www.verywellfamily.com/what-is-motor-planning-1256903. Accessed 8 Jan. 2019.

Holland, Suzanne, Karen Lebacqz, and Laurie Zoloth, editors. *The Human Embryonic Stem Cell Debate: Science, Ethics, and Public Policy*. MIT Press, 2001.

Holt, N. L., et al. "Physical Education and Sport Programs at an Inner-City School: Exploring Possibilities for Positive Youth Development." *Physical Education & Sport Pedagogy*, vol. 17, 2012, pp. 97-113.

Hoppenfeld, J. D. *Fundamentals of Pain Medicine: How to Diagnose and Treat Your Patients*. Lippincott Williams & Wilkin, 2014.

Horsfall, Joseph T., and Jon E. Sprague. "The Pharmacology and Toxicology of the 'Holy Trinity.'" *Basic & Clinical Pharmacology & Toxicology*, vol. 120, no. 2, 2016, pp. 115-19, doi:10.1111/bcpt.12655.

Horstman, Judith. *The Scientific American Day in the Life of Your Brain: A Twenty-four-Hour Journal of What's Happening in Your Brain*. Jossey-Bass, 2009.

"How an Anti-Inflammatory Diet Can Relieve Pain as You Age." *Health Essentials from Cleveland Clinic*, 7 Oct. 2019, health.clevelandclinic.org/anti-inflammatory-diet-can-relieve-pain-age/. Accessed 26 May 2022.

"How Dietary Factors Influence Disease Risk." *National Institutes of Health*, 14 Mar. 2017, www.nih.gov/news-events/nih-research-matters/how-dietary-factors-influence-disease-risk. Accessed 24 Aug. 2020.

"How Much Physical Activity Do Adults Need?" *Centers for Disease Control and Prevention*, 2 Jun. 2022, www.cdc.gov/physicalactivity/basics/adults/index.htm. Accessed 6 Jun. 2022.

"How to Use Food to Help Your Body Fight Inflammation." *Mayo Clinic*, 13 Aug. 2019, www.mayoclinic.org/healthy-lifestyle/nutrition-and-healthy-eating/in-depth/how-to-use-food-to-help-your-body-fight-inflammation/art-20457586. Accessed 26 May 2022.

Hruby, Patrick. "The NCAA Is Running Out of Excuses on Brain Injuries." *Deadspin*, 24 May 2018, deadspin.com/the-ncaa-is-running-out-of-excuses-on-brain-injuries-1819854361.

Hudita, Ariana, et al. "In Vitro Effects of Cetylated Fatty Acids Mixture from Celadrin on Chondrogenesis and

Inflammation with Impact on Osteoarthritis." *Cartilage*, vol. 11, no. 1, 2018, pp. 88-97.

Humphrey, James H. *Stress Among Older Adults: Understanding and Coping*. Charles C Thomas, 1992.

Hunt, K. *Beginner's Guide to Weight Lifting: Simple Exercises and Workouts to Get Strong*. Rockridge Press, 2020.

———. *Bodybuilding for Beginners: A 12-Week Program to Build Muscle and Burn Fat*. Rockridge Press, 2019.

———. *Strength Training for Beginners: A 12-Week Program to Get Lean and Healthy at Home*. Rockridge Press, 2020.

"Hyaluronic Acid (Injection Route)." *Mayo Clinic*, 1 Feb. 2022, www.mayoclinic.org/drugs-supplements/hyaluronic-acid-injection-route/description/drg-20074557. Accessed 8 June 2022.

Hyman, John, et al. "Valgus Instability of the Elbow in Athletes. *Clinics in Sports Medicine*, vol. 20, no. 1, 2001, pp. 25-45.

Hyman, Lindsay. "The Performance Benefits of Lactate Threshold Testing and Training." *CTS*, trainright.com/the-performance-benefits-of-lactate-threshold-testing-and-training/. Accessed 11 June 2019.

Igwebuike, A., et al. "Lack of DHEA Effect on a Combined Endurance and Resistance Exercise Program in Postmenopausal Women." *The Journal of Clinical Endocrinology and Metabolism*, vol. 93, 2008, pp. 534-38.

Ingle, Sean. "IOC Delays New Transgender Guidelines after Scientists Fail to Agree." *The Guardian*, 24 Sept. 2019, www.theguardian.com/sport/2019/sep/24/ioc-delays-new-transgender-guidelines-2020-olympics. Accessed 27 Nov. 2019.

———. "Russia Banned from Winter Olympics Over State-Sponsored Doping." *The Guardian*, 5 Dec. 2017, www.theguardian.com/sport/2017/dec/05/russian-olympic-committee-banned-winter-games-doping.

"Inguinal Hernia," *Johns Hopkins Medicine*, n.d., https://www.hopkinsmedicine.org/health/conditions-and-diseases/hernias/inguinal-hernia.

"Injections That May Ease Your Joint Pain." *Cleveland Clinic*, 2 Apr. 2021, health.clevelandclinic.org/injections-that-could-ease-your-joint-pain/. Accessed 8 June 2022.

Insel, Paul, et al. *Nutrition*. 6th ed., Jones, 2016.

"Introduction to Stem Cells." *NIH Stem Cell Information*. National Institutes of Health, 1 Feb. 2021, stemcells.nih.gov/info/basics.

"Iron-Deficiency Anemia." *American Society of Hematology*, 2022, www.hematology.org/education/patients/anemia/iron-deficiency.

"Iron-Deficiency Anemia." *Mayo Clinic*, 4 Jan. 2022, www.mayoclinic.org/diseases-conditions/iron-deficiency-anemia/symptoms-causes/syc-20355034.

Irvin, Richard, et al. *Sports Medicine: Prevention, Evaluation, Management, and Rehabilitation of Athletic Injuries*. 2nd ed., Allyn & Bacon, 1998.

Isaacs, Scott, and Neil Shulman. *The Hormonal Balance: Understanding Hormones, Weight, and Your Metabolism*. Bull, 2007.

Ive, Frances. *One Step Ahead of Osteoarthritis*. Hammersmith Health Books, 2019.

Iyer, K. Mohan. *Orthopedics of the Upper and Lower Limb*. 2nd ed., Springer, 2020.

James, David. "Design Engineering-Managing Technology: Slight Advantage." *Engineer*, 5 May 2008, p. 34.

Jarvis, Matt. *Sport Psychology: A Student's Handbook*. Rev. ed., Routledge, 2006.

Jelkman, Wolfgang, and Carsten Lundby. "Blood Doping and Its Detection." *Blood Journal*, vol. 118, no. 9, 2013, pp. 2395-402.

Jeurgens, Jeffrey, and Theresa Parisi. "Morphine Addiction and Abuse." *Addiction Center*, 12 Sept. 2019, www.addictioncenter.com/opiates/morphine/.

———. "Oxycodone Addiction and Abuse." *Addiction Center*, 16 July 2019, www.addictioncenter.com/opiates/oxycodone/.

———. "Tramadol Addiction and Abuse." *Addiction Center*, 16 July 2019, www.addictioncenter.com/opiates/tramadol/.

Jobe, Frank, W., et al. "Reconstruction of the Ulnar Collateral Ligament in Athletes." *Journal of Bone & Joint Surgery*, vol. 68, no. 8, 1986, pp. 1158-63.

Johnson, Greg W. "Treatment of Lateral Epicondylitis." *American Family Physician*, vol. 76, no. 6, 15 Sept. 2007, pp. 843-48.

Jones, Marion, and Kate Sekules. *Marion Jones: Life in the Fast Lane*. Warner Books, 2004.

Jonkman, Kelly, et al. "Ketamine for Pain." *F1000Research*, vol. 6, 20 Sept. 2017, p. 1711, doi:10.12688/f1000research.11372.1.

Joseph, Andrew. "New Details Revealed about Purdue's Marketing of OxyContin." *STAT*, 18 Jan. 2019, www.statnews.com/2019/01/15/massachusetts-purdue-lawsuit-new-details/.

Joubert, Dustin P., Gary L. Oden, and Brent C. Estes. "The Effects of Elliptical Cross Training on VO2max in Recently Trained Runners." *International Journal of Exercise Science*, vol. 4 no. 1, 2011, pp. 4-12.

Joyce, Christopher, and Eric Stover. *Witnesses from the Grave: The Stories Bones Tell*. Little Brown & Co., 1991.

Józsa, László, and Pekka Kannus. *Human Tendons: Anatomy, Physiology, and Pathology*. Human Kinetics, 1997.

Juhn, Mark S. "Ergogenic Aids in Aerobic Activity." *Current Sports Medicine Reports*, vol. 1, no. 4, 2002, pp. 233-38.

Juth, Niklas, and Christian Munthe. *The Ethics of Screen in Healthcare and Medicine: Serving Society or Serving the Patient?* Springer, 2012.

Kail, Robert V., and John C. Cavanaugh. *Human Development: A Life-Span View*. 6th ed., Wadsworth Cengage Learning, 2013.

Kaiser, D. A. "Using Reflective Journals in Athletic Training Clinical Education." *Athletic Therapy Today*, vol. 9, 2004, pp. 41.

Kalat, James W. *Biological Psychology*. 11th ed., Wadsworth, 2013.

Kalverboer, Alex F., et al., editors. *Motor Development in Early and Later Childhood: Longitudinal Approaches*. Cambridge UP, 1993.

Kambis, K. W., and S. K. Pizzedaz. "Short-Term Creatine Supplementation Improves Maximum Quadriceps Contraction in Women." *International Journal of Sport Nutrition and Exercise Metabolism*, vol. 13, 2003, pp. 97-111.

Kaminsky, David. *The Netter Collection of Medical Illustrations: Respiratory System*. 2nd ed., Saunders, 2011.

Kandel, Eric, et al. *Principles of Neural Science*. 5th ed., McGraw Hill Professional, 2012.

Karachalios, Theofilos, et al. "Total Hip Arthroplasty." *EFORT Open Reviews*, vol. 3, no. 5, 2018, pp. 232-39, doi:10.1302/2058-5241.3.170068.

Karcher, Susan J., and Richard P. Capriccioso. "Human Genetic Engineering." *Applied Science*, edited by Donald R. Franceschetti, Salem Press, 2012, pp. 987-95.

Karsenty, Gerard. *Translational Endocrinology of Bone: Reproduction, Metabolism, and the Central Nervous System*. Elsevier/Academic, 2013.

Kawasaki, T., et al. "Additive Effects of Glucosamine or Risedronate for the Treatment of Osteoarthritis of the Knee Combined with Home Exercise." *Journal of Bone and Mineral Metabolism*, vol. 26, 2008, pp. 279-87.

Kelikian, Armen S., and Shahan K. Sarrafian. *Sarrafian's Anatomy of the Foot and Ankle: Descriptive, Topographic, Functional*. 4th ed., Lippincott Williams & Wilkins, 2022.

Kelley, Lorrie L., and Connie Petersen. *Sectional Anatomy for Imaging Professionals*. 4th ed., Mosby, 2018.

Kendrick, I. P., et al. "The Effects of Ten Weeks of Resistance Training Combined with Beta-Alanine Supplementation on Whole Body Strength, Force Production, Muscular Endurance, and Body Composition." *Amino Acids*, vol. 34, no. 4, 2008, pp. 547-54.

Kennedy, Jan, et al. "A Survey of Mild Traumatic Brain Injury Treatment in the Emergency Room and Primary Care Medical Clinics." *Military Medicine*, vol. 171, no. 6, 2006, pp. 516-21.

Kenney, W. Larry, et al. *Physiology of Sport and Exercise*. 6th ed., Human Kinetics, 2015.

Kerkhoffs, G. M., et al. "A Double-Blind, Randomised, Parallel-Group Study on the Efficacy and Safety of Treating Acute Lateral Ankle Sprain with Oral Hydrolytic Enzymes." *British Journal of Sports Medicine*, vol. 38, 2004, pp. 431-35.

Kerksick, Chad M., editor. *Nutrient Timing: Metabolic Optimization for Health, Performance, and Recovery*. CRC Press, 2012

Kerr, Mary, and Elizabeth Crago. "Acute Intracranial Problems." In *Medical-Surgical Nursing*, edited by Sharon Lewis, Margaret Heitkemper, and Shannon Dirksen, 6th ed., Mosby, 2004.

Kerr, Zachary Y., et al. "College Sports-Related Injuries United States, 2009-10 through 2013-14 Academic Years." *Morbidity and Mortality Weekly Report (MMWR)*, vol. 64, no. 48, 2015, pp. 1330-36, www.cdc.gov/mmwr/preview/mmwrhtml/mm6448a2.htm. Accessed 16 May 2021.

Khadilkar, A., et al. "Transcutaneous Electrical Nerve Stimulation (TENS) for Chronic Low Back Pain." *The Cochrane Database of Systematic Reviews*, vol. 3, no. CD003008, 2005, doi:10.1002/14651858.CD003008.pub2.

Khan, Karim M., et al. "Overuse Tendinosis, Not Tendinitis: A New Paradigm for a Difficult Clinical Problem." *Physician and Sports Medicine*, vol. 28, no. 5, 2000, pp. 38-45.

———. "Time to Abandon the 'Tendinitis' Myth: Painful, Overuse Tendon Conditions Have a Non-inflammatory Pathology." *British Medical Journal*, vol. 324, no. 7338, 2002, pp. 626-27.

Kidson, Ruth. *Acupuncture for Everyone: What It Is, Why It Works, and How It Can Help You*. Inner Traditions International, 2001.

Kille, L. W. "Performance-enhancing Drugs in Athletics: Research Roundup." *The Journalist's Resource*, 9 May 2013, journalistsresource.org/studies/society/culture/athletic-academic-performance-enhancing-drugs-research-roundup.

Kilner, John F., R. D. Pentz, and F. E. Young, editors. *Genetic Ethics: Do the Ends Justify the Genes?* Wm. B. Eerdmans, 1997.

Kim, Daniel H., et al. *Atlas of Peripheral Nerve Surgery*. Elsevier/Saunders, 2013.

Kimball, Bob, and Beau Dure. "BALCO Investigation Timeline." *USAToday.com*, 27 Nov. 2007, usatoday30.usatoday.com/sports/balco-timeline.htm.

Kirkaldy-Willis, et al., editors. *Managing Low Back Pain*. 4th ed., Churchill Livingstone, 1999.

Kisner, Carolyn, et al., editors. *Therapeutic Exercise: Foundations and Techniques*. 7th ed.,? F. A. Davis Company, 2017.

Kivlan, B. R., et al. "The Effect of Astym® Therapy on Muscle Strength: A Blinded, Randomized, Clinically Controlled Trial." *BMC Musculoskeletal Disorders*, vol. 16, 2015, p. 325.

Klavora, P. *Foundations of Kinesiology: Studying Human Movement and Health*. Sport Books, 2007.

———. *Introduction to Kinesiology: A Biophysical Perspective*. Sport Books, 2009.

Klein, David R. *Organic Chemistry and a Second Language*. 5th ed., Wiley, 2019.

Klein, Penelope, et al. "Meditative Movement, Energetic, and Physical Analyses of Three Qigong Exercises: Unification of Eastern and Western Mechanistic Exercise Theory." *Medicines*, vol. 4, no. 4, 23 Sept. 2017, p. 69, doi:10.3390/medicines4040069.

Klein, Sarah. "13 Reasons to Start Lifting Weights." *Huffington Post*, 12 Jan. 2015, www.huffingtonpost.com/2015/01/12/benefits-of-lifting-weights_n_6432632.html.

Knapp, Rose. *Respiratory Care Made Incredibly Easy*. 2nd ed., Lippincott Williams & Wilkins, 2018.

Koba, T., et al. "Branched-Chain Amino Acids Supplementation Attenuates the Accumulation of Blood Lactate Dehydrogenase During Distance Running." *Journal of Sports Medicine and Physical Fitness*, vol. 47, 2007, pp. 316-22.

Kolata, Gina. "Perks of Cross-Training May End Before Finish Line." *New York Times*, 15 Aug. 2011, www.nytimes.com/2011/08/16/health/16best.html.

Konofal, E., et al. "Effects of Iron Supplementation on Attention Deficit Hyperactivity Disorder in Children." *Pediatric Neurology*, vol. 38, 2008, pp. 20-26.

Kornspan, Alan S. *Fundamentals of Sport and Exercise Psychology*. Human Kinetics, 2009.

Krane, V., and K. S. Barak. "Current Events and Teachable Moments: Creating Dialog About Transgender and Intersex Athletes." *JOPERD: The Journal of Physical Education, Recreation & Dance*, vol. 83, no. 4, 2012, pp. 38-43.

Krans, Brian. "Performance Enhancers: The Safe and the Deadly." *Healthline*, 5 Feb. 2021, www.healthline.com/health/performance-enhancers-safe-deadly.

Kravitz, Len, and Lance Dalleck. "Lactate Threshold Training." *University of New Mexico*, www.unm.edu/~lkravitz/Article%20folder/lactatethreshold.html. Accessed 11 June 2019.

Kreider, Richard B., et al., editors. *Overtraining in Sport*. Human Kinetics, 1998.

Kremkau, Frederick W. *Diagnostic Ultrasound: Principles and Instruments*. 7th ed., Saunders/Elsevier, 2006.

Krohmer, Jon R., editor. *American College of Emergency Physicians First Aid Manual*. 2nd ed., DK, 2004.

Kronenberg, Henry M., et al., editors. *Williams Textbook of Endocrinology*. 12th ed., Saunders/Elsevier, 2011.

Kucera, Jane. *Reverse Osmosis: Design, Processes, and Applications for Engineers*. Wiley, 2010.

Kuebler, Karen M. "Using Morphine in End-of-Life Care." *Nursing*, vol. 44, no. 4, 2014, p. 69, doi:10.1097/01.nurse.0000444548.72595.ac.

Kulish, Peter. *Conquering Pain: The Art of Healing with BioMagnetism*. 6th ed., BioMag Science, 2016.

Kumar, Vinay, et al., editors. *Robbins and Cotran: Pathologic Basis of Disease*. 8th ed., Saunders/Elsevier, 2010.

Kwong, Yune, and Vikram V. Desai. "The Use of a Tantalum-Based Augmentation Patella in Patients with a Previous Patellectomy." *Knee*, vol. 15, no. 2, 2008, pp. 91-94.

"Lactate Threshold 101." *Bicycling*, 30 Apr. 2010, www.bicycling.com/training/a20017067/lactate-threshold-101/. Accessed 12 June 2019.

"Lactate Threshold Testing." *Exercise Physiology Core Laboratory*. University of Virginia Health System, med.virginia.edu/exercise-physiology-core-laboratory/fitness-assessment-for-community-members/lactate-threshold-testing/. Accessed 12 June 2019.

Lafferty, Peter, and Julian Rowe, editors. *The Hutchinson Dictionary of Science*. 2nd ed., Helicon, 1998.

Landau, Elaine. *Head and Brain Injuries*. Enslow, 2002.

Landesa-Martínez, L., and R. Leirós-Rodríguez. "Physiotherapy Treatment of Lateral Epicondylitis: A Systematic Review." *Journal of Back and Musculoskeletal Rehabilitation*, 4 Aug. 2021, doi:10.3233/BMR-210053. PMID:34397403.

Landolfi, E. "Exercise Addiction." *Sports Medicine*, vol. 43, 2012, pp. 111-19.

Landry, Gregory L., and David T. Bernhardt. *Essentials of Primary Care Sports Medicine*. Human Kinetics, 2003.

Lane, Andrew M., editor. *Mood and Human Performance: Conceptual, Measurement, and Applied Issues*. Nova, 2007.

Lane, Nancy E., and Daniel J. Wallace. *All About Osteoarthritis: The Definitive Resource for Arthritis Patients and Their Families*. Oxford UP, 2002.

Laursen, Paul B., and David G. Jenkins. "The Scientific Basis for High-Intensity Interval Training: Optimizing Training Programs and Maximizing Performance in Highly Trained Endurance Athletes." *Sports Medicine*, vol. 32, no. 1, 2002, pp. 53-73.

Lawrence, Glen D. *The Fats of Life: Essential Fatty Acids in Health and Disease*. Rutgers UP, 2010.

Layden, Tim. "Running Amok." *Sports Illustrated*, vol. 93, no. 14, 2000, pp. 39-45.

Leach, Robert E., and Teresa Briedwell. "Tendinopathy." *Health Library*, 18 Mar. 2013.

Leddy, John J., et al. "Rehabilitation of Concussion and Post-concussion Syndrome." *Sports Health*, vol. 4, no. 2, 2012, pp. 147-54, www.ncbi.nlm.nih.gov/pmc/articles/PMC3435903/.

LeDoux, Joseph. *Synaptic Self: How Our Brains Become Who We Are*. 2nd ed., Penguin Books, 2003.

Lee, Myeong Soo, et al. "Is Cupping an Effective Treatment? An Overview of Systematic Reviews." *Journal of Acupuncture and Meridian Studies*, vol. 4, no. 1, 2011, pp. 1-4, doi:10.1016/S2005-2901(11)60001-0.

Lee, Yong Seuk. "Comprehensive Analysis of Pain Management after Total Knee Arthroplasty." *Knee Surgery & Related Research*, vol. 29, no. 2, 2017, pp. 80-86, doi:10.5792/ksrr.16.024.

Leibenluft, Ellen. "Neuropathology of Bipolar Disorder." *Cold Spring Harbor Laboratory*, www.cshl.edu/dnalcmedia/neuropathology-of-bipolar-disorder/. Accessed 4 May 2020.

Lentillon-Kaestner, V. "The Development of Doping Use in High-Level Cycling: From Team-Organized Doping to Advances in the Fight against Doping." *Scandinavian Journal of the Medical Sciences in Sports*, vol. 23, 2013, pp. 189-97.

Lesk, Arthur. *Introduction to Genomics*. 3rd ed., Oxford UP, 2017.

Lesondak, David. *Fascia: What it is and Why it Matters*. Handspring Pub. Ltd., 2017.

Lewis, Tanya. "Human Brain: Facts, Functions & Anatomy." *Live Science*, 25 Mar. 2016, www.livescience.com/29365-human-brain.html. Accessed 11 Jan. 2017.

Lichtenstein, Alice H., et al. "Diet and Lifestyle Recommendations Revision 2006: A Scientific Statement from the American Heart Association Nutrition Committee." *Circulation*, vol. 114, no. 1, 2006, pp. 82-96.

Lichtin, Alan E. "Components of Human Blood." *Merck Manuals*, www.merckmanuals.com/home/blood-disorders/biology-of-blood/components-of-blood. Accessed 11 Mar. 2017.

Lieberman, Michael A., and Alisa Peet. *Marks' Basic and Medical Biochemistry*. 6th ed., Lippincott Williams & Wilkins, 2022.

Lieberman, Shari, and Nancy Bruning. *Real Vitamin and Mineral Book*. 4th ed., Avery, 2007.

Linden, Wolfgang. "The Autogenic Training Method of J. H. Schultz." *Principles and Practice of Stress Management*, edited by Paul M. Lehrer and Robert L. Woolfolk, 4th ed., Guilford Press, 2021, pp. 527-52.

Lindquist, Susan B. "Case Report: Stem Cells a Step Toward Improving Motor, Sensory Function after Spinal Cord Injury." *Mayo Clinic News Network*, 27 Nov. 2019, newsnetwork.mayoclinic.org/discussion/case-report-stem-cells-a-step-toward-improving-motor-sensory-function-after-spinal-cord-injury/. Accessed 31 Dec. 2019.

Lindsay, Mark. *Fascia: Clinical Applications for Health and Human Performance*. Delmar Cengage Learning, 2008.

Liou, Stephanie. "Neuroplasticity." *Huntington's Outreach Project for Education at Stanford*, web.stanford.edu/group/hopes/cgi-bin/hopes_test/neuroplasticity/. Accessed 11 Jan. 2017.

Lipner, Shari R. "Rethinking Biotin Therapy for Hair, Nail, and Skin Disorders." *Journal of the American Academy of Dermatology*, vol. 78, no. 6, 2018, pp. 1236-38.

Lippert, Frederick G., and Sigvard T. Hansen. *Foot and Ankle Disorders: Tricks of the Trade*. Thieme, 2003.

Lippert, Lynn S. *Clinical Kinesiology and Anatomy*. 6th ed., F. A. Davis Company, 2017.

Lisi, Clemente Angelo. *A History of the World Cup: 1930-2006*. Scarecrow Press, 2007.

Liska, Ken. *Drugs and the Human Body, with Implications for Society*. 8th ed., Pearson/Prentice Hall, 2009.

Litin, Scott C., editor. *Mayo Clinic Family Health Book*. 4th ed., Harper Resource, 2009.

Little, Jonathan P., et al. "A Practical Model of Low-Volume High-Intensity Interval Training Induces Mitochondrial Biogenesis in Human Skeletal Muscle: Potential Mechanisms." *Journal of Physiology*, vol. 588, no. 6, 2010, pp. 1011-22.

Liu, Joseph, N., et al. "Outcomes in Revision Tommy John Surgery in Major League Baseball Pitchers." *Journal of Shoulder and Elbow Surgery*, vol. 25, no. 1, 2016, pp. 90-97.

Lodish, Harvey, et al. *Molecular Cell Biology*. 9th ed., W. H. Freeman, 2021.

Loeys, B. L., H. C. Dietz, A. C. Braverman, et al. "The Revised Ghent Nosology for the Marfan Syndrome." *Journal of Medical Genetics*, vol. 47, no. 7, pp. 476-85, doi:10.1136/jmg.2009.072785.

Logsdon, Ann. "Learn about Gross Motor Skills Development." *VeryWell Family*, 30 Aug. 2017, www.verywellfamily.com/what-are-gross-motor-skills-2162137. Accessed 8 Jan. 2019.

Lorimer, Donald L., et al., editors. *Neale's Disorders of the Foot*. 7th ed., Churchill Livingstone/Elsevier, 2006.

Low, Michael Sze Yuan, et al. "Daily Iron Supplementation for Improving Anaemia, Iron Status and Health in Menstruating Women." *The Cochrane Database of Systematic Reviews*, vol. 4, CD009747, 2016, doi:10.1002/14651858.CD009747.pub2.

Ludlow, Ruth, and Mike Phillips. *The Little Book of Gross Motor Skills*. Featherstone Education, 2012.

Lumpkin, A., et al. *Practical Ethics in Sport Management*. McFarland and Company, 2012.

Lundon, Katie. *Orthopedic Rehabilitation Science: Principles for Clinical Management of Nonmineralized Connective Tissue*. Butterworth-Heinemann, 2003.

MacAuley, Domhnall. *Oxford Handbook of Sport and Exercise Medicine*. 2nd ed., Oxford UP, 2012.

Mackenna, B. R., and R. Callander. *Illustrated Physiology*. 6th ed., Churchill Livingstone, 1997.

"Madness, Inc.: How College Sports Can Leave Athletes Broken and Abandoned." *Chris Murphy, US Senator for Connecticut*, 2019, www.murphy.senate.gov/imo/media/doc/Madness%203...pdf. Accessed 17 May 2021.

Mafetoni, Reginaldo Roque, and Antonieta Keiko Kakuda Shimo. "The Effects of Acupressure on Labor Pains during Child Birth: Randomized Clinical Trial." *Revista Latino-Americana De Enfermagem*, vol. 24, no. 8, 2016, doi:10.1590/1518-8345.0739.2738.

Magill, R. A. "Motor Learning is Meaningful for Physical Educators." *QUEST*, vol. 42, 1990, pp. 126-33.

"Magnets for Pain." *National Center for Complementary and Integrative Health*. US Department of Health and Human Services, 27 Dec. 2017, nccih.nih.gov/Health/magnets-for-pain.

Mahoney, T. Q., et al. "Progress for Transgender Athletes: Analysis of the School Success and Opportunity Act." *JOPERD: The Journal of Physical Education, Recreation & Dance*, vol. 86, no. 6, 2015, pp. 45-47.

Maina, M. P., et al. "Muscle Building Activities for Elementary and Middle School Children." *Teaching Elementary Physical Education*, vol. 12, 2001, pp. 13-18.

"Majority of Russian Athletes Doping, Alleges German Documentary." *CNN*, 5 Dec. 2014, www.cnn.com/2014/12/05/sport/russia-doping-allegations/index.html.

Makhni, Eric C., et al. "Performance, Return to Competition, and Reinjury After Tommy John Surgery in Major League Baseball Pitchers." *The American Journal of Sports Medicine*, vol. 42. no. 6, 2014, pp. 1323-32.

Malcolm, Dominic. *The Sage Dictionary of Sports Studies*. Sage, 2008.

Malcolm, Estelle, et al. "The Impact of Exercise Projects to Promote Mental Wellbeing." *Journal of Mental Health*, vol. 22, no. 6, 2013, pp. 519-27.

Manaka, Yoshio, Kazuko Itaya, and Stephen Birch. *Chasing the Dragon's Tail: The Theory and Practice of Acupuncture in the Work of Yoshio Manaka*. Paradigm, 1997.

Mann, Felix. *Reinventing Acupuncture: A New Concept of Ancient Medicine*. Butterworth-Heinemann, 2000.

Mann, Jim, and A. S. Truswell. *Essentials of Human Nutrition*. Oxford UP, 2012.

Manning, George, et al. *Stress: Living and Working in a Changing World*. Whole Person Associates, 1999.

Maradona, Diego, et al. *Maradona: The Autobiography of Soccer's Greatest and Most Controversial Star*. Skyhorse, 2007.

Marcus, Robert, David Feldman, and Jennifer Kelsey, editors. *Osteoporosis*. 3rd ed., Academic Press/Elsevier, 2008.

Marder, Victor J., et al., editors. *Disorders of Thrombosis and Hemostasis: Basic Principles and Clinical Practice*. 6th ed., Lippincott Williams & Wilkins, 2012.

Marieb, Elaine N., and Suzanne Keller. *Essentials of Human Anatomy and Physiology*. 13th ed., Pearson, 2021.

Marsh, J. L., et al. "Fracture and Dislocation Classification Compendium-2007: Orthopaedic Trauma Association Classification, Database and Outcomes Committee." *Journal of Orthopedic Trauma*, vol. 21, Nov./Dec. 2007, pp. 1-133.

Marshall, Keri. *User's Guide to Protein and Amino Acids*. Basic Health Publications, 2005.

Martin, B. R., et al. "Exercise and Calcium Supplementation: Effects on Calcium Homeostasis in Sportswomen." *Medicine and Science in Sports and Exercise*, vol. 39, no. 9, 2007, pp. 1481-86.

Martini, Frederic H., et al. *Fundamentals of Anatomy & Physiology*. 11th ed., Pearson, 2017.

Masdeu, J. C., et al. "Special Review: Brain Single Photon Emission Tomography." *Neurology*, vol. 44, 1994, pp. 1970-77.

Mastaloudis, A., et al. "Antioxidants Did Not Prevent Muscle Damage in Response to an Ultramarathon Run." *Medicine and Science in Sports and Exercise*, vol. 38, 2006, pp. 72-80.

Masters, J., and E. McKirdy. "Olympic Doping Ban Overturned for 28 Russian Athletes." *CNN*, 1 Feb. 2018, www.cnn.com/2018/02/01/europe/russia-doping-ban-lifted-on-28-athletes-intl/index.html.

Masterson, Kathleen. "A New Spinal Cord Injury Treatment is Getting Patients Back on Their Feet." *MedicalXpress*, 10 Sept. 2018, medicalxpress.com/news/2018-09-spinal-cord-injury-treatment-patients.html. Accessed 31 Dec. 2019.

Matthews, Mike. "Does Blood Flow Restriction (Occlusion) Training Really Work?" *Legion Athletics*, legionathletics.com/blood-flow-restriction-occlusion-training/. Accessed 22 Oct. 2018.

Maugham, R. J., and R. Murray. *Sports Drinks: Basic Science and Practical Aspects*. CRC Press, 2001.

Maury, Bertrand. *The Respiratory System in Equations*. Springer, 2013.

Mayo Clinic. "Historically 'Safer' Tramadol More Likely than Other Opioids to Result in Prolonged Use." *ScienceDaily*, 14 May 2019, www.sciencedaily.com/releases/2019/05/190514090953.htm.

Mayo, Cris. *LGBTQ Youth and Education: Policies and Practices*. Teachers College Press, 2013.

Mazzone, Nicholas. "Blood Flow Restriction Training: What Is It and Will It Work for My Patients?" *New Grad Physical Therapy*, 8 May 2017, newgradphysicaltherapy.com/blood-flow-restriction-training/. Accessed 22 Oct. 2018.

McArdle, William, Frank I. Katch, and Victor L. Katch. *Exercise Physiology: Nutrition, Energy, and Human Performance*. 9th ed., Wolters Kluwer, 2022.

McCarthy, Jeanette, and Bryce Mendelsohn. *Precision Medicine: A Guide to Genomics in Clinical Practice*. McGraw Hill/Medical, 2016.

McColl. Janice. "An Introduction to Essential Fatty Acids in Health and Nutrition." *Bioriginal Food & Science Corporation*, 2017, www.bioriginal.com/page-articles/an-introduction-to-essential-fatty-acids-in-health-and-nutrition/

McDermott, Annabel. "Constraint-Induced Movement Therapy-Upper Extremity." *Heart & Stroke Foundation Canadian Partnership for Stroke Recovery*, 22 Sept. 2016, www.strokengine.ca/intervention/constraint-induced-movement-therapy-upper-extremity/. Accessed 29 Nov. 2017.

McDuff, David R. *Sports Psychiatry: Strategies for Life Balance and Peak Performance*. American Psychiatric Publishing, 2012.

McGill, Stuart. *Low Back Disorders: Evidence-Based Prevention and Rehabilitation*. Human Kinetics, 2002.

McGraw-Hill Encyclopedia of Science and Technology. 11th ed., McGraw-Hill, 2012.

McKee, Ann C., et al. "Chronic Traumatic Encephalopathy in Athletes: Progressive Tauopathy after Repetitive Head Injury." *Journal of Neuropathology and Experimental Neurology*, vol. 68, no. 7 (2009): 709-35.

McKenzie, Robin, and Craig Kubey. *Seven Steps to a Pain-Free Life: How to Rapidly Relieve Back and Neck Pain Using the McKenzie Method*. Dutton, 2000.

McKenzie, Shelley. *Getting Physical: The Rise of Fitness Culture in America*. UP of Kansas, 2013.

McKinley, Michael P., et al. *Human Anatomy*. 4th ed., McGraw, 2015.

McPherson, R. "Inflammation and Coronary Artery Disease: Insights from Genetic Studies." *The Canadian Journal of Cardiology*, vol. 28, no. 6, 2012, pp. 662-66.

Medeiros, Joao. "Game Your Brain: The New Benefits of Neuroplasticity." *Wired*, 16 May 2014, www.wired.co.uk/article/game-your-brain. Accessed 11 Jan. 2017.

Megan, Kathleen. "Transgender Sports Debate Polarizes Women's Advocates." *The CT Mirror*, 22 July 2019, ctmirror.org/2019/07/22/transgender-issues-polarizes-womens-advocates-a-conundrum/. Accessed 27 Nov. 2019.

Meggs, William Joel, and Carol Svec. *The Inflammation Cure*. Contemporary Books, 2004.

Mehta, Piyush, et al. "Contemporary Acupressure Therapy: Adroit Cure for Painless Recovery of Therapeutic Ailments." *Journal of Traditional and Complementary Medicine*, vol. 7, no. 2, 2017, pp. 251-63, doi:10.1016/j.jtcme.2016.06.004.

Meisner, Robert C. "Ketamine for Major Depression: New Tool, New Questions." *Harvard Health Blog*. Harvard Medical School, 20 May 2019, www.health.harvard.edu/blog/ketamine-for-major-depression-new-tool-new-questions-2019052216673.

Melmed, Shlomo, et al., editors. *Williams Textbook of Endocrinology*. 14th ed., ? Elsevier, 2019.

"Meniscus Tears." *OrthoInfo*, Mar. 2021, orthoinfo.aaos.org/topic.cfm?topic=A00358.

Merino, Noël. *Genetic Engineering: Opposing Viewpoints*. Greenhaven Press, 2013.

Mestre, L. S. "Matching Up Learning Styles with Learning Objects: What's Effective?" *Journal of Library Administration*, vol. 50, no. 7/8, 2010, pp. 808-29.

Metzl, Jordan. "Concussion in the Young Athlete." *Pediatrics*, vol. 117, no. 5., 2006, p. 1813.

Mez, Jesse, et al. "Clinicopathological Evaluation of Chronic Traumatic Encephalopathy in Players of American Football." *Journal of the American Medical Association*, vol. 319, no. 4, 2017, pp. 360-70.

Michel, S. "Not Quite a First Place Finish: An Argument That Recent Title IX Policy Clarification from the United States Department of Education Does Not Adequately Protect Transgender Interscholastic Athletes." *Law & Sexuality: A Review of Lesbian, Gay, Bisexual & Transgender Legal Issues*, vol 25, 2016, pp. 145-69.

Migala, J. "The Strange Effect of Your Sports Drink." *Men's Health*, 19 May 2014, www.menshealth.com.

Mihalka, Matthew. "Pushing the Limits: Ultramarathons, Ironman, and the Modern Athlete." *American History through American Sports: From Colonial Lacrosse to Extreme Sports*, edited by Danielle Sarver Coombs and Bob Batchelor, vol. 3, Praeger, 2013, pp. 279-93.

Millet, G. P., et al. "Modeling the Transfers of Training Effects on Performance in Elite Triathletes." *International Journal of Sports Medicine*, vol. 1, 2002, pp. 55-63.

Milligan, Eleanor. *The Ethics and Choice in Prenatal Screening*. Cambridge Scholars Publishing, 2011.

Millington, B., and R. Millington. "'The Datafication of Everything': Toward a Sociology of Sport and Big Data." *Sociology of Sport Journal*, vol. 32, no. 2, 2015, pp. 140-60.

Milunsky, Aubrey, and Jeff M. Milunsky. *Genetic Disorders and the Fetus: Diagnosis, Prevention, and Treatment*. 7th ed., Wiley, 2015.

"Mind, Body and Sport: Post-Concussion Syndrome." *National Collegiate Athletic Association*, n.d., www.ncaa.org/sport-science-institute/mind-body-and-sport-post-concussion-syndrome.

Mitchell, George. *The Negotiator: A Memoir*. Simon & Schuster, 2015.

———. *Report to the Commissioner of Baseball of an Independent Investigation into the Illegal Use of Steroids and Other Performance Enhancing Substances by Players in Major League Baseball*. Office of the Commissioner of Baseball, 2007.

"Mixed Connective Tissue Disease." *Mayo Clinic*, 25 May 2022, www.mayoclinic.org/diseases-conditions/mixed-connective-tissue-disease/symptoms-causes/syc-20375147.

Moake, Joel L. "Bruising and Bleeding." *Merck Manual Consumer Version*, Nov. 2021, www.merckmanuals.com/home/blood-disorders/blood-clotting-process/bruising-and-bleeding. Accessed 30 May 2022.

Mock, Donald M. "Biotin: From Nutrition to Therapeutics." *The Journal of Nutrition*, vol. 147, no. 8, 2017, pp. 1487-92.

Mohiyeddini, Changiz. *Contemporary Topics and Trends in the Psychology of Sports*. Nova Science, 2013.

Molassiotis, A., et al. "A Randomized, Controlled Trial of Acupuncture Self-Needling as Maintenance Therapy for Cancer-Related Fatigue after Therapist-Delivered Acupuncture." *Annals of Oncology*, vol. 24, no. 6, 2013, pp. 1645-52.

Monroe, Judy. *Steroids, Sports, and Body Image: The Risks of Performance-Enhancing Drugs*. Enslow, 2004.

Moore, Heather. "Static vs. Dynamic Stretching." *Philly.com*. Interstate General Media, LLC., 28 Jan. 2014, www.philly.com/philly/blogs/sportsdoc/Static-vs-dynamic-stretching.html?c=r. Accessed 24 Mar. 2015.

Moore, Jack. "The Limits of Football Helmets." *The Atlantic*, 5 Feb. 2016, www.theatlantic.com/health/archive/2016/02/super-bowl-football-helmet-concussion/460092/. Accessed 28 Nov. 2021.

Moore, Keith L., and Anne M. R. Agur. *Essential Clinical Anatomy*. 4th ed., Lippincott Williams & Wilkins, 2011.

Moradi, Mohammad, et al. "Use of Oxycodone in Pain Management." *Anesthesiology and Pain Medicine*, vol. 1, no. 4, 2012, pp. 262-64, doi:10.5812/aapm.4529.

Moran, Aidan P. *Sport and Exercise Psychology: A Critical Introduction*. Routledge, 2004.

Morgan, W. J., and L. S. Slowman. "Acute Hand and Wrist Injuries in Athletes: Evaluation and Management." *Journal of the American Academy of Orthopaedic Surgeons*, vol. 9, no. 6, 2001, pp. 389-400.

Moriarty-Craige, S. E., et al. "Multivitamin-Mineral Supplementation Is Not as Efficacious as Is Iron Supplementation in Improving Hemoglobin Concentrations in Nonpregnant Anemic Women Living in Mexico." *American Journal of Clinical Nutrition*, vol. 80, 2004, pp. 1308-11.

Moritz, Eckehard Fozzy, and Steve Haake, editors. *The Engineering of Sport 6: Developments for Disciplines*. Vol. 2. Springer, 2006.

"Morphine." *MedlinePlus*, 15 Oct. 2019, medlineplus.gov/druginfo/meds/a682133.html.

Morris, R. G. M., and Richard G. M. *Elements of a Neurobiological Theory of the Hippocampus: The Role of Activity-Dependent Synaptic Plasticity in Memory*. Amsterdam UP, 2005.

Morton, David, et al. *The Big Picture: Gross Anatomy*. 2nd ed., McGraw Hill/Medical, 2018.

Moser, E. I., et al. "Place Cells, Grid Cells, and the Brain's Spatial Representation System." *Annual Review of Neuroscience*, vol. 31, 2008, pp. 69-89.

Mosley, Michael, and Peta Bee. "A Few Workouts and Tips." *Fast Exercise*. Author, n.d. Accessed 24 Aug. 2016.

"Motor Control and Learning." *Physiopedia*, n.d., www.physio-pedia.com/Motor_Control_and_Learning. Accessed 8 Jan. 2019.

"Motor Control & Motor Learning." *Trek Education*, n.d., exercise.trekeducation.org/motor-learning. Accessed 8 Jan. 2019.

"Motor Control and Movement Disorders." *AllPsychologyCareers*, n.d., www.allpsychologycareers.com/topics/motor-control.htmltest. Accessed 8 Jan. 2019.

"Motor Skills." *Pathways*, pathways.org/topics-of-development/motor-skills-2. Accessed 8 Jan. 2019.

"MRI (Magnetic Resonance Imaging)." *US Food and Drug Administration*, 29 Aug. 2018, www.fda.gov/radiation-emitting-products/medical-imaging/mri-magnetic-resonance-imaging. Accessed 12 June 2022.

"MRI Scans." *MedlinePlus*, 22 Dec. 2016, medlineplus.gov/mriscans.html. Accessed 12 June 2022.

Mulcahey, Mary K. "Sprains, Strains and Other Soft-Tissue Injuries." *OrthoInfo*, June 2020, orthoinfo.aaos.org/en/diseases—conditions/sprains-strains-and-other-soft-tissue-injuries/.

Mulholland, Michael W., et al., editors. *Greenfield's Surgery: Scientific Principles and Practice*. 4th ed., Lippincott Williams & Wilkins, 2006.

Murphy, Andrew. "Knee Bursae." *Radiopaedia*, 9 Nov. 2021, radiopaedia.org/articles/knee-bursae.

Murphy, Joseph G., and Margaret A. Lloyd. *Mayo Clinic Cardiology: Concise Textbook*. 4th ed., Mayo Clinic Scientific Press, 2012.

Murphy, M., et al. "Whole Beetroot Consumption Acutely Improves Running Performance." *Journal of the Academy of Nutrition and Dietetics*, vol. 112, no. 4, 2012, 548-52.

Murray, Michael. *The Pill Book Guide to Natural Medicines: Vitamins, Minerals, Nutritional Supplements, Herbs, and Other Natural Products*. Bantam, 2002.

Murray-Kolb, L. E., and J. L. Beard. "Iron Treatment Normalizes Cognitive Functioning in Young Women." *American Journal of Clinical Nutrition*, vol. 85, 2007, pp. 778-87.

Muscolino, Joseph E. *Kinesiology: The Skeletal System and Muscle Function*. 4th ed., Elsevier, 2022.

"Muscular Dystrophy." *Mayo Clinic*, 11 Feb. 2022, www.mayoclinic.org/diseases-conditions/muscular-dystrophy/symptoms-causes/syc-20375388. Accessed 8 June 2022.

Muzyk, Andrew, et al. "Clinical Effectiveness of Baclofen for the Treatment of Alcohol Dependence: A Review." *Clinical Pharmacology: Advances and Applications*, vol. 5, 2013, p. 99, doi:10.2147/cpaa.s32434.

Myers, Betsy, and June Hanks. *Management of Common Orthopaedic Disorders: Physical Therapy Principles and Methods*. 5th ed., Lippincott Williams & Wilkins, 2022.

Nabili, Siamak N. "Erythropoietin (EPO, the EPO test)." *Medicine Net*, 1 Sept. 2016, www.medicinenet.com/erythropoietin/page3.htm. Accessed 11 Mar. 2017.

Nathanson, Laura Walther. *The Portable Pediatrician: A Practicing Pediatrician's Guide to Your Child's Growth, Development, Health, and Behavior from Birth to Age Five*. 2nd ed., HarperCollins, 2002.

National Center for Injury Prevention and Control. *Report to Congress on Mild Traumatic Brain Injury in the United States: Steps to Prevent a Serious Public Health Problem*. Centers for Disease Control and Prevention, 2003.

National Institute of Biomedical Imaging and Bioengineering. NIH US Department of Health and Human Services, www.nibib.nih.gov/.

"Naturally Produced Testosterone Gives Female Athletes 'Significant' Competitive Edge." *BMJ*, 7 July 2018, www.bmj.com/company/newsroom/naturally-produced-testosterone-gives-female-athletes-significant-competitive-edge. Accessed 21 Nov. 2019.

Neighmond, Patti. "Is the Warning That Creatine's Not for Teens Getting Through?" *NPR*, 2 Jan. 2017, www.npr.org/sections/health-shots/2017/01/02/507478762/is-the-warning-that-creatines-not-for-teens-getting-through. Accessed 25 June 2020.

Neiman, D. *Exercise Testing and Prescription: A Health-Related Approach*. 7th ed., McGraw-Hill, 2011.

Nelms, Marcia, and Kathryn P. Sucher. *Nutrition Therapy and Pathophysiology*. 3rd ed., Brooks Cole, 2015.

Nelson, David L., and Michael M. Cox. *Lehninger Principles of Biochemistry*. 8th ed., W.H. Freeman, 2021.

Nelson, M., et al. "Proof of Homologous Blood Transfusion through Quantification of Blood Group Antigens." *Heamatologica*, vol. 88, no. 11, 2003, pp. 1284-95.

Nelson, Miriam E., and Sarah Wernick. *Strong Women, Strong Bones: Everything You Need to Know to Prevent, Treat, and Beat Osteoporosis*. Rev. ed., Berkley Books, 2006.

Nerem, R. M., et al., editors. *Principles of tissue engineering*. 4th ed., Academic Press, 2013.

Netter, Frank H. *The CIBA Collection of Medical Illustrations*. CIBA Pharmaceutical, 1995.

Neumann, Donald A. *Kinesiology of the Musculoskeletal System: Foundations for Rehabilitation*. 3rd ed., Mosby, 2016.

"Neurological Rehabilitation." *Johns Hopkins Medicine*, www.hopkinsmedicine.org/healthlibrary/conditions/physical_medicine_and_rehabilitation/neurological_rehabilitation_85,P01163. Accessed 29 Nov. 2017.

Neuwirth, Michael, and Kevin Osborn. *The Scoliosis Sourcebook*. 2nd ed., McGraw-Hill, 2008.

Newell, K. M. "Motor Skill Acquisition." *Annual Review of Psychology*, vol. 42, 1991, pp. 213-37.

Newton, Tim, et al. *Managing Stress: Emotion and Power at Work*. Sage, 1996.

Nichols, Hannah. "The Research-Backed Benefits of Yoga." *Medical News Today*, 23 Sept. 2019, www.medicalnewstoday.com/articles/326414.php.

NIDA. "Fentanyl." *National Institute on Drug Abuse*, 6 June 2016, www.drugabuse.gov/drugs-abuse/fentanyl.

Niemisto, L., et al. "Radiofrequency Denervation for Neck and Back Pain." *The Cochrane Database of Systematic Reviews*, vol. 1, no. CD004058, 2003, doi:10.1002/14651858.CD004058.

"NINDS Repetitive Motion Disorders Information Page." *National Institute of Neurological Disorders and Stroke*, 11 July 2013, www.ninds.nih.gov/disorders/repetitive_motion/repetitive_motion.htm. Accessed 30 Jan. 2015.

Nishimura, R. A., H. Seggewiss, and H. V. Schaff. "Hypertrophic Obstructive Cardiomyopathy." *Circulation Research*, vol. 121, no. 7, 2017, pp. 771-83, doi:10.1161/circresaha.116.309348.

Noelle, B. *Weight Training for Women: Exercises and Workout Programs for Building Strength with Free Weights*. Rockridge Press, 2020.

Noll, Eric, et al. "Efficacy of Acupressure on Quality of Recovery After Surgery: Randomised Controlled Trial." *European Journal of Anaesthesiology*, vol. 36, no. 8, 2019, pp. 557-65, doi:10.1097/EJA.0000000000001001.

"Nonopioid Drugs for Pain." *Medical Letter on Drugs and Therapeutics*, vol. 64, no. 1645, 2022, pp. 33-40.

"Non-Steroidal Anti-Inflammatory Drugs (NSAIDs)." *Cleveland Clinic*, 25 Jan. 2020, my.clevelandclinic.org/health/drugs/11086-non-steroidal-anti-inflammatory-medicines-nsaids. Accessed 7 June 2022.

Nordqvist, Christian. "What Is Repetitive Strain Injury (RSI)? What Causes Repetitive Strain Injury?" *Medical News Today*. MediLexicon International Limited, 19 Jan. 2010, www.medicalnewstoday.com/articles/176443.php. Accessed 19 Jan. 2010.

Norkin C. C. *Joint Structure and Function*. 4th ed., F. A. Davis, 2005.

Norton, Amy, "Can High-Protein, Low-Carb Diet Boost Fertility Treatment?" *MedicalXpress*, 6 May 2013, medicalxpress.com/news/2013-05-high-protein-low-carb-diet-boost-fertility.html.

Nosaka, K., et al. "Effects of Amino Acid Supplementation on Muscle Soreness and Damage." *International Journal of Sport Nutrition and Exercise Metabolism*, vol. 16, 2006, pp. 620-35.

"NSAIDs." *National Health Service (UK)*, 27 Feb. 2019, www.nhs.uk/conditions/nsaids/. Accessed 7 June 2022.

"NSAIDs: Do They Increase My Risk of Heart Attack and Stroke?" *Mayo Clinic*, 10 Dec. 2020, www.mayoclinic.org/diseases-conditions/heart-attack/expert-answers/nsaids-heart-attack-stroke/faq-20147557. Accessed 7 June 2022.

Ntoumanis, N., and S. J. H. Biddle. "A Review of Motivational Climate in Physical Activity." *Journal of Sport Sciences*, vol. 17, 1999, pp. 643-65.

O'Connor, T. E., L. J. Skinner, P. Kiely, and J. E. Fenton. "Return to Contact Sports Following Infectious Mononucleosis: The Role of Serial Ultrasonography." *Ear, Nose & Throat Journal*, vol. 90, no. 8, Aug. 2011, pp. E21-24, doi:10.1177/014556131109000819. PMID: 21853428.

O'Keefe, J., and L. Nadel. *The Hippocampus as a Cognitive Map*. Clarendon Press, 1978.

O'Sullivan, Susan B., et al., editors. National Physical Therapy Examination Review and Study Guide, 2022. 25th ed.,? TherapyEd, 2022.

Oatis, Carol A. *Kinesiology: The Mechanics of Human Movement*. 3rd ed., Lippincott Williams & Wilkins, 2016.

"Occupational Outlook Handbook: Physical Therapy." *US Bureau of Labor Statistics*, 18 Apr. 2022, www.bls.gov/ooh/healthcare/physical-therapists.htm.

Offit, Paul A. *Do You Believe in Magic?: The Sense and Nonsense of Alternative Medicine*. Harper, 2012.

Ogal, Hans P., and Wolfram Stor. *Pictorial Atlas of Acupuncture: An Illustrated Manual of Acupuncture Points*. H. F. Ullman Publishing, 2012.

Okabe, Keisuke, et al. "Oral Administration of Nicotinamide Mononucleotide Is Safe and Efficiently Increases Blood Nicotinamide Adenine Dinucleotide Levels in Healthy Subjects." *Frontiers in Nutrition*, vol. 9, 2022, 868640, doi:10.3389/fnut.2022.868640.

Oliver, Zayne. *Physical Medicine and Rehabilitation*. Larsen and Keller Education, 2017.

Olson, Kenneth A. Manual Physical Therapy of the Spine. 3rd ed., Elsevier, 2021.

Olson, Steve, and Institute of Medicine (US). *Integrating Large-Scale Genomic Information into Clinical Practice: Workshop Summary*. National Academies Press, 2012.

Olthof, M. R., et al. "Choline Supplemented as Phosphatidylcholine Decreases Fasting and Postmethionine-Loading Plasma Homocysteine Concentrations in Healthy Men." *American Journal of Clinical Nutrition*, vol. 82, 2005, pp. 111-17.

"Opioids for Pain." *Medical Letter on Drugs and Therapeutics*, vol. 60, no. 1544, 2018, pp. 57-64.

Orhurhu, Vwaire, et al. "Ketamine Infusions for Chronic Pain." *Anesthesia & Analgesia*, vol. 129, no. 1, 2019, pp. 241-54, doi:10.1213/ane.0000000000004185.

Ornstein, Robert. *The Right Mind: Making Sense of the Hemispheres*. Harcourt, 1997.

Ornstein, Robert, and Richard F. Thompson. *The Amazing Brain*. Houghton, 1984.

"Orthopedic Services." *MedlinePlus*, n.d., medlineplus.gov/ency/article/007455.htm.

Osborne, Sue. "It's Not About the Bike: A Critique of Themes Identified in Lance Armstrong's Narrative." *Urologic Nursing*, vol. 29, no. 6, 2009, pp. 415-43.

Ostojic, S. M., et al. "Glucosamine Administration in Athletes: Effects on Recovery of Acute Knee Injury." *Research in Sports Medicine*, vol. 15, 2007, pp. 113-24.

Owen, Liz, and Holly Lebowitz Rossi. *Yoga for a Healthy Lower Back: A Practical Guide to Developing Strength and Relieving Pain*. Shambhala, 2013.

"Oxycodone." *MedlinePlus*, US National Library of Medicine, 15 Oct. 2019, medlineplus.gov/druginfo/meds/a682132.html.

Pagana, Kathleen Deska, and Timothy J. Pagana. *Mosby's Diagnostic and Laboratory Test Reference*. 15th ed., Mosby, 2020.

"Pain Management Programs." *American Chronic Pain Association*, 2021, www.theacpa.org/pain-management-programs/.

"Pain Treatment." *Leukemia and Lymphoma Society*, n.d., www.lls.org/treatment/managing-side-effects/pain/pain-treatment.

Palermo, Elizabeth. "Does Magnetic Therapy Work?" *LiveScience*. Future US, Inc., 12 Feb. 2015, www.livescience.com/40174-magnetic-therapy.html.

Pangotra, Aditi, et al. "Effectiveness of Progressive Muscle Relaxation, Biofeedback and L-Theanine in Patients Suffering from Anxiety Disorder." *Journal of Psychosocial Research*, vol. 13, no. 1, 2018, pp. 219-28, doi:10.32381/jpr.2018.13.01.21.

Panno, Joseph. *Gene Therapy: Treating Disease by Repairing Genes*. Facts On File, 2005.

Paoletti, Serge. *The Fasciae: Anatomy, Dysfunction, and Treatment*. Eastland Press, 2006.

Papaionnou, A. G., et al. "Motivational Climate and Achievement Goals at the Situational Level of Generality." *Journal of Applied Sport Psychology*, vol. 19, 2007, pp. 16-37.

Papaioannou, Athanasios G., and Dieter Hackfort. *Routledge Companion to Sport and Exercise Psychology: Global Perspectives and Fundamental Concepts*. Taylor, 2014.

Park, Myung K., and Mehrdad Salamat. *Park's the Pediatric Cardiology Handbook*. 6th ed., Mosby/Elsevier, 2021.

Parsaik, Ajay K., et al. "Efficacy of Ketamine in Bipolar Depression." *Journal of Psychiatric Practice*, vol. 21, no. 6, 2015, pp. 427-35, doi:10.1097/pra.0000000000000106.

"Parts of the Brain That Slow Down or Speed up in Depression." *McGill University*, thebrain.mcgill.ca/flash/i/i_08/i_08_cr/i_08_cr_dep/i_08_cr_dep.html. Accessed 4 May 2020.

Pasternak, Jack J. *An Introduction to Human Molecular Genetics*. 2nd ed., Wiley-Liss, 2005.

Patel, Deepa P., et al. "A Review of the Use of Biotin for Hair Loss." *Skin Appendage Disorders*, vol. 3, no. 3, 2017, pp. 166-69.

"Patella Fracture." *Cleveland Clinic*, 12 Nov. 2021, my.clevelandclinic.org/health/diseases/22081-patella-fracture. Accessed 9 June 2022.

"Patellar Tendon Tear." *OrthoInfo*, Sept. 2021, orthoinfo.aaos.org/en/diseases—conditions/patellar-tendon-tear/.

Paul, Gunchan, et al. "Carisoprodol Withdrawal Syndrome Resembling Neuroleptic Malignant Syndrome: Diagnostic Dilemma." *Journal of Anaesthesiology Clinical Pharmacology*, vol. 32, no. 3, 2016, p. 387, doi:10.4103/0970-9185.173346.

The PDR Family Guide to Nutritional Supplements: An Authoritative A-to-Z Resource on the One Hundred Most Popular Nutritional Therapies and Nutraceuticals. Ballantine Books, 2001.

Pelletier, Kenneth. *The Best Alternative Medicine*. Fireside, 2002.

Pelliccia, A., F. M. Di Paolo, E. De Blasiis, et al. "Prevalence and Clinical Significance of Aortic Dilatation in Highly Trained Competitive Athletes." *Circulation*, vol. 122, 2010, pp. 698-706.

"Performance-Enhancing Drugs: Know the Risks." *Mayo Clinic*, 4 Dec. 2020, www.mayoclinic.org/healthy-lifestyle/fitness/in-depth/performance-enhancing-drugs/art-20046134.

Perlmutter, David. "Making New Connections: The Gift of Neuroplasticity." *Integrative Practitioner*, 19 Apr. 2010, www.integrativepractitioner.com/topics/brain-health/making-new-connections-the-gift-of-neuroplasticity/. Accessed 11 Jan. 2017.

Perna, F. M., et al. "Cognitive-Behavioral Stress Management Effects on Injury and Illness Among Competitive Athletes." *Annals of Behavioral Medicine*, vol. 25, 2003, pp. 66-73.

Perrin, David H. *Athletic Taping and Bracing*. 3rd ed., Human Kinetics, 2012.

Perry, Laura, et al. "Cardiovascular Risks Associated with NSAIDs and COX-2 Inhibitors." *US Pharmacist*, vol. 39, no. 3, 2014, pp. 35-38.

"Personal Trainer Job Description." Workable Technology Limited, n.d., resources.workable.com/personal-trainer-job-description.

Peterson, Lynne S. *Mayo Clinic Guide to Arthritis: Managing Joint Pain for an Active Life*. Mayo Clinic Press, 2020.

Petraglia, Anthony L., Julian E. Bailes, and Arthur L. Day. *Handbook of Neurological Sports Medicine: Concussion and Other Nervous System Injuries in the Athlete*. Human Kinetics, 2015.

Pevsner, Jonathan. *Bioinformatics and Functional Genomics*. 3rd ed., Wiley-Blackwell, 2015.

Pfeiffer, Ronald P., and Brent C. Mangus. *Concepts of Athletic Training*. 6th ed., Jones and Bartlett, 2012.

Pham, Phuc Van, editor. *Bone and Cartilage Regeneration*. Springer, 2016.

"Physiatry-Rehabilitation Medicine." *Johns Hopkins Medicine*, n.d., www.hopkinsmedicine.org/physical_medicine_rehabilitation/. Accessed 14 Jun. 2022.

"Physical Education." *Play and Playground Encyclopedia*, 2022, www.pgpedia.com/p/physical-education. Accessed 27 May 2022.

"Physical Medicine and Rehabilitation." *Mayo Clinic*, 20 Nov. 2021, www.mayoclinic.org/departments-centers/physical-medicine-rehabilitation/overview. Accessed 21 Nov. 2016.

"Physical Medicine and Rehabilitation." *MedlinePlus*, 8 Oct. 2015, medlineplus.gov/ency/article/007448.htm. Accessed 21 Nov. 2016.

Piccolino, Marco. "Biological Machines: From Mills to Molecules." *Nature Reviews: Molecular Cell Biology*, vol. 1, 2000, pp. 149-53.

Pietrangelo, Ann. "What Causes Muscle Wasting?" *Healthline*, 23 Aug. 2019, www.healthline.com/health/muscle-atrophy. Accessed 8 Jun. 2022.

Piscatella, Joseph, and Barry Franklin. *Prevent, Halt & Reverse Heart Disease: 109 Things You Can Do*. Rev. ed., Workman, 2011.

Pittler, Max H., et al. "Static Magnets for Reducing Pain: Systematic Review and Meta-Analysis of Randomized Trials." *CMAJ: Canadian Medical Association Journal = Journal de l'Association Medicale Canadienne*, vol. 177, no. 7, 2007, pp. 736-42, doi:10.1503/cmaj.061344.

"Plantar Fasciitis." *MedlinePlus*, 20 Jan. 2022, www.mayoclinic.org/diseases-conditions/plantar-fasciitis/symptoms-causes/syc-20354846. Accessed 8 Jun. 2022.

"Play and Playground Encyclopedia." *National Association for Sport and Physical Education*, 2022, www.pgpedia.com/n/national-association-sport-and-physical-education.

Plezbert, J. A., and J. R. Burke. "Effects of the Homeopathic Remedy Arnica on Attenuating Symptoms of Exercise-Induced Muscle Soreness." *Journal of Chiropractic Medicine*, vol. 4, 2005, pp. 152-61.

Plosser, Liz. "A WH Fitness Face Off." *Women'sHealth*, 2 Aug. 2007, www.womenshealthmag.com/fitness/cardio-vs-strength-training-workouts.

Pluim, B. M., et al. "The Effects of Creatine Supplementation on Selected Factors of Tennis Specific Training." *British Journal of Sports Medicine*, vol. 40, 2006, pp. 507-11.

Poewe, Werner, and Joseph Jankovic, editors. *Movement Disorders in Neurologic and Systemic Disease*. Oxford UP, 2014.

Ponorac, Nenad, et al. "Professional Female Athletes Are at a Heightened Risk of Iron-Deficient Erythropoiesis Compared with Nonathletes." *International Journal of Sport Nutrition and Exercise Metabolism*, vol. 30, no. 1, 2020, pp. 48-53, doi:10.1123/ijsnem.2019-0193.

Porter, J. L., and M. Varacallo. "Osteoporosis." *StatPearls*, 12 Feb. 2022, www.ncbi.nlm.nih.gov/books/NBK441901/. Accessed 28 May 2022.

Porter, Robert S., et al., editors. *The Merck Manual Home Health Handbook*. Merck Research Laboratories, 2009.

Porter, Roy. *Blood and Guts: A Short History of Medicine*. W. W. Norton, 2002.

———. *The Greatest Benefit to Mankind*. W. W. Norton, 1998.

"Post-Concussion Syndrome." *Mayo Clinic*, 6 Oct. 2020, www.mayoclinic.org/diseases-conditions/post-concussion-syndrome/symptoms-causes/syc-20353352. Accessed 30 Oct. 2017.

"Post-Concussion Syndrome." *WebMD*, 19 Apr. 2021, www.webmd.com/brain/post-concussion-syndrome. Accessed 30 Oct. 2017.

"Postconcussive Syndrome in the ED." *MedScape*, 24 Sept. 2018, emedicine.medscape.com/article/828904-overview?pa=KwZqvW%2FA7DuAHx67PMGl7hi9c58jxFhRd2Zx%2BUzZm%2FaYsSfkvLYCg1JVxbMrw1SmBxE%2FchwRMJ0Z5P4D5Tj5%2FQ8oyMK1o%2FrQdMeQkhfWxCQ%3D. Accessed 30 Oct. 2017.

Pound, Richard W. *Inside the Olympics: A Behind-the-Scenes Look at the Politics, the Scandals, and the Glory of the Games*. John Wiley & Sons Canada, 2004.

"A Powerful Duo; HPC and Graphene Paving the Way for Cutting-Edge Sports Gear Design." *NIMBIX*, 21 Sept. 2021, www.nimbix.net/blog-graphene-hpc-sports-gear. Accessed 28 Nov. 2021.

Powers, Michael E. "The Safety and Efficacy of Anabolic Steroid Precursors: What Is the Scientific Evidence?" *Journal of Athletic Training*, vol. 37, no. 3, 2002, pp. 300-305.

Powers, Pauline S., and Ron Thompson. *The Exercise Balance: What's Too Much, What's Too Little, What's Just Right for You!* Gurze, 2008.

Powers, Scott K., and Edward T. Howley. *Exercise Physiology: Theory and Application to Fitness and Performance*. 11th ed., McGraw-Hill, 2021.

Preddy, Victor R., and Ronald R. Watson. *Bioactive Food as Interventions and Related Inflammatory Diseases*. Elsevier/Academic Press, 2013.

Preidt, Robert. "Too Little Vitamin D May Hasten Disability as You Age." *HealthDay*, 17 July 2013, consumer.healthday.com/senior-citizen-information-31/misc-aging-news-10/too-little-vitamin-d-may-hasten-disability-as-you-age-678337.html.

Prentice, William E. *Arnheim's Principles of Athletic Training*. 14th ed., McGraw-Hill, 2011.

Prescribers Digital Reference, www.pdr.net. A resource to look up specific drugs.

Preston, David C., and Barbara Ellen Shapiro. *Electromyography and Neuromuscular Disorders: Clinical-electrophysiologic Correlations*. 3rd ed., Elsevier/Saunders, 2013.

"Prevent RSI." *National Health Service*. Gov.UK, 10 Oct. 2013, www.nhs.uk/Livewell/workplacehealth/Pages/rsi.aspx.

"Preventing RSI." *Harvard RSI Action*. Harvard University, www.rsi.deas.harvard.edu/preventing.html. Accessed 2 Feb. 2015.

Price, Sylvia Anderson, and Lorraine McCarty Wilson, editors. *Pathophysiology: Clinical Concepts of Disease Processes*. Mosby, 2003.

Price-Mitchell, M. "The Psychology of Youth Sports." *Psychology Today*, 8 Jan. 2012, www.psychologytoday.com/us/blog/the-moment-youth/201201/the-psychology-youth-sports. Accessed 28 May 2022.

Primrose, S. B., R. M. Twyman, and R. W. Old. *Principles of Genetic Manipulation: An Introduction to Genetic Engineering*. 6th ed., Blackwell Science, 2001.

Pringle, A., et al. "Cognitive Mechanisms of Diazepam Administration: A Healthy Volunteer Model of Emotional Processing." *Psychopharmacology*, vol. 233, no. 12, 6 May 2016, pp. 2221-28, doi:10.1007/s00213-016-4269-y.

Pringle, Michael. "Some Thoughts on Fire Cupping." *Journal of Chinese Medicine*, vol. 83, 2007, pp. 46-51.

Pritchard, Sarah, and Andrew Croysdale. *Tui Na: A Manual of Chinese Massage Therapy*. Singing Dragon, 2015, eBook Collection (EBSCOhost). Accessed 27 Jan. 2016.

"Protein in Diet." *MedlinePlus*, n.d., medlineplus.gov/ency/article/002467.htm.

"Quadriceps Tendon Tear." *OrthoInfo*, Oct. 2021, orthoinfo.aaos.org/en/diseases—conditions/quadriceps-tendon-tear/.

Quinn, Elizabeth. "Lactate Threshold Training for Athletes." *VeryWell Fit*, 19 Nov. 2018, www.verywellfit.com/lactate-threshold-training-3120092. Accessed 11 June 2019.

Raak, Christa K., et al. "*Hypericum perforatum* to Improve Postoperative Pain Outcome After Monosegmental Spinal Sequestrectomy (HYPOS): Results of a Randomized, Double-Blind, Placebo-Controlled Trial." *Journal of Integrative and Complementary Medicine*, vol. 28, no. 5, 2022, pp. 407-17, doi:10.1089/jicm.2021.0389.

Radenkovic, Dina, et al. "Clinical Evidence for Targeting NAD Therapeutically." *Pharmaceuticals (Basel, Switzerland)*, vol. 13, no. 9, 2020, p. 247, doi:10.3390/ph13090247.

Rader, B. *American Sports: From the Age of Folk Games to the Age of Televised Sports*. Prentice-Hall, 2009.

Radnedge, Keir. *The Complete Encyclopedia of Soccer*. Carlton Books, 2007.

Radomski, Kirk. *Bases Loaded: The Inside Story of the Steroid Era in Baseball by the Central Figure in the Mitchell Report*. Hudson, 2009.

"Raducan Tests Positive for Stimulant." *Associated Press*, 26 Sept. 2000, assets.espn.go.com/oly/summer00/news/2000/0925/776388.html. Accessed 8 Jun. 2022.

Raffa, R. B., et al. "Oxycodone Combinations for Pain Relief." *Drugs of Today*, vol. 46, no. 6, 2010, p. 379, doi:10.1358/dot.2010.46.6.1470106.

Raleigh, M. D., et al. "Safety and Efficacy of an Oxycodone Vaccine: Addressing Some of the Unique Considerations Posed by Opioid Abuse." *PLOS One*, vol. 12, no. 12, 2017, doi:10.1371/journal.pone.0184876.

Ramirez, S., et al. "Creating a False Memory in the Hippocampus." *Science*, vol. 341, 2013, pp. 387-91.

Ramos-Matos, et al. "Fentanyl." *StatPearls*, 8 May 2022, https://www.ncbi.nlm.nih.gov/books/NBK459275/. Accessed 8 June 2022.

Rapoport, Ron. *See How She Runs: Marion Jones and the Making of a Champion*. Algonquin Books, 2000.

Ray, Richard, and Konin, Jeff. *Management Strategies in Athletic Training*. 4th ed., Human Kinetics, 2011.

Reddy, Luke. "Larry Johnson: Ex-NFL Player on Battle with What He Thinks Is Chronic Traumatic Encephalopathy." *BBC Sport*, 15 Dec. 2017, www.bbc.com/sport/american-football/42364622. Accessed 3 Jan. 2018.

Reece, Jane B., et al. *Campbell Biology: Concepts & Connections*. 8th ed., Pearson, 2020.

Reeves, Roy R., et al. "Carisoprodol." *Southern Medical Journal*, vol. 105, no. 11, 2012, pp. 619-23, doi:10.1097/smj.0b013e31826f5310.

"Repetitive Strain Injury (RSI)." *NHS Choices*. Gov.UK, 27 Jan. 2016, www.nhs.uk/conditions/repetitive-strain-injury-rsi/. Accessed 23 Feb. 2018.

"Request Denied: Arbitrators Uphold Decision to Strip Raducan of Gold." *CNN Sports Illustrated*, 13 Nov. 2000, web.archive.org/web/20040928011117/http://sportsillustrated.cnn.com/olympics/2000/gymnastics/news/2000/09/27/raducan_decision_ap/. Accessed 8 Jun. 2022.

Reynolds, Gretchen. "One Minute of All-Out Exercise May Have Benefits of 45 Minutes of Moderate Exertion." *New York Times*, 27 Apr. 2016.

———. "Stretching: The Truth." *Play Magazine*, 31 Oct. 2008, www.nytimes.com/2008/11/02/sports/playmagazine/112pewarm.html.

"Rheumatoid Arthritis." Cleveland Clinic, 18 Feb. 2022, my.clevelandclinic.org/health/diseases/4924-rheumatoid-arthritis. Accessed 8 June 2022.

Ridgeway, Neale, and Roger McLeod, editors. *Biochemistry of Lipids, Lipoproteins, and Membranes*. Elsevier, 2015.

Roberts, Melanie, and Stephanie Kaiser. "The Different Types of Stretching." *Idiot's Guides: Stretching*. Alpha Books, 2013.

Robertson, V. J., and K. G. Baker. "A Review of Therapeutic Ultrasound: Effectiveness Studies." *Physical Therapy*, vol. 81, 2001, pp. 1339-50.

Robles, J., et al. "The Impact of Preceptor and Student Learning Styles on Experiential Performance Measures." *American Journal of Pharmaceutical Education*, vol. 76, 2012, pp. 1-7.

Rock, C. L., and C. Thomson, et al. "American Cancer Society Guideline for Diet and Physical Activity for Cancer Prevention." *CA: A Cancer Journal for Clinicians*, 9 June 2020, acsjournals.onlinelibrary.wiley.com/doi/full/103322/caac.21591. Accessed 24 Aug. 2020.

Roe, Shirley. *The Natural Philosophy of Albrecht von Haller*. Arno Press, 1981.

Rogerson, S., et al. "The Effect of Five Weeks of *Tribulus terrestris* Supplementation on Muscle Strength and Body Composition During Preseason Training in Elite Rugby League Players." *The Journal of Strength and Conditioning Research*, vol. 21, no. 2, 2007, pp. 348-53.

Rogol, Alan D., and Lindsay Parks Pieper. "Genes, Gender, Hormones, and Doping in Sport: A Convoluted Tale." *Frontiers in Endocrinology*, 12 Oct. 2017, doi:10.3389/fendo.2017.00251. Accessed 27 Nov. 2019.

Rohen, Johannes W., Chihiro Yokochi, and Elke Lütjen-Drecoll. *Color Atlas of Anatomy: A Photographic Study of the Human Body*. 7th ed., Lippincott Williams & Wilkins, 2006.

Romain, Meeusen, et al. "Prevention, Diagnosis, and Treatment of the Overtraining Syndrome." *European Journal of Sport Science*, vol. 6, no. 1, 2006, pp. 1-14.

Romeo, Jim. "Using 3D Printing to Improve Sports Equipment." *GrabCAD*, 6 July 2020, blog.grabcad.com/blog/2020/07/06/3d-printing-sports-equipment/. Accessed 28 Nov. 2021.

Ropper, Allan H., et al. *Adams and Victor's Principles of Neurology*. 11th ed., McGraw Hill / Medical, 2019.

Rosen, Clifford J., Julie Glowacki, and John P. Bilezikian. *The Aging Skeleton*. Academic Press, 1999.

Rosenberg, Roger N., and Juan Pascual, editors. *Rosenberg's Molecular and Genetic Basis of Neurological and Psychiatric Disease*. 6th ed., Academic Press, 2020.

Rosenfeld, Arthur. *The Truth About Chronic Pain: Patients and Professionals on How to Face It, Understand It, Overcome It*. Rev. ed., Basic Books, 2005.

Rosse, Cornelius, and Penelope Gaddum-Rosse. *Hollinshead's Textbook of Anatomy*. 5th ed., Lippincott-Raven, 1997.

"Rotator Cuff Repair." *MedlinePlus*, n.d., www.nlm.nih.gov/medlineplus/ency/article/007207.htm.

"Rotator Cuff Tears." *American Academy of Orthopedic Surgeons*, June 2022, orthoinfo.aaos.org/topic.cfm?topic=A00064.

"Rotator Cuff Tears." *Cleveland Clinic*, 28 Jan. 2021, my.clevelandclinic.org/health/diseases/8291-rotator-cuff-tears-overview.

Rothschuh, Karl. *History of Physiology*. Robert E. Krieger, 1973.

Rouzier, Pierre A. *The Sports Medicine Patient Advisor*. 3rd ed., Sports Med Press, 2010.

Royce, Peter M., and Beat Steinmann, editors. *Connective Tissue and Its Heritable Disorders: Molecular, Genetic, and Medical Aspects*. Wiley-Liss, 2002.

Rozendaal, R. M., et al. "Effect of Glucosamine Sulfate on Hip Osteoarthritis." *Annals of Internal Medicine*, vol. 148, 2008, pp. 268-77.

Ruiz, R. R. "Report Shows Vast Reach of Russian Doping: 1,000 Athletes, 30 Sports." *The New York Times*, 9 Dec. 2016, www.nytimes.com/2016/12/09/sports/russia-doping-mclaren-report.html.

Ruiz, R. R., and M. Schwirtz. "Russian Insider Says State-Run Doping Fueled Olympic Gold." *The New York Times*, 12 May 2016, www.nytimes.com/2016/05/13/sports/russia-doping-sochi-olympics-2014.html.

Ryan, Dennis J., and Arthur Remillard. "From Purity to Pollution: The Transformation of Baseball in the Steroid Era." *Journal of Student Research at Saint Francis University*, vol. 5, no. 1, 2014, p. 4.

Ryan, S. L., and P. Wallace. "Use of Astym® Treatment to Improve Contractures and Dyskinesia in an Individual with Anoxic Encephalopathy." *Combined Sections Meeting*, APTA, Feb. 2009.

Sage, G., and D. S. Eitzen. *Sociology of North American Sport*. 10th ed., Oxford UP, 2015.

Sahay, A. et al. "Increasing Adult Hippocampal Neurogenesis Is Sufficient to Improve Pattern Separation." *Nature*, vol. 472, 2011, pp. 466-70.

Salter, Robert Bruce. *Textbook of Disorders and Injuries of the Musculoskeletal System*. 3rd ed., Williams & Wilkins, 1999.

Saltin, Bengt, et al., editors. *Exercise and Circulation in Health and Disease*. Human Kinetics, 2000.

Sandoiu, Ana. "Treating Pain with Magnetic Fields." *Medical News Today*. MediLexicon International, 9 Aug. 2018, www.medicalnewstoday.com/articles/322718.php#1.

Sandrock, Michael. *Running with the Legends*. Human Kinetics, 1996.

Sankaranarayanan, S., et al. "Daily Iron Alone but Not in Combination with Multimicronutrients Increases Plasma Ferritin Concentrations in Indonesian Infants with Inflammation." *Journal of Nutrition*, vol. 134, 2004, pp. 1916-22.

Santiago, J. A., et al. "Elementary Physical Education Teachers' Content Knowledge of Physical Activity and Health-Related Fitness." *Physical Educator*, vol. 69, 2012, pp. 395-412.

Satel, Sally, and Scott O. Lilienfield. *Brainwashed: The Seductive Appeal of Mindless Neuroscience*. Basic Books, 2013.

Sato, Y. "The History and Future of KAATSU Training." *International Journal of Kaatsu*, 2005, www.kaatsu-global.com/Assets/Files/Presentations/The_history_and_future_of_KAATSU_Training.pdf. Accessed 22 Oct. 2018.

Schafer, Walt, and Sharrie A. Herbold. *Stress Management for Wellness*. 4th ed., Thomson/Wadsworth, 2000.

Scheer, N. A., et al. "Astym(r) Therapy Improves Bilateral Hamstring Flexibility and Achilles Tendinopathy in a Child with Cerebral Palsy: A Retrospective Case Report." *Clinical Medicine Insights: Case Reports*, vol. 9, 2016, pp. 95-98, doi:10.4137/CCRep.S40623.

Schinke, Robert J. *Innovative Writings in Sport and Exercise Psychology*. Nova Science, 2014.

Schleip, Robert. *Fascia in Sport and Movement*. 2nd ed., Handspring Publishing, 2021.

Schmidt-Hansen, Mia, et al. "Oxycodone for Cancer-Related Pain." *Cochrane Database of Systematic Reviews*, 2017, doi:10.1002/14651858.cd003870.pub6.

Schmotzer, Brian, et al. "'The Natural'? The Effects of Steroids on Offensive Performance in Baseball." *Chance*, vol. 22, no. 2, 2009, pp. 21-32.

Schneider, M. B., and H. J. Benjamin. "Sports Drinks and Energy Drinks for Children and Adolescents: Are They Appropriate?" *American Academy of Pediatrics*, vol. 127, no. 6, 2011, pp. 1182-1189.

Schoen, Delores Christina. *Adult Orthopaedic Nursing*. Lippincott Williams & Wilkins, 2000.

Schwartz, Jeffrey M., and Sharon Begley. *The Mind and the Brain: Neuroplasticity and the Power of Mental Force*. HarperCollins, 2002, pp. 138-62.

"Scope of Practice for NFPT Personal Trainers." National Federation of Personal Trainers, n.d., www.nfpt.com/the-role-of-a-personal-trainer.

Scott, Celicia. *Doping: Human Growth Hormone, Steroids, and Other Performance-Enhancing Drugs*. Mason Crest, 2015.

Scoville, W. B., and Milner, B. "Loss of Recent Memory After Bilateral Hippocampal Lesions." *Journal of Neurology, Neurosurgery, and Psychiatry*, vol. 20, no. 1, Feb. 1957, pp. 11-21.

Scuderi, Giles R. *Sports Medicine: A Comprehensive Approach*. 2nd ed., Mosby/Elsevier, 2005.

Scuderi, Giles R., and Peter D. McCann, editors. *Sports Medicine: A Comprehensive Approach*. 2nd ed., Mosby/Elsevier, 2005.

Seaward, Brian L. *Managing Stress: Principles and Strategies for Health and Well-Being.* 6th ed., Jones and Bartlett, 2009.

Selhub, Eva. "The Alexander Technique Can Help You (Literally) Unwind." *Harvard Health,* 19 Nov. 2015, www.health.harvard.edu/blog/the-alexander-technique-can-help-you-literally-unwind-201511238652.

Sellami, Maha, et al. "Herbal Medicine for Sports: A Review." *Journal of the International Society of Sports Nutrition,* vol. 15, no. 14, 2018, doi:10.1186/s12970-018-0218-y.

Selva, Joaquin. "Progressive Muscle Relaxation (PMR): A Positive Psychology Guide." *PositivePsychology.com,* 4 July 2019, positivepsychology.com/progressive-muscle-relaxation-pmr/.

Senchina, David. "Athletics and Herbal Supplements." *American Scientist,* vol. 101, no. 2, Mar.-Apr. 2013, doi:10.1511/2013.101.134.

Serafini, Gianluca, et al. "The Role of Ketamine in Treatment-Resistant Depression: A Systematic Review." *Current Neuropharmacology,* vol. 12, no. 5, 12 Sept. 2014, pp. 444-61, doi:10.2174/1570159x12666140619204251.

Sevier, T. L., and C. W. Stegink-Jansen. "Astym® Treatment vs. Eccentric Exercise for Lateral Elbow Tendinopathy: A Randomized Controlled Clinical Trial." *PeerJ,* vol. 3, 2015, p. e967, doi.org/10.7717/peerj.967.

Shah, Seema, and Vivek Mehta. "Controversies and Advances in Non-Steroidal Anti-Inflammatory Drug (NSAID) Analgesia in Chronic Pain Management." *Postgraduate Medical Journal,* vol. 88, no. 1036, 2012, pp. 73-78.

Shannon, Joyce Brennfleck, editor. *Sports Injuries Sourcebook.* 4th ed., Omnigraphics, 2012.

Sharieff, W., et al. "Is Cooking Food in Iron Pots an Appropriate Solution for the Control of Anaemia in Developing Countries? A Randomised Clinical Trial in Benin." *Public Health Nutrition,* vol. 9, 2008, pp. 971-77.

Sharpe, Neil F., and Ronald F. Carter. *Genetic Testing: Care, Consent, and Liability.* Wiley-Liss, 2006.

Sheftel, Alex D., et al. "The Long History of Iron in the Universe and in Health and Disease." *Biochimica et Biophysica Acta,* vol. 1820, no. 3, 2012, pp. 161-87, doi:10.1016/j.bbagen.2011.08.002.

Shehab, Ramsey, and Mark H. Mirabelli. "Evaluation and Diagnosis of Wrist Pain: A Case-Based Approach." *American Family Physician,* vol. 87, no. 8, 2013, pp. 568-73.

Shekelle, Paul G., et al. "Efficacy and Safety of Ephedra and Ephedrine for Weight Loss and Athletic Performance: A Meta-analysis." *Journal of the American Medical Association,* vol. 289, no. 12, 2003, pp. 1537-45.

Shelton, C. D. *Vitamins, Minerals & Supplements: Essential or Over-Hyped?* Amazon Digital Services Inc., 2013.

Shields, D. L., and B. J. Bredemeier. *Character Development and Physical Activity.* Human Kinetics, 1995.

Shils, Maurice E., et al. *Modern Nutrition in Health and Disease.* 10th ed., Lippincott Williams & Wilkins, 2005.

Shixi, Huang, and Cao Yu. "Cupping Therapy." *Journal of Chinese Medicine,* vol. 82, 2006, pp. 52-57.

Shlotzhauer, Tammi L. *Living with Rheumatoid Arthritis.* 3rd ed., Johns Hopkins UP, 2014.

Shmerling, Robert H. "Are You Taking Too Much Anti-Inflammatory Medication?" *Harvard Health Blog,* 23 Mar. 2018, www.health.harvard.edu/blog/are-you-taking-too-much-anti-inflammatory-medication-2018040213540. Accessed 26 May 2022.

———. "Is Tramadol a Risky Pain Medication?" *Harvard Health Blog.* Harvard Medical School, 16 Aug. 2019, www.health.harvard.edu/blog/is-tramadol-a-risky-pain-medication-2019061416844.

"Shoulder Joint Replacement." *OrthoInfo,* Sept. 2021, orthoinfo.aaos.org/en/treatment/shoulder-joint-replacement.

"Shoulder Problems and Injuries." *WebMD,* 16 Jan. 2015, www.webmd.com/a-to-z-guides/shoulder-problems-and-injuries-topic-overview.

Shumway-Cook, Anne, and Marjorie Woollacott. *Motor Control: Translating Research into Clinical Practice.* 4th ed., Philadelphia: Lippincott Williams & Wilkins, 2012.

Silva, John M., and Diane E. Stevens, editors. *Psychological Foundations of Sport.* 2nd ed., Allyn, 2002.

Silverman, S. "Thinking Long Term: Physical Education's Role in Movement and Mobility." *QUEST,* vol. 57, 2005, pp. 138-47.

Simmons, John. *The Scientific One Hundred: A Ranking of the Most Influential Scientists, Past and Present.* Carol, 1996.

Simons, Stephen M., and Michael Roberts. "Patient Education: Rotator Cuff Tendinitis and Tear (Beyond the Basics)." *UpToDate,* May 2022, www.uptodate.com/contents/rotator-cuff-tendinitis-and-tear-beyond-the-basics.

Sims, S. E., et al. "Non-surgical Treatment of Lateral Epicondylitis: A Systematic Review of Randomized Controlled Trials." *HAND,* vol. 9, no. 4, 2014, pp. 419-46.

Singer, Robert N., et al., editors. *Handbook of Sport Psychology.* 2nd ed., Wiley, 2001.

Singh, N. K., and R. C. Prasad. "A Pilot Study of Polyunsaturated Phosphatidyl Choline in Fulminant and Subacute Hepatic Failure." *Journal of the Association of Physicians of India*, vol. 46, 1998, pp. 530-32.

Singh, Simon, and Ernst, Edzard. *Trick or Treatment: The Undeniable Facts about Alternative Medicine*. W. W. Norton and Company, 2008.

Sinkler, Jen. "4 Myths about Strength-Training Busted!" *Women'sHealth*, 24 Dec. 2013, www.womenshealthmag.com/fitness/strenght-training-myths.

Skinner-Thompson, S., and I. M. Turner. "Title IX's Protections for Transgender Student-Athletes." *Wisconsin Journal of Law, Gender & Society*, vol. 28, no. 3, 2013, pp. 271-300.

Slovik, David M. *Osteoporosis: A Guide to Prevention and Treatment*. Harvard Health Publishing, 2019.

Small, Eric, et al. *Kids and Sports: Everything You and Your Child Need to Know About Sports, Physical Activity, and Good Health*. Newmarket Press, 2002.

Smith, Cooper. "Codeine: Drug Effects, Addiction, Abuse and Treatment-Rehab Spot." *RehabSpot*, 9 July 2019, www.rehabspot.com/opioids/codeine.

Smith, Karen E., and Greg J. Norman. "Brief Relaxation Training Is Not Sufficient to Alter Tolerance to Experimental Pain in Novices." *PLOS One*, vol. 12, no. 5, 2017, doi:10.1371/journal.pone.0177228.

Smith, Lori. "How Can Physical Therapy Help?" Medical News Today, 6 Jan. 2022, www.medicalnewstoday.com/articles/160645.

Smith, Stephen A. "Falls from Grace: What Young Black Athletes Should Learn from the Michael Vick and Marion Jones Dramas." *Ebony*, vol. 63, no. 3, 2008, p. 40.

Smith, W. A., et al. "Effect of Glycine Propionyl-L-Carnitine on Aerobic and Anaerobic Exercise Performance." *International Journal of Sport Nutrition and Exercise Metabolism*, vol. 18, no. 1, 2008, pp. 19-36.

Smolin, Lori A., and Mary B. Grosvenor. *Nutrition: Science and Applications*. 3rd ed., Wiley, 2013.

Snyder, Michael. *Genomics and Personalized Medicine: What Everyone Needs to Know*. Illustrated ed., Oxford UP, 2016.

"Sociology of Sport." *UNI.edu*. Dec. 1998, www.uni.edu/greenr/soc/sportsoc.htm.

Solloway, Michele R., et al. "An Evidence Map of the Effect of Tai Chi on Health Outcomes." *Systematic Reviews*, vol. 5, no. 1, 27 July 2016, doi:10.1186/s13643-016-0300-y.

Solomon, Daniel H. "Non-Steroidal Anti-Inflammatory Drugs (NSAIDs) (Beyond the Basics)." *UpToDate*, 8 Mar. 2022, www-uptodate-com.arbor.idm.oclc.org/contents/nonsteroidal-antiinflammatory-drugs-nsaids-beyond-the-basics?search=NSAIDs&topicRef=7989&source=see_link. Accessed 7 June 2022.

Solon-Biet, Samantha M., et al. "Branched-Chain Amino Acids Impact Health and Lifespan Indirectly via Amino Acid Balance and Appetite Control." *Nature Metabolism*, vol. 1, no. 5, 2019, pp. 532-45.

Sosin, Kate. "USA Powerlifting Agrees to Meditate Dispute with Trans Athlete." *NewNowNext*. Viacom International, 1 Nov. 2019, www.newnownext.com/usa-powerlifting-to-mediate-lawsuit-jaycee-cooper-trans-athlete/11/2019/. Accessed 18 Nov. 2019.

Sotas, Pierre-Edouard, et al. "Prevalence of Blood Doping in Samples Collected from Elite Track and Field Athletes." *Clinical Chemistry*, vol. 57, no. 5, 2011, pp. 762-69.

Sparacino, Alyssa. "How to Improve Your Lactate Threshold." *Shape*, 4 Apr. 2019, www.shape.com/fitness/tips/how-improve-lactate-threshold-workouts. Accessed 12 June 2019.

Sparks, S. D. "Suicidality, Self-Harm, and Body Dissatisfaction in Transgender Adolescents and Emerging Adults with Gender Dysphoria." *Education Week*, vol. 36, no. 3, 2016, p. 5.

Spector, Jesse. "Will Colleges Cover Medical Bills for Athletes Who Get COVID-19? Don't Count on It." *Deadspin*, 2 July 2020, deadspin.com/will-colleges-cover-medical-bills-for-athletes-who-get-1844251705. Accessed 20 May 2021.

"Spinal Cord Injury: Hope Through Research." *National Institute of Neurological Disorders and Stroke*, 13 Aug. 2019, www.ninds.nih.gov/disorders/patient-caregiver-education/hope-through-research/spinal-cord-injury-hope-through-research. Accessed 31 Dec. 2019.

"Spinal Cord Research." *Christopher & Dana Reeve Foundation*, 2019, www.christopherreeve.org/research/spinal-cord-research. Accessed 31 Dec. 2019.

"Sprained Thumb." *American Society for the Surgery of the Hand*, 2015, www.assh.org/handcare/condition/sprained-thumb.

Spranger, Marty D., et al. "Blood Flow Restriction Training and the Exercise Pressor Reflex: A Call for Concern." *American Journal of Physiology-Heart and Circulatory Physiology*, Nov. 2015, www.physiology.org/doi/full/10.1152/ajpheart.00208.2015. Accessed 22 Oct. 2018.

Spritzler, Franziska. "The 13 Most Anti-Inflammatory Foods You Can Eat." *Healthline*, 19 Dec. 2019, www.healthline.com/nutrition/13-anti-inflammatory-foods. Accessed 26 May 2022.

St. Laurent, Christine. "Static Stretching Advantages." *Livestrong.com*. Demand Media, Inc., 20 Oct. 2013, www.livestrong.com/article/437963-static-stretching-advantages/. Accessed 24 Mar. 2015.

Stacy, Jason J., Thomas R. Terrell, and Thomas D. Armsey. "Ergogenic Aids: Human Growth Hormone." *Current Sports Medicine Reports*, vol. 3, no. 4, 2004, pp. 229-33.

Staehler, Richard A. "What Is a Physiatrist?" *Spine-health.com*, 29 Sept. 2011, www.spine-health.com/treatment/spine-specialists/what-a-physiatrist. Accessed 21 Nov. 2016.

Standish, William D., et al. *Tendinitis: Its Etiology and Treatment*. Oxford UP, 2000.

Standring, Susan, et al., editors. *Gray's Anatomy*. 40th ed., Churchill Livingstone/Elsevier, 2008.

Stanhope, K. L., and P. J. Havel. "Fructose Consumption: Considerations for Future Research on Its Effects on Adipose Distribution, Lipid Metabolism, and Insulin Sensitivity in Humans." *Journal of Nutrition*, vol. 139, no. 6, 2009, pp. 1236S-41S.

Stanish, William D., et al. *Tendinitis: Its Etiology and Treatment*. Oxford UP, 2000.

Stanley, Theodore H. "The Fentanyl Story." *The Journal of Pain*, vol. 15, no. 12, 2014, pp. 1215-26, doi:10.1016/j.jpain.2014.08.010.

Starkey, Chad, editor. *Athletic Training and Sports Medicine: An Integrated Approach*. American Academy of Orthopaedic Surgeons, 2013.

Steinke, Hubert, and Claudia Profos. *Bibliographia Halleriana*. Schwabe Verlag, 2004.

Stevinson, C., et al. "Homeopathic Arnica for Prevention of Pain and Bruising." *Journal of the Royal Society of Medicine*, vol. 96, 2003, pp. 60-65.

"The Story of Erythropoietin." *American Society of Hematology*, www.hematology.org/About/History/50-Years/1532.aspx. Accessed 11 Mar. 2017.

Strandness, D. Eugene, Jr. *Duplex Scanning in Vascular Disorders*. 4th ed., Lippincott Williams & Wilkins, 2009.

Street, Scott, Runkle, Deborah. *Athletic Protective Equipment: Care, Selection, and Fitting*. McGraw-Hill, 2000.

Stremmel, W., et al. "Phosphatidylcholine for Steroid-Refractory Chronic Ulcerative Colitis." *Annals of Internal Medicine*, vol. 147, 2007, pp. 603-10.

"Strength Training." *Salem Press Encyclopedia of Health*. Salem Press. Accessed 15 May 2021.

"Strength Training: Get Stronger, Leaner, Healthier." *Mayo Clinic*. Mayo Foundation for Medical Education and Research, www.mayoclinic.org/healthy-living/fitness/in-depth/strength-training/art-20046670.

"Stretching: Focus on Flexibility." *Mayo Clinic*, 23 Mar. 2015, www.mayoclinic.org/healthy-living/fitness/in-depth/stretching/art-20047931.

Stux, Gabriel, and Bruce Pomeranz. *Basics of Acupuncture*. 5th ed., Springer, 2003.

Subbarao, Italo, et al., editors. *American Medical Association Handbook of First Aid and Emergency Care*. Rev. ed., Random House Reference, 2009.

Subedi, Muna, et al. "An Overview of Tramadol and Its Usage in Pain Management and Future Perspective." *Biomedicine & Pharmacotherapy*, vol. 111, 2019, pp. 443-51, doi:10.1016/j.biopha.2018.12.085.

Sugden, David, and Michael G. Wade. *Typical and Atypical Motor Development*. Mac Keith Press, 2013.

Sutton, H. "Transgender College Students More at Risk for Suicide When Denied Bathroom, Housing Rights." *Campus Security Report*, vol. 13, no. 2, 2016, p. 9.

Swaab, D. F. *We Are Our Brains: A Neurobiography of the Brain, from the Womb to Alzheimer's*. Translated by Jane Hedley-Prôle. Random, 2014.

Swanton, R. H. *Cardiology*. 6th ed., Blackwell Science, 2008.

Szabo, Attila. "Acute Psychological Benefits of Exercise: Reconsideration of the Placebo Effect." *Journal of Mental Health*, vol. 22, no. 5, 2013, pp. 449-55.

Szalay, Jessie. *What Is Inflammation?* LiveScience, 19 Oct. 2018, www.livescience.com/52344-inflammation.html. Accessed 26 May 2022.

Tabata, I., et al. "Effects of Moderate-Intensity Endurance and High-Intensity Intermittent Training on Anaerobic Capacity and VO2max." *Medicine and Science in Sports and Exercise* vol. 28, no. 10, 1996, pp. 1327-30.

Tal, J. "Adeno-Associated Virus-Based Vectors in Gene Therapy." *Journal of Biomedical Science*, vol. 7, 2000, pp. 279-91.

Tapley, Donald F., et al., editors. *The Columbia University College of Physicians and Surgeons Complete Home Medical Guide*. Rev. 3rd ed., Crown, 1995.

Taub, Edward. "The Behavior-Analytic Origins of Constraint-Induced Movement Therapy: An Example of Behavioral Neurorehabilitation." *Behavioral Analysis*, vol. 35, no. 2, Fall 2012.

Taylor, Jim, and Gregory S. Wilson, editors. *Applying Sport Psychology: Four Perspectives*. Human Kinetics, 2005.

Taylor, William N. *Anabolic Steroids and the Athlete*. 2nd ed., McFarland, 2002.

Teichler-Zallen, Doris. *To Test or Not to Test: A Guide to Genetic Screening and Risk*. Rutgers UP, 2008.

"Tendinitis and Bursitis." *American College of Rheumatology*, Dec. 2021, www.rheumatology.org/I-Am-A/Patient-Caregiver/Diseases-Conditions/Tendinitis-Bursitis.

"Tendinitis." *MedlinePlus*, 16 Mar. 2017, medlineplus.gov/tendinitis.html.

"Tendon Repair." *MedlinePlus*, n.d., medlineplus.gov/ency/article/002970.htm.

Tenoschok, M. "The Intramural Handbook." *Teaching Elementary Physical Education*, vol. 14, 2003, p. 32.

Tenoschok, M., et al. "How Good Is Your Intramural Program?" *Teaching Elementary Physical Education*, vol. 13, 2002, pp. 30-31.

Testa, G., et al. "Extracorporeal Shockwave Therapy Treatment in Upper Limb Diseases: A Systematic Review." *Journal of Clinical Medicine*, vol. 9, no. 2, 6 Feb. 2020, doi:10.3390/jcm9020453. PMID: 32041301; PMCID: PMC7074316.

Tétreault, Patrice, and Hugue Ouellette. *Orthopedics Made Ridiculously Simple*. MedMaster, 2014.

Teut, Michael, et al. "Qigong or Yoga Versus No Intervention in Older Adults with Chronic Low Back Pain-A Randomized Controlled Trial." *The Journal of Pain*, vol. 17, no. 7, 2016, pp. 796-805, doi:10.1016/j.jpain.2016.03.003.

Thaler, Alison I., and Malcolm S. Thaler. *The Only Neurology Book You'll Ever Need*. Lippincott Williams & Wilkins, 2022.

Thanasas, Christos, et al. "Platelet-Rich Plasma Versus Autologous Whole Blood for the Treatment of Chronic Lateral Elbow Epicondylitis: A Randomized Controlled Clinical Trial." *American Journal of Sports Medicine*, vol. 39, no. 10, 2011, pp. 2130-34.

Thelen, Esther, and Linda B. Smith. *A Dynamic Systems Approach to the Development of Cognition and Action*. 5th ed., MIT Press, 2002.

Thiels, Cornelius A., et al. "Chronic Use of Tramadol after Acute Pain Episode: Cohort Study." *BMJ*, vol. 365, 2019, doi:10.1136/bmj.l1849.

Thomas, E. Donnall. "Facts." *Nobel Prize Outreach AB 2022*, NobelPrize.org, 24 June 2022, www.nobelprize.org/prizes/medicine/1990/thomas/facts/.

Thompson, Janice J., and Melinda Manore. *Nutrition: An Applied Approach*. 5th ed., Pearson, 2017.

Thompson, Janice, et al. *The Science of Nutrition*. 5th ed., Pearson, 2019.

Thompson, Jon C. *Netter's Concise Orthopaedic Anatomy*. 2nd ed., Elsevier, 2015.

Thordarson, David B., editor. *Foot and Ankle*. 2nd ed., Lippincott Williams & Wilkins, 2013.

Thorpe, H., et al. "Toward New Conversations Between Sociology and Psychology." *Sociology of Sport Journal*, vol. 31, no. 2, 2014, pp. 131-38.

Thygerson, Alton L. *First Aid and Emergency Care Workbook*. Jones and Bartlett, 1987.

Tierney, Lawrence M., et al., editors. *Current Medical Diagnosis and Treatment 2007*. McGraw-Hill Medical, 2006.

Today's Dietitian, www.todaysdietitian.com/newarchives/092208p66.shtml.

Todorovich, J. R., and E. D. Model. "The TARGET Approach to Motivating Students." *Teaching Elementary Physical Education*, vol. 16, 2005, pp. 8-10.

Todorovich, John, editor. "Influence of Sports and Physical Activity Programs on the Activity of High School Youths and Young Adults." *JOPERD: The Journal of Physical Education, Recreation & Dance*, vol. 83, no. 4, 2012, p. 49.

Tortora, Gerard J., and Bryan Derrickson. *Principles of Anatomy and Physiology*. 16th ed., John Wiley & Sons, 2020.

Townsend, Courtney M., Jr., et al., editors. *Sabiston Textbook of Surgery*. 19th ed., Saunders/Elsevier, 2012.

"Tramadol." *MedlinePlus*, 15 Jan. 2019, medlineplus.gov/druginfo/meds/a695011.html.

"Traumatic Brain Injury." *MedlinePlus*, 21 Feb. 2020, medlineplus.gov/traumaticbraininjury.html. Accessed 30 May 2022.

Treasure, D. C., and G. C. Roberts. "Applications of Achievement Goal Theory to Physical Education: Implications for Enhancing Motivation." *QUEST*, vol. 47, 1995, pp. 475-89.

Tveiten, D., and S. Bruset. "Effect of Arnica D30 in Marathon Runners." *Homeopathy*, vol. 92, 2003, pp. 187-89.

Twomey, Lance T., and James R. Taylor, editors. *Physical Therapy of the Low Back*. Churchill Livingstone, 2000.

Tyler, T. F., et al. "The Effect of Creatine Supplementation on Strength Recovery After Anterior Cruciate Ligament (ACL) Reconstruction." *American Journal of Sports Medicine*, vol. 32, 2004, pp. 383-88.

"Ultrasound." *MedlinePlus*, 15 Dec. 2020, medlineplus.gov/lab-tests/sonogram/.

Underwood, M., et al. "Advice to Use Topical or Oral Ibuprofen for Chronic Knee Pain in Older People: Randomized Control Trial and Patient Preference Study." *British Medical Journal*, vol. 336, no. 138, 2007, pp. 1-12, doi:10.1136/bmj.39399.656331.25.

Urhausen, Axel, and Wilfried Kindermann. "Diagnosis of Overtraining: What Tools Do We Have?" *Sports Medicine*, vol. 32, no. 2, 2002, pp. 95-102.

Urry, Lisa A., et al. *Campbell Biology*. 12th ed., Cummings, 2020.

US Department of Health and Human Services. *Physical Activity Guidelines for Americans*. 2nd ed., US Department of Health and Human Services, 2018.

US Department of Health and Human Services and US Department of Agriculture. *Dietary Guidelines for Americans 2005*. 6th ed., Government Printing Office, 2005.

Usha, P. R., and M. U. Naidu. "Randomised, Double-Blind, Parallel, Placebo-Controlled Study of Oral Glucosamine, Methylsulfonylmethane, and Their Combination in Osteoarthritis." *Clinical Drug Investigation*, vol. 24, 2004, pp. 353-63.

Vacanti, Joseph P., editor. *Tissue Engineering and Regenerative Medicine*. Cold Spring Harbor Laboratory Press, 2017.

Vad, Vijay. "Hyaluronic Acid Injections for Knee Osteoarthritis." *Arthritis-health*, 28 Mar. 2019, www.arthritis-health.com/treatment/injections/hyaluronic-acid-injections-knee-osteoarthritis. Accessed 8 June 2022.

Vadalà, Maria, et al. "Mechanisms and Therapeutic Effectiveness of Pulsed Electromagnetic Field Therapy in Oncology." *Cancer Medicine*, vol. 5, no. 11, 17 Oct. 2016, pp. 3128-39, doi:10.1002/cam4.861.

Valentine, Raymond C., and David L. Valentine. *Human Longevity: Omega-3 Fatty Acids, Bioenergetics, Molecular Biology, and Evolution*. CRC Press, 2015.

"Valium: Side Effects, Addiction, Symptoms & Treatment: What Is Valium?" *American Addiction Centers*, 14 Nov. 2019, americanaddictioncenters.org/valium-treatment.

Van De Graaff, Kent M. *Human Anatomy*. 6th ed., McGraw-Hill, 2002.

Van Dusen, Duncan P. "Associations of Physical Fitness and Academic Performance Among Schoolchildren." *Journal of School Health*, vol. 81, no. 12, 2011, pp. 733-40.

Van Heertum, R. L., et al. "Single Photon Emission CT and Positron Emission Tomography in the Evaluation of Neurologic Disease." *Radiologic Clinics of North America* vol. 39, no. 5, 2001, pp. 1007-33, doi:10.1016/s0033-8389(05)70326-2.

Van Raalte, Judy L., and Britton W. Brewer, editors. *Exploring Sport and Exercise Psychology*. 3rd ed., APA, 2014.

Vanderah, Todd, and Douglas Gould. *Nolte's The Human Brain: An Introduction to its Functional Anatomy*. 8th ed., Elsevier, 2020.

Vandusseldorp, Trisha, et al. "Effect of Branched-Chain Amino Acid Supplementation on Recovery Following Acute Eccentric Exercise." *Nutrients*, vol. 10, no. 10, 2018, p. 1389.

VanPutte, Cinnamon, et al. *Seeley's Anatomy and Physiology*. 13th ed., McGraw Hill, 2022.

Vasic, Goran, et al. "Blood Doping and Risks." *Sports Montreal*, vol. 43, 2015, pp. 189-94.

Verdon, F., et al. "Iron Supplementation for Unexplained Fatigue in Non-anaemic Women." *British Medical Journal*, vol. 326, 2003, p. 1124.

Verducci, Tom. "Reason to Believe." *Sports Illustrated*, vol. 102, no. 8, 2005, pp. 39-45.

Vertosick, Frank T., Jr. *Why We Hurt: The Natural History of Pain*. Harcourt, 2000.

Vickers, A. J., et al. "Homeopathic Arnica 30x Is Ineffective for Muscle Soreness After Long-Distance Running." *Clinical Journal of Pain*, vol. 14, 1998, pp. 227-31.

———. "Homeopathy for Delayed Onset Muscle Soreness." *British Journal of Sports Medicine*, vol. 31, 1997, pp. 304-7.

Virén, Lasse, et al. *Lasse Virén: Olympic Champion*. Continental, 1978.

"Viscosupplementation Treatment for Knee Arthritis." *OrthoInfo*, Feb. 2021, orthoinfo.aaos.org/en/treatment/viscosupplementation-treatment-for-knee-arthritis/. Accessed 8 June 2022.

"Vitamins and Minerals." *Centers for Disease Control and Prevention*, 11 Apr. 2022, www.cdc.gov/nutrition/infantandtoddlernutrition/vitamins-minerals/index.html. Accessed 8 June 2022.

Vorvick, Linda J. "Tendon vs. Ligament." *MedlinePlus*, 13 Aug. 2020, medlineplus.gov/ency/imagepages/19089.htm.

Waddell, Gordon. *The Back Pain Revolution*. 2nd ed., Churchill Livingstone/Elsevier, 2004.

Wade, Christopher H., et al. "Effects of Genetic Risk Information on Children's Psychosocial Wellbeing: A Systematic Review of the Literature." *Genetics in Medicine*, vol. 12, no. 6, 2010, pp. 317-26.

Wadehra, Sunali, and Charles F. van Gunten. "Ketamine for Chronic Pain Management." *Practical Pain Management*, 4 Dec. 2018, www.practicalpainmanagement.com/patient/treatments/medications/ketamine-chronic-pain-management-current-role-future-directions.

Wahlert, L., and A. Fiester. "Gender Transports: Privileging the 'Natural' in Gender Testing Debates for Intersex and Transgender Athletes." *American Journal of Bioethics*, vol. 12, no. 7, 2012, pp. 19-21.

Waldman, Steven D. *Atlas of Uncommon Pain Syndromes*. Elsevier, 2014.

Walker, Brad. *The Anatomy of Stretching*. Atlantic Books, 2007.

Wall, Patrick David. *Pain: The Science of Suffering*. Columbia UP, 2013.

Wallechinsky, David, and Jaime Loucky. *The Complete Book of the Olympics: 2008 Edition*. Aurum Press, 2008.

Walrod, Bryant James. "Lateral Epicondylitis." *Medscape*, 8 Mar. 2021, emedicine.medscape.com/article/96969-overview. Accessed 19 Aug. 2017.

Walsh, Meghan. "'I Trusted 'Em': When NCAA Schools Abandon Their Injured Athletes." *The Atlantic*, 1 May 2013, www.theatlantic.com/entertainment/archive/2013/05/i-trusted-em-when-ncaa-schools-abandon-their-injured-athletes/275407/. Accessed 20 May 2021.

Walther, David S. *Applied Kinesiology: Synopsis*. 2nd ed., Systems DC, 2000.

Wann, Daniel L. *Sport Fans: The Psychology and Social Impact of Spectators*. Routledge, 2001.

Ward, Jeremy P. T., Jane Ward, and Richard M. Leach. *The Respiratory System at a Glance*. 4th ed., Wiley, 2015.

Warren, M. P., and N. E. Perlroth. "The Effects of Intense Exercise on the Female Reproductive System." *Journal of Endocrinology*, vol. 170, July 2001, pp. 3-11, doi:10.1677/joe.0.1700003. PMID:11431132.

Warwick, Hunter, et al. "Immediate Physical Therapy Following Total Joint Arthroplasty: Barriers and Impact on Short-Term Outcomes." *Advances in Orthopedics*, vol. 2019, 8 Apr. 2019, pp. 1-7, doi:10.1155/2019/6051476.

Watson, James C. "Evaluation of Pain." *Merck Manual Consumer Version*, Apr. 2020, www.merckmanuals.com/home/brain,-spinal-cord,-and-nerve-disorders/pain/evaluation-of-pain. Accessed 7 June 2022.

Watson, Ronald Ross, and Fabien De Meester, editors. *Handbook of Lipids in Human Function: Fatty Acids*. Academic Press and ACCS Press, 2015.

———. *Omega-3 Fatty Acids in Brain and Neurological Health*. Academic, 2014.

Weber C., et al. "Efficacy of Physical Therapy for the Treatment of Lateral Epicondylitis: A Meta-analysis." *BMC Musculoskeletal Disorders*, vol. 16, no. 1, 2015, p. 223, doi:10.1186/s12891-015-0665-4.

Weber, Markus, et al. "Predicting Outcome after Total Hip Arthroplasty: The Role of Preoperative Patient-Reported Measures." *BioMed Research International*, vol. 2019, 2019, pp. 1-9, doi:10.1155/2019/4909561.

Wedro, B. "Steroids Types, Side Effects, and Treatment." *emedicinehealth*, 29 July 2014, www.emedicinehealth.com/steroids/article_em.htm.

Wei, Liping, et al. "Comparative Genomics Approaches to Study Organism Similarities and Differences." *Journal of Biomedical Informatics*, vol. 35, 2002, pp. 142-50.

"Weight Training: Improve Your Muscular Fitness." *Mayo Clinic*, 14 Aug. 2015, www.mayoclinic.org/healthy-lifestyle/fitness/in-depth/weight-training/art-20047116.

Weil, Andrew. *Eight Weeks to Optimum Health: A Proven Program for Taking Full Advantage of Your Body's Natural Healing Power*. Rev. ed., Ballantine Books, 2007.

Weinberg, Robert S., and Daniel Gould. *Foundations of Sport and Exercise Psychology*. 4th ed., Human Kinetics, 2007.

Weintraub, Karen. "Advances Bring First True Hope to Spinal Cord Injury Patients." *leapsmag*. Future Frontiers, 12 Nov. 2018, leapsmag.com/advances-bring-first-true-hope-to-spinal-cord-injury-patients. Accessed 31 Dec. 2019.

Weintraub, William. *Tendon and Ligament Healing: A New Approach to Sports and Overuse Injury*. 2nd Rev. ed., Paradigm, 2003.

Weiss, M. R., and E. Ferrer-Caja. "Motivational Orientations in Sport Behavior." *Advances in Sport Psychology*, edited by T. Horn, Human Kinetics, 2002, pp. 101-84.

"Welcome to the British Autogenic Society." *British Autogenic Society*, 2022, britishautogenicsociety.uk/. Accessed 28 May 2022.

Wells, Cherie, et al. "The Effectiveness of Pilates Exercise in People with Chronic Low Back Pain: A Systematic Review." *PLOS One*, vol. 9, no. 7, 1 July 2014, doi:10.1371/journal.pone.0100402.

Welsh, Charles, and Cynthia Prentice-Craver. *Hole's Human Anatomy & Physiology*. 16th ed., McGraw-Hill Education, 2021.

Westhoff, Ben. *Fentanyl, Inc.: How Rogue Chemists Are Creating the Deadliest Wave of the Opioid Epidemic*. Atlantic Monthly Press, 2019.

"What Are Heritable Connective Tissue Disorders?" *The ILC Foundation*, 2022, www.theilcfoundation.org/what-are-heritable-connective-tissue-disorders/.

"What Are Shoulder Problems?" *National Institute of Arthritis and Musculoskeletal and Skin Diseases*. National Institutes of Health, June 2010, www.niams.nih.gov/

Health_Info/Shoulder_Problems/shoulder_problems_ff.asp.

"What Is a Concussion?" *Brain Injury Research Institute*, 2021, www.protectthebrain.org/Brain-Injury-Research/What-is-a-Concussion-.aspx. Accessed 19 May 2021.

"What Is PCS?" *Concussion Legacy Foundation*, n.d., concussionfoundation.org/PCS-resources/what-is-PCS. Accessed 30 Oct. 2017.

"What Is Sociology?" *Department of Sociology*. University of North Carolina at Chapel Hill, 2015, sociology.unc.edu/undergraduateprogram/sociology-major/what-is-sociology/.

"What Is a Total Artificial Heart?" *NIH National Heart, Lung, and Blood Institute*, 24 Mar. 2022, www.nhlbi.nih.gov/health/total-artificial-heart. Accessed 8 June 2022.

"What Occupational Therapists (OTs) Do." *College of Occupational Therapists of Ontario*, 2017, www.coto.org/you-and-your-ot/what-occupational-therapists-do. Accessed 13 June 2022.

Wichmann, S., and D. R. Martin. "Exercise Excess: Treating Patients Addicted to Fitness." *Physiological Sports Medicine*, vol. 20, 1992, pp. 193-200.

Willems, Mark. *Skeletal Muscle: Physiology, Classification, and Disease*. Nova Biomedical, 2013.

Williams, Jean M., editor. *Applied Sport Psychology: Personal Growth to Peak Performance*. 5th ed., McGraw, 2006.

Wilner, Barry, and Ken Rappoport. *Harvard Beats Yale 29-29, and Other Great Comebacks from the Annals of Sports*. Taylor Trade, 2008.

Wilson, J. K., et al. "Comparison of Rehabilitation Methods in the Treatment of Patellar Tendinitis." *Journal of Sport Rehabilitation*, vol. 9, no. 4, 2000, pp. 304-14.

Wilson, Jacob. "Your Complete Guide to Blood Flow Restriction Training." *Body Building*, 27 July 2018, www.bodybuilding.com/content/your-complete-guide-to-blood-flow-restriction-training.html. Accessed 22 Oct. 2018.

Wilson, Jacque. "Lance Armstrong's Doping Drugs." *CNN*, 18 Jan. 2013, www.cnn.com/2013/01/15/health/armstrong-ped-explainer/. Accessed 11 Mar. 2017.

Wilson, M. L. "Learning Styles, Instructional Strategies, and the Question of Matching: A Literature Review." *International Journal of Education*, vol. 4, 2012, pp. 67-87.

Wilson, Wayne, and Ed Derse. *Doping in Elite Sport: The Politics of Drugs in the Olympic Movement*. Human Kinetics, 2001.

Winter, Arthur. *Organic Chemistry for Dummies*. 2nd ed., For Dummies, 2016.

Wolf, Steven L., et al. "The EXCITE Stroke Trial: Comparing Early and Delayed Constraint-Induced Movement Therapy." *Stroke*, vol. 41, no. 10, Oct. 2010, pp. 2309-15.

Wolfe, Robert R. "Branched-Chain Amino Acids and Muscle Protein Synthesis in Humans: Myth or Reality?" *Journal of the International Society of Sports Nutrition*, vol. 14, no. 1, 2017, doi.org/10.1186/s12970-017-0184-.

Won, A. C., and A. Ethell. "Spontaneous Splenic Rupture Resulted from Infectious Mononucleosis." *International Journal of Surgery Case Reports*, vol. 3, no. 3, 2012, pp. 97-99, doi.org/10.1016/j.ijscr.2011.08.012.

Wong, Cathy. "The Health Benefits of Cetyl Myristoleate." *Verywell Health*, 25 Nov. 2019, www.verywellhealth.com/the-benefits-of-cetyl-myristoleate-89434.

Woolsey, Thomas A., et al. *Brain Atlas: A Visual Guide to the Human Central Nervous System*. 4th ed., Wiley, 2017.

Woolston, C. "Human Growth Hormone." *HealthDay*, 11 Mar. 2015, consumer.healthday.com/encyclopedia/substance-abuse-38/illicit-drugs-news-217/human-growth-hormone-647257.html.

"The World of Applied Kinesiology." *International College of Applied Kinesiology*, 2022, www.icak.com. Accessed 27 May 2022.

Wright, Thomas. *William Harvey: A Life in Circulation*. Oxford UP, 2013.

Wrightson, Philip, and Dorothy Gronwall. *Mild Head Injury: A Guide to Management*. Oxford UP, 1999.

"Wrist Sprains." *OrthoInfo*, Apr. 2018, orthoinfo.aaos.org/en/diseases—conditions/wrist-sprains.

Wu, C. L., and C. Williams. "A Low Glycemic Index Meal Before Exercise Improves Endurance Running Capacity in Men." *International Journal of Sport Nutrition and Exercise Metabolism*, vol. 16, no. 5, 2006, pp. 510-27.

Wyatt, Frank B., Alissa Donaldson, and Elise Brown. "The Overtraining Syndrome: A Meta-Analytic Review." *Journal of Exercise Physiology*, vol. 16, no. 2, 2013, pp. 12-23.

Yaksh, Tony L., et al. "Development of New Analgesics: An Answer to Opioid Epidemic." *Trends in Pharmacological Sciences*, vol. 39, no. 12, 2018, pp. 1000-1002, doi:10.1016/j.tips.2018.10.003.

Yao, G., J. Chen, Y. Duan, and X. Chen. "Efficacy of Extracorporeal Shock Wave Therapy for Lateral Epicondylitis: A Systematic Review and Meta-Analysis." *BioMed Research International*, 18 Mar. 2020, p. 2064781, doi:10.1155/2020/2064781. PMID: 32309425; PMCID: PMC7106907.

Yao, Reina, et al. "Does Patellectomy Jeopardize Function after TKA?" *Clinical Orthopaedics & Related Research*, vol. 471, no. 2, 2013, pp. 544-53.

Yesalis, C. E., and M. S. Bahrke. "Doping Among Adolescent Athletes." *Baillieres Best Practice and Research in Clinical Endocrinology and Metabolism*, vol. 14, no. 1, 2000, pp. 25-35.

Yesalis, Charles E. *Anabolic Steroids in Sport and Exercise*. 2nd ed., Human Kinetics, 2000.

Yesalis, Charles E., and Michael S. Bahrke. "Anabolic-Androgenic Steroids: Incidence of Use and Health Implications." *President's Council on Physical Fitness and Sports Research Digest*, vol. 5, no. 5, 2005, pp. 1-8.

Yian, Gu, and Nikolas Scarmeas. "Dietary Inflammation Factor Rating System and Risk of Alzheimer Disease in Elder." *Alzheimer Disease and Associated Disorders*, vol. 25, no. 2, 2011, pp. 149-54.

Youngson, R. M. *First Aid*. HarperCollins, 2003.

"Your Guide to Living Well with Heart Disease." *National Heart, Lung, and Blood Institute*, Nov. 2015, www.nhlbi.nih.gov/files/docs/public/heart/living_well.pdf.

Zaret, Barry L., et al., editors. *Yale University School of Medicine Heart Book*. William Morrow, 1992.

Zasler, Nathan D., et al. *Brain Injury Medicine*. 2nd ed., Demos Medical Publishing, 2013.

Zeigler, C. *Fair Play: How LGBT Athletes Are Claiming Their Rightful Place in Sports*. Akashic Books, 2016.

Zhang, Zhen-Yu, et al. "Branched-Chain Amino Acids as Critical Switches in Health and Disease." *Hypertension*, vol. 72, no. 5, 2018, pp. 1012-22.

Ziegler, E. M., and T. I. Huntley. ""It Got Too Tough to Not Be Me': Accommodating Transgender Athletes in Sport." *Journal of College & University Law*, vol. 39, no. 2, 2013, pp. 467-509.

Zimlich, Rachael, and Donald Collins. "Concussion: Symptoms, Causes, Diagnosis, & Treatment." Healthline, 1 Mar. 2022, www.healthline.com/health/concussion.

Zirin, D. "Calling Sports Sociology Off the Bench." *Contexts.org*, 1 July 2008, contexts.org/articles/calling-sports-sociology-offthe-bench/.

Zollman, Felise S. *Manual of Traumatic Brain Injury: Assessment and Management*. 2nd ed., Springer Publishing, 2016.

Zoumbaris, Sharon K., editor. *Encyclopedia of Wellness*. Greenwood, 2012.

Glossary

α-linolenic acid (ALA): an essential fatty acid (EFA) from which EPA and DHA are synthesized

γ-linolenic acid (GLA): an essential fatty acid from which other fatty acids are synthesized

abdomen: the rib-free part of the trunk, below the diaphragm

abdominal binders: a compression belt that facilitates recovery after abdominal surgeries

abrasion: an injury that results from scraping that removes or damages the skin layer

abuse-deterrent formulations: drug preparation intended to prevent, impede, or discourage physical and chemical tampering (e.g., crushing, chewing, extraction, smoking, snorting, injecting) while still being able to provide safe and accurate delivery of the opioid for therapeutic benefit

accreditation: the process of review and certification for athletic training programs

acetabulum: the portion of the pelvic bone joining the femoral head to create the hip joint

Achievement Goal Theory: a theory of motivation that considers the individual's concept of ability as well as personal and situational factors that influences the meaning that is attached to successful or unsuccessful experiences

Achilles tendon: the tendon connecting calf muscles to the heel

acromion: the outward end of the spine of the scapula or shoulder blade

action: type of movement made by a muscle contraction

action potential: an electrochemical event that nerve cells use to send signals along their cellular extensions in the nervous system

acute: referring to the sudden onset of a disease process

acute pain: sudden, extreme pain that is short-term; serves as a warning of damage or disease

adaptive task practice: a training method in which a motor or behavioral objective is approached in small steps by successive approximations or by making the task more difficult per the patient's motoric capabilities

addiction: a neuropsychological disorder characterized by persistent use of a drug, despite substantial harm and other negative consequences

adenosine triphosphate (ATP): an important biological molecule that represents the energy currency of the cell; the energy in a special high-energy bond in ATP is used to drive almost all cellular processes that require energy

adipocyte: a cell whose specific function is to store fats and associated nutrients, hormones, etc.

adipose tissue: tissue that stores fat; occurs in humans beneath the skin, usually in the abdomen or in the buttocks

adventure races: a multidisciplinary team sport involving navigation over an unmarked wilderness course with races extending anywhere from two hours up to two weeks in length

aerobic: metabolism involving the breakdown of energy substrates using oxygen

aerobic exercise: any type of cardiovascular conditioning that increases the heart rate

aerodynamics: the study of the properties of moving air and the interaction between the air and solid bodies moving through it

agonist muscle: the muscle contracting during an activity

Alexander technique: a process that teaches how to properly coordinate body and mind to release harmful tension and to improve posture, coordination, and general health

alpha-amylase: an enzyme that hydrolyses alpha-linked polysaccharides, such as starch and glycogen, yielding shorter sugar chains

alternating pole devices: magnets that expose the skin to both north and south magnetic fields

alveoli: the tiny, clustered, air-filled sacs in the lungs where the exchange of oxygen and carbon dioxide takes place

American Occupational Therapy Association (AOTA): the national professional association was established in 1917 to represent the interests and concerns of occupational therapy practitioners and students and improve the quality of occupational therapy service

amino group: a functional group containing a nitrogen atom bonded to two hydrogen atoms (-NH2)

amnesia: partial or total memory loss

amyotrophic lateral sclerosis: a nervous system disease that weakens muscles and impacts physical function

anabolic steroid: a synthetic steroid hormone that resembles testosterone and promotes muscle growth; used medicinally to treat some forms of weight loss and illegally by some athletes and others to enhance physical performance

anabolic-androgenic steroids (AAS): natural androgens like testosterone as well as synthetic androgens that are structurally related and have similar effects to testosterone

anabolism: the metabolic activity through which complex substances are synthesized from simpler substances

anaerobic: metabolism involving the breakdown of energy substrates without using oxygen

analgesic: a drug or medication that alleviates pain by blocking pain receptors

androstenedione: a naturally occurring steroid hormone, also available as a dietary supplement, believed to increase serum testosterone levels.

anemia: a condition in which the blood doesn't have enough healthy red blood cells

anesthesia: a state characterized by loss of sensation, caused by or resulting from the pharmacological depression of normal nerve function

anesthetic: medicines that induce an anesthetic state

aneurysm: a localized enlargement of a vessel, usually an artery

anisocytosis: a condition in which red blood cells are unequal in size

annular bulge: protrusion of a disk beyond its normal circumference, usually because of compression caused by gravity, the strain on the spine, or aging

anorexia nervosa: an eating disorder characterized by abnormally low body weight, an intense fear of gaining weight, and a distorted perception of weight

antagonist: a muscle that has an opposite action from its paired muscle and limits its action

antagonist muscle: the muscle relaxing or lengthening during an activity

anticonvulsants: a diverse group of pharmacological agents used to treat epileptic seizures

antidepressant: medications that alleviate depression

anxiolytic: a drug used to reduce anxiety

applied kinesiology: a dubious diagnostic technique used in chiropractic medicine

arachnoid mater: the fine, delicate membrane, the middle one of the three membranes or meninges that surround the brain and spinal cord, situated between the dura mater and the pia mater

Arnica: a genus of perennial, herbaceous plants in the sunflower family that are used to make homeopathic preparations

arteries: vessels that take blood away from the heart and toward the tissues

arthralgia: joint pain

arthritis: a painful condition that involves inflammation of one or more joints

arthrofibrosis: scar tissue in a joint that develops after surgery, implant, or joint replacement

arthropathy: disease of a joint in the body

arthroscopy: minimally invasive surgical procedure on a joint in which an examination and sometimes treatment of damage is performed using an arthroscope, an endoscope that is inserted into the joint through a small incision

articulation: a joint between two bones of the skeleton; also called an "arthrosis"

aspiration: breathing in foreign objects, such as sucking food particles or saliva into the airway

ASTYM®: a tool used to break up scar tissue and damaged soft tissue to promote regeneration of healthy tissue to improve one's function

atherosclerosis: accumulation of plaque within the arteries

athletic competition: a contest between athletes

athletic injury: injuries that occur when engaging in sports or exercise

athletic trainer: an allied health professional who provides health care in the areas of physical medicine and rehabilitation services by preventing, assessing, and treating injuries

athletic training programs (ATEPs)-collegiate education programs professionally and academically preparing athletic trainers

atria: the upper receiving chambers of the heart that lie above the ventricles

atrioventricular (A-V) node: a small region of specialized heart muscle cells that receives the electrical impulse from the atria and begins its transmission to the ventricles

atrophy: the wasting of tissue, an organ, or an entire body as the result of a decrease in the size or number of the cells within that tissue, organ, or body

autonomic nervous system: the part of the nervous system responsible for the control of the bodily functions not consciously directed, such as breathing, the heartbeat, and digestive processes

autosuggestion: the hypnotic or subconscious adoption of an idea that one has originated oneself, sometimes by repeating verbal statements to oneself to change behavior

avulsion: a wound caused by tearing of the skin and underlying tissue

axon: the part of a neuron responsible for sending information to other neurons

B vitamins: a class of water-soluble vitamins that play important roles in cell metabolism and synthesis of red blood cells and tend to coexist in the same foods

back braces: an orthopedic device that limits spinal motion after a bone fracture or spinal fusion surgery.

basal metabolic rate (BMR): the standardized measure of metabolism in warm-blooded organisms

behavioral medicine: an interdisciplinary field of research and practice that focuses on how people's thoughts and behavior affect their health

belladonna: a drug prepared from the leaves and root of deadly nightshade, containing atropine

benzodiazepine: a class of psychoactive drugs whose core chemical structure is the fusion of a benzene ring and a diazepine ring that lower brain activity and are prescribed to treat conditions such as anxiety, insomnia, and seizures

beta-oxidation: the catabolic process by which fatty acid molecules are broken down

bile acids: steroid acids, synthesized in the liver, found predominantly in the bile of mammals and other vertebrates, conjugated with taurine or glycine residues to give anions

biodegradability: the artificial scaffold used to support the growth of bioengineered tissue should dissolve once the transplanted tissue takes hold

bioflavonoids: a group of compounds occurring mainly in citrus fruits and black currants, formerly regarded as vitamins

bioinformatics: a computational discipline that provides the tools needed to study whole genomes and proteomes

biological scaffold-made of polyester (plastic), collagen (protein), or other sources, is used as a structural framework for tissue engineering

biomaterials: replacements for body tissues, sometimes used as implants. Examples are engineered skin tissue, renal tissue, or cardiac implants; biomaterials can be made of metal alloys, plastic polymers, and living tissues like collagen

biomechanical considerations: environmental (space) considerations conducive to cellular growth and development; effective tissue engineering may occur when combined with a biological scaffold and a blend of growth factors

biomechanics: the study of the anatomical principles of human movement

blood clots: an important process that prevents excessive bleeding when a blood vessel is injured

blood doping: the injection of oxygenated blood into an athlete before an event in an attempt to enhance athletic performance

blood pressure: the pressure in the circulatory system, often measured for diagnosis since it is closely related to the force and rate of the heartbeat and the diameter and elasticity of the arterial walls

body composition: proportion of lean muscle mass to fat mass

body weight: the use of the person's natural weight as the form of resistance while exercising

bone marrow: the soft, spongy tissue with many blood vessels found in the center of most bones

Bouchard's nodes: osteophytes or bony spurs that develop as a result of the destruction of joint cartilage in proximal interphalangeal joints

brain: an organ of soft nervous tissue contained in the skull of vertebrates, functioning as the coordinating center of sensation and intellectual and nervous activity

brain herniation: a phenomenon that occurs when increased pressure inside the skull due to bleeding, a stroke, head injury, or tumor moves brain tissues, causing neurological dysfunction or neuronal death

brain lobes: structural divisions of the cerebrum into four divisions or lobes-the frontal, parietal, temporal, and occipital lobes-each with distinct functions; the frontal lobe houses cognitive functions and control of voluntary movement or activity; the parietal lobe processes temperature, taste, touch, and movement information; the occipital lobe is primarily responsible for vision; and the temporal lobe processes memories, integrating them with taste, sound, sight, and touch sensations

brain parenchyma: the functional tissue of the brain consisting of cells for cognition and controlling the rest of the body and stroma, or supportive tissue

bronchioles: branches of the primary bronchus

bulimia nervosa: an emotional disorder involving distortion of body image and an obsessive desire to lose weight, in which bouts of extreme overeating are followed by depression and self-induced vomiting, purging, or fasting

bursa: a connective tissue sac filled with fluid that reduces friction at joints

bursitis: inflammation of the fluid-filled pads (bursae) that act as cushions at the joints

calcification: the deposit of lime salts in organic tissue, leading to calcium in the arterial wall

calcitonin: a hormone made and released by the thyroid gland that lowers the level of calcium in the blood by stimulating the formation of bone

callus: a hard, bone-like substance made by osteocytes found in and around the ends of a fractured bone; it temporarily maintains bony alignment and is resorbed after complete healing or union of a fracture occurs

calorie: a measurement of heat, particularly in measuring the value of foods for producing energy and heat in an organism

capillaries: hairlike vessels that connect the ends of the smallest arteries to the beginnings of the smallest veins

carbohydrate: one of three macronutrients; foods that provide carbohydrates are starches, sugars, fruit, vegetables, and milk products

carboxyl group: a functional group containing a carbon atom double-bonded to an oxygen atom and single-bonded to a hydroxyl group (-OH); has the formula CO_2H, typically written -COOH

cardiac muscle: a type of muscle found only in the heart that makes up the major portion of the heart; involved in the movement of blood through the body

cardiovascular: activities or conditions that affect the heart and blood vessels

cardiovascular disease: circulatory conditions that include diseased vessels, heart and blood vessel structural problems, and blood clots

carpus: the wrist

cartilage: a smooth material covering the ends of bone joints that cushions the bone, allowing the joint to move easily

catabolism: damage to muscles

catalyst: a chemical species that initiates or speeds up a chemical reaction but is not consumed in the reaction

cellular respiration: a complex series of chemical reactions by which chemical energy stored in the bonds of food molecules is released and used to form ATP

central nervous system: the brain and spinal cord, which process incoming information from the peripheral nervous system and form the main network of coordination and control in advanced organisms

cerebral cortex: the outer layer of the cerebrum. composed of folded gray matter and plays an important role in consciousness

cerebral hemispheres: either of the rounded halves of the brain's cerebrum, divided laterally by a deep fissure and connected at the bottom by the corpus callosum

cerebral lobes: cerebral cortex is divided lengthways into two cerebral hemispheres connected by the corpus callosum; each hemisphere is divided into four lobes-frontal, parietal, temporal, and occipital

cerebrum: the largest part of the brain, divided into two hemispheres, or halves, called the "cerebral hemispheres"

cervical collars: also known as a "neck brace," this device supports a person's neck and protects the neck after a traumatic head or neck injury, and can be used to treat chronic medical conditions

cervical spine: the highest of three parts of the spine, consisting of seven vertebrae, named C1 (top of the neck) to C7, in a natural lordosis

cetyl alcohol: C-16 fatty alcohol with the formula CH3(CH2)15OH

Ch'i: Chinese concept of the vital essence; when Ch'i is unbalanced, disease results

character development: the possession of those personal qualities or virtues that facilitate the consistent display of moral action or choosing the moral ideal over competing values

chemical energy: the energy locked up in the chemical bonds that hold the atoms of a molecule together; food molecules, such as glucose, contain much energy in their bonds

chemotaxis: movement of white blood cells toward a gradient of increasing or decreasing concentration of a particular substance

chondrocyte: the cell type responsible for secreting the collagen and elastin components of the cartilage matrix

chondromalacia: degeneration of cartilage in the knee, usually caused by excessive wear between the patella and lower end of the femur

chronic: referring to a lingering disease process

chronic pain: a deeper, aching pain that comes on slowly and lasts longer than the normal course for a specific injury or condition; it may be constant or intermittent

chylomicrons: lipoprotein particles that consist of triglycerides, phospholipids, cholesterol, and proteins and transport dietary lipids from the intestines to other locations in the body

cisgender: a person whose gender identity matches the sex assigned to them at birth; contrast with transgender

classism: social inequalities based on class that favor or privilege wealthier or more affluent individuals or families over those less affluent; also refers to elitist attitudes that disparage or devalue the poor and working class

claudication: muscle cramps that occur when arterial blood flow does not meet the muscles' demand for oxygen

closed head injury: an injury to the brain that arises from a problem within the cranium

coenzymes: a nonprotein compound that is necessary for the functioning of an enzyme

cognitive functions: mental functions such as reasoning, language, memory, and problem-solving

cognitive sequential: a learning style that prefers structured, physical hands-on tasks

collagen: the main structural protein found in skin and other connective tissues, widely used in purified form for cosmetic surgical treatments

colorectal: refers to cancers of the lower digestive tract consisting of the colon and the rectum

Commission on Accreditation of Athletic Training Education (CAATE): the organization responsible for accrediting athletic training preparation programs and curricula

compensatory hypertrophy: an increase in the size of a tissue or an organ in response to an increased workload placed upon it

complete protein: proteins that provide all eight essential amino acids

computational fluid dynamics: a branch of fluid mechanics that uses numerical analysis and data structures to analyze and solve problems that involve fluid flows

computer-aided design (CAD): the use of computers to aid in the creation, modification, analysis, or optimization of a design

computerized tomography (CT) scan: a visual diagnostic technology using X-rays that can detect brain abnormalities

concentration gradient: the gradual change in the concentration of solutes in a solution across a specific distance

concussion: temporary unconsciousness or confusion caused by a blow on the head

conditioning: the process of training to become physically fit through a regimen of exercise, diet, and rest

condyle: a rounded protuberance at the end of a bone that is part of an articulated joint

conflict theory: a theoretical framework within sociology that envisions tensions, divisions, and inequalities as a basic feature of society due to unequal access to education, wealth, and other valuable social resources

connective tissue: tissue throughout the body that develops from mesoderm, the middle embryological layer, and serves various functions in stability and anatomic structure

contraction: the process in which a muscle becomes or is made shorter and tighter

contusion: a wound that typically does not break the skin but causes bruising

coronary arteries: the arteries that supply blood to the heart muscle

corticosteroid: a fatlike molecule (or steroid), produced by the adrenal gland or made synthetically, that can be used to treat inflammation

creatine: a compound formed in protein metabolism and present in much living tissue; it is involved in the supply of energy for muscular contraction

creatine kinase: an enzyme expressed by various tissues and cell types that catalyzes the conversion of creatine and uses adenosine triphosphate (ATP) to create phosphocreatine and adenosine diphosphate (ADP)

creatine phosphate: an energy-containing molecule present in significant quantities in muscle tissue; energy is stored in a high-energy bond like that of ATP

creatinine: a breakdown product of creatine phosphate from muscle and protein metabolism. It is released at a constant rate by the body

crepitus: the scraping or grinding sound heard or felt when bone rubs over bone in joint spaces

cutaneous: pertaining to the skin

cutaneous pain: caused by injuries to the skin or superficial tissues; brief and localized

cyclooxygenase: an enzyme that is responsible for the formation of prostanoids, including thromboxane and prostaglandins such as prostacyclin, from arachidonic acid

cytokine: a broad category of small, secreted proteins and glycoproteins, such as interferon, interleukin, and growth factors, secreted by certain cells of the immune system and other tissues that influence other cells

DASH diet: a low-sodium diet promoted by the US-based National Heart, Lung, and Blood Institute to prevent and control hypertension

degenerative: marked by progression to a state below what is considered normal or desirable

dehydration: loss of body fluid caused by illness, sweating, or inadequate intake

deltoid muscle: the muscle forming the rounded contour of the human shoulder

dendrite: a branching nerve cell extension that receives and processes the effects of action potentials from other nerve cells

diastole: the period of relaxation of the heart between beats

dietary supplement: a manufactured product that, when consumed, provides nutrients above the recommended daily requirements

diffusion: the process by which different particles, such as atoms and molecules, gradually become intermingled due to random motion caused by thermal energy

disorder: an illness that disrupts normal physical and mental functions

disorientation: lack of comprehension of reality

dissociative states: mental disorders that involve experiencing a disconnection and lack of continuity between thoughts, memories, surroundings, actions, and identity

distal: farther away from the base or attached end

distal interphalangeal joints: the distal joints of the fingers

diuretics: drugs that increase urine production

dizziness: a sensation of spinning around and losing one's balance

DNA microarrays: solid supports which contain many or all genes from a given genome, enabling the expression of these genes to be monitored simultaneously

DNA sequencing: determining the order of deoxyribonucleic acid (DNA) bases in a particular unit of genetic information

docosapentaenoic acid (DHA): an omega-3 fatty acid with 22 carbons and six carbon-carbon double bonds

doping: administration of drugs to inhibit or enhance sporting performance

Doppler effect: the relationship of the apparent frequency of waves, such as sound waves, to the relative motion of the source of the waves and the observer or instrument; the frequency increases as the two approach each other and decreases as they move apart; an effect also known as the "Doppler shift"

double-blinded: a test or trial, especially of a drug, in which any information that may influence the tester's behavior or subject is withheld until after the test

ductus arteriosus: a bypass vessel in fetal circulation connecting the pulmonary artery with the aorta that allows blood to skip circulating through the lungs

duodenum: the first part of the small intestine; it is located between the stomach and the middle part of the small intestine, or jejunum

duplex scan: an ultrasound representation of echo images of tissues and blood vessels combined with a Doppler representation of blood flow patterns

dura mater: the tough outermost membrane enveloping the brain and spinal cord

dysfunction: the disordered or impaired function of a body system, organ, or tissue

dyskinesia: a neurologic disorder causing difficulty in the performance of voluntary movements

dysmorphia: deformity or abnormality in the shape or size of a specified part of the body

East Germany: officially the German Democratic Republic, was a state that existed from 1949 to 1990 in middle Germany as part of the Eastern Bloc in the Cold War

ecchymosis: a purplish patch on the skin caused by bleeding; the spots are easily visible to the naked eye

edema: the accumulation of an excessive amount of fluid in cells or tissues

eicosanoids: any of a class of compounds (such as the prostaglandins) derived from polyunsaturated fatty acids (such as arachidonic acid) and involved in cellular activity

eicosapentaenoic acid (EPA)-an omega-3 fatty acid with 20 carbons and five carbon-carbon double bonds

elbow: the joint between the upper arm and the forearm

electrocardiogram (ECG): a graphic record of electrical currents of the heart

electroencephalograph: a physiological instrument used to record electrical activity from the scalp

electrolytes: minerals in your blood and other body fluids that carry an electric charge

electromagnetic waves: a convenient way of understanding energy as a wave; visible light, X-rays, and radio waves, which have the longest wavelength and lowest energy, are the most familiar examples

electromyography: an electrodiagnostic technique for recording the extracellular activity (action and evoked potentials) of skeletal muscles at rest, during voluntary contractions, and during electrical stimulation

electrophysiology: the study of the electrical properties of cells

embolus: an obstruction or occlusion of a vessel (most commonly, an artery or vein) caused by a transported blood clot, vegetation, mass of bacteria, or other foreign material

eminence: a projection or prominence in the shape of a bone

endocrine glands: glands that release hormones directly into the bloodstream

endorphins: brain chemicals released by the body that act as natural painkillers

endurance: denoting or relating to a race or other sporting event that takes place over a long distance or otherwise demands great physical stamina

enzyme: a biological catalyst that speeds up a chemical reaction without itself being used up; enzymes are made of protein, and a single enzyme can usually only catalyze a single chemical reaction

epicondylitis: inflammation of the tendons surrounding the elbow, typically due to overuse and repetitive motions of the forearm

epidural: the injection of an anesthetic into the fluid around the spine or into the epidural space in the back

epiphysis: the part of a long bone from which growth or elongation occurs

episodic memory (relational): memory of events, the associated temporal and spatial relationships, and the context in which an event occurs

equilibrium: the state that exists when the forward activity is exactly equal to the reverse activity of that process

ergonomics: the science of the relationship between the human form and its biomechanical environment

erythropoiesis: a tightly regulated, complex process originating in the bone marrow from a multipotent stem cell and terminating in a mature, enucleated erythrocyte

erythropoietin: a hormone secreted by the kidneys that increases the rate of production of red blood cells in response to falling levels of oxygen in the tissues

essential amino acids: amino acids that cannot be synthesized by an organism and must come from diet

essential fatty acid (EFA): a fatty acid that humans cannot synthesize

essential nutrients: molecules that an organism needs for survival but cannot manufacture itself

ester: an organic compound formed by reacting a carboxylic acid with an alcohol with the elimination of a water molecule. Many naturally occurring fats and essential oils are esters of fatty acids; they are among the most fragrant organic molecules

ethnocentrism: a biased perspective in which one assumes that the social or cultural understandings that are familiar to them are inherently "natural," "normal," "best," or "right"

euphoria: a feeling or state of intense excitement and happiness

eustress: a positive response one has to a stressor, which can depend on one's current feelings of control, desirability, location, and timing of the stressor

excitation: one consequence of the binding of neurotransmitters to the dendrite of a neuron; when the neuron receives enough excitation in its dendrite, the cell will release the neurotransmitter from its axon onto other cells

exercise: activity requiring physical effort, carried out to sustain or improve health and fitness

exercise recovery: the period between the end of a bout of exercise and the subsequent return to a resting or recovered state

exercise routine: physical exertion to improve one's fitness for athletic competition, ability, or performance that consists of regularly doing a series of things in a fixed order

expression: the action of cell biochemistry to produce and release a particular hormone in response to a stimulus

extensor: any of the muscles that increase the angle between members of a limb, as by straightening the elbow or knee or bending the wrist or spine backward

extracorporeal: pertaining to something occurring outside the body, such as therapy

fair play: conformity to established rules, upright conduct, and equitable conditions in and around the playing field

fascia: a thin layer of connective tissue that surrounds each structural component of a body like a protective coating

fat: one of three macronutrients; foods that provide fat are oils, margarine, butter, meat, and dairy

fat-soluble vitamins: vitamins that, because of their structure and solubility, migrate to fatty tissues in the body, where they are stored

Feldenkrais method: a system of gentle movements that promote flexibility, coordination, and self-awareness

femur: the leg bone extending from the knee to the hip

ferritin: a protein produced by mammalian cells that stores iron

fibrocartilage: a type of cartilage in which the matrix contains thick bundles of collagen fibers, making it appear white

fibula: the smaller of the two bones in the lower leg, on the lateral side

fitness training: regular, structured activity designed to promote health in human beings

flexor: any of the muscles that decrease the angle between bones on two sides of a joint, as in bending the elbow or knee

forearm: the region from the elbow joint to the wrist; also called the "antebrachium"

forebrain: the anterior of the three primary divisions of the brain in the embryo of a vertebrate, or the part of the adult brain derived from this tissue, including the diencephalon and telencephalon; the prosencephalon

Fourier transform: a mathematical method that allows magnetic resonance imaging (MRI) to utilize one radio frequency pulse and thereby examine all wavelengths, as opposed to examining each wavelength individually with a continuous wave

free weight: a freestanding object whose weight is used as resistance while exercising

frequency: the number of complete cycles, such as sound cycles, produced by an alternating energy source; sound is measured in cycles per second, and one cycle per second is equal to 1 hertz

friction: the force resisting the relative motion of solid surfaces, fluid layers, and material elements sliding against each other

functionalist theory: a sociology theory that envisions society as a living organism, with its institutions serving as the organs, each of which has its niche to perform to ensure the maintenance and survival of society; functionalist theory seeks to explain how unity and cohesion are maintained within society

fundamental motor skills: motor skills that are the building blocks of movement, including, for example, skipping, running, catching, throwing, bending and swaying

gamma rays: electromagnetic radiation emitted during radioactive decay with short wavelengths

gamma-aminobutyric acid (GABA): the chief inhibitory neurotransmitter in the mammalian central nervous system; its principal role is reducing neuronal excitability throughout the nervous system

gangrene: necrosis (tissue death) caused by the obstruction of the blood supply; may be localized in a small area or may involve an entire extremity

gas chromatography-a common laboratory procedure used in analytical chemistry for separating and analyzing compounds that can be vaporized without decomposition

gender identity: one's inner conception of their gender, whether female, male or something else

gene cloning: the development of a line of genetically identical organisms that contain identical copies of the same gene or deoxyribonucleic acid (DNA) fragments

gene therapy: the insertion of a functional gene or genes into a cell, tissue, or organ to correct a genetic abnormality

genetic disorder: a disorder caused by a mutation in a gene or chromosome

genetic marker: a distinctive deoxyribonucleic acid (DNA) sequence that shows variation in the population and can therefore potentially be used for identification of individuals and discovery of disease genes

ginseng: an herbal remedy used in Asian countries to help develop strength, also helps reduce fatigue

glycogen: the form that glucose takes when it is stored in the muscles and liver

glycolysis: the breakdown of glucose by enzymes, releasing energy and pyruvic acid

gonads: a collective term referring to the testes and ovaries

goniometry: the measurement of angles, particularly those for the range of motion of a joint

Gregorc mind styles: theory of learning styles that focuses on the cognitive skills of perception and organization

grid cells: specialized cells found in the entorhinal cortex that encode a specific region in space and are involved in allowing for spatiotemporal navigation

growth: the increase in the size of an organism or any of its parts during the developmental process; caused by increases in both cell numbers and cell size

growth hormone (GH): a peptide hormone that stimulates growth, cell reproduction, and cell regeneration

head: the part of the body containing the major sense organs (such as the eyes and ears) and the brain

headaches: a continuous pain in the head

heart attack: the common term for a myocardial infarction

heart failure: a condition in which the heart pumps inefficiently, allowing fluid to back up into the lungs or body tissue

heart rate: the number of times the heart contracts, or beats, per minute

hematoma: a pool of mostly clotted blood that forms in an organ, tissue, or body space

hematopoiesis: the formation of blood cellular components

hemoglobin: a protein inside red blood cells that carries oxygen from the lungs to tissues and organs in the body and carries carbon dioxide back to the lungs

herb: a plant or plant part used for its scent, flavor, or therapeutic properties

Herberden's nodes: osteophytes or bony spurs that develop as a result of the destruction of joint cartilage in distal interphalangeal joints

herniated disk: prolapse of the nucleus through a rupture or weakness in the annulus

HIF-1: hypoxia-inducible factor; a transcription factor that responds to decreases in available oxygen in the cellular environment, or hypoxia

hindbrain: the most posterior of the three primary divisions of the brain in the embryo of a vertebrate or the part of the adult brain derived from this tissue, including the cerebellum, pons, and medulla oblongata; rhombencephalon

histamine: a small molecule released by cells in response to injury and allergic and inflammatory reactions, causing contraction of smooth muscle and dilation of capillaries

homeopathy: the treatment of disease by minute doses of natural substances that in a healthy person would produce symptoms of the disease

hormone: a class of signaling molecules in multicellular organisms that are transported to distant organs to regulate physiology and behavior

human growth hormone (HGH): a peptide hormone that stimulates growth, cell reproduction, and cell regeneration in humans and other animals. It is thus important in human development

humeral: relating to the humerus bone, the bone of the upper arm or forelimb, forming joints at the shoulder and the elbow

humerus: the bone that forms the structural beam of the upper arm

hyaline cartilage: a type of cartilage that is smooth and glassy in appearance

hyaluronan: a naturally occurring gel-like material that is found primarily in synovial fluid

hyaluronic acid: a substance present in body tissues, such as skin and cartilage. In joints, it serves to help lubricate the joints

hydration: drinking water to replace bodily water lost through perspiration after intense exercise

hydrotherapy: exercises in a pool as part of treatment for conditions such as arthritis or partial paralysis

hydroxymethyl butyrate (HMB): a dietary supplement and ingredient in certain medical foods that promote wound healing and provide nutritional support for people with muscle wasting due to cancer or human immunodeficiency virus (HIV) infections

hyperplasia: the increase in size or growth of a tissue or an organ as a result of an increase in cell numbers, with the size of the cells remaining constant

hypertension: a blood pressure higher than what is normal

hypertonic: describes a solution with a greater concentration of solutes than the solution to which it is being compared; in biology, a solution with a greater solute concentration than the cytoplasm of a cell

hypotonic: describes a solution with a lower concentration of solutes than the solution to which it is being compared; in biology, a solution with a lower solute concentration than the cytoplasm of a cell

immune rejection: natural antibody response to foreign transplanted tissue; tissues engineered from the patient's own cells will not have this type of rejection

incision: a wound or injury that results from the slicing motion of a sharp edge

incomplete protein: proteins that are missing at least one essential amino acid

inflammation: a condition of tenderness and disturbed function of an area of the body, caused by a reaction of tissue to injury or infection

inflammatory: irritation that causes swelling, heat, and discomfort

injury: hurt, damage, or loss of function due to some event or illness

injury risk: a state in which a person has the potential for being physically harmed due to participation in certain athletic competitions or practices

insertion: point of muscle attachment on the bone that moves

instability: excessive mobility of two or more bones caused by damage to ligaments, the joint capsule, or fracture of one or more bones

intensity: the difficulty of an exercise, typically based on the amount of weight you lift

interleukins: any of various cytokines of low molecular weight that are produced by lymphocytes, macrophages, and monocytes and that function especially in the regulation of the immune system and especially cell-mediated immunity

International Association of Athletics Federation (IAAF): the organization that sets rules and regulations for international track-and-field events

International Olympic Committee (IOC): the organization that sets the rules and regulations that govern, among other things, the criteria for participation in the Olympic Games

intersex: a broad term used to describe natural variations in which individuals have sex characteristics that are not typically male or female; chromosomal differences or unusual hormone levels may cause intersex variations

intervertebral disk: the flexible, cylindrical pad between every two vertebrae, consisting of the nucleus pulposis (gelatinous center) and the annulus fibrosis (concentric rings of cartilage); the flexibility, moistness, and thickness of the disk decreases naturally with age

intra-articular: occurring within a joint

intracellular: refers to the space between cells in a tissue structure

intramural sports/activities: recreational sports or activities that primary and secondary schools provide and are held before or after the school day and, in some schools, during recess.

iron-deficiency anemia: too few healthy red blood cells resulting from insufficient bodily iron levels

ischemia: local anemia or area of diminished or insufficient blood supply due to a mechanical obstruction, commonly narrowing of an artery

isokinetic machine: an instrument that measures the strength of muscles through the joint's full range of motion

isoleucine: an essential hydrophobic amino acid that is one of three branch-chain amino acids and a constituent of most proteins; it is an essential nutrient in the diet of vertebrates

isotonic: describes a solution with the same concentration of solutes as the solution to which it is being compared; in biology, a solution with the same solute concentration as the cytoplasm

joint: a specialized structure in the body where bones come together, and motion occurs

joint effusion: a collection or buildup of fluid in a joint

Kaatsu training: a patented exercise method developed by Dr. Yoshiaki Sato that is based on blood flow moderation exercise involving compression of the vasculature proximal to the exercising muscles

ketogenesis: the biochemical process through which organisms produce ketone bodies by breaking down fatty acids and ketogenic amino acids

kinesiology: the study of the mechanics of body movements

knee: the complex articulated joint between the thigh and the lower leg

knee cartilage defect: an area of damaged cartilage in the knee

Krebs cycle: the sequence of reactions by which most living cells generate energy during aerobic respiration. It takes place in the mitochondria, consuming oxygen, producing carbon dioxide and water as waste products, and converting adenosine diphosphate (ADP) to energy-rich adenosine triphosphate (ATP)

kwashiorkor: a disease caused by severe protein deficiency; symptoms include apathy, diarrhea, inactivity, failure to grow, fatty liver, and edema

kyphoplasty: similar to vertebroplasty but uses a special balloon to restore vertebral height and lessen spinal deformity

kyphosis: backward curvature of the spine or a section of the spine

lactate: an organic acid the body forms when it breaks down carbohydrates to use for energy, while oxygen levels are low

lateral: on the outer side; toward the little toe when in reference to the leg

lateral epicondyle: a large eminence on the lateral side of the proximal end of the humerus that is an attachment site for the radial collateral ligament at the elbow joint and the common tendon of the supinator and extensor muscles

learned nonuse: a motor learning phenomenon whereby limb movement is suppressed initially due to adverse reactions and failure of any activity attempted with the affected limb, resulting in the suppression of motor behavior

learning style: differences in how individuals successfully acquire knowledge, that is, visual, tactile, auditory

leg: the lower extremity, excluding the foot; the lower leg runs from the knee to the ankle

leucine: a hydrophobic amino acid that is one of three branch-chain amino acids and a constituent of most proteins; it is an essential nutrient in the diet of vertebrates

leukocytes: colorless, nucleated, amoeboid cells that circulate throughout the blood and body fluids and destroy or isolate foreign substances and infectious agents, including lymphocytes, granulocytes, monocytes, and macrophages

leukotriene: fatty acid-derived compounds that mediate inflammation and cause constriction of the bronchioles

ligament: a membranous fold that supports an organ and keeps it in position.

long jump: a track and field event in which athletes combine speed, strength, and agility in an attempt to leap as far as possible from a takeoff point

lordosis: forward curvature of the spine or a section of the spine

lower extremities: the thigh, lower leg, and foot

lumbar spine: the lowest of three parts of the spine, consisting of five vertebrae, named L1 to L5 (just above the sacrum), in a natural lordosis

lumen: the space within an artery, vein, or other tubes

macronutrients: materials ingested in large amounts to supply the energy and materials for physical bodies

magnetic resonance imaging (MRI): a visual diagnostic technology that can create high-resolution pictures of brain structures

Major League Baseball (MLB): a professional baseball organization and the oldest major professional sports league in the world

Major League Baseball Players Association (MLBPA): the collective bargaining representative for all current MLB players

matrix: in bone, the matrix is a solid nonliving material that is a composite of protein fibers and mineral crystals

maximal oxygen uptake: the maximum rate of oxygen consumption during exercise

medial: on the side toward the midline of the body; toward the big toe when in reference to the leg

megadose: ten or more times the recommended daily allowance of a nutrient

meniscus: a crescent- or lens-shaped structure composed of fibrocartilage found especially in the knee joint

menstruation: the process in a woman of discharging blood and other materials from the lining of the uterus at intervals of about one lunar month from puberty until menopause, except during pregnancy

mental health: a person's condition concerning their psychological and emotional well-being

meridians: designated pathways in the body with points that react to acupuncture stimulation

metabolic equivalent (MET): a unit used to estimate the metabolic cost of physical activity; 1 MET is equal to 3.5 milliliters of oxygen consumed per kilogram of body weight per minute

metabolism: the biochemical processes in our bodies by which it degrades food, converts it to energy, and uses that energy to carry out the processes of life

microcytosis: a condition in which red blood cell size smaller than the normal range

micronutrients: substances of which only milligrams are needed in the daily diet, such as vitamins and minerals

midbrain: the middle of the three primary divisions of the brain in the embryo of a vertebrate or the part of the adult brain derived from this tissue; mesencephalon

mineral: an inorganic salt of particular metals or elements needed for good health

minerals: inorganic substances that are essential for body processes; the major minerals include calcium, phosphorus, magnesium, sodium, chloride, and potassium

mission statement: brief description of an organization's purpose.

mitochondria: an organelle found in large numbers in most cells, in which the biochemical processes of respiration and energy production occur; it has a double membrane, the inner layer being folded inward to form layers (cristae)

monosaccharide: any of the class of sugars such as glucose that cannot be hydrolyzed to give a simpler sugar

motivation: choice, effort and persistence to engage in a particular activity or task

motor: relating to or involving movements of a muscle

motor control: the nature and cause of movement, which focuses on stability and movement of the body, and the manipulation of objects, which is achieved through the coordination of many structures organized both hierarchically and in a parallel manner

motor development: the study of changes in motor behavior which reflects the interaction of maturation and the environment

motor learning: the acquisition and modification of movement as a result of practice and experience, which leads to relatively permanent intrinsic changes in the ability to perform skilled activities; not directly measurable but inferred from measures of motor performance

motor nerve: a nerve carrying impulses from the brain or spinal cord to a muscle or gland

motor performance: the directly measurable extent to which the objective of a motor task is met, the scientific study of which originated as a branch of experimental psychology

motor skills: skills in which both movement and the outcome of actions are emphasized

moxibustion: a traditional Chinese medicine therapy that consists of burning dried mugwort at particular points on the body

mucosa: the moist, inner lining of some organs and body cavities (such as the nose, mouth, lungs, and stomach

muscle: a band or bundle of fibrous tissue in a human or animal body that can contract, move in, or maintain the position of parts of the body

muscle contraction: the shortening of a muscle, which may result in the movement of a particular body part

muscle fibers: elongated muscle cells that make up skeletal, cardiac, and smooth muscles

muscle fitness: having muscles that can lift heavier objects or muscles that will work longer before becoming exhausted

muscle relaxant: a class of medications that reduce skeletal muscle function and decrease muscle tone, and treat muscle spasms, pain, and hyperreflexia

muscle soreness: muscle pain commencing after a workout

muscle testing: an alternative medical technique that purports to diagnose illness or select treatments by testing muscles for strength and weakness

muscular endurance: the ability for a muscle group to perform, or contract, repeatedly at resistance below the maximum resistance the muscle can move

muscular strength: the force that a muscle can produce or exert in a maximal effort one time, in other words, the greatest amount of weight or resistance a muscle can move or lift for one repetition only; this measure of strength is also known as the "one rep max" or 1 rm

musculature: the arrangement of skeletal muscles in the body

musculoskeletal: a term used to describe the relationship between bones and muscles within the framework of the body and how they provide stability and locomotion

musculotendinous unit: a structure that consists of a muscle that provides motion of a bone and its attachment to the bone, the tendon, which is a tough, inelastic fibrous structure

myocardial perfusion imaging (MPI): a type of cardiac stress test

myofascial release: an alternative medicine therapy claimed to be useful for treating skeletal muscle immobility and pain by relaxing contracted muscles, improving blood and lymphatic circulation, and stimulating the stretch reflex in muscles

myopathies: neuromuscular disorders in which the primary symptom is muscle weakness due to dysfunction of muscle fiber

narcotics: psychoactive compounds with numbing or paralyzing properties

National Athletic Trainers Association (NATA): professional association for members who are certified athletic trainers and other individuals who are interested in the athletic training career

National Board for Certification in Occupational Therapy (NBCOT): a professional organization that administers the national exam for occupational therapy certification

National Collegiate Athletic Association (NCAA): the regulatory body for intercollegiate athletics for over 1,200 participating institutions (divided into three divisions)

National Standards: content standards for physical education curricula set forth by the National Association of Sport and Physical Education (NASPE)

nervous system: a highly complex part of an animal that coordinates its actions and sensory information by transmitting signals to and from different parts of its body

neural tube: a tube formed by the closure of ectodermal tissue in the early vertebrate embryo that later develops into the brain, spinal cord, nerves, and ganglia

neurodegeneration: the death and destruction of neurons and neuronal fibers that often occurs as a direct result of many diseases that target the nervous system

neurogenesis: the development or growth of new neuronal cells

neuron: the basic cell of the nervous system; commonly referred to as a "brain cell"

neuropathic pain: pain caused by a lesion or disease of the somatosensory nervous system

neurotransmitter: a chemical that communicates nerve impulses from one nerve cell to another

nicotinamide: a compound that is the form in which nicotinic acid often occurs in nature

nicotinamide adenine dinucleotide (NAD): a molecule used to hold pairs of electrons when they have been removed from a molecule by some biological process; the empty molecule is denoted by NAD@Glossary = +, while it is denoted as NADH when it is carrying electrons

N-methyl-D-aspartate (NMDA) receptors: a glutamate receptor and ion channel found in neurons

nociception: the process of transmitting pain messages to the brain through the spinal cord by sensitive nerve endings in skin and tissues

nonsteroidal anti-inflammatory drugs (NSAIDs): compounds that inhibit the synthesis of prostaglandins and thromboxanes

nucleus: a collection of nerve cell bodies in the brain, separable from other groups by their cellular form or by surrounding nerve cell extensions

occupational therapy programs: certified training programs at high learning institutes that train students to work as licensed occupational therapists

Olympics: a major international multisport event normally held once every four years

omega-3 fatty acids: being or composed of polyunsaturated fatty acids that have the final double bond in the hydrocarbon chain between the third and fourth carbon atoms from the end of the molecule opposite that of the carboxyl group and that are found especially in fish, fish oils, green leafy vegetables, and some nuts and vegetable oils

opiate: a substance derived from opium that relieves pain and induces sleep

opioid: substances that act on opioid receptors to relieve pain, including anesthesia, suppress diarrhea, reverse opioid overdose, and suppress coughs

origin: point of muscle attachment on the bone that remains stationary

orthologues: similar genes from different species that are thought to be related by evolution

orthopedic bracing: medical devices designed to properly align, correct the position, support, stabilize, and protect certain parts of the body

orthopedic surgery: the field of surgery that deals with the musculoskeletal system

orthopedics: the surgical or manipulative treatment of any disorder of the skeletal system and the associated motor organs

orthotic device: a podiatric appliance or prosthesis that is used to correct a foot deformity

oscilloscope: an instrument that displays a visual representation of electrical variations on the fluorescent screen of a cathode-ray tube

osmotic pressure: the pressure that would have to be applied to a solution to prevent the flow of solvent through a semipermeable membrane

osteoarthritis: a progressive disorder of the joints caused by gradual loss of cartilage which can result in the development of bone spurs and cysts at the margins of joints

osteoblast: a bone cell that can produce and form bone matrix; osteoblasts are responsible for new bone formation

osteoclast: a large bone cell that can destroy bone matrix by dissolving the mineral crystals

osteocyte: the primary living cell of mature bone tissue

overexertion: any case in which a person works or exerts themselves beyond their physical capabilities

overload: the body must undergo a level of stress that is greater than the norm in order for the body to undergo physiological adaptations that increase muscular strength, muscular endurance, and aerobic endurance

oxidation: a chemical process that removes electrons from molecules or atoms

oxidative phosphorylation: the metabolic pathway in which cells use enzymes to oxidize nutrients, thereby releasing chemical energy to produce adenosine triphosphate

pai mater: the delicate innermost membrane enveloping the brain and spinal cord

pain: physical suffering or discomfort caused by illness or injury

pain relief: alleviation of pain, typically through medication

palliative treatments: therapies that reduce symptoms without completely eradicating a disorder

paralysis: the loss of power of voluntary movement or other function of a muscle as a result of disease or injury to its nerve supply

parasympathetic nervous system: part of the autonomic nervous system that restores and conserves the body's resources

patella: the flat, triangular bone in the front of the knee; also called the "kneecap"

patellar tendon: a structure that attaches the bottom of the kneecap (patella) to the top of the shinbone (tibia)

patent ductus arteriosus: a persistent connection between two major blood vessels, the aorta, and the pulmonary artery, that lead from the heart

pathogen: any disease-causing microorganism

peptide bond: a covalent bond that links the carboxyl group of one amino acid to the amine group of another, enabling the formation of proteins and other polypeptides

performance-enhancing drugs (PEDs): substances used to improve any form of activity performance in humans

peripheral nervous system: the system of nerves that link the central nervous system to the rest of the body; consists of twelve pairs of cranial nerves, thirty-one pairs of spinal nerves, and the autonomic nervous system

petechiae: minute spots caused by hemorrhage or bleeding into the skin; the spots are the size of pinheads

pharmacology: the aspect of biomedical science that studies therapeutic drugs, their administration, and their bioproperties

phosphatidylcholine: a class of phospholipids that incorporate choline as a headgroup and a major component of biological membranes; it is easily obtained from a variety of readily available sources, such as egg yolk or soybeans

photons: particles that travel at the speed of light

photonutrients: any chemical or nutrient derived from a plant source that absorbs light

physiatry: the branch of medicine dealing with the prevention, diagnosis, and treatment of disease or injury and the rehabilitation from resultant impairments and disabilities; uses physical agents such as light, heat, cold, water, electricity, therapeutic exercise, mechanical apparatus, and pharmaceutical agents

physical activity: physical exercise forces the body to undergo physiological adaptations related to an increase in cardiovascular and musculoskeletal health

physical ailment: a physical disorder or illness, especially of a minor or chronic nature

physical fitness: a state of health and well-being through proper nutrition, moderate-vigorous physical exercise, and sufficient rest, along with a formal recovery plan so that someone can perform aspects of sports, occupations, and daily activities

physical rehabilitation: a set of interventions designed to optimize functioning and reduce disability in individuals with health conditions in interaction with their environment

physiology: a branch of biology that deals with the normal functions of living organisms and their parts

phytonutrients: a substance found in certain plants which is believed to be beneficial to human health and help prevent various diseases

Pilates: a system of physical conditioning involving low-impact exercises and stretches designed to strengthen muscles of the torso and often performed with specialized equipment

place cells: specialized cells found in the hippocampus that encode a specific point in space and seem to encode an animal's position or perceived position in a given setting

placebo: a harmless pill, medicine, or procedure prescribed more for the psychological benefit to the patient than for any physiological effect

plasticity: a characteristic of brain cells that allows them to change as a result of stimulation or changes in activity

platelets: blood cells that help your body form clots to stop bleeding

pleura: a pair of moist and slippery membranes that surround the lungs; the outer, or parietal, pleura lines the inside of the rib cage and the diaphragm, and the inner, or visceral, pleura covers the lungs; the space between the two pleura is the intrapleural space that contains fluid secreted by the pleura

pluripotent stem cells: stem cells that can differentiate into any adult cell type

polycythemia: an abnormally increased concentration of hemoglobin in the blood, through either reduction of plasma volume or increase in red cell numbers; it may be a primary disease of unknown cause or a secondary condition linked to respiratory or circulatory disorder or cancer

polymerase chain reaction (PCR): an in vitro process by which specific parts of a DNA molecule or a gene can be made into millions or billions of copies within a short time

polysaccharide: a carbohydrate whose molecules consist of many sugar molecules bonded together

positive competition: competition that focuses on respecting the opponent and putting forth effort.

pressure points: a point on the surface of the body sensitive to pressure

prone: the position of the body when face downward, on one's stomach and abdomen

prostacyclin: a fatty acid-derived compound that inhibits platelet aggregation and blood clotting and acts as a vasodilator

prostaglandins: a large group of biologically active unsaturated, twenty-carbon fatty acids that represent some of the metabolites of arachidonic acid

protein: a biological polymer consisting of one or more long chains of amino acids linked by peptide bonds in a sequence specified by an organism's deoxyribonucleic acid (DNA)

proteoglycan: a compound found in connective tissue, and other places in the body, composed of a protein to which chains of sugar-based groups are attached

proteolytic enzymes: enzymes that catalyze proteolysis by breaking down proteins into smaller polypeptides or single amino acids and spurring the formation of new protein products

proteomics: the study of proteomes; a proteome is the complete set of proteins in a particular cell type

proximal: closer to the base or attached end

proximal interphalangeal joints: the proximal joints in the fingers

pseudoephedrine: a drug obtained from plants of the genus *Ephedra* (or prepared synthetically) and used as a nasal decongestant

psoriatic arthritis: a chronic, inflammatory disease of the joints and the places where tendons and ligaments connect to bone, usually associated with plaque psoriasis that affects the skin

psychotherapy: treatment using the mind to remedy problems related to disordered behavior or thinking, emotional problems, or disease

pulse: the rhythmical dilation of an artery, produced by the increased volume of blood forced into the vessel by the contraction of the heart

pulsed electromagnetic field therapy: uses electromagnetic fields in an attempt to heal nonunion fractures and depression

qi: the circulating life energy that in Chinese philosophy is thought to be inherent in all things; in traditional Chinese medicine, the balance of negative and positive forms in the body is believed to be essential for good health

qigong: a Chinese system of breathing exercises, body postures, movements, and mental concentration intended to maintain good health and control the flow of vital energy

quadriceps muscle: a hip flexor and a knee extensor; it consists of four individual muscles; three vastus muscles and the rectus femoris; they form the main bulk of the thigh and collectively are one of the most powerful muscles in the body; it is located in the anterior compartment of the thigh

radial: toward the edge of the forearm and hand containing the radius and thumb

radiculopathy: also called "nerve root entrapment" or "pinched nerve"; irritation or compression of the root of a spinal nerve between vertebrae, caused by an annular bulge, herniated disk, or spinal injury

radius: the shorter of the two forearm bones on the thumb side

recombinant DNA: a hybrid DNA molecule created in the test tube by joining a DNA fragment of interest with a carrier DNA

recommended daily (or dietary) allowance (RDA): the intake levels of the essential nutrients that are considered adequate to meet the known nutritional needs of most healthy persons

recovery: the period between the end of a bout of exercise and the subsequent return to a resting or recovered state

reduction: a chemical reaction that adds electrons to molecules or atoms

referred pain: any pain whose origin is elsewhere in the body from where it is felt; with radiculopathy in the lumbar spine, the pain is typically in the leg

regenerative medicine: another term for tissue engineering, where biological properties are employed to maintain, repair, replace or enhance tissue function

rehabilitation: restoring someone to health or normal life through training and therapy after imprisonment, addiction, or illness

repetitive strain injury: injuries to muscles, nerves, ligaments, and tendons caused by improper technique or overuse that most commonly affect the elderly

repetitive transcranial magnet therapy: a form of brain stimulation therapy used to treat depression and anxiety

resistance training: the performance of physical exercises that are designed to improve strength and endurance, often associated with the lifting of weights

reverse osmosis: the application of pressure to a solution to overcome the osmotic pressure of a semipermeable membrane and force water to pass through it in the direction opposite to normal osmotic flow

rheumatoid arthritis: a chronic progressive disease, causing inflammation in the joints and resulting in painful deformity and immobility, especially in the fingers, wrists, feet, and ankles

rib belt: a device applied to the thoracic and upper abdominal region to compress and bind the rib cage during rib fractures and postoperative care while allowing flexibility and comfortable breathing

risk management: the forecasting and evaluation of injury risks and the identification of procedures to avoid or minimize injury probability or impact

rotator cuff: a capsule with fused tendons that supports the arm at the shoulder joint and is often subject to athletic injury

salicylates: a group of drugs (including aspirin) derived from salicylic acid, used to relieve pain, reduce inflammation, and lower fever

saturated fatty acid: a fatty acid with no carbon-carbon double bonds

sciatica: intense pain in one buttock and down the back of that leg, caused by inflammation of the sciatic nerve, the largest nerve in the body; in some cases, this inflammation is referred pain from radiculopathy where the sciatic nerve originates between L4 and the sacrum

sclera: the white part of the eyeball that is visible when the eyelids are withdrawn

scoliosis: sideways curvature of the spine or a section of the spine

selective awareness: the process of directing our awareness to relevant stimuli while ignoring other stimuli in the environment

self-esteem: confidence in one's own worth or abilities; self-respect

self-hypnosis: putting oneself in a highly suggestive state to focus, motivate, become more self-aware, and make the best use of innate skills

semipermeable membrane: a membrane that allows the passage of a material, such as water or another solvent, from one side to the other while preventing the passage of other materials, such as dissolved salts or another solute

semisynthetic: about compounds that are obtained by altering or augmenting the molecular structure of a compound obtained from a natural source

sex: refers to a person's reproductive characteristics, including chromosomes, hormones, and internal and external organs

shin splints: pain caused by overuse along the shinbone, the large front bone in the lower leg

shoulder impingement: a common cause of shoulder pain, often caused by the repeated activity of the shoulder; also called "swimmer's shoulder"

sinoatrial (S-A) node: a small region of specialized heart muscle cells that spontaneously generates and sends an electrical signal that gives the heart an automatic rhythm for contraction

skeletal muscle: a type of muscle that attaches to bone and causes movement of body parts; the only type that is under conscious, voluntary control

skill variations: different movement patterns or action characteristics that can be produced from the same movement pattern

smooth muscle: a type of muscle found in the walls of internal organs such as the stomach, intestines, and urinary bladder; involved in the movement of food through the digestive tract

sodium: a mineral found in many foods, required by the human body for normal muscle and nerve functions

soft tissue massage: a form of manual physical therapy involving hands-on techniques on muscles, ligaments, and fascia to break adhesions and optimize muscle function

solute: any material dissolved in a liquid or fluid medium, usually water

solvent: any fluid, most commonly water, that dissolves other materials

soma: the body of a cell, where the cell's genetic material and other vital structures are located

somatosensory system: the system by which muscle, joint, and cutaneous sensory receptors contribute to the perception and control of movement through ascending pathways

Southern blot: a procedure used to transfer DNA from a gel to a nylon membrane, which in turn allows the finding of genes that are complementary to particular DNA sequences called "probes"

spasm: a sudden contraction of a muscle or group of muscles, such as a cramp

spectator: the effect on performance when a task is carried out in the presence of others

spinal cord injury: damage to the tight bundle of cells and nerves that sends and receives signals from the brain to and from the rest of the body

sport & exercise psychology: the study of the psychological aspects of human movement

sports: an activity involving physical exertion and skill in which an individual or team competes against another or others for entertainment

spotter: a person who assists with a person exercising to ensure proper technique and injury prevention; this can be hands-on, by being in a physical position to prevent accidents, or hands-off by watching the exercising person and being ready to assist as needed

sprain: injury to a ligament, typically from overstretching it along its length that may cause pain, swelling, and instability

standard metabolic rate (SMR): the standardized measure of metabolism in cold-blooded organisms

starch: a glucose polymer consisting of numerous glucose units joined by glycosidic bonds and is the major storage carbohydrate in plants and photosynthetic bacteria

static magnets: a magnet that retains its magnetism after being removed from a magnetic field

stenosis: the constriction or narrowing of a passage

steroids: a class of hormones produced by the adrenal glands; can also be made synthetically

stimulant: a substance that raises levels of physiological or nervous activity in the body

storage compounds: areas in the body that store nutrients not immediately required by an organism

strain: a stretching or tearing of a muscle or a tissue connecting muscle to bone

strength: the measure of a human's exertion of force on physical objects; increasing physical strength is the goal of strength training

stress: physical, environmental, or psychological strain experienced by an individual that requires adjustment

stretchable tubing: elastic workout object with little to no weight that uses tension to create resistance for exercise

substance P: a peptide found in nerve cells in the body, which serves as a chemical messenger (neurotransmitter) that carries pain messages along pathways to the brain

sudden cardiac death: a situation in which the heart stops beating or beats irregularly, stopping blood flow

supplement: a nutritional product, such as vitamin, mineral, herb, amino acid, or enzyme, taken orally that augments someone's diet to ensure that their nutritional needs are satisfactorily met

surfactant: compounds that reduce the surface tension of fluid into which they are dissolved

suture: also known as a "stitch" or "stitches," is a medical device used to hold body tissues together and approximate wound edges after an injury or surgery

symbolic interaction theory: a theoretical approach within sociology that examines the shared symbolic meanings that members of a society attach to certain objects, behaviors, or cultural phenomena, as well as how these meanings shape individuals' and collective groups' behaviors

Symphytum: a genus of flowering plants in the borage family, Boraginaceae, used to make homeopathic preparations

synapse: an area of close contact between nerve cells that is the functional junction where one cell communicates with another

synaptic plasticity: the cellular process in the nervous system where connections between neurons, known as "synapses," strengthen or weaken in an activity-dependent manner; this process is believed to underlie learning in the brain

synovial: referring to the lubricating fluid in the joints or the membrane surrounding the joints

synovial fluid: a clear fluid that serves as a lubricant in a joint, tendon sheath, or bursa

synovium: fluid-filled sacs in joint margins

synteny: when whole regions of chromosomes from different species are similar in structure

synthetic: about compounds that are produced entirely by synthesis reactions carried out in the laboratory from simple starting materials

systole: the period of contraction of the heart when blood moves out of the heart chambers and into the arteries

Tai Chi: Chinese martial art and form of stylized, meditative exercise characterized by methodically slow circular and stretching movements and positions of bodily balance

tarsus: the ankle

telencephalon: an early embryological structure in the developing nervous system that ultimately develops into the cortex, basal ganglia, and hippocampus, among other mature brain regions

tendinopathy: a general term referring to any tendon disorder

tendinosis: degeneration of the tendon's collagen in response to chronic overuse

tendon: a flexible but inelastic cord of strong fibrous collagen tissue attaching a muscle to a bone

tendonitis: inflammation of a tendon, most commonly from overuse but also from infection or rheumatic disease

testosterone: a sex hormone, a type of androgen, an anabolic steroid that affects sexual characteristics and physical strength; typically produced in greater quantities by male bodies, testosterone can be used for hormone therapy and as a performance-enhancing drug

therapeutic exercise: movement prescribed to correct impairments, restore muscular and skeletal function and maintain a state of well-being

therapeutic massage: manipulation of the body's soft tissues to treat body stress or pain

therapeutic treatments: therapeutics, treatment, and care of a patient for both preventing and combating disease or alleviating pain or injury

thigh: the upper segment of the leg, from the hip joint to the knee

thoracic cavity: the space within the body between the diaphragm and the neck; it contains the lungs and heart and is enclosed by the ribs

thoracic spine: the middle of three parts of the spine, consisting of twelve vertebrae, named T1 (top of the chest) to T12, in a natural kyphosis

thorax: the part of the trunk above the diaphragm, containing the ribs; the chest

thromboxane: fatty acid-derived compounds that are vasodilators and promote platelet aggregation and blood clotting

thrombus: a blood clot that commonly obstructs a vein but may also occur in an artery or the heart

tibia: the larger of the two bones in the lower leg, on the medial side

tissue: a collection of similar cells that perform a specific function

Title IX: the portion of federal education law that forbids discrimination based on gender in education programs that receive federal funding

trace elements: elements needed in the diet at levels of less than 100 milligrams per day

tracer: a substance that is injected into the body and releases energy that allows it to be followed along its path through the circulatory system and metabolism pathways

tract: a collection of nerve fibers (axons) in the brain or spinal cord that all have the same place of origin and the same place of termination

traction-test devices: measures the length of time that rats can keep their front paws on a horizontally suspended bar

traditional Chinese medicine: an alternative medical practice drawn from traditional medicine in China

Trager approach: a combination of hands-on tissue mobilization, relaxation, and movement reeducation called "Mentastics"

transcutaneous electrical nerve stimulation (TENS): the use of electric current produced by a device to stimulate the nerves for therapeutic purpose

transducer (probe): a device designed to transfer ultrasound waves into the body noninvasively, receive the returning echoes, and transform those echoes into electrical voltages

transection: a partial or complete severance of the spinal cord

trans-fatty acid: a fatty acid with at least one carbon-carbon double bond where the hydrogens attached to the carbons that participate in the double bond are on opposite sides of the double bond

transgender: a person whose gender identity differs from the sex assigned to them at birth; a trans man was born female and has transitioned to male; a trans woman was born male and has transitioned to female

traumatic brain injury: an injury to the brain caused by blunt force

triathlete: an athlete who competes in a multisport race that involves swimming, biking, and running across long distances

triathlon: an athletic contest consisting of three different events, typically swimming, cycling, and long-distance running

trigger point: a sensitive area of the body, stimulation or irritation of which causes a specific effect in another part, especially a tender area in a muscle that causes generalized musculoskeletal pain when overstimulated

trunk: the central part of the body to which the extremities are attached

tuberosity: an elevated round process in the shape of a bone

ulcerative colitis: a chronic, inflammatory bowel disease that causes inflammation in the large intestine of the digestive tract

ulna: the larger of the two forearm bones, forming the principal part of the elbow joint with the humerus

ulnar: toward the edge of the forearm and hand containing the ulna and little finger

ulnar collateral ligament: a ligament that runs on the inner side of the elbow to help support it when performing certain motions, such as throwing

ultrasonic: referring to any frequency of sound that is higher than the audible range-that is, higher than 20,000 cycles per second (20 kilohertz)

ultrasound therapy: an ultrasonic procedure that uses ultrasound for therapeutic benefit

unconsciousness: lack of awareness of one's surroundings

unipolar magnets: magnets with north on one side and south on the other; the north (or negative) side is typically applied to the skin

unsaturated fatty acid: a fatty acid with at least one carbon-carbon double bond

upper arm: the region from the shoulder joint to the elbow joint; also called the "brachium"

upper extremities: the arm, forearm, and hand

valgus: a deformity involving oblique displacement of part of a limb away from the midline

valine: a hydrophobic a-amino acid used in the biosynthesis of proteins that is a member of the branch chain amino acids; in humans, valine must be obtained from the diet

vascular: relating to or containing blood vessels

vasoconstriction: a decrease in the diameter of a blood vessel

vasodilation: an increase in the diameter of a blood vessel

veins: vessels that take blood to the heart and from the tissues

ventricles: the lower pumping chambers of the heart located below the atria; they force blood into the arteries

vertebroplasty: a medical procedure where acrylic cement is injected into the body of the vertebra for stabilization

very low-density lipoproteins: one of the major groups of lipoproteins that enable fats and cholesterol to move within the water-based solution of the bloodstream

visceral pain: throbbing or aching pain that originates in the deeper body tissues and organs; of longer duration than cutaneous pain

viscosupplementation injections: injections to add lubrication into the joint to make joint movement less painful

vitamin: a nutrient that the body needs in small amounts to function and stay healthy

water-soluble vitamins: vitamins that, because of their structure, show strong solubility in water; they normally pass through the body in a relatively short time

weight machine: a stationary machine used for exercise that uses attached weights and gravity to offer resistance

workout: a session of vigorous physical exercise or training

yang: Chinese concept of the positive, male element of the universe

yin: Chinese concept of the negative, female element of the universe

yoga: comes from a Sanskrit word meaning "union;" yoga combines physical exercises, mental meditation, and breathing techniques to strengthen the muscles and relieve stress

youth sports: any sports event where competitors are younger than adult age, whether children or adolescents

zeugmatography: a name applied to MRI characterizing the close relationship of nuclear magnetic forces and electromagnetic waves (from the Greek *zeugma*, meaning "to yoke together")

ORGANIZATIONS

Academy of Nutrition and Dietetics
120 South Riverside Plaza
Suite 2190
Chicago, IL 60606
312-899-0040
eatrightpro.org

Academy for Sports Dentistry (ASD)
PO Box 358
Isanti, MN 55040
612-440-7125
academyforsportsdentistry.org

American Academy of Family Physicians
11400 Tomahawk Creek Parkway
Leawood, KS 66211
800-274-2237
aafp.org

American Academy of Pediatrics (AAP)
345 Park Boulevard
Itasca, IL 60143
800-433-9016
aap.org

American College of Sports Medicine (ACSM)
401 West Michigan St.
Indianapolis, IN 46202-3233
317-637-9200
acsm.org

American Medical Society for Sports Medicine
4000 West 114th St.
Suite 100
Leawood, KS 66211
913-327-1415
amssm.org

American Orthopaedic Society of Sports Medicine (AOSSM)
9400 West Higgins Road
Suite 300
Rosemont, IL 60018
847-292-4900
sportsmed.org

American Osteopathic Academy of Sports Medicine (AOASM)
2424 American Lane
Madison, WI 53704
608-443-2477
aoasm.org

Centers for Disease Control and Prevention
1600 Clifton Rd.
Atlanta, GA
800-232-4636
cdc.gov

Gatorade Sports Science Institute (GSSI)
gssiweb.org

Hockey Equipment Certification Council, Inc. (HECC)
29 Pioneer St.
Cooperstown, NY 13326
607-282-4447
hecc.org

Joint Commission on Sports Medicine and Science
2952 North Stemmons Freeway
Dallas, TX 75247
214-637-6282
jcsmsonline.org

National Athletic Trainers' Association (NATA)
1620 Valwood Parkway
Suite 115
Carrollton, TX 75006
727-497-5972
nata.org

National Collegiate Athletic Association
NCAA Health and Safety
700 W. Washington St.
Indianapolis, IN 46206
ncaa.org

National Operating Committee on Standards for Athletic Equipment (NOCSAE)
11020 King St.
Suite 215
Overland Park, KS 66210
913-888-1340
nocsae.org

Sports and Fitness Industry Association (SFIA)
962 Wayne Ave.
Suite 300
Silver Spring, MD 20910
301-495-6321

Subject Index

2018 Winter Olympics, 487, 488, 489

abdominal binders, 356, 358
abrasion, 321, 322, 360
abuse-deterrent formulations, 445, 446
Accreditation Council for Occupational Therapy Education (ACOTE), 581
acetaminophen, 84, 151, 155, 270, 290, 297, 368, 442, 443, 445, 446, 447
Achievement Goal Theory, 564, 567
Achilles tendon, 56, 58, 289, 308, 380, 603
acquired immune deficiency syndrome (AIDS), 464
acupressure, 387-390
acupuncture, 390-395
adaptive task practice, 361, 363
adenosine diphosphate (ADP), 99, 125, 127, 214
adenosine triphosphate (ATP), 92, 93, 94, 99, 100, 101, 102, 103, 104, 105, 117, 118, 125, 127, 129, 131, 134, 182, 183, 214, 223, 229, 246, 251, 466, 570, 573
adipose tissue, 5, 31, 109, 124, 181, 240
aerobic exercise, 93, 94, 96, 102, 105, 169, 170, 177, 178, 570, 571, 574
aerodynamics, 528, 529, 530
agonist muscle, 189, 191, 573
Alexander technique, 364, 365, 366
a-linolenic acid (ALA), 126, 219, 222, 223
alternative medicine, 153, 194, 213, 255, 257, 267, 364, 390, 404, 414, 447, 468
American Academy of Medical Acupuncture, 389
American Academy of Neurology, 277, 278
American Association of Acupuncture and Oriental Medicine, 389
American Board of Physical Medicine and Rehabilitation (ABPMR), 593
American Board of Podiatric Medicine, 602
American Board of Podiatric Public Health, 602
American Board of Podiatric Surgery, 602
American College of Sports Medicine (ACSM), 96, 98, 303, 590, 591
American Council on Exercise (ACE), 590, 591
American Massage Therapy Association, 389
American Medical Association (AMA), 262, 272, 344, 514, 551, 593, 602
American Occupational Therapy Association (AOTA), 578, 581
American Physical Therapy Association (APTA), 598

American Podiatric Medical Association, 600
American Society of Exercise Physiologists, 565, 592
amino acid, 126, 201-205
amnesia, 19, 44, 276, 277, 292, 316, 319, 432, 436, 453
amputation, 30, 61, 84, 281, 282, 323, 324, 586, 587, 594, 596
amyotrophic lateral sclerosis (ALS) (also Lou Gehrig's disease), 61, 77, 209, 210, 216, 218, 272, 406, 412
anabolic steroids, 111, 163, 165, 166, 183, 246, 253, 455, 457, 467, 478, 483, 484, 487, 489, 492, 493, 494, 496
anabolic-androgenic steroids (AAS), 181, 484, 494, 495
androstenedione, 161, 162, 181, 182, 253, 254, 466, 467, 484, 495
anemia, 116-121, 133, 163, 220, 221, 228, 229, 230, 231, 238, 259, 279, 353, 371, 463, 464, 465, 469, 470
anesthesia, 91, 279, 282, 353, 370, 374, 378, 379, 388, 390, 392, 393, 434, 436, 437, 438, 447, 451, 587
anesthesiology, 152, 156, 267, 351, 389, 390, 434, 436, 447
Anesthesiology and Pain Medicine, 389
aneurysm, 26, 28, 138, 318, 339, 608
angiotensin-converting enzyme (ACE), 40, 230, 562
anisocytosis, 116, 118, 119
anorexia nervosa, 511
antagonist muscle, 189, 191, 573
anterior cruciate ligament (ACL), 50, 53, 358
anticonvulsants, 452
anti-inflammatory diets, 205-207
anti-inflammatory drugs, 427-430
applied kinesiology (AK), 395-397
arachnoid mater, 312, 318
Armstrong, Lance, 461-463
arthrofibrosis, 367
arthropathy, 367, 369
arthroplasty, 351-354
arthroscopy, 367, 376, 378, 585
Astym(r) therapy, 354-356
atherosclerosis, 7, 26, 28, 29, 38, 39, 94, 165, 166, 224, 237, 239, 251, 557, 562
athletic competition, 175, 460, 483, 494, 505, 512, 539, 542, 543, 575
athletic drug testing, 458
athletic injury, 273, 276, 282, 308, 376, 512
athletic trainer, 97, 121, 176, 430, 551, 552, 553, 554, 556, 574, 604, 605, 607, 609, 610
athletic training, 551-556

679

athletic training programs (ATEPs), 551, 553, 554, 556
atrioventricular (A-V) node, 36, 38, 66, 557
autogenic training (or AT), 171-174
automated external defibrillator (AED), 590
autonomic nervous system, 28, 34, 38, 139, 155, 172, 173, 186, 188, 288, 391
autosuggestion, 171, 172
avulsion, 321

B vitamins, 207, 219, 236, 238, 258
back pain, 267-269
baclofen, 430-431
basal metabolic rate (BMR), 124, 522
baseball finger (or mallet finger), 299
Bay Area Laboratory Co-Operative (BALCO), 479, 496
behavioral medicine, 186, 188
belladonna, 402, 403, 419, 420
benzodiazepine, 194, 452
bicipital tendinitis, 307
biochemistry, 30, 98, 121, 124, 147, 157, 181, 201, 207, 209, 211, 214, 222, 235, 241, 331, 336, 387, 440, 457, 468, 475, 478, 483, 486, 489, 494, 496, 570, 601
biocytin, 207
biodegradability, 421, 422
bioflavonoids, 241, 285, 286, 287
bioinformatics, 331, 332
biological scaffolds, 421
biotechnology, 157, 331, 336, 468, 469, 483
biotin, 207-209
blood doping, 182, 458-461
blood flow restriction (BFR) training, 174-175
Boerhaave, Herman, 106
Bouchard's nodes, 150, 151
Boutonniere deformity, 300
brain herniation, 313, 318
brain parenchyma, 313, 317, 318
bronchioles, 45, 47, 222, 224, 288
bulimia nervosa, 511, 512
bursitis, 83, 273, 276, 294, 297, 377, 388, 427, 586

cardiology, 557-564
cardiopulmonary resuscitation (CPR), 590
cardiovascular disease, 110, 174, 182, 186, 237, 238, 239, 240, 399, 400, 450, 484, 602
carisoprodol (brand name Soma), 431-432
carpal tunnel syndrome (CTS), 34, 35, 77, 294, 355, 409, 586, 594
cartilage, 23-26
catabolism, 124, 125, 127, 133, 134, 301
cellular respiration, 99, 104, 127, 129

Centers for Disease Control and Prevention (CDC), 276, 364, 508, 513
central nervous system (CNS), 4, 6, 16, 33, 106, 135, 139, 140, 142, 143, 145, 161, 163, 252, 259, 284, 349, 361, 392, 430, 433, 434, 437, 439, 452
cerebral hemispheres, 15, 17, 19, 21, 22, 42, 68, 69, 89, 318
cerebral lobes, 69
Cerrini, Daniel, 489, 490
cervical spine, 267, 314, 317, 409
cetyl alcohol, 213
cetylated fatty acids, 213-214
character development, 516, 517, 518, 519, 521
chemotaxis, 113, 114, 115
chiropractor, 35, 395, 574
cholesterol, 30, 39, 40, 94, 126, 131, 157, 158, 159, 160, 161, 162, 163, 165, 166, 216, 217, 228, 233, 239, 242, 250, 400, 401, 484, 495, 557, 562, 563
chondrocytes, 23, 25, 26, 225, 583
chondroitin, 151, 152, 214, 225, 226, 227, 228, 418
chondromalacia, 369, 370
chorionic villus sampling (CVS), 327, 470
chronic degenerative diseases, 205
chronic pain, 153, 154, 155, 156, 157, 173, 195, 393, 397, 412, 414, 434, 448, 449, 594
chronic traumatic encephalopathy (CTE), 270-273
cisgender, 539, 541, 542, 543, 544
classism, 523
closed wounds, 322
codeine, 432-434
collagen, 5, 9, 23, 25, 31, 32, 33, 34, 50, 53, 54, 55, 81, 82, 115, 150, 189, 192, 298, 304, 305, 306, 307, 323, 354, 380, 414, 416, 418, 421, 422, 423, 582, 583
colostrum, 249, 250
Commission on Accreditation of Athletic Training Education (CAATE), 551, 553
common shoulder injuries, 273-276
comparative genomics, 333
compartment syndrome, 34, 309, 359
compensatory hypertrophy, 108, 109, 110, 112
complementary and alternative medicine (CAM), 157, 227, 364
computational fluid dynamics, 528, 530
computed tomography (CT), 8, 21, 84, 95, 151, 277, 338-340, 561, 587
computer-aided design (CAD), 528
concentration gradient, 129, 147, 148
concussion, 276-279
conflict theory, 523, 526
connective tissue, 30-33

680

constraint-induced movement therapy (CIMT), 361-364
contusion, 269, 285, 289, 313, 317, 318, 319, 321
coronary artery bypass graft (CABG) surgery, 389
coronary care unit (CCU), 562
corticosteroid, 35, 81, 85, 160, 164, 165, 216, 233, 234, 289, 290, 305, 306, 311, 381, 427, 429, 430, 443, 448, 600, 602
COVID-19 crisis, 471, 515
creatine kinase, 214
creatine phosphate, 94, 99, 102, 103, 182, 214
creatinine, 214
cross-training, 175-177
cupping therapy, 397-399
cutaneous pain, 153, 155
cyclooxygenase (or COX), 151, 427, 428, 429, 440, 449
cytokines, 116, 205, 522
cytology, 98, 124, 331, 334

dehydration, 130, 149, 150, 163, 164, 183, 243, 244, 245, 289, 401
dehydroepiandrosterone (DHEA), 161, 182, 252, 484
dementia pugilistica ("punch drunk syndrome"), 271
dendrites, 6, 87, 88, 135, 144, 145
deoxyribonucleic acid (DNA), 33, 160, 201, 204, 229, 327, 328, 331, 334, 469
DeQuervain's syndrome, 299
dermatology, 367, 420, 427, 468, 600
diabetes mellitus, 7, 97, 104, 105, 182, 212, 240, 353, 471, 484, 600, 602
Diack, Lamine, 487, 488
Diagnostic and Statistical Manual of Mental Disorders (DSM-5), 508
Dietary Approaches to Stop Hypertension (DASH) diet, 400
dietary carbohydrates, 132, 134, 211-213
dietary supplements, 199, 221, 227, 250, 255, 256, 495
diet-based therapy, 399-401
dietetics, 116, 205, 207, 209, 213, 214, 219, 228, 241, 242, 245, 399, 416
dislocations, 81, 82, 84, 273, 275, 282, 285, 299
distal interphalangeal joints, 150, 151
diuretics, 40, 319, 440, 443, 562, 563
Division of Special Hospitals and Physical Reconstruction, 372
DNA and RNA molecules, 204
DNA sequencing, 331, 332
docosahexaenoic acid (DHA), 126, 223, 239
docosapentaenoic acid (DHA), 222
doctor of podiatric medicine (DPM), 600
Doppler effect, 341, 345

Doppler shift, 341, 342, 343, 344
DREAM (downstream regulatory element antagonistic modulator), 448
Dreschler, Heike, 500-502
drug doping, 183, 256, 455-502
Drug Enforcement Administration (DEA), 436, 437
duplex scan, 341, 344, 345
dynamic stretching, 97, 189, 191, 192, 193
dyskinesia, 86, 90, 210, 234
dysmorphia, 508, 510

ecchymoses, 269
ecchymosis, 279, 281, 314
edema, 7, 49, 241, 242, 260, 286, 317, 318, 359, 361, 371, 374, 443, 450, 559, 560, 561, 563, 606
eicosanoids, 205, 222, 224
eicosapentaenoic acid (EPA), 126, 222, 223, 239
electrocardiograph (ECG), 41, 94
electroencephalogram (EEG), 89
electroencephalograph, 89, 576, 577
electrolytes, 237, 242, 243, 244
electromagnetic therapy, 404, 405, 406, 410, 411
electromagnetic waves, 336
electromyography (EMG), 371, 372, 595
electrophysiology, 107, 576, 599
electrotherapy, 296, 596, 597
embryology, 107, 331, 341, 468
emergency medicine, 15, 36, 45, 135, 267, 269, 276, 279, 312, 321, 359, 447, 512, 557, 604, 610
endocrine glands, 5, 157
endocrinology, 108, 157, 181, 211, 257, 427, 539, 542
endorphins, 153, 154, 178, 510, 511
endurance training, 177-180
energy drinks, 242-245
environmental engineering, 569
environmental health, 194
epicondylitis, 294, 304, 307, 309-312, 609
epiphysis, 279, 283
episodic memory (relational), 42, 44
ergogenic aids, 181-184
erythrocytes, 5, 32, 116, 464
erythropoiesis, 116, 117
erythropoietin (EPO), 463-466
essential fatty acid (EFA), 126, 219, 222, 223, 401
ethnocentrism, 523
exercise addiction, 508-510
exercise physiology, 92-98
exercise recovery, 416, 466
exercise science, 564-570
extensor carpi ulnaris (ECU), 74, 75, 299, 310

681

fair play, 516, 517, 519
family medicine, 36, 92, 108, 113, 181, 255, 257, 267, 269, 287, 304, 321, 359, 367, 427, 604, 608, 610
fascia, 33-36
Federation of State Boards of Physical Therapy (FSBPT), 598
Feldenkrais method, 364, 365, 366
feminist theory, 523, 526
fentanyl, 434-436
fibrocartilage, 50
fibromyalgia, 34, 297, 407, 412, 413, 414, 511, 594
follicle-stimulating hormone (FSH), 162, 609
Food and Drug Administration (FDA), 13, 165, 245, 256, 261, 395, 437, 444, 451, 465, 475, 484
forensic medicine, 468, 472, 473
functionalist theory, 523, 526

gamma oryzanol, 251
gamma-aminobutyric acid (GABA), 430, 432, 452, 453
gas chromatography, 457
gastroenterology, 124, 219, 420
gastrointestinal disturbances, 84
Gatorade, 243, 244
gender identity, 539, 541, 542, 543, 544, 545, 546
gene cloning, 335, 469, 475
gene splicing, 468
gene therapy, 469, 471, 472, 474
general surgery, 152, 267, 351, 359, 380, 539, 542
genetic counseling, 327, 329, 470
genetic disorder, 132, 327, 328, 329, 469, 470, 472, 474, 475
genetic engineering, 468-475
genetic marker, 290, 327, 329
genetic testing, 327-331
genetics, 134, 139, 147, 152, 238, 240, 327, 331, 332, 468
genomics, 331-335
geriatrics, 23, 81, 267, 351, 447, 575, 599
gerontology, 81, 267, 301, 351, 447
Gerschler's technique, 185
ginseng, 245, 246, 248, 249, 253, 256
Glasgow Coma Scale, 277, 314
glucocorticoids, 161, 163, 165, 427, 428
glucosamine, 225-228
glycolysis, 98-105
goniometry, 371, 372
Gregorc mind styles, 551, 555
gynecology, 228, 327, 341

Hackett, George, 414
Haikkola, Rolf, 481

hand fracture, 299
Handbook of Physical Medicine and Rehabilitation, 593
Harrison Narcotics Tax Act, 438
Harvey, William, 8, 41, 77
health-care providers, 119, 120, 305, 311, 317, 366, 447, 449
heart attack, 28, 29, 30, 38, 39, 97, 98, 151, 164, 166, 178, 224, 231, 427, 429, 441, 443, 445, 449, 450, 459, 492, 495, 557, 558, 559, 562, 563, 574
heart failure, 39, 40, 67, 110, 111, 120, 216, 217, 239, 443, 557, 559, 560, 562, 563
hematology, 26, 30, 36, 116, 181, 228, 269, 458, 463
hematoma, 7, 269, 313, 314, 317, 318, 319, 320, 322, 343, 359
  epidural, 313, 317, 318, 320
  subdural, 313, 317, 318, 320
hematopoiesis, 116
hemoglobin, 47, 102, 103, 104, 116, 117, 118, 119, 120, 162, 229, 231, 237, 238, 252, 260, 459, 460, 570, 573
Herberden's nodes, 150, 151
herniated disk, 267
high-intensity intermittent exercise (HIIE), 184
high-intensity interval training (HIIT), 184-186
hippocampus, 42-45
homeopathy, 402-403, 418-420
homophobia, 523, 527
Human Genome Project, 332, 334, 335
human growth hormone (HGH), 181, 246, 253, 471, 483, 484, 487, 489, 494, 499
human immunodeficiency virus (HIV), 91, 163, 230, 246, 464, 471
human physiology, 106, 107
human respiratory system, 45-50
hyaline cartilage, 24, 25, 50
hyaluronic acid, 367-369
hydrotherapy, 194, 371, 373, 374, 375, 595, 596, 597
hydroxymethyl butyrate (HMB), 217, 246, 247, 248
hyperplasia, 108, 110, 165
hypertrophic cardiomyopathy, 560, 607, 608

immune system, 33, 113, 163, 165, 205, 206, 242, 256, 257, 365, 397, 417, 422, 440, 463, 472
immunoassay, 457, 458
immunology, 157, 194
incision, 85, 321, 352, 353, 358, 370, 376, 378, 379, 381, 392, 408, 586, 602
inflammatory biomarkers, 205, 207
injury risk, 175, 512
interleukins, 113, 205

internal medicine, 108, 113, 152, 181, 255, 257, 321, 341, 359, 427, 593, 604, 610
International Association of Athletics Federation (IAAF), 487, 539, 540
International Olympic Committee (IOC), 183, 252, 457, 459, 468, 475, 477, 478, 479, 487, 494, 539, 543
intersex, 539, 542, 544
intervertebral disk, 267
intramural sports, 516-521
iron-deficiency anemia, 116-121
ischemia, 279, 282, 320, 338, 339, 359, 371, 557, 558, 560, 562

Jersey finger, 300
Jones, Marion, 478-481
Journal of the American Medical Association, 262, 272, 344, 514
Jumper's knee (or patellar tendinitis), 305, 308

kaatsu training, 174
Kentucky Spinal Cord Injury Research Center, 349
ketamine, 436-438
ketogenesis, 125, 129, 130
kinesiology, 570-575
knee cartilage defect, 367
kneecap (or patella), 11, 56, 57, 308, 351, 369-371, 380
Krebs cycle, 117, 125, 128, 129, 131
kwashiorkor, 241, 242
kyphoplasty, 279, 284
kyphosis, 267, 268

lactate threshold, 121-124
lateral collateral ligament (LCL), 50, 52
leadership skills, 505, 507, 516, 517, 519, 555, 575
lecithin, 233-234
leukocytes, 5, 31, 32, 113, 114, 115
LGBTQ (lesbian, gay, bisexual, transgender, and queer), 542, 543, 546
ligaments, 52-55
lordosis, 267, 269
lower extremities, 55-62
lumbar spine, 57, 267, 268, 269, 318, 420

macronutrients, 219, 236, 238, 240, 241, 257, 258, 259
magnet therapy, 403-414
magnetic resonance imaging (MRI), 336-338
major depressive disorder (MDD), 437
Major League Baseball (MLB), 183, 466, 467, 468, 486, 493, 496
Major League Baseball Players Association (MLBPA), 466

Maradona, Diego, 489-492
mass spectrometry, 457
Mayo Clinic News Network, 350
McGwire, Mark, 466-468
McLaren, Richard, 487, 488
medial collateral ligament (MCL), 50
Medicaid, 601
Medical College Admissions Test (MCAT), 601
medical laboratory testing, 475, 478
Medicare, 601
medicinal chemistry, 457
Menem, Carlos, 489, 491
menorrhagia, 229, 230, 231
menstruation, 14, 229, 230, 231
mental health, 510-512
metabolic equivalent (MET), 92, 95, 96
methylmorphine, 432
microbiology, 201, 331
microcytosis, 116
micronutrients, 219, 258, 261
minor sprains, 286
Mitchell report, 183, 468, 497, 498, 499
Mitchell, George, 497
mitochondria, 94, 109, 111, 112, 125, 128, 129, 131, 132, 161, 216, 223, 251, 288, 443
molecular biology, 55, 147
monosaccharide, 131, 211
morphine, 438-439
morphine methyl ester, 432
motor control, 135-138
motor skill development, 139-144
motor vehicle accidents (MVAs), 276, 299, 349
moxibustion, 387, 397
multiple sclerosis (MS), 7, 138, 178, 362, 410, 428, 430, 594
muscle contraction, 28, 40, 62, 63, 68, 88, 90, 99, 102, 106, 219, 237, 373, 570, 573, 574
muscle fitness, 196
muscle relaxant, 267, 268, 297, 425, 430, 431, 432, 452
muscle soreness, 94, 192, 193, 226, 402, 403, 409, 416, 417, 418, 419, 420, 521, 522
muscle testing, 395, 396, 602
muscular dystrophy, 7, 61, 66, 67, 77, 111, 112, 210, 216, 290, 329, 469, 579, 580, 594, 596, 597
myocardial perfusion imaging (MPI), 338, 339
myofascial release, 414
myopathies, 287, 288, 289, 560, 563, 607, 608

narcotics, 155, 359, 393, 431, 432, 438, 447, 448
National Academy of Sports Medicine (NASM), 590, 591

National Association of Sport and Physical Education (NASPE), 565
National Athletic Trainers Association (NATA), 551
National Board for Certification in Occupational Therapy (NBCOT), 578
National Center for Injury Prevention and Control, 276
National Collegiate Athletic Association (NCAA), 457, 493, 513, 514, 515, 537, 542, 543, 545, 546
National Commission for Certifying Agencies (NCCA), 591
National Institute of Neurological Disorders and Stroke (NINDS), 349
National Institutes of Health (NIH), 157, 261, 395, 400, 437, 565
National Physical Therapy Examination (NPTE), 598
National Standards for Physical Education, 565, 567, 569
National Strength and Conditioning Association (NSCA), 591
neonatology, 139
nephrology, 181
nerve conduction studies (NCS), 595
neural tube, 15, 16, 220
neuroanatomy, 68
neurodegeneration, 42, 44
neurogenesis, 42, 44, 303
neurology, 15, 33, 35, 42, 55, 71, 86, 105, 107, 135, 139, 144, 152, 156, 267, 270, 276, 292, 312, 349, 361, 430, 512, 533, 575, 576, 592, 594, 599, 601
neuromuscular disorders, 61, 76, 288, 365
neuropathic pain, 447
neuroplasticity, 144-147
neuroscience, 575-578
neurosurgery, 15, 135, 155, 312, 316, 320, 349
neurotransmitter, 38, 64, 65, 66, 133, 138, 153, 234, 290, 303, 338, 340, 430, 434, 436, 437, 443, 446, 451, 452, 453, 576, 577
nicotinamide adenine dinucleotide (NAD), 234-235
N-methyl-D-aspartate (NMDA) receptors, 436, 437
nociception, 153
nonsteroidal anti-inflammatory drugs (NSAIDs), 439-445
nuclear magnetic resonance (NMR) imaging, 336
nutritional medicine, 205

obesity, 97, 111, 150, 151, 178, 186, 206, 207, 212, 238, 239, 240, 242, 243, 388, 399, 511, 586
obsessive-compulsive disorder, 19, 340, 412
occupational health, 194, 267, 304, 307, 380
Occupational Therapist Registered (OTR), 581
occupational therapists, 578-582

occupational therapy, 15, 55, 68, 71, 135, 144, 150, 151, 186, 189, 191, 273, 296, 297, 312, 354, 361, 364, 369, 414, 564, 578, 579, 580, 581, 598
occupational therapy programs, 578, 579, 581
omega-3 fatty acids, 205, 206, 239
oncology, 81, 152, 327, 432, 438, 447, 451, 463
open wounds, 323, 389
ophthalmology, 427
opioids, 395, 425, 431, 432, 433, 434, 435, 436, 437, 438, 439, 441, 445, 446, 447, 449, 451
oral homeopathic remedies, 402, 403, 419
organic chemistry, 201, 601
orthodontics, 8
orthologues, 331, 333
orthopedic braces, 356-358
orthopedic surgery, 50, 68, 298, 367, 376, 587, 604
orthopedics, 582-588
orthotic device, 290, 600, 602, 603
osmosis, 147-150
osmotic pressure, 147, 148, 149
osteoarthritis (OA), 150-152
osteoblast, 9, 10, 12, 13, 32, 81, 82, 84, 279, 283
osteoclast, 5, 9, 10, 12, 13, 32, 81, 82, 83, 84
osteocyte, 5, 9, 279, 583, 584, 588
osteopathic medicine, 8, 33, 62, 267, 287, 371
osteopetrosis, 12, 82
osteoporosis, 12, 13, 14, 33, 81, 84, 153, 163, 206, 221, 237, 238, 240, 241, 253, 262, 284, 287, 353, 365, 429, 495, 505, 583, 584, 585, 588, 594
osteotomy, 152
Oswald, Denis, 487, 488
otolaryngology, 23
otorhinolaryngology, 427
overexertion, 151, 267, 288, 289, 290, 521, 558
overtraining syndrome, 521-522
oxidative phosphorylation, 125, 127, 129
oxycodone, 445-447

pain management, 447-448
pain medicine, 156, 186, 353, 449, 451, 592, 594
pain relief, 151, 296, 297, 320, 364, 368, 413, 433, 434, 436, 442, 446, 447, 451
palliative treatments, 194
parasympathetic nervous system, 34, 38
Parkinson's disease, 18, 211, 216, 234, 235, 272, 334, 406, 412, 429, 470, 594
patellar tendon, 51, 55, 308, 355, 370, 380
pathology, 11, 105, 113, 139, 373, 379, 553
pathophysiology, 79, 309, 344, 609

pediatrics, 139, 269, 327, 359, 539, 542, 575, 593, 599, 610
peer-assisted learning, 551, 555
peptide bond, 201, 203
performance-enhancing drugs (PEDs), 483-486
perinatology, 139, 327
peripheral nervous system (PNS), 135, 139, 349, 433
peripheral neuropathy, 133, 407, 408, 412, 413
personal trainer, 588-592
personal training, 177, 184, 186, 196, 214, 245, 309, 416, 496, 500, 564, 574, 590, 591, 592
pharmacology, 98, 124, 157, 181, 331, 430, 431, 432, 436, 438, 445, 447, 449, 451, 452, 468, 475, 478, 553, 575, 600, 601, 604
phencyclidine (PCP), 436
phosphatidylcholine, 233, 234
phosphatidylserine, 250, 252, 418
phosphocreatine, 214, 215, 217, 246
photonutrients, 255
physical exercise, 105, 124, 196, 249, 291, 301, 364, 365, 409, 508, 511, 516, 562, 588, 596
physical fitness, 96, 98, 121, 176, 192, 364, 493, 508, 516, 517, 518, 565, 566, 568, 588
physical medicine and rehabilitation (PM&R, also "physiatry"), 592-595
physical rehabilitation, 371-376
physical therapists (PTs), 595-600
physical therapy, 15, 33, 35, 50, 52, 55, 62, 71, 92, 135, 139, 144, 150, 151, 152, 153, 155, 174, 186, 189, 191, 196, 267, 268, 269, 273, 275, 286, 287, 289, 290, 296, 297, 298, 304, 305, 307, 309, 311, 312, 349, 350, 351, 353, 354, 359, 361, 364, 368, 369, 370, 371, 372, 376, 378, 379, 382, 392, 397, 414, 416, 447, 448, 512, 538, 553, 564, 581, 582, 585, 592, 593, 595, 596, 597, 598, 599, 602, 604, 605, 606
physical training, 121, 364, 416
physiology, 8, 33, 35, 36, 37, 62, 68, 79, 92-98, 105-108, 117, 120, 124, 135, 139, 147, 150, 157, 165, 169, 181, 243, 267, 287, 301, 304, 371, 387, 492, 521, 533, 552, 565, 566, 568, 570, 572, 573, 574, 580, 581, 589, 598, 601, 604
physiotherapy, 186, 403, 419, 595
phytonutrients, 255
pilates, 364, 365, 366, 589, 592
pituitary gland, 5, 12, 18, 161, 162, 163, 164, 182, 471, 494
podiatrists, 600, 601, 602, 603, 604
podiatry, 600-604
policosanol, 250
polycythemia, 459

polymerase chain reaction (PCR), 469, 470
polysaccharide, 5, 131, 211
positive competition, 516, 518
positron emission tomography (PET), 339, 561
post-concussion syndrome (PCS), 292-294
postmenopausal osteoporosis, 13
postpolio syndrome, 407
post-traumatic stress disorder, 292, 412
prefrontal cortex (PFC), 68-71
prenatal diagnosis, 327, 330, 470, 474, 475
prescription NSAIDs, 449-450
preventive medicine, 41, 92, 194, 235, 267, 304, 390, 468, 557, 563, 604
professional physical therapy (PT) license, 598
progressive muscle relaxation (PMR), 186-189
prolotherapy, 414-416
prostacyclin, 222, 440
prostaglandins, 113, 114, 115, 151, 205, 222, 224, 427, 440, 441, 443, 449
proteoglycan, 23, 25, 26, 31, 54
proteolytic enzymes, 285, 286, 297
proteomics, 331, 332, 333
proximal interphalangeal joints, 150, 151
pseudoephedrine, 475, 476, 477
psoriatic arthritis, 83, 85, 273
psychiatry, 15, 68, 86, 152, 188, 194, 270, 292, 312, 338, 436, 445, 447, 452, 492, 508, 512, 533, 575
psychology, 15, 42, 68, 86, 139, 144, 171, 181, 186, 188, 194, 270, 292, 312, 361, 445, 447, 492, 503, 508, 511, 512, 521, 523, 533-538, 565, 566, 567, 568, 570, 572, 573, 575, 576, 580, 581, 597, 598, 604
psychotherapy, 194, 195
public health, 235, 255, 435
pulmonology, 45, 106, 420
pulsed electromagnetic field therapy (PEMF), 404, 409
pyruvate, 101, 102, 103, 127, 128, 131, 132, 133, 250
pyruvic acid, 125, 250

qigong, 364, 365, 366, 387
Quick Disabilities of the Arm, Shoulder and Hand (QuickDASH), 379

radiculopathy, 267, 268
radiology, 8, 15, 23, 267, 336, 338, 341, 601
Raducan, Andreea, 475-478
recombinant DNA technology, 468
recommended daily allowance (RDA), 221, 229, 257, 258, 261
reflective journaling/learning log, 551, 556
regenerative medicine, 349, 351, 421, 469, 470

Subject Index

registered clinical dietitian, 400, 401
rehabilitation, 52, 68, 71, 93, 95, 97, 98, 144, 146, 156, 265, 283, 303, 347, 349, 354, 356, 358, 359, 361, 362, 371-376, 379, 380, 383, 395, 415, 452, 512, 538, 551, 553, 566, 571, 573, 574, 575, 578, 579, 581, 587, 592-595, 596, 597, 605, 606, 607, 610
relaxation techniques, 151, 187
repetitive strain injury (RSI), 294-297
repetitive transcranial magnet therapy, 404
reproductive specialist, 327
resistance training, 96, 196, 248, 250, 252, 253, 301, 568, 571
respiratory therapy, 45, 48
reverse osmosis, 147, 149
rheumatism, 153
rheumatoid arthritis, 25, 33, 35, 83, 84, 85, 115, 206, 214, 224, 226, 273, 351, 374, 406, 407, 428, 430, 586, 587, 594
rheumatologist, 586
rheumatology, 23, 30, 36, 81, 113, 152, 205, 267, 351, 427, 439, 449, 582, 604
risk management, 512, 553
Rodchenkov, Grigory, 487, 488
Röntgen, Wilhelm Conrad, 8, 336, 587
rotator cuff, 273, 274, 275, 276, 294, 297, 305, 376-380
Russian Olympic team, 486, 487

salicylates, 427, 430, 441, 443, 444
sarcomeres, 192
saturated fatty acid, 205, 222, 223, 239, 259
schizophrenia, 22, 45, 188, 216, 340, 406, 411
sciatica, 153, 267, 268, 414
sclera, 31
sclerotherapy, 414
scoliosis, 83, 267, 268
selective awareness, 171, 172
selective estrogen receptor modulator (SERM), 14, 84
self-esteem, 141, 375, 376, 388, 507, 516, 517, 518, 534, 535, 536, 537
self-hypnosis, 171, 172, 187, 195
semipermeable membrane, 147, 148, 149
shin splints, 307, 308, 309, 609
shoulder impingement, 376
single-photon emission computed tomography (SPECT), 338-340
sinoatrial (S-A) node, 36, 38
social identity, 534, 536
soft tissue pain, 297-298
somatic motor system (SMS), 136
somatosensory system, 139, 142

spinal cord injury (SCI), 349-351
sports drinks, 243, 244, 245
sports engineering, 528-533
Sports Illustrated, 462
sports medicine, 604-611
sports psychology, 533-538
sports sociology, 523, 524, 525, 527
sprint interval training (SIT), 184
standard metabolic rate (SMR), 125
static stretching, 189-191
steroids, 157-166, 492-500
strength training (also "resistance training" or weight lifting), 301-304
stress reduction, 194-196
stretchable tubing, 301, 303
stretching, 191-194
substance use, 157, 207, 233
sudden cardiac death, 557, 559, 563, 608
supraspinatus tendinitis (or swimmer's shoulder), 307, 308
symbolic interaction theory, 523, 526
symphytum, 402, 403, 419, 420
synaptic cleft, 63, 64
synovial fluid, 51, 150, 152, 367, 368
synovial joint, 50, 52
synovium, 150

Tai Chi, 35, 296, 364, 365, 366, 387
tendinitis, 304-306
tendinopathy, 304, 305, 306, 312, 354, 355
tendinosis, 298, 299, 304, 305, 306
tendon disorders, 307-309
tendon injuries, 226, 299, 377, 380
tendon overuse syndrome, 304
tendon repair, 380-382
tendonitis, 35, 226, 294, 297, 304, 354, 376, 377, 414, 427, 594, 603
tennis elbow (or lateral epicondylitis), 309-312
therapeutic exercise, 297, 371, 375, 553, 595, 596, 597
therapeutic massage, 186, 297, 596
therapeutic treatments, 578
thinspiration addiction, 508
thoracic cavity, 45, 47, 49
thoracic spine, 267
thromboxane, 222, 224, 440, 441
tissue development, 421, 423
tissue engineering, 420-423
Title IX, 505, 542, 546
Tommy John surgery, 382-383
topical combination homeopathic remedy, 402
toxicology, 181, 316, 575

traction-test devices, 528, 530
traditional Chinese medicine (TCM), 387, 397
traditional homeopathic remedies, 402
Trager approach, 364, 365, 366
tramadol, 451-452
transcutaneous electrical nerve stimulation (TENS), 155, 297, 448
transection, 279, 284
trans-fatty acid, 222
transgender, 539-547
traumatic brain injury (TBI), 312-321
treatment-resistant depression (TRD), 411, 437
triathlete, 461
triathlon, 177, 179, 244, 461
tribulus terrestris, 252
trigger point, 35, 407, 409, 412, 593, 595
trimethylglycine, 233, 251, 252
type 1 diabetes, 7, 104, 208, 212, 240
type 2 diabetes, 186, 208, 212, 240, 399, 400, 444

ulcerative colitis, 119, 233, 428
ulnar collateral ligament (UCL), 298, 382
ultrasonography, 341-345
ultrasound therapy, 308, 596, 597
unsaturated fatty acid, 205, 222, 223, 239, 259
upper extremities, 71-78
uridine triphosphate (UTP), 131
urology, 341, 420

US Anti-Doping Agency (USADA), 183, 460, 463, 479, 487, 494

valium, 452-453
vascular medicine, 26, 36, 269, 341, 427, 557, 600
vasodilation, 26, 28, 113, 114, 186, 188
vertebroplasty, 279, 284
Virén, Lasse, 481-483
visceral pain, 153, 155
viscosupplementation injections, 351, 353
vitamin deficiency diseases, 262
von Haller, Albrecht, 105-108

water-soluble vitamins, 207, 258
weight training, 196-198
whiplash, 322
World Anti-Doping Agency (WADA), 183, 487, 494
World Health Organization, 388
World Journal of Psychiatry, 389
wound medicine, 269
wrist fractures, 299
wrist guards, 300
wrist sprain, 298, 412

y-linolenic acid (GLA), 222, 223
yoga, 35, 191, 268, 296, 364, 365, 366, 589, 592

zeugmatography, 336, 337

The Principles of... Series

Principles of Science

Principles of Anatomy
Principles of Astronomy
Principles of Behavioral Science
Principles of Biology
Principles of Biotechnology
Principles of Botany
Principles of Chemistry
Principles of Climatology
Principles of Computer Science
Principles of Computer-Aided Design
Principles of Ecology
Principles of Energy
Principles of Fire Science
Principles of Geology
Principles of Information Technology
Principles of Marine Science
Principles of Mathematics
Principles of Microbiology
Principles of Modern Agriculture
Principles of Pharmacology
Principles of Physical Science
Principles of Physics
Principles of Programming & Coding
Principles of Robotics & Artificial Intelligence
Principles of Scientific Research
Principles of Sports Medicine & Kinesiology
Principles of Sustainability
Principles of Zoology

The Principles of... Series

Principles of Health
Principles of Health: Allergies & Immune Disorders
Principles of Health: Anxiety & Stress
Principles of Health: Depression
Principles of Health: Diabetes
Principles of Health: Nursing
Principles of Health: Obesity
Principles of Health: Pain Management
Principles of Health: Prescription Drug Abuse

Principles of Business
Principles of Business: Accounting
Principles of Business: Economics
Principles of Business: Entrepreneurship
Principles of Business: Finance
Principles of Business: Globalization
Principles of Business: Leadership
Principles of Business: Management
Principles of Business: Marketing

Principles of Sociology
Principles of Sociology: Group Relationships & Behavior
Principles of Sociology: Personal Relationships & Behavior
Principles of Sociology: Societal Issues & Behavior

SALEM PRESS   https://salempress.com   (800) 221-1592